Photographic Atlas of Rhinoplasty

Süreyya Şeneldir

Photographic Atlas of Rhinoplasty

Problem-solving and Troubleshooting

Second Edition 2024

Springer

Süreyya Şeneldir
Rhinoplasty School
Istanbul, Türkiye

ISBN 978-3-031-65621-7 ISBN 978-3-031-65619-4 (eBook)
https://doi.org/10.1007/978-3-031-65619-4

This Springer imprint is published by the registered company Springer Nature Switzerland AG
The registered company address is: Gewerbestrasse 11, 6330 Cham, Switzerland

For my father who was always there for me and who will continue to be…

Preface

I often look back on my life, remember what I passed through, and think of where I am right now. Just like it was yesterday, I remember what I wanted to learn and where I started. Currently, books are not the initial choice for learning, perhaps because tablets, phones, and computers are more convenient and faster. Videos attract more attention because they are dynamic. Everyone has a history that they want to be respected. Writing this book is proof of my respect for the belief that books are the best teachers and friends.

I learned everything from books. When I started my career, few people were well trained in rhinoplasty, and it was difficult to contact other professionals. Therefore, I took advantage of the books I read and meetings I attended. I spent much time experimenting with what I learned, keeping up with new techniques, and identifying key points. Sometimes it took me years to answer the questions in my head. Now, it is much simpler to obtain the information that we need. However, with this excess "infollution," we have trouble determining which information to use or where to use it.

I asked myself "What type of book should I write?" I decided that it should be like an atlas and include everything about rhinoplasty. The language should flow and be organized and readable. It should be a guide for my colleagues, conveying everything that I show them when practicing with them face to face. In addition, every example should be real, not hypothetical.

That is why this *Atlas* includes extensive pictures and drawings that are in order and follow each other sequentially. The pictures and drawings took 2 years to complete. The videos of the examples of the described subjects were prepared for colleagues using an augmented reality technique. I am aware of what I needed to learn when I was at the beginning of my career, and my current colleagues have the same requirements.

Jacob Riis said "When nothing seems to help, I go look at a stonecutter hammering away at his rock perhaps a hundred times without as much as a crack showing in it. Yet at the hundred and first blow it will split in two, and I know it was not that blow that did it, but all that had gone before." This book reflects not just my most recent work but the first hundred that went into that work.

In the *Photographic Atlas of Rhinoplasty*, each chapter is supported by related examples. However, these examples do not simply show techniques. Each pre-, intra-, and postoperative example is real and refers to specific subjects. Therefore, there are no hypothetical examples in this book.

I went to the effort of supporting every detail with real examples and interpreting them clearly and accurately. It was very important that I make them understandable for everyone, at any level of training. As I always highlighted in my "Rhinoplasty School" meetings and other meetings at which I spoke, there is no such thing as a miracle rhinoplasty technique. Therefore, considering many techniques is always more helpful because one technique may lead to different conclusions in different cases. That is why every step and detail in rhinoplasty should be explained.

I did my best to convey my experiences and knowledge in my book. Rhinoplasty improves with sharing, and sharing my own experiences in this book brought me great satisfaction. I hope that it will be as helpful and as satisfying for my colleagues, and I hope they can obtain the information that they need.

Thank you to everyone who has helped me through my journey in rhinoplasty. I am grateful for everyone who contributed material aid and spiritual support. Special thanks to Omer Faruk Guven, who was with me in this from the beginning to the end and who gave meaning to the book with his original drawings.

Istanbul, Turkey Süreyya Şeneldir

Contents

1 Radix: Definition and Analysis

The deepest point of the nose (where the upper nose joins the forehead) is the radix, which is both the root and the starting point of the nose. "Radix" is a clinical definition. Other structures of the nasal root, such as the nasofrontal suture and sellion, are anatomical definitions that do not correspond to the radix; we do not need to know these structures. When analyzing the nose, it is necessary to commence at the radix; this is the starting point of the nasal structure. Radix position and height determine the nasal profile. If this is to be ideal (well-proportioned), the radix must be in the right place. Meticulous analysis is necessary using two descriptive parameters.

1.1 One: The Vertical Position of the Radix

The ideal position of the radix is where an imaginary line commencing in the middle of the upper eyelid and running parallel to the ground intersects the nose (Fig. 1.1). This affects the length of the nose. A radix that is slumped caudally makes the nose look short (usually in revision cases); a radix located in the cephalic region makes the nose appear longer.

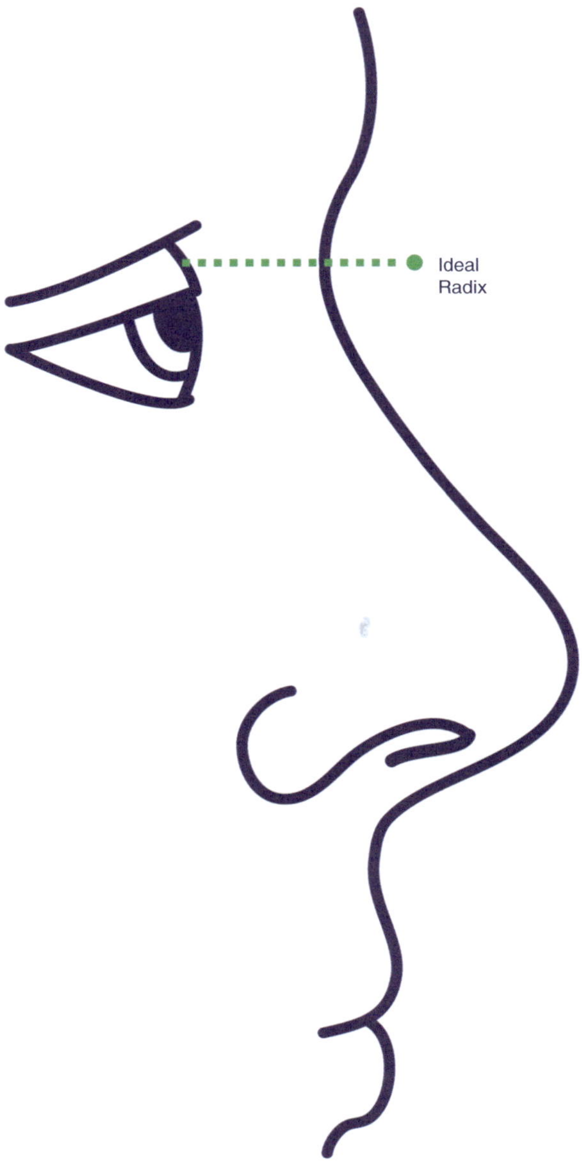

Fig. 1.1 Ideal position of the radix

S. Şeneldir, *Photographic Atlas of Rhinoplasty*, https://doi.org/10.1007/978-3-031-65619-4_1

1.2 Two: The Projection (Height) of the Radix

The height of the radix, measured in the anterior corneal plane, defines the nasal projection. The ideal projection is 9–14 mm (Fig. 1.2). This projection critically affects the dorsum and tip projections. The radix, dorsum, and tip projections must be balanced. To this end, we must first ensure that the radix projection is ideal. The acceptable range of projections is wide. How do we choose the projection?

A projection of 9–11 mm is adequate for females. The radix projection should be near the upper limit in males when a strong dorsum is required and when the nasal tip is large or droopy. Otherwise, the nasal tip will remain relatively large, despite ideal radix projection and rotation (the next case is a good example).

Consequently, a radix projection within the ideal dimensions does not mean that we will not modify the radix.

In this case, for example, the principal complaint is the width of the nose tip. The radix position is ideal; the projection is normal but lies close to the lower limit (Fig. 1.3). It is very unlikely that the patient will be satisfied if the nose tip (only) is reduced and the radix is neglected. Moving the ideal radix projection to its upper limit by placement of a small graft will improve the effect of tip-plasty.

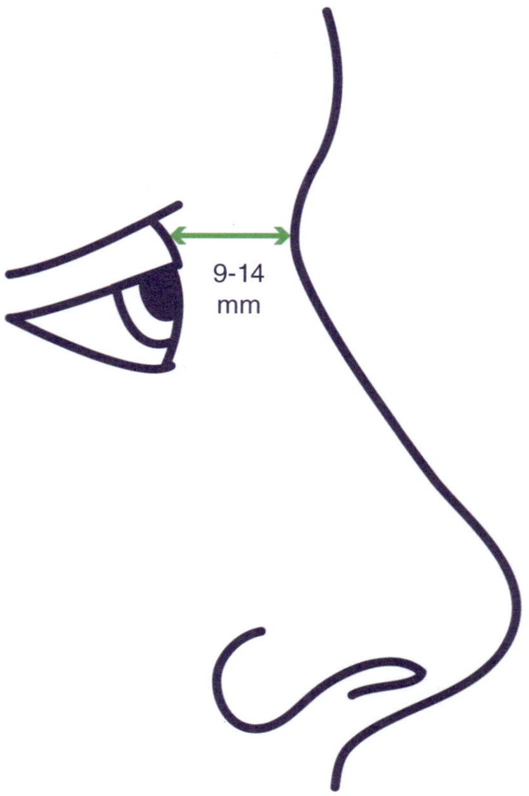

Fig. 1.2 Ideal projection of the radix

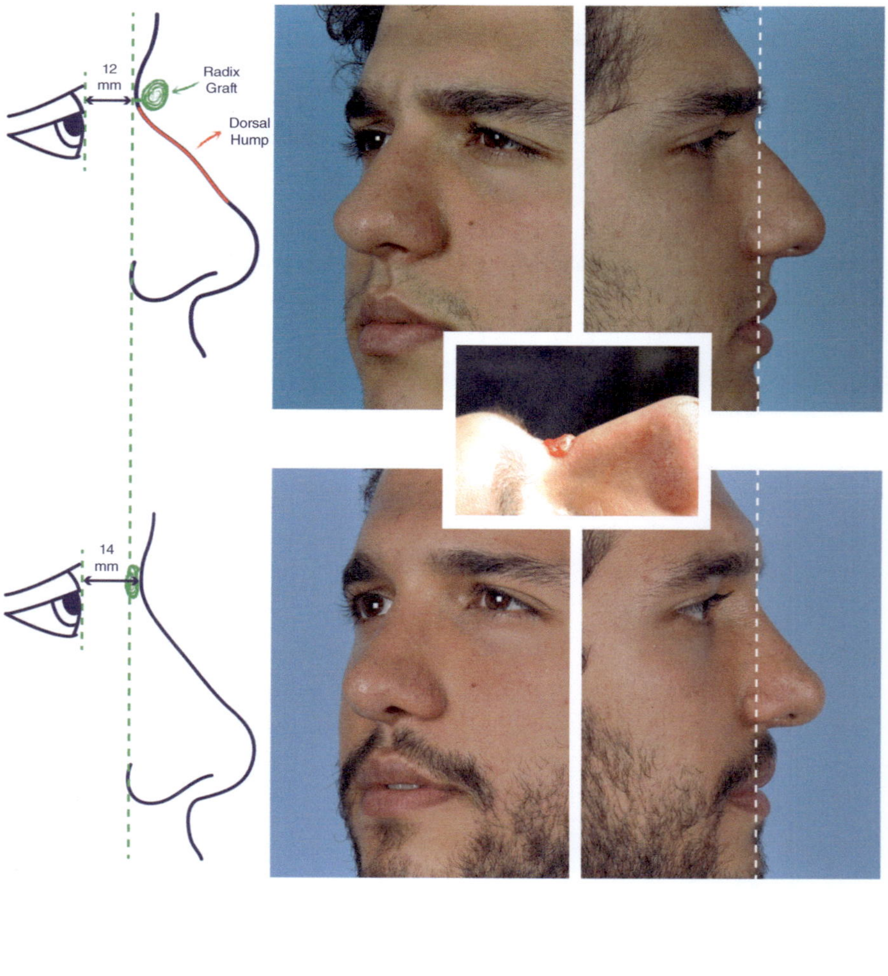

Fig. 1.3 If we look at the schematic above, moving the radix projection to the upper limit in a patient with a large nose tip will make the tip appear smaller even though the nose volume has not changed

If you fail to understand ideal radix positioning and projection, problems will arise both during planning and after surgery. In 80% of patients seeking rhinoplasty, the radix is ideal in terms of both projection and position; the remaining 20% have one of two major problems, which are high radix and low radix.

Disclosures The author reports no conflicts of interest or funding requiring disclosure.

Further Reading

Azizzadeh B, Mashkevich G. Middle Eastern rhinoplasty. Facial Plast Surg Clin North Am. 2010;18(1):201–6.

Constantian MB. Four common anatomic variants that predispose to unfavorable rhinoplasty results: a study based on 150 consecutive secondary rhinoplasties. Plast Reconstr Surg. 2000;105(1):316–31; discussion 332–3.

Daniel RK. Middle Eastern rhinoplasty: anatomy, aesthetics, and surgical planning. Facial Plast Surg. 2010;26(2):110–8.

Eskandarlou M, Motamed S. Evaluation of frequency of four common nasal anatomical deformities in primary rhinoplasty in a Tehran plastic surgery center. World J Plast Surg. 2014;3(2):122–8.

Guyuron B. Precision rhinoplasty. Part I: the role of life-size photographs and soft-tissue cephalometric analysis. Plast Reconstr Surg. 1988;81(4):489–99.

Lazovic GD, Daniel RK, Janosevic LB, Kosanovic RM, Colic MM, Kosins AM. Rhinoplasty: the nasal bones—anatomy and analysis. Aesthet Surg J. 2015;35(3):255–63.

McKinney P, Sweis I. A clinical definition of an ideal nasal radix. Plast Reconstr Surg. 2002;109(4):1416–8. discussion 1419–20

Naini FB, Cobourne MT, Garagiola U, McDonald F, Wertheim D. Nasofacial angle and nasal prominence: a quantitative investigation of idealized and normative values. J Craniomaxillofac Surg. 2016;44(4):446–52.

Sheen JH. The radix as a reference in rhinoplasty. Semin Plast Surg. 1987;1:33–50.

Steiger JD, Baker SR. Nuances of profile management: the radix. Facial Plast Surg Clin North Am. 2009;17(1):15–28.

2 High Radix

2.1 Introduction

If projection of radix is higher than 14 mm the case is considered high radix. The position may be normal, but may also lean caudally (Fig. 2.1a, b).

In high radix cases:

- The nose appears long and the dorsal hump appears less than the actual size.
- In the profile view, the angle between the nose and the base of the forehead is wide.
- The nose seems to be a continuation of the forehead (the "avatar" nose).
- In the frontal view, the eyes appear too far apart, because the nasal bones are widely spaced.
- The cranium of a nose with a high radix is more prominent than usual (a "top-heavy" nose).

In a patient with a high radix, the projection is more than 14 mm. However, the position varies. In profile, the radix should be the deepest part of the nose and may be ideally positioned in a patient with a high radix, but it may also be below or above that position. As can be seen in this patient, the deepest point of the nose is displaced from the dorsal to the caudal direction. It is necessary to adjust the nose starting point when lowering the radix. In this patient, for example, the radix projection should be adjusted; the current radix point must be moved to the ideal position (Fig. 2.2a, b).

Technical Pearl: Excessive dorsum and tip projections can be easily overlooked, and must be carefully considered during surgical planning. Otherwise, the projections remain unacceptably high after surgery.

The highest point of the nose can appear different when lying down due to changes in lymph drainage. It suggests that despite seeing an ideal radix during surgery, if diagnosed preoperatively as a high radix case, the diagnosis should not change. This could imply the importance of maintaining consistency in diagnosis based on preoperative assessments despite intraoperative observations (Fig. 2.3a, b).

Supplementary Information The online version contains supplementary material available at https://doi.org/10.1007/978-3-031-65619-4_2.

S. Şeneldir, *Photographic Atlas of Rhinoplasty*, https://doi.org/10.1007/978-3-031-65619-4_2

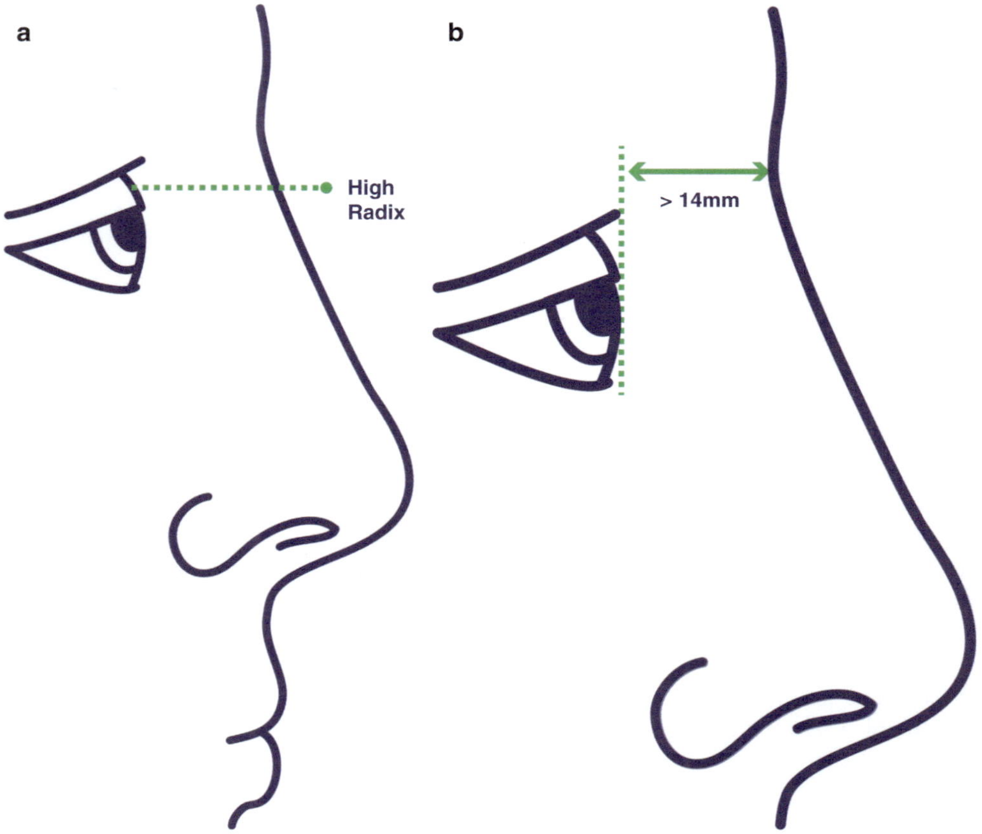

Fig. 2.1 (**a**, **b**) The illustration shows high radix

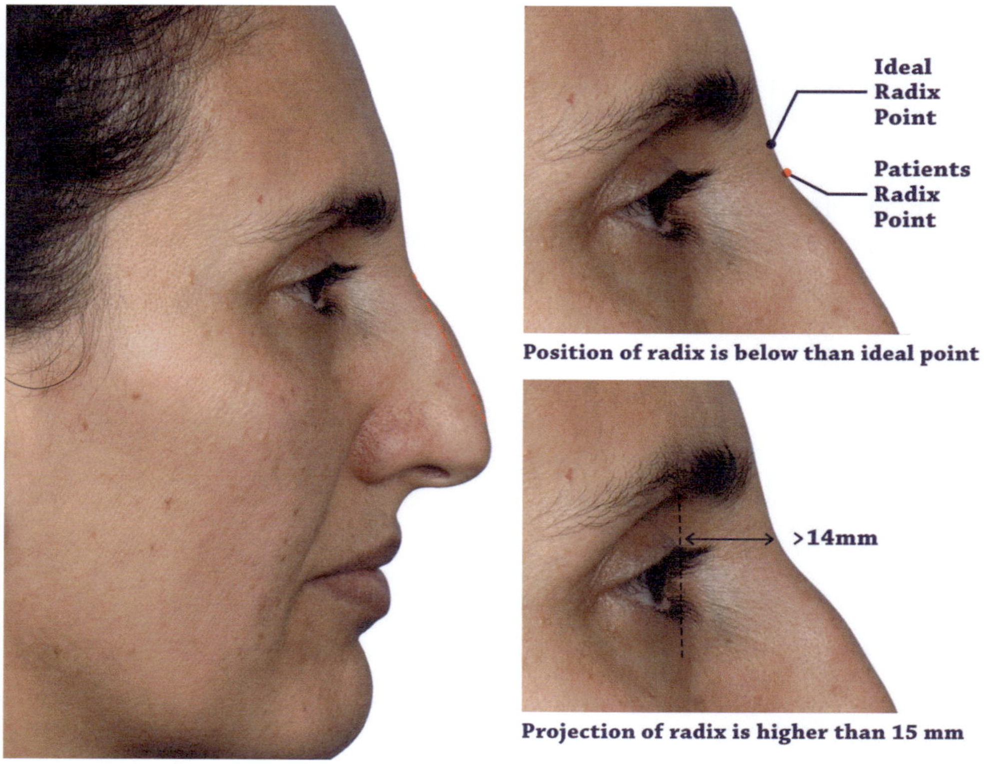

Fig. 2.2 (**a**, **b**) The upper right image shows that the position of radix is below the ideal point, while the lower right image shows that projection of radix is higher than 14 mm

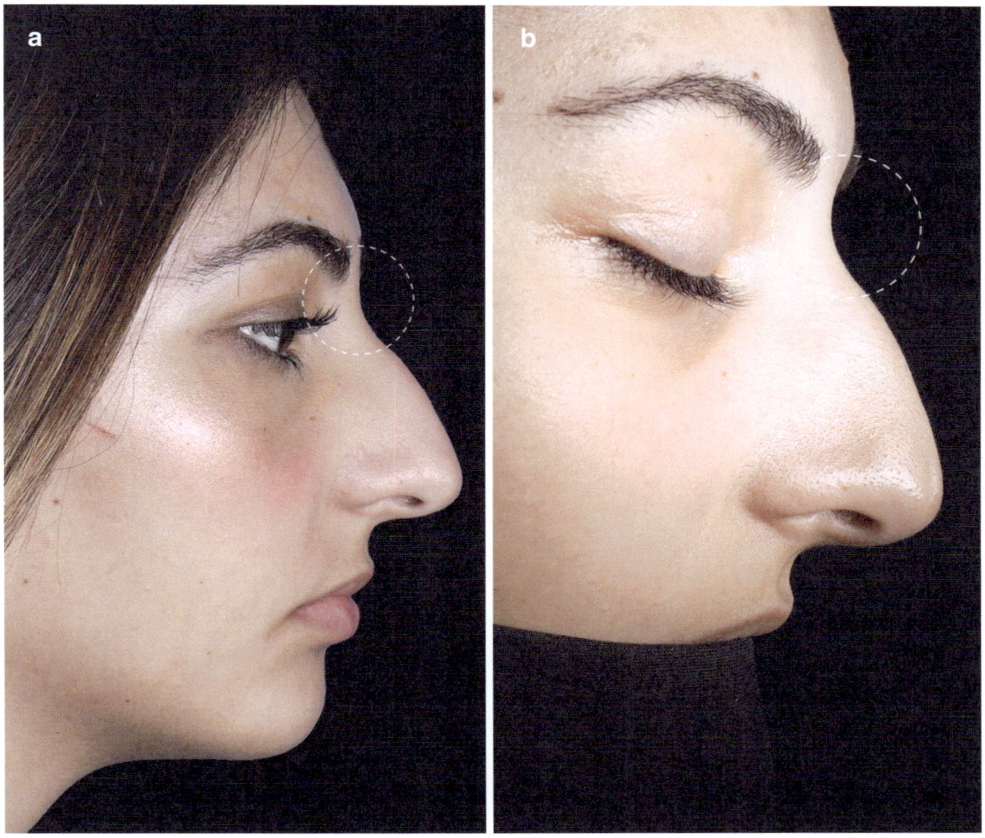

Fig. 2.3 (**a**, **b**) In the same patient, the presurgery image indicated a high radix, yet during the operation, it appeared normal. However, relying solely on the view from the surgical table may not provide a complete assessment

2.2 Treatment Strategy

In a patient with a high radix, the radix and dorsum modifications should be performed in three stages:

- The first step is to work on the primary dorsum and remove the hump (Fig. 2.4a).
- The next step is to lower the radix and work on the secondary dorsum (Fig. 2.4b).
- After the radix is lowered, a hidden hump appears. Finally, continue working to reduce this to the ideal projection (Fig. 2.4c).

It is necessary to adhere to this order of work. The dorsum and radix should not be deepened simultaneously. Separate osteotomies are used to remove excess bone from the radix and reduce radix projection. For this purpose, flat osteotomy combined with the use of a radix saw is highly effective and affords a clean and safe resection with clear boundaries (Fig. 2.5). **The ideal radix position is marked on the skin, prior to induction of anesthesia, with the patient sitting. Do not mark the radix position when the patient is lying on the operating table. A recent study has found the nasofrontal angle to be larger in supine position.** When the primary hump is removed, and radix lowering is to commence, the radix saw is used to perform a transverse osteotomy immediately below the marked area. The location of this osteotomy roughly determines the final radix position.

The upper limit of the bone to be removed is clearly defined and cut.

A straight osteotome is then placed in the radix region at an angle of 40/60° and the bone is incised toward the transverse osteotomy described above.

After these incisions are created, a wedge-shaped section of bone is removed (Fig. 2.6). The incisions and the resection are meticulously controlled via combined osteotomy and sawing. If more bone needs to be removed, further rasping is possible using the radix saw (Fig. 2.6; Supplementary Video 2.1).

Technical Pearl: To avoid septal collapse, aggressive septal surgery should be avoided in a patient with a high radix.

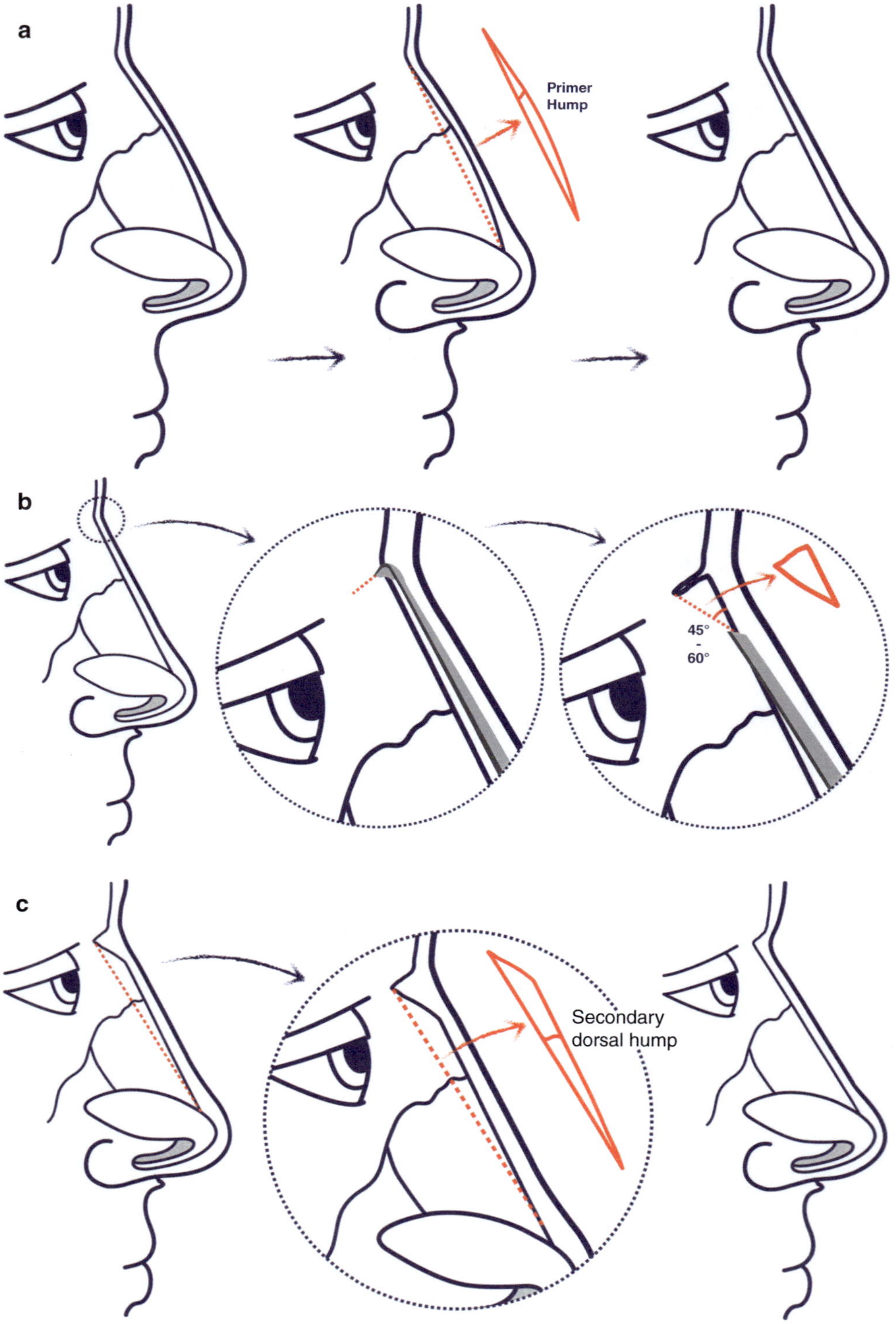

Fig. 2.4 (**a**) Primary dorsal reduction. (**b**) Lowering the radix. (**c**) Secondary dorsal reduction

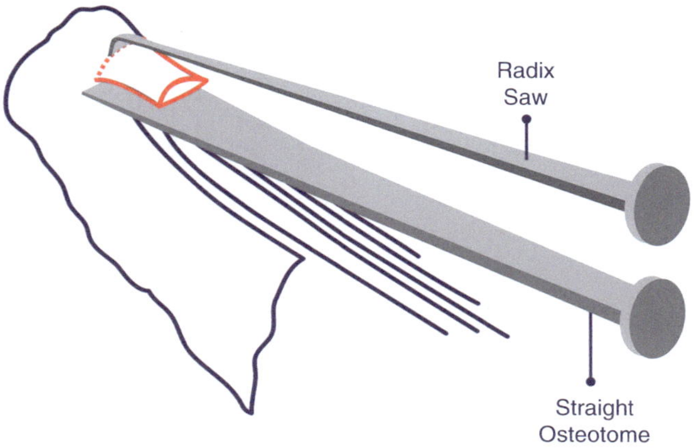

Fig. 2.5 For radix reduction flat osteotomy is combined with radix saw

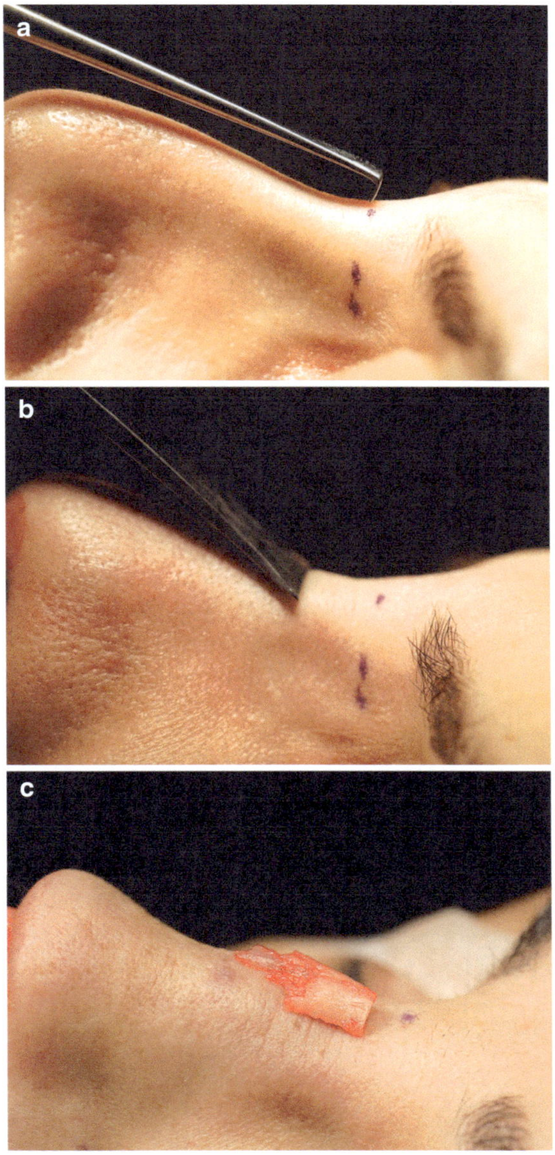

Fig. 2.6 (**a**–**c**) The proper angles of tools are shown over the skin

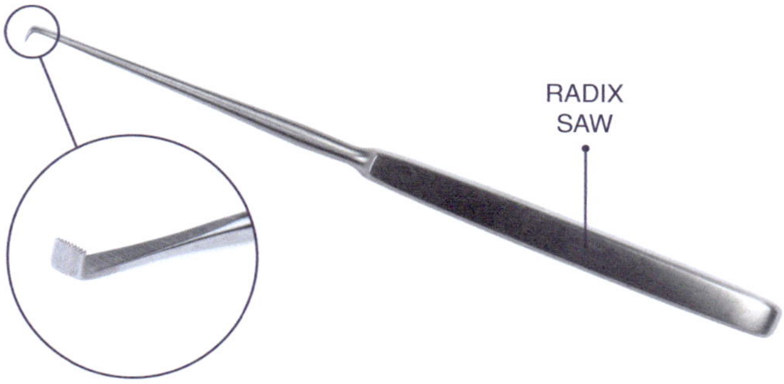

Fig. 2.7 Radix saw

2.3 What Is the Radix Saw?

The radix saw is made of hardened stainless steel; it has a tip with a width of 4 mm and a depth of 7 mm, a gear angle of 90°, and a shank length of 12 cm. The head of the instrument is small; elevation is not excessive, and skin bruising/reddening is not of concern (Fig. 2.7).

2.4 Clinical Outcomes

Visual demonstrations of high radix surgeries are discussed in cases for better understanding.

2.4.1 Case 1

- At first the ideal radix point is marked (Fig. 2.8).
- Secondly the primary hump is removed via osteotomy (Fig. 2.9).
- Then the ideal radix projection marked on the skin is cut transversely with a saw (Fig. 2.10).
- After incision, a wedge-shaped section of bone is removed via flat osteotomy (Fig. 2.11).
- A secondary hump develops after removal of excess bone in the radix region. Then the secondary hump is removed. Finally, irregularities are eliminated using the radix saw as a rasp (Fig. 2.12).

The clinical outcome of the case is shown 2 years after surgery (Fig. 2.13).

2.4.2 Case 2

Another high radix case that suffered from a large nose is shown. Overall, nasal size won't be reduced unless the high radix is fixed. Excessive radix part has been removed with radix saw using the method previously discussed (Fig. 2.14a, b).

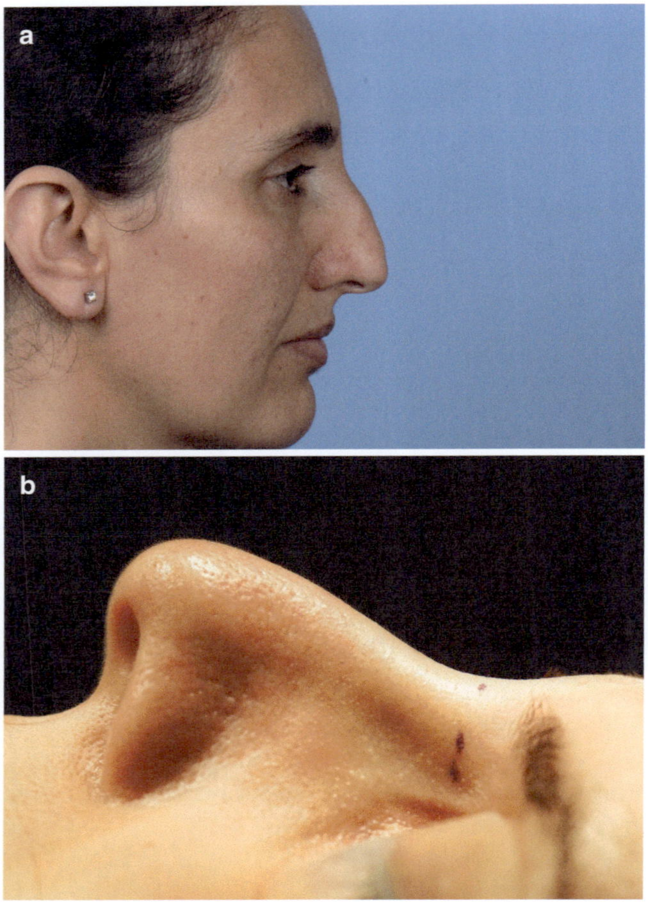

Fig. 2.8 (**a**, **b**) As seen in preoperative and intraoperative photographs, the projection of radix is high

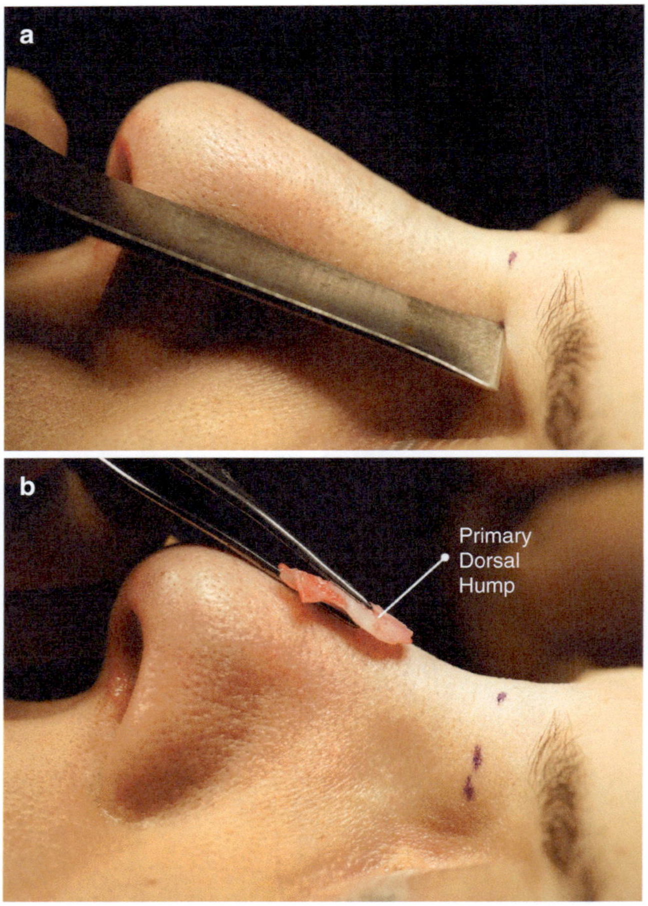

Fig. 2.9 (**a**, **b**) Primary hump removal with straight osteotome

The desired improvement of nose shape can be seen in 1-year postop photos (Fig. 2.15; Supplementary Video 2.2).

2.4.3 Case 3

High radix inevitably causes a large nose. Another example is shown in which the patient's complaint was a large nose. If the surgical aim is to reduce the nose size, lowering the radix must be the first step. Reducing the nasal volume without addressing the radix won't be sufficient (Fig. 2.16a–e; Supplementary Video 2.3).

2.4.4 Case 4

There is a relationship between the radix and chin projection. Therefore, the surgeon has to examine the face in its entirety. Deficiency of the chin makes the dorsum appear higher. For this reason, in cases with low chin projection, treating the chin intraoperatively will strengthen the nasal profile; hence less radix reduction is needed (Fig. 2.17).

2.4.5 Case 5

It is well known that long-term results are much valuable for examining the surgeon's work. Last case of this chapter is an example of long-term results (Fig. 2.18).

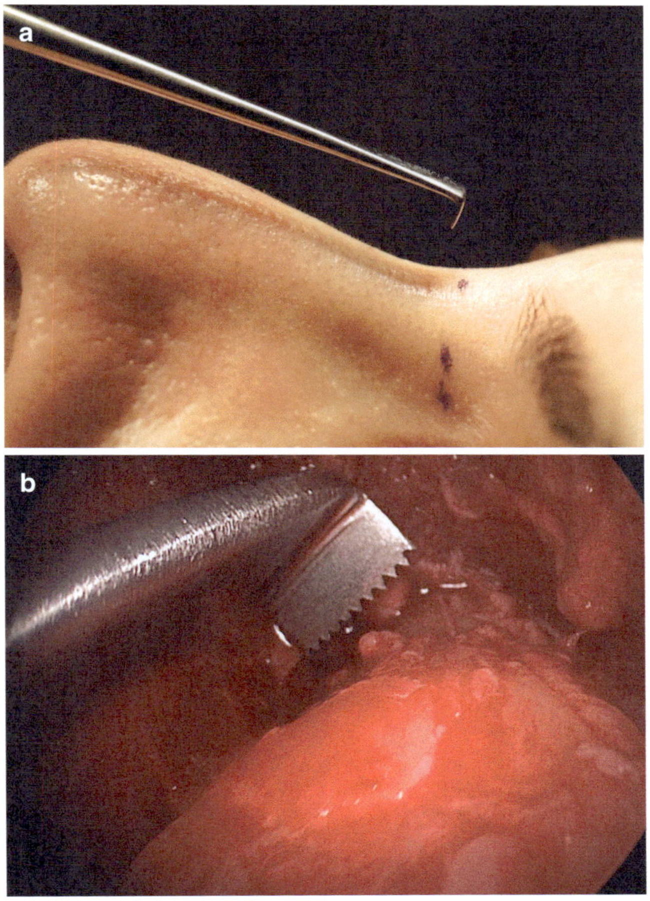

Fig. 2.10 (**a**) The placement of radix saw is shown extracorporally. (**b**) The depth of the cut varies individually

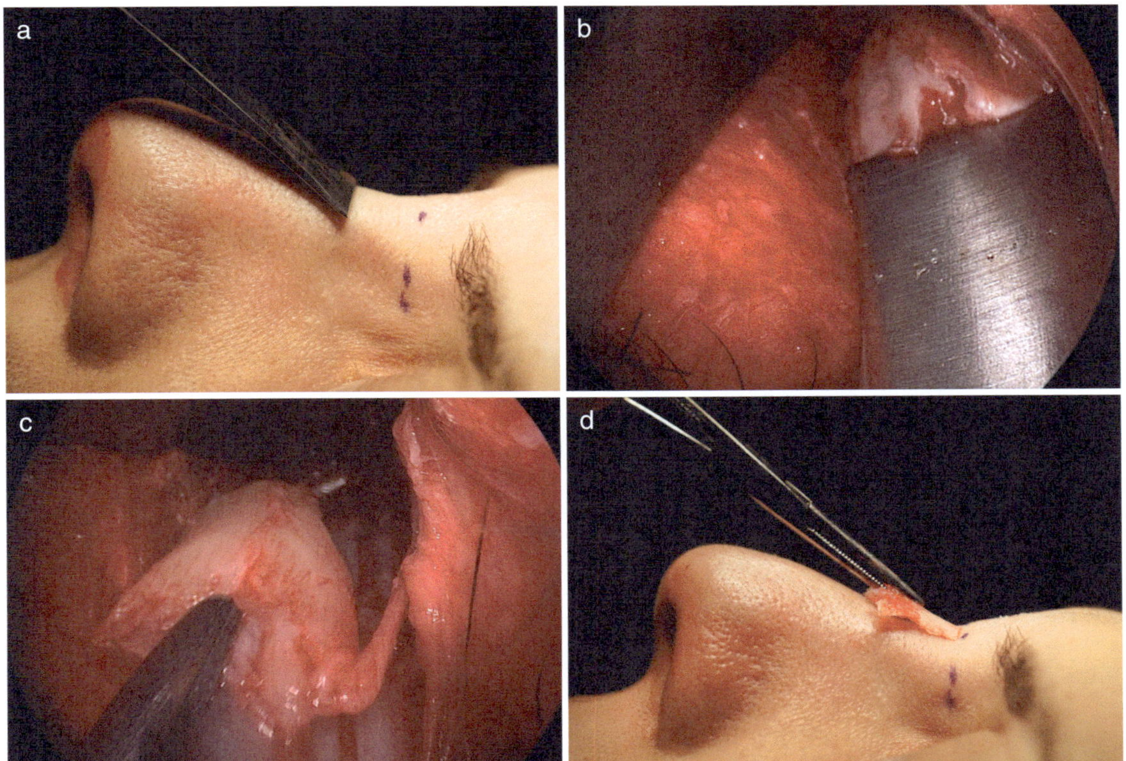

Fig. 2.11 (**a–d**) After defining upper border of the cut, straight osteotome is used for resection

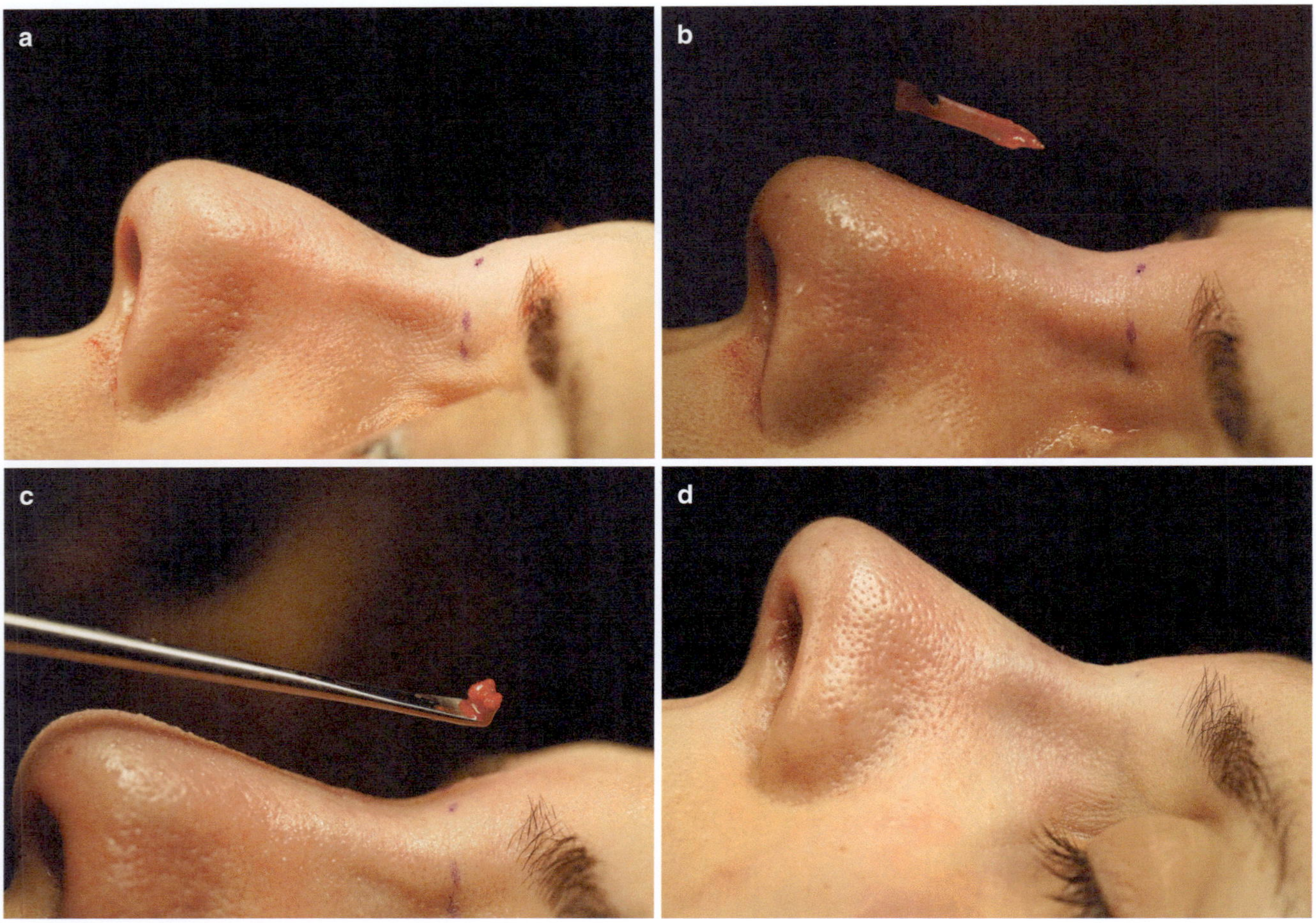

Fig. 2.12 (**a**–**d**) The ideal nasal projection is achieved intraoperatively

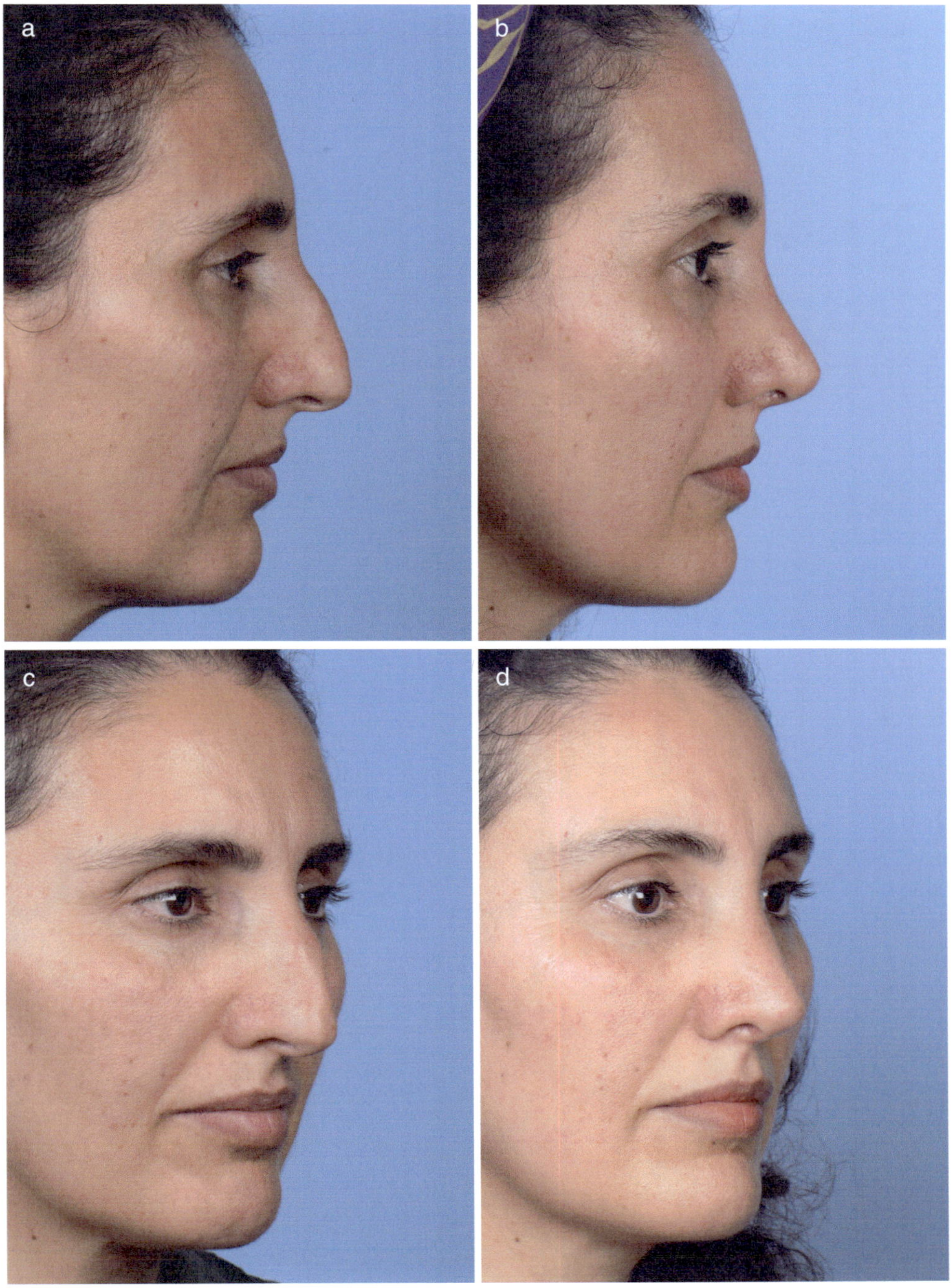

Fig. 2.13 (**a**–**h**) In our first case a high dorsum and a prominent tip projection are evident, in combination with a high radix (a "tension nose"). The dorsum, tip projection, and radix are reduced using an endonasal approach. Vertical alar resection (VAR) is used to reduce the tip projection. The reductions in both the radix and dorsum are evident in the lateral and oblique images; the reduced tip projection is also observed in the baseline image

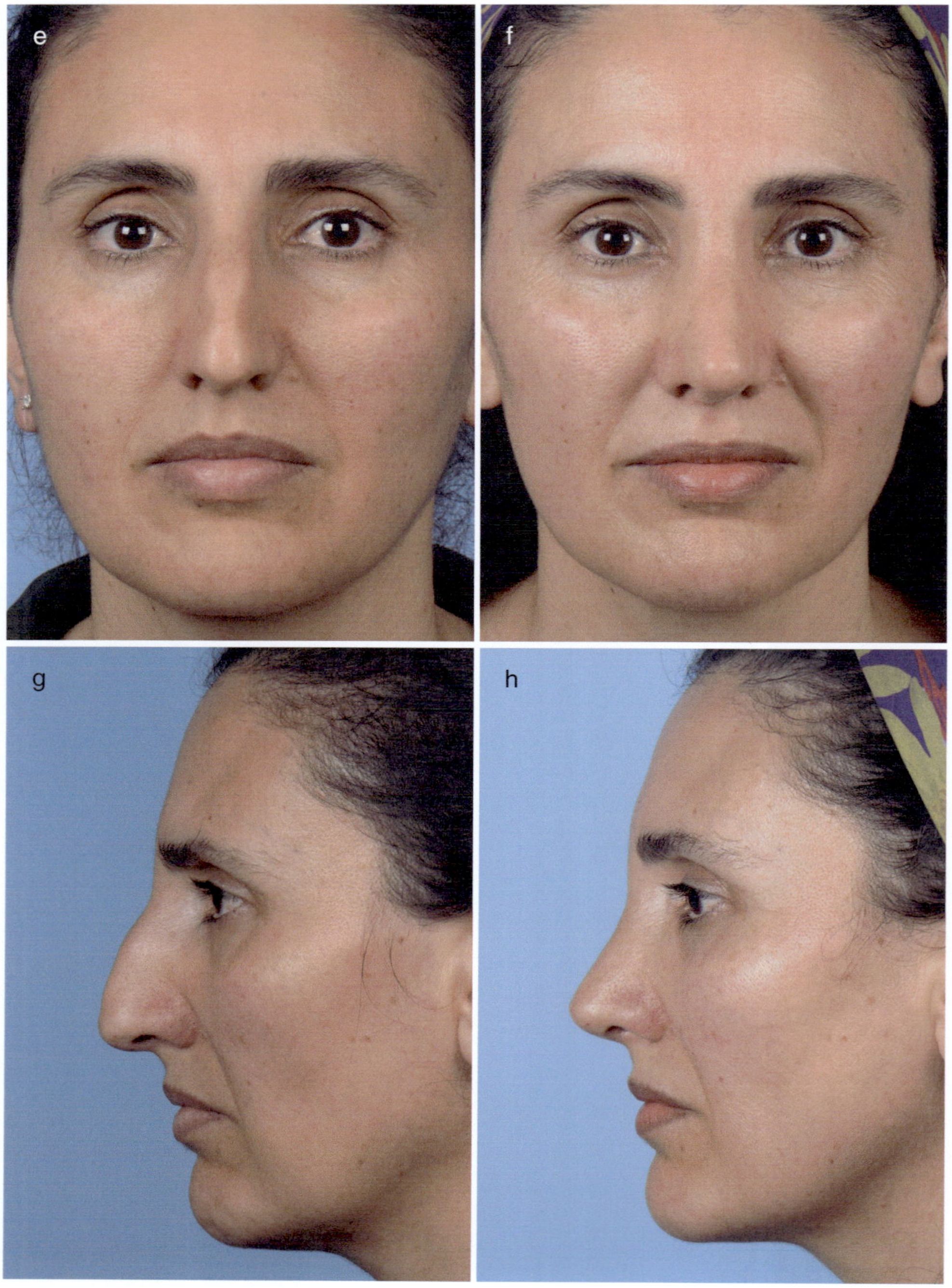

Fig. 2.13 (continued)

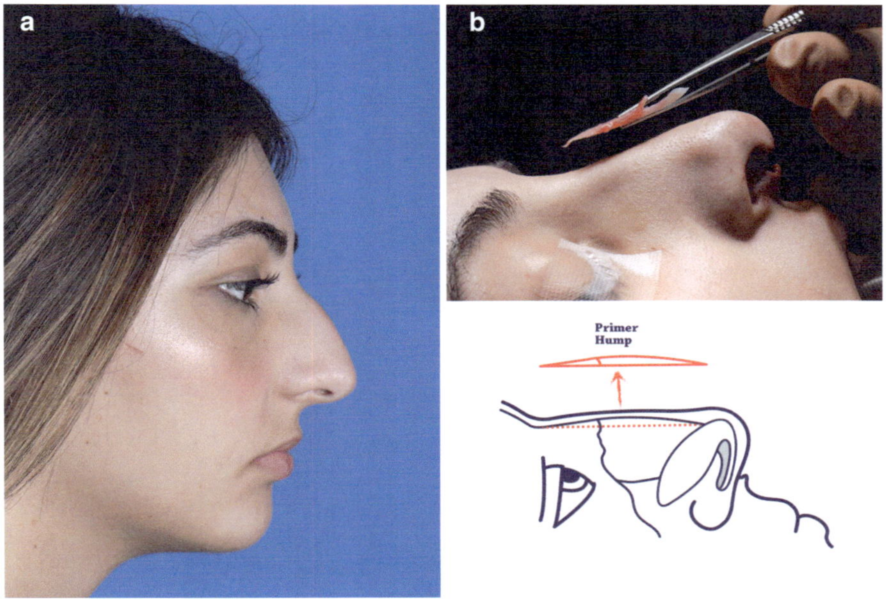

Fig. 2.14 (**a**) Preoperative photograph of the patient with high radix. (**b**) First primary hump is removed

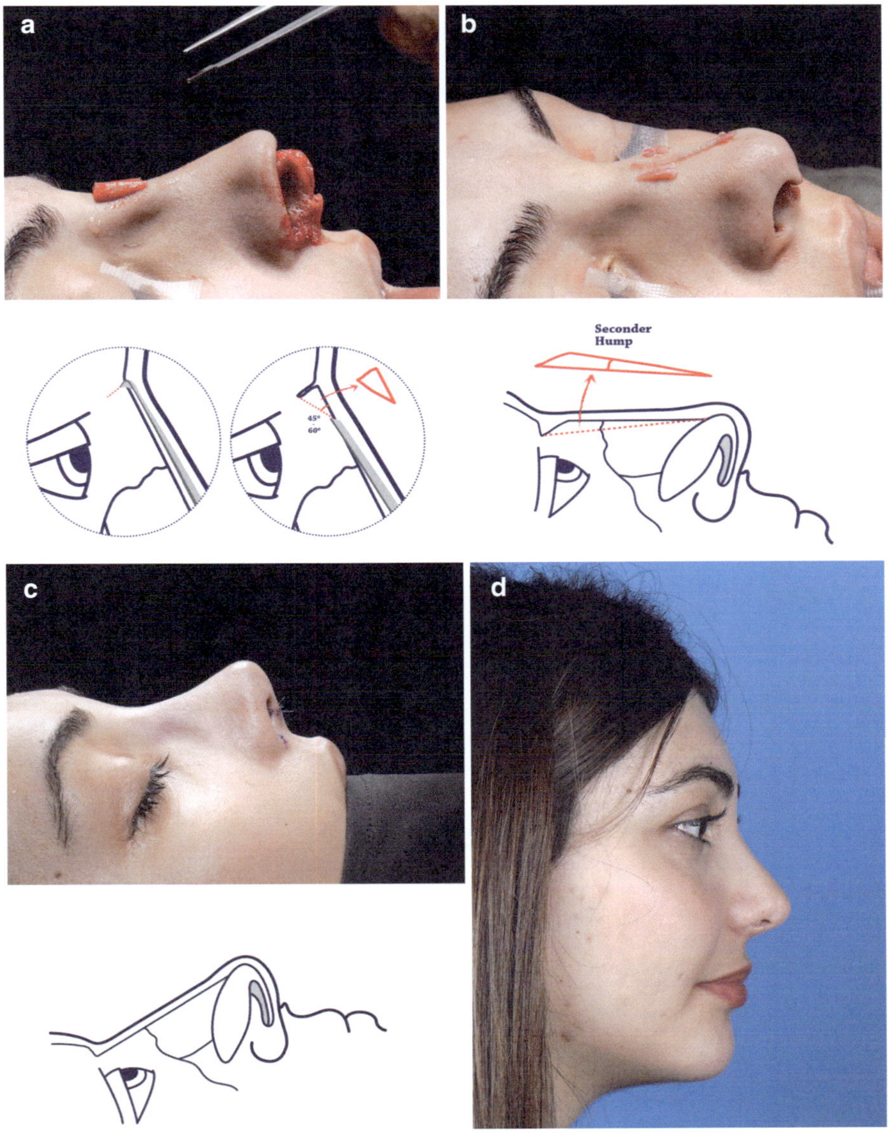

Fig. 2.15 (**a**–**d**) A high radix that breaks the eyebrow-to-nose-tip aesthetic line, and a large nose tip, were the main concerns of this patient. The dorsum and radix projections are reduced using an open approach. We attempted to move the radix to an ideal position. A two-sided autospreader flap is used to reconstruct the eyebrow-tip aesthetic line. Suture-tip plasty was used to remove the large nasal tip

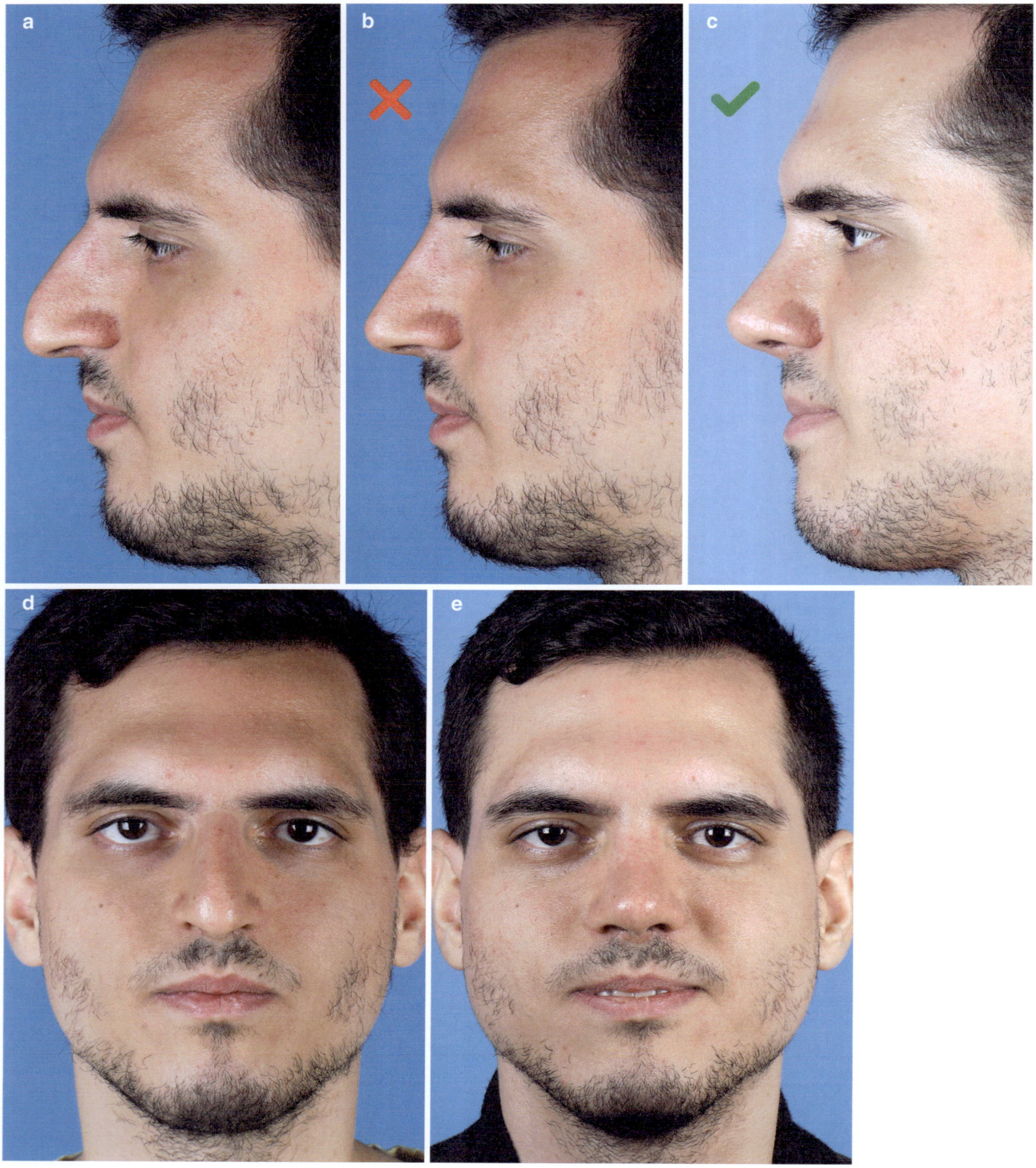

Fig. 2.16 (**a**) The overall size of the nose must be reduced starting from dorsum to tip. (**b**) This illustration exhibits the result when only the primary hump is removed without deprojecting the radix, which is not the desired dorsal view for this patient. (**c**) Real result. The dorsum and radix projection are lowered with the surgical technique mentioned before. At the same time, vertical alar resection (VAR) is used to reduce the tip projection. (**d**) Preoperative frontal view and (**e**) 1 year after. See Supplementary Video 2.3

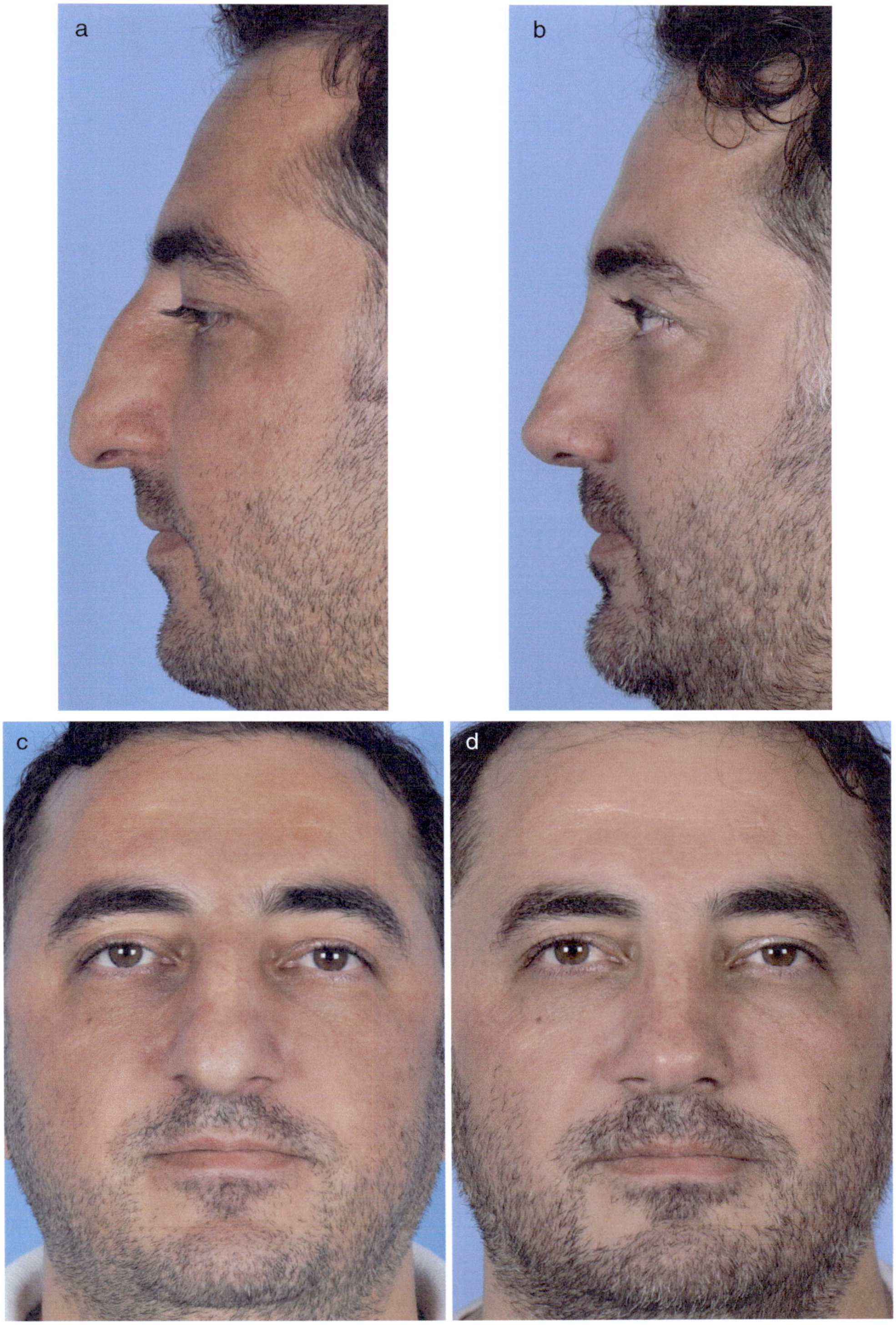

Fig. 2.17 (**a–d**) Two years after rhinoplasty and chin augmentation, the strong dorsal profile is still preserved. Under favor of chin augmentation, less radix reduction is sufficient

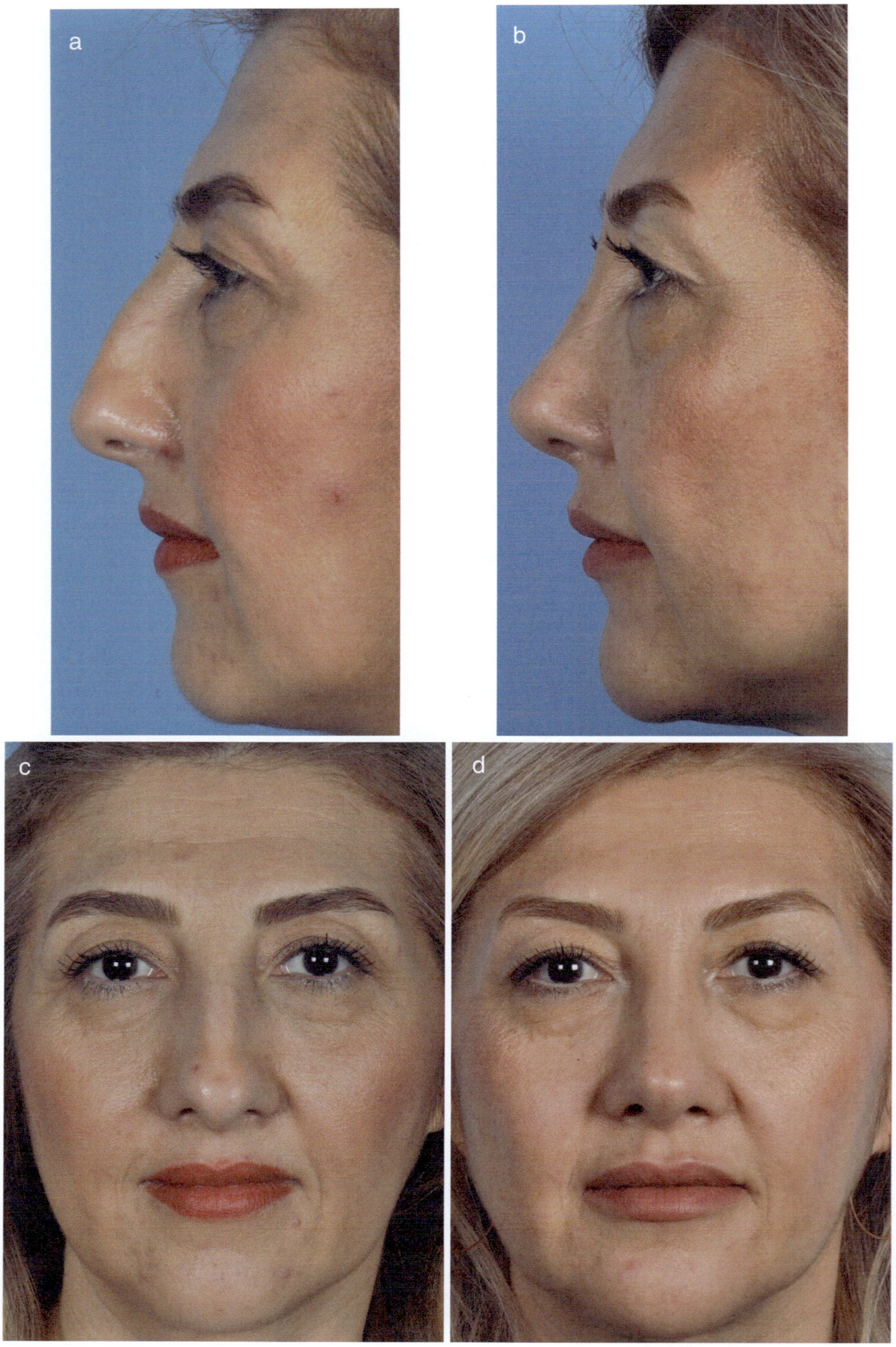

Fig. 2.18 (**a**–**d**) This patient's projections were high and in the cranial position. Additionally, the nose tip was slightly wide. The nose appeared to emerge smoothly from the forehead, (the "avatar" appearance). Primary dorsum and wedge-shaped radix were removed intraoperatively. The radix was lowered using an open technique and shaped via suture tip-plasty. Five years later, the "avatar" appearance was much less marked. However, although the radix was adjusted to its ideal projection and position, soft tissue (skin and subcutaneous and muscle tissues) prevented attainment of a perfect outcome

2.5 Conclusion

A number of rhinoplasty surgeons have developed techniques to lower the radix, but no procedures capable of thinning the skin envelope over the radix have yet been reported. Although minor reductions in the caudal portion of the radix may be achieved using a rasp, substantial reduction requires a more aggressive approach. The use of an osteotome with radix saw to perform a wedge resection of the nasofrontal bones may effectively reduce the projection of the radix and deepen the nasofrontal angle. The radix saw has a number of advantages; for example, it is possible to mark the upper limit with respect to the amount of bone to be removed, by using osteotomes, and the bone can be smoothly removed, and the ideal radix position precisely determined. It is crucial to know that removal of nasofrontal bone at the level of the radix leads to a visible reduction in bone height of only approximately 25%. Patients must therefore be informed that an ideal projection may not be achieved after surgery.

Disclosures The author reports no conflicts of interest or funding requiring disclosure.

Further Reading

Apaydin F. Rhinoplasty in the Middle Eastern nose. Facial Plast Surg Clin North Am. 2014;22(3):349–55.

Eskandarlou M, Motamed S. Evaluation of frequency of four common nasal anatomical deformities in primary rhinoplasty in a Tehran plastic surgery center. World J Plast Surg. 2014;3(2):122–8.

Kayabaşoğlu G, Dizdar D. An effective technique for nasal radix reduction in septorhinoplasty: procerus muscle resection. J Craniofac Surg. 2017;28(8):2143–4.

Kim SJ, Ryu IY, Kim SW, Lee KH. Does the supine position affect the nasal profile in rhinoplasty patients? A comparison of nasal anthropometric measurements in different body positions. Aesthet Surg J. 2017;37(10):1098–102.

Lazovic GD, Daniel RK, Janosevic LB, Kosanovic RM, Colic MM, Kosins AM. Rhinoplasty: the nasal bones: anatomy and analysis. Aesthet Surg J. 2015;35(3):255–63.

Pousti SB, Jalessi M, Asghari A. Management of nasofrontal angle in rhinoplasty. Iran Red Crescent Med J. 2010;12:7–11.

Şeneldir S, Dizdar D, Tuna A. Radix saw: a useful tool for rhinoplasty to correct high radix. Braz J Otorhinolaryngol. 2021;87(1):59–65. https://doi.org/10.1016/j.bjorl.2019.06.013.

Sheen JH. The radix as a reference in rhinoplasty. Semin Plast Surg. 1987;1:33–50.

Steiger JD, Baker SR. Nuances of profile management: the radix. Facial Plast Surg Clin North Am. 2009;17(1):15–28.

3 Low Radix

3.1 Introduction

An under-projected radix is usually low (≤9 mm from the corneal plane) (Fig. 3.1). The position may be ideal, but the radix may also be too caudal.

Low Radix:

- A deeply set radix makes the nose appear short.
- The hump looks bigger than its actual size (a "pseudo overhump").
- On the frontal view, the root of the nasal cavity appears to be light-toned; the nose looks like it is divided into two parts and the facial expression is harsh and angry ("angry face syndrome").
- If a deep radix, a flat dorsum, and a high projection are accompanied by a prominently projected glabella, the overall nasal balance shifts caudally (a "bottom-heavy" nose) (Fig. 3.2).

During traditional rhinoplasty, a convex dorsum (high bridge) is lowered to a plane in the direction of the radix. If the radix is low, this approach becomes problematic. When the hump is resected in a patient without augmenting the radix the dorsum becomes under-projected and the tip appears over-projected. Overall, the facial balance is very poor. To avoid this, a deep radix should be carefully examined, and surgical planning must be meticulous (Fig. 3.3).

Supplementary Information The online version contains supplementary material available at https://doi.org/10.1007/978-3-031-65619-4_3.

S. Şeneldir, *Photographic Atlas of Rhinoplasty*, https://doi.org/10.1007/978-3-031-65619-4_3

Fig. 3.1 Low radix

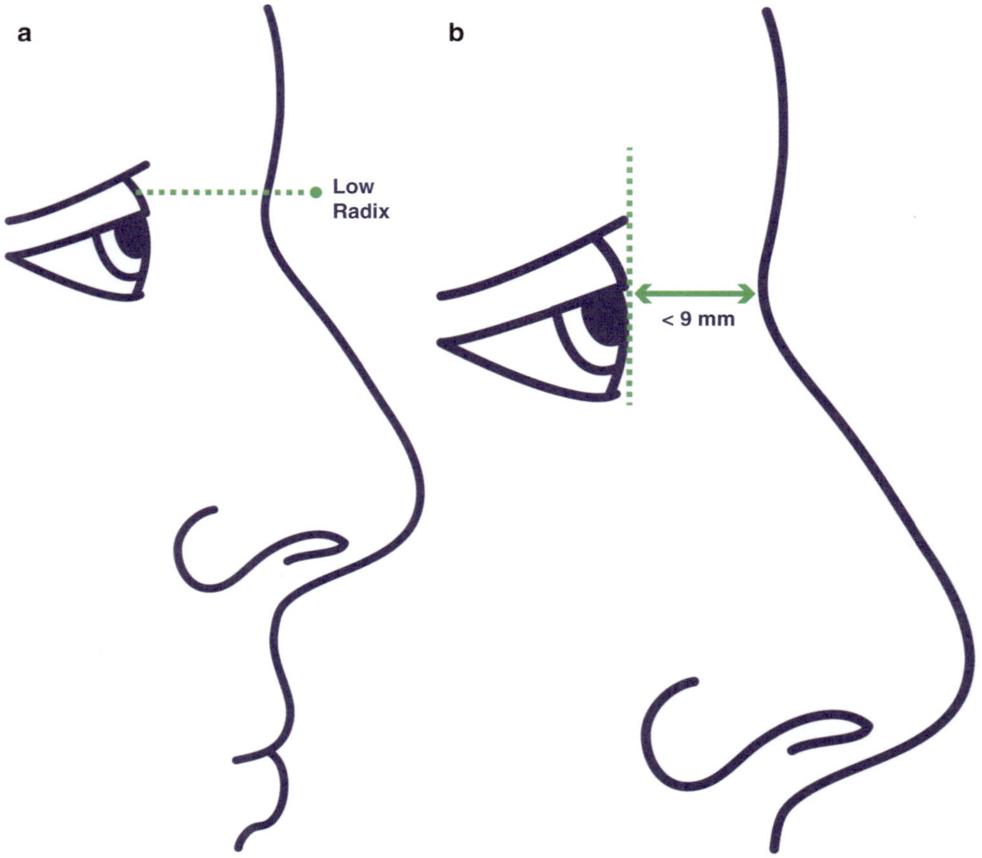

Fig. 3.2 A patient with low radix, angry face syndrome

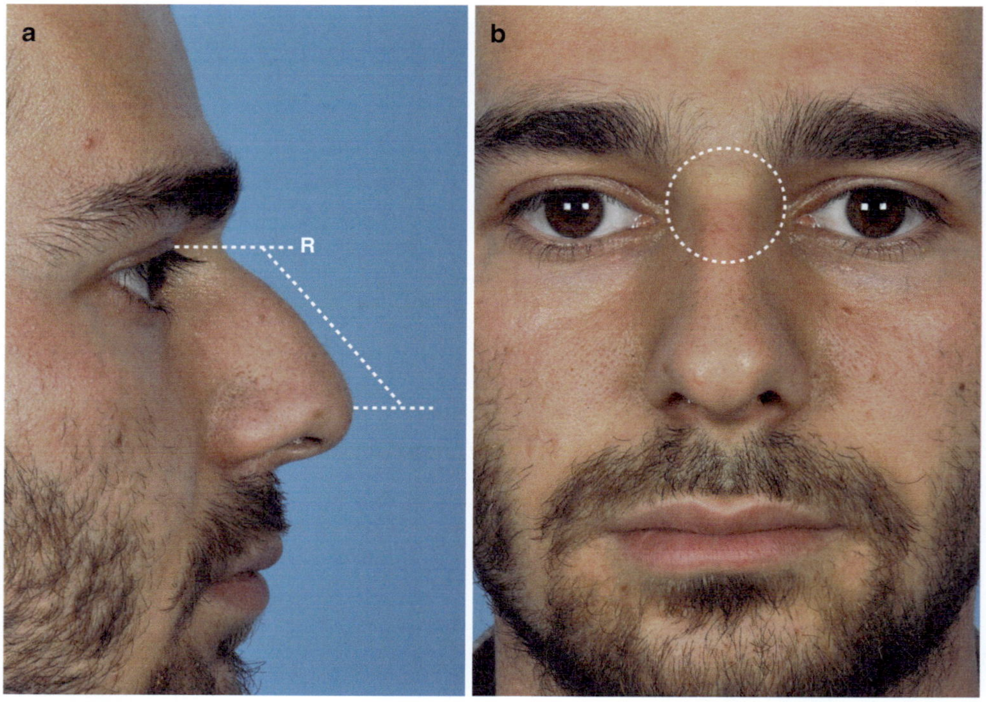

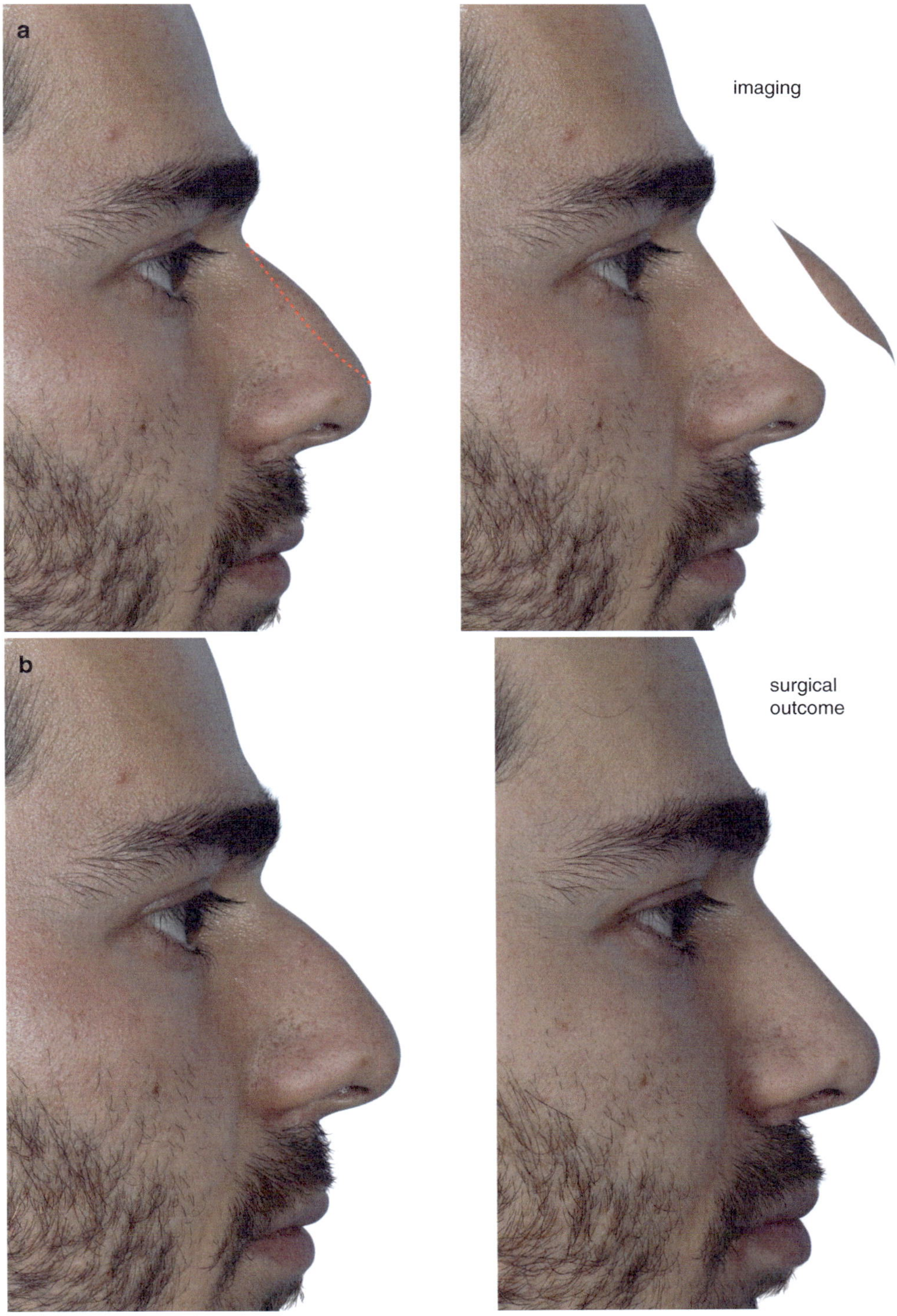

Fig. 3.3 (**a**) This patient with a low radix is at risk of an unsatisfactory outcome if the surgeon seeks to align the base projection with the low nose root. (**b**) Postoperatively, you can see that the nose was balanced by filling the radix and minimizing the dorsum

3.2 Treatment Strategy

Surgery should be performed in three stages for a patient with a low radix.

Stage 1: Primary dorsum work: Before radix augmentation, the dorsal hump must be removed, but aggressive hump resection should be avoided in a patient with a low radix. If the hump is reevaluated on the operating table (assuming that the radix is now in the ideal position), it will be observed that any hump surplus is minimal (Fig. 3.4).

Stage 2: Radix augmentation: The radix is adjusted to an ideal position and any excessive projection is corrected by grafting (Fig. 3.5).

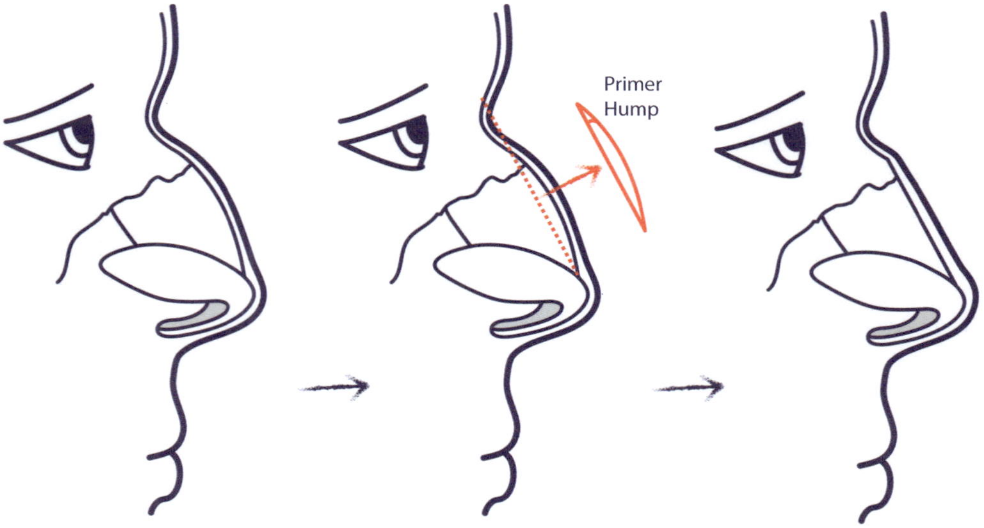

Fig. 3.4 Primer hump removal

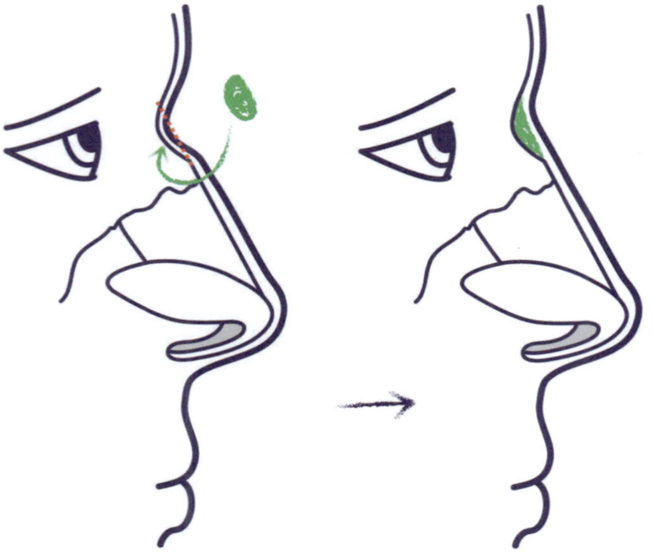

Fig. 3.5 Radix augmentation by inserting graft material

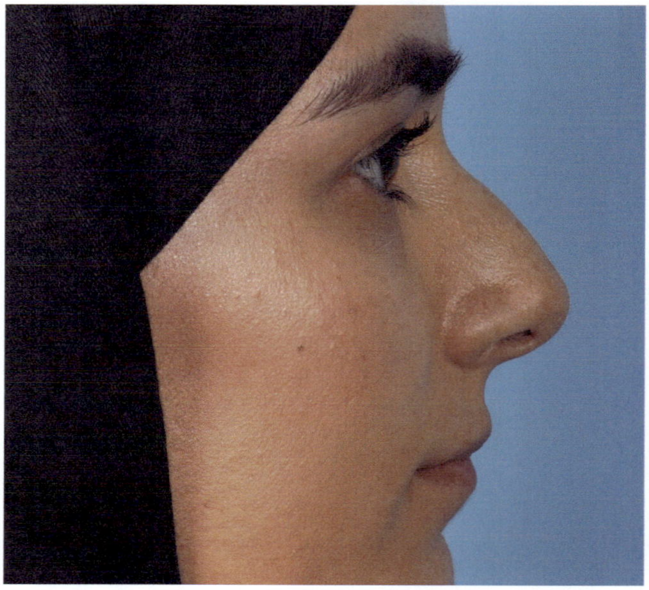

Fig. 3.6 Preoperative photograph of the patient

Grafts used to increase radix projection should have the fallowing three features:

- They should not be resorbed in the long term.
- They must adapt well.
- They must be invisible and nonpalpable.

Technical Pearl: If cartilage is to be used as a graft material, it should be softened by gentle crushing and the excess removed; the cartilage is then placed in the envelope created earlier in the radix. The envelope should not be too wide; if it is, the graft may slip. An external bandage affords adequate fixation.

Stage 3: Secondary dorsum work: The dorsum should be revisited after radix adjustment. If necessary, minimal hump resection should be performed.

3.3 Clinical Outcomes

Visual demonstrations of low radix surgeries are discussed in cases for better understanding.

3.3.1 Case 1

The first case is characterized by a prominent dorsal bridge. If low radix is not considered, it gives us a false impression that aggressive dorsal resection is needed (Fig. 3.6).

The endonasal approach is used in this case.

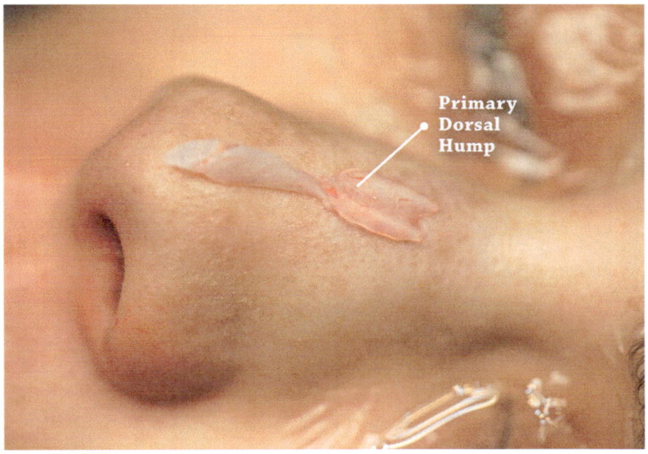

Fig. 3.7 Primary hump was removed

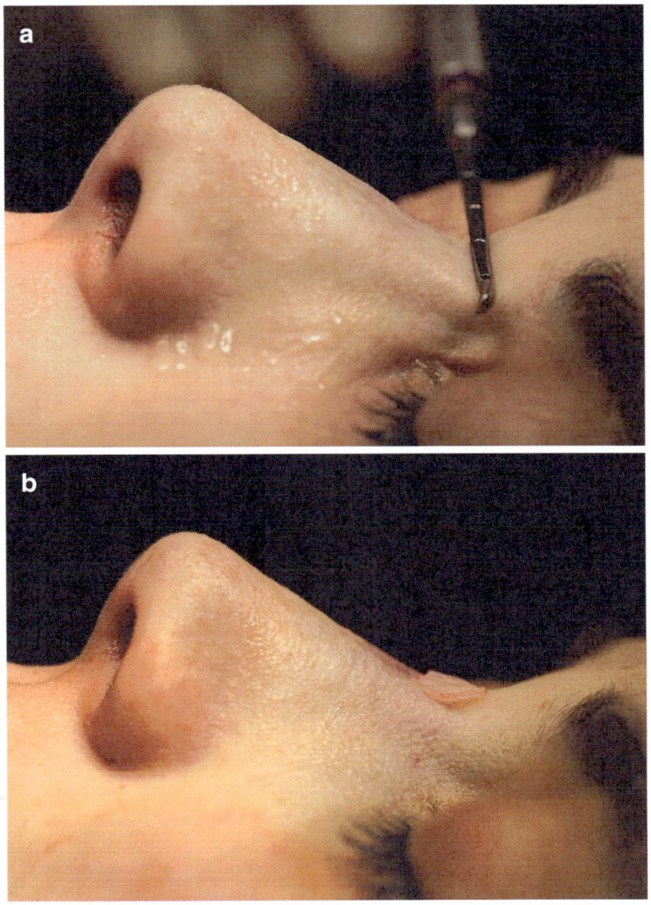

Fig. 3.8 The graft size was determined intraoperatively

- At first the primary hump is removed (Fig. 3.7).
- Then the size of the septal cartilage graft is approximately determined and the radix is augmented using morselized septal cartilage inside an envelope created earlier in the radix (Fig. 3.8).

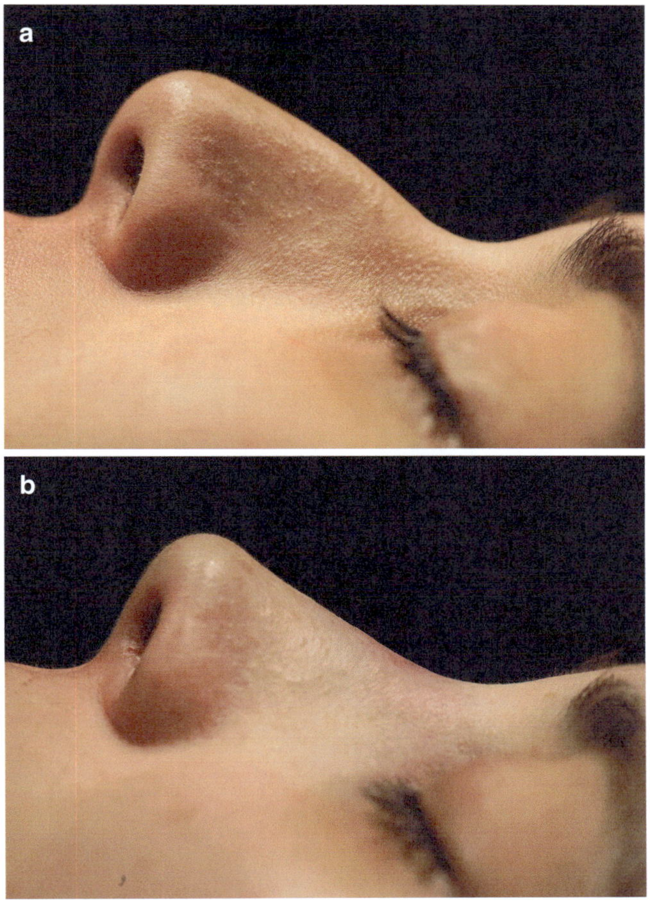

Fig. 3.9 Before and after graft placement during surgery

- The hump has been lowered slightly and radix has been augmented, achieving a more pleasing dorsal profile (Fig. 3.9).

The Clinical outcomes of the case is shown 2 years after surgery (Fig. 3.10).

3.3.2 Case 2

The main complain of the second case is about her tip, which the patient found too wide. When profile view is analyzed, her radix is low. Augmenting her radix, in addition to performing tip plasty, will provide a narrow-appearing tip (Fig. 3.11).

Overall, the tip is narrower and the ideal proportion between the tip and dorsum has been established under favor of tip plasty and radix graft (Fig. 3.12).

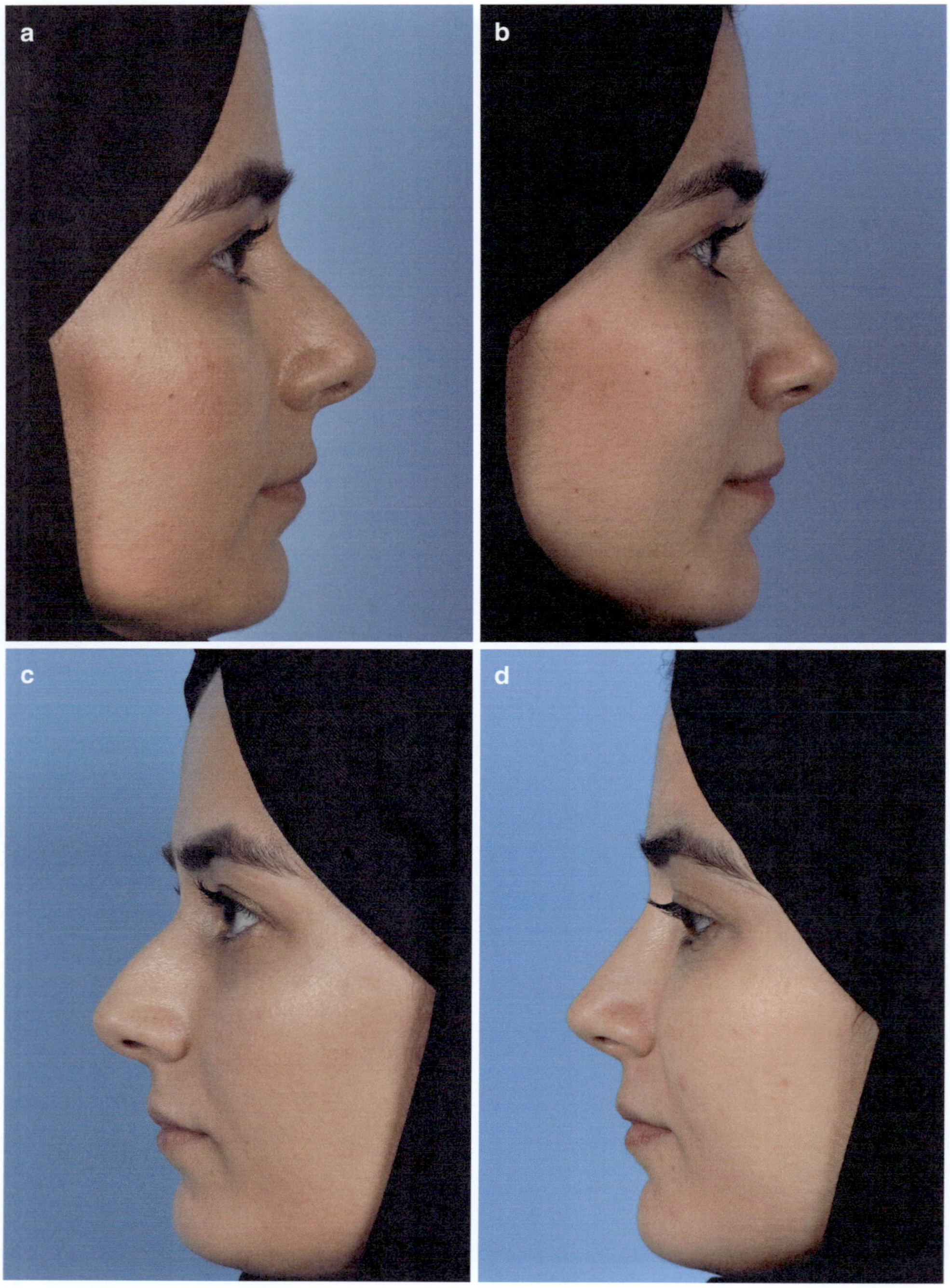

Fig. 3.10 (**a**–**h**) If carefully examined, the preoperative photographs of this patient, whose principal concern is a high dorsum bridge, demonstrate that the radix projection is low and that the radix is caudally positioned. To attain the ideal (proportional) dorsal profile, the radix projection is increased, and the dorsum projection lowered; the projections meet in the middle. Using an endonasal approach, suture tipplasty is sufficient to remodel the nose tip

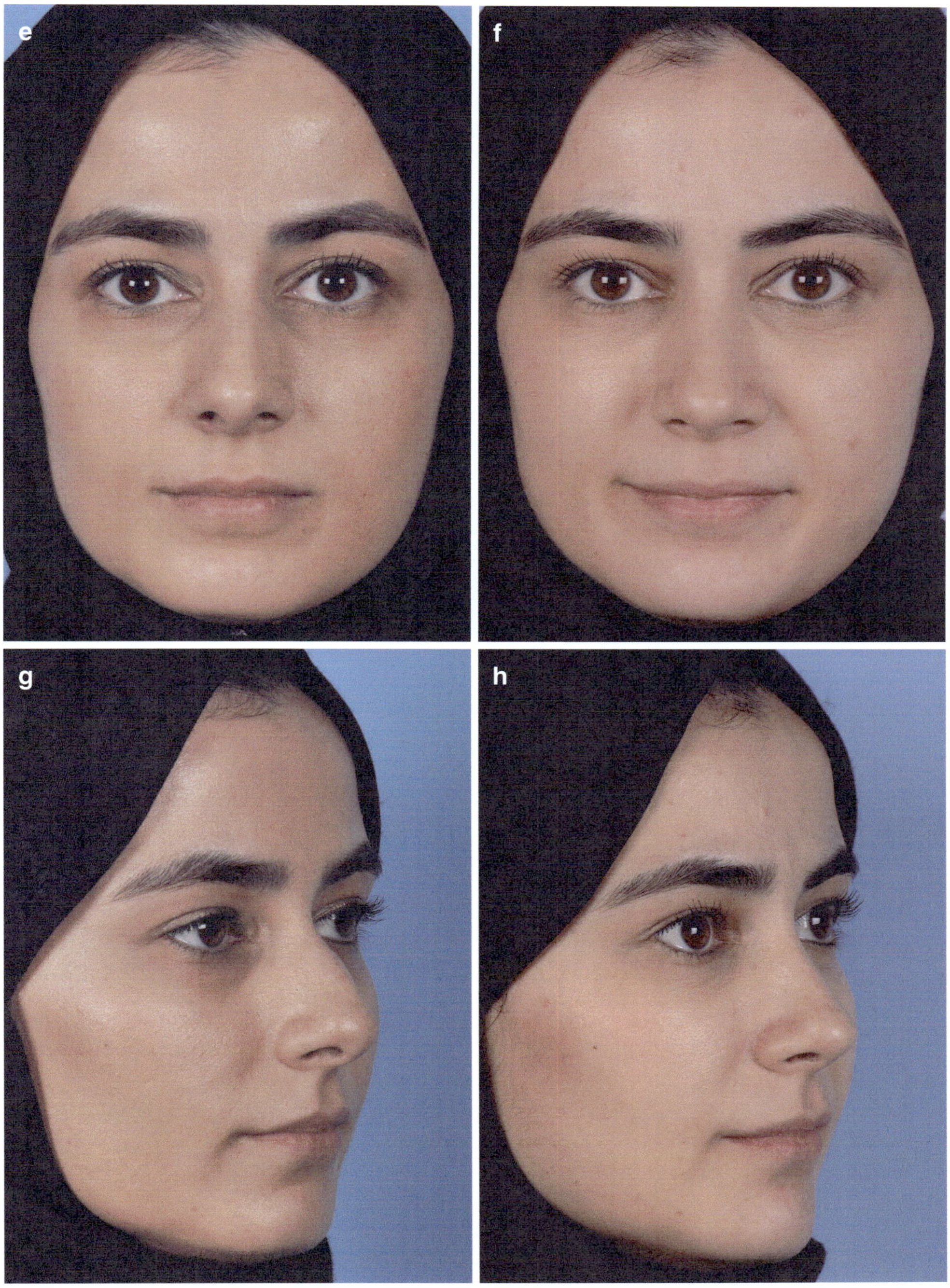

Fig. 3.10 (continued)

3.3.3 Case 3

If the radix requires less graft material as in this case, bone powder obtained during hump rasping can serve as a graft. Bone shavings are particularly useful; they can be placed anywhere on the dorsum. Shavings collected by the nurse into a separate serum-filled container can also be used as radix grafts. After rasping, the accumulated shavings are placed on a cutting board and pressed under gauze; the granules then adhere/integrate to form a cartilage-like material that is 1–2 mm in thickness; the edges can even be cut to shape. When a graft of the desired shape is formed, this is placed into the radix using a bayonet (non-serrated if possible). If a deeply serrated bayonet is used, the graft may lose its integrity and placement becomes difficult. The slightly low radix is augmented using bone powder (Fig. 3.13). Figure 3.14 shows preoperative and 1-year postoperative photographs of the patient (Fig. 3.14).

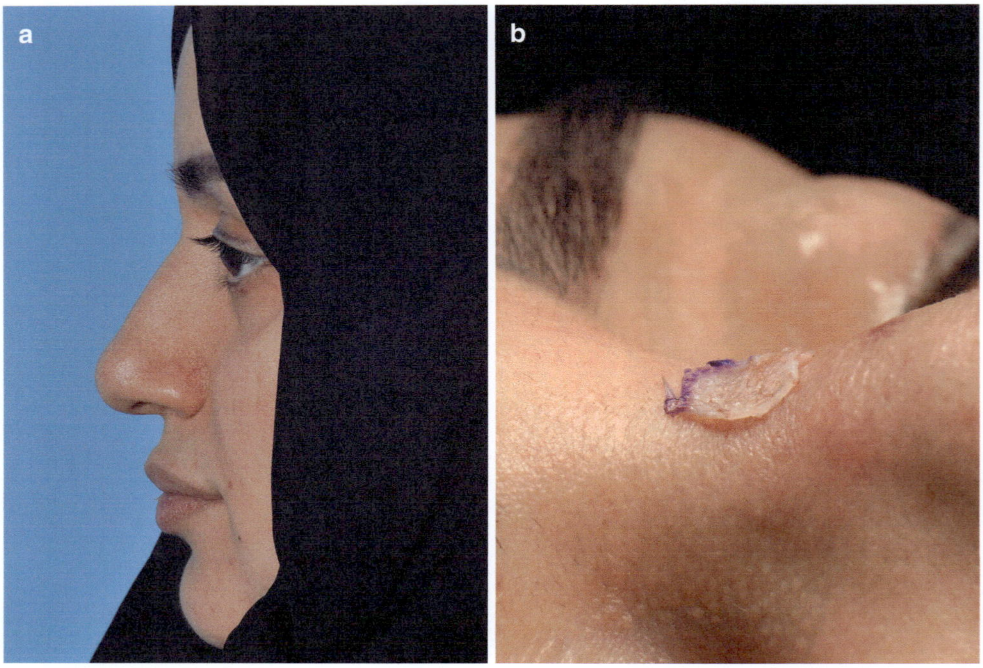

Fig. 3.11 Preoperative lateral view shows radix augmentation is needed. Intraoperative graft placement is shown externally

3.3.4 Case 4

Cephalic excess of alar cartilage is also suitable for radix augmentation if slight augmentation is needed (Fig. 3.15). As shown in preoperative and postoperative photographs an ideal dorsum profile is achieved 1 year after the surgery (Fig. 3.16).

3.3.5 Case 5

If more radix projection is required, precut cartilages can serve as a graft material. Cartilage cubes 0.5–1 mm in size can be used to elevate the radix. The ideal source of cartilage is the patient's nasal septum. Alternatively, auricular cartilage can be considered. Costal cartilage should be used only as a last resort. The cartilage should be mixed with the patient's blood before placement (to avoid graft migration); the mixture is placed into an insulin syringe and injected into the previously prepared envelope. Be careful not to inject too much; any cartilage injected remains in the envelope and an excess may later become palpable (which is undesirable). Intraoperative photographs of the case, demonstrating injection of the precut cartilages (Fig. 3.17). Preoperative and 1 year postoperative photographs of the patient are shown (Fig. 3.18).

Temporal fascia is another safe radix graft material that is a useful alternative to precut cartilage. The greatest advantage of temporal fascia is that the tissue adapts very well to the radix; no medium- or long-term irregularities are evident. The disadvantage is that temporal fascia placement requires a separate incision associated with some medium-term volume loss.

Technical Pearl: If temporal fascia is used alone, the graft will lose up to 20% of its volume in the medium term; this should never be forgotten, and over-grafting by 20% is essential. Over the first few months after surgery, the radix may thus seem overlarge. This should be explained to the patient prior to surgery. Later, the dorsum becomes completely flat.

3.3.6 Case 6

The patient was complaining about her prominent bridge, which is caused by dorsal hump and low radix (Fig. 3.19). Radix augmentation was planned and temporal fascia was preferred as a graft material. During the surgery 20% graft volume loss is not calculated, therefore the patient was unsatisfied with the result (Fig. 3.20). A revision surgery was performed and the radix is augmented (Fig. 3.21).

3.3.7 Case 7

Radix augmentation by temporal fascia graft is shown in this case. Surgery commences with collection of temporal fascia via a z-shaped scalp incision. Ideally, a 5 × 5-cm area of fascia should be harvested; this will increase the radix projection by 5 mm. A 4/0 resorbable suture is placed into the fascia, which is then curved at the sides, shaped into a roll, and secured to the radix using the suture. Then the needle is pushed through the skin and the free end of the suture is taped to the forehead (Fig. 3.22). Preoperative and 3-year postoperative photographs of the patient is shown (Fig. 3.23).

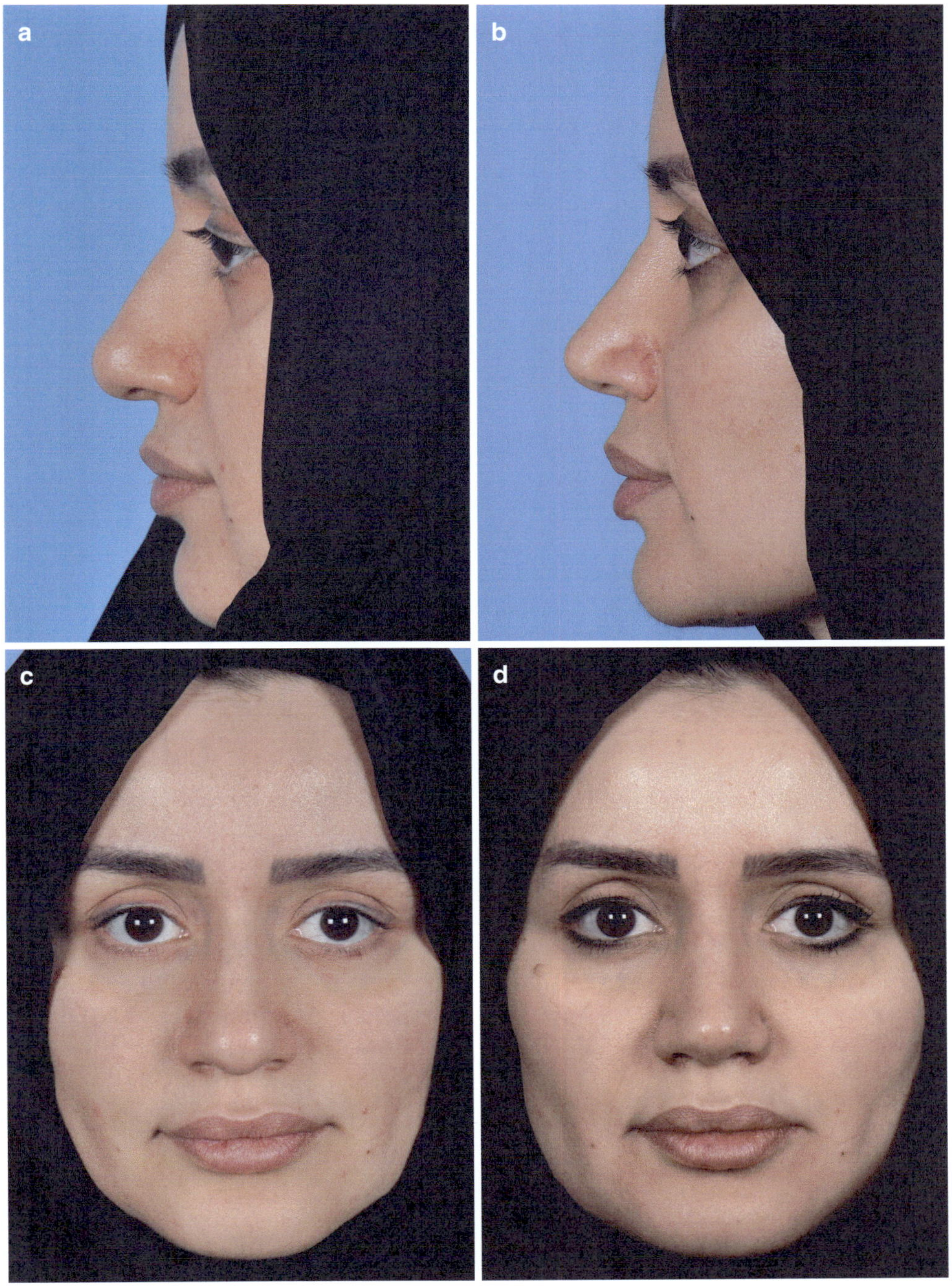

Fig. 3.12 (**a**–**f**) Endonasal approach is used in this case. For her tip, vertical alar resection (VAR) technique is used. Morselized septal cartilage is used as a radix graft

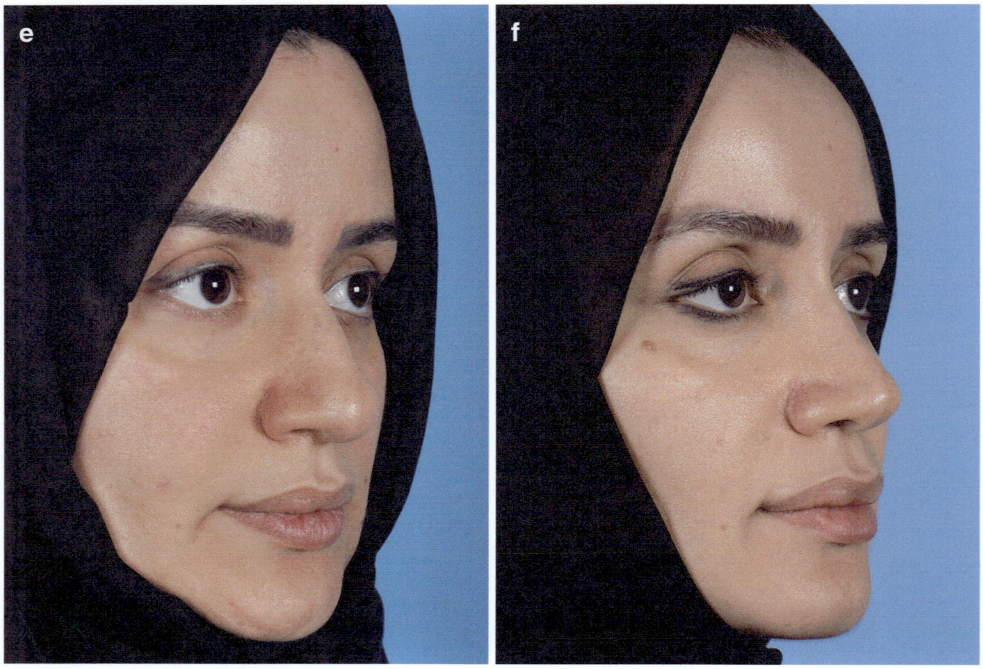

Fig. 3.12 (continued)

3.3.8 Case 8

Liquid rhinoplasty should be kept in mind for patients who do not require surgery to treat the low radix as in this case. Liquid (or filler) rhinoplasty uses an injectable filler to shape the nose safely and effectively, without any need for surgery. The results are extremely reliable and repeatable in patients with low radixes and ideal nasal tips. A hydroxyapatite filler is injected into the radix and bony dorsum and massaged to assume a fan-like shape, narrowing caudally toward the dorsal hump. Our purpose was to raise the level of the radix to the upper eyelash line to better proportion the nose (which, prior to surgery, was curved and bottom-heavy). The fan shape also created a gentle ("hourglass") curvature from the brow to the nose. Injection can be slightly more caudal if a very prominent dorsal hump requires smoothing (Fig. 3.24). Before and after photographs of the case is shown which liquid injection is performed (Fig. 3.25).

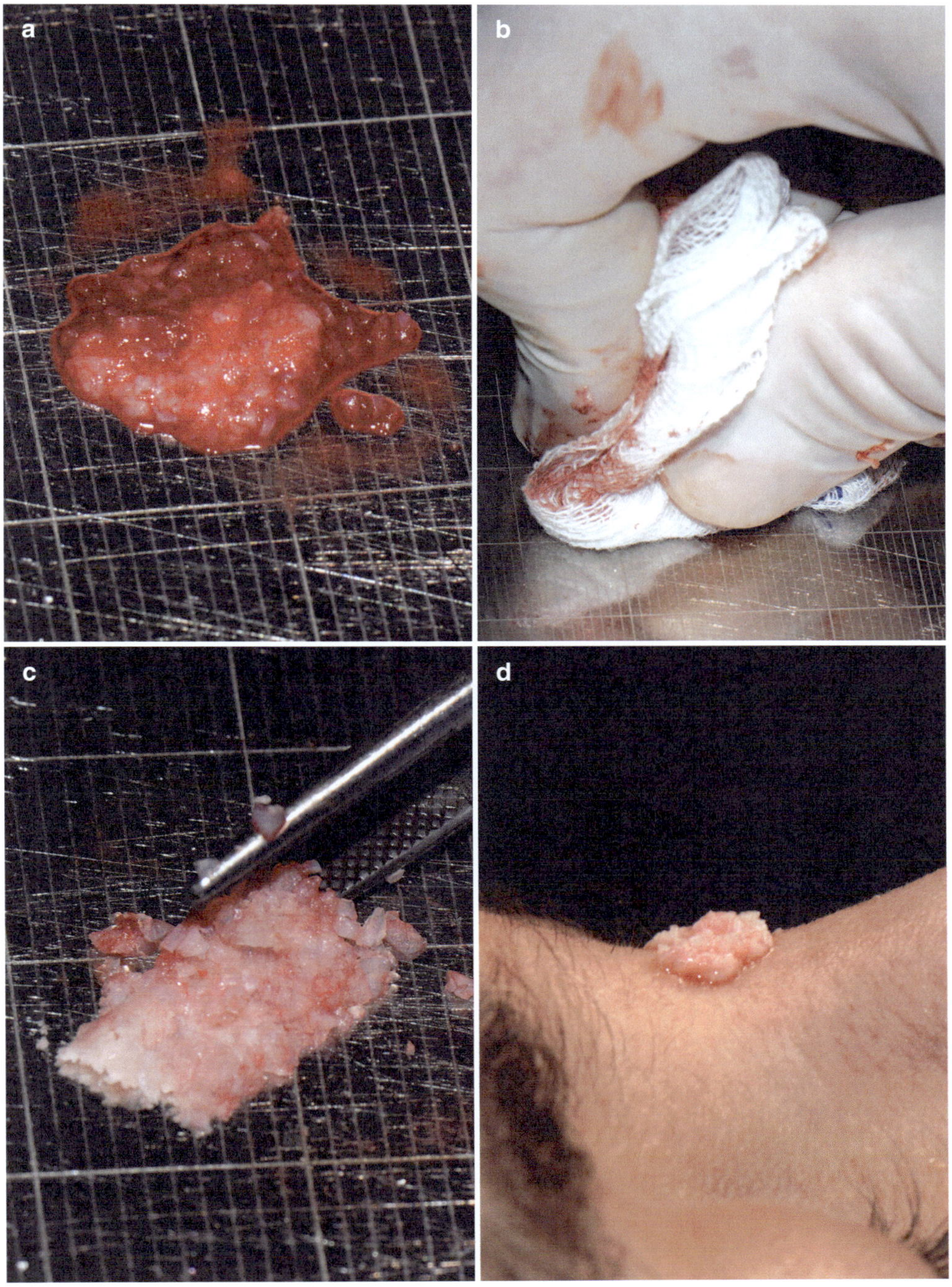

Fig. 3.13 Bone dust graft preparation is shown

Fig. 3.14 (**a** and **b**) Preoperative and postoperative photos of the patient

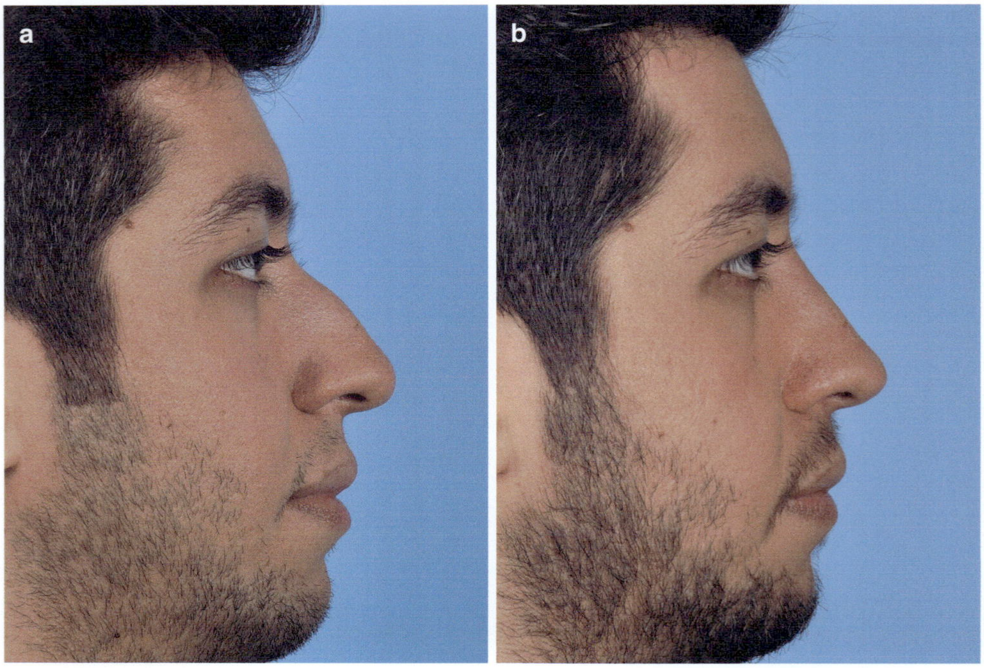

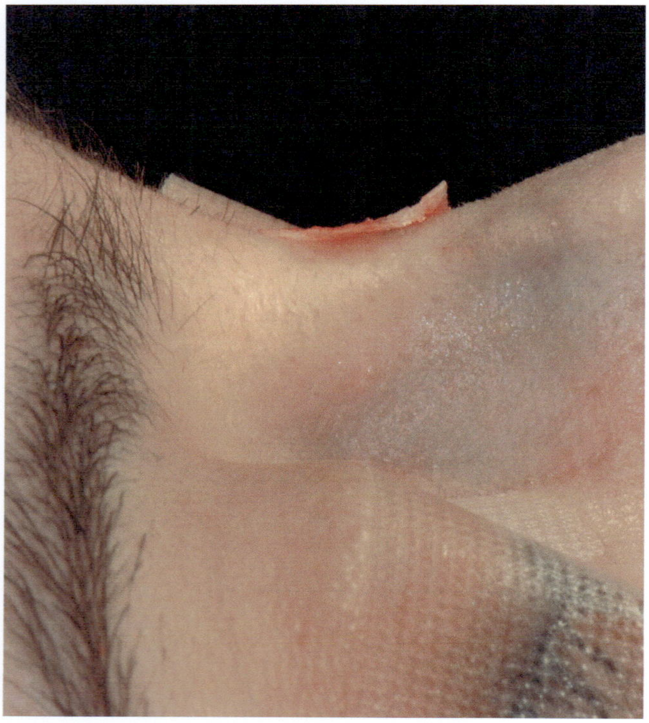

Fig. 3.15 Graft placement is shown externally

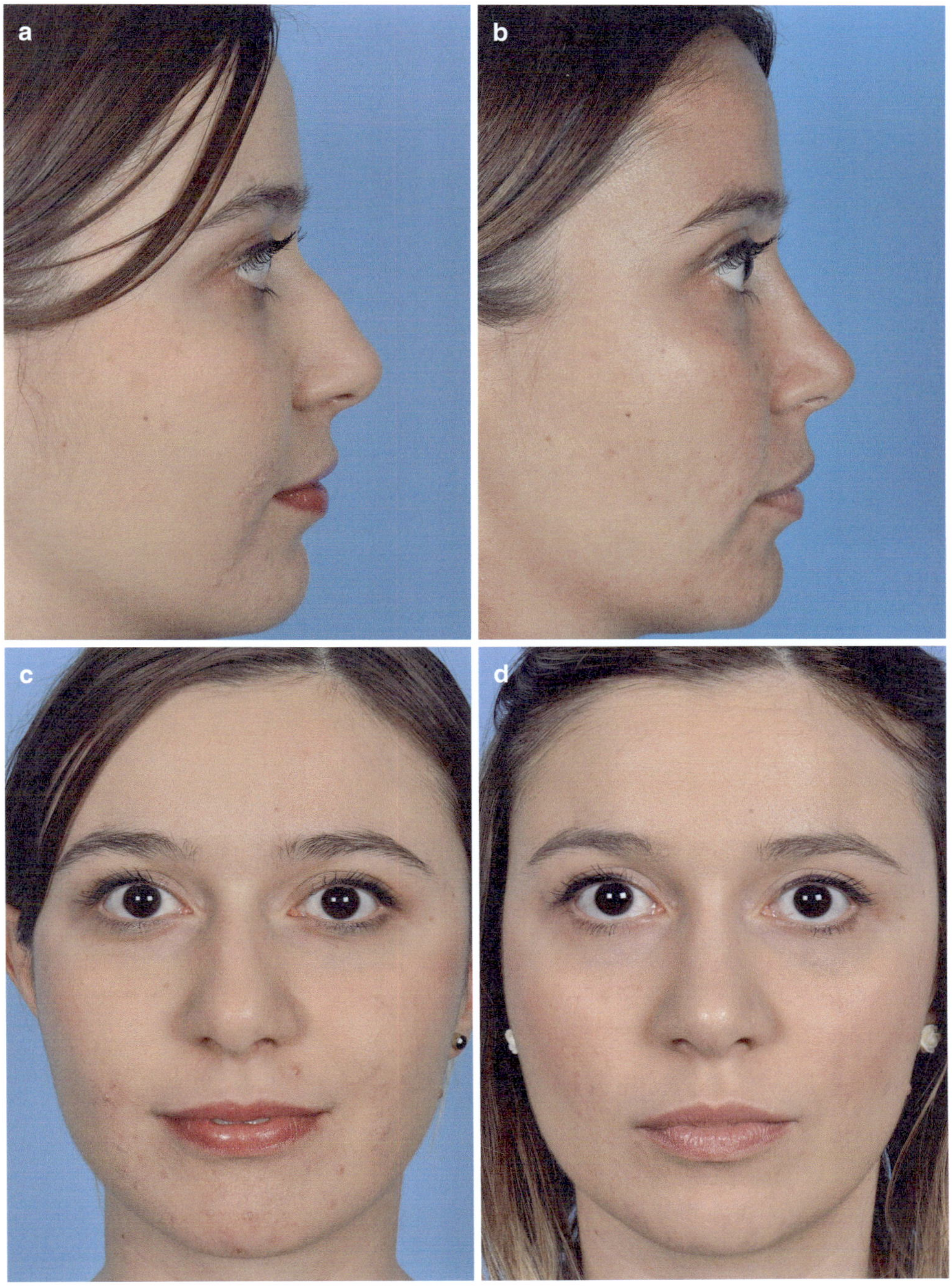

Fig. 3.16 (**a**–**d**) Preoperative and postoperative photos of the patient

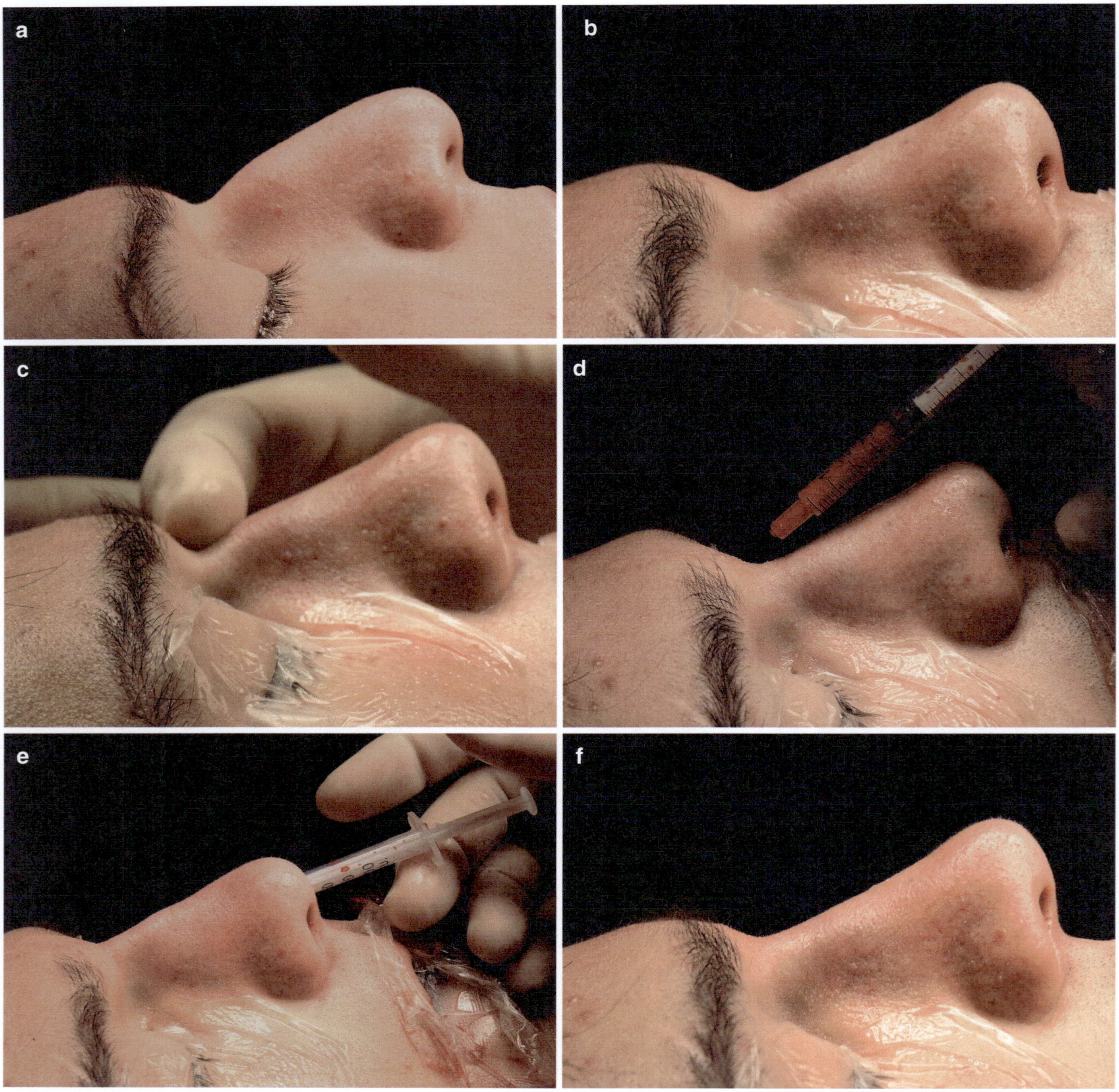

Fig. 3.17 (**a**) Commence surgery. (**b**) Remove the primer hump. (**c**) Graft the radix zone. (**d**) Fill an insulin syringe with cartilage/blood. (**e**, **f**) Fill the radix with cartilage/blood to achieve an ideal dorsal profile; use of an endonasal technique is appropriate

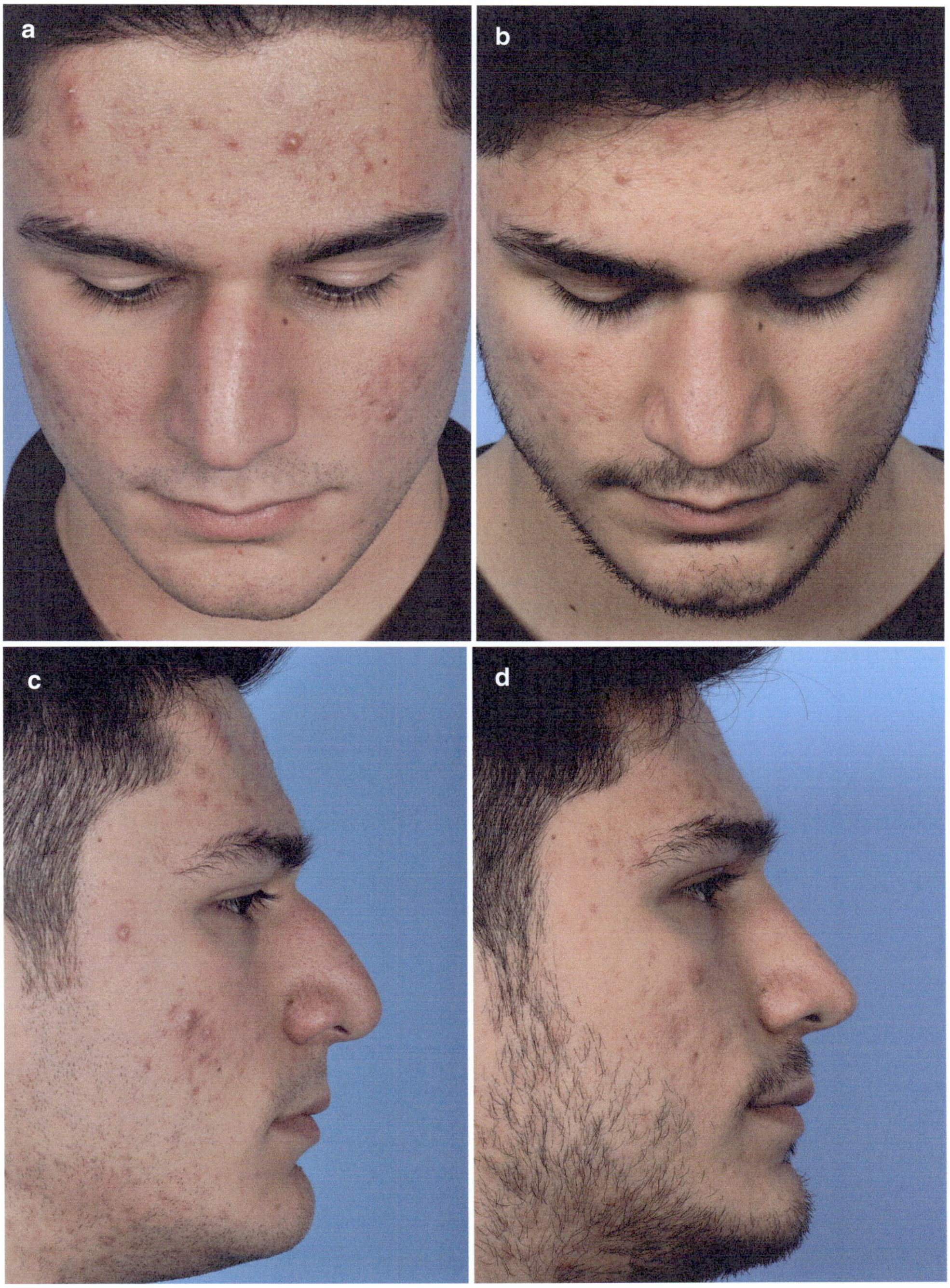

Fig. 3.18 (**a**–**d**) The major complaints of this patient were a nasal hump and deviations in the nasal axes. However, as can be seen on the preoperative lateral photograph, the principal dorsal problem is the low radix. Together with minimal hump removal, a balanced dorsal profile was achieved by filling the radix. To correct the nose roof axes, a right-side double lateral osteotomy and a left-side single osteotomy were performed. Thus, the bony roof was moved to the midline. Suture tip-plasty adequately reconstructed the nose tip

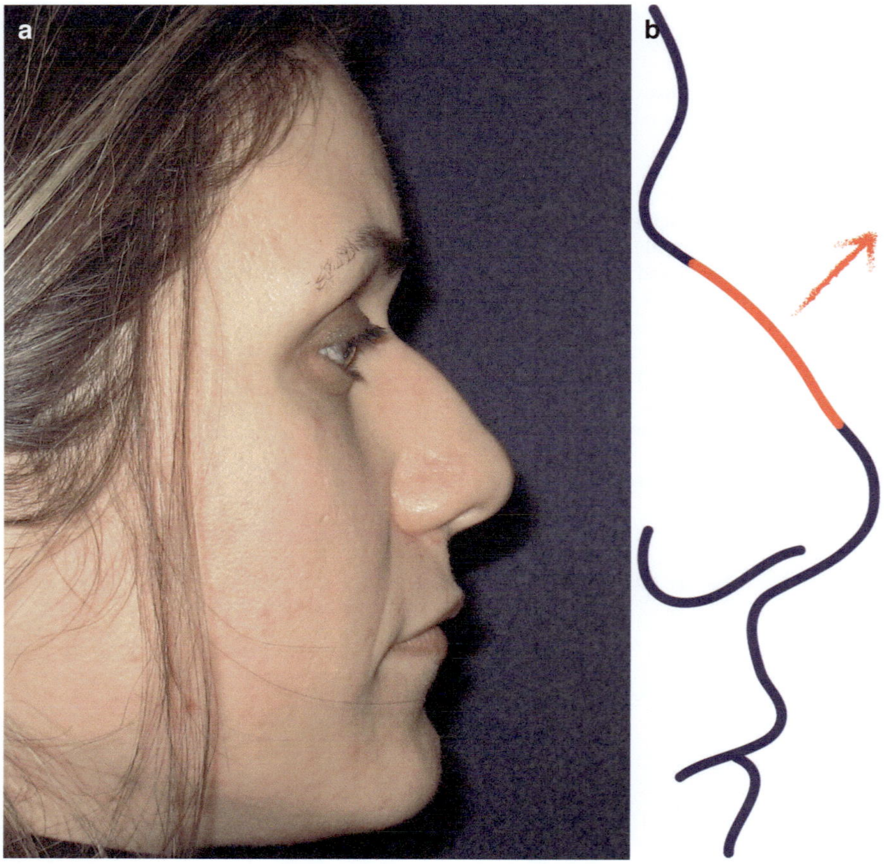

Fig. 3.19 (**a**, **b**) Before using temporal fascia to augment low radix

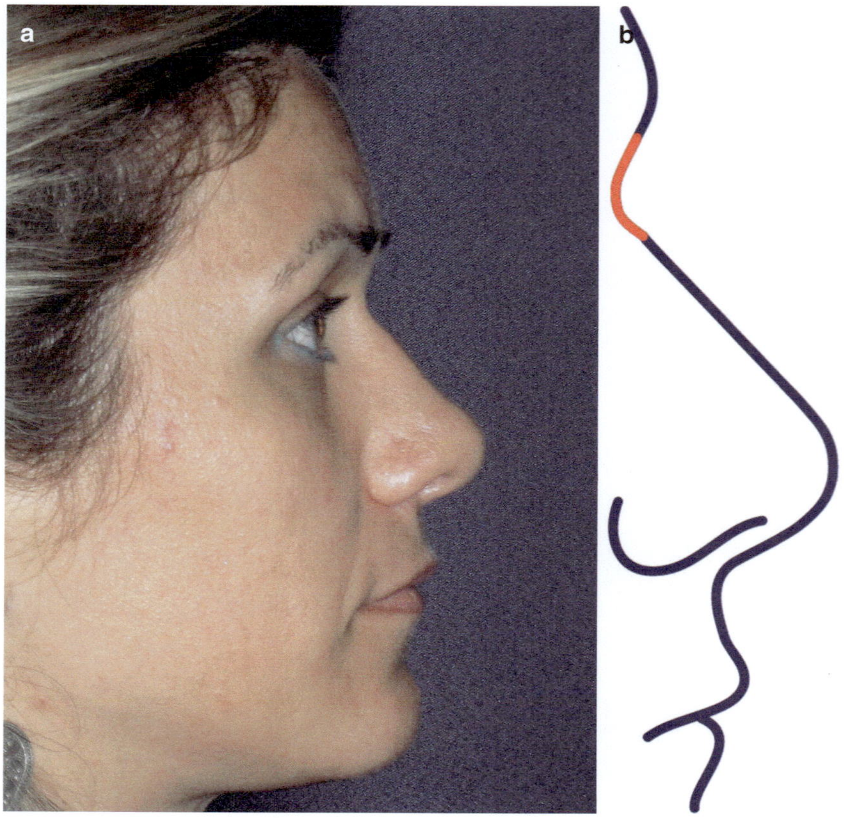

Fig. 3.20 (**a**, **b**) Patient still has low radix postop 2 months because over-grafting was not done with temporal fascia

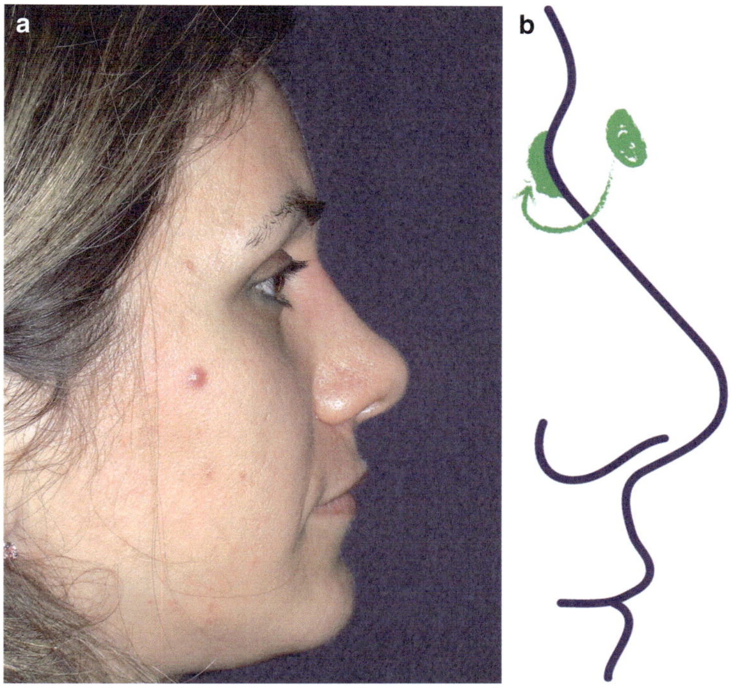

Fig. 3.21 (**a**, **b**) After revision surgery, radix is now in its ideal projection via cartilage grafting in revision surgery

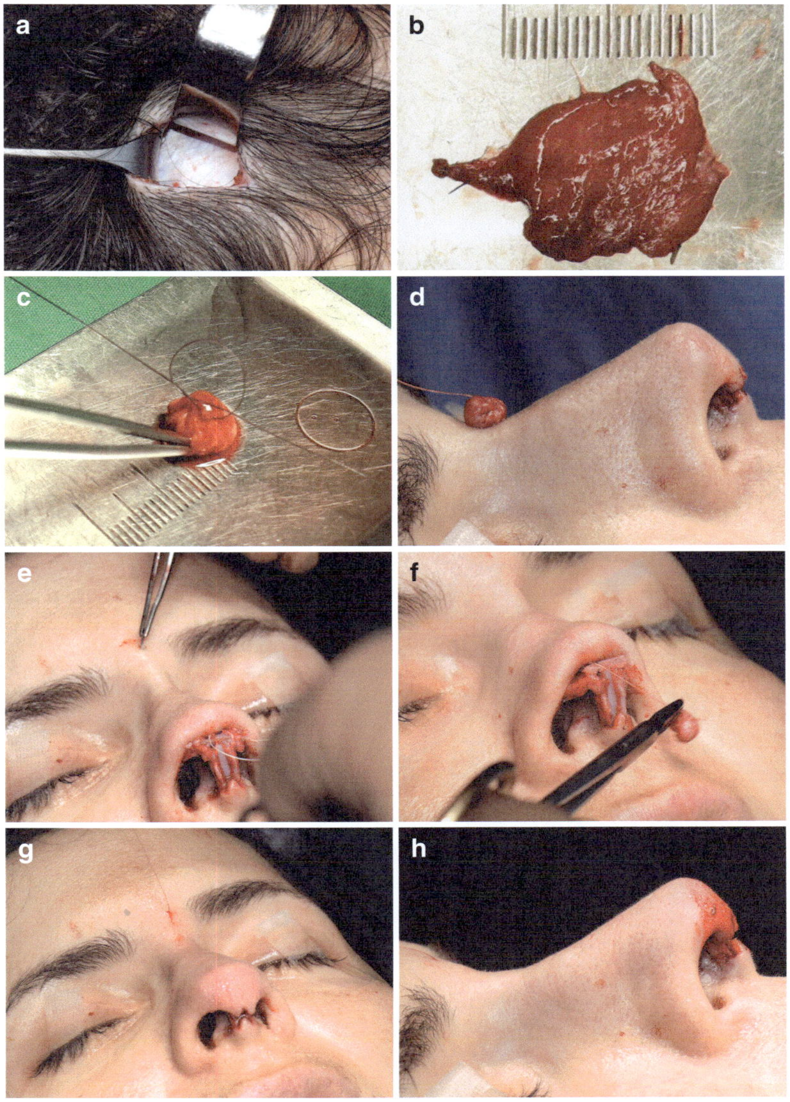

Fig. 3.22 (**a**, **b**) A 5 × 5-cm area of temporal fascia is removed through a scalp incision created above the ear. (**c**) The fascia is shaped into a roll. (**d**) The location where the graft is to be placed is externally determined. (**e**, **f**) The graft, containing a resorbable suture, is guided into position. (**g**) The guiding thread that exits the skin is not cut but is, rather, taped to the skin using a sterile bandage. (**h**) Note that some over-grafting is appropriate

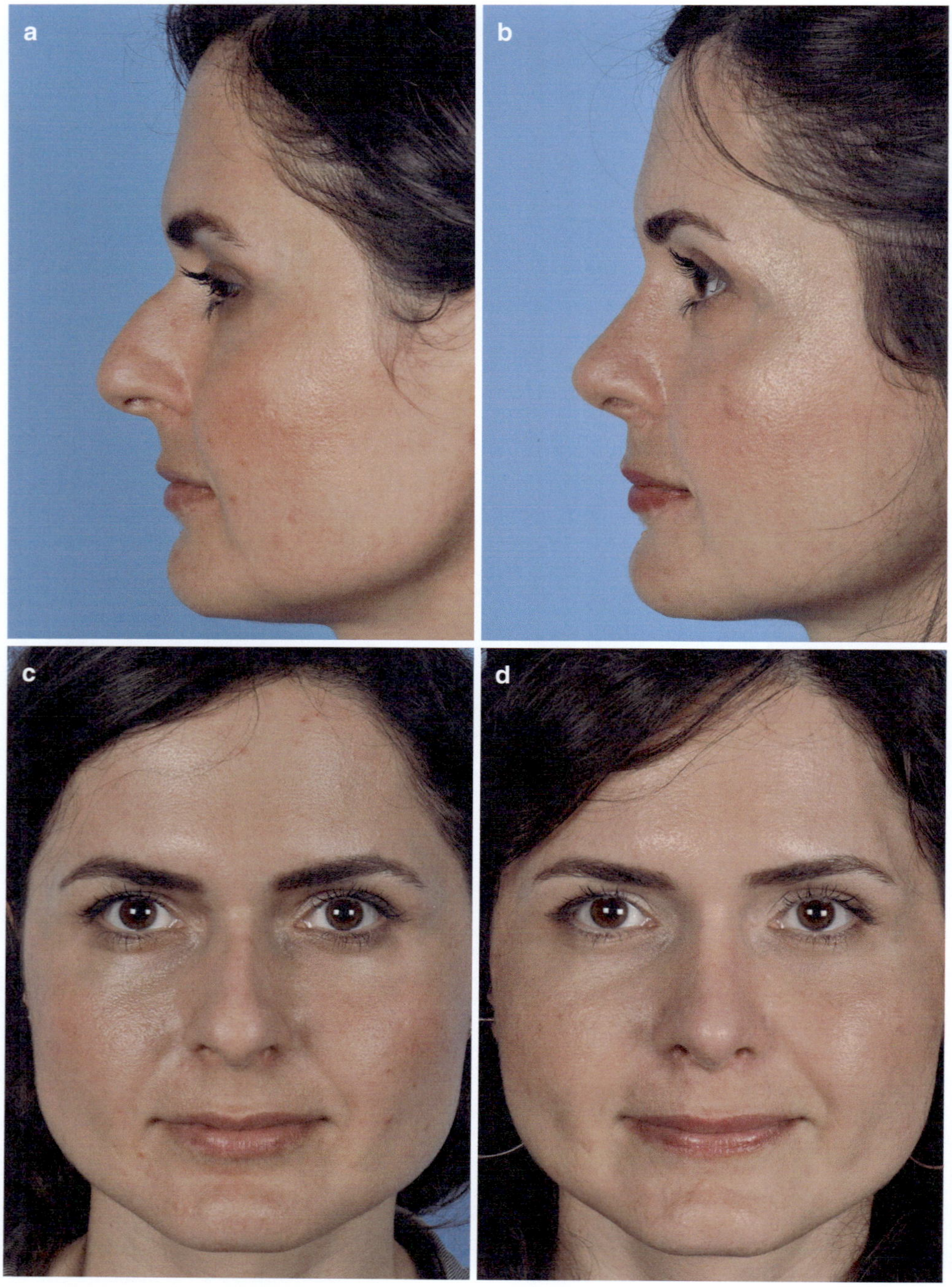

Fig. 3.23 (**a**–**h**) This patient had a prominent nasal dorsum, a slightly wide nasal tip, and a hanging infratip lobule; we used an open technique. The ideal dorsum was achieved via nasal hump resection and radix grafting. As the surgical steps are demonstrated before, temporal fascia served as a radix graft. The nose tip was reconstructed via vertical alar resection (VAR)

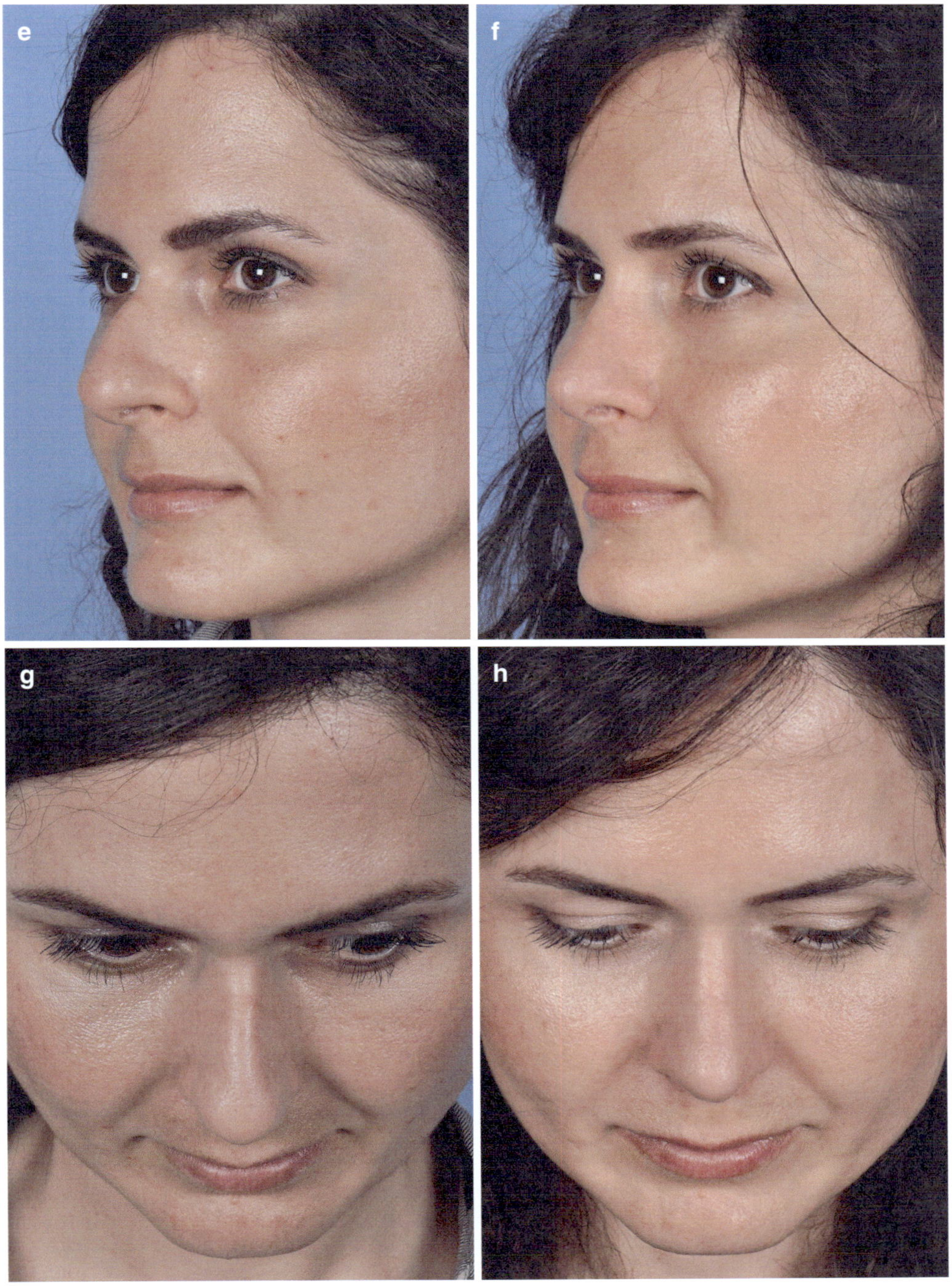

Fig. 3.23 (continued)

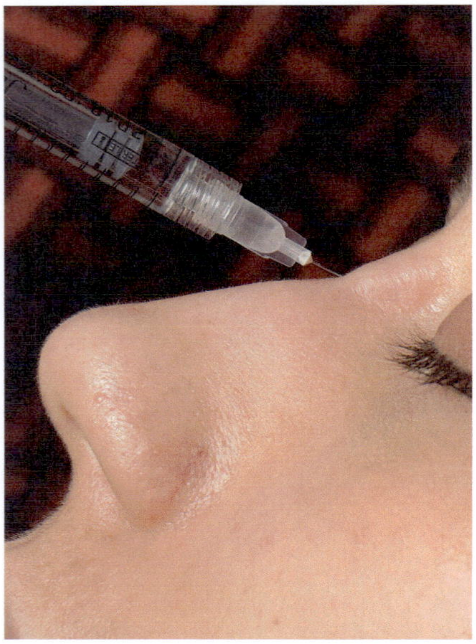

Fig. 3.24 This is a nonsurgical office procedure with virtually no downtime

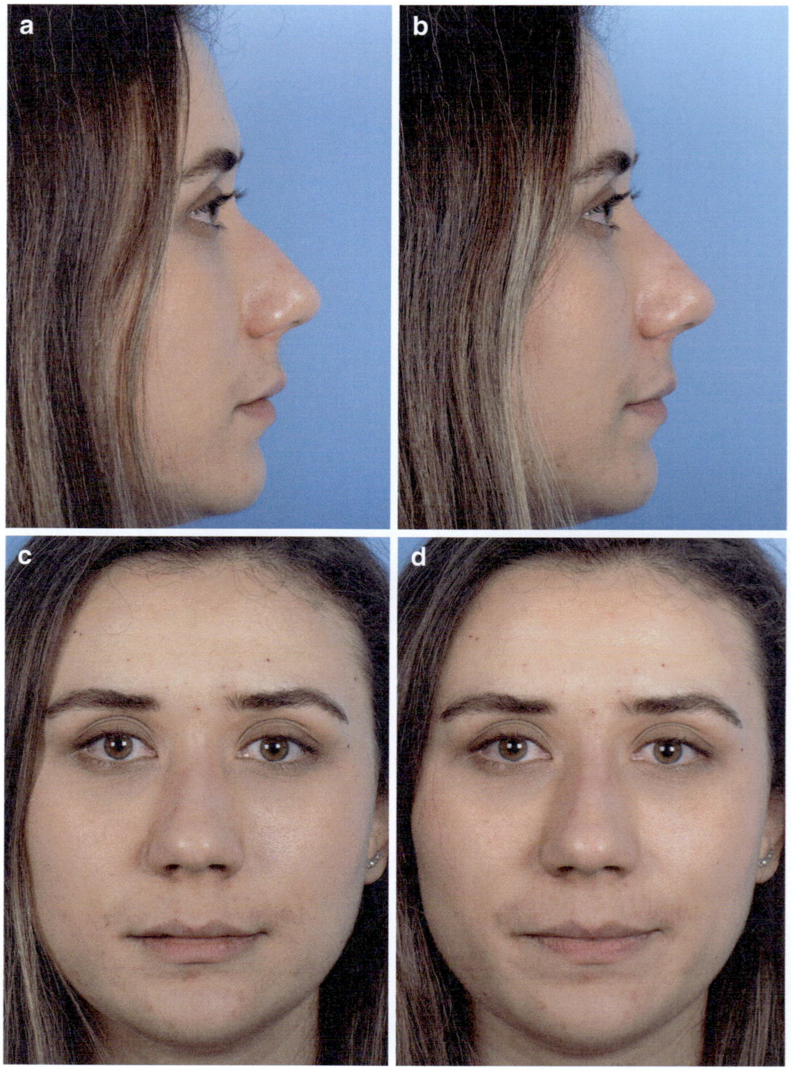

Fig. 3.25 (**a**–**d**) Before and after hydroxyapatite injection

3.4 Conclusion

Radix grafts are used for increasing low radix projection and moving the radix position superiorly. Augmentation of the radix may be performed with autogenous materials obtained from one of several sources: septal cartilage, alar cartilage, bone powder, or temporal fascia. In the meantime, for patients who do not require surgery to treat low radix, liquid fillers might be used. Alar cartilage, septum (crushed or not crushed), or bone powder (rasping material) are used for mild low radix cases, while diced cartilage from the septum can serve as a graft if moderate radix projection is needed. Finally, temporal fascia is a useful graft for severe cases. Each graft material has its own advantage and disadvantage, so the surgeon must decide wisely. Crushed or non-crushed alar cartilage or septal cartilage is suitable for mild cases but insufficient for others. While diced septal cartilage as a graft is nonvisible and provides more projection, the possibility of a graft migration is a risky disadvantage (mixing cartilage with the patient's blood and using an external bandage for better fixation is discussed in this chapter. Although temporal fascia is a more difficult graft to apply because it shrinks by 20% after surgery, it adapts very well to the radix and no medium- or long-term irregularities are evident (Fig. 3.26).

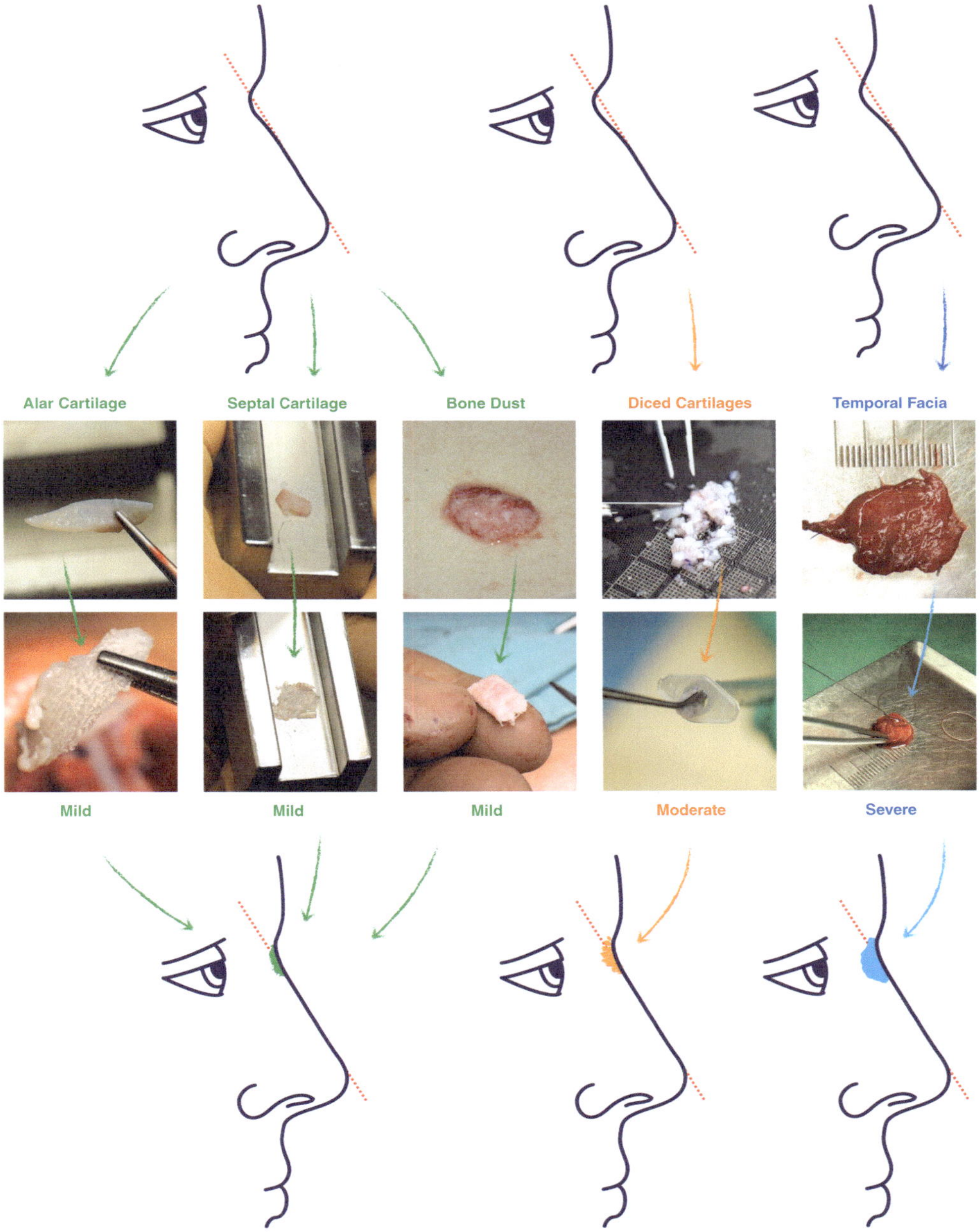

Fig. 3.26 Alar cartilages, septal cartilages, and bone dust are the ideal graft material in mildly low radix cases, whereas in moderate cases diced cartilage is a more suitable graft material. For severe low radix cases, temporalis fascia can be used

Disclosures The author reports no conflicts of interest or funding requiring disclosure.

Further Reading

Bohluli B, Varedi P, Bagheri SC, Rezazade M. Nasal radix augmentation in rhinoplasty: suggestion of an algorithm. Int J Oral Maxillofac Surg. 2017;46(1):41–5.

Cohen JC, Pearlman SJ. Radix grafts in cosmetic rhinoplasty: lessons from an 8-year review. Arch Facial Plast Surg. 2012;14(6):456–61.

Daniel RK. Middle eastern rhinoplasty: anatomy, aesthetics, and surgical planning. Facial Plast Surg. 2010;26(2):110–8.

Eskandarlou M, Motamed S. Evaluation of frequency of four common nasal anatomical deformities in primary rhinoplasty in a Tehran plastic surgery center. World J Plast Surg. 2014;3(2):122–8.

Guyuron B, Precision rhinoplasty. Part I: the role of life-size photographs and soft-tissue cephalometric analysis. Plast Reconstr Surg. 1988;81(4):489–99.

Lazovic GD, Daniel RK, Janosevic LB, Kosanovic RM, Colic MM, Kosins AM. Rhinoplasty: the nasal bones: anatomy and analysis. Aesthet Surg J. 2015;35(3):255–63.

Sheen JH. The radix as a reference in rhinoplasty. Perspect Plast Surg. 1987;1:33–50.

Steiger JD, Baker SR. Nuances of profile management: the radix. Facial Plast Surg Clin North Am. 2009;17(1):15–28. v

Tasman AJ, Suárez GA. The diced cartilage glue graft for radix augmentation in rhinoplasty. JAMA Facial Plast Surg. 2015;17(4):303–4.

4 Dorsum: Definition and Analysis

Achieving an aesthetically pleasing dorsal profile is one of the most common goals of patients seeking rhinoplasty. Surgical treatment should not be performed without a comprehensive knowledge of the dorsal anatomy. The essence of this surgery is to improve the relationship of the dorsum with the other structures of the nose and face.

The nasal dorsum, a complex structure consisting of bone, cartilage, and overlying skin, has an upper and middle nasal vault. The upper nasal vault (bony vault) consists of two nasal bones, which are attached to the frontal bone superiorly and to the maxillary bones laterally. The middle nasal vault (upper cartilaginous vault) is comprised of two upper lateral cartilages and the dorsal nasal septum (Fig. 4.1).

In the lateral view, the nasal dorsum begins at the deepest point of the nasofrontal angle (radix) and ends at the tip-defining point. In an ideal nasal profile, a slight depression (or break) is observed between the nasal dorsum and the nasal tip, which is known as the supratip break. The supratip break provides a slight distinction between the nasal dorsum and the nasal tip and contributes to the natural nasal profile (Fig. 4.2).

In females, the dorsal shape is generally straight or slightly concave, whereas it is straight or slightly convex in males. Figure 4.3 shows some examples of natural and ideal noses.

In the frontal view, the nasal dorsum appears as an even curved line from the medial portion of the eyebrow to the tip-defining point (Fig. 4.4).

The nasal profile is influenced by both the internal and external components (skin, soft tissue envelope) of the nasal anatomy. Also, adjacent structures, such as the forehead (glabella) and the upper lip and chin, play major roles in determining the nasal profile. Therefore, patients must be informed about their other facial issues to ensure realistic expectations and satisfactory results.

The goals of dorsal surgery should be to maintain the ideal dorsal profile view and establish a symmetrical and smooth dorsal aesthetic line in the frontal view.

S. Şeneldir, *Photographic Atlas of Rhinoplasty*, https://doi.org/10.1007/978-3-031-65619-4_4

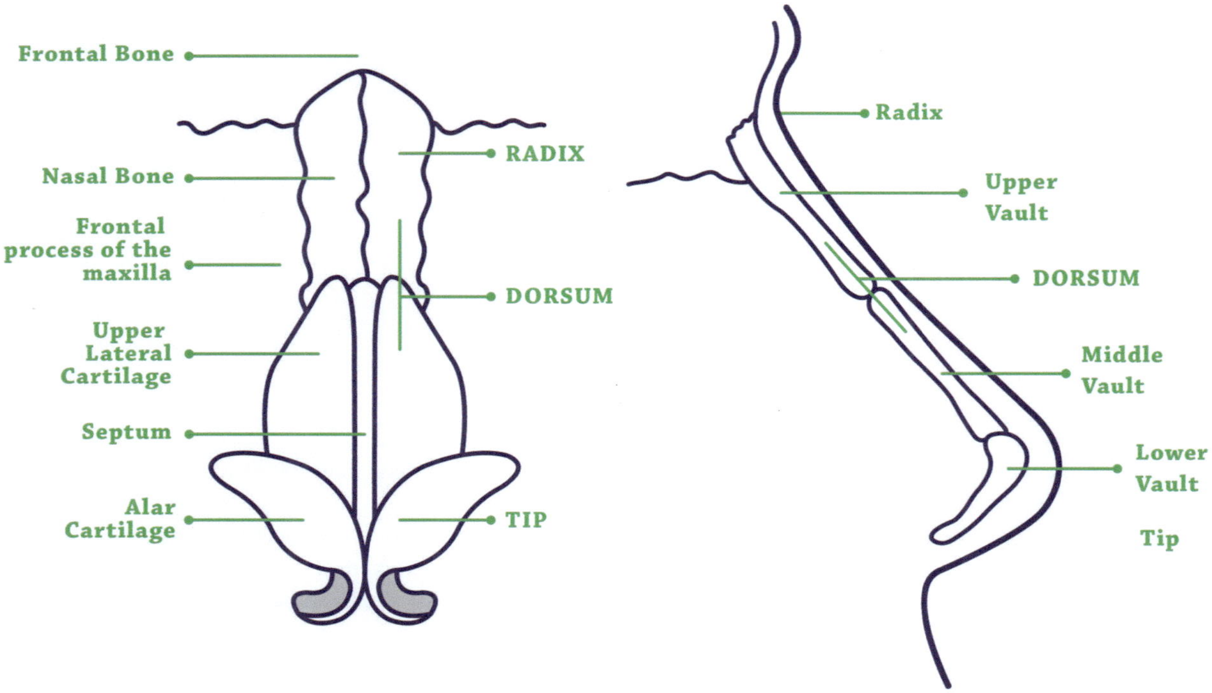

Fig. 4.1 The primary anatomy of the nasal skeleton and clinically important landmarks

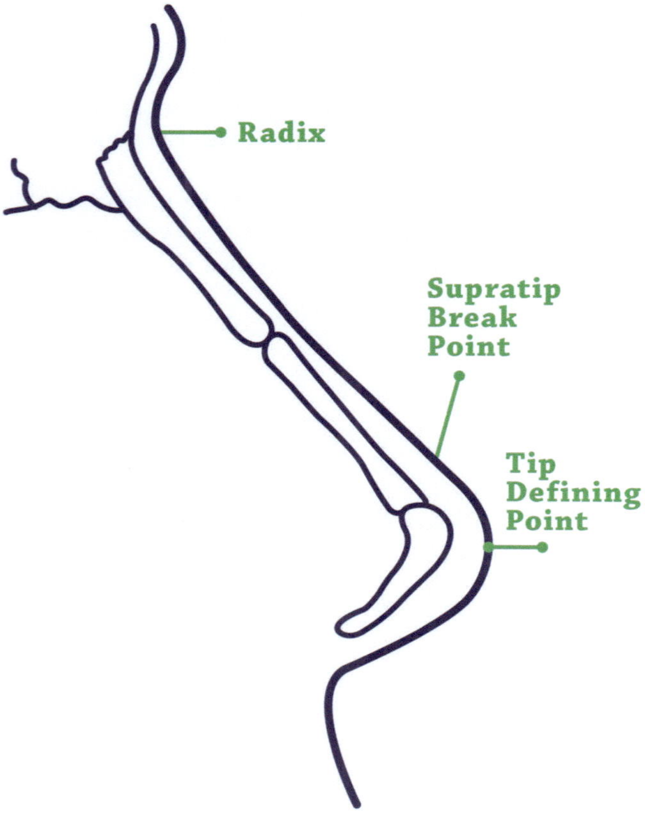

Fig. 4.2 Supratip break

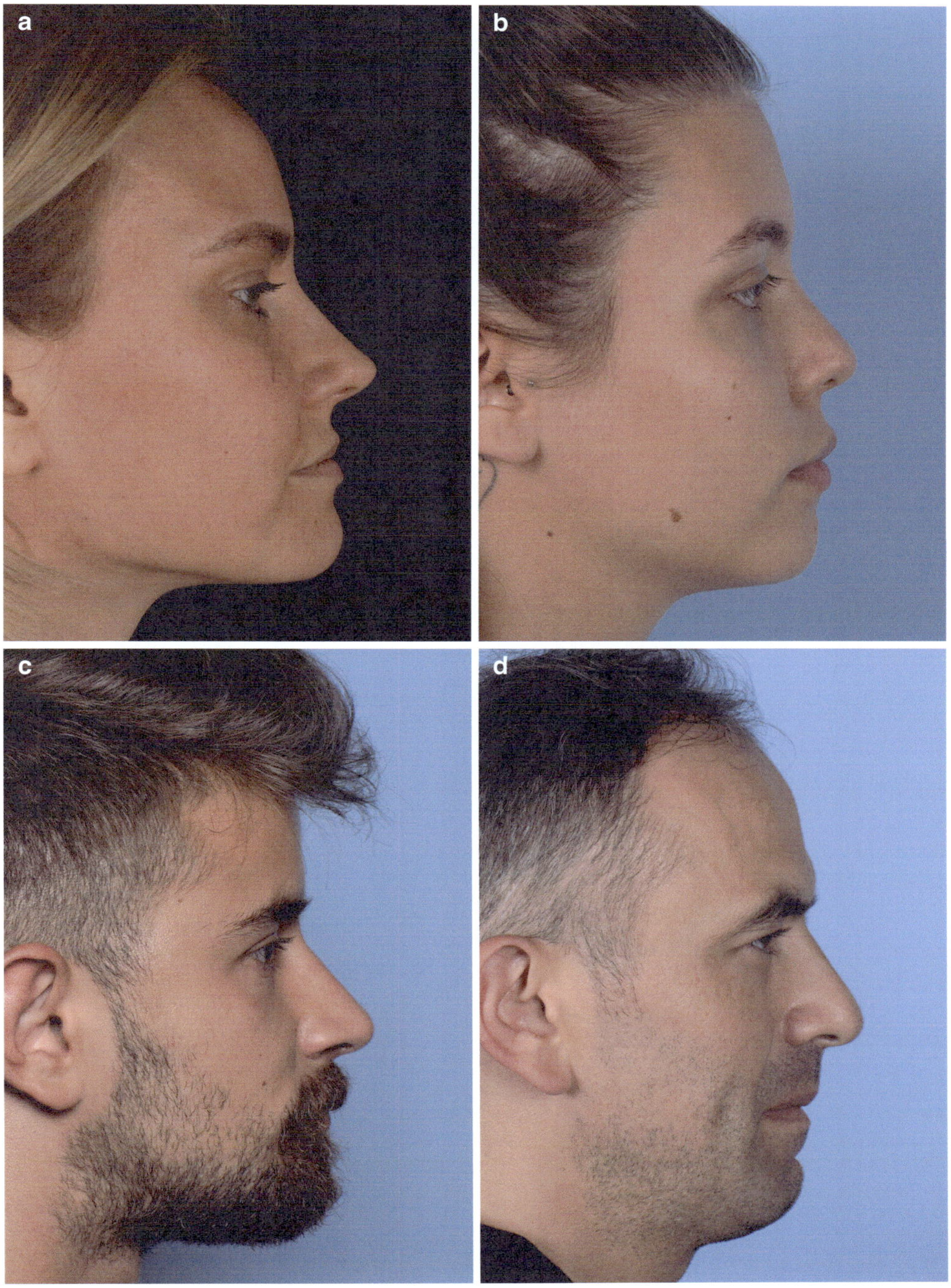

Fig. 4.3 (**a**) Slightly concave dorsum. (**b**) Straight dorsum. (**c**) Straight dorsum. (**d**) Slightly convex dorsum

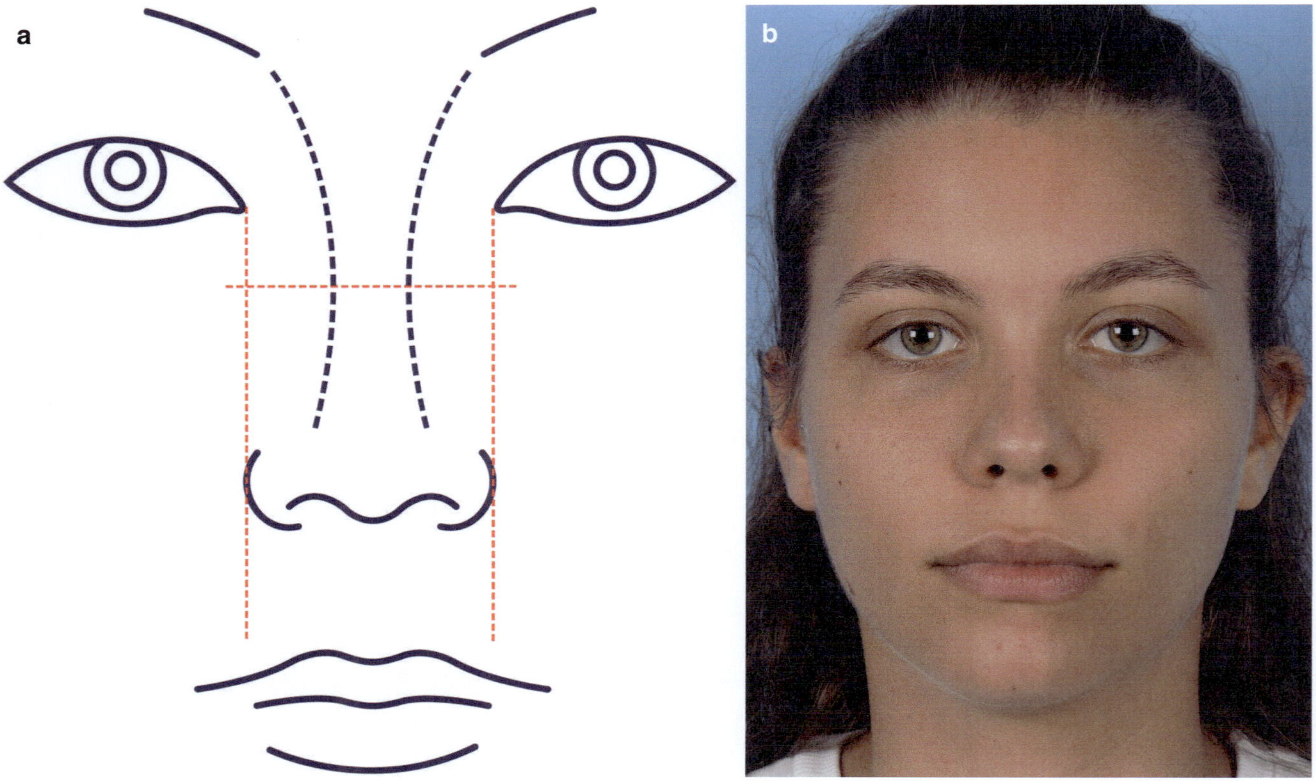

Fig. 4.4 (**a**, **b**) Brow-tip aesthetic line

Disclosures The author reports no conflicts of interest or funding requiring disclosure.

Further Reading

Afrooz PN, Rohrich RJ. The keystone: consistency in restoring the aesthetic dorsum in rhinoplasty. Plast Reconstr Surg. 2018;141(2):355–63.

Allak A, Park SS. Surgical treatment of the middle nasal vault. Clin Plast Surg. 2016;43(1):85–94.

Berkowitz RL, Gruber RP. Management of the nasal dorsum: construction and maintenance of a barrel vault. Clin Plast Surg. 2016;43(1):59–72.

Daniel RK, Pálházi P. Osseocartilaginous vault. In: Rhinoplasty: an anatomical and clinical atlas. Cham: Springer International; 2018. p. 113–63.

Fedok FG. Primary rhinoplasty. Facial Plast Surg Clin North Am. 2016;24(3):323–35.

Harris MO, Baker SR. Management of the wide nasal dorsum. Arch Facial Plast Surg. 2004;6(1):41–8.

Krane NA, Markey JD, Moneta LB, Kim MM. Aesthetics of the nasal dorsum: proportions, light, and shadow. Facial Plast Surg. 2017;33(2):120–4.

Lee MR, Unger JG, Rohrich RJ. Management of the nasal dorsum in rhinoplasty: a systematic review of the literature regarding technique, outcomes, and complications. Plast Reconstr Surg. 2011;128(5):538e–50e.

Roostaeian J, Unger JG, Lee MR, Geissler P, Rohrich RJ. Reconstitution of the nasal dorsum following component dorsal reduction in primary rhinoplasty. Plast Reconstr Surg. 2014;133(3):509–18.

Sykes JM, Tapias V, Kim JE. Management of the nasal dorsum. Facial Plast Surg. 2011;27(2):192–202.

5 Dorsum: Dorsal Reduction

In planning for hump resection, the reference point must be the starting point of the dorsum, i.e., the radix. In cases in which the radix is high or low, i.e., there is a problem with the radix, *any hump resection performed without solving these problems will not achieve an ideal dorsum*. In addition, if the chin projection is low, it gives a false impression that further dorsal reduction is needed (Fig. 5.1).

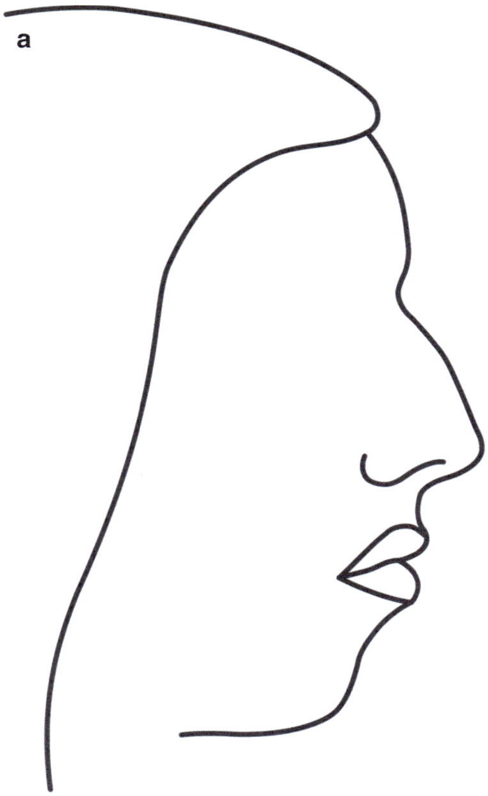

Fig. 5.1 (**a**) Dorsal hump appears greater when chin projection is low. (**b**) Comparing to figure **a**, the dorsal hump appears more realistic with an ideal chin projection

Supplementary Information The online version contains supplementary material available at https://doi.org/10.1007/978-3-031-65619-4_5.

S. Şeneldir, *Photographic Atlas of Rhinoplasty*, https://doi.org/10.1007/978-3-031-65619-4_5

5.1 Introduction

- A large nose is a common complaint among patients seeking rhinoplasty, and dorsal hump is the major reason for the large appearance of the nose from the lateral view.
- While hump resection provides the ideal dorsal line in cases with dorsal hump, hump resection allows us to make alterations to the appearance in the frontal view. Any irregularity or asymmetry at the brow-tip aesthetic line, or even a wide nasal base, must be resolved by hump resection.

Dorsal hump resection can be performed with either an open or closed approach.

Technical Pearl: The closed technique allows more controlled resection because the skin flap is distorted in the open technique.

Regardless of the approach used, two types of resection can be performed; en bloc resection of the excess dorsum or separate resection of each segment of the nasal dorsum. Both resection types are applicable in all cases (Figs. 5.2, 5.3 and 5.4).

One technique may be preferred over the other depending on the patient. For example, segmental resection is preferred in cases where excess upper lateral cartilage will be used as a spreader flap, while en bloc resection is preferred in cases where the whole hump will be used as a graft (Fig. 5.5).

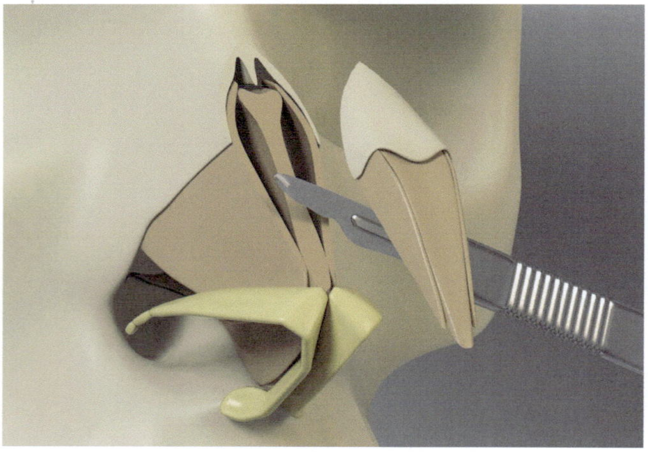

Fig. 5.2 En bloc hump resection

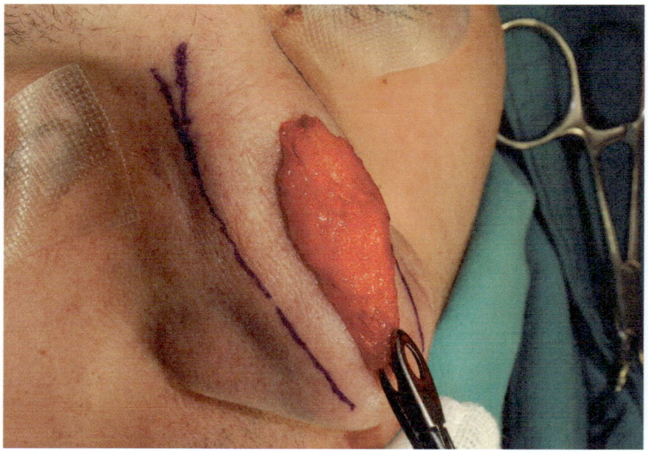

Fig. 5.3 En bloc hump resection

Fig. 5.4 (**a**, **b**) Separate hump resection

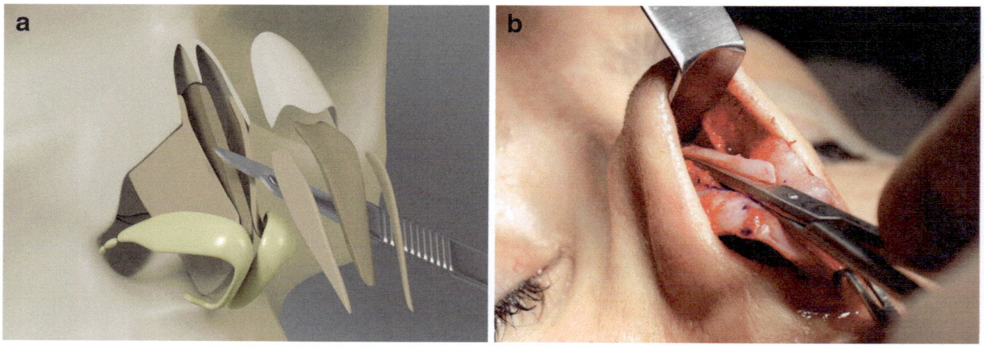

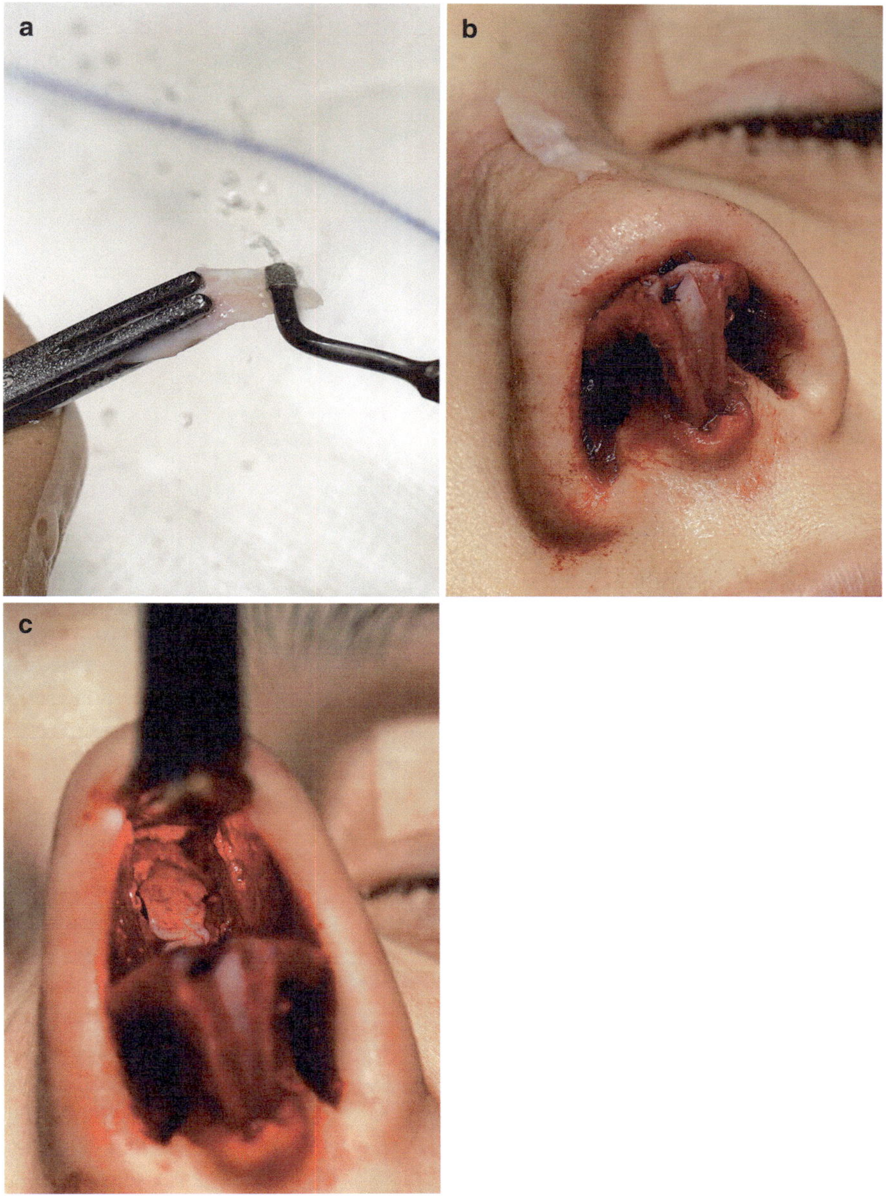

Fig. 5.5 (**a**) Dorsal hump is reshaped. (**b**) Exact location of the dorsal hump graft shown externally. (**c**) A dorsal hump graft is used for reconstruction of the dorsum

5.2 Treatment Strategies

5.2.1 En Bloc Resection

En bloc resection starts with cutting of the starting point of the hump with a scalpel parallel to the dorsum. The scalpel is advanced to the K-point, i.e., the osseocartilaginous junction (Fig. 5.6).

The osteotome is then placed parallel to the dorsum at this point (Fig. 5.7).

The assistant strikes the back of the osteotome in a rhythmic manner, and the bone is cut up to the radix (Fig. 5.8).

The edges of the osteotome are palpated under the skin with the other hand. The surgeon must pay attention to avoid penetrating too deeply. Wide dorsum elevation is vital before removing the hump to allow the osteotome to move easily in the skin. Otherwise, the skin may be incised from the lateral sides (Fig. 5.9).

Technical Pearl: There is no need to panic if skin incision occurs during osteotomy. In such cases, appropriate postsurgical taping to approximate the scar surfaces would be adequate. Closing the skin with a suture increases the likelihood of scar formation (Fig. 5.10).

Technical Pearl: After completing the resection, the resected pieces must be removed. The surgeon must check whether the bone is fully cut or the hump is fully elevated from the skin, and not forcefully remove the resected pieces (Fig. 5.11).

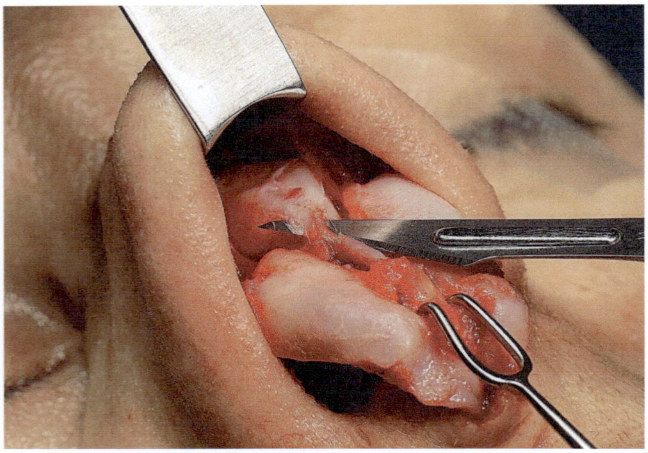

Fig. 5.6 A No. 11 scalpel is suitable for dorsal hump removal

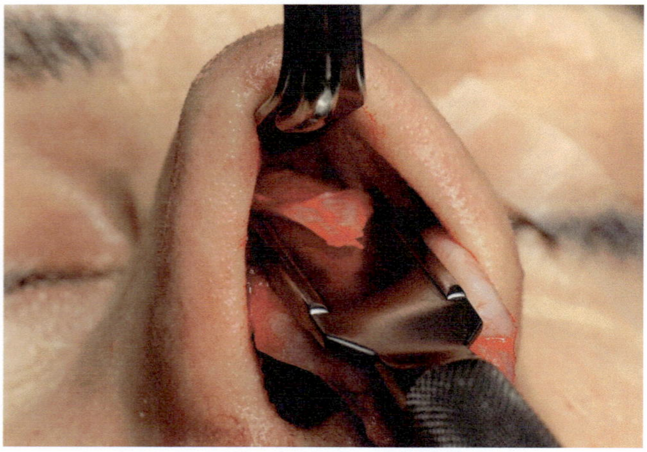

Fig. 5.7 A flat osteotome is placed to remove the dorsal hump

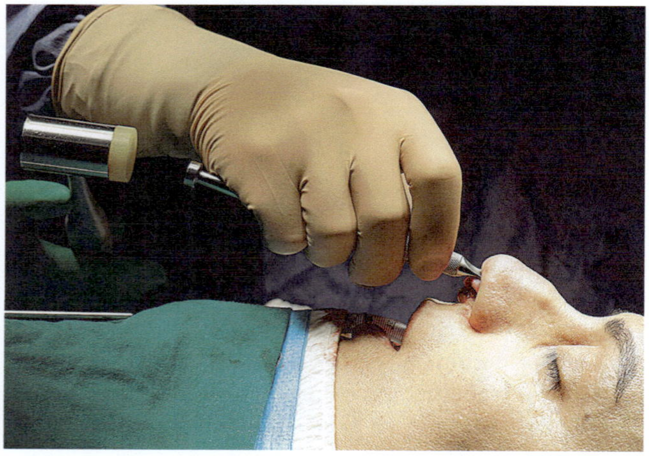

Fig. 5.8 Axis of the osteotome is seen on the profile view

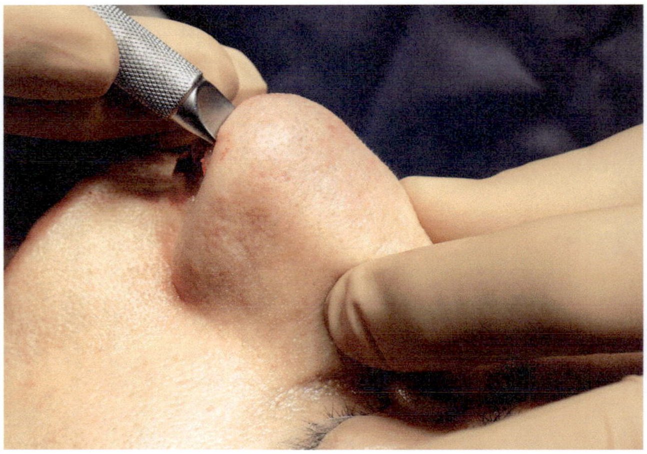

Fig. 5.9 Axis of the osteotome is seen

5.2.2 Segmental Resection

In cases in which segmental resection is preferred, the septum is separated from the upper lateral cartilages, first from one side and then from the contralateral side, with an incision starting from the anterior septal angle parallel to the septum. The incision is advanced up to the bony dorsum (Fig. 5.12).

The excess septum is removed, preferably with an angled scissor (Fig. 5.13).

The upper lateral cartilages are saved if they are to be used as spreader grafts.

Otherwise, excess segments are also resected. Over-resection of the upper lateral cartilages should be avoided. The upper lateral cartilages should be 1–2 mm above the septum after dorsal resection (Fig. 5.14).

Finally, the bony portion of the hump is lowered to the ideal height. A rasp can be used for this purpose; an osteotome may also be used to resect the excess bone. Gentle rather than aggressive rasping is preferred in cases where a rasp is used to reduce the bony hump. Aggressive rasping at the sides may cause the upper lateral cartilage to detach from the nasal bone, and aggressive rasping at the midline may reduce the septal integrity such that the septum may collapse to the base (Fig. 5.15).

After the dorsum is lowered to the required level, septoplasty is performed. **Septoplasty must not be performed before hump resection**. The dorsum must be checked again, as minor alterations may occur at the dorsum after septoplasty (Fig. 5.16).

It is essential to leave a smooth surface at the dorsum after hump resection.

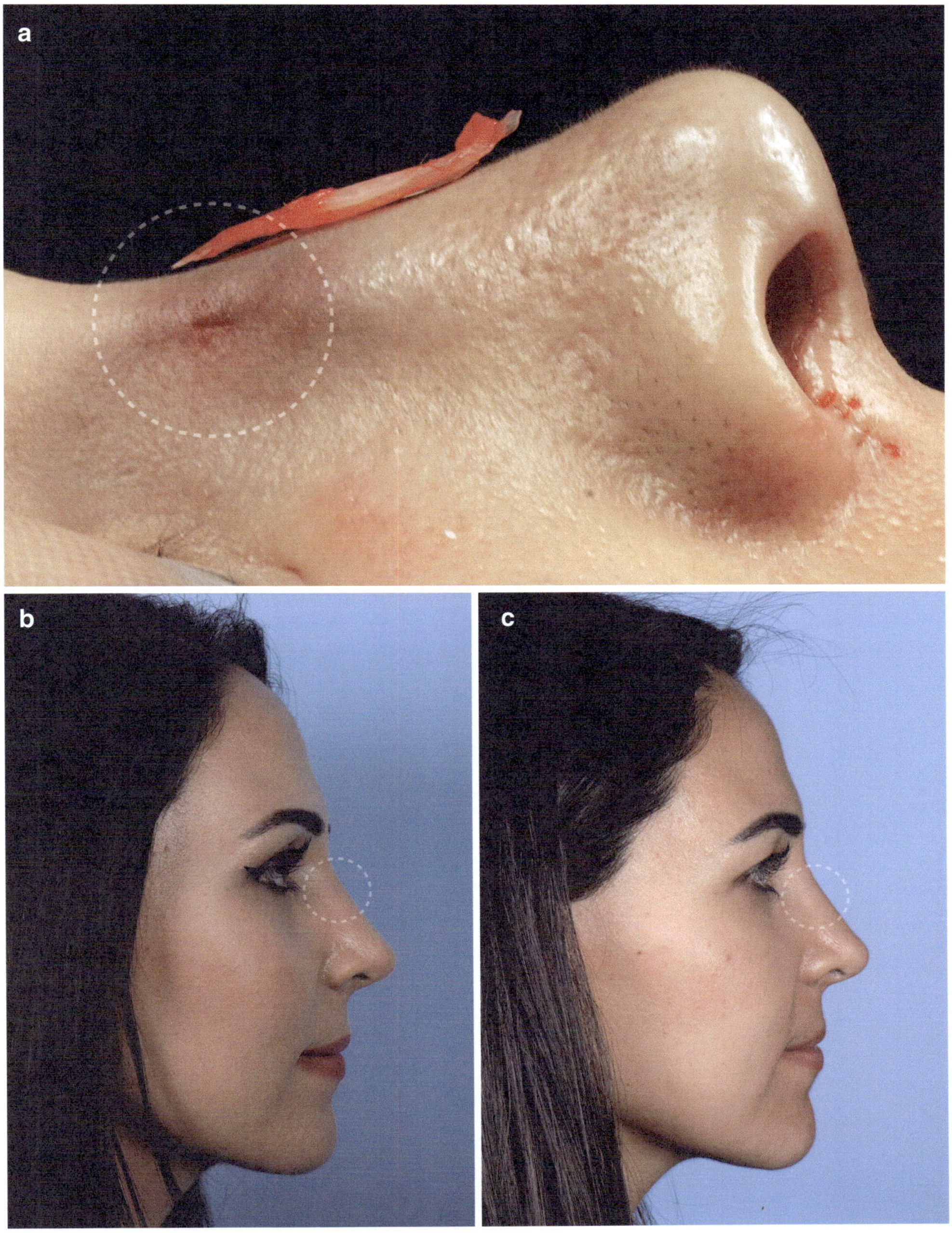

Fig. 5.10 (**a**) Skin perforation due to the osteotome. (**b**) Shadowing in the early postoperative period. (**c**) Healed skin without scar formation

Minor irregularities are identified by palpation. Wetting the glove during palpation improves the tactile sense and prevents missing any irregularities. It is important to notice excess segments at the junction between the upper laterals and the nasal bone, i.e., the lateral nasal hump; this can be easily overlooked. Blunt scissors can be used as an alternative to a rasp for removing the palpable excess pieces, in particular at the bony segment (Fig. 5.17).

How do we know that we have reached the ideal dorsum level after following these steps, and how should we define the surgical relationship between the tip and the dorsum, to achieve an ideal dorsal profile?

Two points are helpful to understand the ideal dorsum level:

- Intraoperatively there must be a difference of 8–11 mm between the new tip-defining point and the anterior-most portion of the dorsum. This is required not as a guarantee of projection, but rather as protection against polly beak deformity associated with the dorsum. This distance should be achieved after stability of the tip projection is realized; if ideal tip stability is not achieved, the distance between the new tip-defining point and the anterior-most portion of the dorsum is irrelevant.

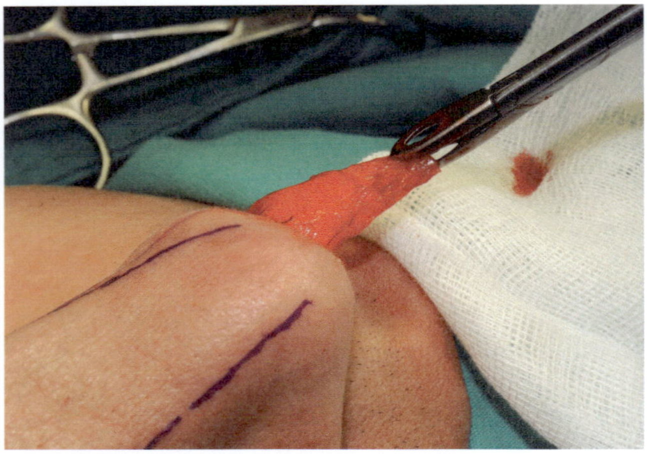

Fig. 5.11 Note that the punch is not fully compressed but rather gently supports the cartilage

- The radix and the anterior dorsum must be at the same level (Fig. 5.18).

Technical Pearl: In cases where there is still a palpable region at the supratip despite bringing the middle and lower vaults to the ideal level, the focus must be turned toward the alar cartilage. The cephalic portion of the alar cartilage may be hump-like. If cephalic resection is not performed, removal of the hump may be attempted by cephalic resection. If there is persistent resistance despite cephalic resection, malposition of the lateral crus must be considered (Fig. 5.19).

Technical Pearl: The hump to be removed should be freed from septal mucosa prior to resection. The septal mucosa is not resected. It is important to spare the septal mucosa, as it can be used as a spreader graft if needed. However, in cases with an excessive hump, non-resected excess mucosa can be resected in a controlled manner. Another alternative to this trimming procedure would be to slightly cauterize the dome using a bipolar device.

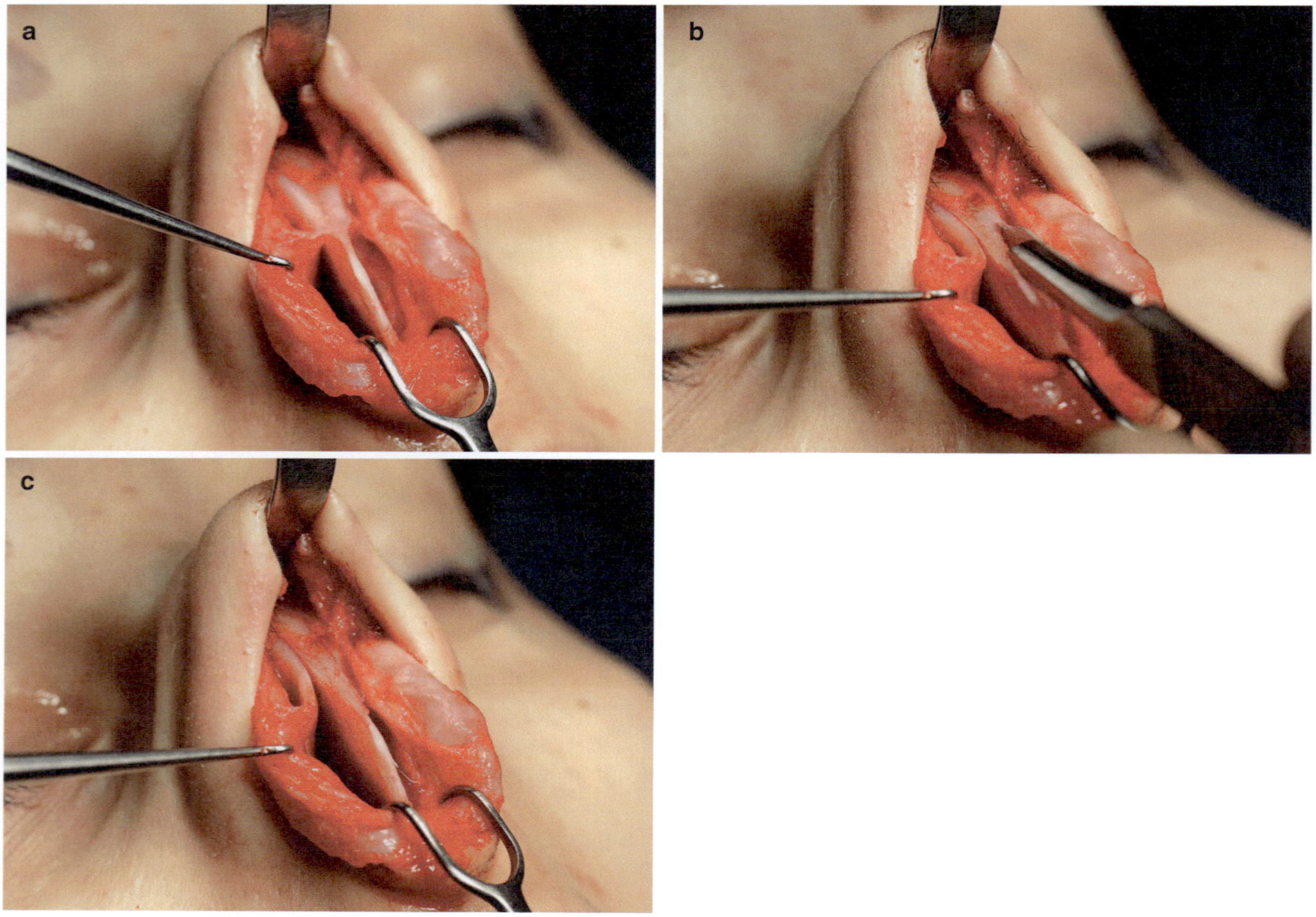

Fig. 5.12 (**a**–**c**) The septum is separated from the upper lateral cartilages

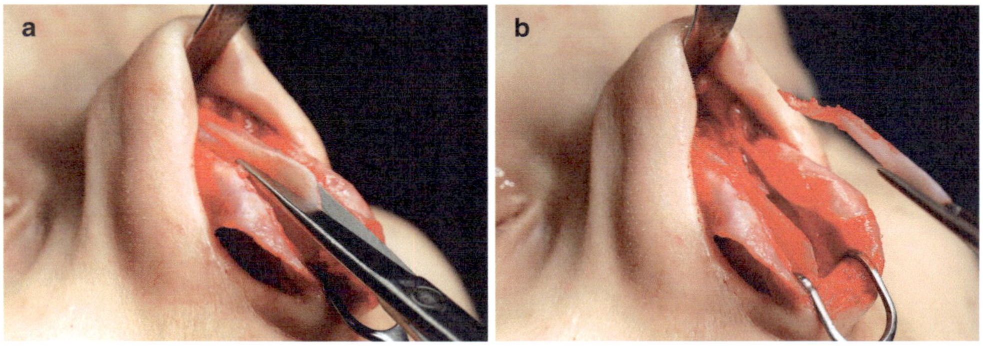

Fig. 5.13 (**a**, **b**) Septal hump is removed

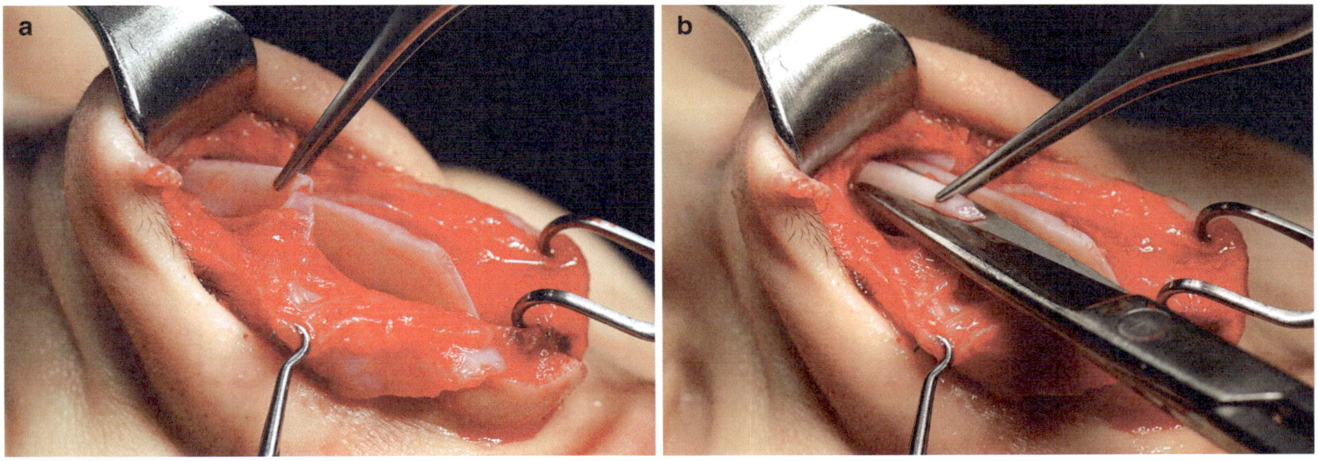

Fig. 5.14 (**a**, **b**) Right excess part of upper lateral cartilage is dissected from its perichondrium and resected

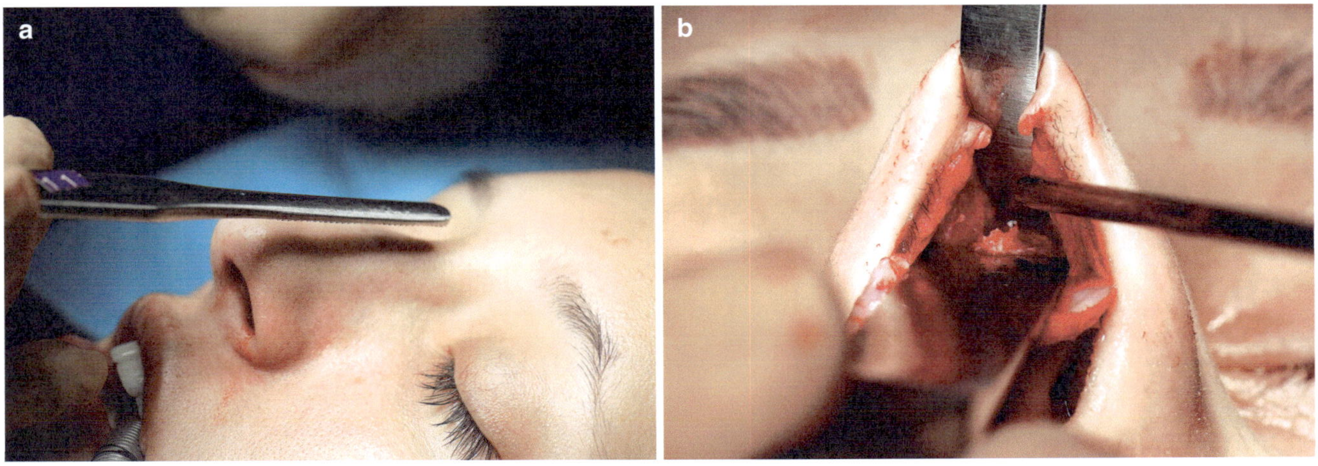

Fig. 5.15 (**a**, **b**) An osteotome or a rasp can be used to reduce bony hump

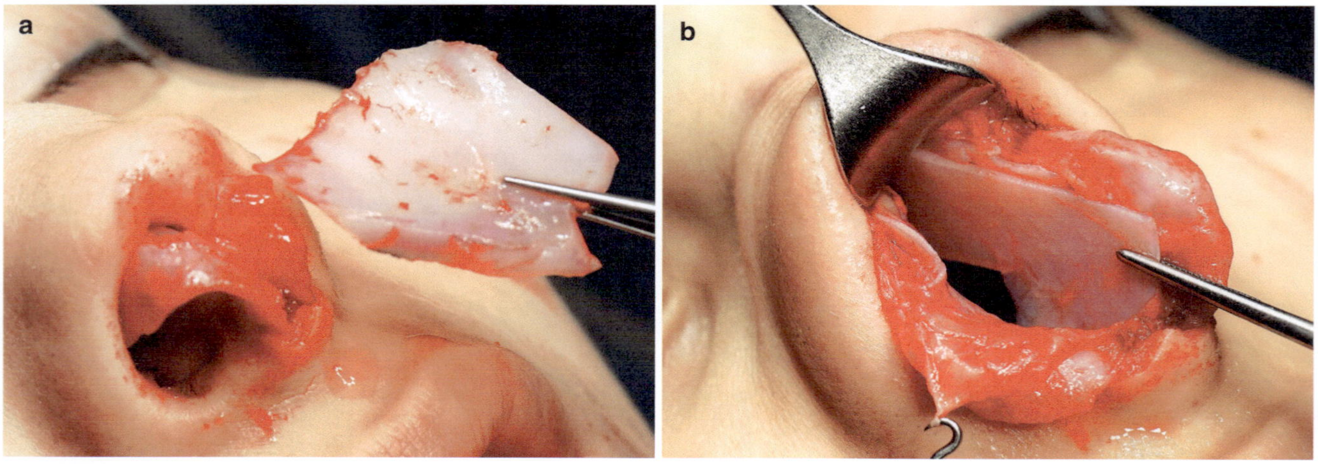

Fig. 5.16 (**a**, **b**) The remaining septum should form an "L" shape (L-strut) at least 1 cm in length, caudally and dorsally

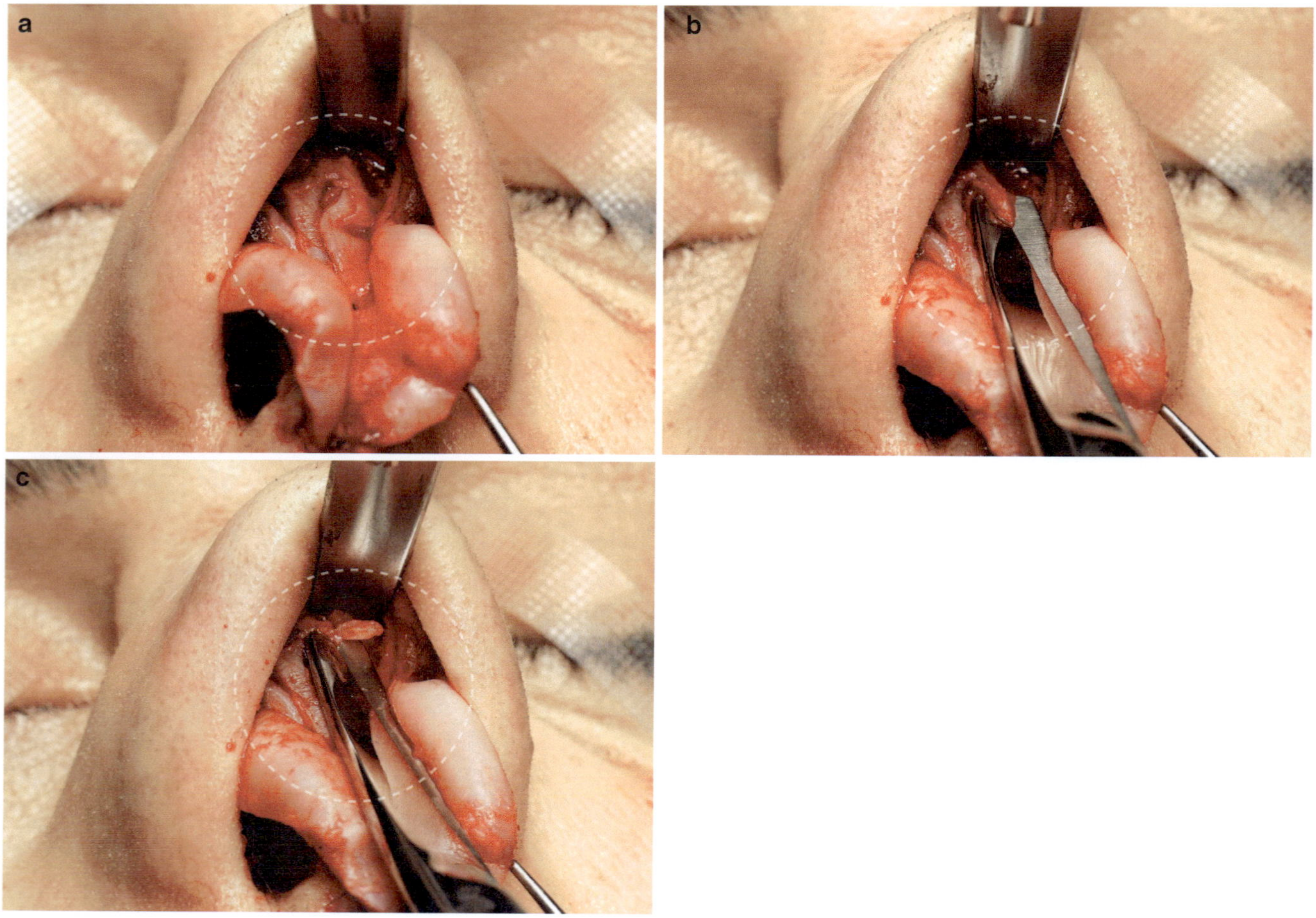

Fig. 5.17 (**a**–**c**) Blunt scissors are used to remove the lateral nasal hump

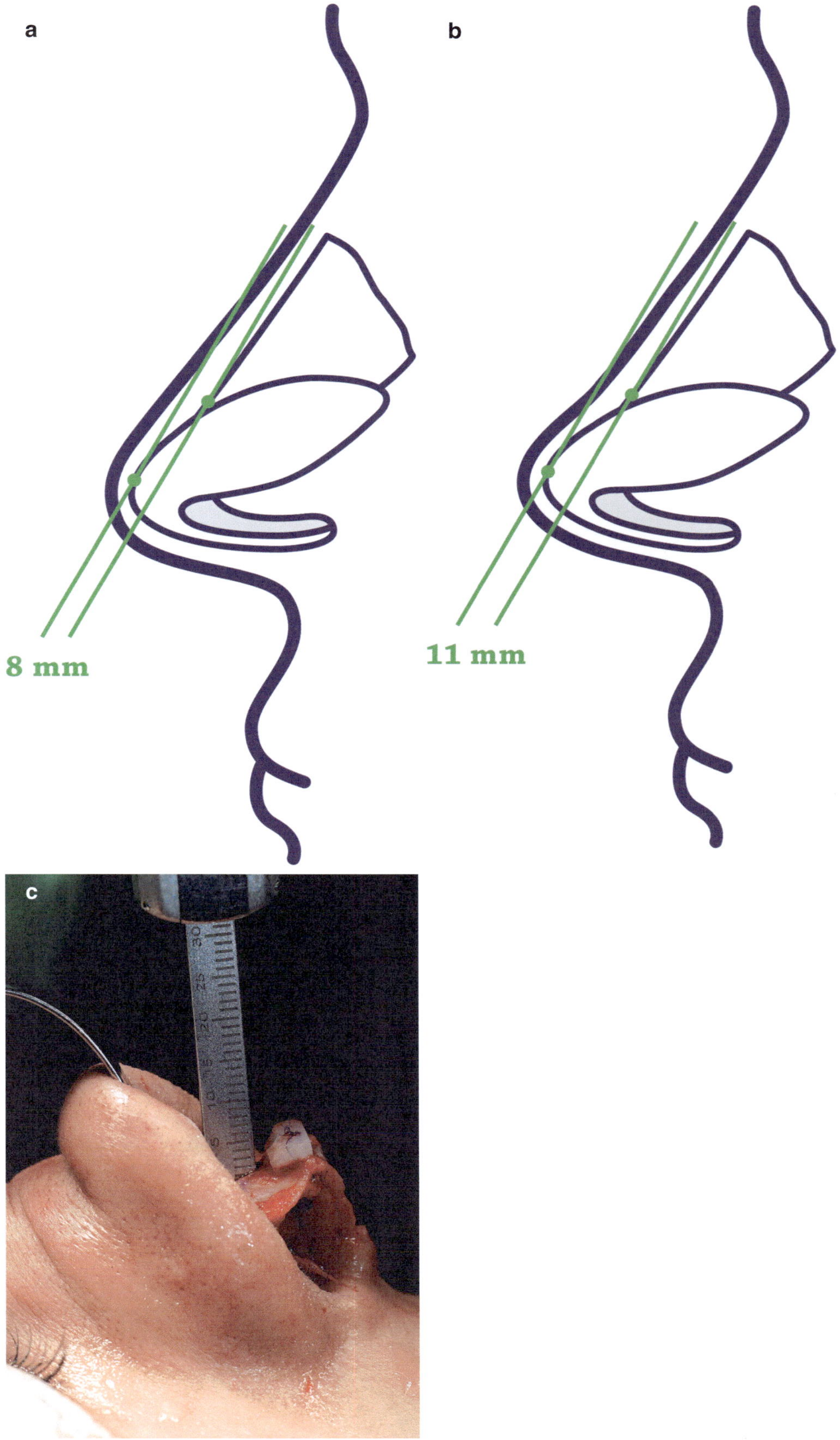

Fig. 5.18 (**a**) If a straight dorsum is required, a distance of 6–8 mm between the nasal tip and the anteriormost part of the dorsum should be present. (**b**) If a curved dorsum is required, a distance of 9–11 mm between the nasal tip and the anterior-most part of the dorsum should be present. (**c**) A tool designed by the author for measuring the distance between the anteriormost part of the dorsum and the tip-defining point

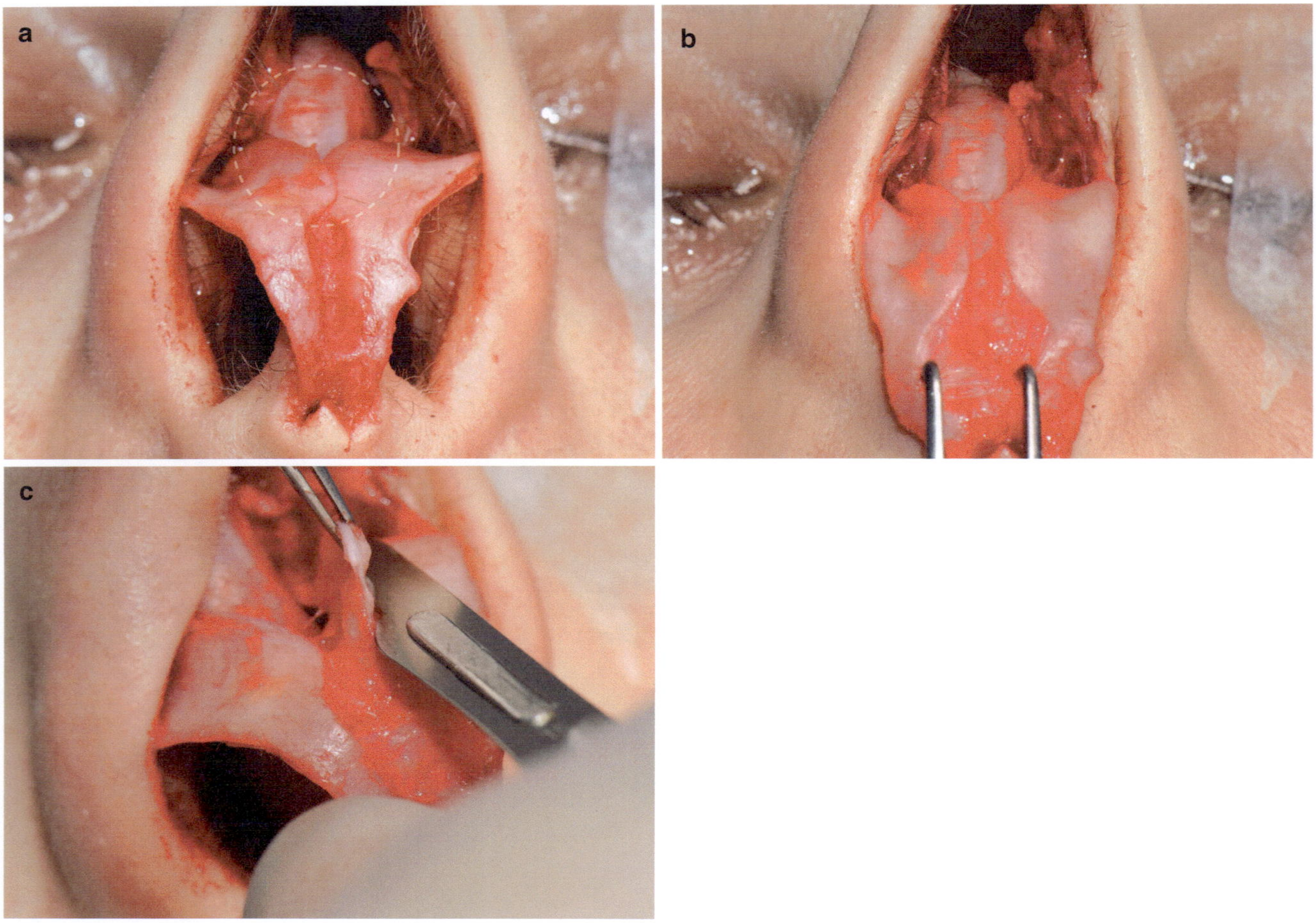

Fig. 5.19 (**a**) The dorsal cartilage in this case is covered by alar cartilages. The alar cartilages covering the dorsal cartilage are responsible for the dorsal hump effect. (**b**, **c**) In some situations, the lower lateral crus may cause the dorsal cartilage to

5.3 Clinical Outcomes

5.3.1 Case 1

Dorsal reduction planning should take into consideration the relationship between the dorsum and other parts of the nose (i.e., the radix, tip, and skin envelope).

The main complaint in this case was the large size of the nose. The over-projected dorsum and tip seemed to be responsible for the large nose. The radix was ideally positioned. When hump reduction is planned, lowering the dorsum without treating the tip would lead to an imbalanced profile view. On the other hand, given the size of the skin/soft tissue envelope, dorsal reduction was limited. Therefore, it may not be possible to achieve ideal reduction of nose size, which must be discussed with the patient prior to surgery (Fig. 5.20).

5.3.2 Case 2

Dorsal reduction planning should take into consideration the relationships between the dorsum and other facial components (i.e., the chin and forehead).

The main complaint in this case was the large nose, which seemed to be due to a dorsal hump and deficient chin. Without augmenting the chin, dorsal reduction would not be sufficient to achieve an ideal profile view. The necessity of chin augmentation should be discussed with the patient prior to surgery (Fig. 5.21).

The main component of the hump should be analyzed well. In most cases with a dorsal hump, the main component of the hump is cartilaginous dorsum, so the aggressive rasping of the bony dorsum should be avoided. Let us look at the following case.

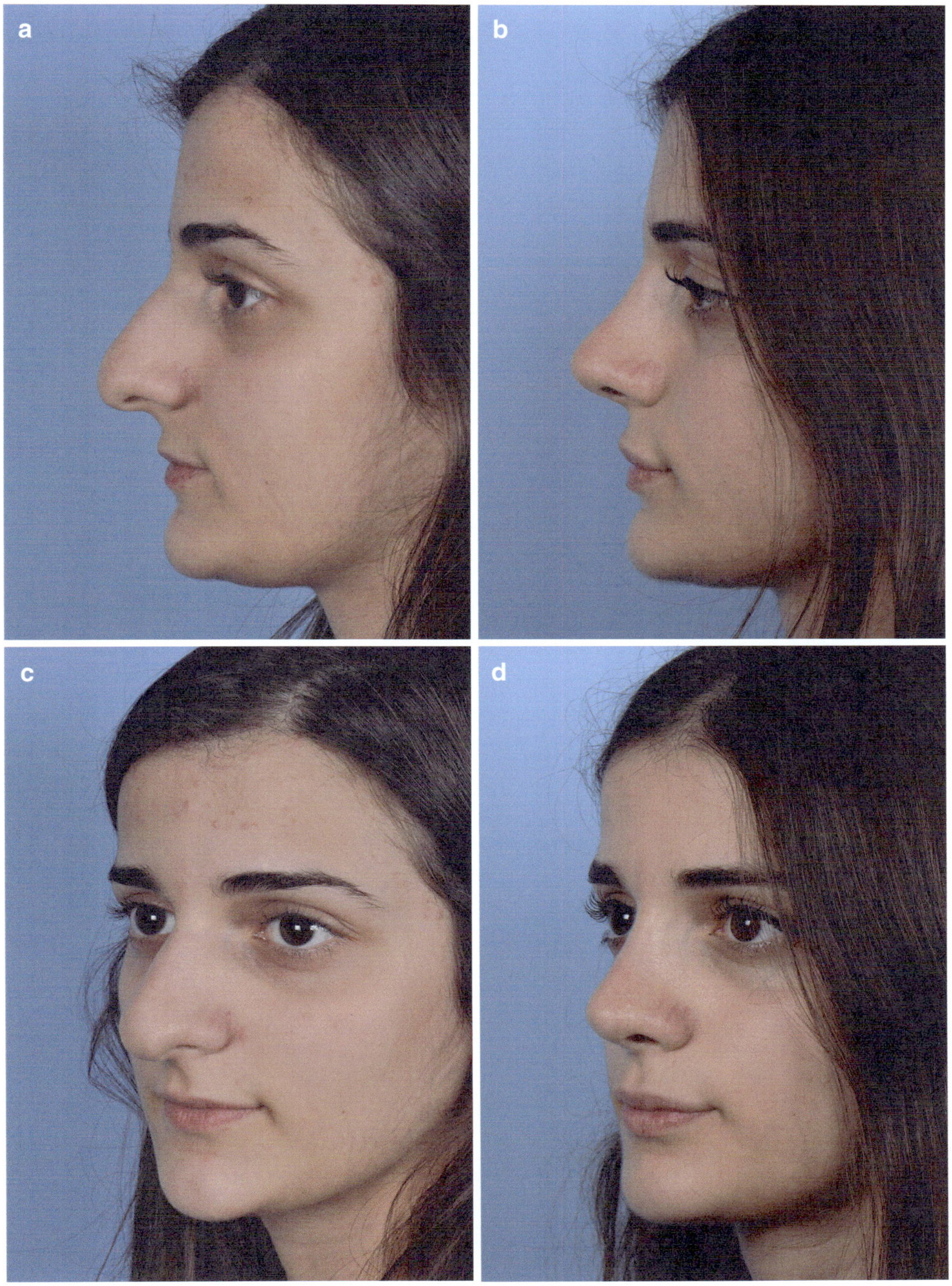

Fig. 5.20 (**a**–**f**) All overdeveloped components (dorsum, tip) of the nose were reduced. A straight dorsum is preferred when lowering an oversized nose

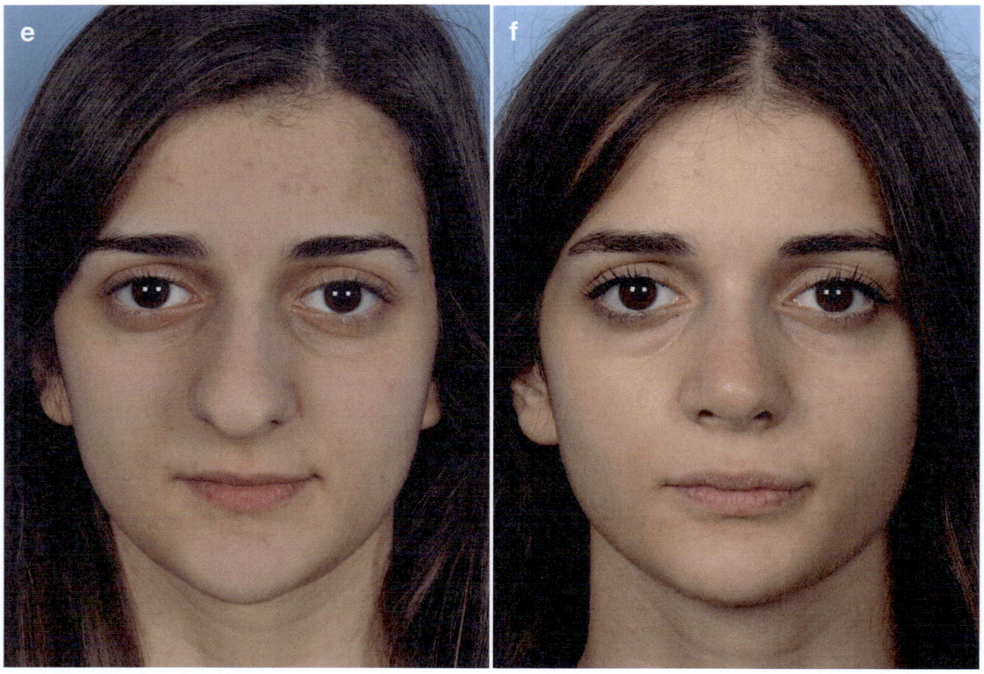

Fig. 5.20 (continued)

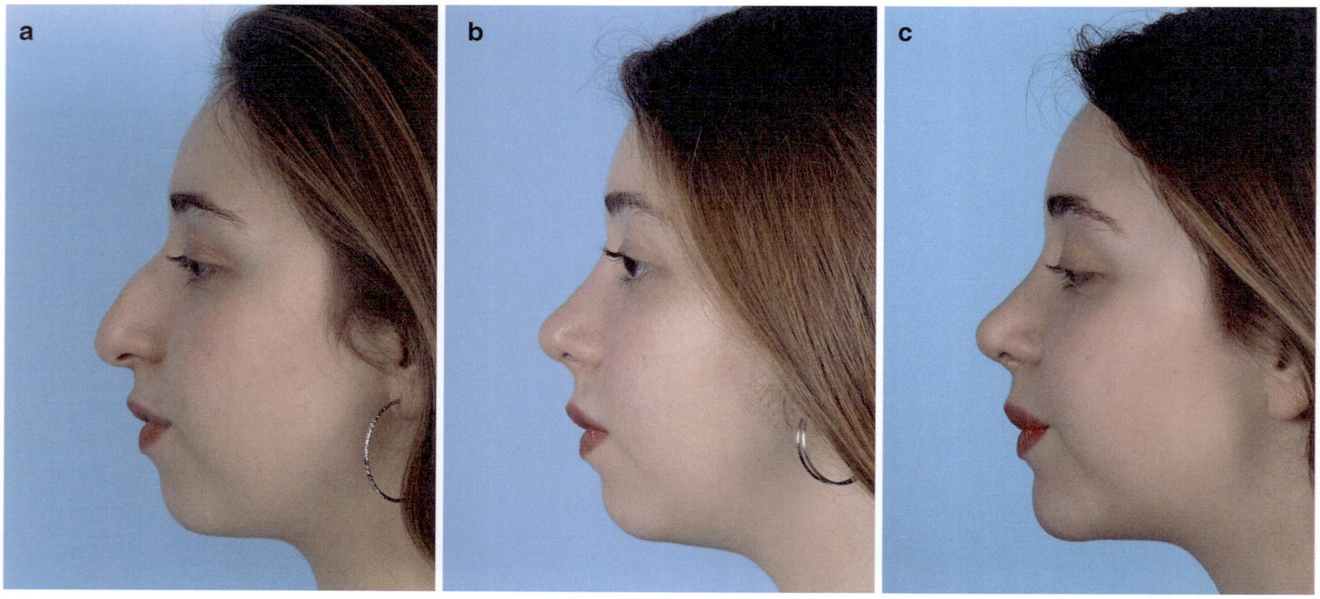

Fig. 5.21 (**a**) Patient's profile view before rhinoplasty. (**b**) Patient's profile view after rhinoplasty without chin augmentation. The nose still has a slightly large appearance. (**c**) After chin augmentation, dorsal profile view is more balanced

5.3.3 Case 3

Intraoperative photos show a patient who is suffering from her high dorsal bridge. The nasal bones, rhinon area, and cartilaginous dorsum are all high (Fig. 5.22).

In photographs taken before the surgery and 2 years after, the dorsal height is reduced with a slight supra tip break. Brow tip aesthetic line has been restored (Fig. 5.23).

5.3.4 Case 4

On the other hand, when the main component of the hump is bony dorsum, the cartilaginous reduction should be performed meticulously.

A 24-year-old woman requested reduction of the size of her nose. The hump was mainly on the bony dorsum, so a limited cartilaginous resection was performed (Fig. 5.24).

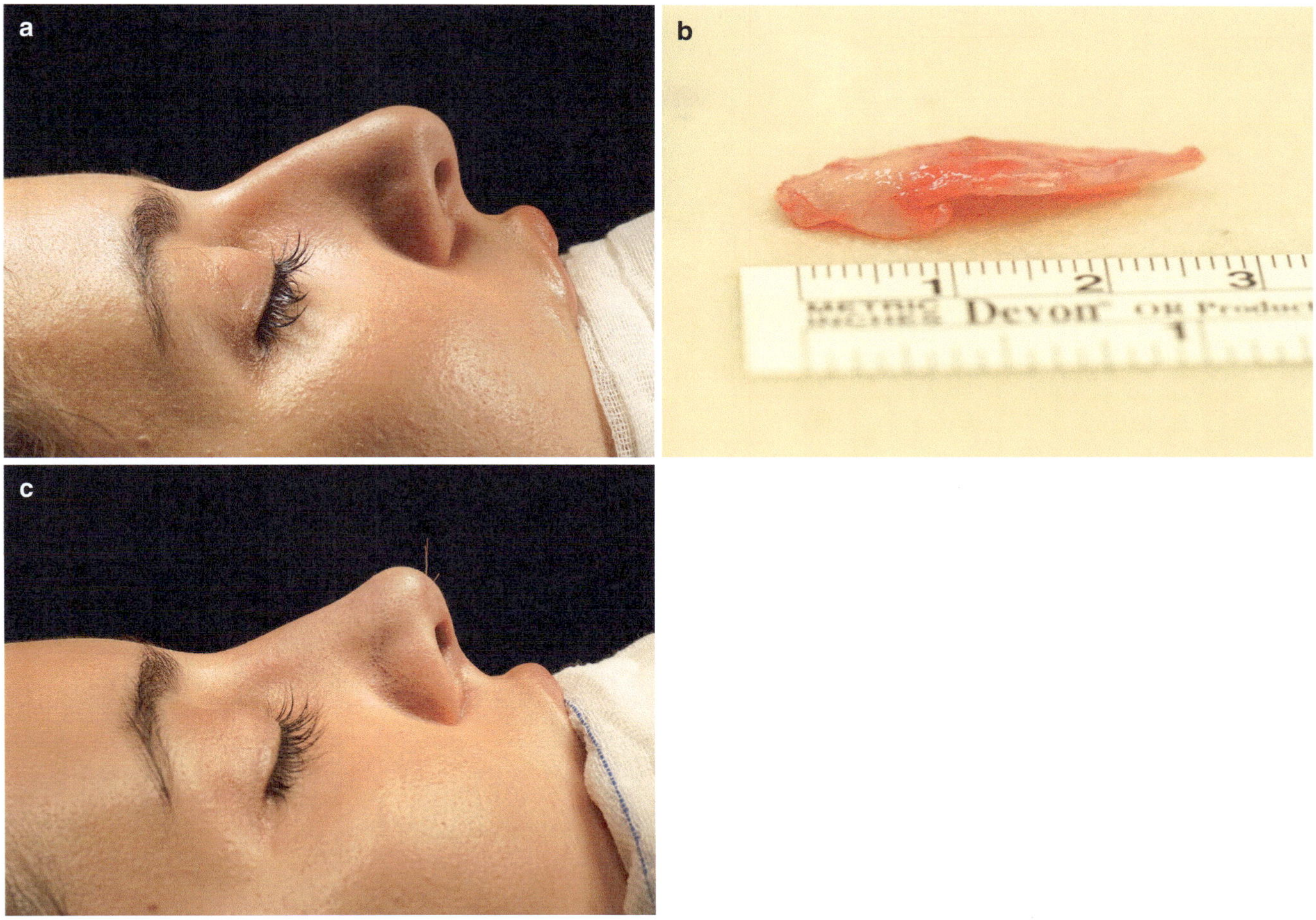

Fig. 5.22 (**a**) Intraoperative profile photograph. (**b**) En block dorsal hump reduction was performed. The main component of dorsal hump was the cartilage. (**c**) Immediately after hump removal

5.3.5 Case 5

In some cases, the alar cartilage behaves like a dorsal hump. Therefore, cephalic resection of the alar cartilage should be performed. Otherwise, even with lowering of the dorsal cartilage hump, it would retain a high appearance.

This 27-year-old patient complained of a prominent dorsum. Intraoperative photographs demonstrate cartilaginous dorsal hump caused by both the cephalic part of alar cartilage and the cartilaginous dorsum (Fig. 5.25).

The dorsal hump was eliminated. To achieve an ideal dorsum, three resections were performed, i.e., of the upper lateral cartilages, dorsal bone, and cephalic parts of the alar cartilages (Fig. 5.26).

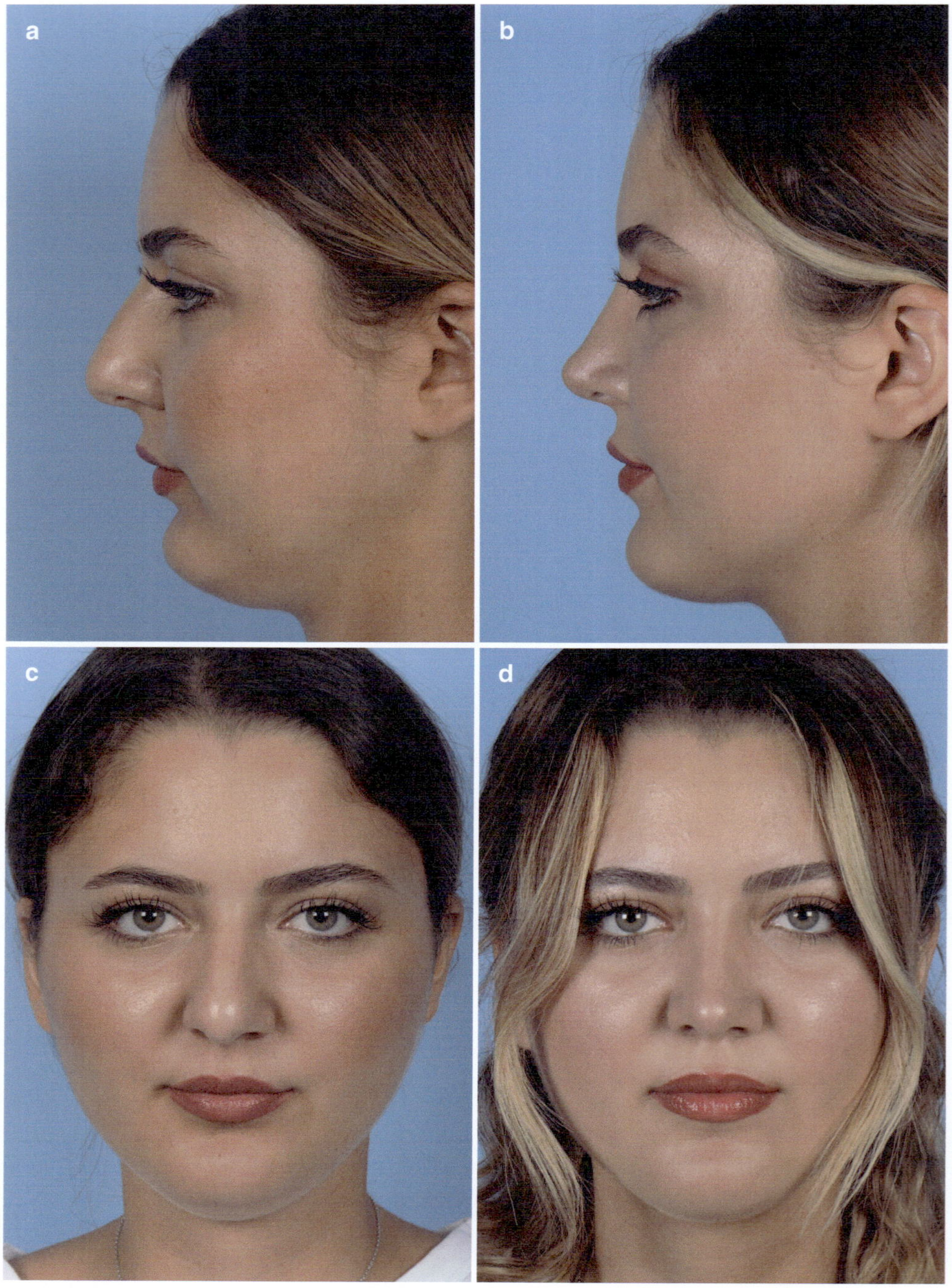

Fig. 5.23 (**a**–**d**) Pre- and 2-year postoperative photographs

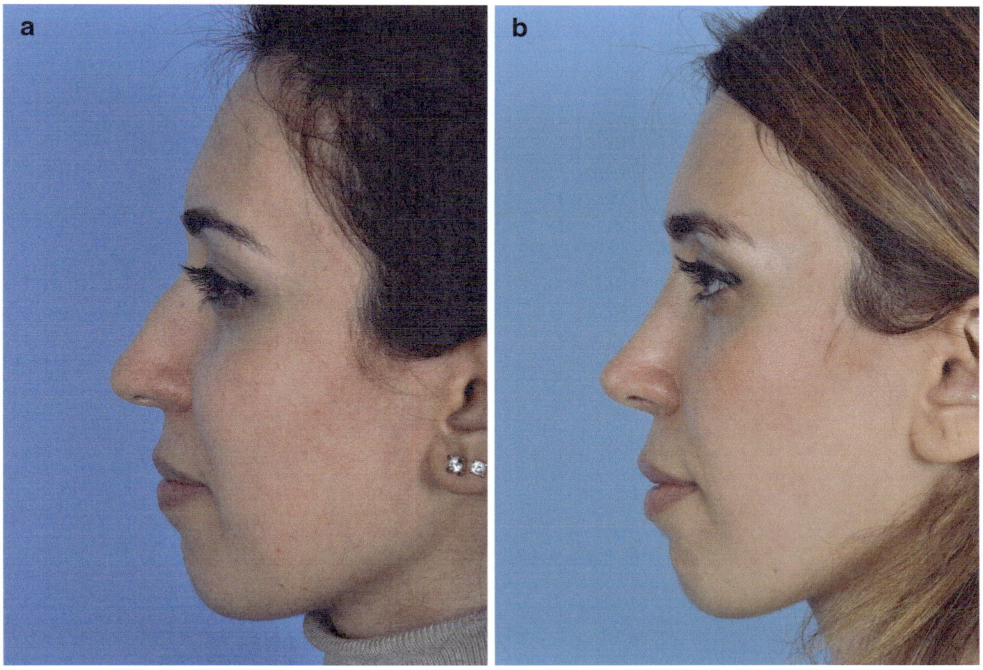

Fig. 5.24 (**a**, **b**) The dorsal height was reduced with a slight supratip break

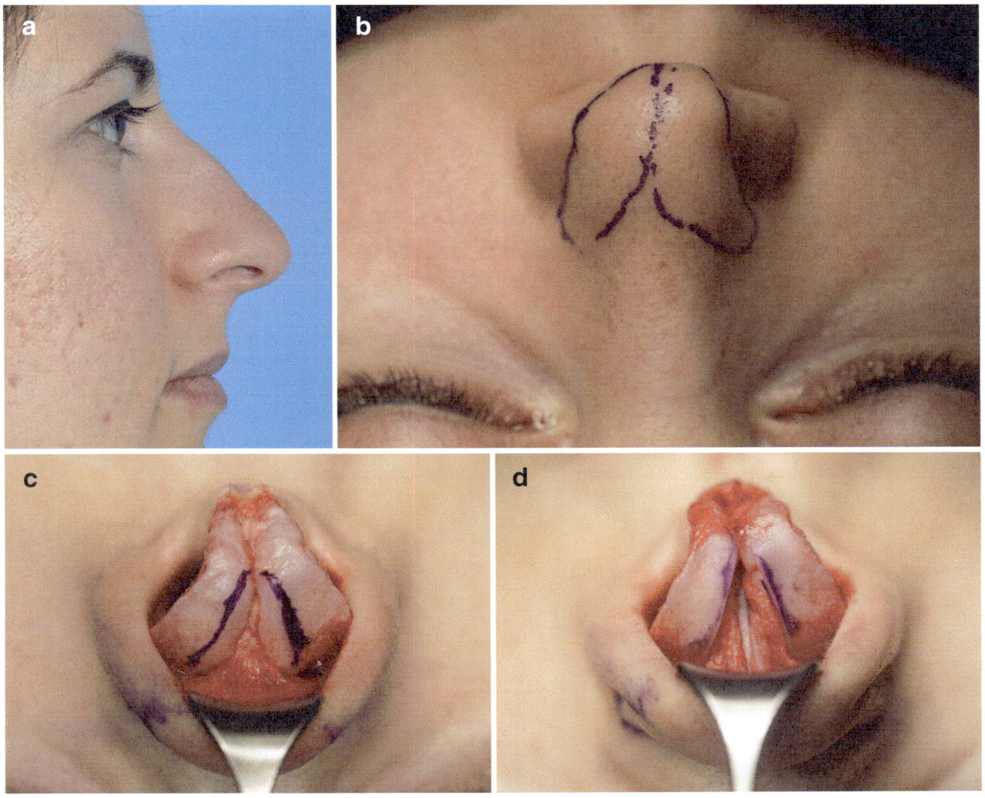

Fig. 5.25 (**a**–**d**) The cephalic part of the alar cartilage covering the cartilaginous dorsum was resected

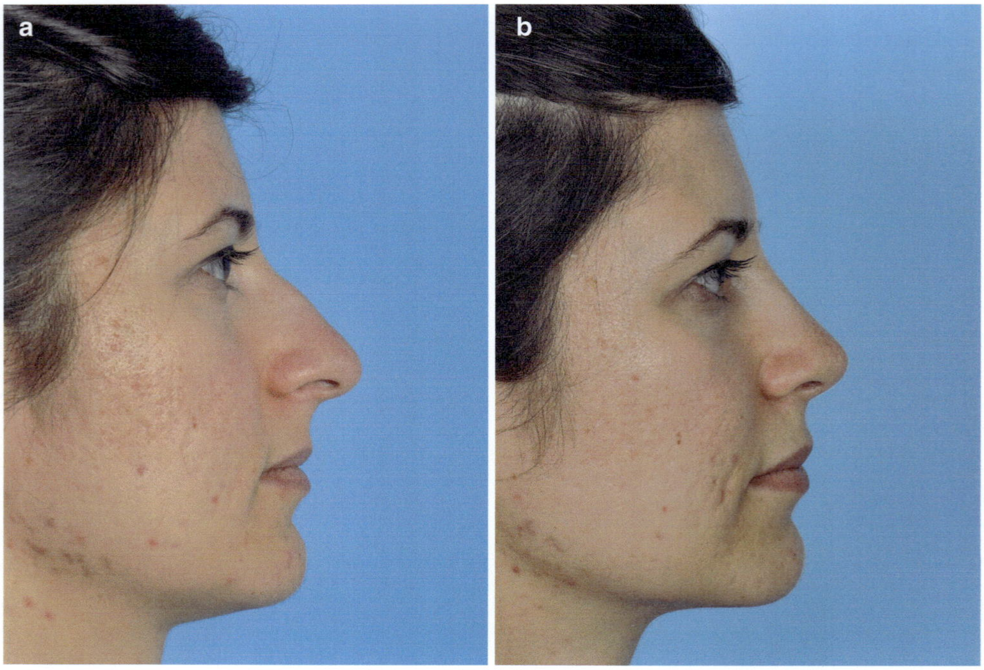

Fig. 5.26 (**a**, **b**) Pre- and 2-year postoperative profile photographs

5.4 Conclusion

Many patients requesting rhinoplasty desire reduction of the dorsum. The main goal of dorsal reduction is to achieve a smooth, straight dorsum without compromising the nasal airway. For this purpose, adequate dorsal resection requires a clear understanding of the aesthetic goals and accurate techniques. In the meantime, the dorsal resection should be analyzed carefully to maintain balance with the tip projection, radix projection, chin projection, and forehead projection.

There are two techniques for dorsal reduction, which are en bloc and segmental. While a cartilaginous hump can be reduced by en bloc or segmental resection, a bony hump may be reduced with rasps if smaller reduction is needed, and a guarded osteotome can be used if a larger amount of bone is to be removed.

Disclosures The author reports no conflicts of interest or funding requiring disclosure.

Further Reading

Davis RE, Raval J. Powered instrumentation for nasal bone reduction: advantages and indications. Arch Facial Plast Surg. 2003;5(5):384–91.

Gruber RP, Perkins SW. Humpectomy and spreader flaps. Clin Plast Surg. 2010;37(2):285–91.

Jin HR, Won TB. Nasal hump removal in Asians. Acta Otolaryngol Suppl. 2007;558:95–101.

Lee MR, Unger JG, Rohrich RJ. Management of the nasal dorsum in rhinoplasty: a systematic review of the literature regarding technique, outcomes, and complications. Plast Reconstr Surg. 2011;128(5):538e–50e.

Lohuis PJ, Faraj-Hakim S, Knobbe A, Duivesteijn W, Bran GM. Split hump technique for reduction of the overprojected nasal dorsum: a statistical analysis on subjective body image in relation to nasal appearance and nasal patency in 97 patients undergoing aesthetic rhinoplasty. Arch Facial Plast Surg. 2012;14(5):346–53.

Neu BR. Use of the upper lateral cartilage sagittal rotation flap in nasal dorsum reduction and augmentation. Plast Reconstr Surg. 2009;123(3):1079–87.

Rohrich RJ, Muzaffar AR, Janis JE. Component dorsal hump reduction: the importance of maintaining dorsal aesthetic lines in rhinoplasty. Plast Reconstr Surg. 2004;114(5):1298–308; discussion 1309–12

Roostaeian J, Unger JG, Lee MR, Geissler P, Rohrich RJ. Reconstitution of the nasal dorsum following component dorsal reduction in primary rhinoplasty. Plast Reconstr Surg. 2014;133(3):509–18.

Sadick H, Rowe-Jones JM, Gassner HG. Nuances in component nasal hump reduction. J Plast Reconstr Aesthet Surg. 2018;71(2):178–84.

Sykes JM, Tapias V, Kim JE. Management of the nasal dorsum. Facial Plast Surg. 2011;27(2):192–202.

6 Middle Vault Reconstruction

6.1 Introduction

After achieving ideal dorsum projection from the lateral view by removing the hump, the second step involves reconstruction of the middle vault. The goal of reconstruction is to reestablish the integrity of the middle vault, which was distorted following hump resection. The aim of middle vault reconstruction is to create a symmetrical, stable middle vault with ideal horizontal width, which also requires an ideal brow-tip aesthetic line (Fig. 6.1).

Middle vault reconstruction is also important for respiratory function because the middle vault contains the internal nasal wall area. The internal nasal wall is an anatomically active area during respiration. The internal valve is defined as the area between the caudal border of the upper lateral cartilages and the dorsal septum. The angle between the upper lateral and dorsal septum should be 10–15° to allow unrestricted airflow. **When reconstructing the middle vault, the goal should be to ensure integrity of the skin, cartilage, and fibrofatty tissue in the nasal valve** (Fig. 6.2).

Various surgical methods are employed to reconstruct the middle nasal vault, including use of structural materials as grafts or reconstructive sutures.

Cartilage is the structural material required for middle vault reconstruction. An ideal middle vault is achieved by using three main grafts prepared from cartilage:

- Spreader graft
- Autospreader graft
- Camouflage graft

While the first two grafts are used for both aesthetic and functional reasons, the third graft, which provides the brow-tip aesthetic line, is used solely for aesthetic purposes. We will discuss spreader grafts in this chapter. You can find more details about the camouflage graft in the final touch chapter.

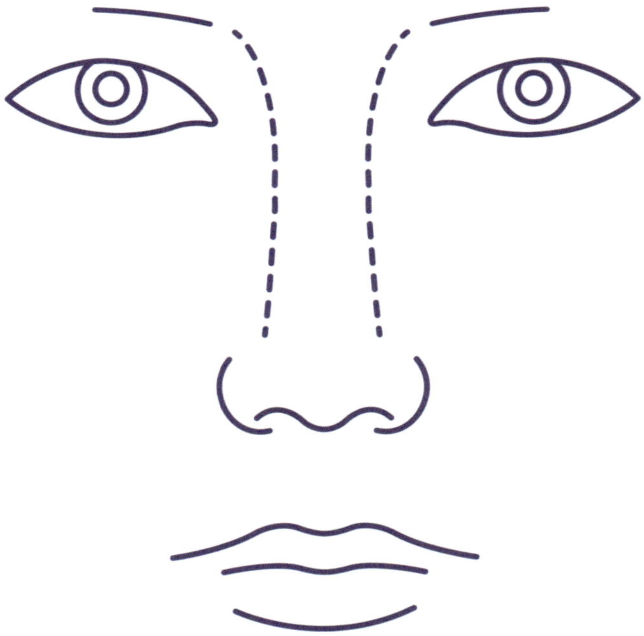

Fig. 6.1 The brow-tip aesthetic line is an imaginary line traced from the medial brow down the lateral wall of the nose to the tip-defining points. The line should be slightly wider at the radix, narrow in the middle third, and then wider at the tip. In the middle third, the dorsum should measure approximately 80% of the width of the base

Supplementary Information The online version contains supplementary material available at https://doi.org/10.1007/978-3-031-65619-4_6.

S. Şeneldir, *Photographic Atlas of Rhinoplasty*, https://doi.org/10.1007/978-3-031-65619-4_6

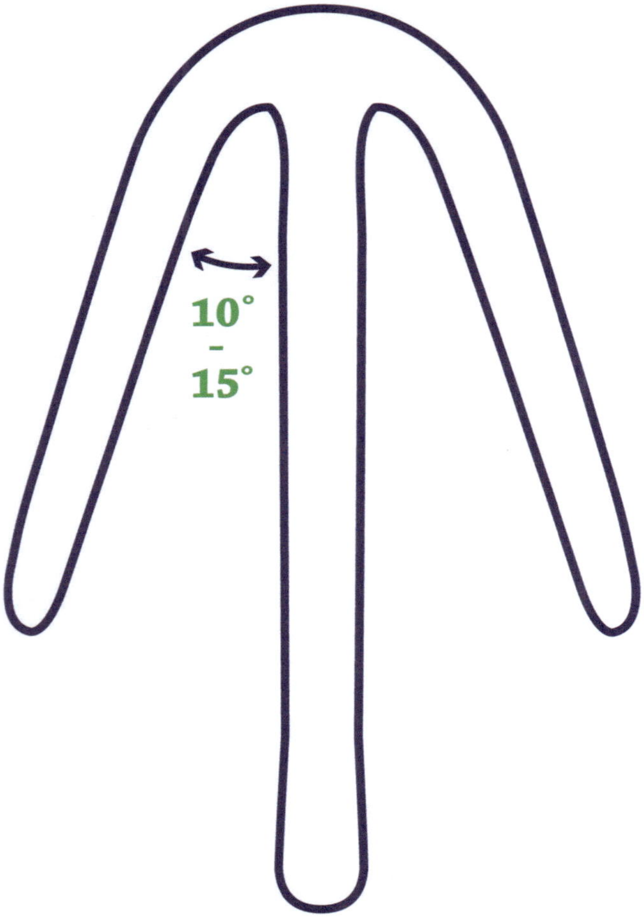

Fig. 6.2 Internal nasal valve. It is formed by the junction of the caudal margin of the upper lateral cartilage, nasal septum, and floor of the nose

6.2 Treatment Strategy and Clinical Outcomes

We will first discuss middle vault reconstruction by using spreader grafts.

6.2.1 Spreader Graft

Spreader grafts are the gold standard for reconstructing the middle vault. The traditional spreader graft is rectangular in shape and may vary in length and thickness from case to case. The length of the graft may vary from 10 mm to 25 mm, and the thickness may vary from 2 mm to 4 mm, while the height always remains the same at 3 mm to 4 mm (Fig. 6.3).

The graft can be modified according to middle vault problems:

- Modification done using thicker portion cephalically or caudally (Fig. 6.4).
- The edges of the graft can be beveled caudally and/or cephalically (Fig. 6.5).
  The graft can also be curved in a "C" shape (Fig. 6.6).
- Spreader graft Source is the septal or costal cartilage. Auricular cartilage is the final resort as a graft source because it is weaker than the others (Figs. 6.7 and 6.8).

The prepared graft is placed between the septum and the upper cartilage in the caudocranial direction. The spreader grafts are sutured to the septal cartilage caudally and cephalically by mattress sutures. Absorbable suture material is preferred. The superior edges of the grafts are at the same height as the septal cartilage. Grafts are generally placed caudally 1–2 mm behind the anterior septal angle and extend cranially to the starting point of the nasal bones. Spreader graft can be placed through an open approach or closed approach (Figs. 6.9 and 6.10).

The indications of spreader grafts are discussed in this section with reference to actual clinical cases.

6.2.2 Spreader Grafts Are Used to Avoid a Narrow Middle Vault

The width of the open roof deformity is in accordance with the size of the hump resection. In cases with excessive dorsal hump resection, use of a spreader graft prevents a pinched look in the middle third of the nose. Let us look at the following example.

6.2.2.1 Case 1

A 29-year-old patient has huge dorsal hump. A pinched look to the middle vault was prevented by placement of bilateral spreader grafts after aggressive dorsal hump reduction (Fig. 6.11). Reconstruction of the middle vault with spreader grafts provided an ideal brow-tip aesthetic line (Fig. 6.12).

6.2.2.2 Case 2

There is an excessive dorsal hump in this case. Closed rhinoplasty approach was preferred. Bilateral spreader grafts after aggressive dorsal reduction were used to prevent an inverted V-shaped appearance in the frontal view (Fig. 6.13).

Attempting to close a wide middle vault without using a spreader would result in the upper laterals falling to a level below the septum. If the surgery is finalized before identifying and correcting this condition, the relationship with the upper vault will be distorted. A narrow middle vault and relatively wider upper vault result in an inverted V-shaped appearance in the frontal view; this not only affects the appearance, but also results in functional respiratory problems associated with narrowing of the internal nasal valve.

Case 3 is a good example of this condition.

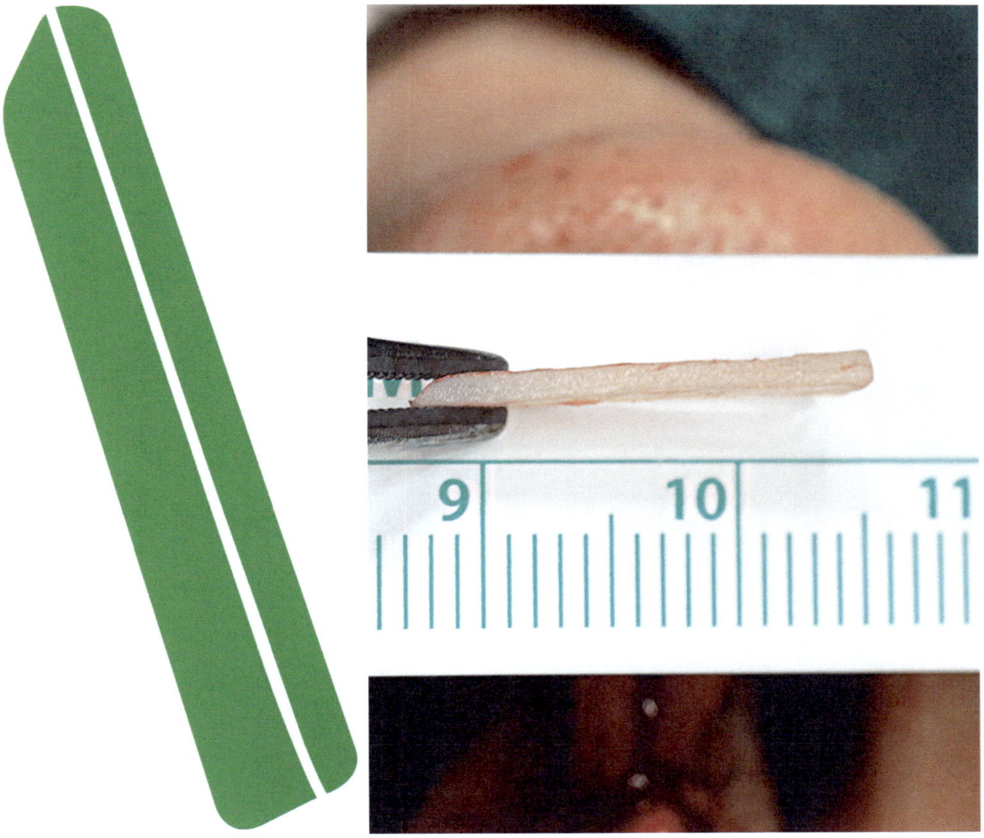

Fig. 6.3 Standard-sized and -shaped spreader graft

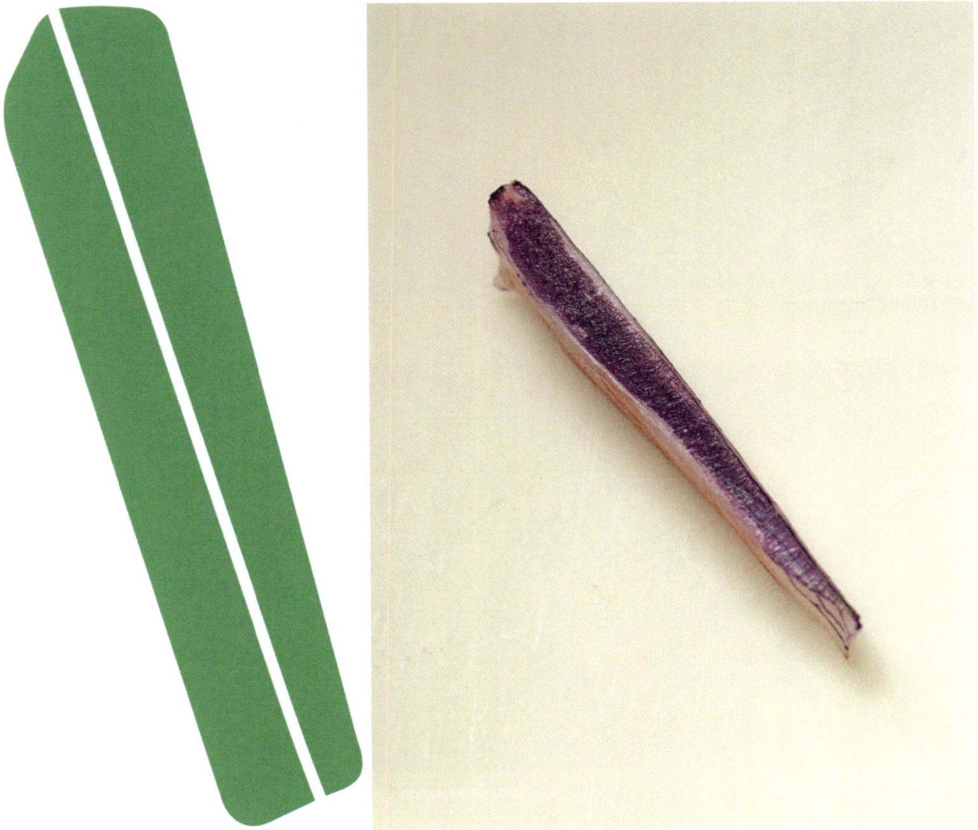

Fig. 6.4 Spreader graft, one end is thicker than the other end

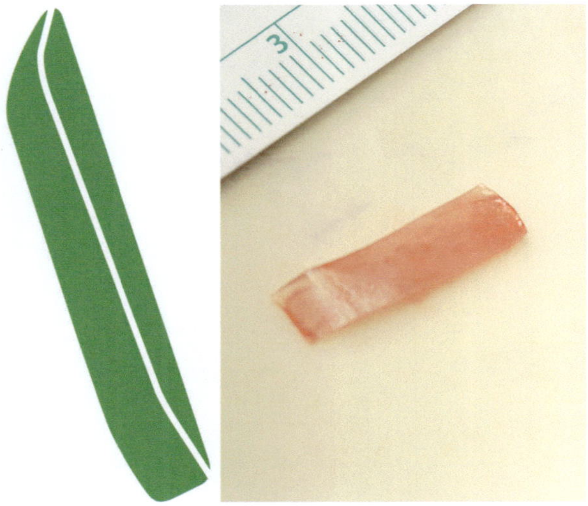

Fig. 6.5 Two ends can be trimmed

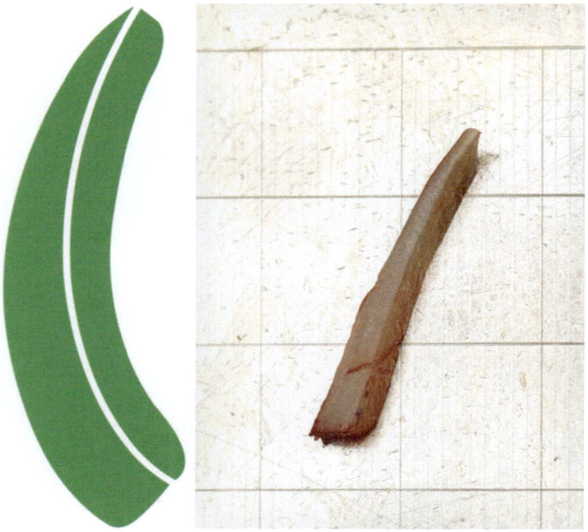

Fig. 6.6 "C"-shaped spreader graft is a handy tool for correcting dorsal septal deviations

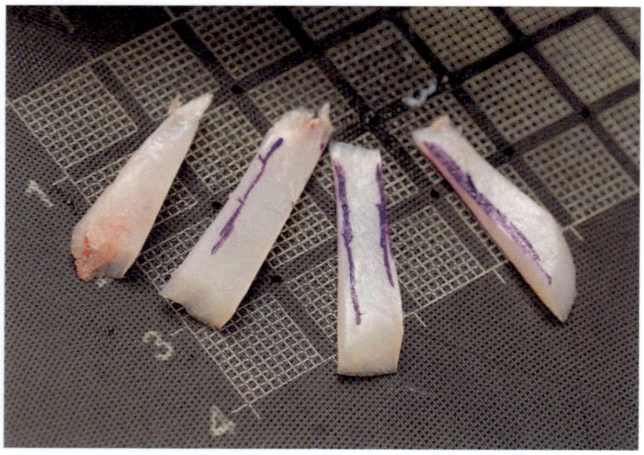

Fig. 6.7 Septal cartilage

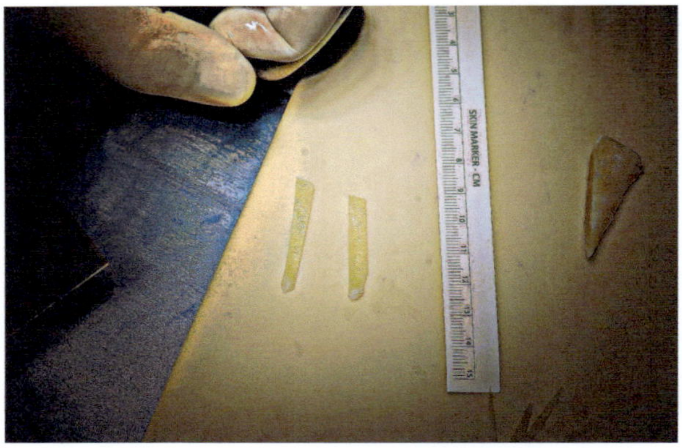

Fig. 6.8 Costal cartilage

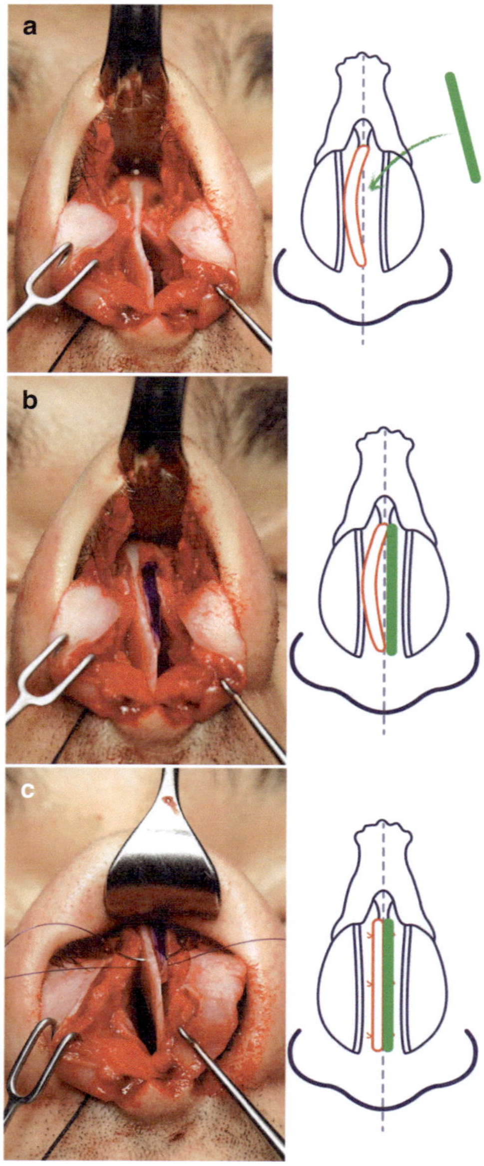

Fig. 6.9 (**a**–**c**) Spreader graft placement via open approach

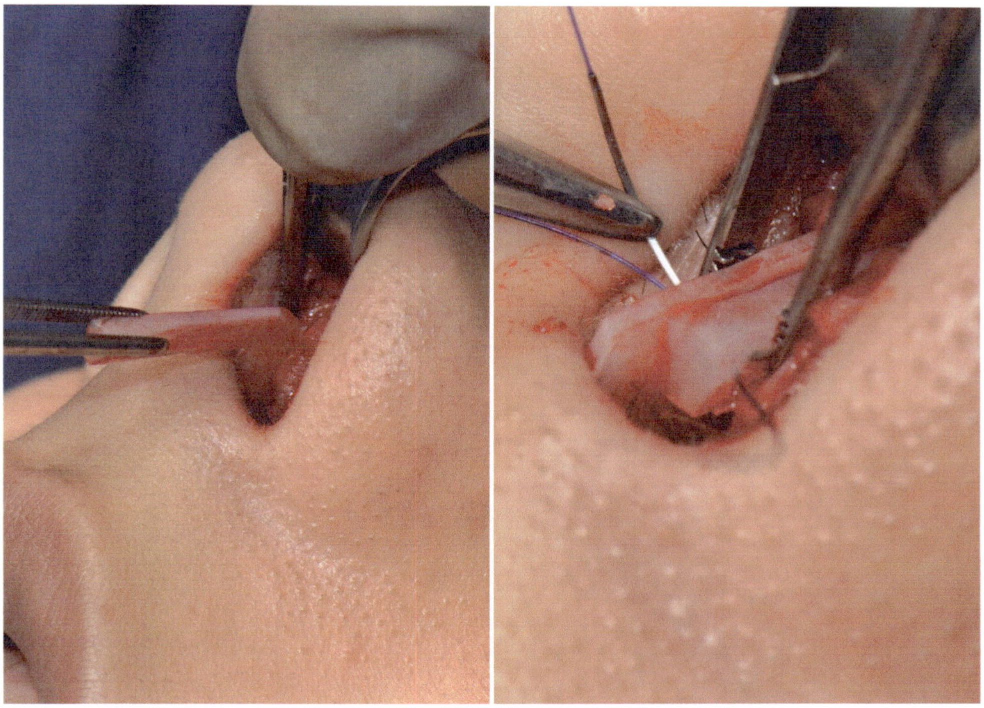

Fig. 6.10 Spreader graft placement via closed approach

6.2.2.3 Case 3

The patient's history includes rhinoplasty 6 years ago performed by another surgeon. She had in the frontal view; an inverted V-shaped appearance was observed because of the narrow middle vault and insufficient medialization of the nasal bones (Fig. 6.14). In this case, bilateral spreader grafts should be used for middle vault reconstruction (Fig. 6.15). Bilateral spreader graft and lateral osteotomy resolved the inverted V-shaped appearance. The pinched nasal tip was also resolved by lateral crural graft (Fig. 6.16).

6.2.3 Correction of Dorsal Septal Deviations Can Also Be Performed with Spreader Grafts

Treatment of the deviated middle vault may include any combination of spreader grafts. Spreader grafts are inserted between the upper lateral cartilages and the dorsal septum for structural reinforcement and straightening of the crooked middle vault. If a unilateral spreader graft is used, it should be positioned on the concave side of the deformity (*see* Case 4).

6.2.3.1 Case 4

This woman with unilateral nasal obstruction and a deviated nose requested septorhinoplasty to improve nasal breathing and shape (Fig. 6.17). Figure 6.18 shows the outcome at 2 years after surgery.

In cases with a moderate C-shaped deviated septum, use of a spreader graft alone is not sufficient for reconstruction of the middle vault. It may be necessary to remove inverted triangles from the convex portion to medialize the septum. Removing such triangles from the most convex portion of the septum brings the convex and concave planes to the same length after septoplasty. This breaks septal resistance, and middle vault symmetry can then be achieved using the spreaders placed unilaterally or bilaterally. Case 5 provides a typical example.

6.2.3.2 Case 5

In helicopter view, a C-shaped middle vault can be seen (Fig. 6.19). The technique described above is performed (Fig. 6.20). Figure 6.21 shows the outcome at 1 year after surgery. The upper and middle vault have been straightened.

As mentioned before, it is essential to think in three dimensions during performance of rhinoplasty. While dorsal resection lowers the dorsum, open roof deformity provides an opportunity for middle vault reconstruction and correction of dorsal irregularities, such as septal deviations.

6.2.3.3 Case 6

This case has a dorsal hump and a narrow asymmetrical middle vault (Fig. 6.22). In this case, after hump removal, inverted triangles were removed from the most convex part of the dorsal septum unilaterally and a spreader graft was placed and sutured to the concave side (Fig. 6.23). Preoperative and 3-years postoperative photographs are seen in Fig. 6.24.

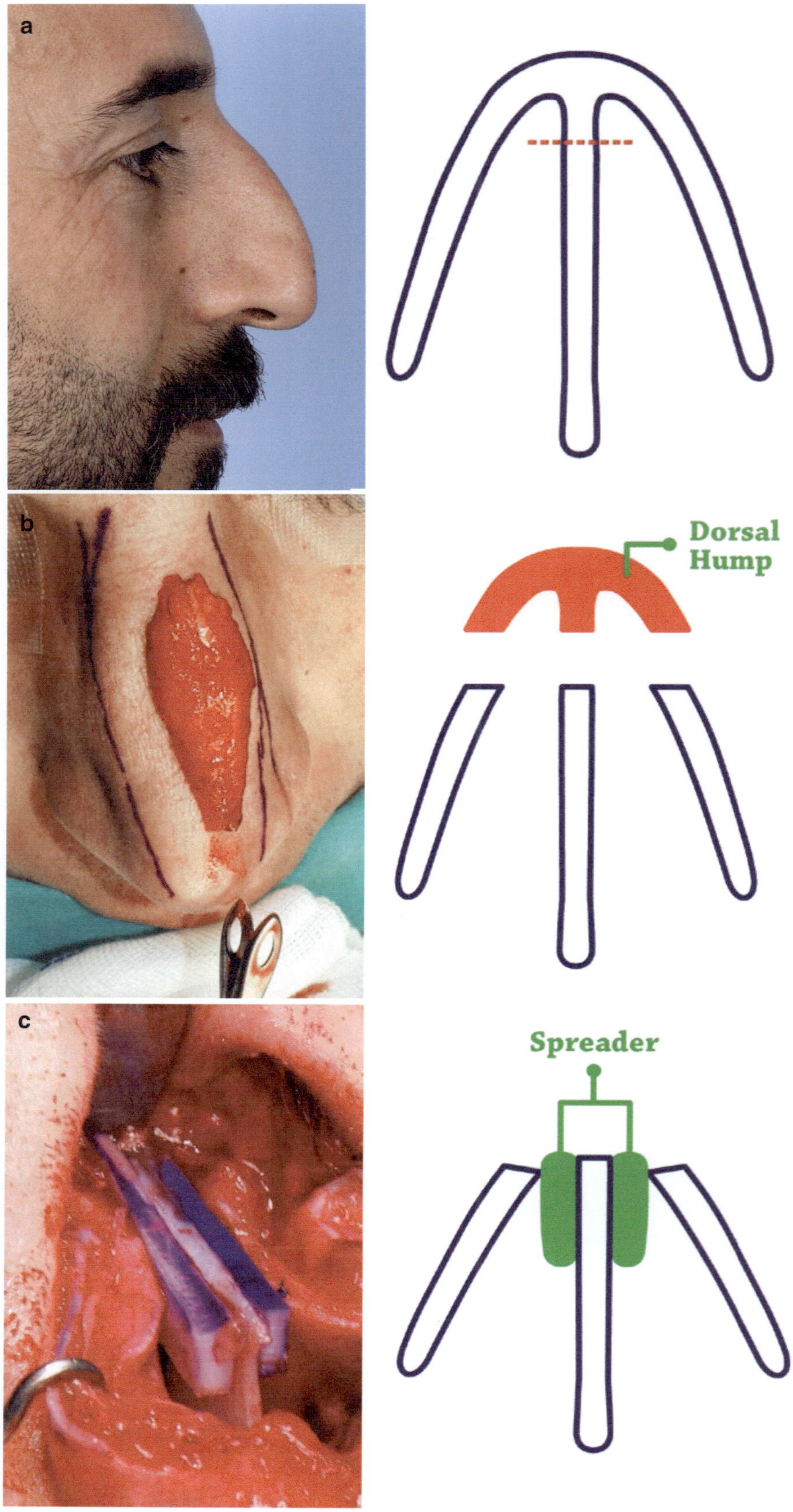

Fig. 6.11 (**a**) Before hump removal. (**b**) Open roof deformity occurs after hump removal. (**c**) Bilateral spreader grafts are used for middle vault reconstruction

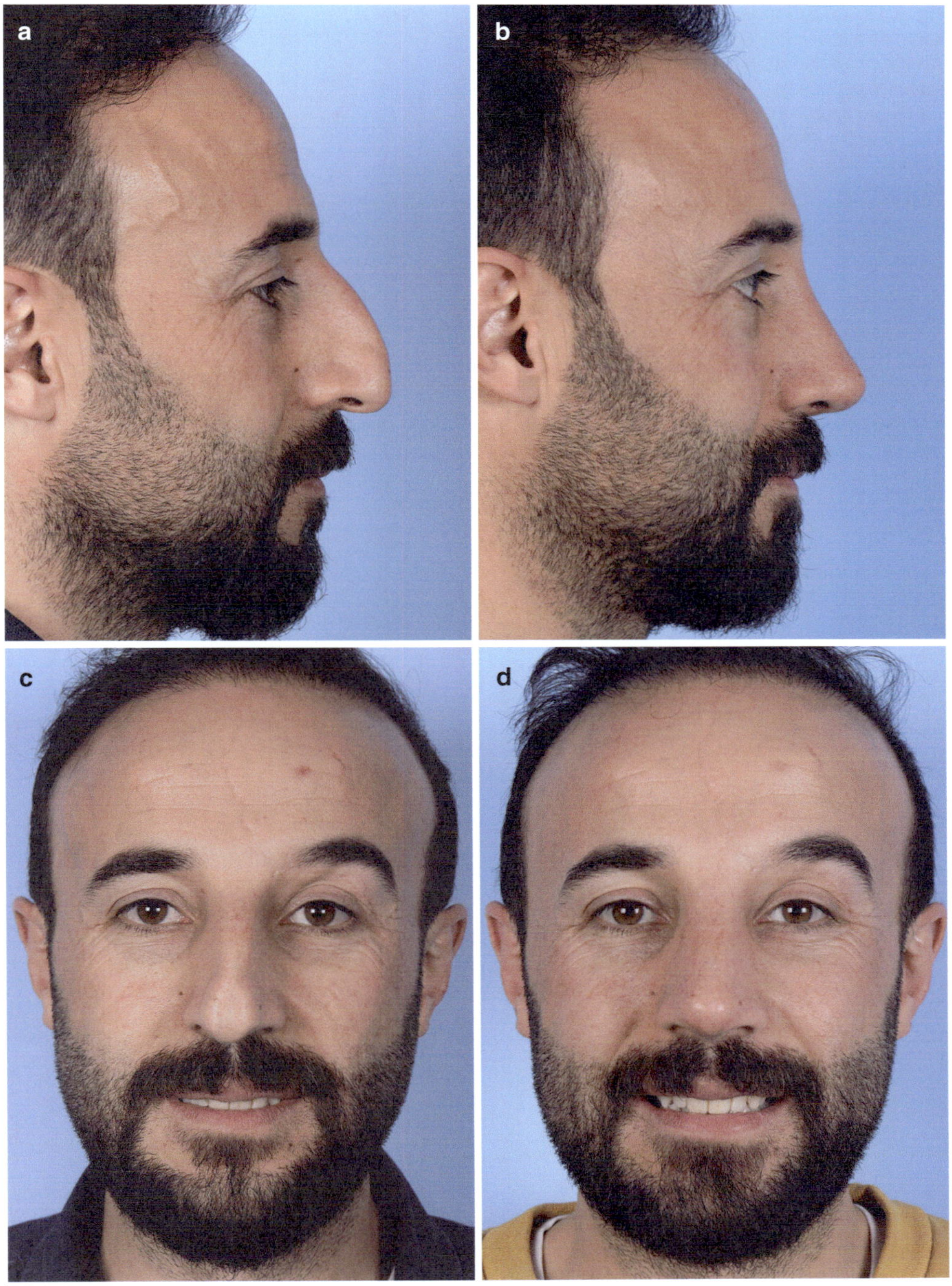

Fig. 6.12 (**a**–**d**) While dorsal hump removal improved the dorsal profile, middle vault reconstruction provided ideal brow tip aesthetic line

6.2.4 Asymmetric Spreader Graft to Reconstruct the Middle Vault

Use of asymmetric spreader graft is sometimes required to reconstruct the middle vault when the spreaders placed to the right and left of the septum are of different length and width.

6.2.4.1 Case 7

As illustrated in the case outlined here, a mild S-shaped septal deviation was observed in the middle vault after nasal hump resection and septoplasty. Failure to correct this mild S-shaped deviation would result in medium- and long-term aesthetic problems. The asymmetric spreader technique is a good solution to avoid this problem, which will later manifest in the form of breaks through the brow-tip aesthetic line (Fig. 6.25).

The surgical outcome at 1 year after surgery is shown in Fig. 6.26.

6.2.4.2 Case 8

Asymmetric spreader grafts were used for constructing the middle vault in another case with an S-shaped septal deviation. **It is important to remember that different asymmet-**

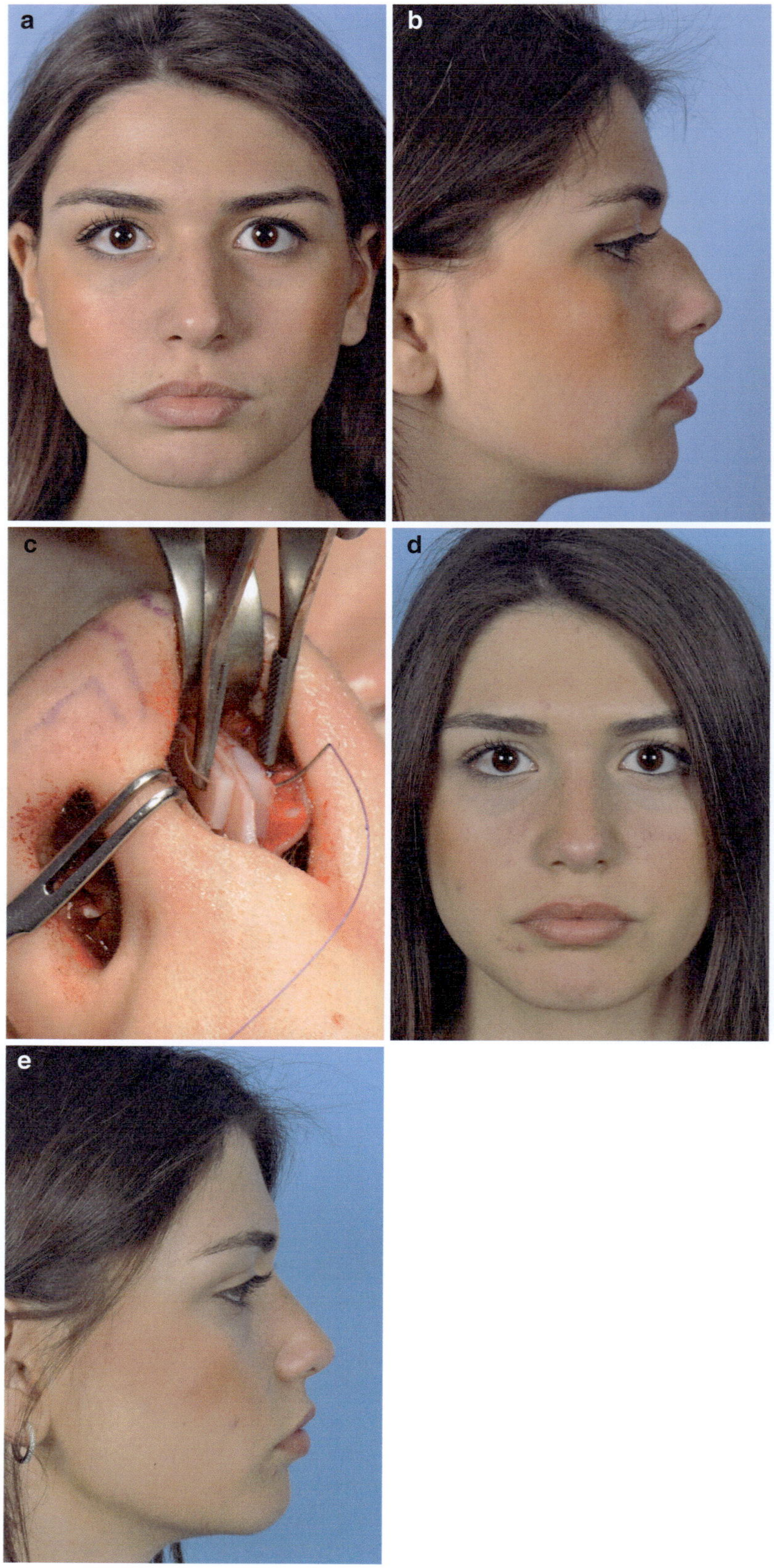

Fig. 6.13 (**a**, **b**) The big hump on her dorsum. (**c**) After hump removal, bilateral spreader grafts were placed via closed approach. (**d**, **e**) The tip and dorsum more defined. There is no problem on her middle vault

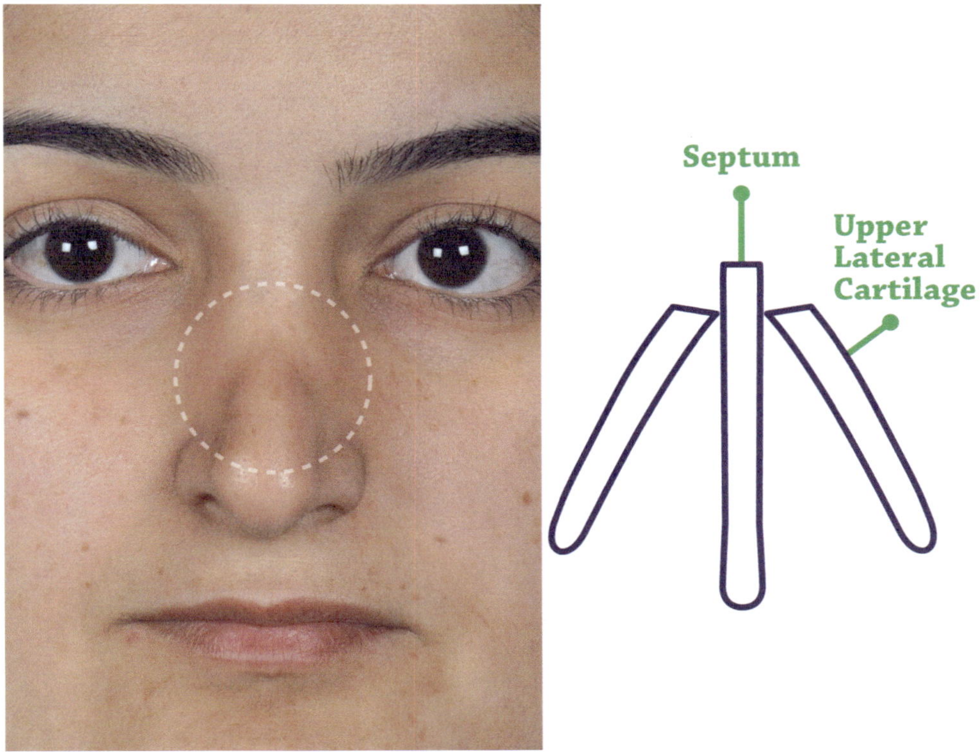

Fig. 6.14 Inverted V-shaped appearance

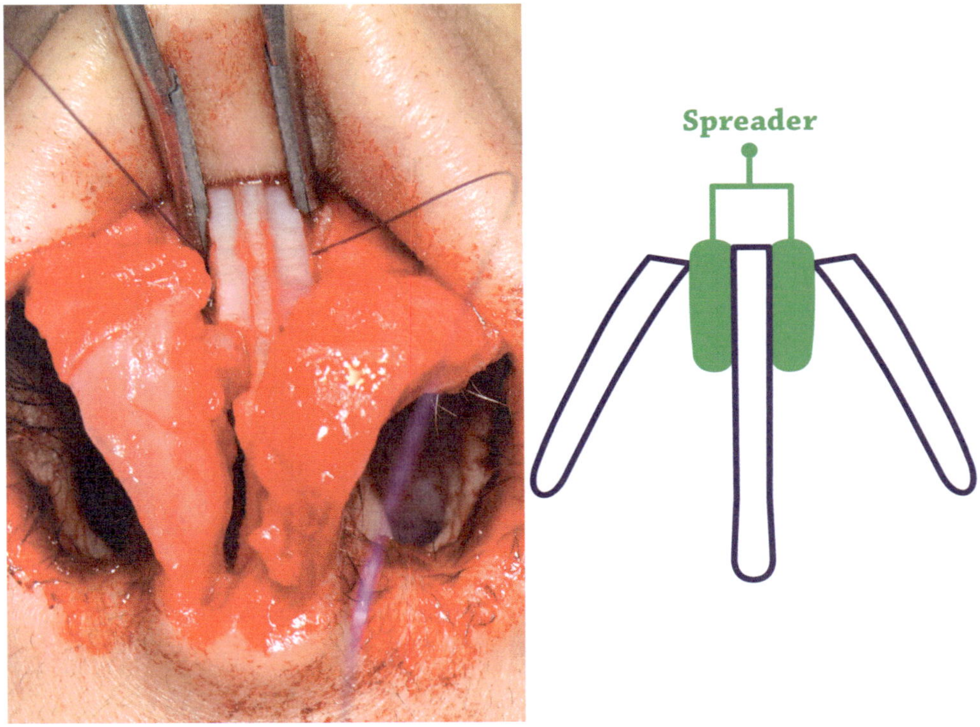

Fig. 6.15 Open rhinoplasty approach and bilateral spreader grafts

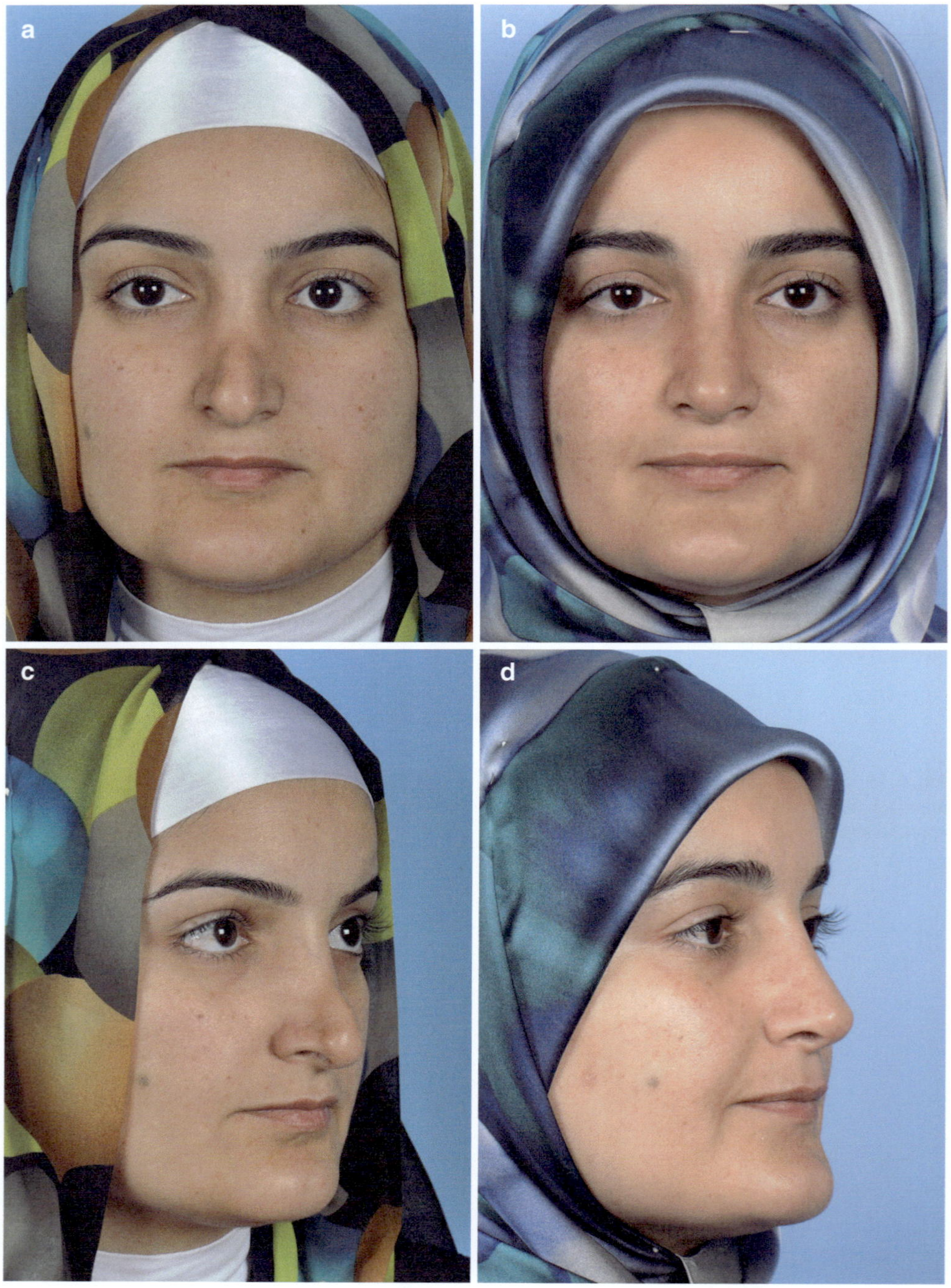

Fig. 6.16 (**a**–**d**) Significant correction of pinched appearance. Increase in the width of the middle third as a result of the spreader grafts. Also, re-osteotomy and spreader grafts solved inverted V deformity

ric spreader grafts are applicable in each case. Therefore, a variety of spreader grafts should be sutured and detached intraoperatively until the septum is straight and stable. Graft replacement in this case is shown in Fig. 6.27. Preoperative and 1-year postoperative photographs are seen in Fig. 6.28.

6.2.5 Collapsed Lateral Nasal Wall

Spreader grafts are also used in the repair of a collapsed lateral nasal wall after osteotomy. In such cases, the spreader graft is placed under the nasal bone and pushes the collapsed bone wall outward.

6.2.5.1 Case 9

In the case outlined here, the left lateral nasal wall had collapsed medially following osteotomies performed on the left side. Insertion of the spreader graft 3–4 mm underneath the nasal bone would be sufficient. However, the surgeon may also need to advance the graft up to the radix. The surgeon must check which position of the spreader best resolves the problem intraoperatively and then place the

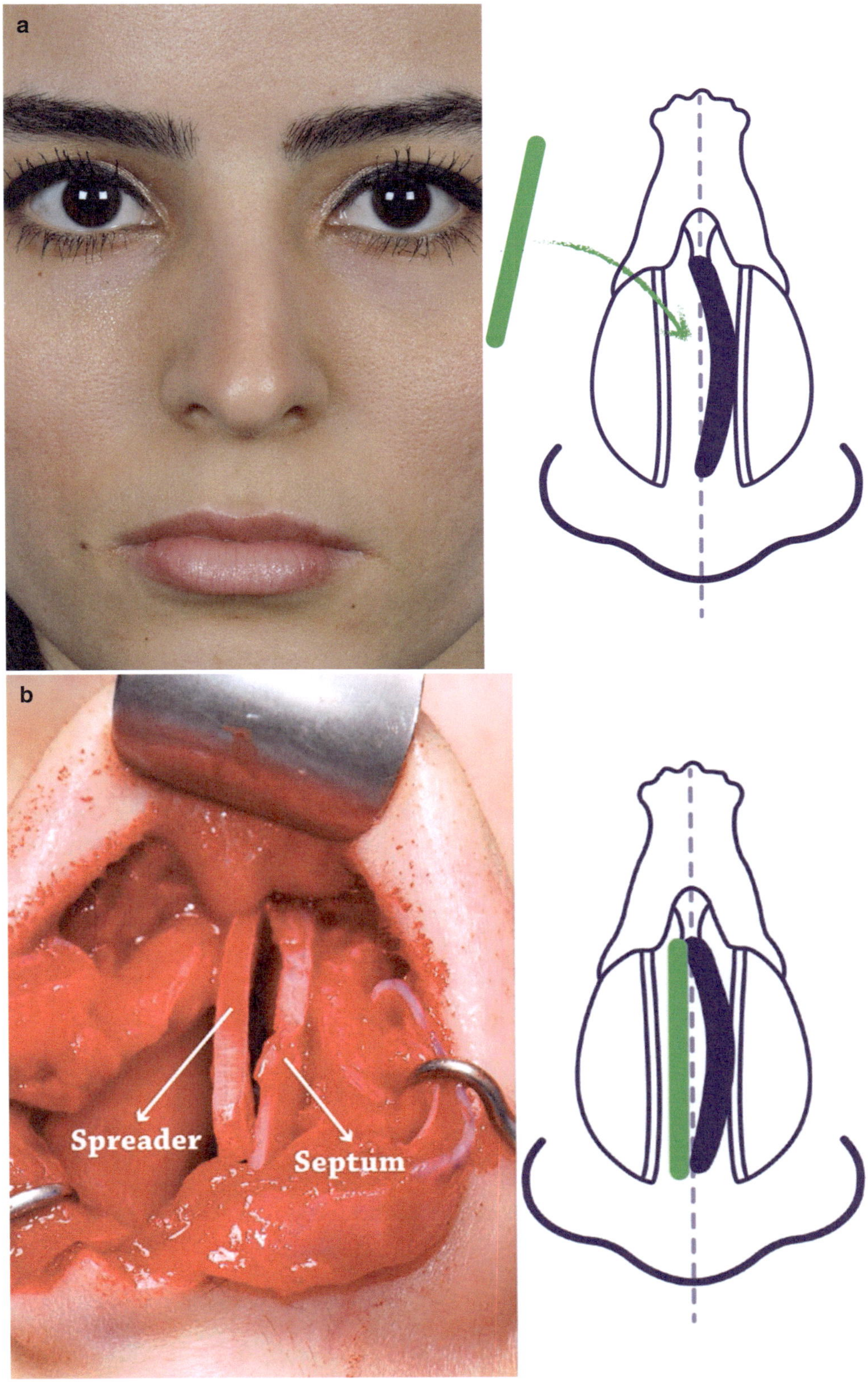

Fig. 6.17 (**a**) This case had a C-shaped septum, which resulted in a mildly deviated dorsum. (**b**) After hump removal, a C-shaped septum could be seen. (**c**) A unilateral spreader graft was placed and sutured on the concave side of the septum. Intraoperatively, a straight septum was achieved. Fixation of the spreader graft to the septum should be performed with 5–0 nonabsorbable sutures

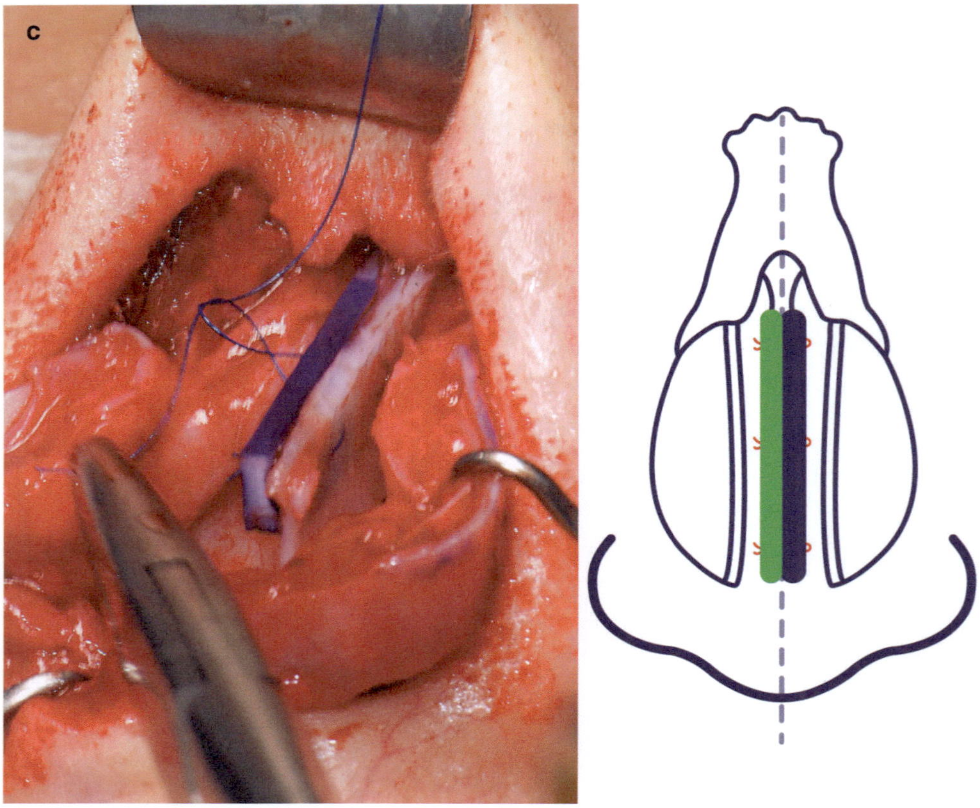

Fig. 6.17 (continued)

spreader at this position. The area is controlled after fixation and checked for minor irregularities and pits, and then corrected by filling with rasping materials or diced cartilage (Fig. 6.29).

One year after surgery, the middle vault and nasal walls were still stable and symmetrical. The collapsed lateral nasal wall was resolved intraoperatively, and postoperative complications due to osteotomy were prevented (Fig. 6.30).

Technical Pearl: In most cases, the cranial edges of spreader grafts end just caudal to the nasal bones. Nevertheless, the surgeon may need to extend the spreader graft through the underside of the bony vault in cases with collapse of the bony vault medially after the osteotomy procedure, or for closure of open roof deformity in cases contraindicated for osteotomy due to short nasal bone.

6.2.5.2 Case 10

In the case outlined here, the nasal wall, which collapsed medially intraoperatively, was not lateralized using a spreader, thus resulting in the illustrated postoperative complication (Fig. 6.31).

6.2.6 Straightening of the Dorsal Septum and the Caudal Septum

Straightening of the dorsal septum will not be sufficient in cases of severe septal deviation, and the caudal septum should also be straightened to achieve a symmetrical middle vault.

6.2.6.1 Case 11

An example of complete septal deviation including both the caudal and dorsal septum is shown here. In the frontal view, the septum was entirely deviated from the cranial to caudal direction. In the base view, the nostrils appeared asymmetrical due to caudal septal deviation.

After middle vault reconstruction, caudal septal work should be performed to achieve symmetry in the entire septum (Fig. 6.32).

A spreader graft was placed on the left side of the dorsal septum. However, caudal deflection remained. An inverted triangle-shaped excision was performed on the convex side of the caudal septum. Then, a bilateral septal batten graft was sutured to strengthen the caudal septum (Fig. 6.33).

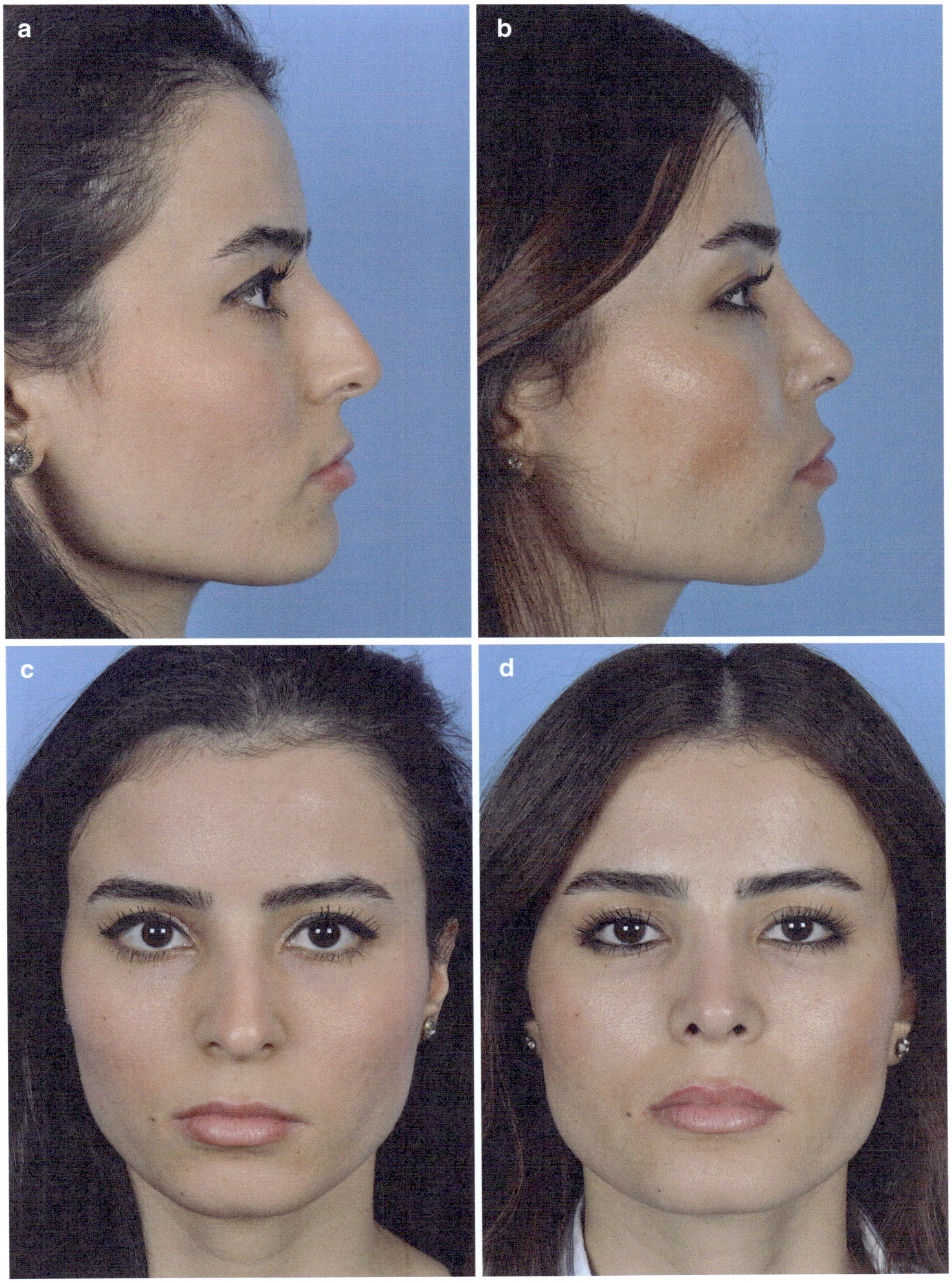

Fig. 6.18 (**a–d**) The hump was removed en bloc. After surgery, a slightly curved dorsum was preferred in this case. In the frontal view, middle vault reconstruction was performed with a unilateral spreader graft. The nose was straight in the frontal view

Figure 6.34 shows 4-year postoperative results. The dorsum is straight with no hump. The caudal septum is straight and the nostrils are symmetric.

6.2.7 Autospreader Graft (Autospreader Flap)

Using autospreader graft as an alternative to spreader graft should be considered.

An autospreader flap involves use of the upper lateral cartilage itself as a spreader graft. The indications for autospreader flap are the same as for the spreader graft. That is, like the spreader graft, an autospreader flap is used to preserve and restore the internal nasal valve angle and establish an aesthetic line at the nasal dorsum.

Figure 6.35 illustrates resection of the dorsal hump without the upper lateral cartilage. Excess upper lateral cartilage had been folded inward against the septum and fixed using 5–0 polydioxanone sutures.

Fig. 6.19 The nose is deviated due to severe dorsal septal deviation

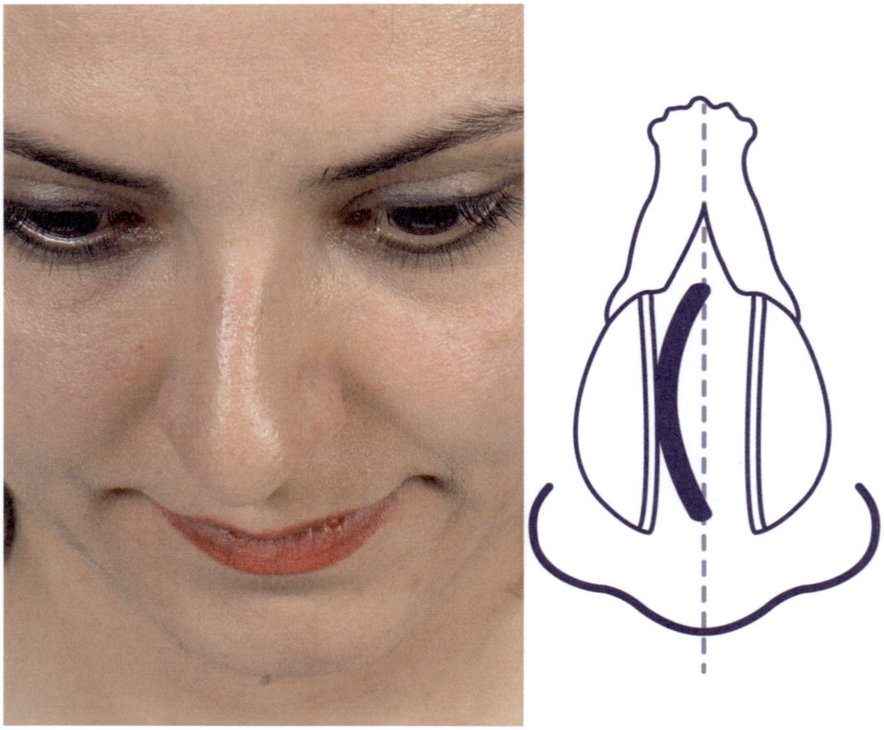

The author prefers to use an autospreader flap rather than a spreader graft in patients with a narrow middle vault owing to its ability to effectively and efficiently open the vault. It also reduces the need for grafting in patients with previous septoplasty.

Technical Pearl: The upper lateral cartilage is used as a flap, provided that its length is sufficient to allow it to be folded inside. Therefore, the autospreader flap can be used in cases with a septal hump.

Use of an autospreader flap is illustrated in the cases described below.

6.2.7.1 Case 12

Autospreader graft for middle vault reconstruction was preferred in this case for two reasons: (1) the patient had an excessive dorsal hump, so the upper lateral cartilages were adequate for folding; (2) her middle vault was narrow, so the autospreader graft would widen the middle vault to a greater extent than a spreader graft (Fig. 6.36).

First, the upper lateral cartilages were separated from the septum (Fig. 6.37). Then incremental reduction of the septum and incremental dorsal reduction were performed (Fig. 6.38).

Different suture techniques are available. One mattress suture would be sufficient to fix the bilateral autospreader graft to the septum. Each upper lateral crus may be fixed to the septum, either separately or together (Fig. 6.39).

At the end of the procedure, a satisfactory dorsal view was achieved via middle vault reconstruction (Fig. 6.40).

One-year postoperative surgical outcomes are shown in Fig. 6.41.

6.2.7.2 Case 13

Figure 6.42 shows another case with a high dorsum and narrow middle vault in which an autospreader graft was suitable. In this case, the upper lateral cartilages were separately fixed to the septum (Fig. 6.43). Middle vault reconstruction was performed using bilateral autospreader grafts, and ideal brow-tip aesthetic line was achieved (Fig. 6.44).

6.2.7.3 Case 14

Another case with a narrow middle vault reconstructed with bilateral autospreader grafts (Fig. 6.45).

The caudal part of the autospreader graft occasionally pushes the cephalic border of the lower lateral cartilage, causing bulbosity. This should be kept in mind when performing autospreader grafting. If this is noticed intraoperatively, the medial-caudal part of the autospreader graft must be excised.

6.2.7.4 Case 15

Intraoperative photographs demonstrate resection of the caudal part of autospreader graft (Fig. 6.46). Long-term results of the case described here are shown in Fig. 6.47.

6.2.8 Unique Situations in Middle Vault Reconstruction

Where severe distortion mainly due to trauma is present, a spreader graft or spreader flap is not sufficient for constructing middle vaults. In severe middle vault distortion, dorsal deflection of the septum should be treated extracorporeally,

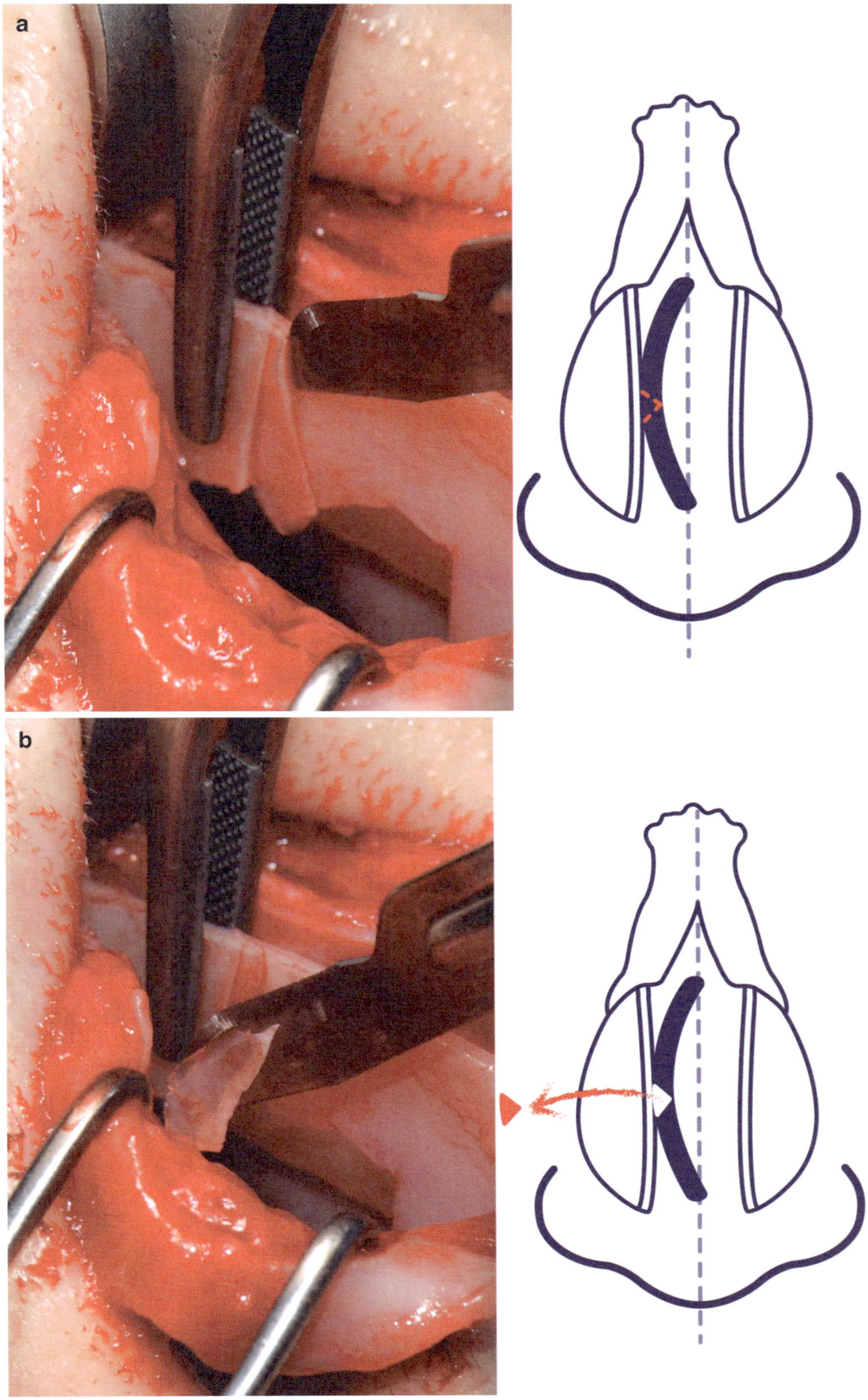

Fig. 6.20 (**a**–**e**) Inverted triangles are removed from the most convex portion of the septum. Then, bilateral spreader grafts are sutured both sides of the septum to reconstruct the middle vault

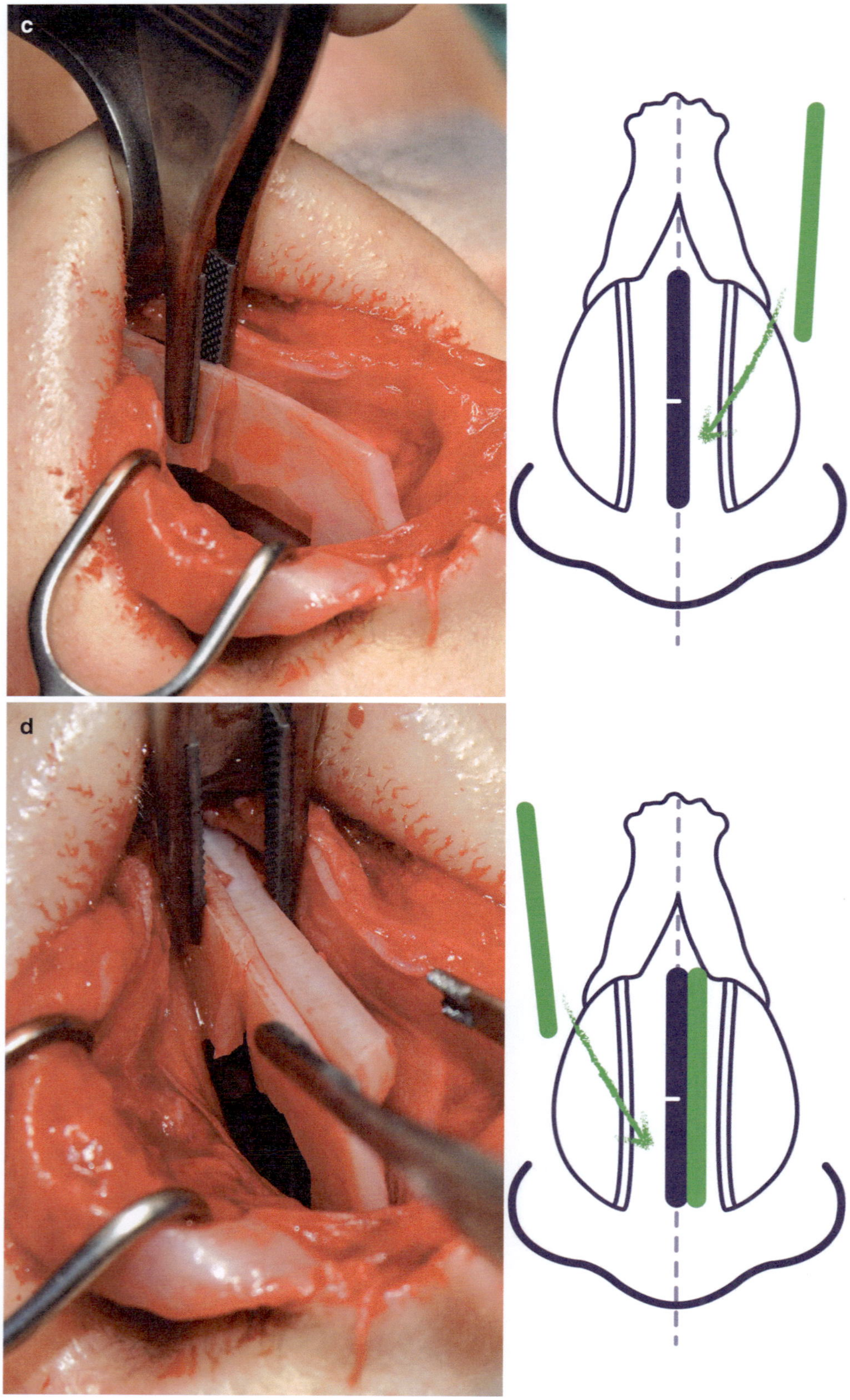

Fig. 6.20 (continued)

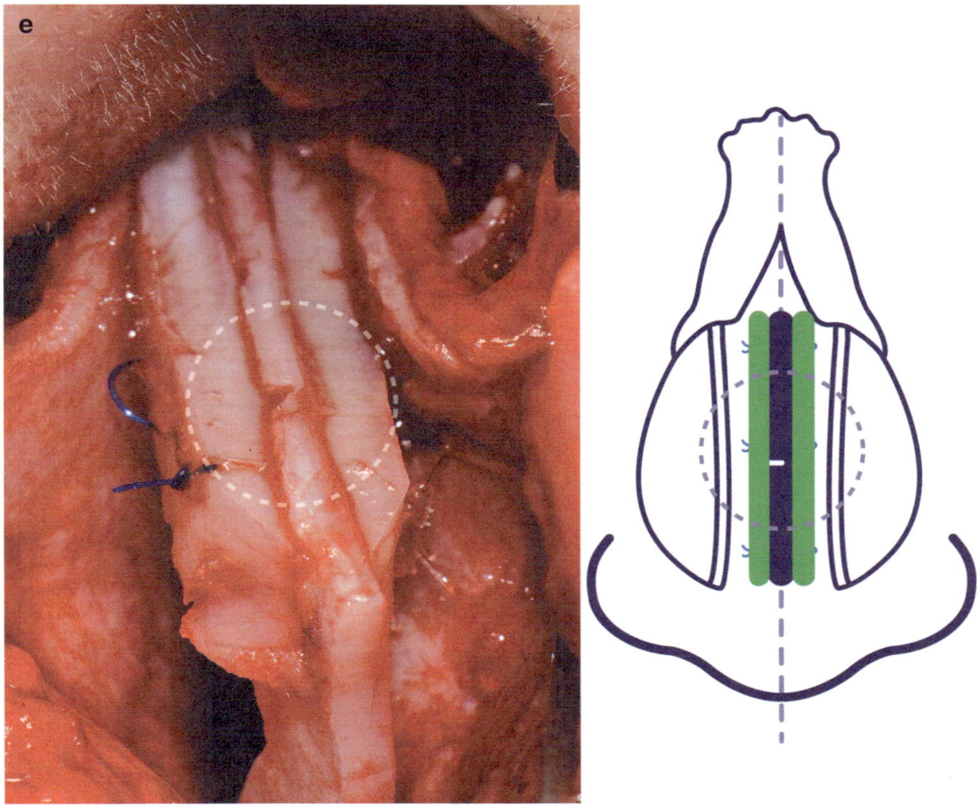

Fig. 6.20 (continued)

which is also called subtotal septal reconstruction. This technique is preferred in cases that cannot be treated using less invasive methods.

With this technique, the entire septum is resected, except a remnant of 1–1.5 cm of the dorsal septum. Septal replacement is prepared from the excised part. Then, a straight septal replacement graft is placed and sutured between the nasal spine and the dorsal remnant part (Fig. 6.48).

6.2.8.1 Case 16

An example of severe septal deviation caused by trauma is shown in Fig. 6.49. The surgical steps for subtotal septal reconstruction are shown in Fig. 6.50. Three-year postoperative results are seen in Fig. 6.51. The middle vault was reconstructed successfully.

6.2.8.2 Case 17

Figure 6.52 shows another case with severe septal deviation caused by childhood trauma.

The intraoperative surgical steps are outlined in Fig. 6.53. Figure 6.54 shows the surgical outcome; the septum was straight, stable, and symmetric.

6.2.8.3 Case 18

Preoperative and intraoperative photographs of another case show a distorted middle vault and severe septal deviation. Subtotal septal reconstruction was performed in this case. One year after surgery, an attractive middle vault was achieved (Fig. 6.55).

6.2.8.4 Case 19

Subtotal septal reconstruction was performed in this case. Five years after surgery, the middle vault reconstruction was still stable, strong, and well balanced in relation to the rest of the nose. The long-term results of this technique were satisfactory (Fig. 6.56).

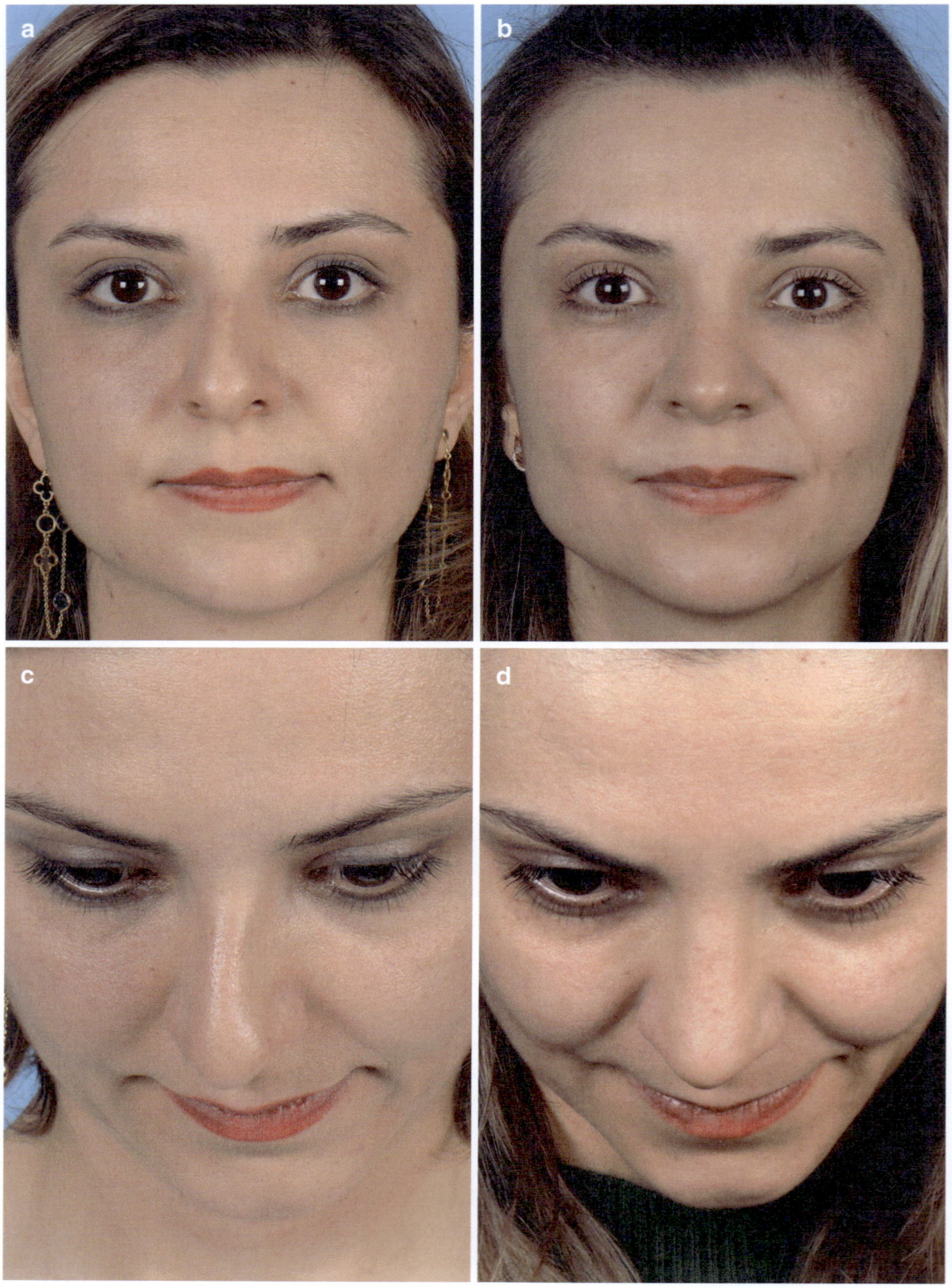

Fig. 6.21 (**a–d**) Preoperative and 1-year postoperative photographs. An ideal brow-tip aesthetic line is achieved after surgery

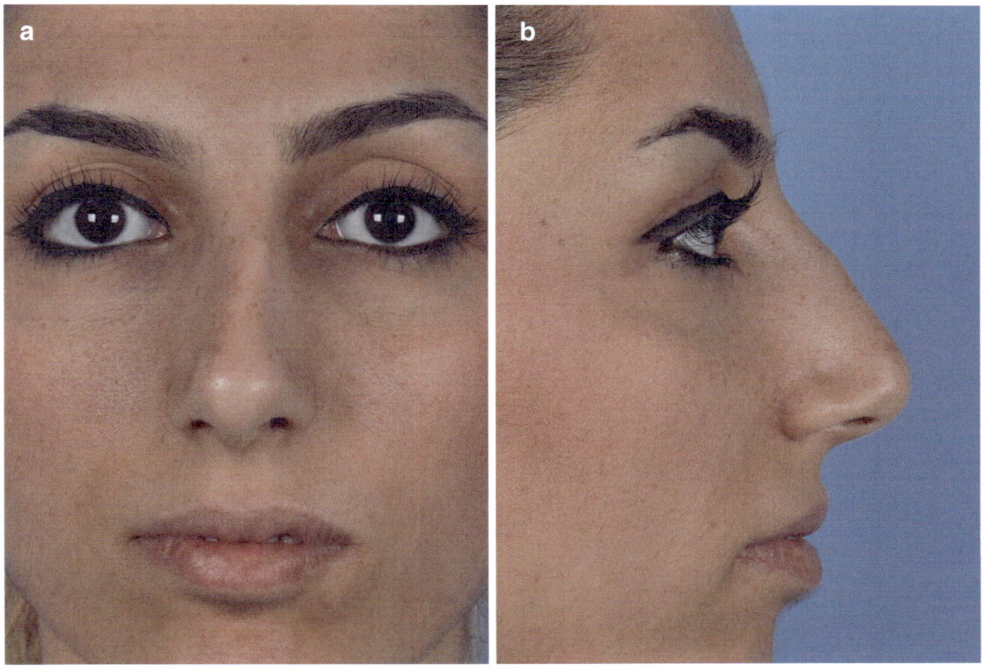

Fig. 6.22 (**a**, **b**) The nose is deviated to the left with angulation at the rhinion. There is a mild dorsal hump

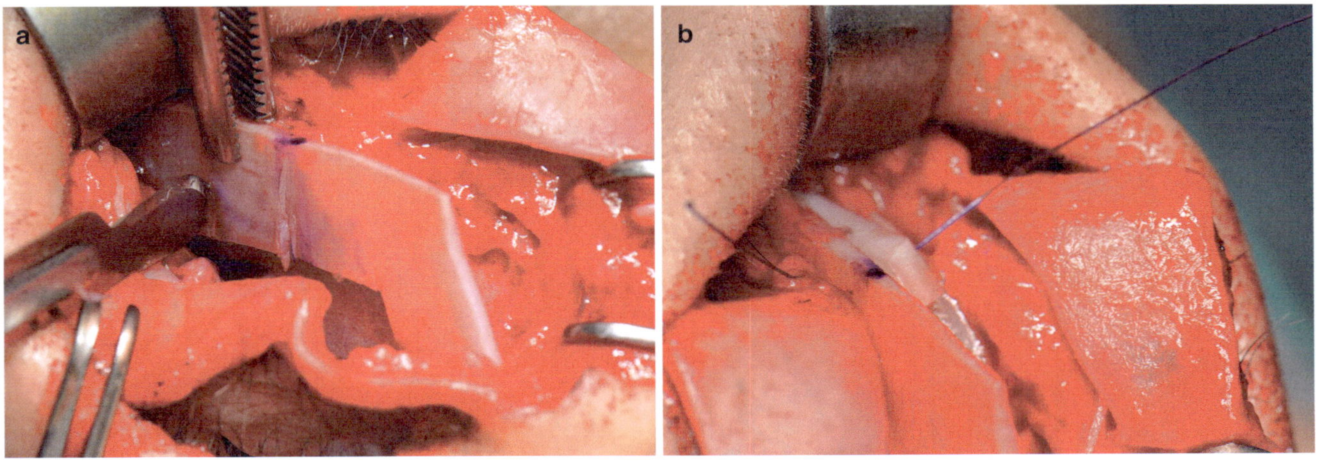

Fig. 6.23 (**a**, **b**) Before spreader graft placement a triangular piece of cartilage was removed from the concave side of the septum

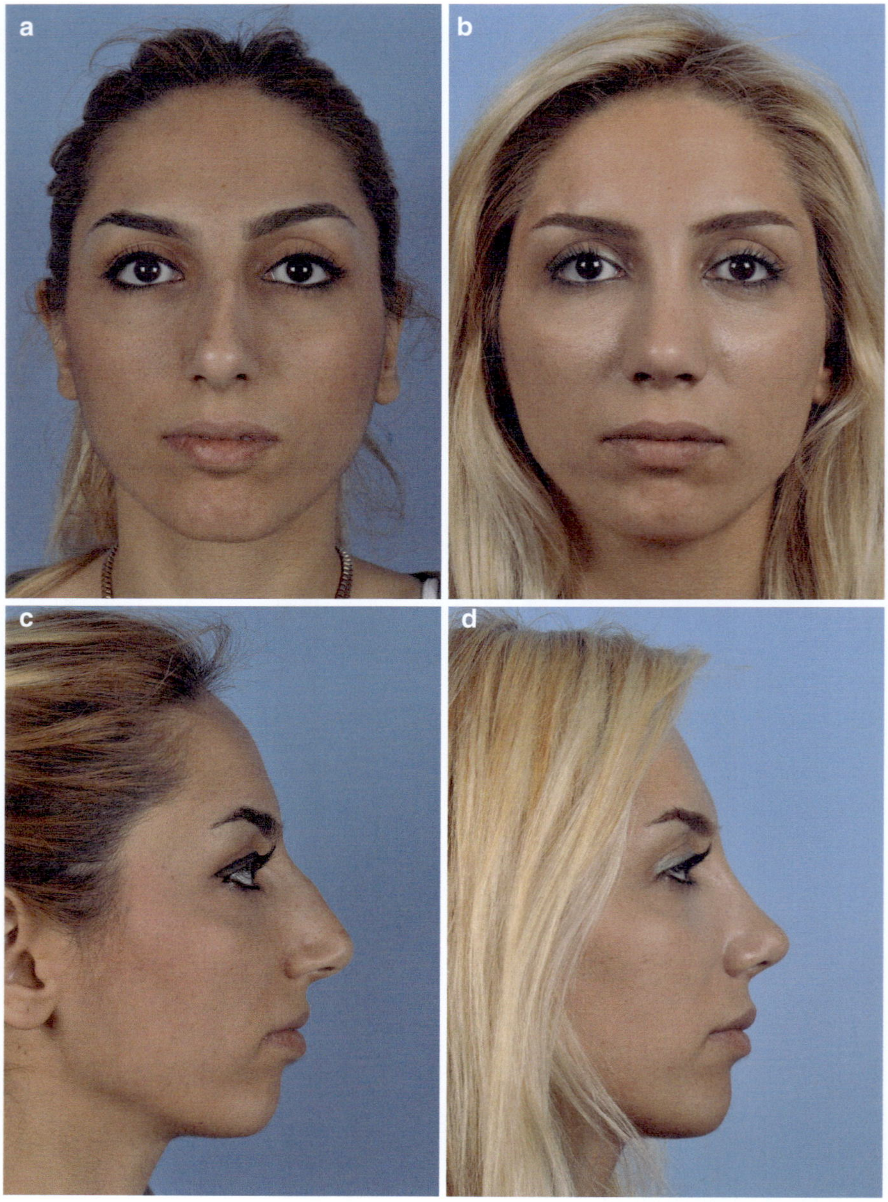

Fig. 6.24 (**a**–**d**) The middle vault was reconstructed with spreader graft. The nose is straighter and the hump has been removed

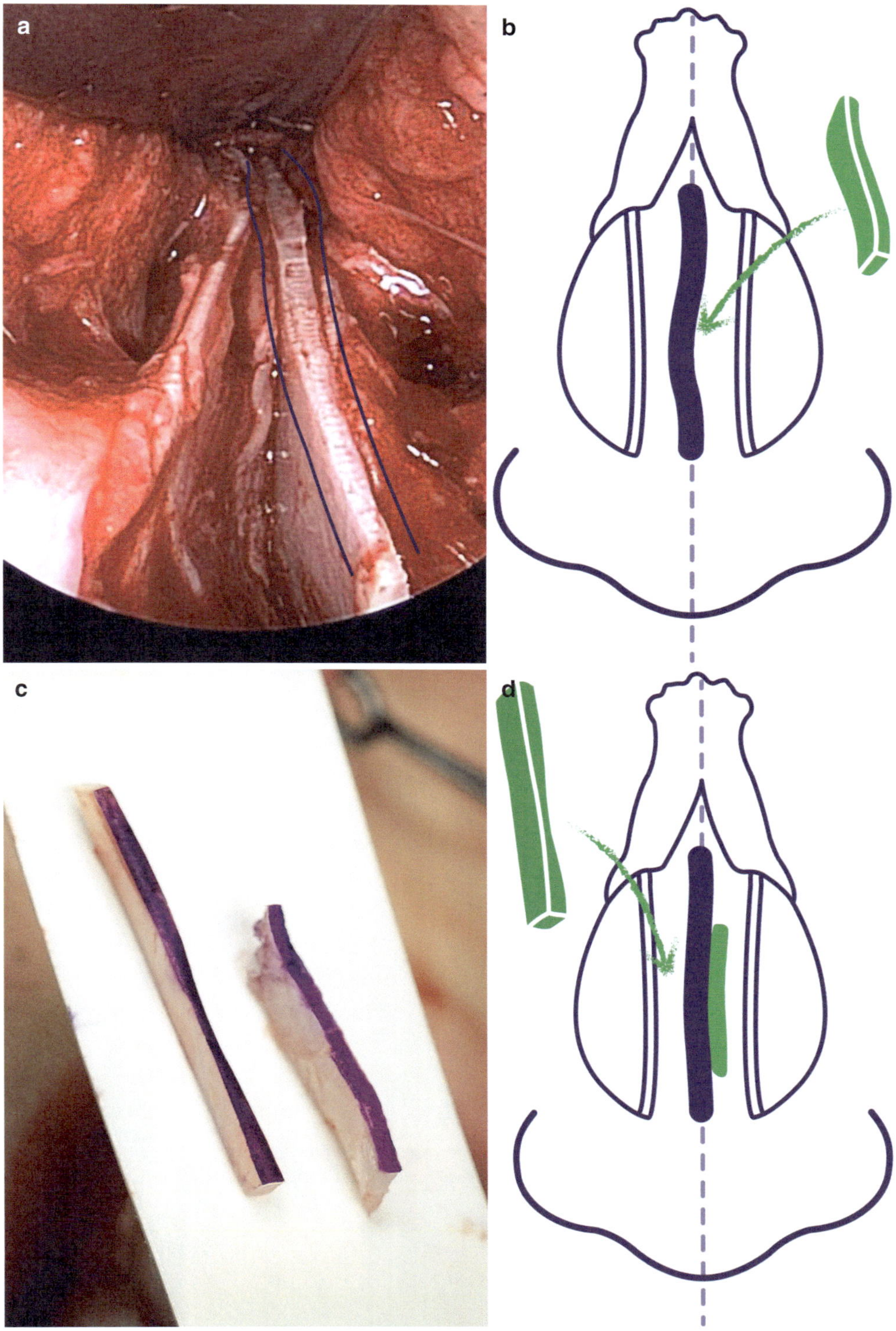

Fig. 6.25 (**a**–**f**) Due to the asymmetrical pathology in this case, the spreader graft was prepared to be thick at the right side cephalically, thin at the bend of the "S," and thick again caudally. Balance was achieved by placing one short, thick spreader at the left side. A symmetrical middle vault appearance was achieved after the grafts were sutured

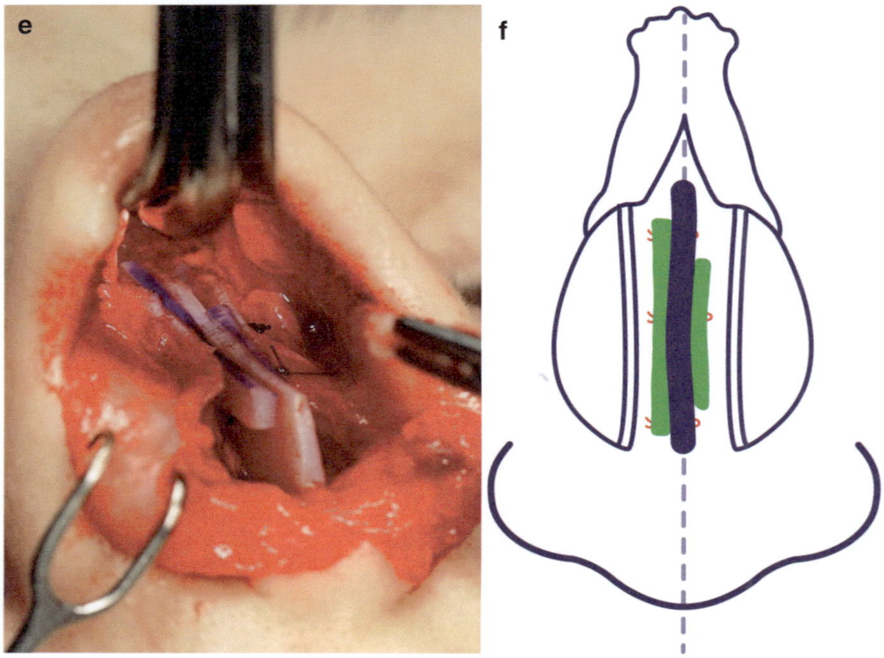

Fig. 6.25 (continued)

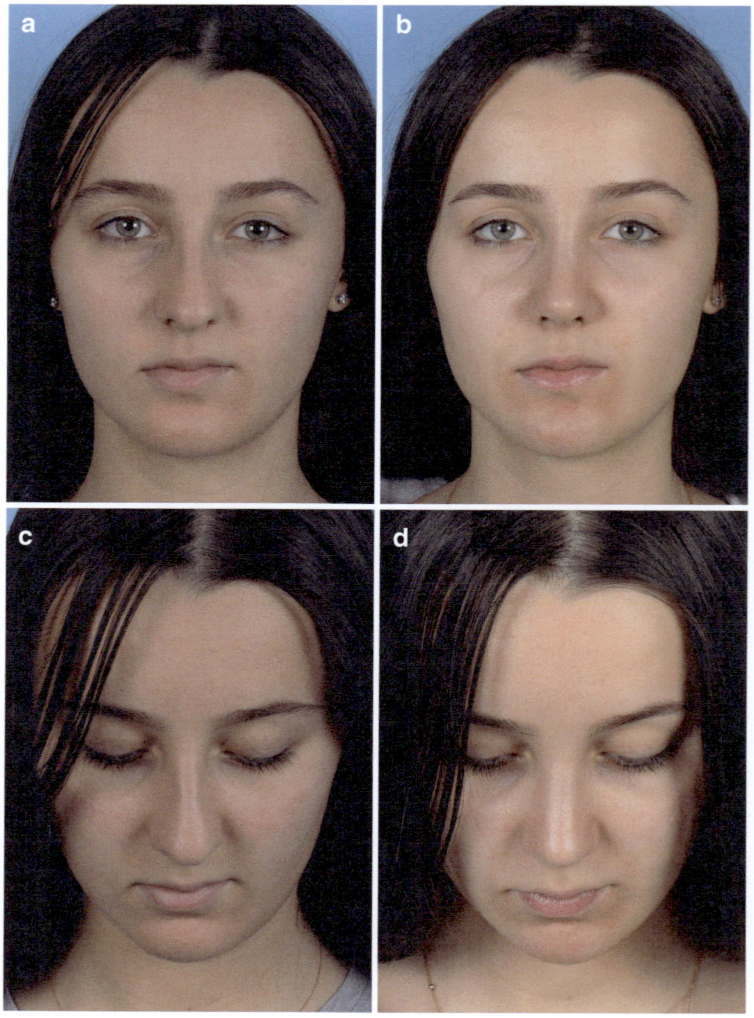

Fig. 6.26 (**a–d**) The middle vault is symmetrical and stable. Eyebrow tip aesthetic line is improved

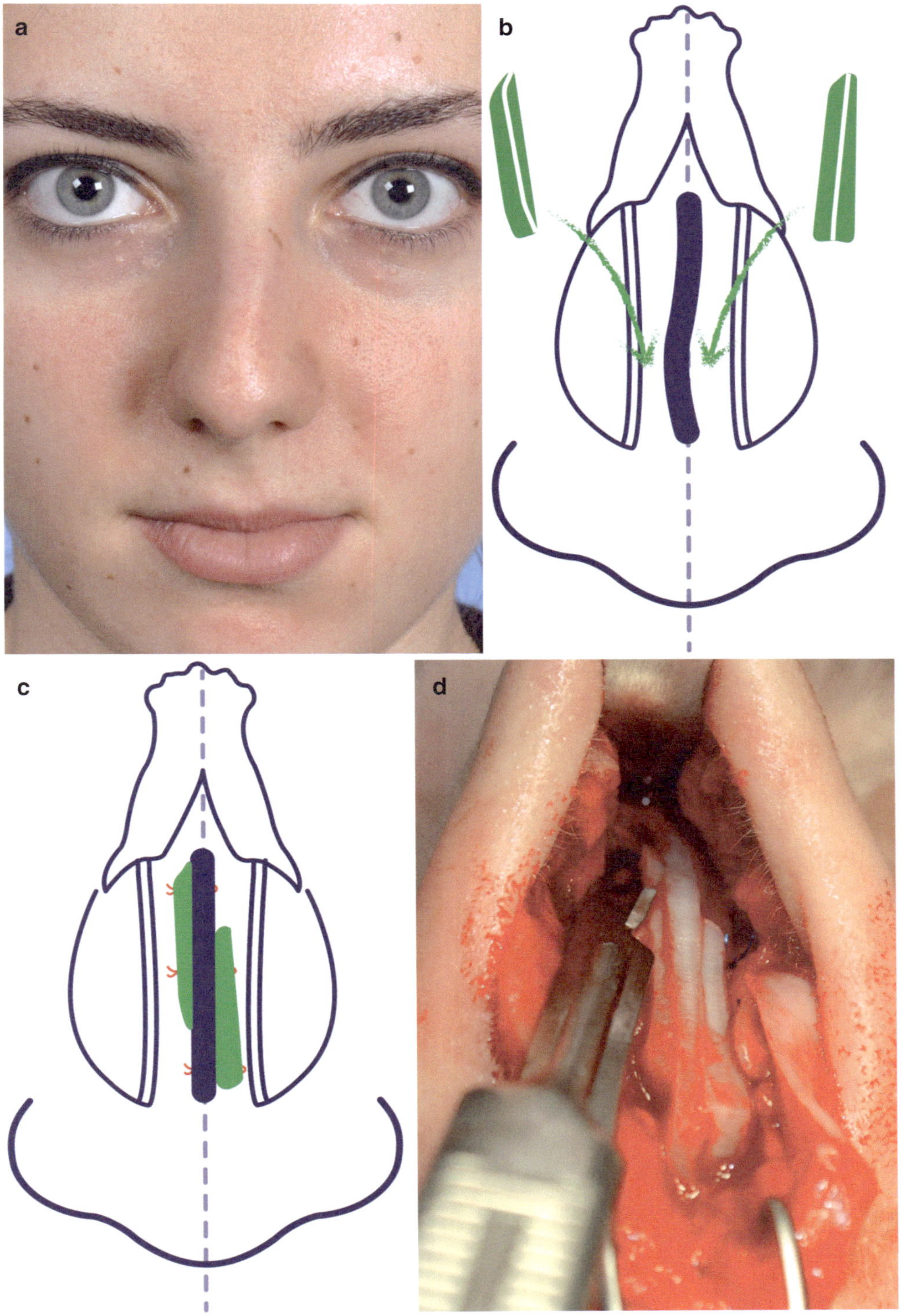

Fig. 6.27 (**a–d**) Bilateral asymmetrical grafts were fixed to the septum and formed a straight septum and middle vault

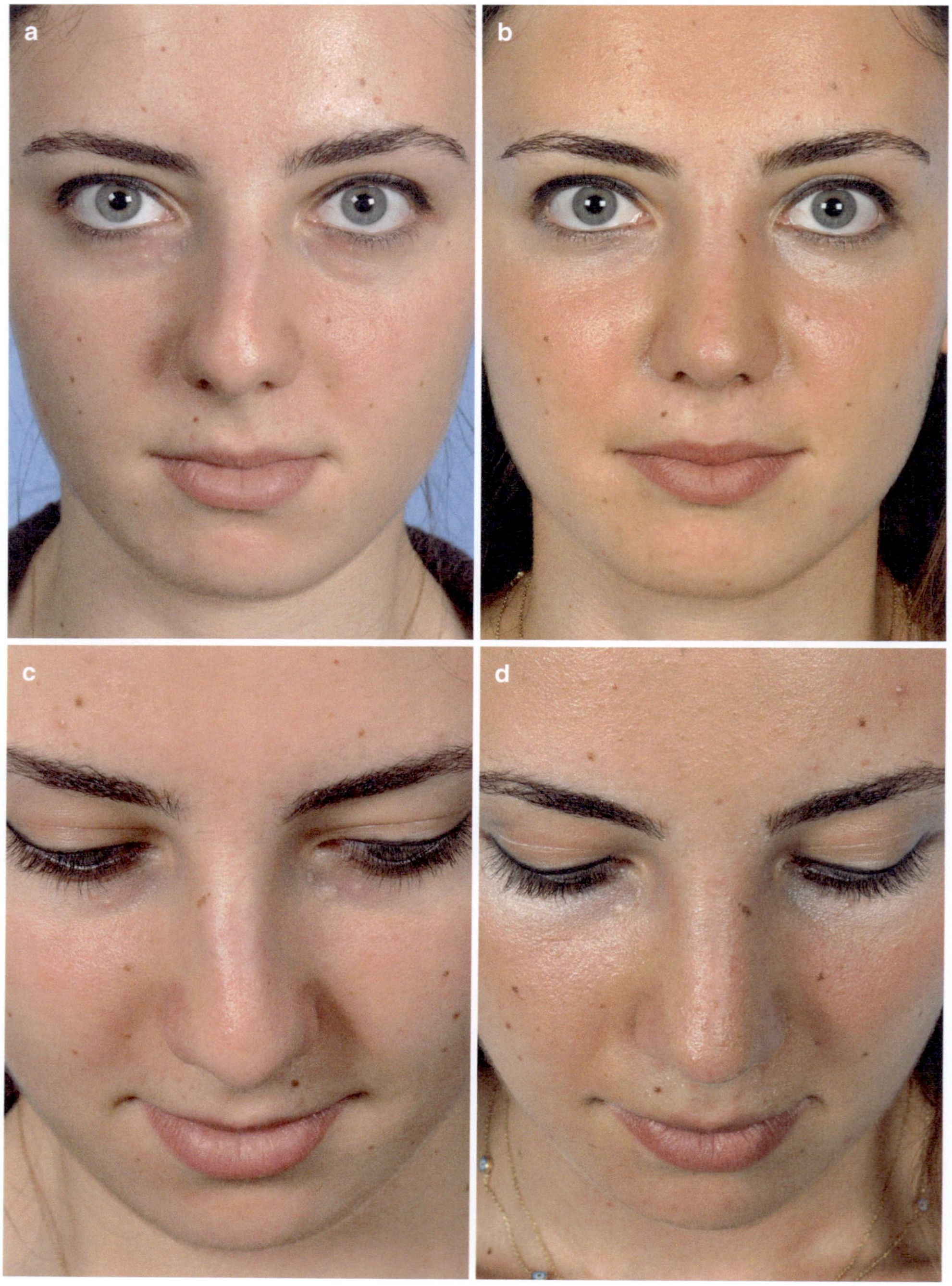

Fig. 6.28 (**a**–**d**) The dorsal hump has been eliminated. The middle vault is more stable and symmetric

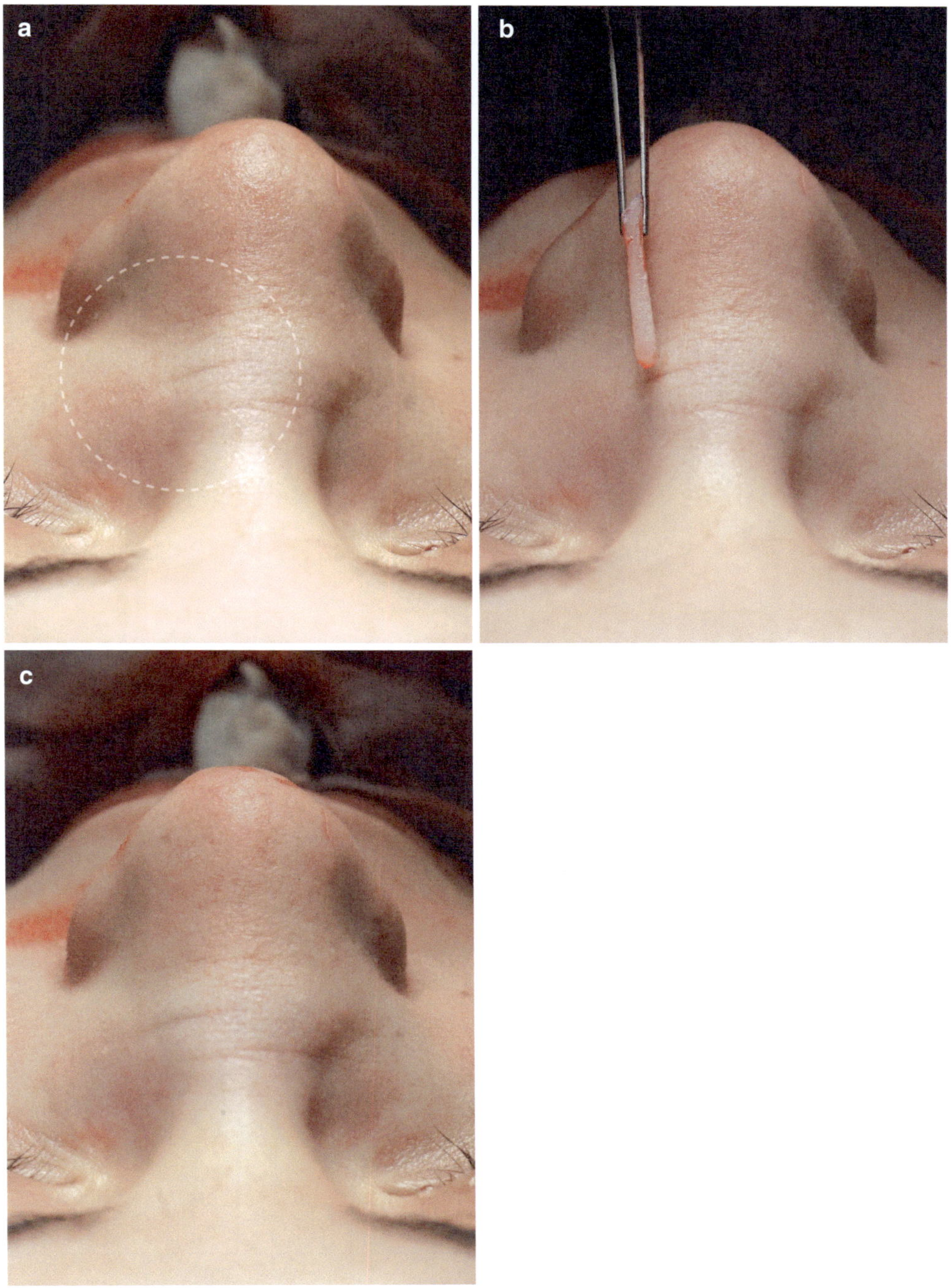

Fig. 6.29 (**a**) Collapsed lateral nasal wall after osteotomy. (**b**) Spreader grafts placed externally. (**c**) The problem was resolved intraoperatively

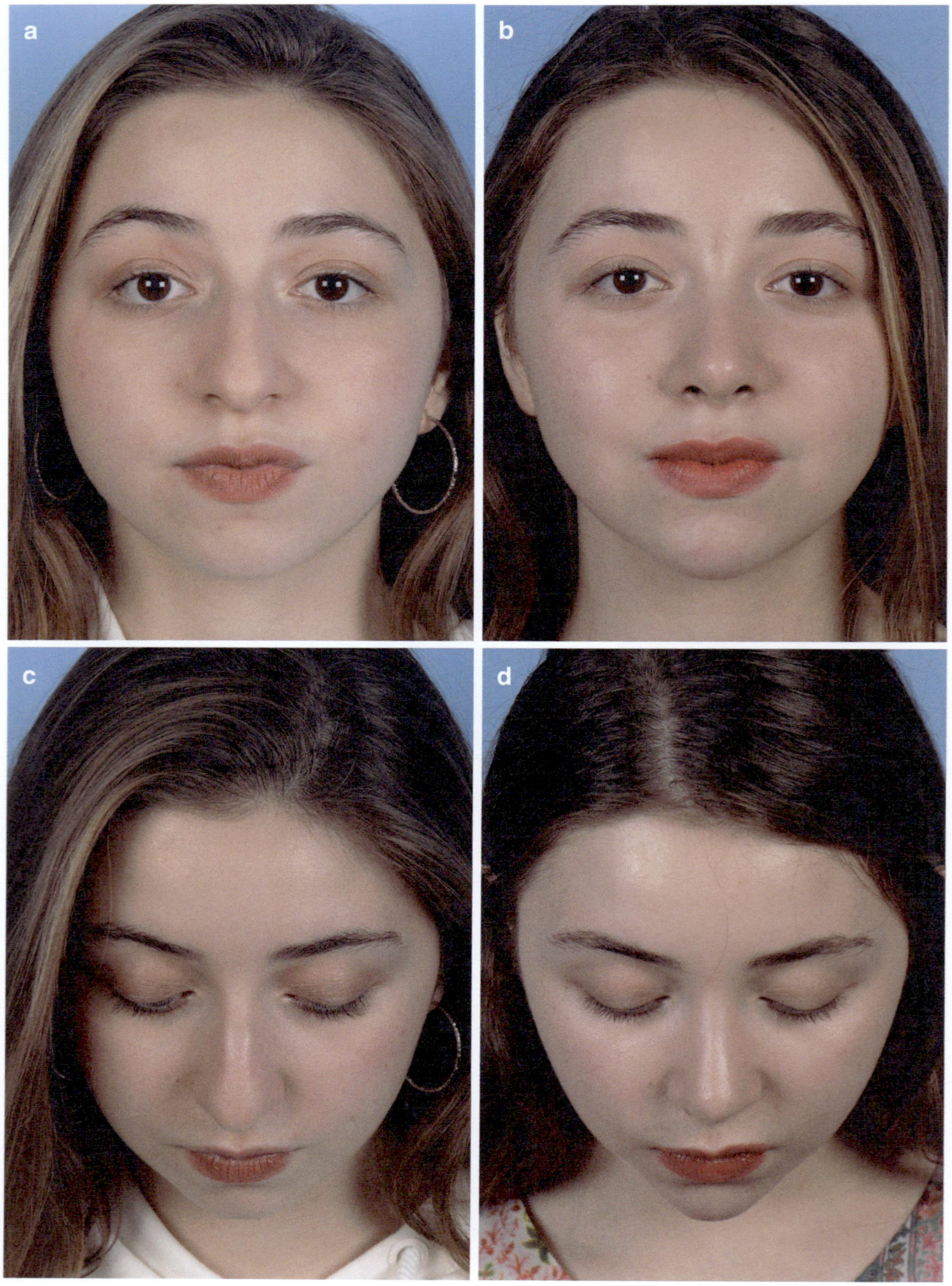

Fig. 6.30 (**a**–**d**) Left nasal bone is still intact due to the spreader effect

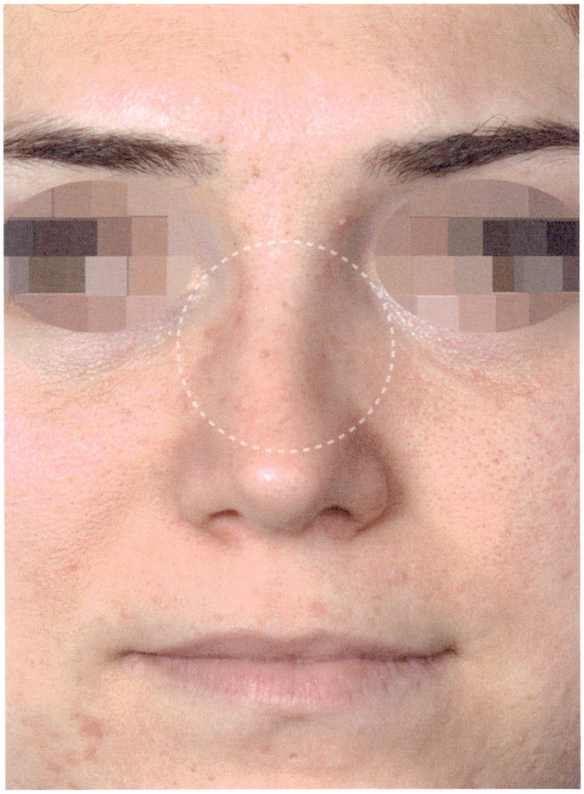

Fig. 6.31 The left nasal wall collapsed due to complications of osteotomy

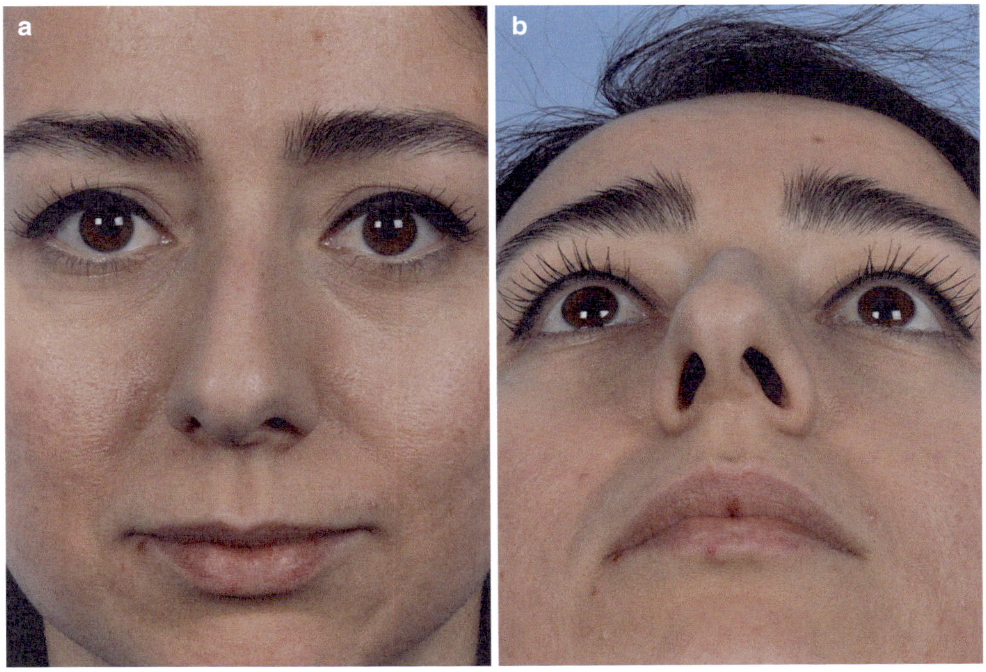

Fig. 6.32 (**a**, **b**) The nose is deviated due to caudal and dorsal septal deflection together

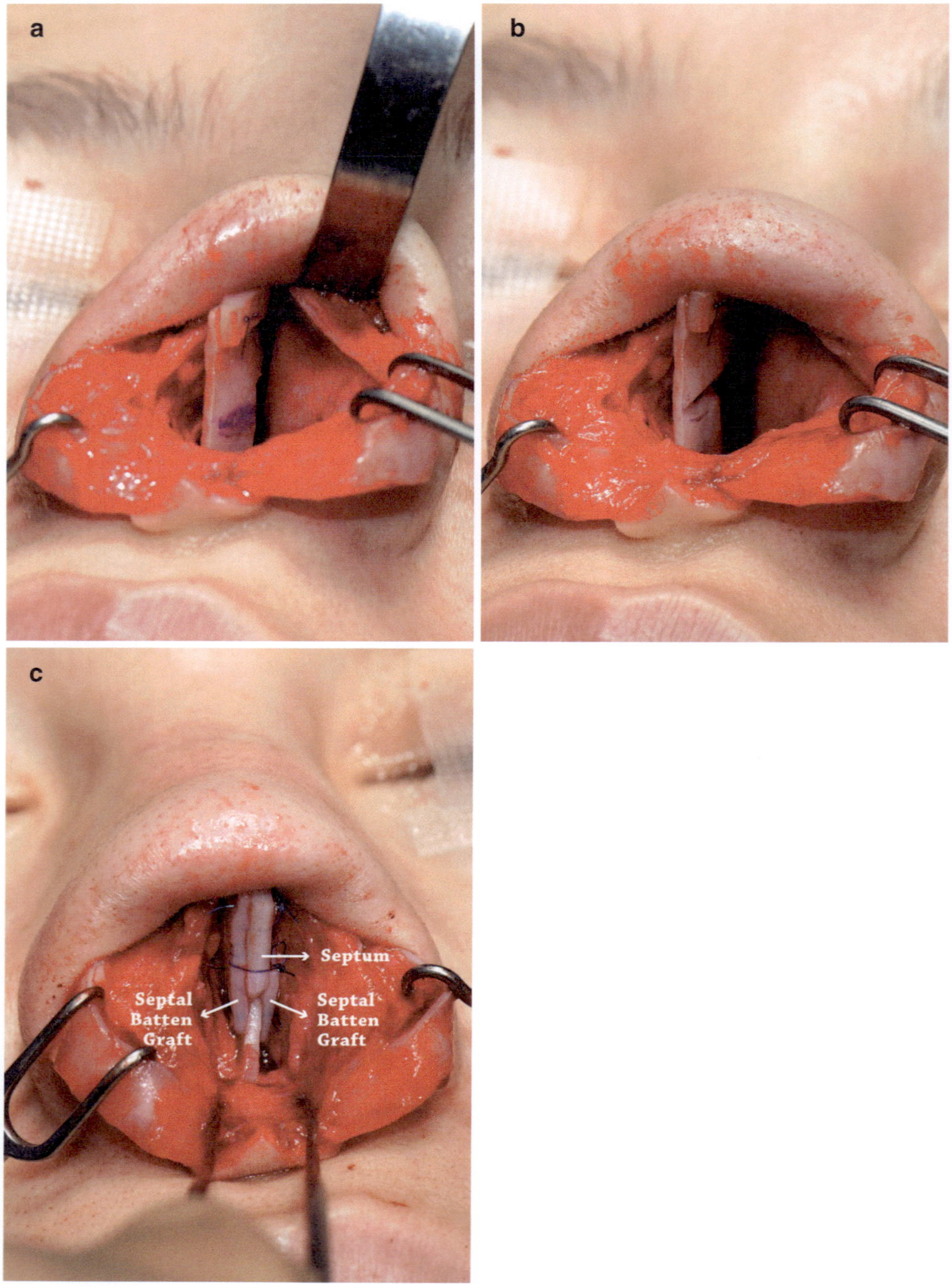

Fig. 6.33 (**a–c**) Single spreader graft sutured to the dorsal septum. Triangular-shaped trimming was done on the convex side of the caudal septum. Placement of bilateral septal batten grafts sutured to the caudal septum

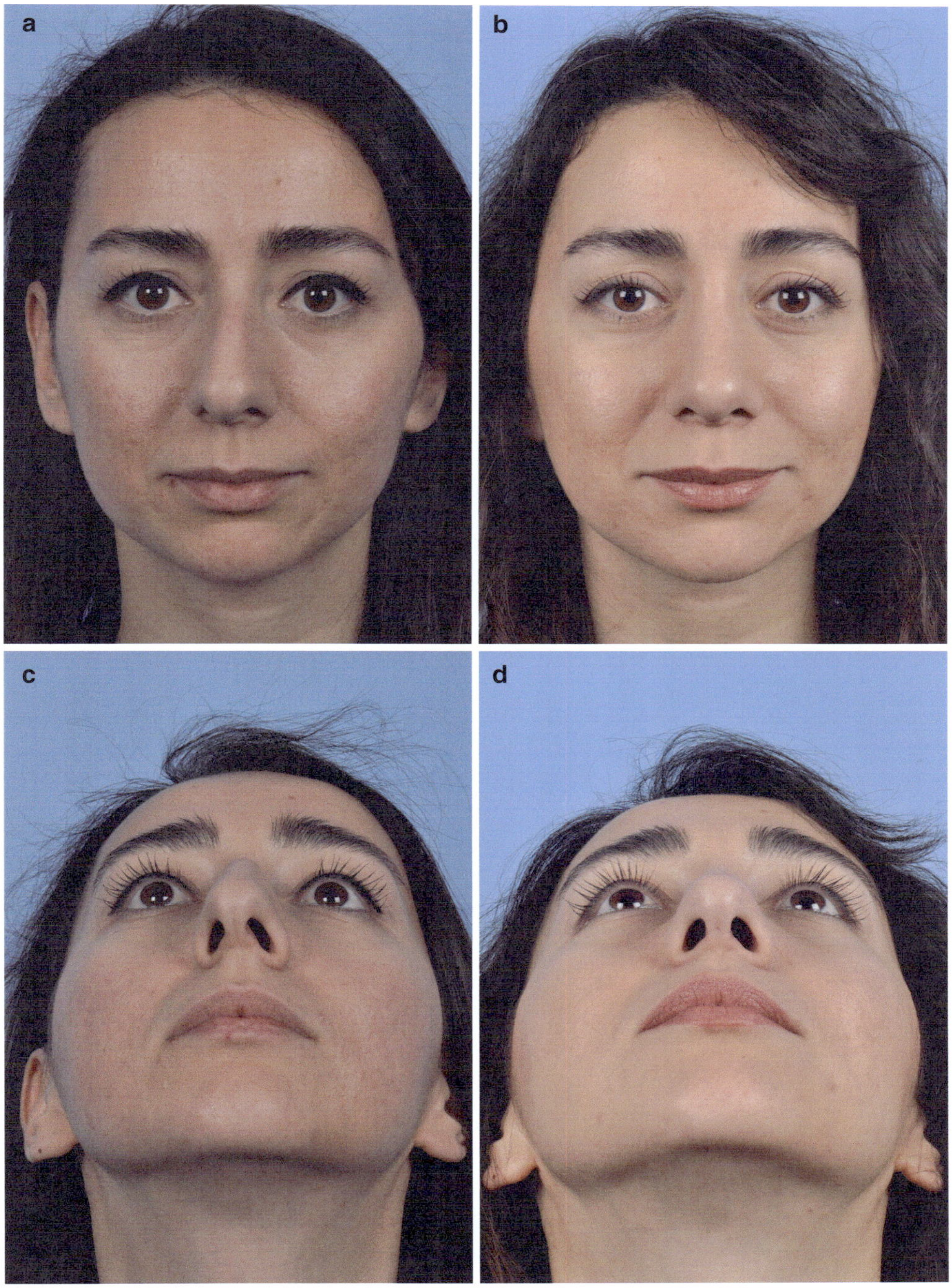

Fig. 6.34 (**a**–**h**) The middle vault and caudal septum were reconstructed simultaneously. The nose is in a more centralized position of the face

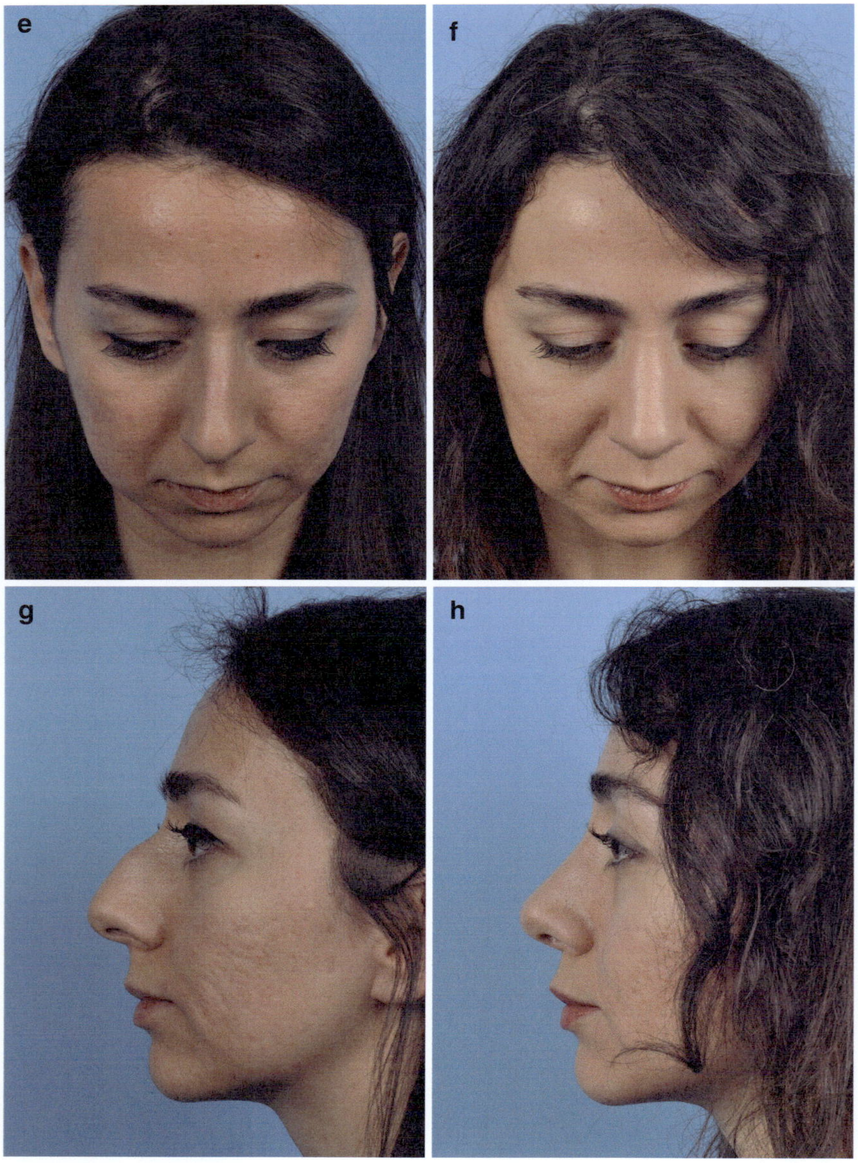

Fig. 6.34 (continued)

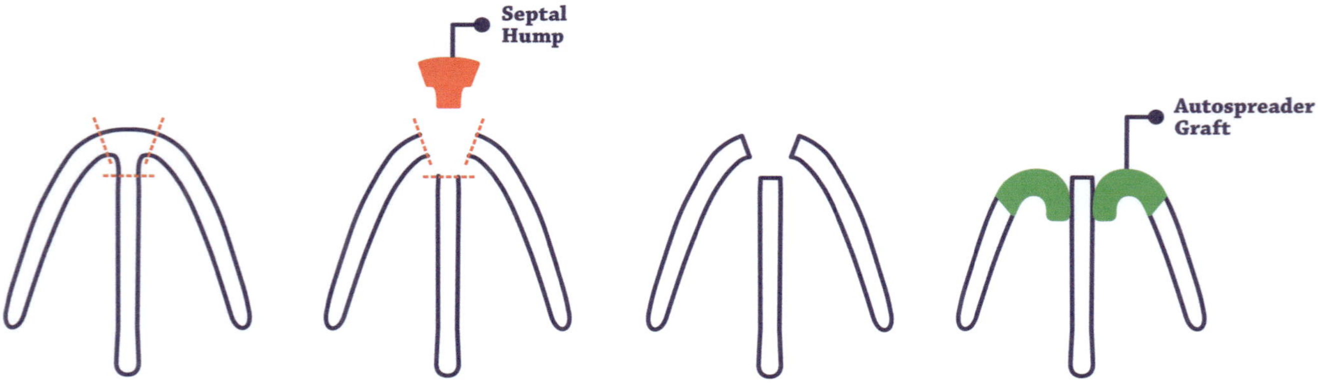

Fig. 6.35 Upper lateral cartilages are separated from septum, septal excess is removed, and then upper lateral cartilages are folded inward and sutured

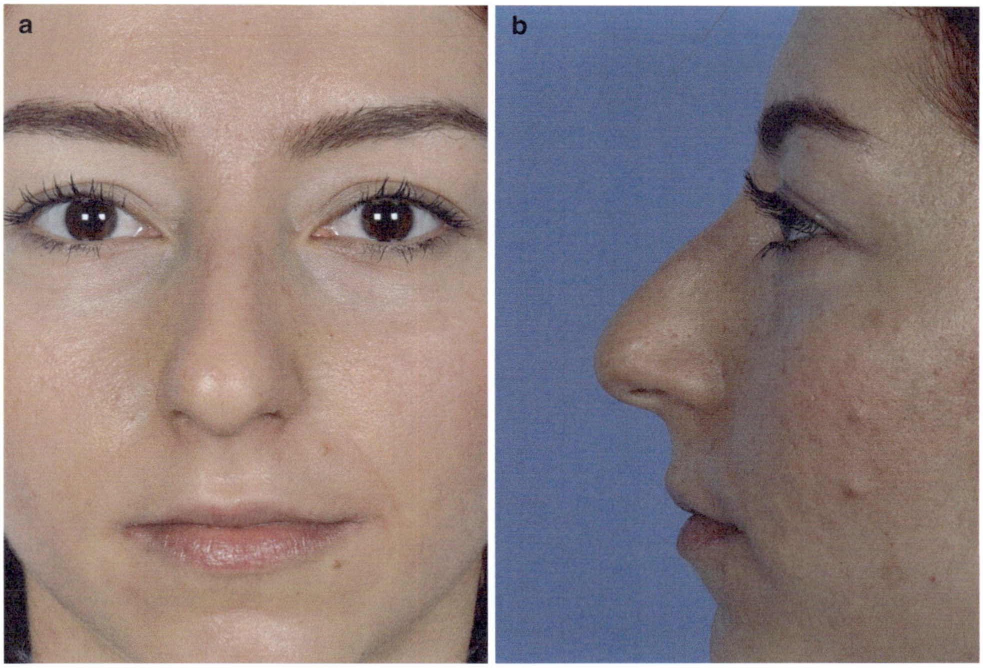

Fig. 6.36 (**a**, **b**) A prominent dorsal hump. The middle vault is too narrow. The ideal candidate for spreader flap

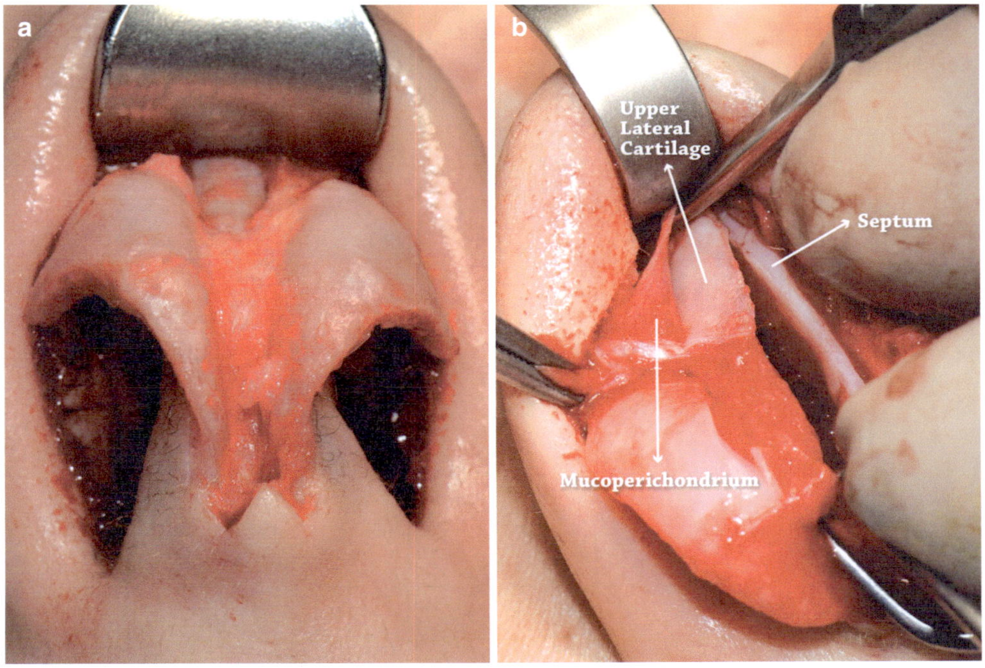

Fig. 6.37 (**a**, **b**) Separation can be performed efficiently using a straight scissor. The mucoperichondrium was peeled from the upper lateral cartilages

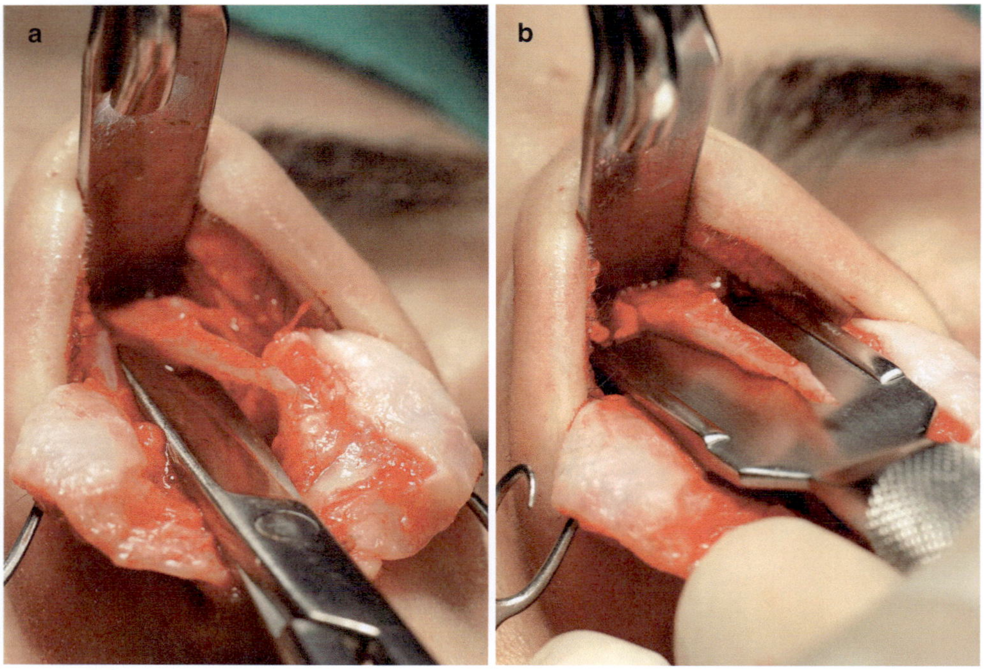

Fig. 6.38 (**a**, **b**) Removal of the septal hump

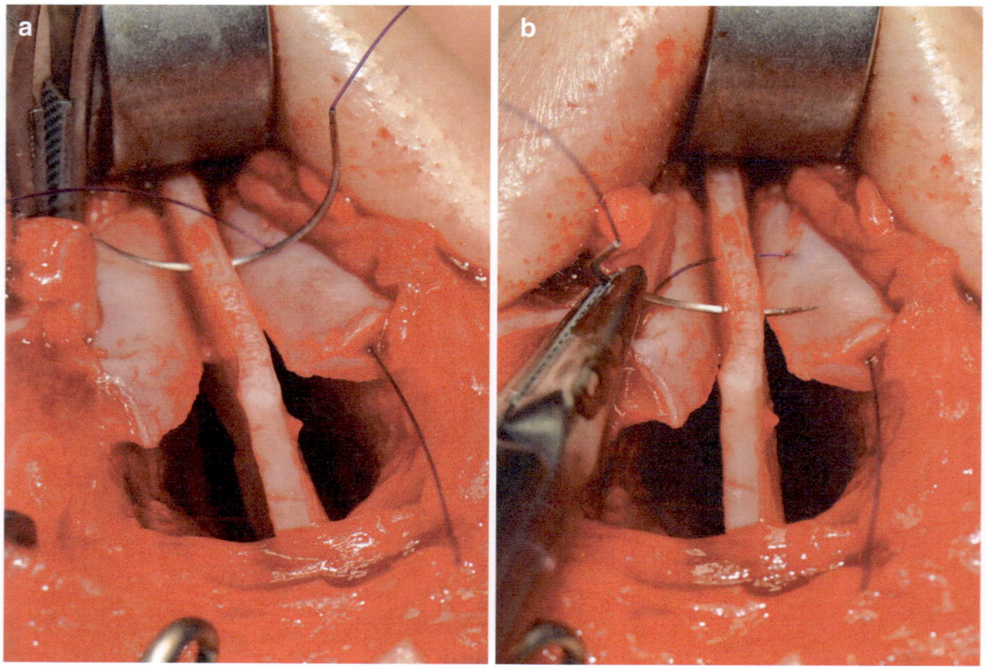

Fig. 6.39 (**a**, **b**) The upper lateral cartilages may fold inward spontaneously

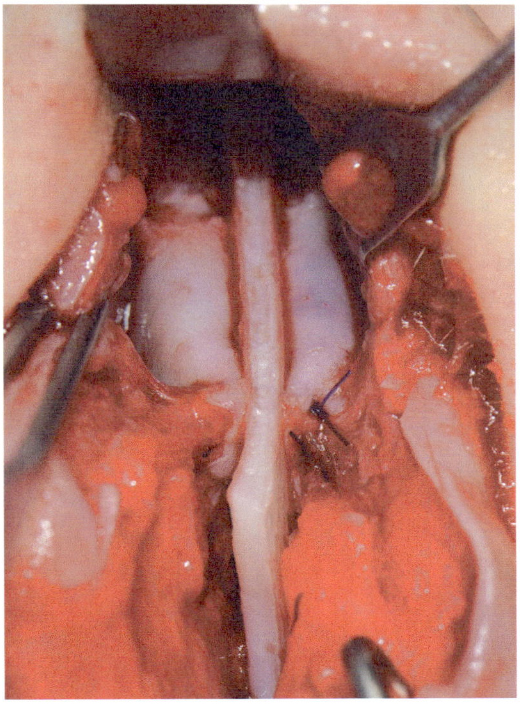

Fig. 6.40 The final intraoperative result should look similar to the anatomical middle vault

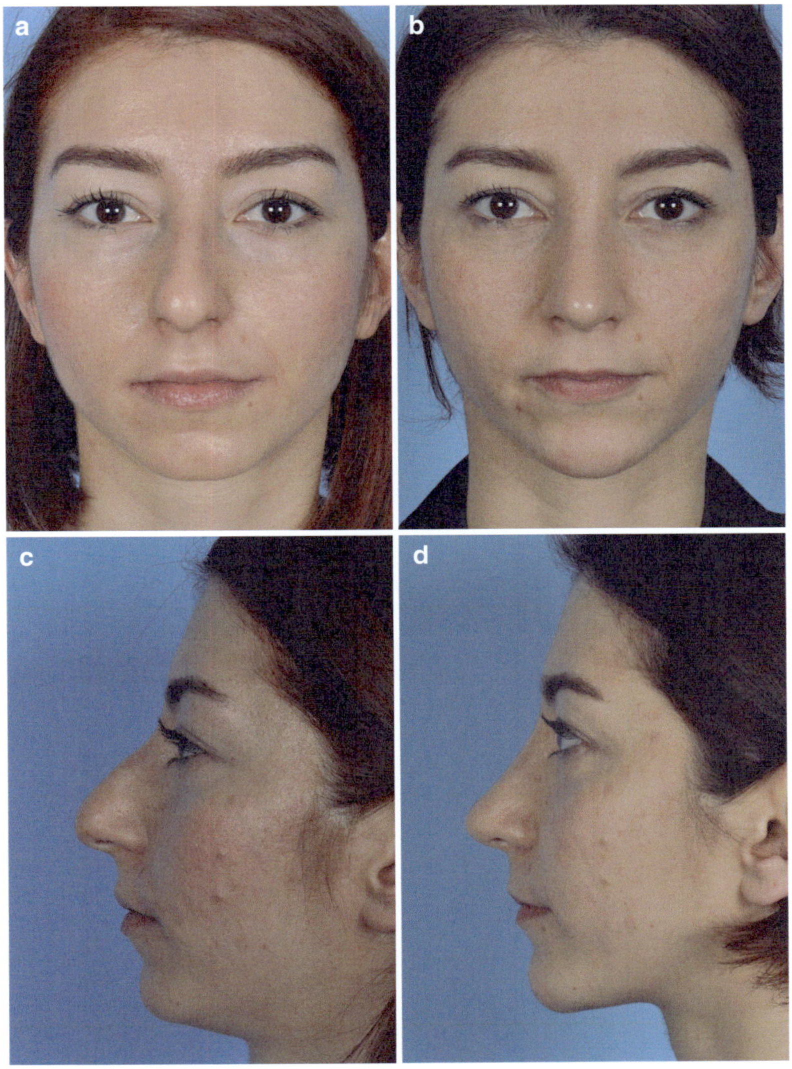

Fig. 6.41 (**a**–**f**) There is an aesthetically pleasing widening of the middle vault. The dorsal profile alignment is improved

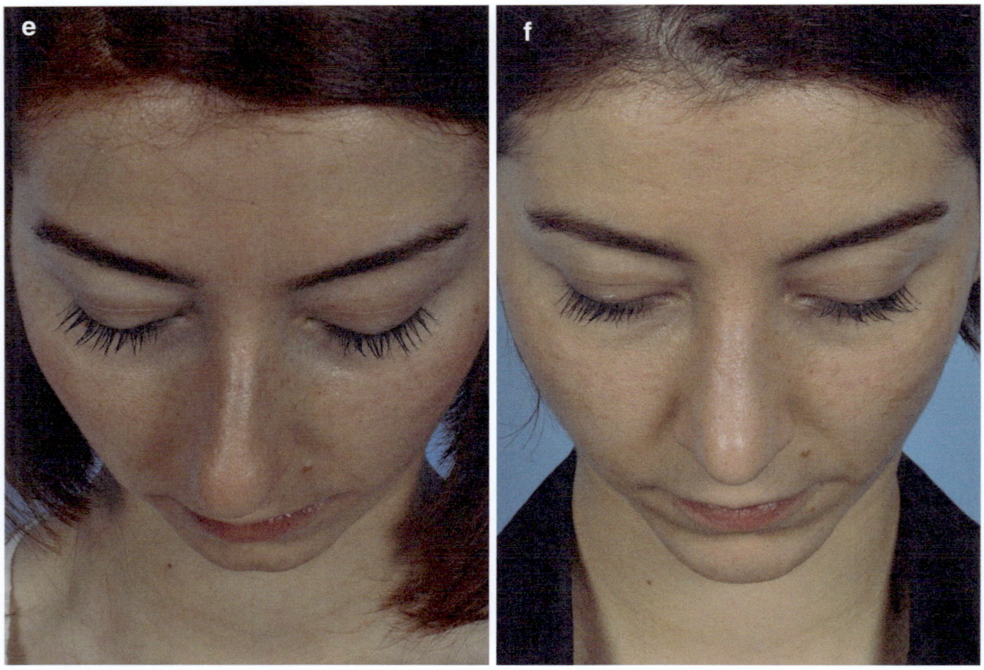

Fig. 6.41 (continued)

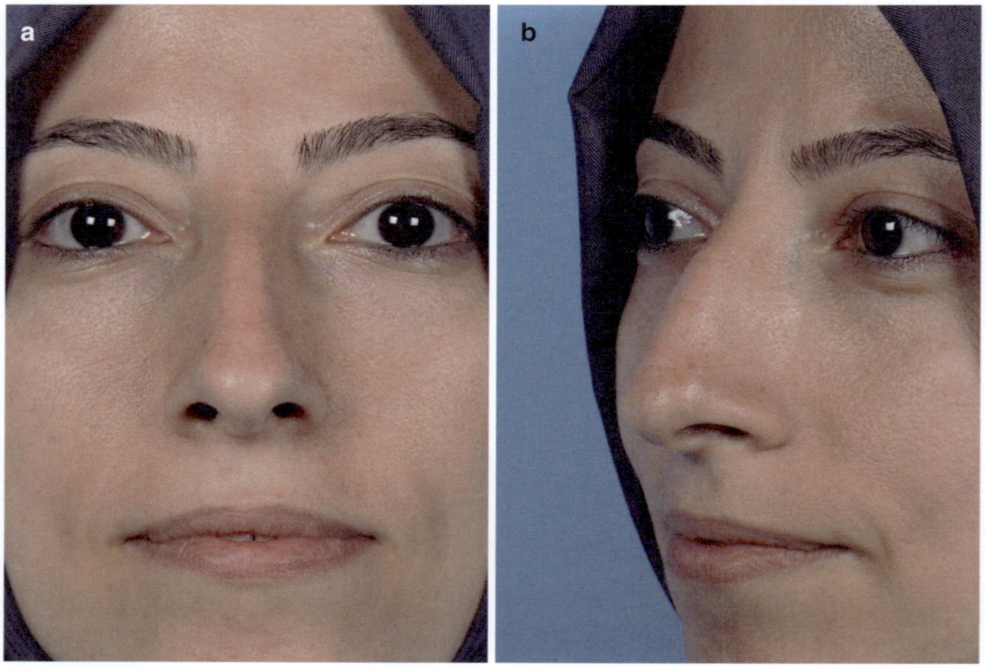

Fig. 6.42 (**a**, **b**) There is large dorsal hump and narrow middle vault

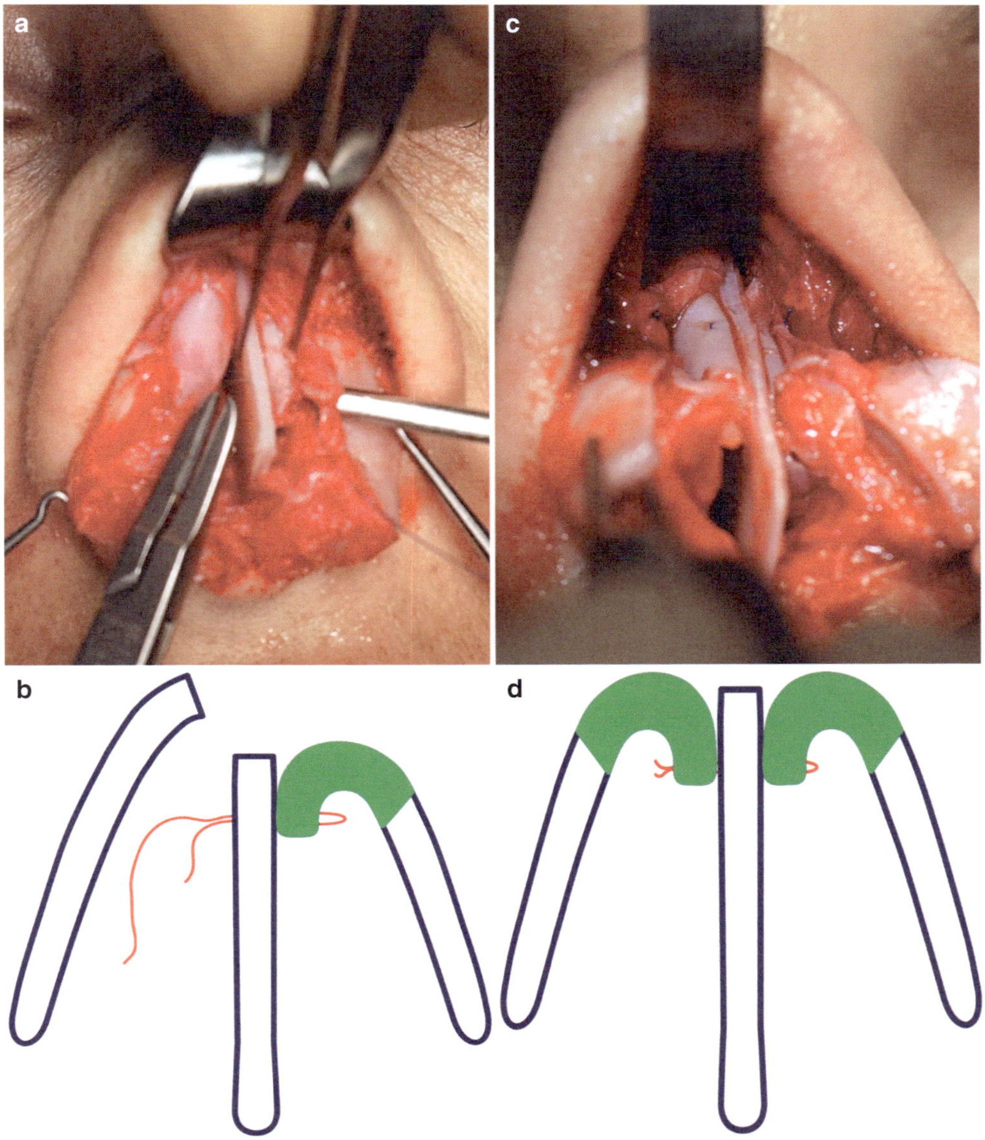

Fig. 6.43 (**a**, **b**) The left upper lateral cartilage was folded inward and fixed to one side of the septum intraoperatively, with the intention of reconstructing the middle vault based on the preoperative frontal view. (**c**) However, placement of the unilateral autospreader graft was not sufficient for middle vault reconstruction. Therefore, the other upper lateral cartilage was folded inward and fixed to the septum. (**d**) Each upper lateral cartilage was separately sutured to the septum

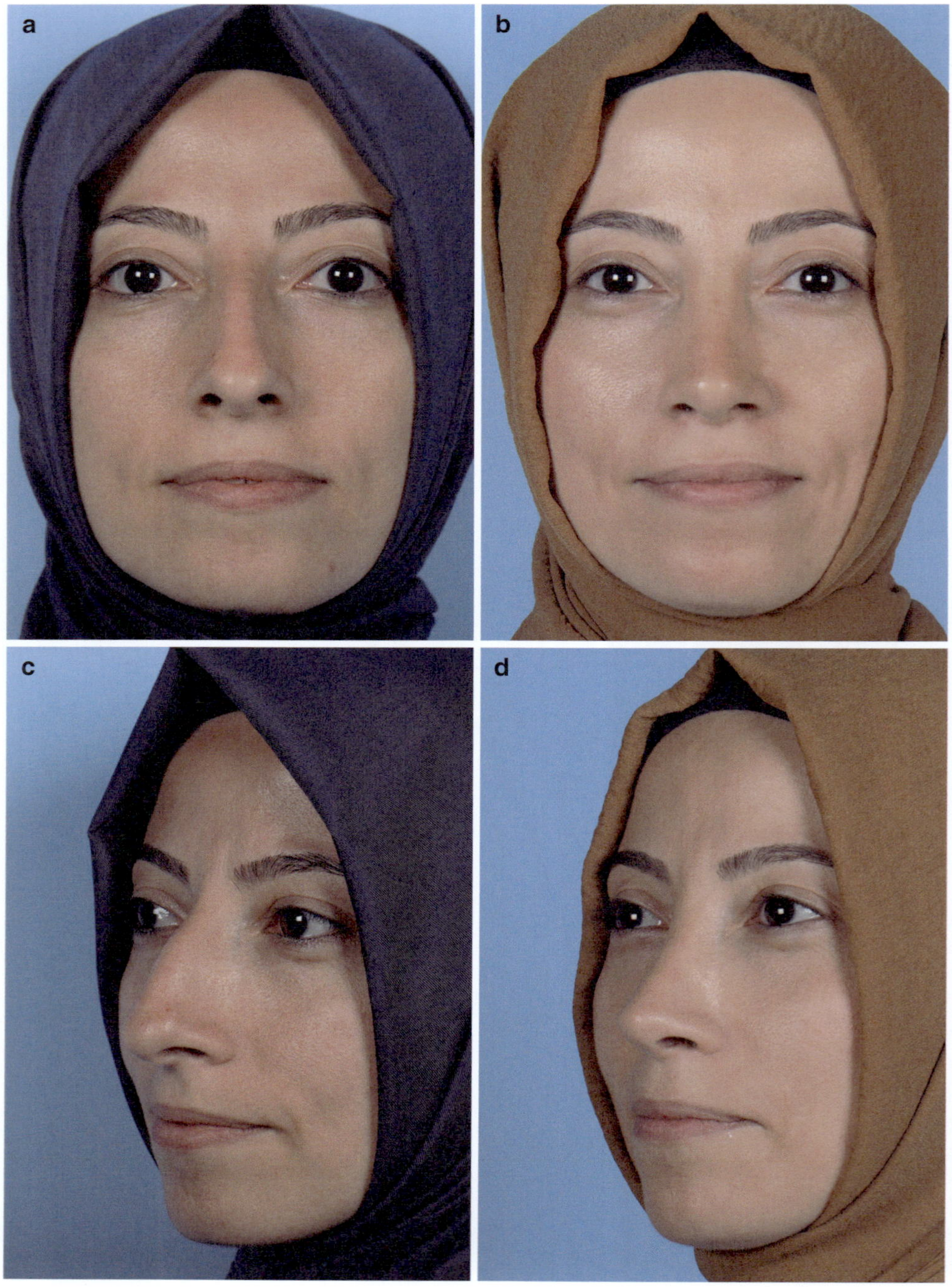

Fig. 6.44 (**a**–**d**) The sizeable dorsal hump has been reduced with a widened middle vault

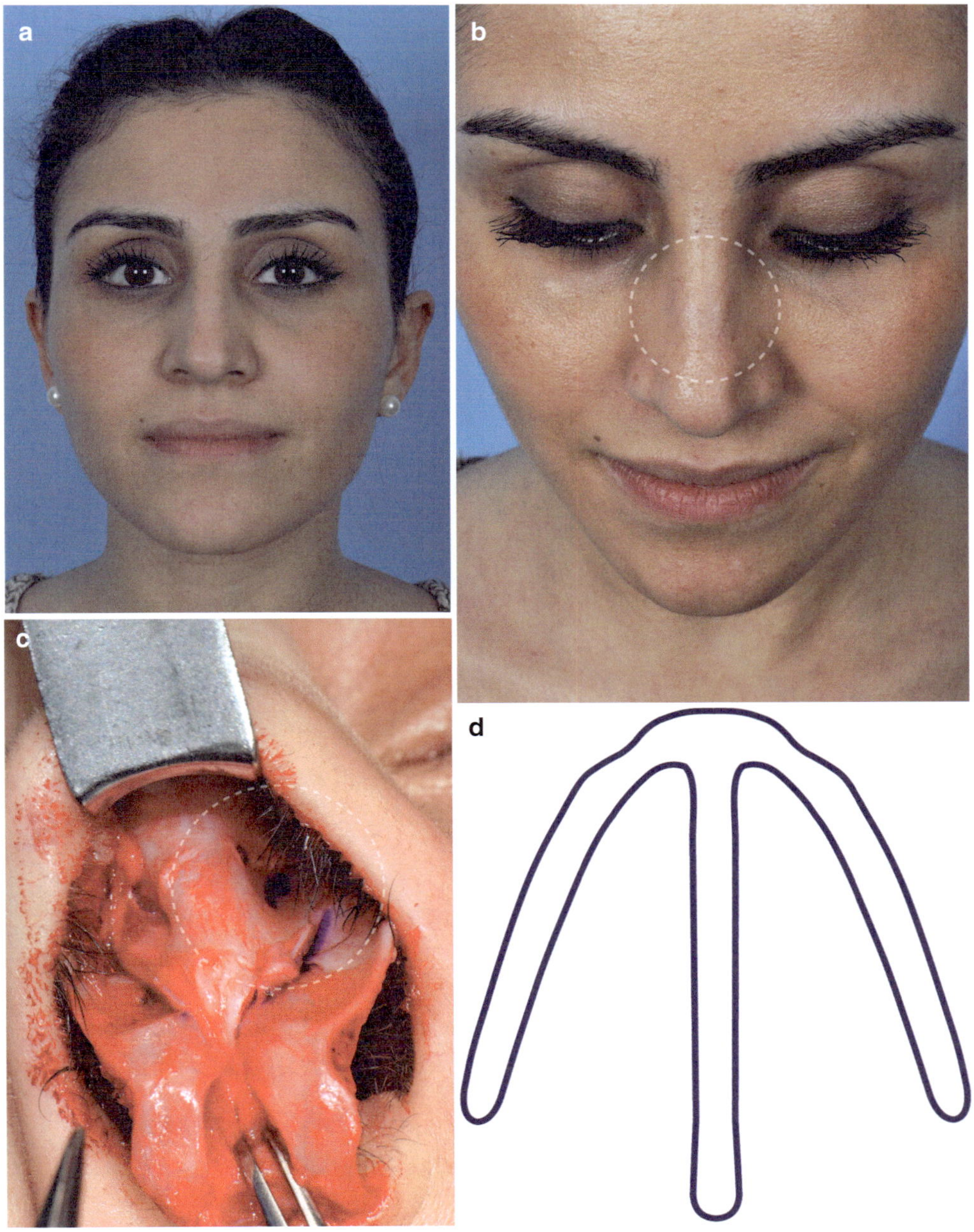

Fig. 6.45 (**a**–**d**) The dotted area shows concavity of the upper lateral cartilage, which caused a narrow middle vault. (**e**–**h**) Bilateral autospreader grafts eliminated the concavity of the middle vault

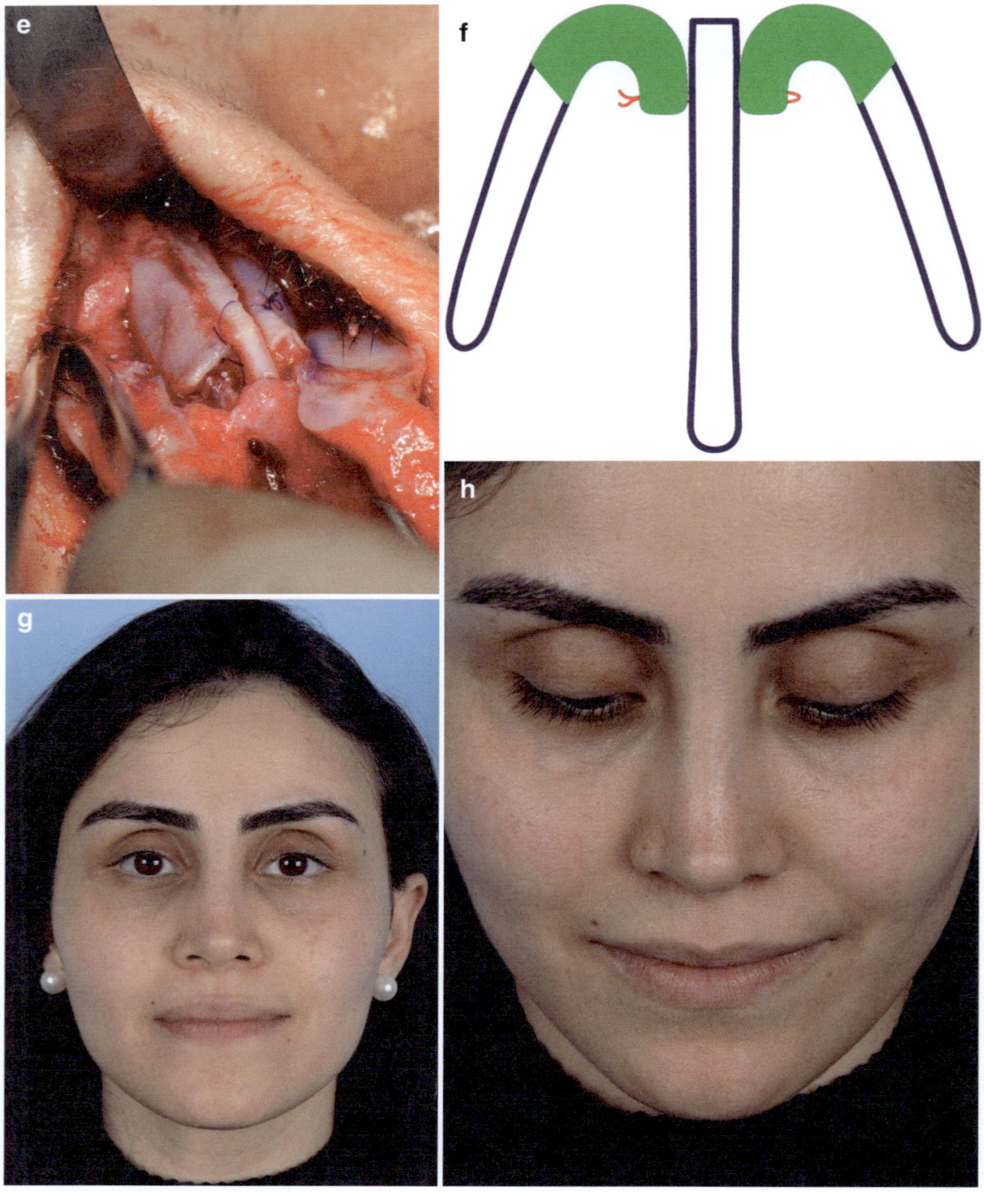

Fig. 6.45 (continued)

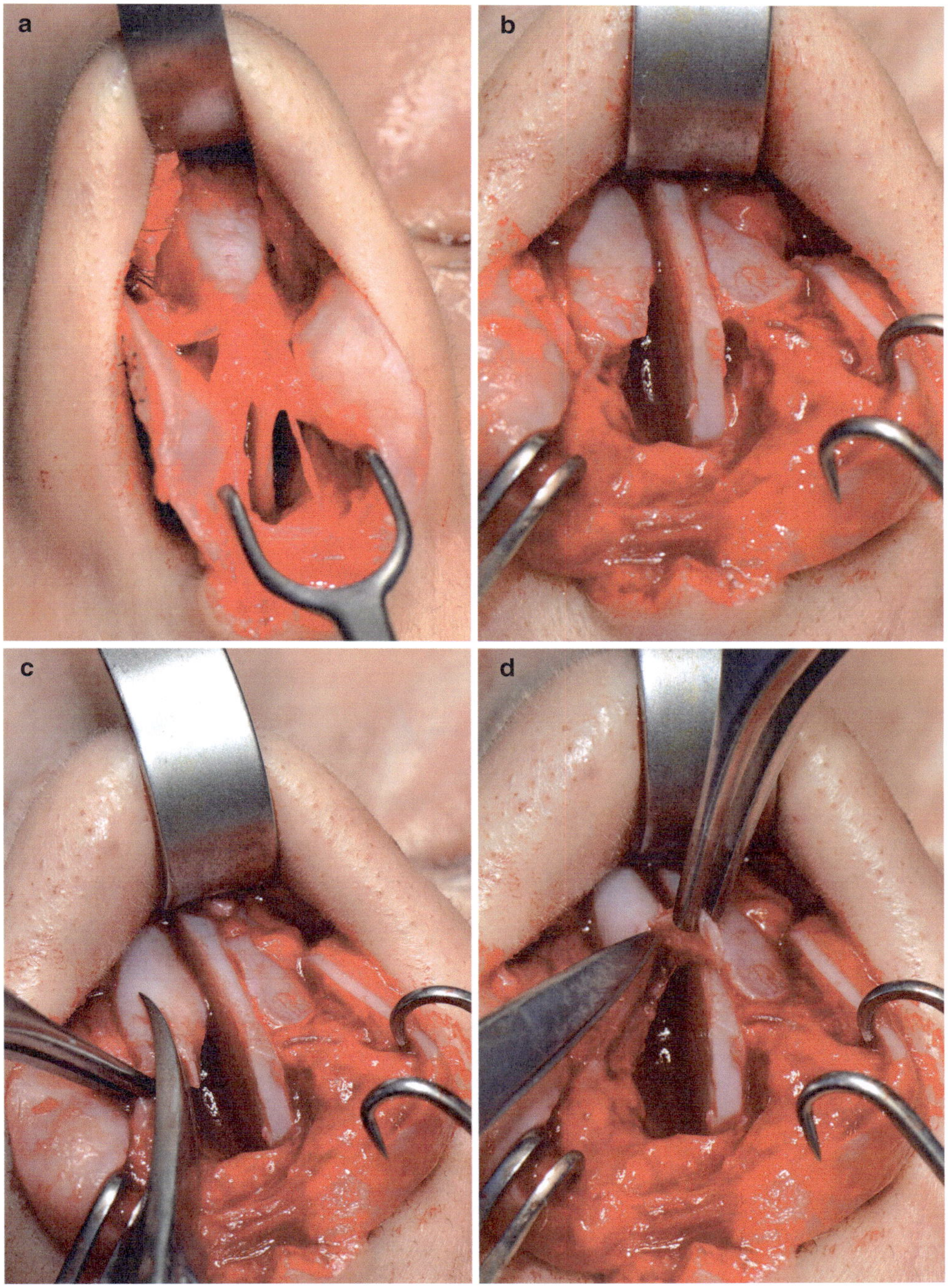

Fig. 6.46 (**a–f**) The excess caudal part of the spreader flap is removed before suturing

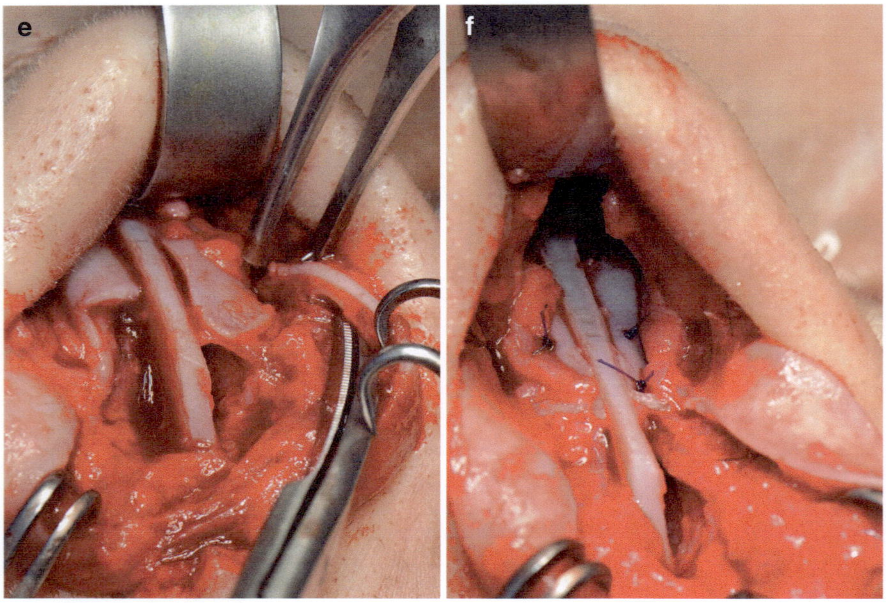

Fig. 6.46 (continued)

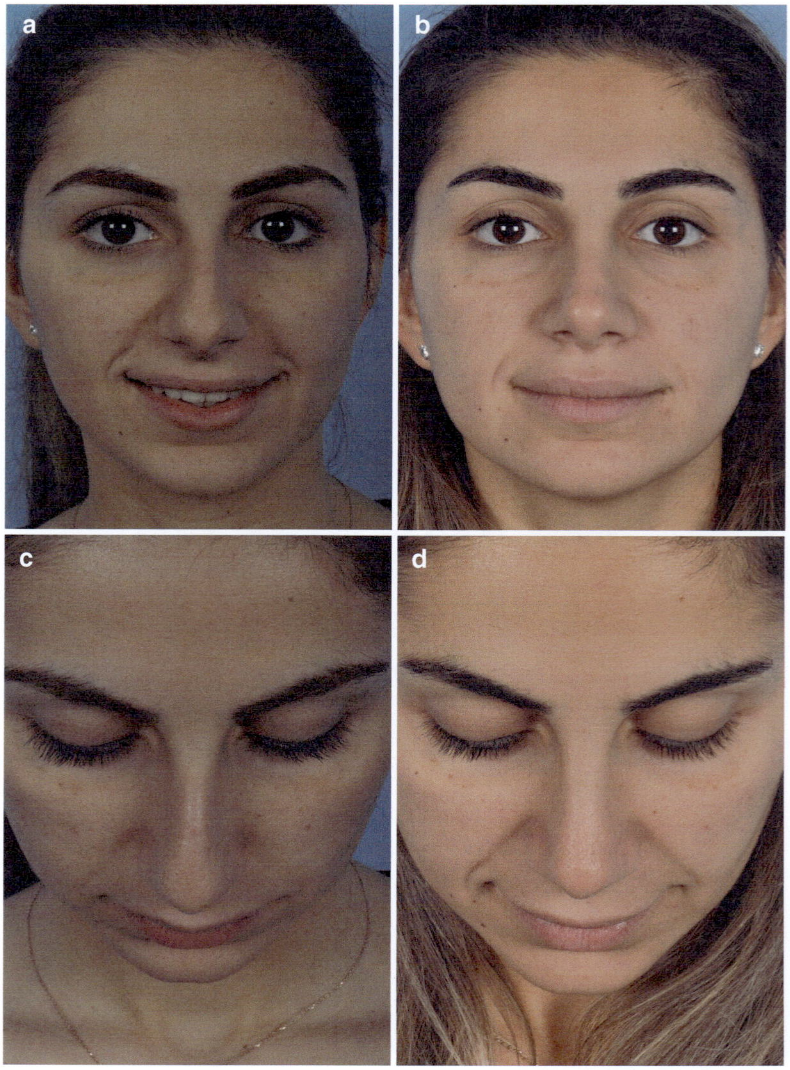

Fig. 6.47 (**a–d**) Preoperative and 5-year postoperative appearance. The middle vault remains stable during these years

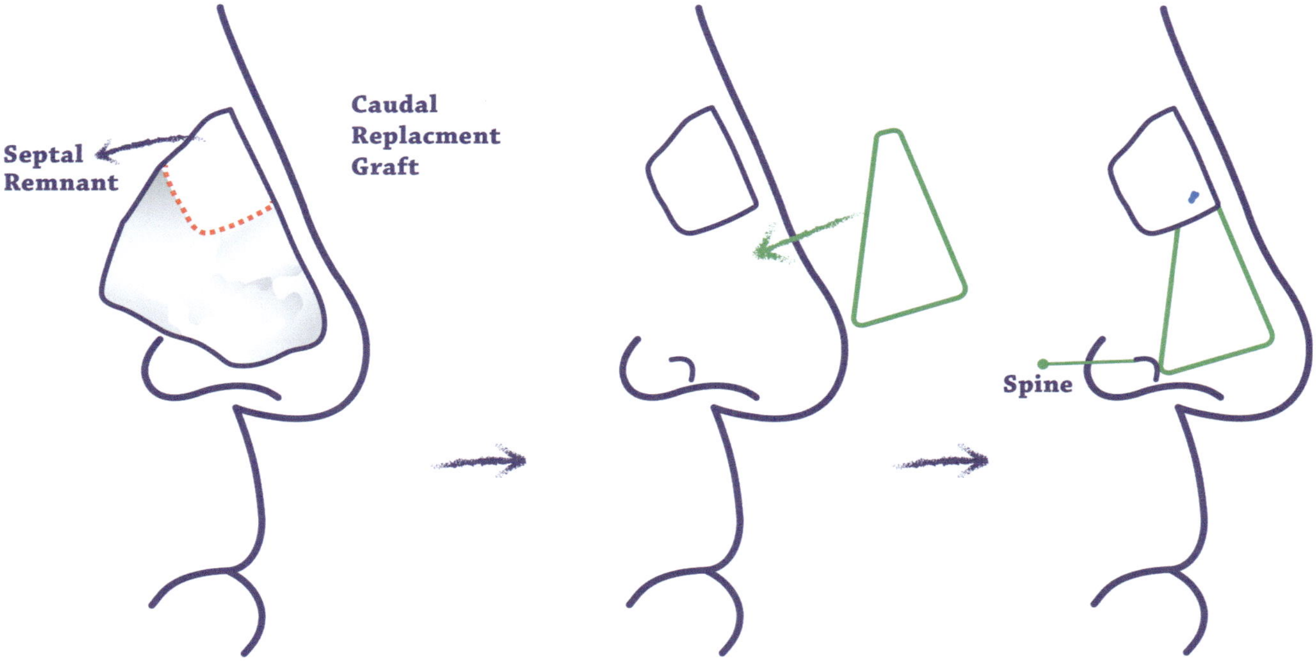

Fig. 6.48 The gray area shows severely deviated septum. First, a severe part of the cartilaginous septum is removed. A straight septal replacement graft is then prepared extracorporeally. Finally, septal replacement graft is placed and sutured to the nasal spine and septal remnant

Fig. 6.49 (**a**, **b**) The nasal bridge and tip are deviated to the right side. Broken brow-tip aesthetic line

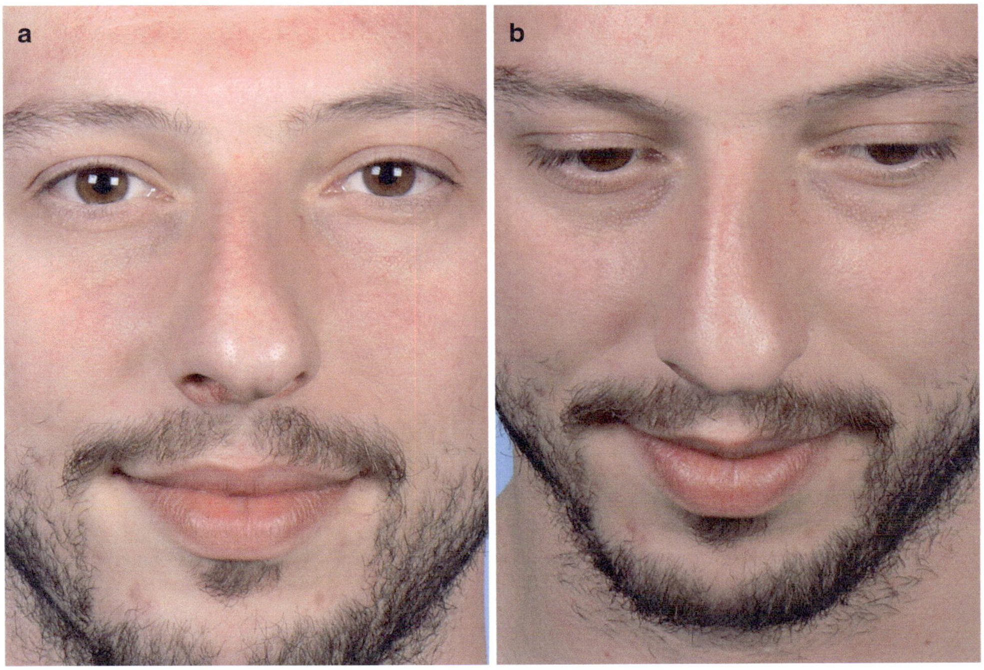

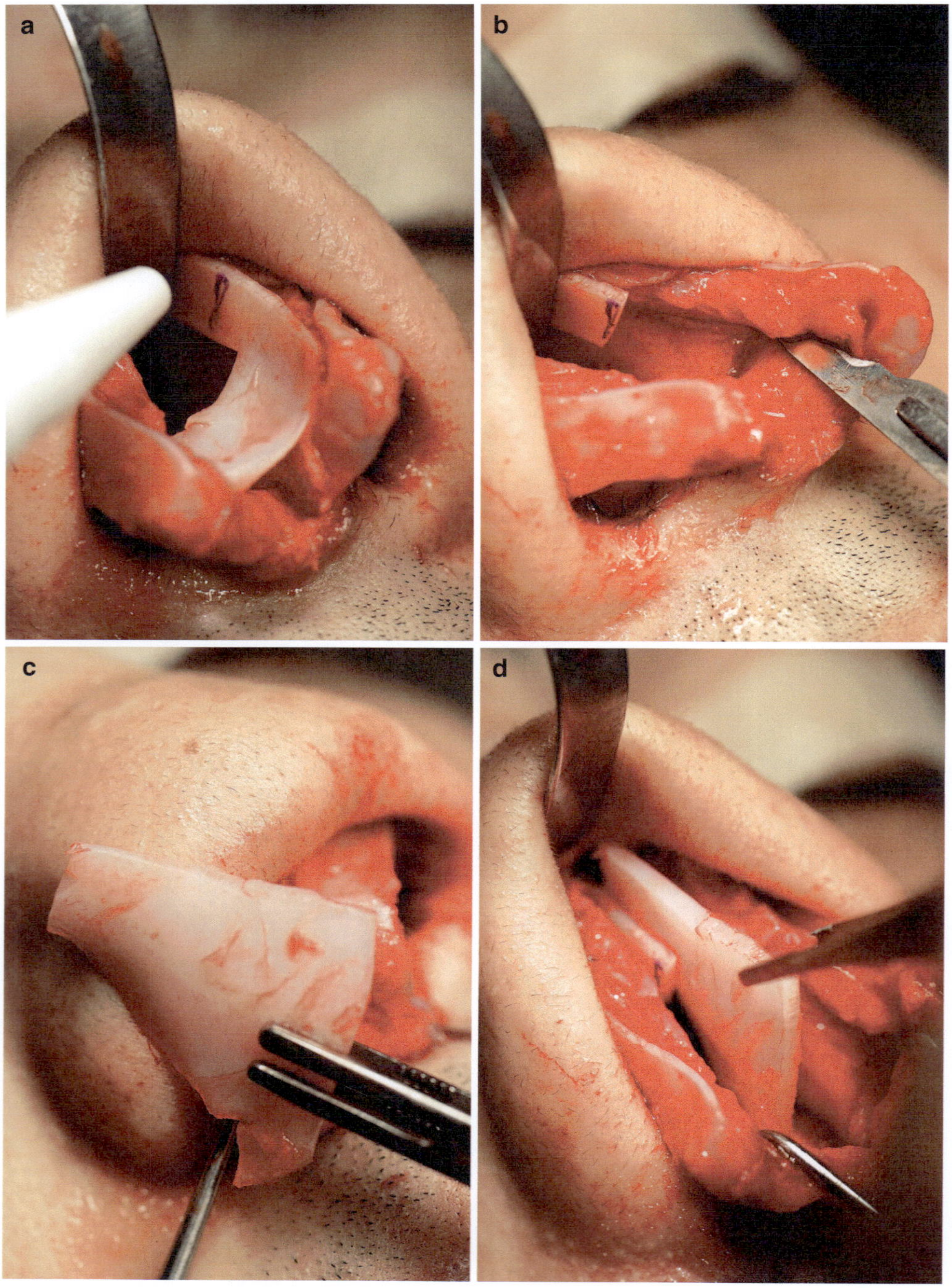

Fig. 6.50 (**a**) Intraoperative view of the L-shaped septal strut after septoplasty. (**b**) The deviated septum was removed, leaving a remnant of 1–1.5 cm of the dorsal septum. (**c**) A caudal septal replacement graft was prepared extracorporeally. (**d**, **e**) The caudal septal replacement graft was placed and sutured between the nasal spine and remnant dorsal septum. (**f**) Subtotal septal reconstruction was performed. The septum was straight and stable

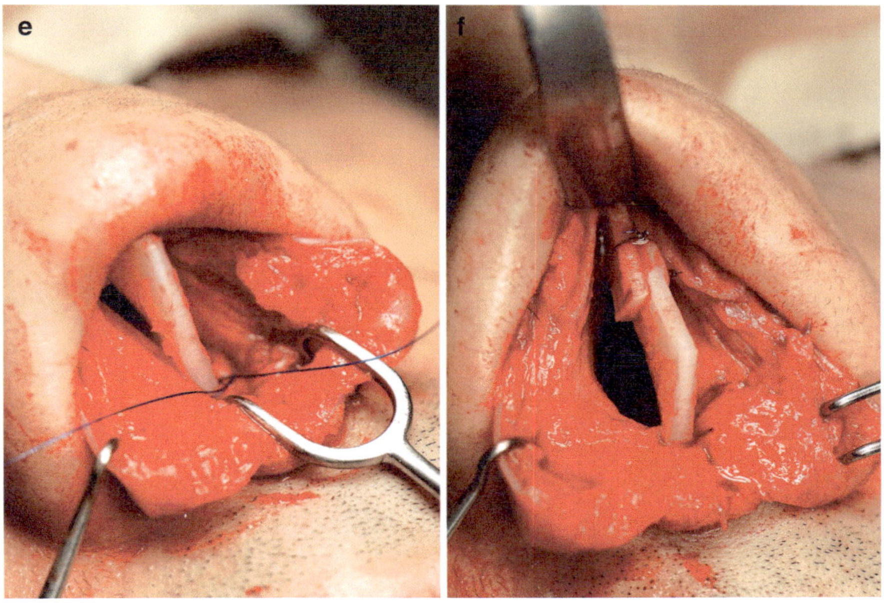

Fig. 6.50 (continued)

Fig. 6.51 (**a**–**f**) The nose appears straight and dorsal aesthetic lines are symmetric

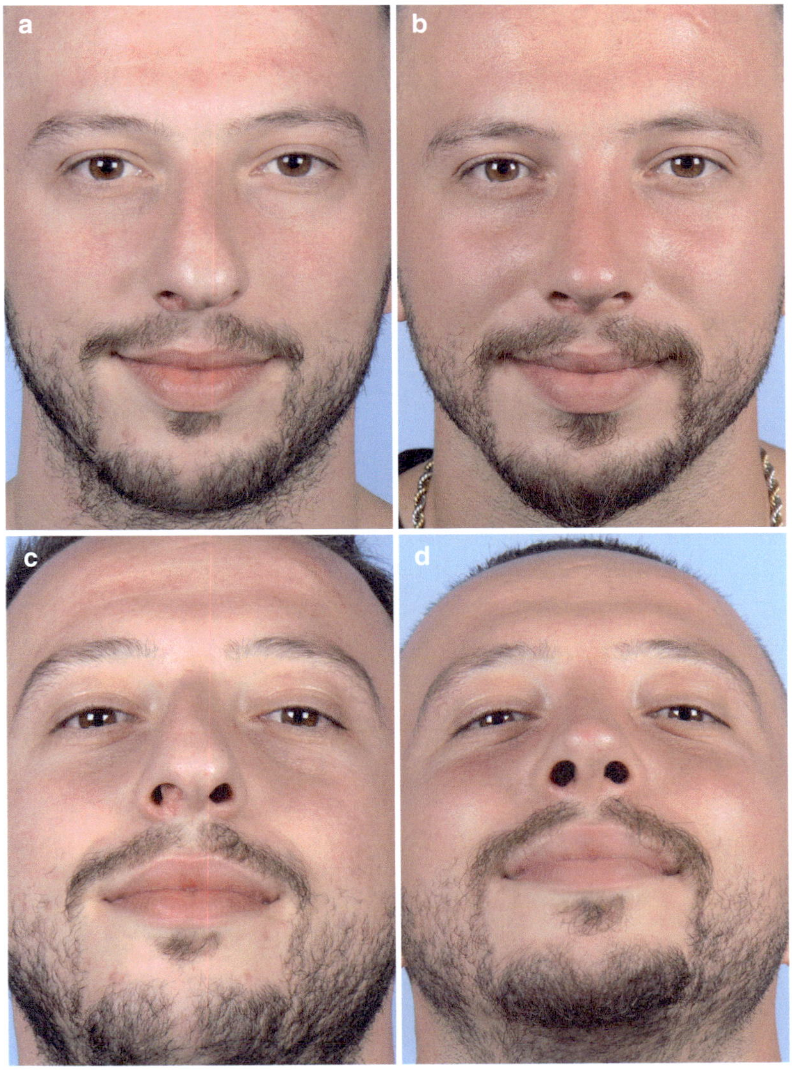

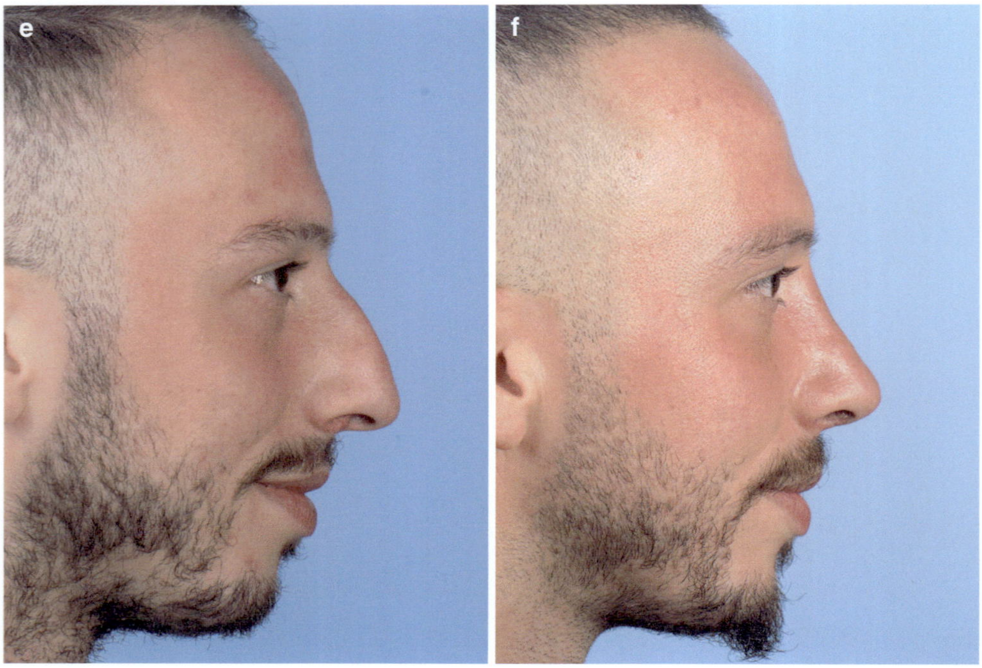

Fig. 6.51 (continued)

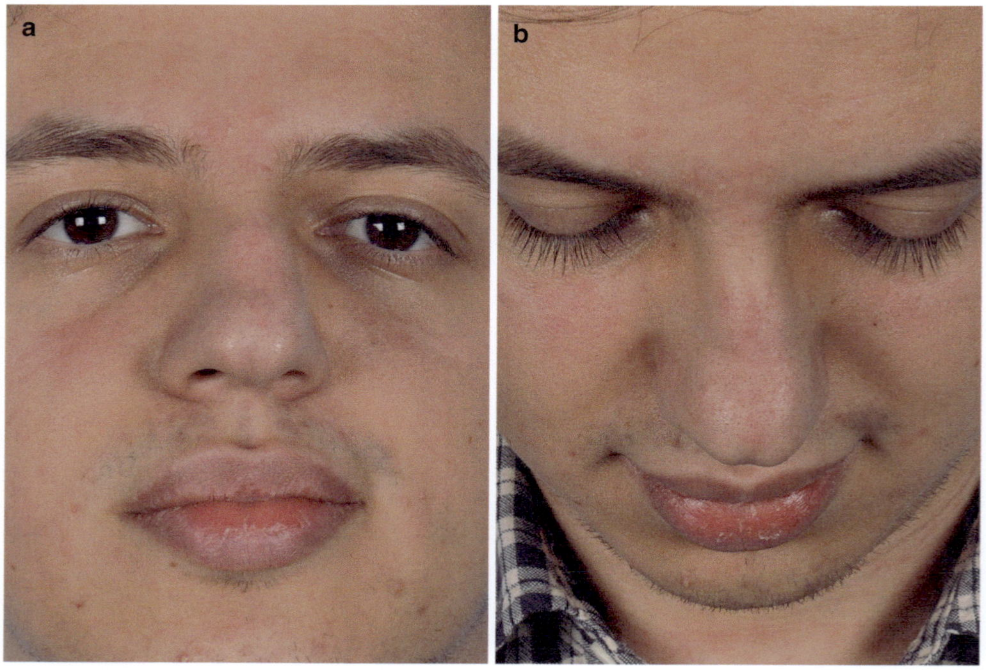

Fig. 6.52 (**a**, **b**) The middle vault is twisted

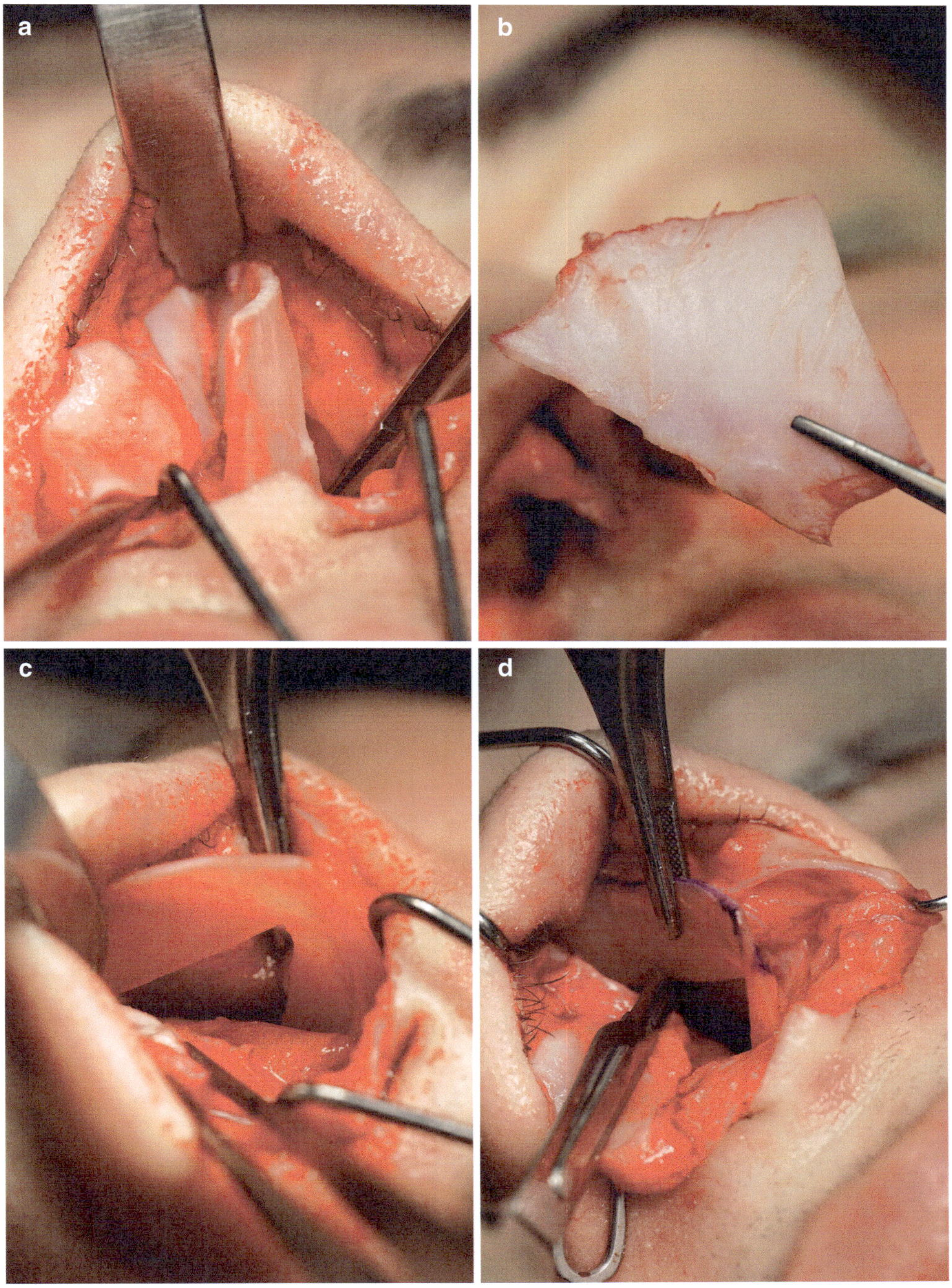

Fig. 6.53 (**a–c**) The septum was severely deviated. L-strut septoplasty was performed. (**d–g**) The septum was cut and excised for subtotal septal reconstruction. (**h**, **i**) The dorsal and caudal parts of the placement site were measured. (**j–l**) The caudal septal replacement graft was prepared for insertion. (**m–o**) The caudal septal replacement graft was sutured to the nasal spine and remnant dorsal septum. Finally, an auto-spreader graft was applied to the right side to provide extra support.

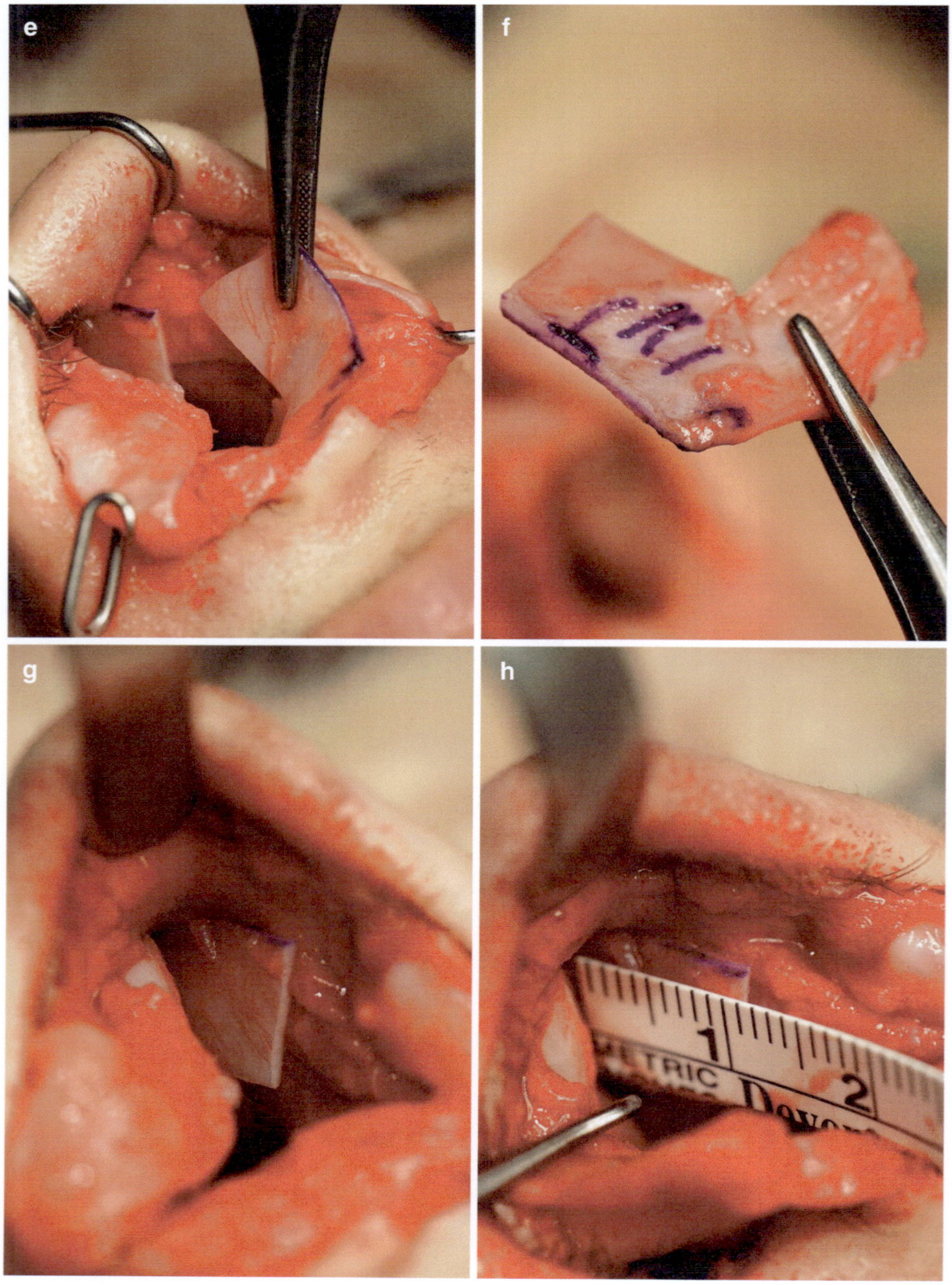

Fig. 6.53 (continued)

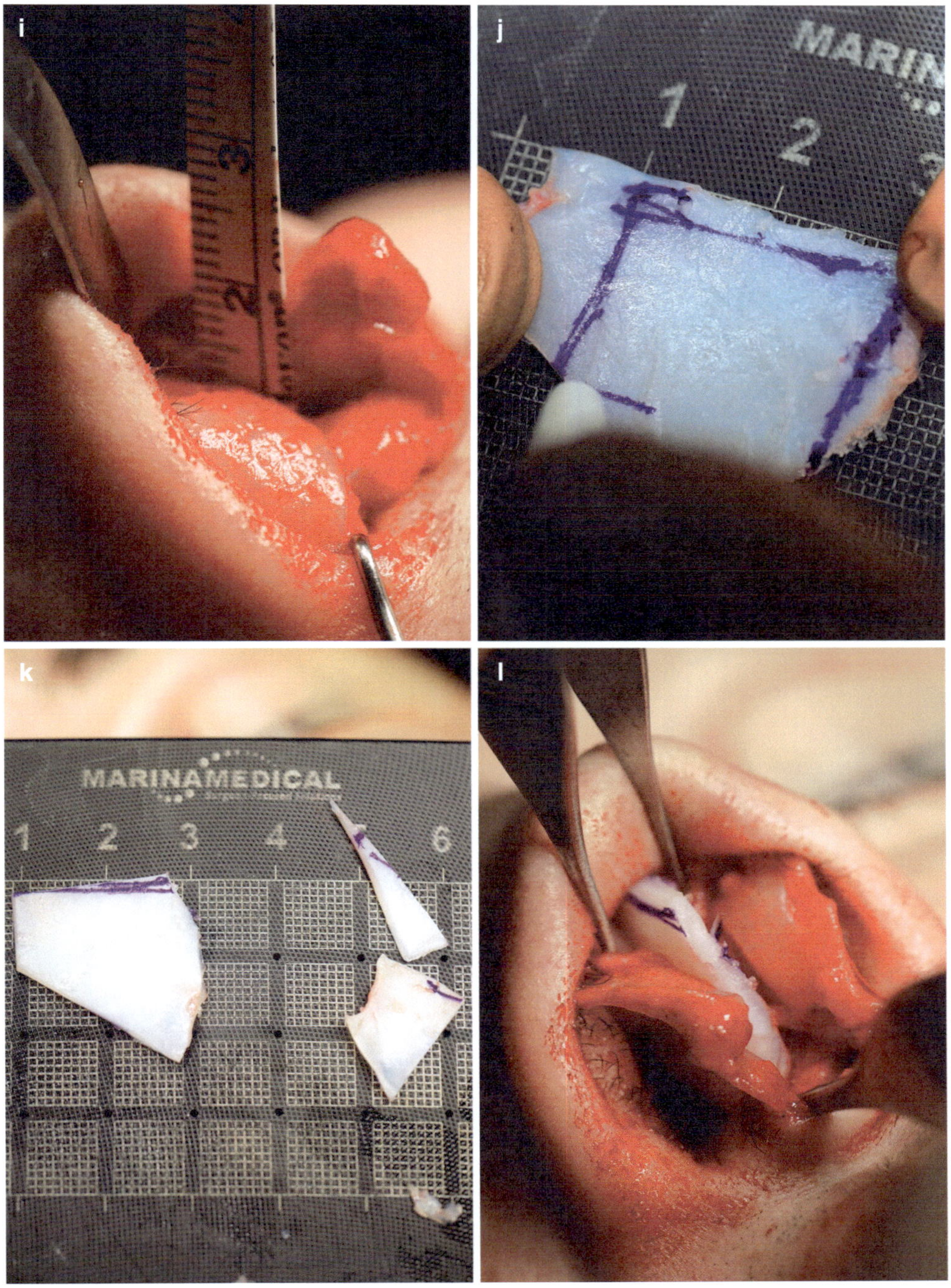

Fig. 6.53 (continued)

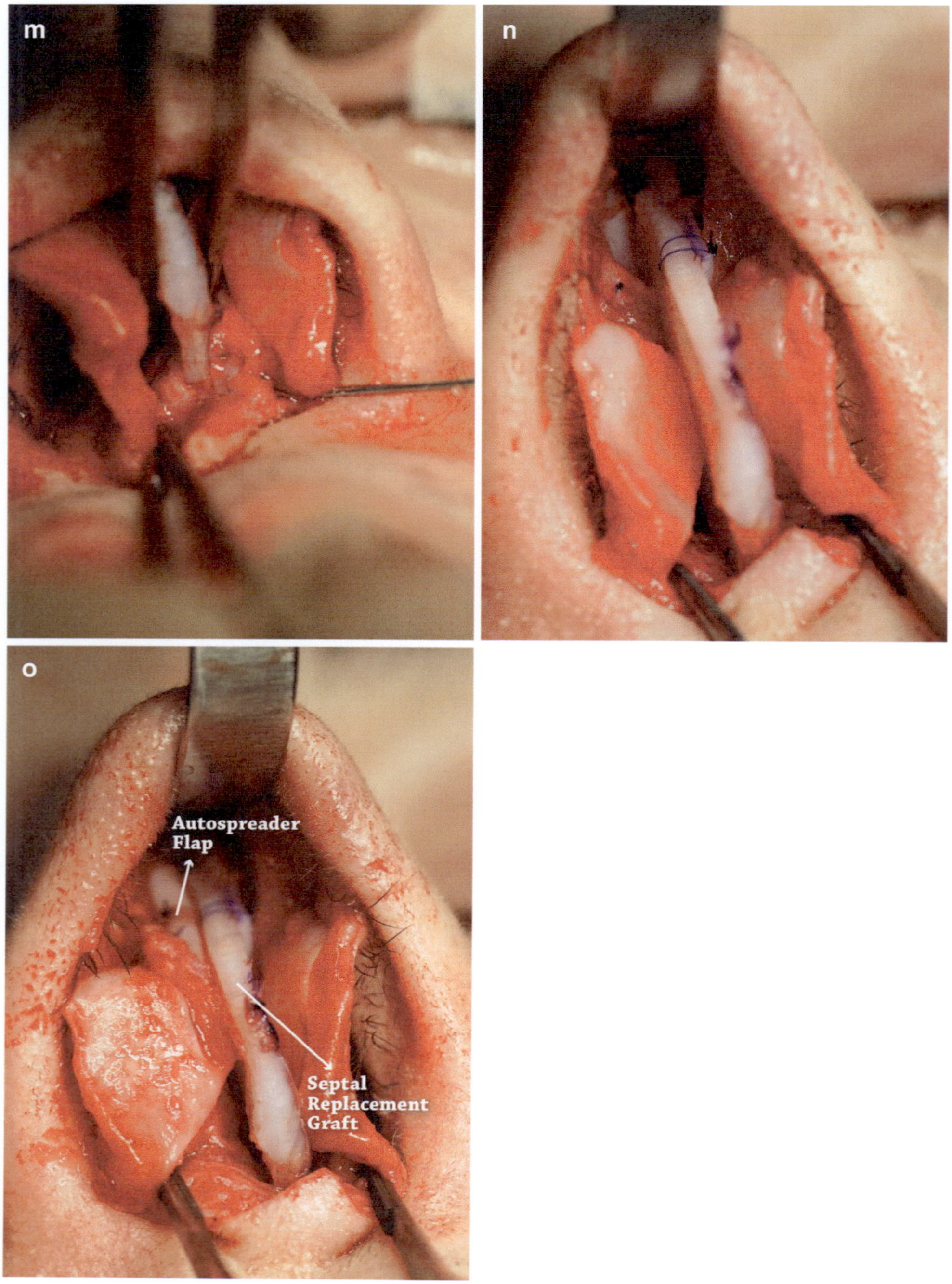

Fig. 6.53 (continued)

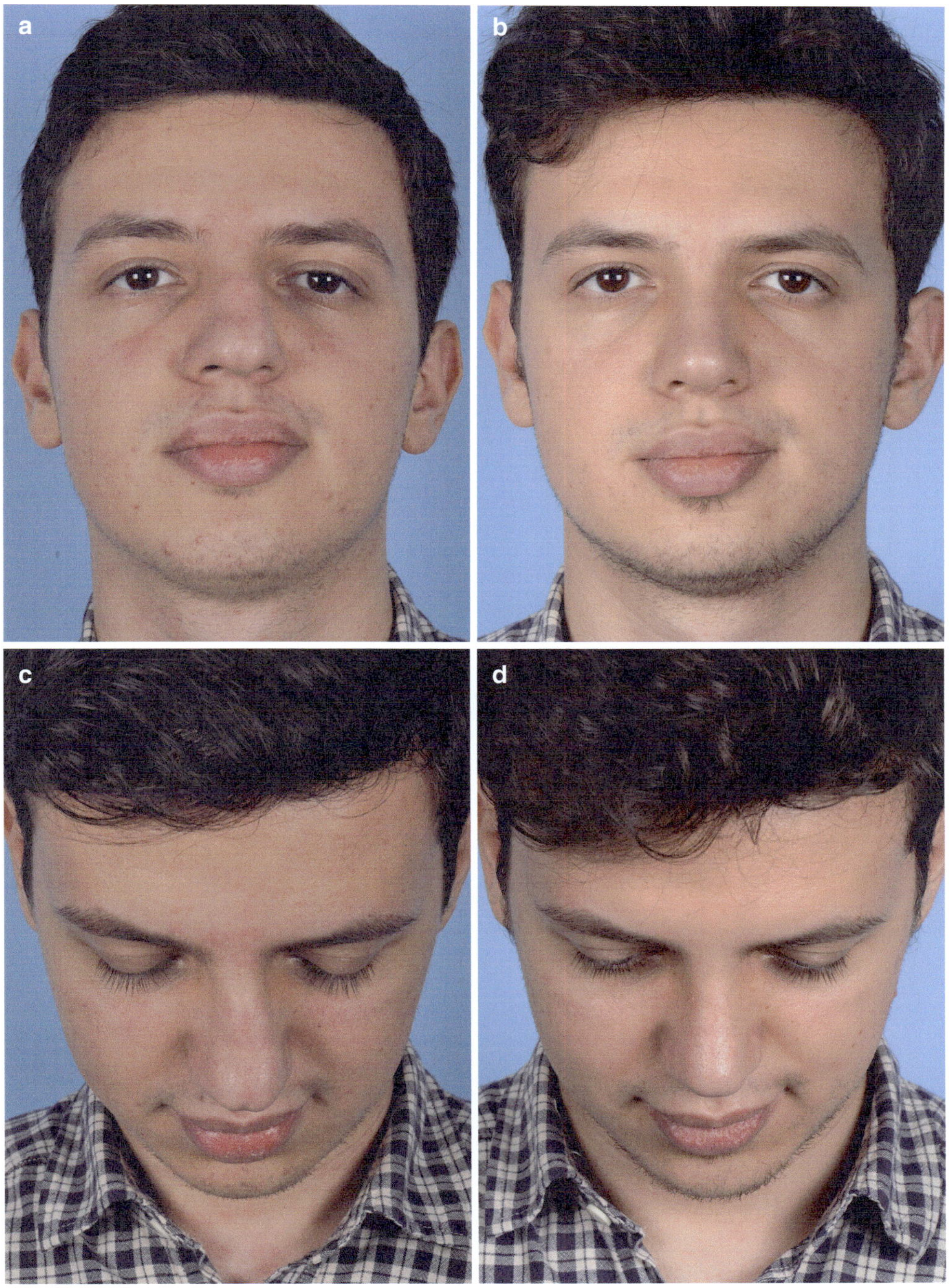

Fig. 6.54 (**a**–**f**) The nasal pyramid is straight and middle vault is more symmetrical

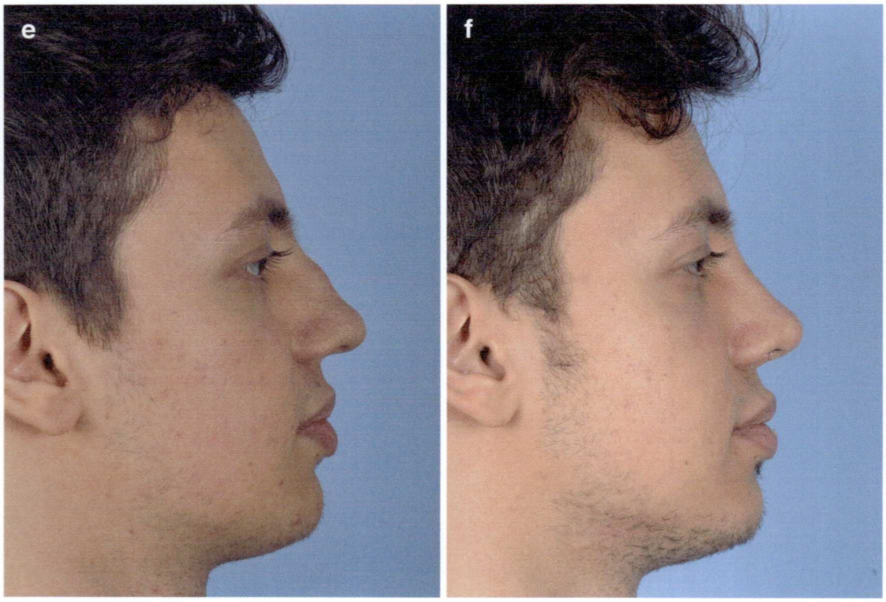

Fig. 6.54 (continued)

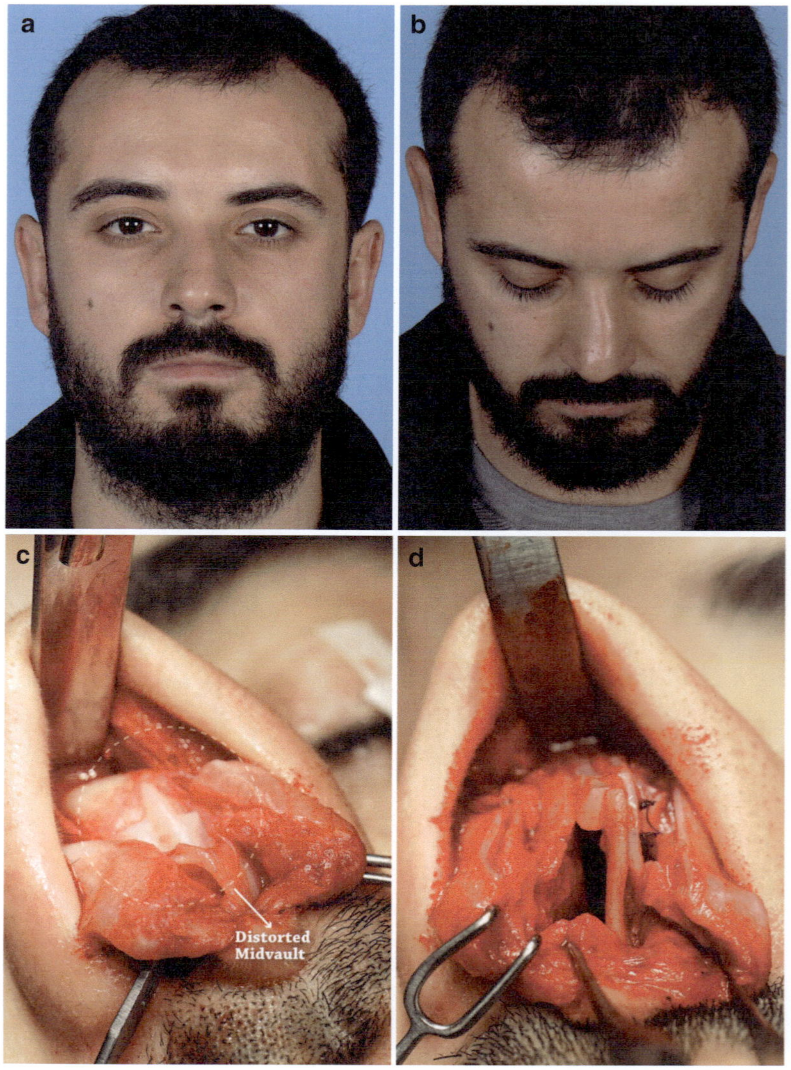

Fig. 6.55 (**a**, **b**) The bony dorsum and midvault are shifted off the right side. (**c**, **d**) Subtotal septal reconstruction was done for middle vault reconstruction. (**e**, **f**) The upper two thirds of the nose have been moved to the midline

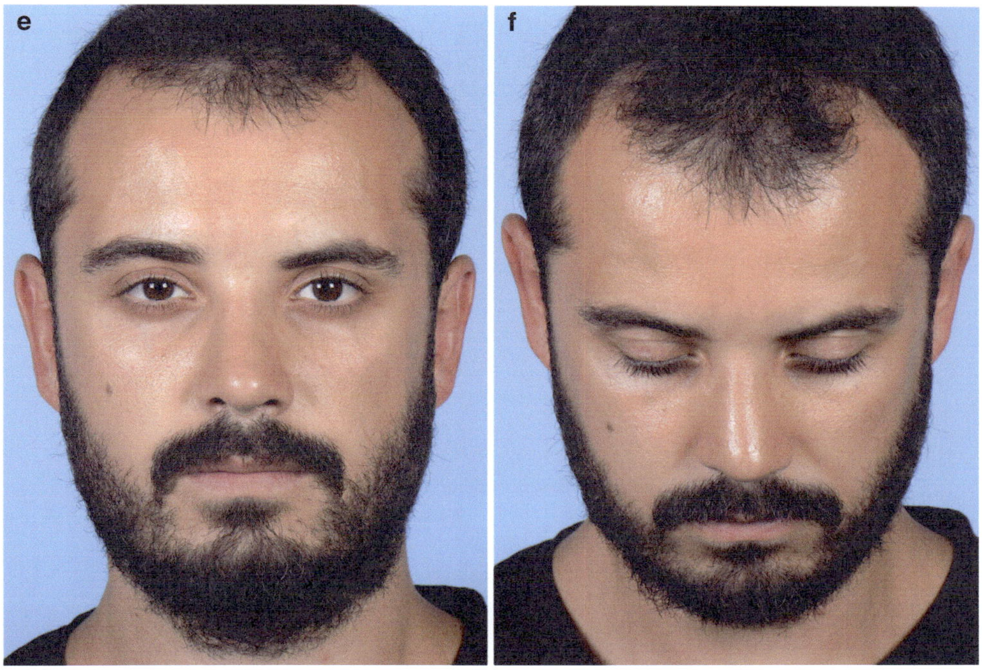

Fig. 6.55 (continued)

Fig. 6.56 (**a**–**d**) The crooked nose looks straight after subtotal septal reconstructions in years

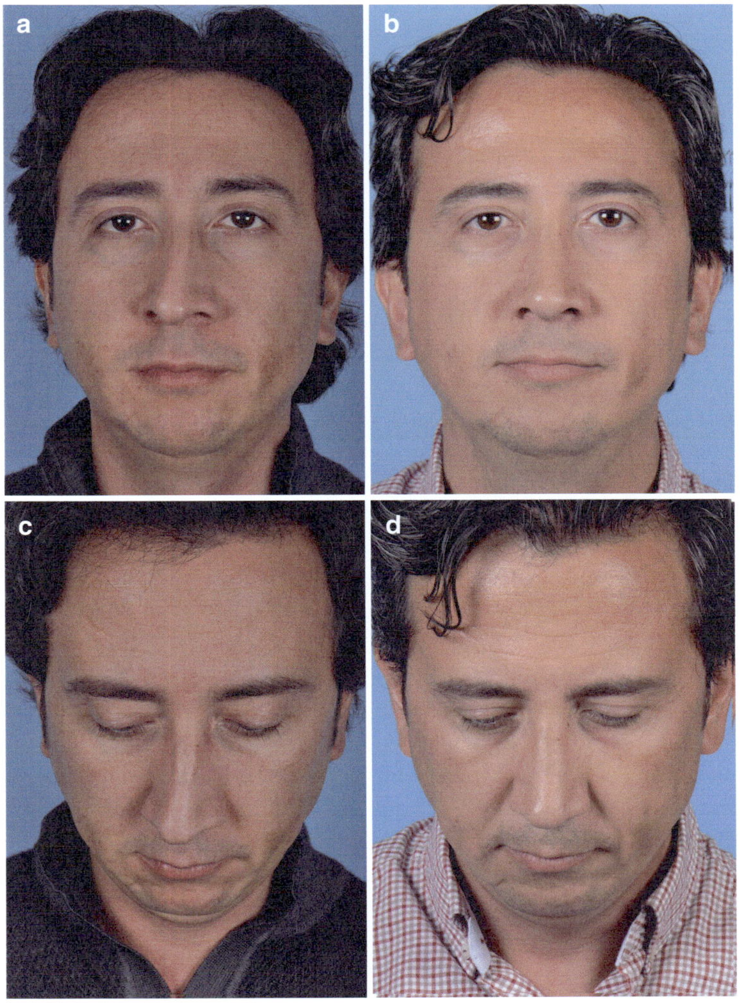

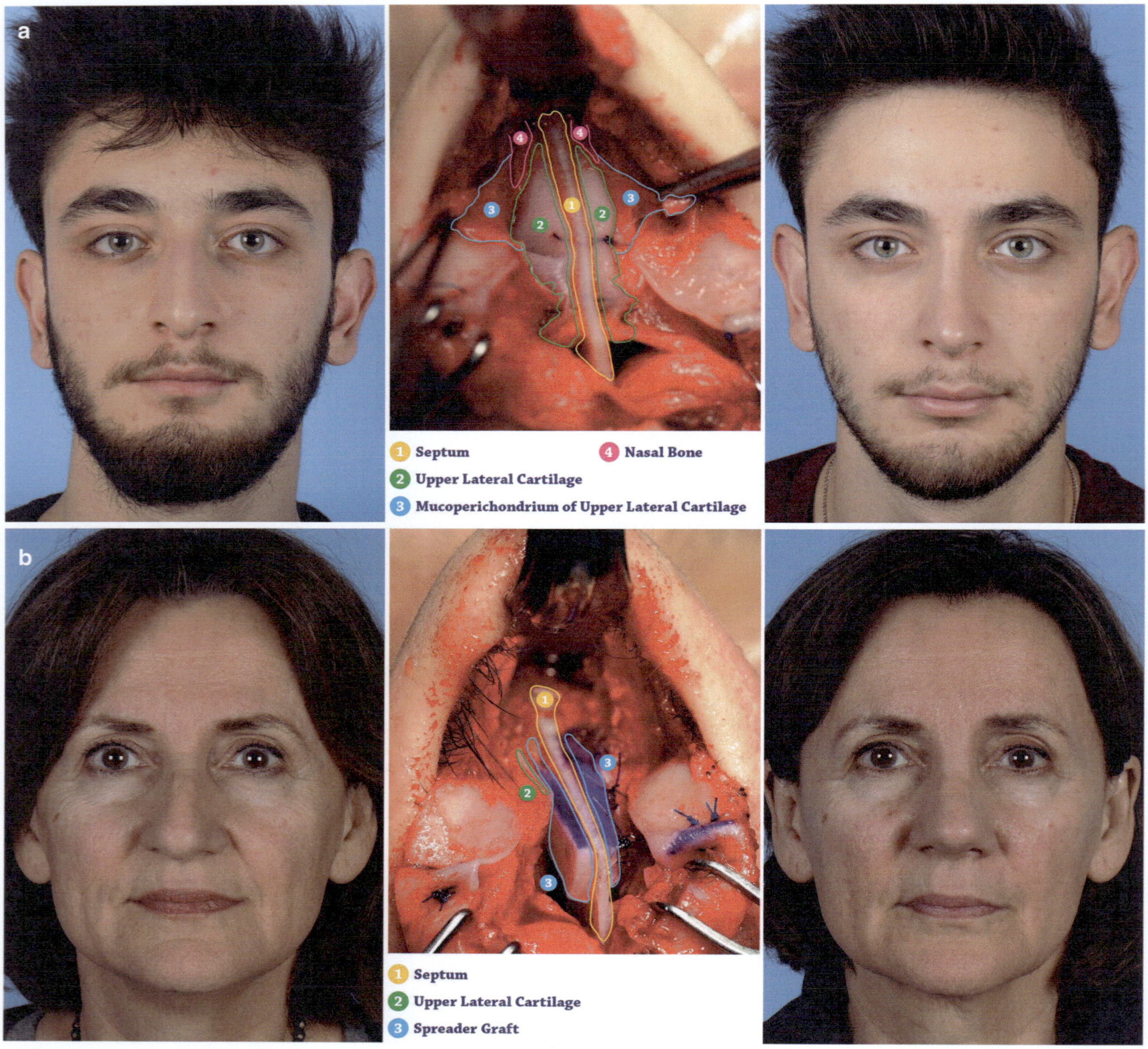

Fig. 6.57 (**a**) Spreader flaps were used for middle vault reconstruction. (**b**) Bilateral spreader grafts were used for middle vault reconstruction

6.3 Conclusion

The creation of an attractive nasal dorsum, as is typical in aesthetic rhinoplasty, involves producing a continuous, uninterrupted form in which the highlights and shadows are harmonious with the rest of the face. This extends beyond the profile, involving symmetry and shape in the frontal view and edge highlights in the oblique view. Middle third grafting techniques are available for this purpose. These grafts contribute to internal nasal valve anatomy and are therefore crucial for respiratory function of the nose. Two main grafts are used for reconstruction of the middle vault, i.e., autospreader and spreader grafts (Fig. 6.57).

There are no specific rules regarding graft placement. Different sizes, shapes, and combinations of grafts can be used in each case as required. The septum is a good source of graft material if available. Alternatively, autologous or homologous costal cartilage may be used as a source material. Finally, subtotal septal reconstruction should be preferred in cases of severe septal deviation that cannot be treated with spreader or autospreader grafts.

Disclosures The author reports no conflicts of interest or funding requiring disclosure.

Further Reading

Afrooz PN, Rohrich RJ. The keystone: consistency in restoring the aesthetic dorsum in rhinoplasty. Plast Reconstr Surg. 2018;141(2):355–63.

Allak A, Park SS. Surgical treatment of the middle nasal vault. Clin Plast Surg. 2016;43(1):85–94.

Apaydin F. Nasal valve surgery. Facial Plast Surg. 2011;27(2):179–91.

Apaydin F. Rebuilding the middle vault in rhinoplasty: a new classification of spreader flaps/grafts. Facial Plast Surg. 2016;32(6):638–45.

Ashrafi AT. Management of upper lateral cartilages (ULCs) in rhinoplasty. World J Plast Surg. 2014;3(2):129–37.

Berkowitz RL, Gruber RP. Management of the nasal dorsum: construction and maintenance of a barrel vault. Clin Plast Surg. 2016;43(1):59–72.

Byrd HS, Meade RA, Gonyon DL. Using the autospreader flap in primary rhinoplasty. Plast Reconstr Surg. 2007;119(6):1897–902.

Daniel RK, Pálházi P. Rhinoplasty: an anatomical and clinical atlas. Cham: Springer International; 2018. p. 113–63.

Gruber RP, Melkun ET, Woodward JF, Perkins SW. Dorsal reduction and spreader flaps. Aesthet Surg J. 2011;31(4):456–64.

Gruber RP, Park E, Newman J, Berkowitz L, Oneal R. The spreader flap in primary rhinoplasty. Plast Reconstr Surg. 2007;119(6):1903–10.

Gruber RP, Perkins SW. Humpectomy and spreader flaps. Clin Plast Surg. 2010;37(2):285–91.

Harris MO, Baker SR. Management of the wide nasal dorsum. Arch Facial Plast Surg. 2004;6(1):41–8.

Hassanpour SE, Heidari A, Moosavizadeh SM, Tarahomi MR, Goljanian A, Tavakoli S. Comparison of aesthetic and functional outcomes of spreader graft and autospreader flap in rhinoplasty. World J Plast Surg. 2016;5(2):133–8.

Kim L, Papel ID. Spreader grafts in functional rhinoplasty. Facial Plast Surg. 2016;32(1):29–35.

Kovacevic M, Riedel F, Göksel A, Wurm J. Options for middle vault and dorsum restoration after hump removal in primary rhinoplasty. Facial Plast Surg. 2016;32(4):374–83.

Kovacevic M, Wurm J. Spreader flaps for middle vault contour and stabilization. Facial Plast Surg Clin North Am. 2015;23(1):1–9.

Lohuis PJ, Faraj-Hakim S, Knobbe A, Duivesteijn W, Bran GM. Split hump technique for reduction of the overprojected nasal dorsum: a statistical analysis on subjective body image in relation to nasal appearance and nasal patency in 97 patients undergoing aesthetic rhinoplasty. Arch Facial Plast Surg. 2012;14(5):346–53.

Moubayed SP, Most SP. The autospreader flap for midvault reconstruction following dorsal hump resection. Facial Plast Surg. 2016;32(1):36–41.

Park SS. Fundamental principles in aesthetic rhinoplasty. Clin Exp Otorhinolaryngol. 2011;4(2):55–66.

Quatela VC, Jacono AA. Structural grafting in rhinoplasty. Facial Plast Surg. 2002;18(4):223–32.

Sykes JM, Tapias V, Kim JE. Management of the nasal dorsum. Facial Plast Surg. 2011;27(2):192–202.

Yoo DB, Jen A. Endonasal placement of spreader grafts: experience in 41 consecutive patients. Arch Facial Plast Surg. 2012;14(5):318–22.

Yoo S, Most SP. Nasal airway preservation using the autospreader technique: analysis of outcomes using a disease-specific quality-of-life instrument. Arch Facial Plast Surg. 2011;13(4):231–3.

7 Dorsum: Osteotomy

7.1 Introduction

The osseous structure of the nose provides the foundation for both nasal shape and function. Alterations in the shape and orientation of the bony framework may be congenital or acquired secondary to previous trauma or surgery. Osteotomy is the process of making controlled incisions on the bone roof of the nose during rhinoplasty. These controlled incisions enable simultaneous closure of the open roof, which forms after hump removal, and correction of asymmetries in the bone.

Nasal anatomy and osteotomy techniques must be adequately understood to achieve good aesthetic and functional results.

While osteotomy is an essential step in rhinoplasty, it is rather challenging mainly because the osteotomy line is not visible. The following outcomes indicate that osteotomy was successful (Fig. 7.1):

- Absence of uncontrolled fracture and collapse.
- Presence of minimal postoperative swelling and ecchymosis.
- Achievement of the desired aesthetic result in the short, medium, and long term.

Osteotomy should be performed after hump removal and preferably after septal surgery. There are many approaches regarding location and method for performing osteotomy. In practice, a wide range of osteotomy patterns may lead to confusion. In fact, the logic is relatively simple:

After hump removal, the left and right bony nasal side walls are cut, mobilized, and then symmetrically reunited in the midline.

The first osteotomy line must be extended to the base of the nose. This line begins at the apertura piriformis (caudally) and extends to the medial canthal ligament line (cranially). The second wall to be mobilized is the line that begins from the cranial edge of the open roof and extends to the base of the nose (Fig. 7.2).

Lateral osteotomy constitutes the incision that mobilizes the nasal base, whereas transverse osteotomy constitutes the incision that joins the base with the open roof (Fig. 7.3).

With the aid of nasal side wall osteotomies, the open roof is closed. This also narrows the base of the nose (Fig. 7.4).

In most patients, transverse and lateral osteotomies are sufficient for mobilization of the nasal wall in the midline. Rarely, it may be necessary to separate the lateral nasal wall from the bony septum; this can be achieved by medial osteotomy (Fig. 7.5).

Osteotomy is mainly performed using one of two methods: internal continuous and external perforation techniques. Other techniques used for osteotomy are modifications of these basic methods.

Supplementary Information The online version contains supplementary material available at https://doi.org/10.1007/978-3-031-65619-4_7.

S. Şeneldir, *Photographic Atlas of Rhinoplasty*, https://doi.org/10.1007/978-3-031-65619-4_7

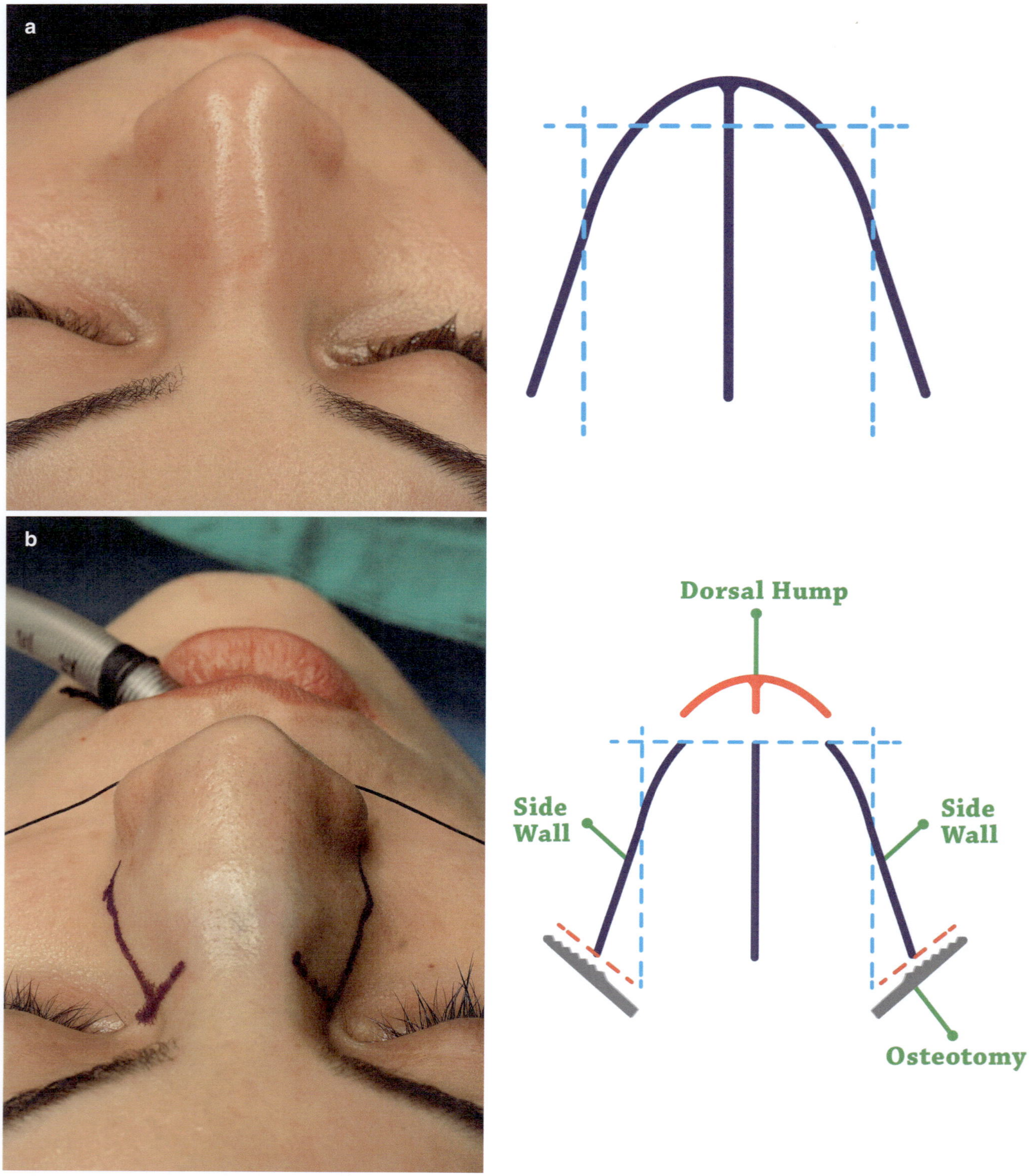

Fig. 7.1 (**a–c**) Compare these illustrations to intraoperative pictures. After hump removal, osteotomy is performed and open roof is closed. In conclusion, bone volume is reduced

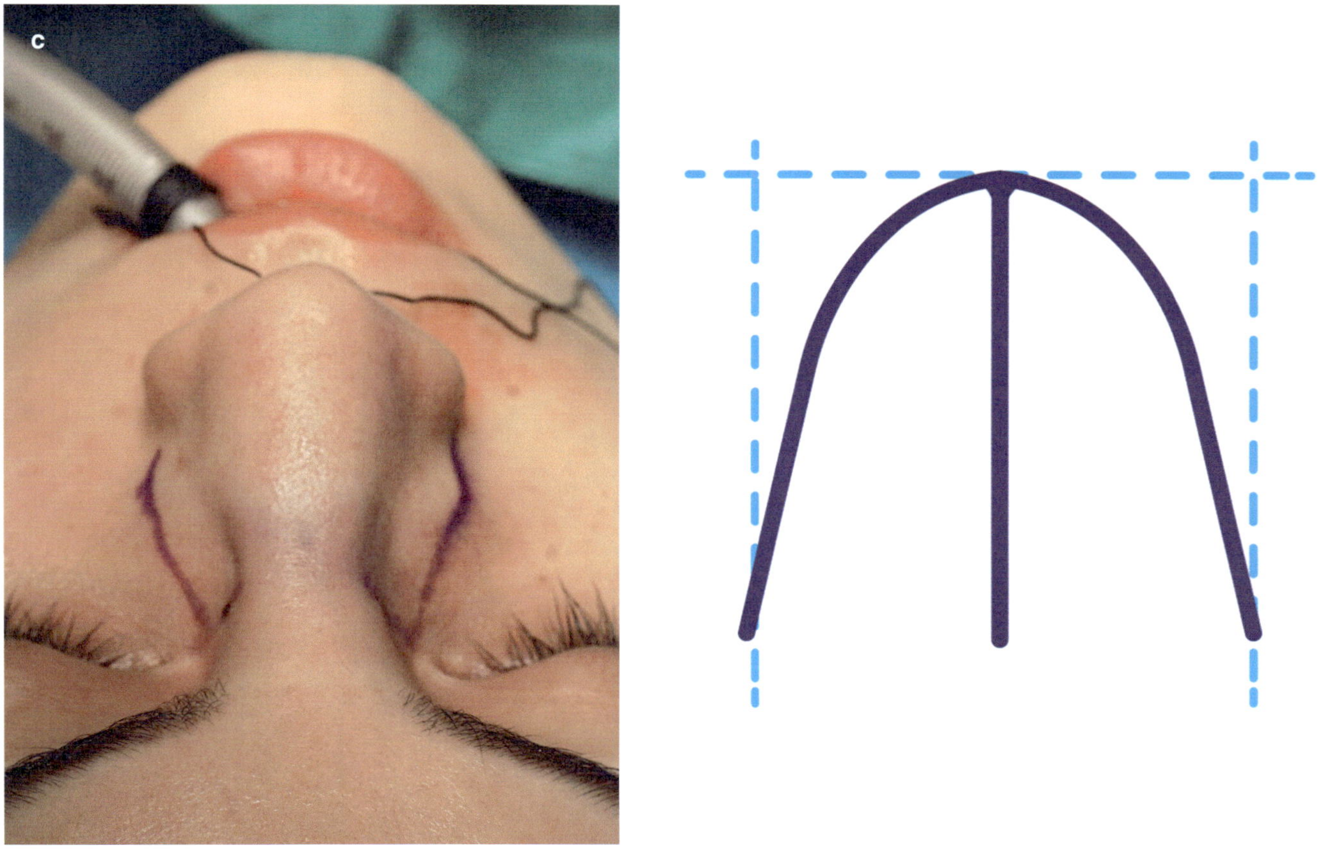

Fig. 7.1 (continued)

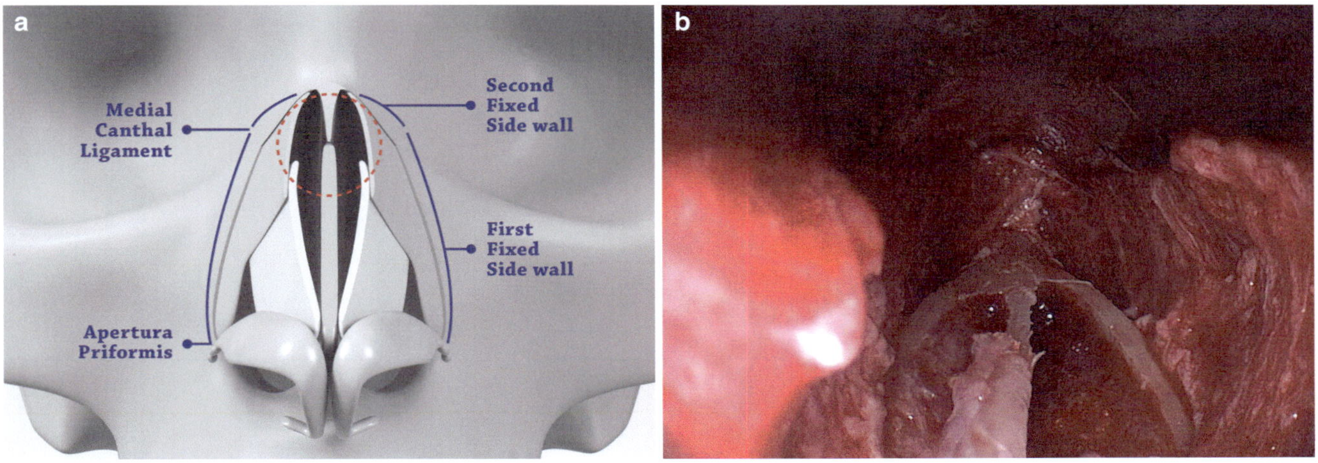

Fig. 7.2 (**a**, **b**) Open roof after hump removal

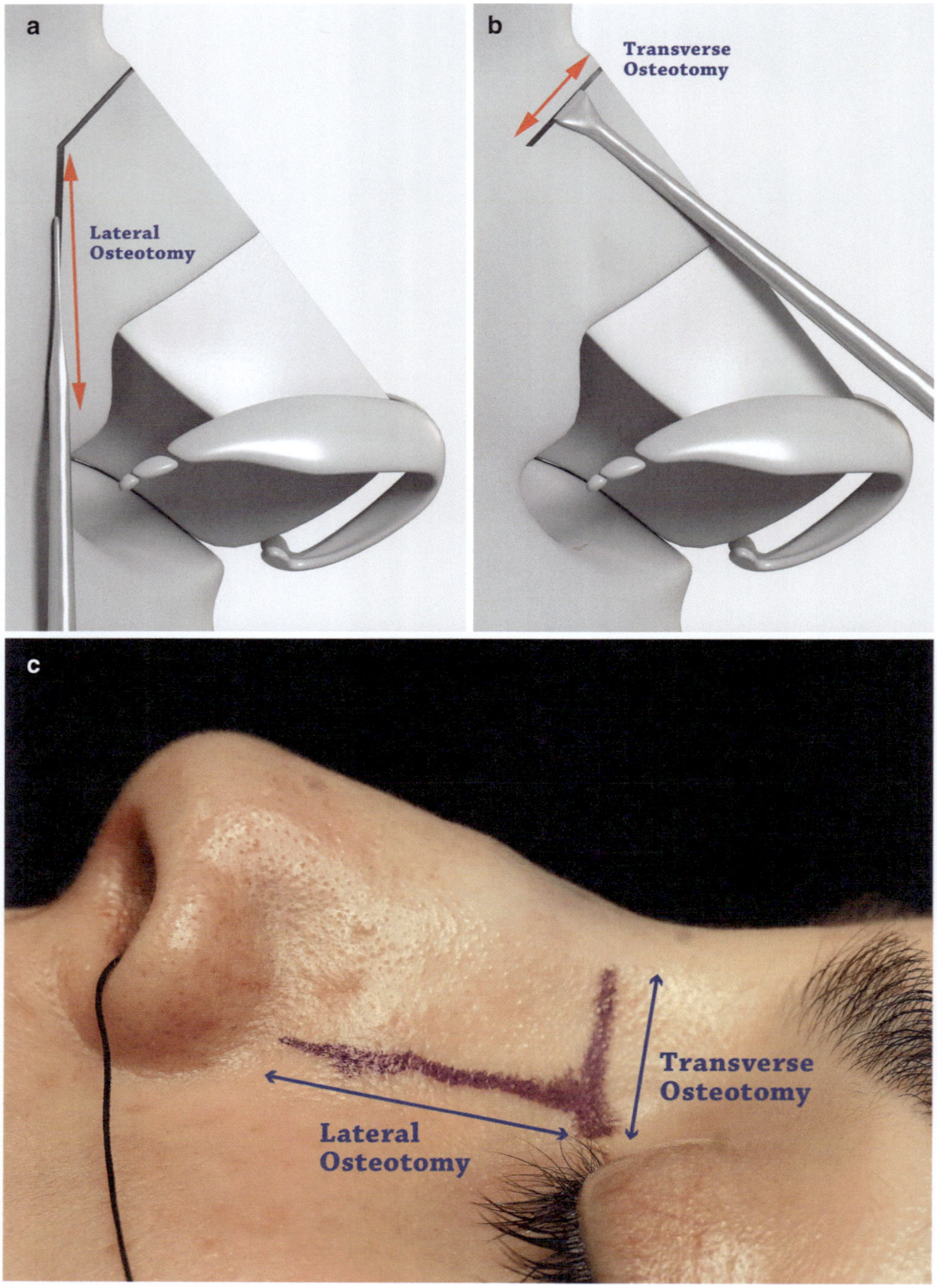

Fig. 7.3 (**a**) Lateral osteotomy line. (**b**) Transverse osteotomy line. (**c**) Lateral and transverse osteotomy line

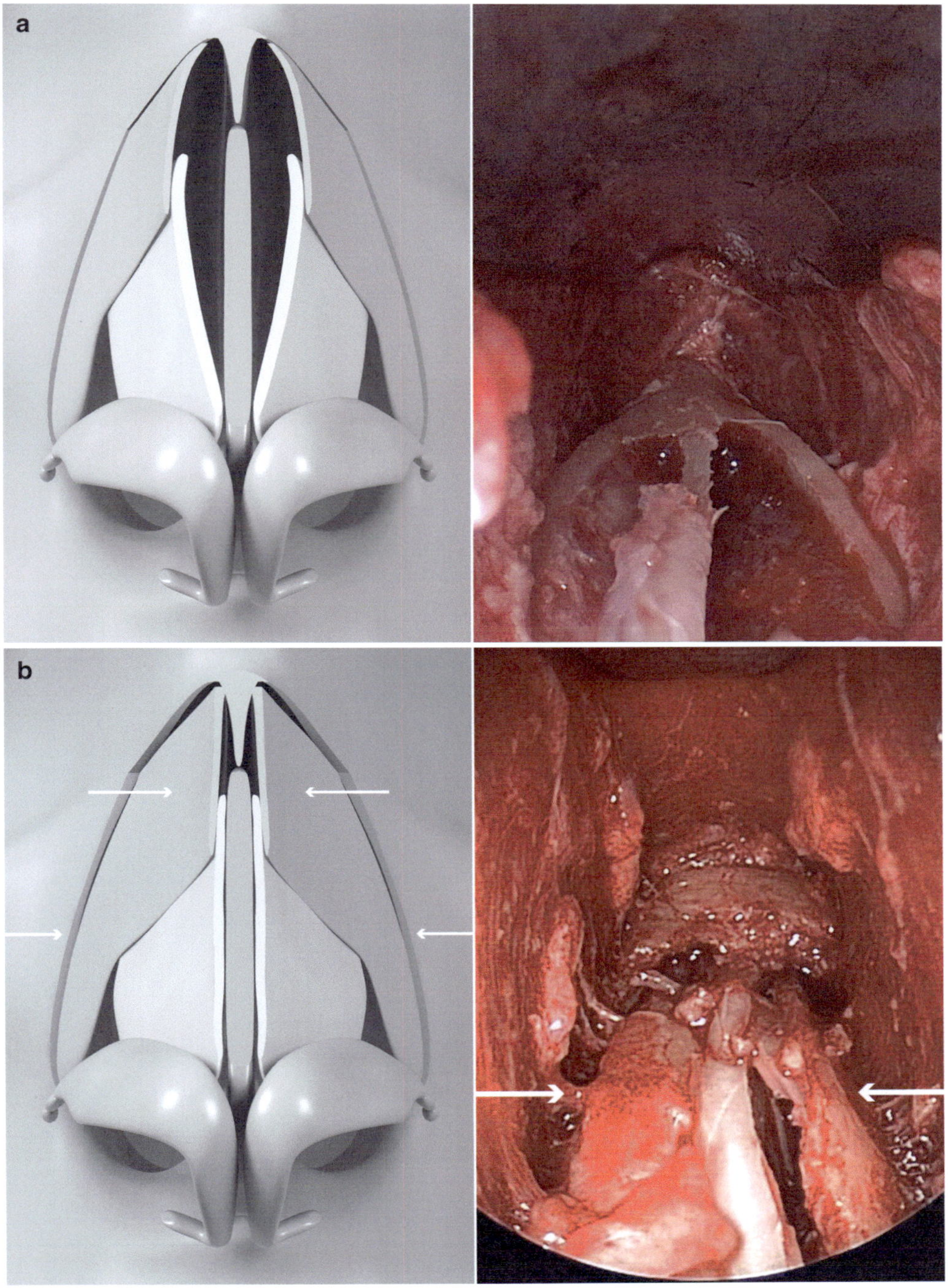

Fig. 7.4 (**a**) Open roof after hump removal. (**b**) Open roof is closed after osteotomies

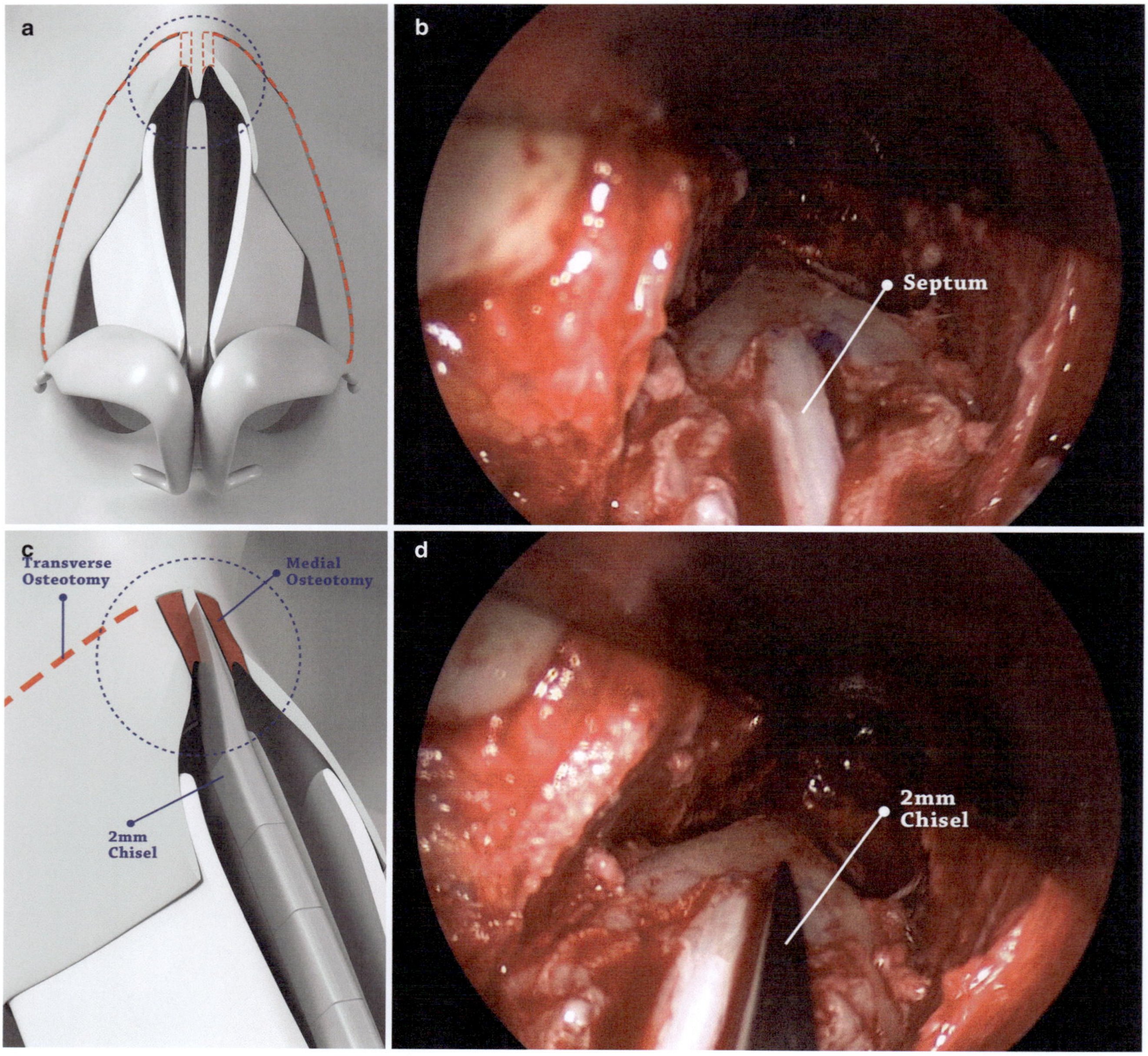

Fig. 7.5 (**a**, **b**) Open roof in wide nasal dorsum after hump removal. (**d**, **e**) Open roof is closed by medial osteotomy

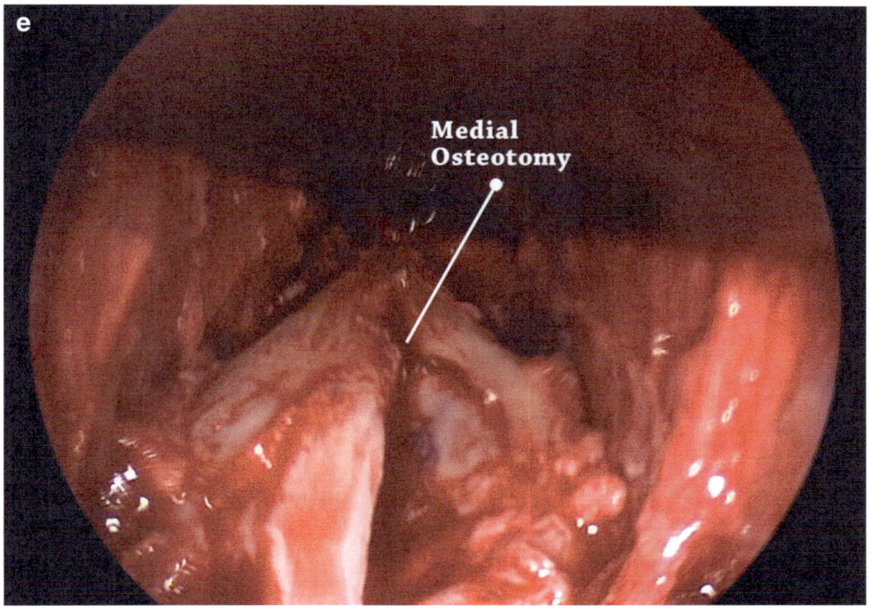

Fig. 7.5 (continued)

7.2 Treatment Strategy

Performing osteotomy types will be discussed.

7.2.1 Transverse Osteotomy

Transverse osteotomy can be performed via the following approaches:

- External perforating osteotomy with a 2-mm chisel
- Internally with small saws (manual or powered saws)

Regardless of the instrument used, the practice of marking the osteotomy line prior to the procedure makes the osteotomy practical and easy. The transverse osteotomy line extends from the cephalic end point of the lateral osteotomy line to the dorsum, to the cephalic part of the open roof.

If external perforating osteotomy is preferred, a small incision is made with the scalpel to the middle of the marked line. Osteotomy is performed with a 2-mm chisel through this incision (Fig. 7.6).

In addition, some surgeons recommend performance of osteotomy after passage through the skin by directly using a 2-mm chisel as a scalpel. However, during this procedure, epithelial cells may be transported under the skin; this may lead to a rigid epidermal cyst that occurs within a few weeks postoperatively and can only be removed by skin excision (Fig. 7.7).

If the internal technique with a saw is used for transverse osteotomy, a specially designed saw is placed just below the peak of the open roof and perpendicular to the nasal bone (Fig. 7.8).

Then, with small movements along the planned transverse line, the blades of the saw pierce the bone. When the saw is placed on the bone, the incision is completed with upward and downward movements along the line. A full-fold incision is not required. With minimal compression after lateral osteotomy, the bone can be mobilized medially (Fig. 7.9).

7.2.1.1 Saw for Transverse Osteotomy

This new instrument, which is used only for transverse osteotomy during rhinoplasty, produces a single, precise cut during osteotomy. It is designed with a slight curve to adapt fully to nasal bones during transverse osteotomy (Fig. 7.10).

7.2.2 Lateral Osteotomy

As in transverse osteotomy, lateral osteotomy can be performed internally or externally. If external perforation is to be performed, as in transverse osteotomy, a straight 2-mm chisel is used. First, an incision is made on the skin in the nasofacial sulcus, typically in the middle of the osteotomy line; the chisel is then passed through this cut. Upward and downward maneuvers are made in the osteotomy area to shift the angular vein and artery. Osteotomy then begins from the pyriform aperture and continues up to the medial canthus by perforation at 2–3 mm intervals on the line, followed by medialization of the bone with slight finger pressure. Determination of the line with a marker before osteotomy is useful (Fig. 7.11).

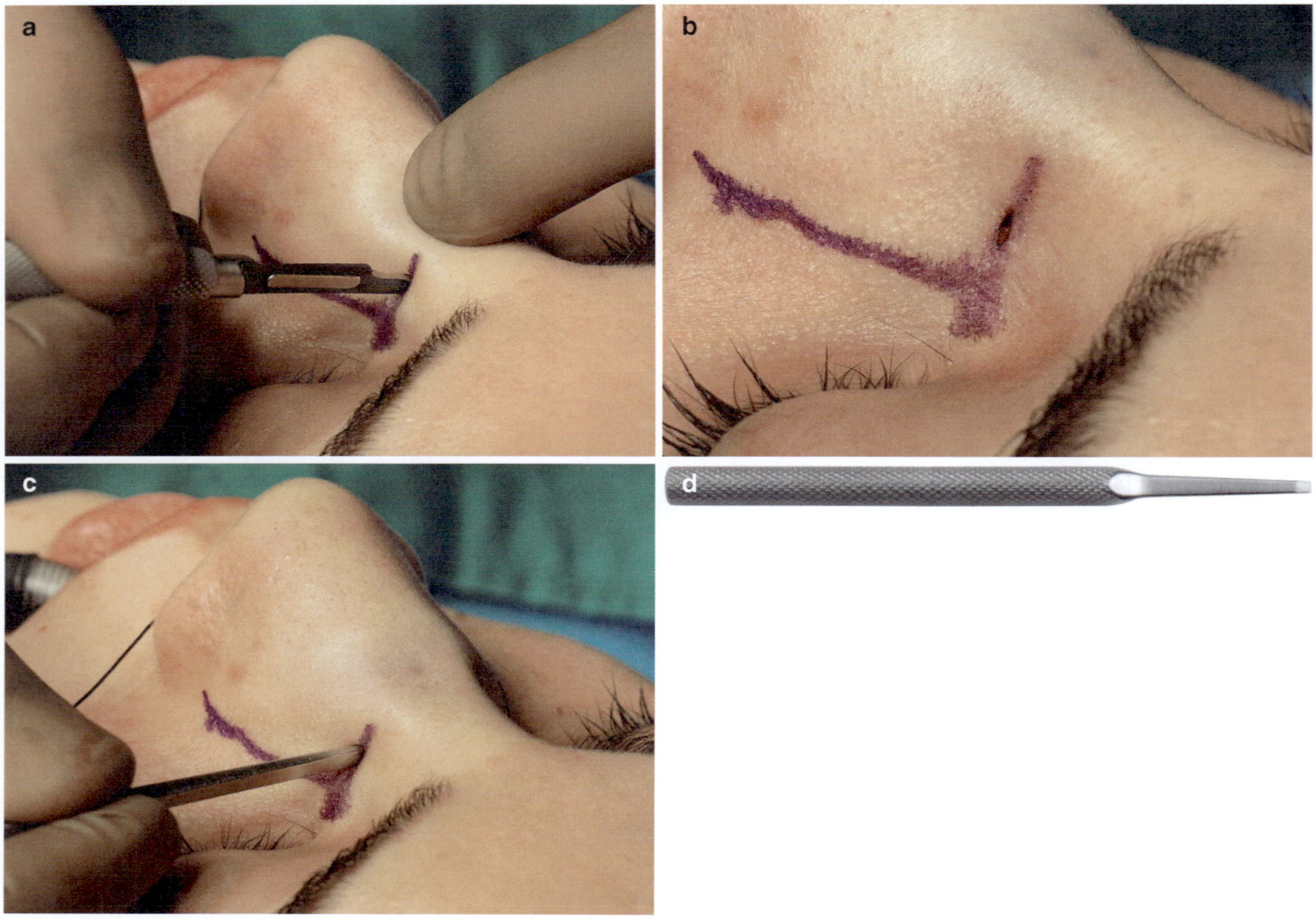

Fig. 7.6 (**a**, **b**) Skin incision for external transverse osteotomy. (**c**) Osteotomy is performed with a 2 mm chisel through the incision. (**d**) 2 mm chisel

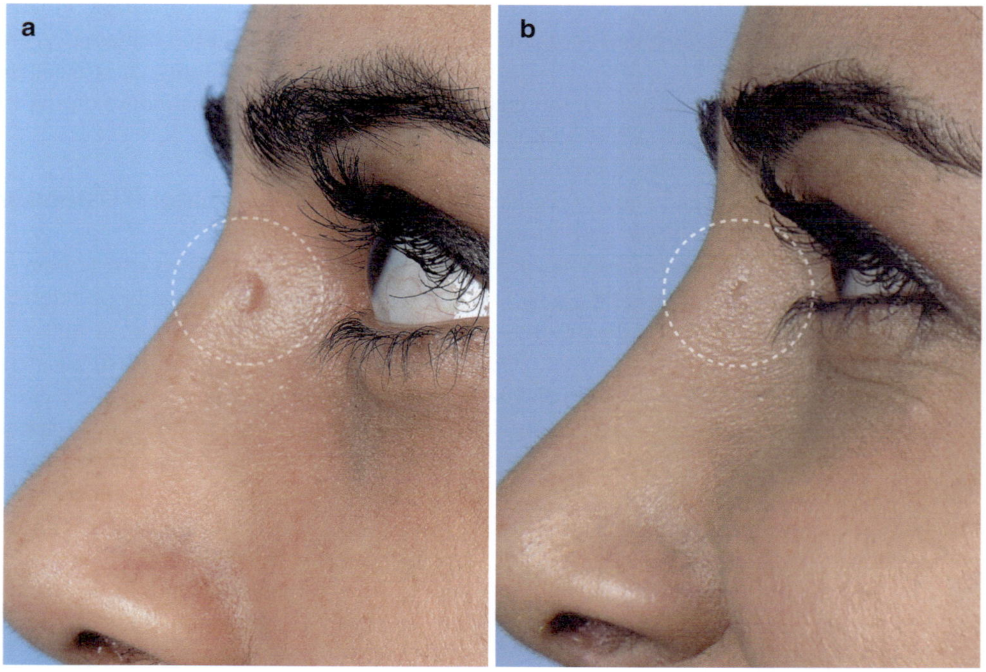

Fig. 7.7 (**a**) Epidermal cyst. (**b**) 6 months after cyst excision

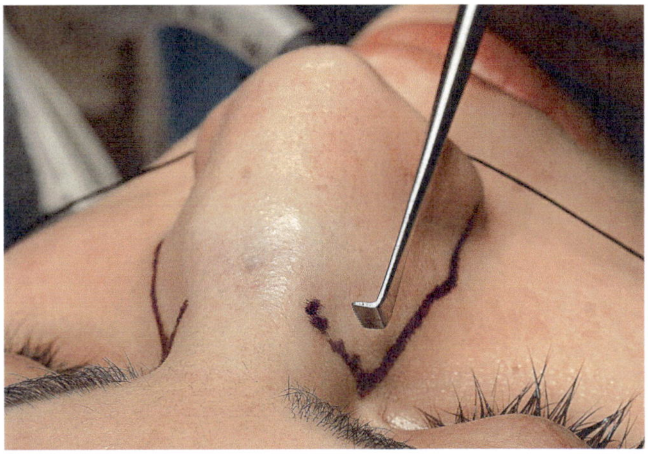

Fig. 7.8 Transverse osteotomy with the saw

If internal continuous osteotomy is preferred, either a guided osteotome or a saw is used in the conventional method (Fig. 7.12).

The starting point of the lateral osteotomy with both instruments is immediately above the anterior attachment point of the inferior concha. Thus, the inferior concha is excluded from the osteotomy line and potential functional problems related to breathing are prevented. A small incision is made immediately above the attachment point of the inferior concha (Fig. 7.13).

If a guided osteotome is to be used, the osteotome inserted into the incision is first directed to the lateral canthus. While in this position, the assistant taps the osteotome with a hammer so that the osteotome fits appropriately into the bone. The osteotome is then directed to the medial canthus. The

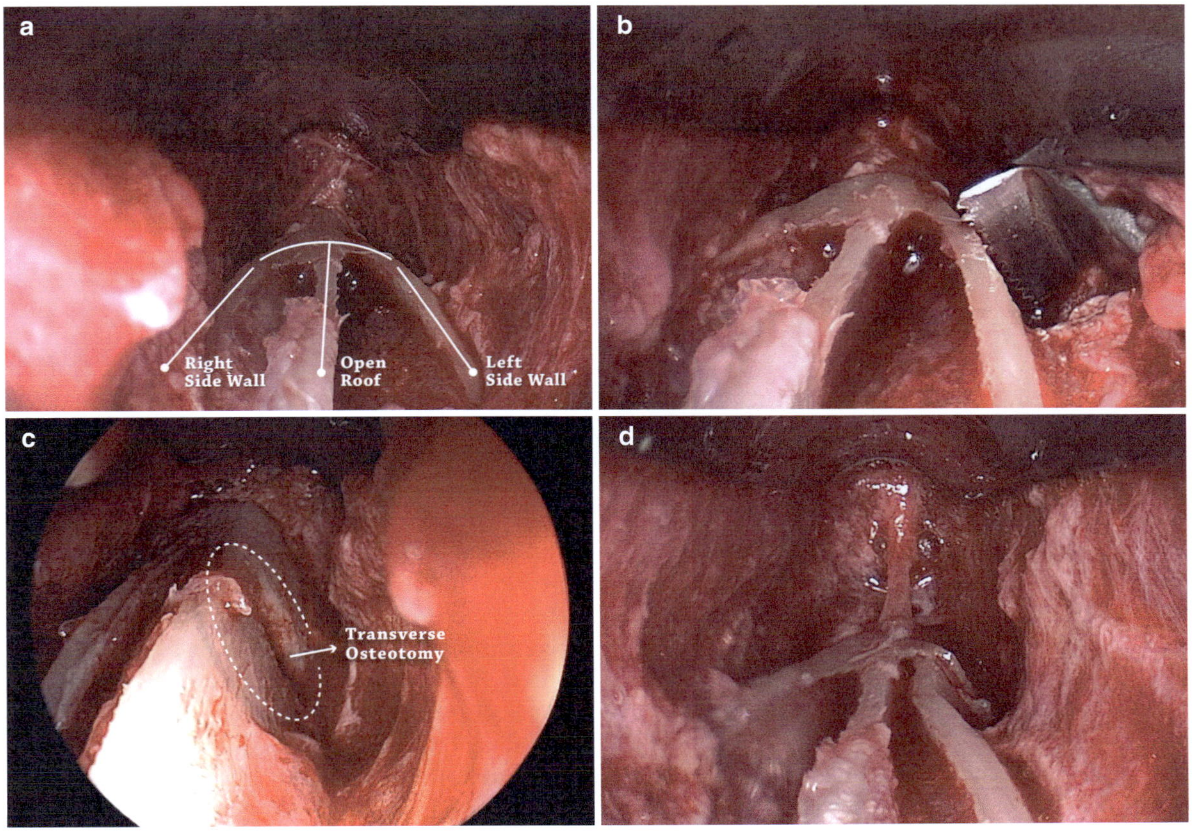

Fig. 7.9 (**a**) Roof of the nose is opened after hump removal. (**b**) Saw is placed to the cephalic part of the open roof. (**c**) Transverse osteotomy is performed. (**d**) Left nasal wall is mobilized and pushed toward to septum

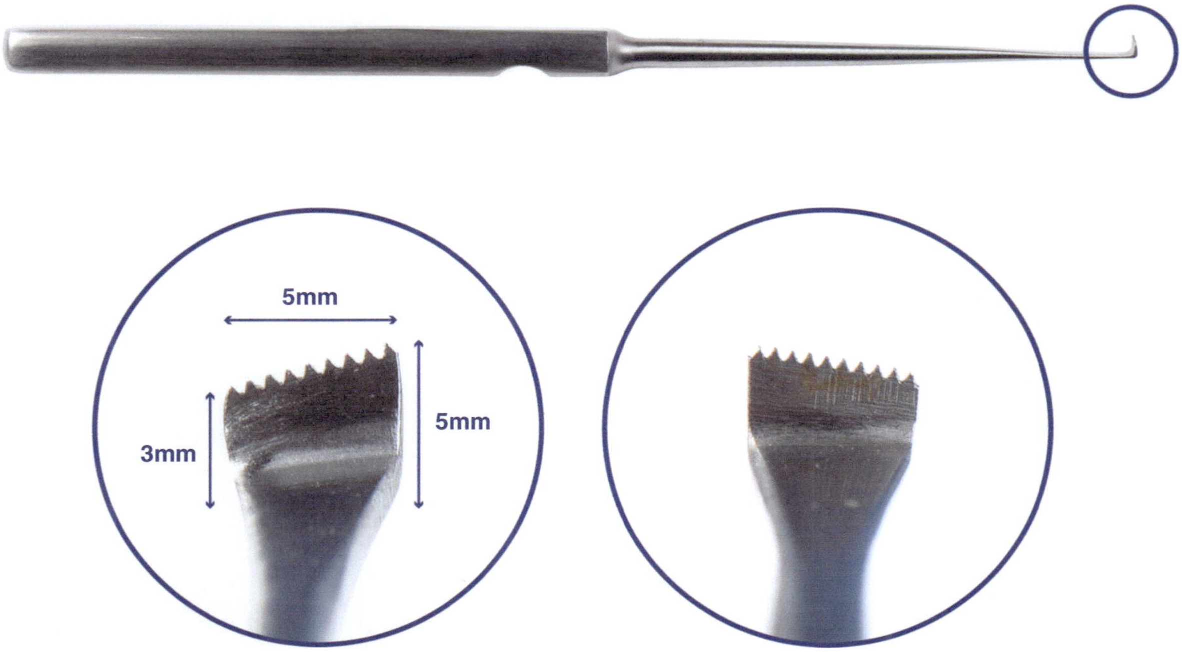

Fig. 7.10 Transverse osteotomy saw

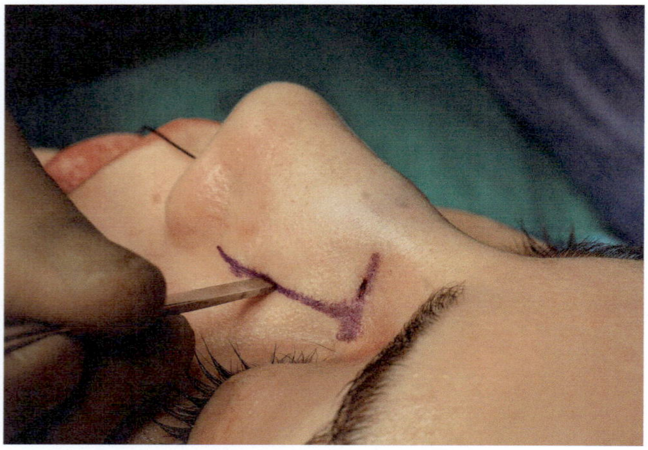

Fig. 7.11 External lateral osteotomy with chisel

lateral osteotomy is completed with an incision that extends to the medial canthus with soft but effective strokes (Fig. 7.14).

7.2.2.1 Saw for Lateral Osteotomy

Traditional saws or specially designed thin lateral osteotomy saws can be used during the procedure. The lateral saw is made of hardened stainless steel, and the distance between its teeth is 1 mm. These saws allow a safer and more predictable approach to lateral osteotomy (Fig. 7.15).

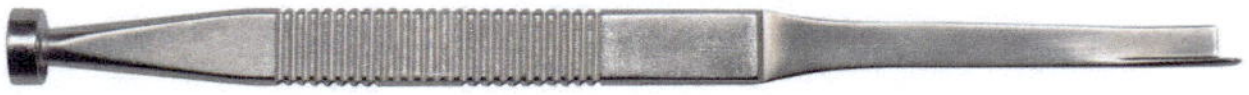

Fig. 7.12 Lateral osteotomy

If a lateral saw is used, its teeth are first placed in the bone by movement backward and forward along the drawn line, and the bone incision is then completed with soft backward and forward movements (Fig. 7.16).

Regardless of the instruments used, the author has found it unnecessary to create a tunnel from the periosteum prior to osteotomy. In the author's clinical practice, he observed that swelling and ecchymosis were more common in patients when a tunnel was created. To reduce postoperative edema and ecchymosis, and to achieve optimum aesthetic results, conventional osteotomy alternatives (e.g., electrical instruments) are widely used in daily practice, depending on the surgeon's preference and experience. Many studies have compared the benefits and limitations of these two methods. Although the indications for lateral osteotomy are clear, the optimal method remains an important point of discussion.

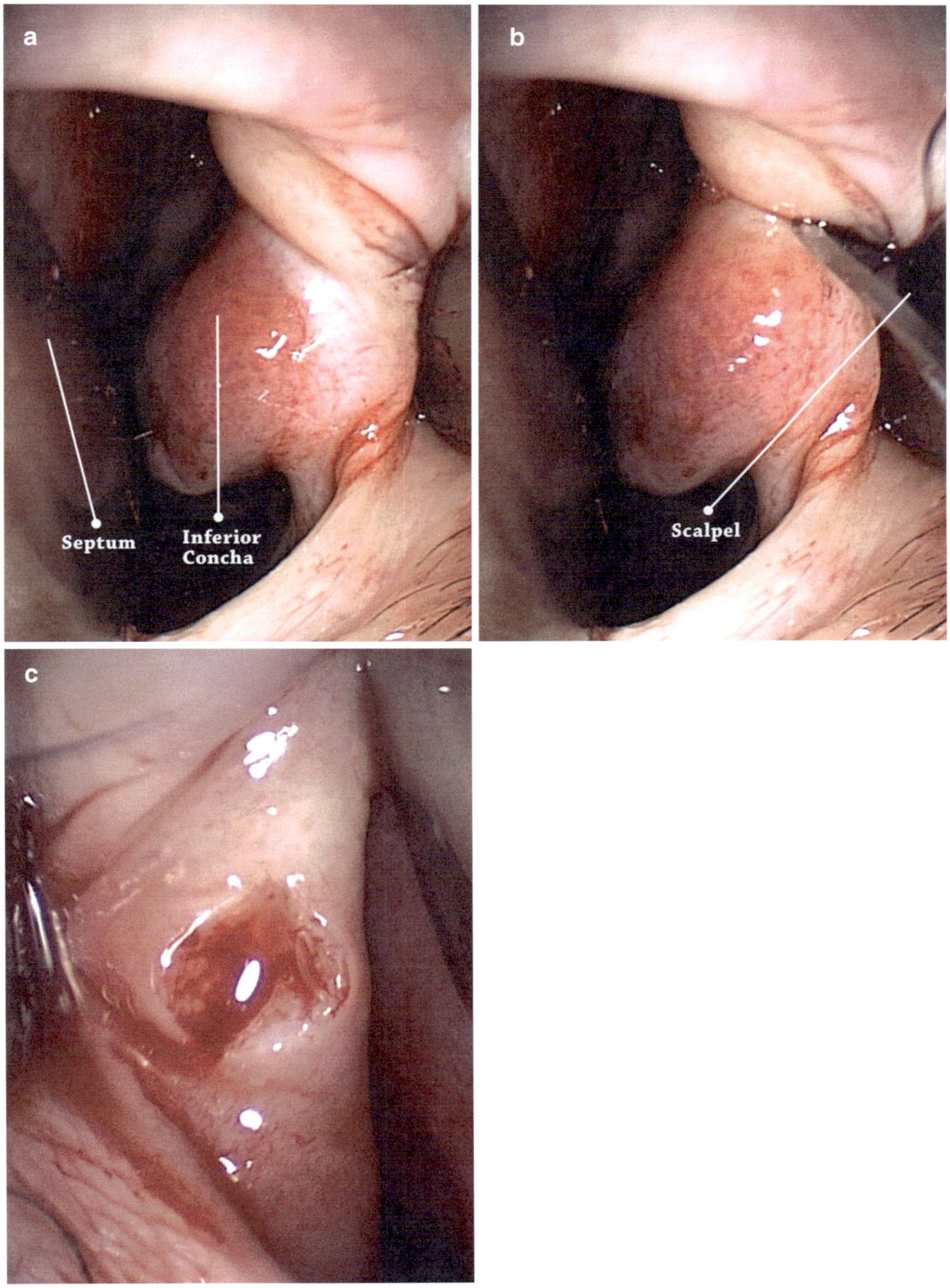

Fig. 7.13 (**a–c**) Lateral osteotomy incision is performed just superior to anterior attachment of the inferior concha

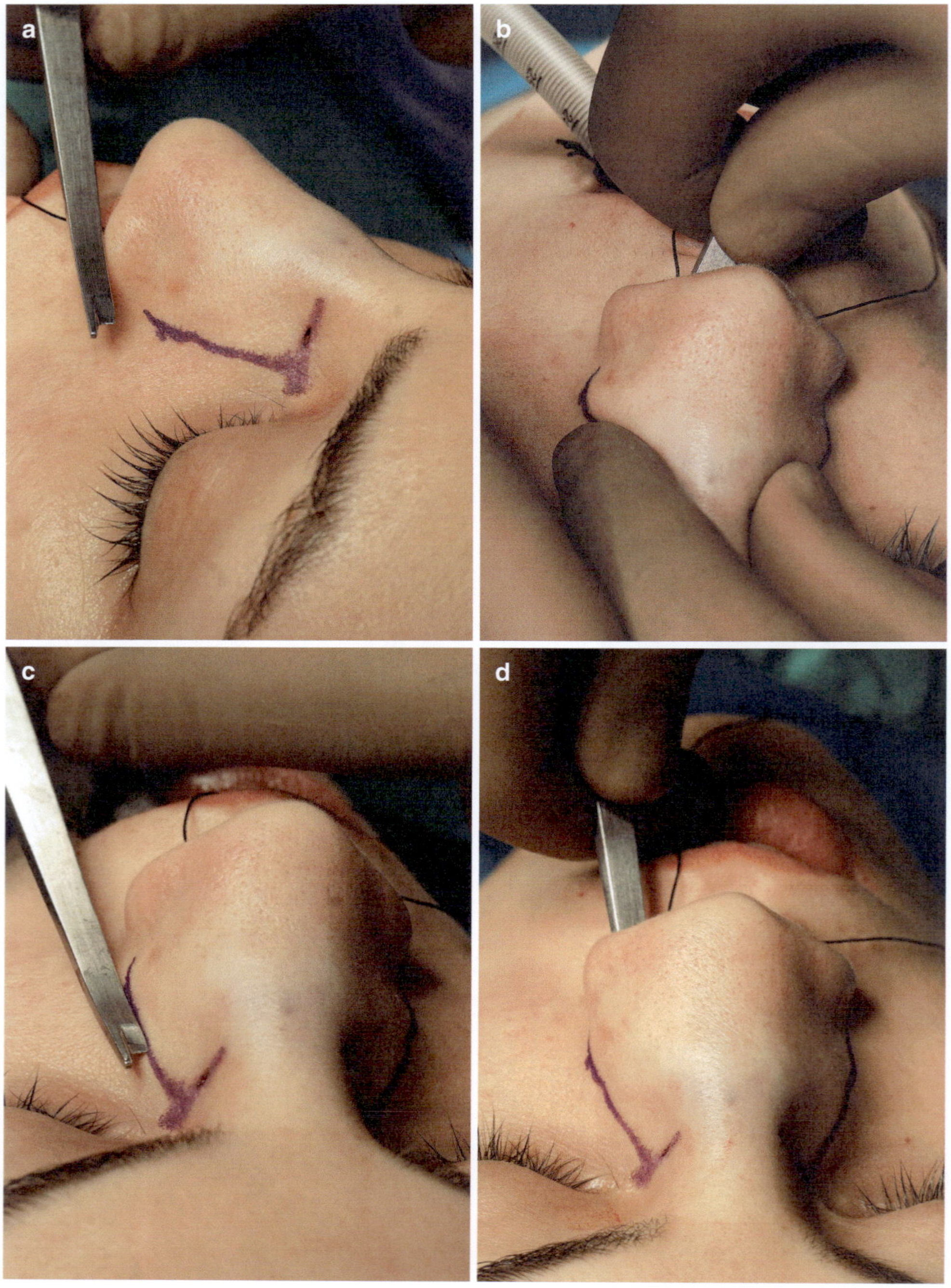

Fig. 7.14 (**a**, **b**) The osteotome is directed to lateral canthus. (**c**, **d**) Preserving the anterior attachment of inferior concha, the osteotome is directed to medial canthus

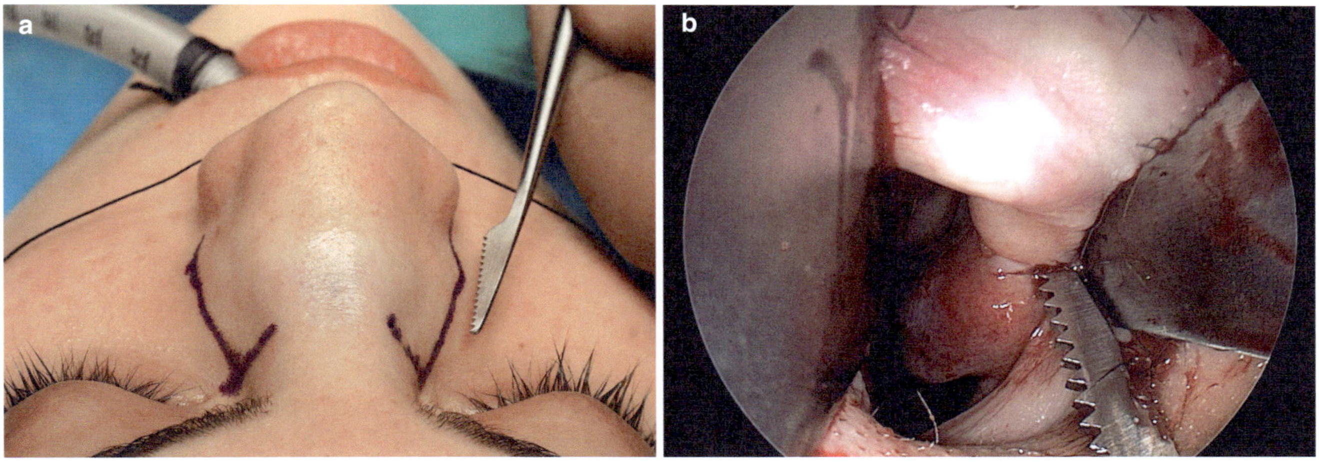

Fig. 7.15 Lateral osteotomy saw

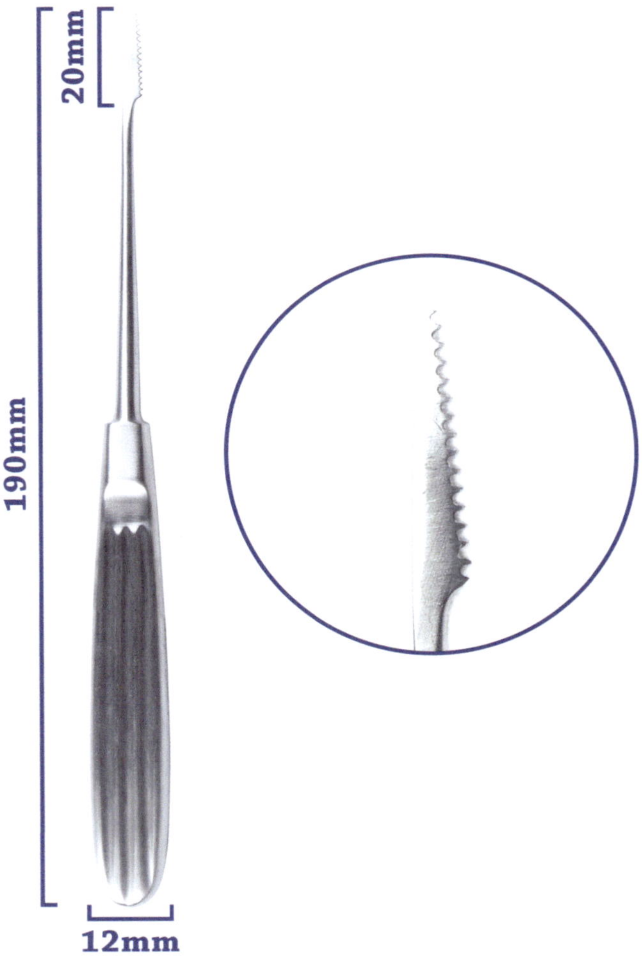

Fig. 7.16 (a, b) Lateral osteotomy with saw

7.3 How Can We Use Osteotomy in Cases?

Because performance of osteotomy is discussed generally, various osteotomy techniques are shown in representative cases.

7.3.1 Wide Nasal Bones

In an ideal nose, the widest part of the bone base should remain within 1–2 mm of the imaginary line drawn perpendicular from the medial canthus. In situations where the medial canthus lines are exceeded, a wide nasal base becomes the focus of the operation; lateral osteotomy is the solution, as it narrows and optimizes the wide nasal base (Fig. 7.17).

In such cases where a lateral osteotomy is needed due to a wide nasal base, the proper base–dorsum relationship should be established. In this context, there are three possible base–dorsum relationships:

- Wide base and uncomplicated dorsum
- Wide base and narrow dorsum
- Wide base and wide dorsum

7.3.2 Wide Base and Uncomplicated Dorsum

In patients who have a wide nasal base without a prominent dorsum problem, lateral and transverse osteotomies are typically sufficient for base narrowing. The open roof is closed

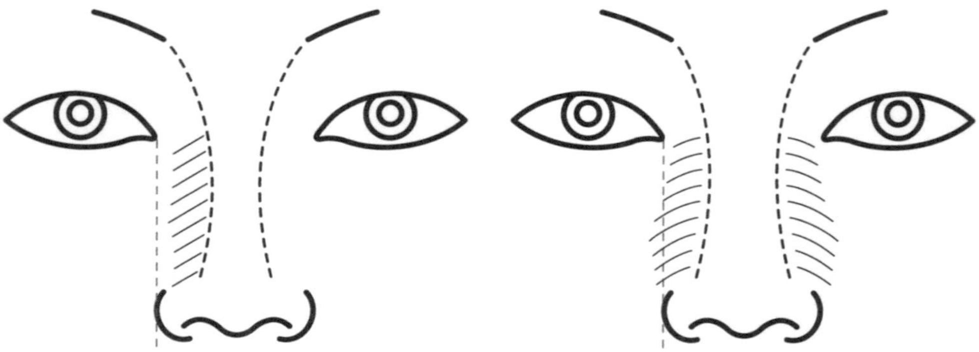

Fig. 7.17 The ideal width of the bony base (*left*); the wide bony base (*right*)

as a result of both osteotomies and the bone is narrowed at the base. *The middle vault is reconstructed before or immediately after osteotomy to provide the ideal dorsum and nasal base balance.*

7.3.2.1 Case 1

In this example with a broad base, the widest part of the bone base is marked with a blue dot. An excess of a few millimeters from the medial canthus line is the source of the broad base. Contraction of the base due to osteotomy is clearly observed. Transverse and lateral osteotomies were sufficient for base narrowing. Cartilage grafts were not used for closing the middle vault. Excess dorsal septal mucosa acted like a spreader graft (Fig. 7.18).

In 7-year postoperative photographs, the pyramid is narrower than before and the brow-tip aesthetic line is in a more aesthetically pleasing position (Fig. 7.19).

7.3.2.2 Case 2

In this case the main problem is the wide base, whereas there is no significant problem in the dorsum. Lateral and transverse osteotomies would be sufficient to narrow the wide base. A thin spreader graft was used for the left side. Two-year postoperative photographs show the outcome (Fig. 7.20).

7.3.2.3 Case 3

In another representative case, there is no problem with dorsal width, but the nasal base exceeds medial canthal lines; therefore, lateral and transverse osteotomies are sufficient to resolve the wide base. A spreader graft was used for the left side. Two-year postoperative photographs show the result (Fig. 7.21).

7.3.3 Wide Base and Narrow Dorsum

Lateral and transverse osteotomies are sufficient for base narrowing in patients with a wide base. However, an already narrow dorsum will be further narrowed by the impact of the osteotomy, which may cause some undesirable aesthetic and functional problems. To avoid this situation, bilateral spreader grafts must be used in patients with a narrow dorsum. The spreader enables the narrow dorsum to expand while narrowing the broad base, resulting in an ideal base–dorsum balance.

7.3.3.1 Case 4

A 25-year-old woman with no previous history of nasal surgery was unhappy with the appearance of her nose. The nasal bones were wide and the middle third was narrow. While the nasal base of osteotomy was narrowed, bilateral spreader grafts widened the middle vault (Fig. 7.22).

Five-year postoperative photographs show that the bony base is narrowed, resulting in osteotomy, and the proportion between the base and dorsum on the frontal view has been established (Fig. 7.23).

7.3.4 Wide Base and Wide Dorsum

The combination of a wide base and wide dorsum is a rare condition that requires adjustment of osteotomy design. *While lateral and transverse osteotomies are sufficient to narrow the broad bone base, medial osteotomy is needed to narrow the wide dorsum.* The septum is separated from the lateral nasal wall by medial osteotomy, while the dorsum is narrowed by the same volume of the separated part (Fig. 7.24).

7.3.4.1 Case 5

In this representative case of a wide base and wide dorsum, medial osteotomy was used to narrow the wide dorsum, while the amount of narrowing in nasal bones was sufficient to achieve the ideal width (Fig. 7.25).

The dorsum also contains the septal cartilage and upper lateral cartilages with nasal bones; therefore, a wide dorsum indicates that one or more of these structures has excessive size.

In patients with a wide base and wide dorsum, the wide cartilaginous dorsum may be caused by the thickness of the septal cartilage and upper lateral cartilage. This should be considered and the excess cartilages must be resected along a vertical line (Fig. 7.26).

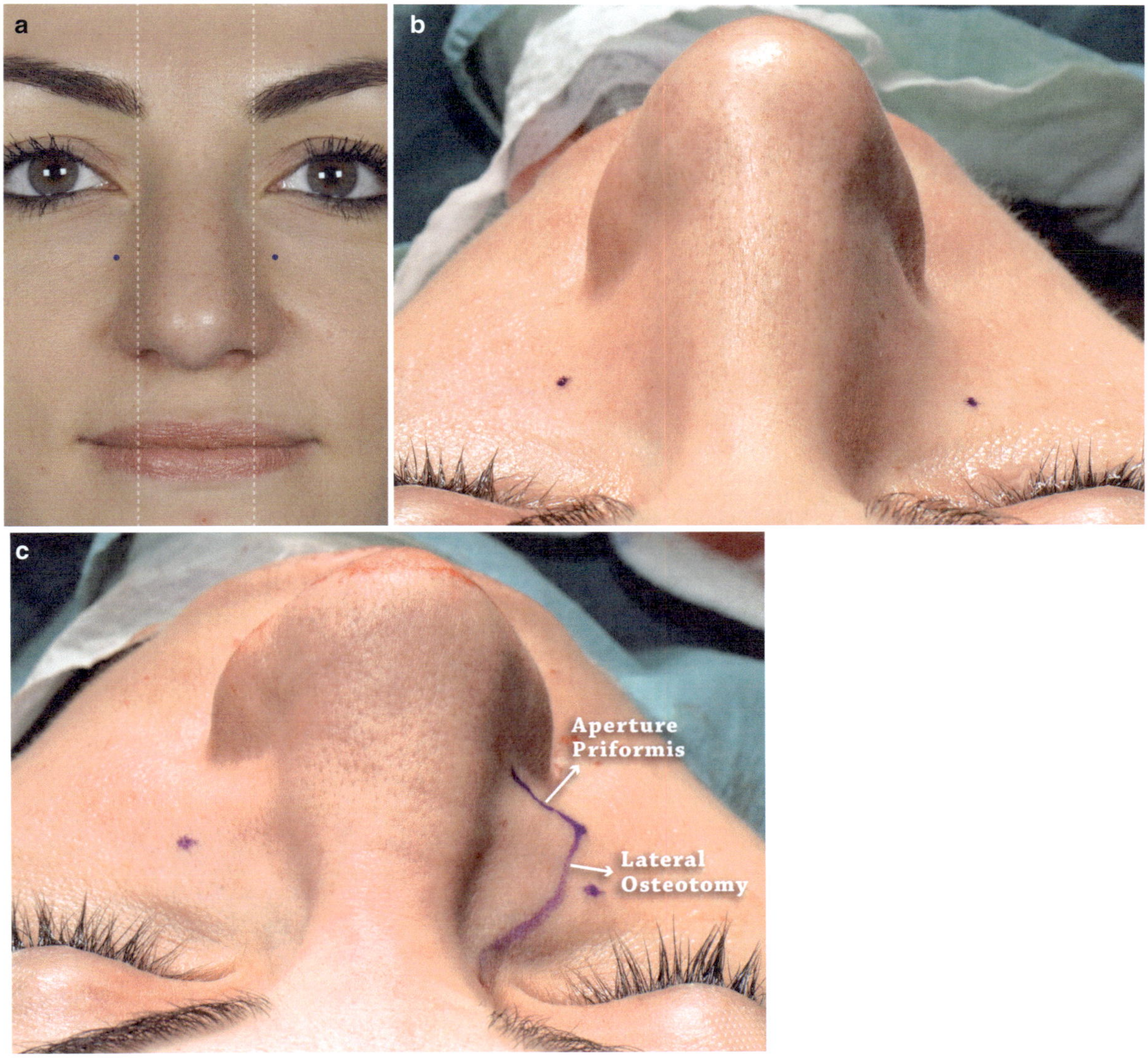

Fig. 7.18 (**a**) *Yellow dotted lines* indicate medial canthal lines; *blue points* indicate the bony base. The bony base is wider than intercanthal lines. Lateral osteotomies are needed to fix that wideness. (**b**) Intraoperative image before osteotomies. (**c**) Immediately after osteotomy, bony base is replaced with osteotomies

7.3.4.2 Case 6

Patient demonstrating overly wide nasal bones and dorsal width. Upper lateral cartilages and septal cartilage thickness cause a wide cartilaginous dorsum look. In this case, while bilateral medial osteotomy was performed to narrow the bony dorsum, excessive septal and upper lateral cartilages were resected to narrow the cartilaginous dorsum (Fig. 7.27).

Narrowing of the bony dorsum may be insufficient, despite the use of medial osteotomy. *In such situations, a second medial osteotomy is performed,* and the wedge-shaped bone piece remaining between the two osteotomies is removed. In this manner, the dorsum is narrowed by a volume equal to that of the bone removed (Fig. 7.28).

7.3.4.3 Case 7

In this case, the ideal dorsal width was achieved by removing the bilateral wedge-shaped bone pieced between the two medial osteotomies (Fig. 7.29).

Technical Pearl: In patients with a wide base and wide dorsum, if the dorsum is not sufficiently narrowed along with the nasal base, the base–dorsum relationship deteriorates. From the frontal view, the dorsum and base are oriented very closely to each other and form a "sausage nose" image.

A case with sausage nose who was operated by another surgeon is shown (Fig. 7.30).

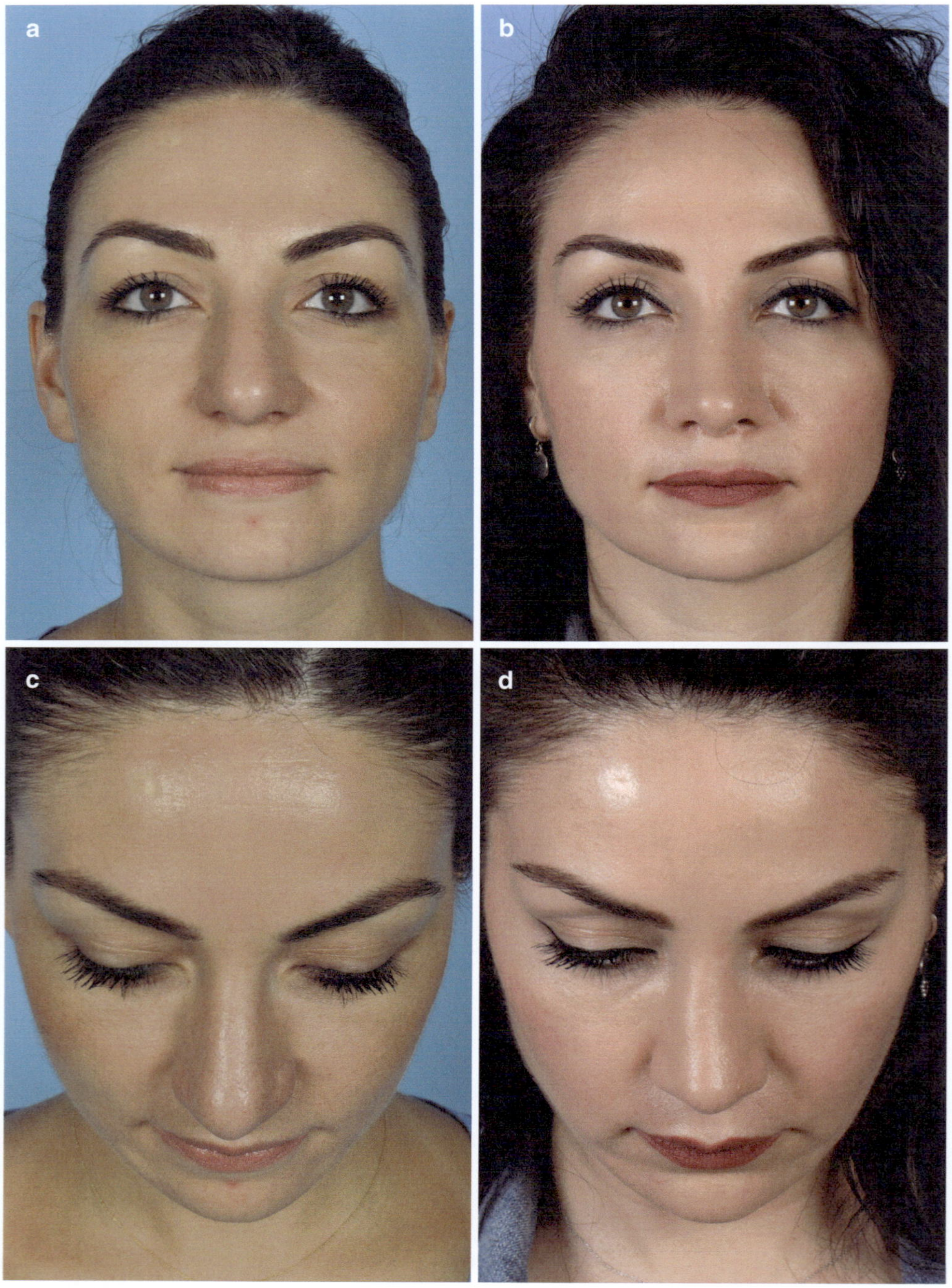

Fig. 7.19 (**a–d**) In this case with both wide nasal tip and wide nasal base, long and strong lateral cruses are the sources of the wide nasal tip. To restructure the wide nasal tip, the vertical alar resection technique was used

7.3.5 Asymmetric Bone Pyramid (Deviated Nasal Bone Pyramid)

If asymmetry is present between both nasal bone walls, symmetry can be achieved via osteotomy. The general rule also applies here. Lateral and transverse osteotomies are standard. To ensure symmetry, an additional lateral osteotomy is added from the asymmetrical wall to the more convex side (in practice, the longer side). Another osteotomy is performed 3–4 mm above and parallel to the lateral osteotomy, which is also known as intermediate osteotomy.

Technical Pearl: *Additional lateral osteotomy is performed on the more convex side wall* (Fig. 7.31).

If conventional osteotomies are preferred, upper osteotomy should be performed first, followed by lower osteotomy.

The double saw should be considered as an alternative to conventional double osteotomy, performed to the more convex side. Both upper and lower bone incisions are performed simultaneously using the saw. The bone piece between the two incisions is easily medialized and symmetry is ensured.

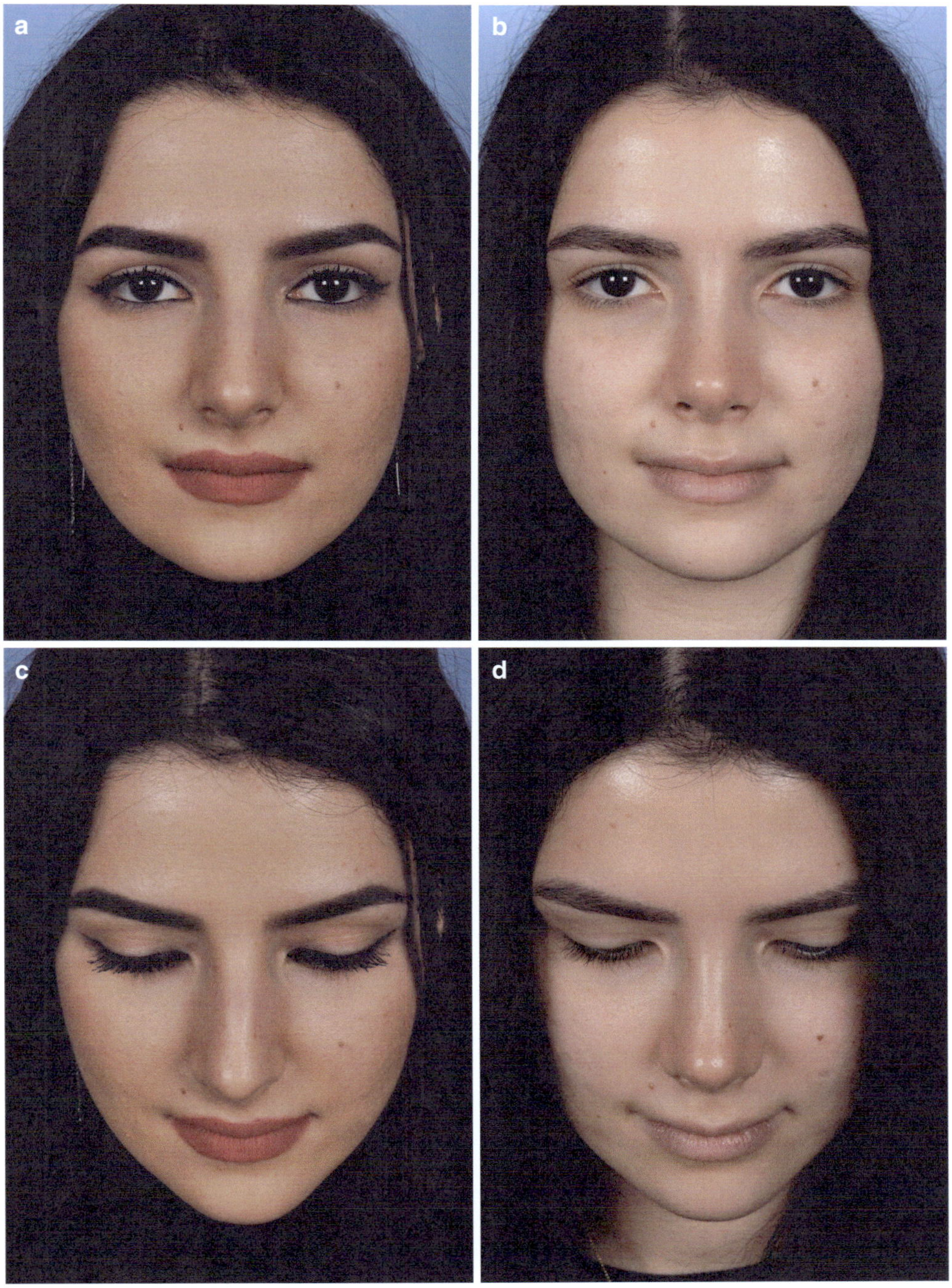

Fig. 7.20 (**a**, **b**) Before and 1 year after, pyramid narrowed. (**c**, **d**) Before and after. Brow-tip aesthetics improved

7.3.6 Double Saw

The double saw is similar to the lateral saw, but has two separate blades separated by a distance of 3 mm. The upper blade is used to perform intermediate osteotomy (Fig. 7.32).

7.3.6.1 Case 8

In this case, asymmetric nasal bone is evident, and left-sided bony deviation was corrected by double osteotomy. Double osteotomy was performed on the convex left side (Fig. 7.33).

After osteotomies, nasal axis deviation was corrected (Fig. 7.34).

7.3.6.2 Case 9

Here is another case of asymmetric nasal bone. Nasal bony deviation was corrected by performing double osteotomy on the convex left side (Fig. 7.35).

In patients with an asymmetric bony roof, particularly at the convex bony wall, if the bone is not mobilized or tends to return to its former position upon mobilization, the problem

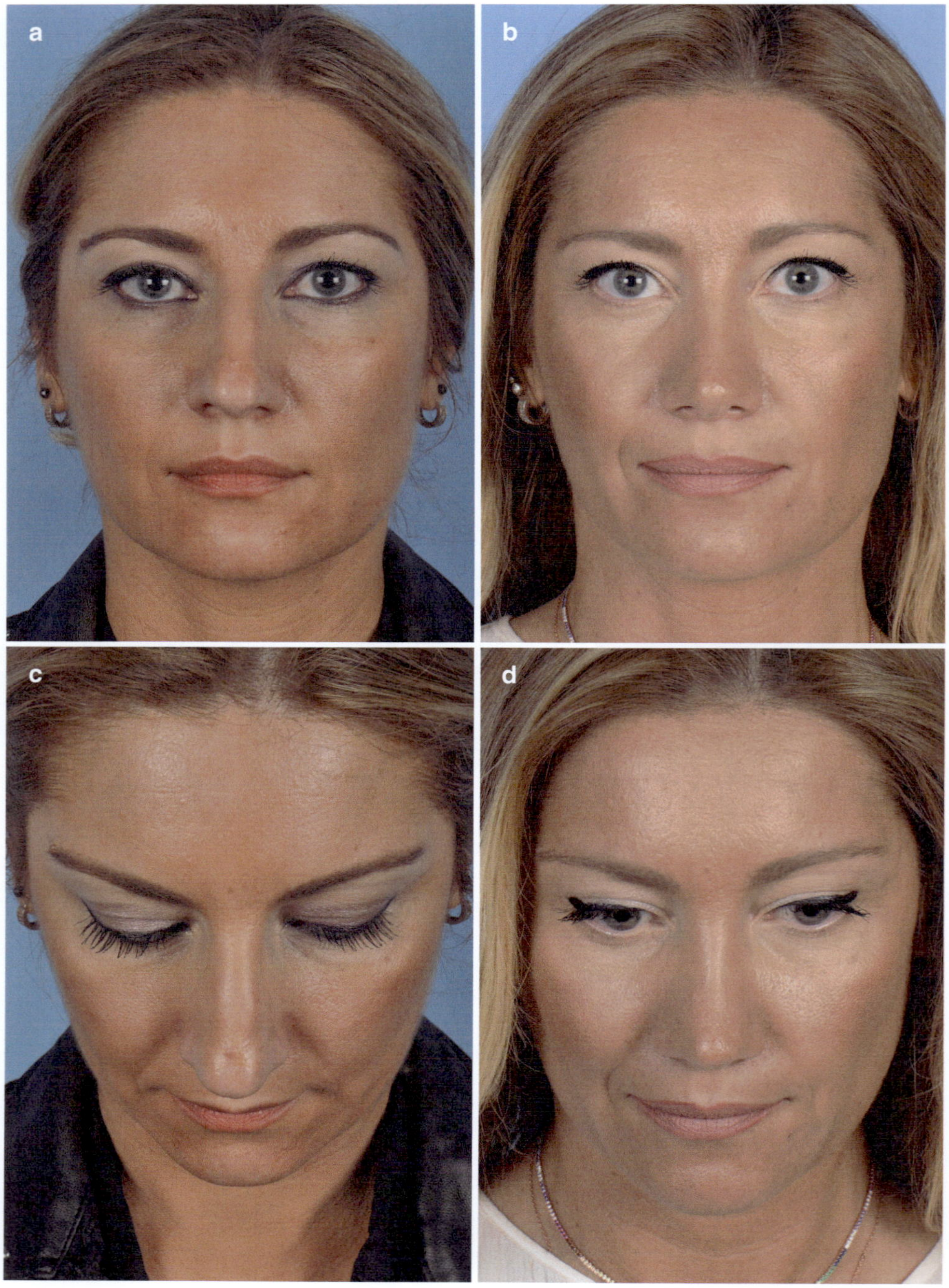

Fig. 7.21 (**a**, **b**) Before and after. The bony base now lies in a more aesthetically pleasing position. (**c**, **d**) Before and after. More favorable dorsal lines

may originate from the septum, despite the completion of osteotomies. High septal deviations, particularly at the middle concha level, prevent the bone in this section from reaching the midline (Fig. 7.36).

In such situations, the most convex part of the septum should be shaved. If the distance procured by shaving is insufficient, the septum should be weakened by multiple incisions parallel to the dorsum and extended to the midline. Scissors can be used for these incisions.

In the intranasal endoscopic view shown in Fig. 7.37a, the lateral nasal wall and septum are in contact and the middle concha is nearly hidden, due to increased septal deviation. In contrast, Fig. 7.37e shows a clearly visible mid-concha, as well as improved lateral nasal wall and septum contact, after surgical procedures (Fig. 7.37).

If high septal deviations are not detected and corrected during primary surgery, they may cause an opening in the osteotomy in the medium term.

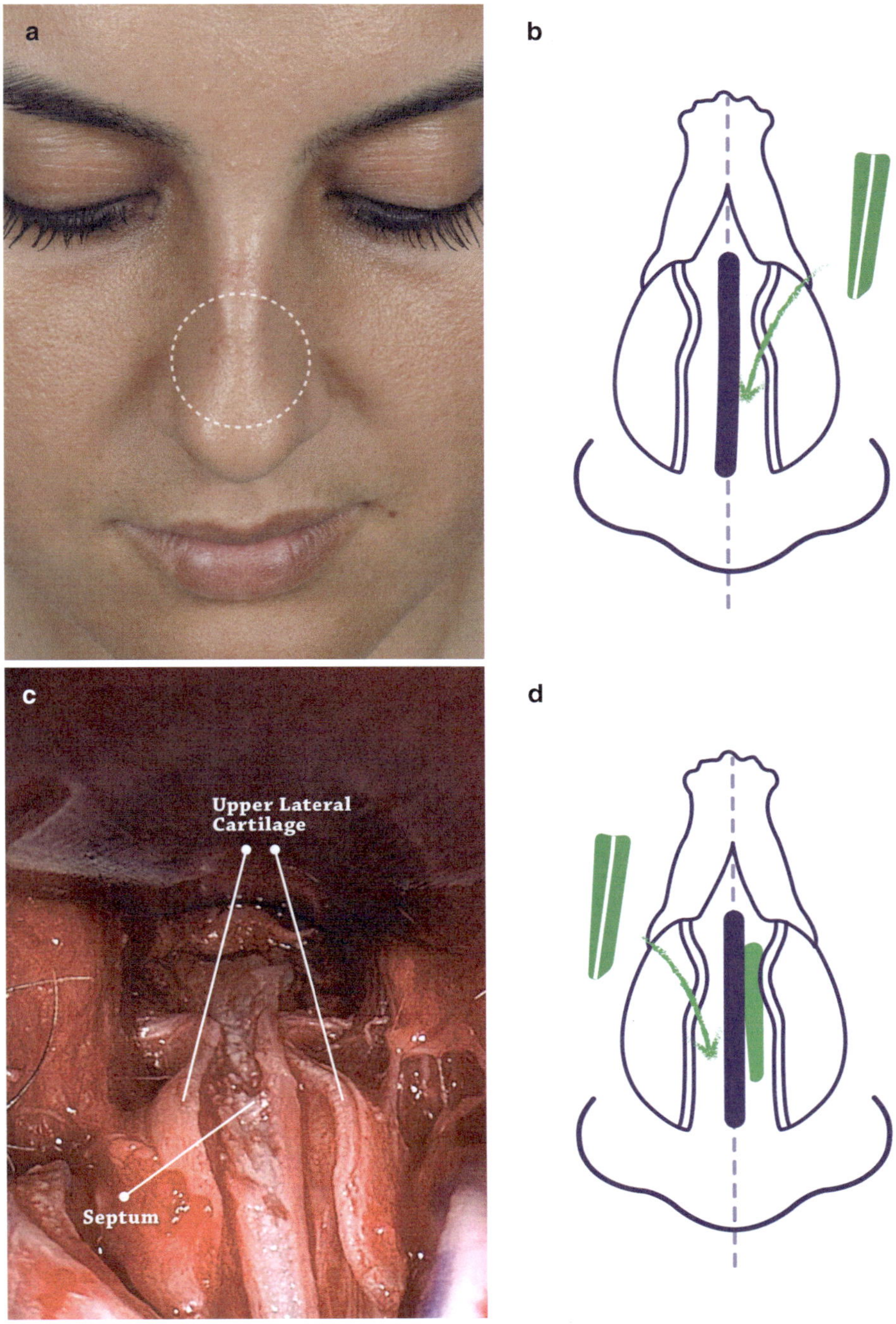

Fig. 7.22 (**a**, **b**) Preoperative frontal photograph and illustration, narrow dorsum is evident. (**c**, **d**) Upper lateral cartilages are concave, causing a narrow look. (**e**, **f**) Spreader grafts are placed bilaterally for an ideal base–dorsum balance

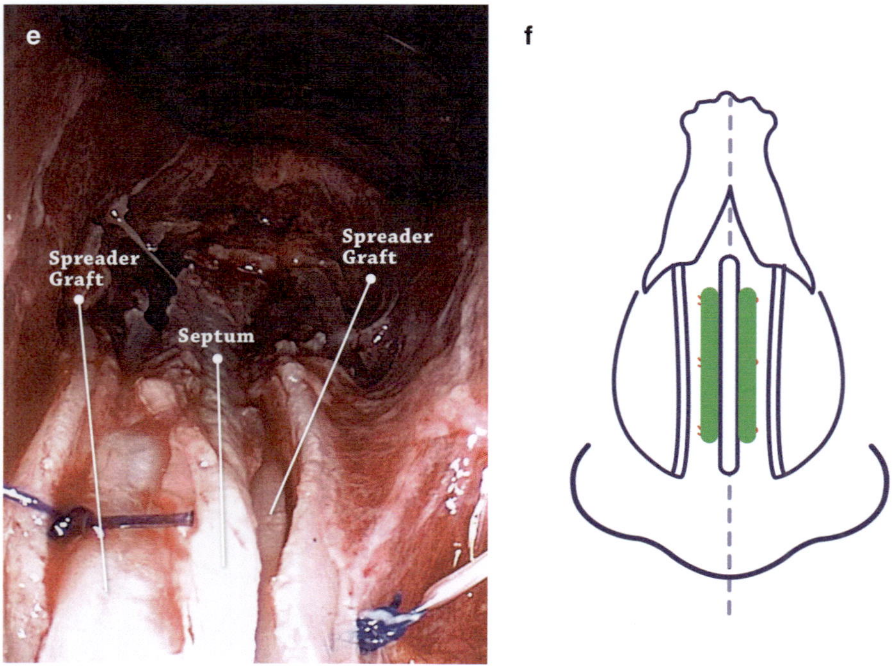

Fig. 7.22 (continued)

Fig. 7.23 (**a–d**) The upper third is narrower and the middle third is widened

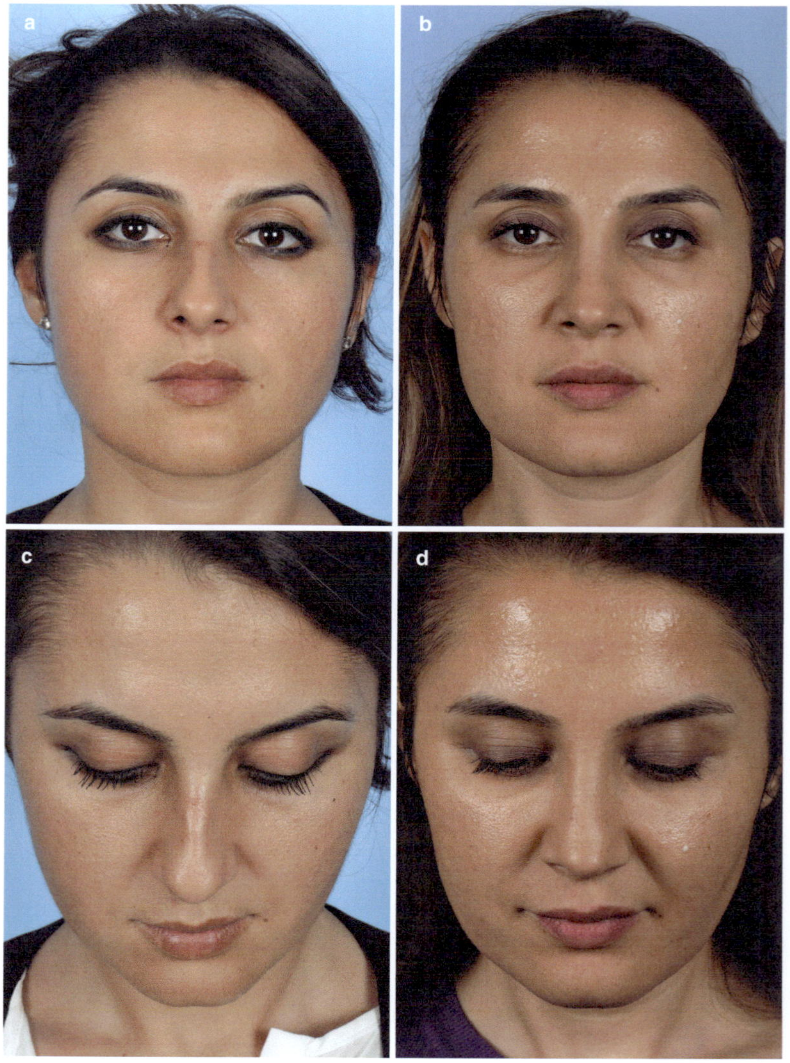

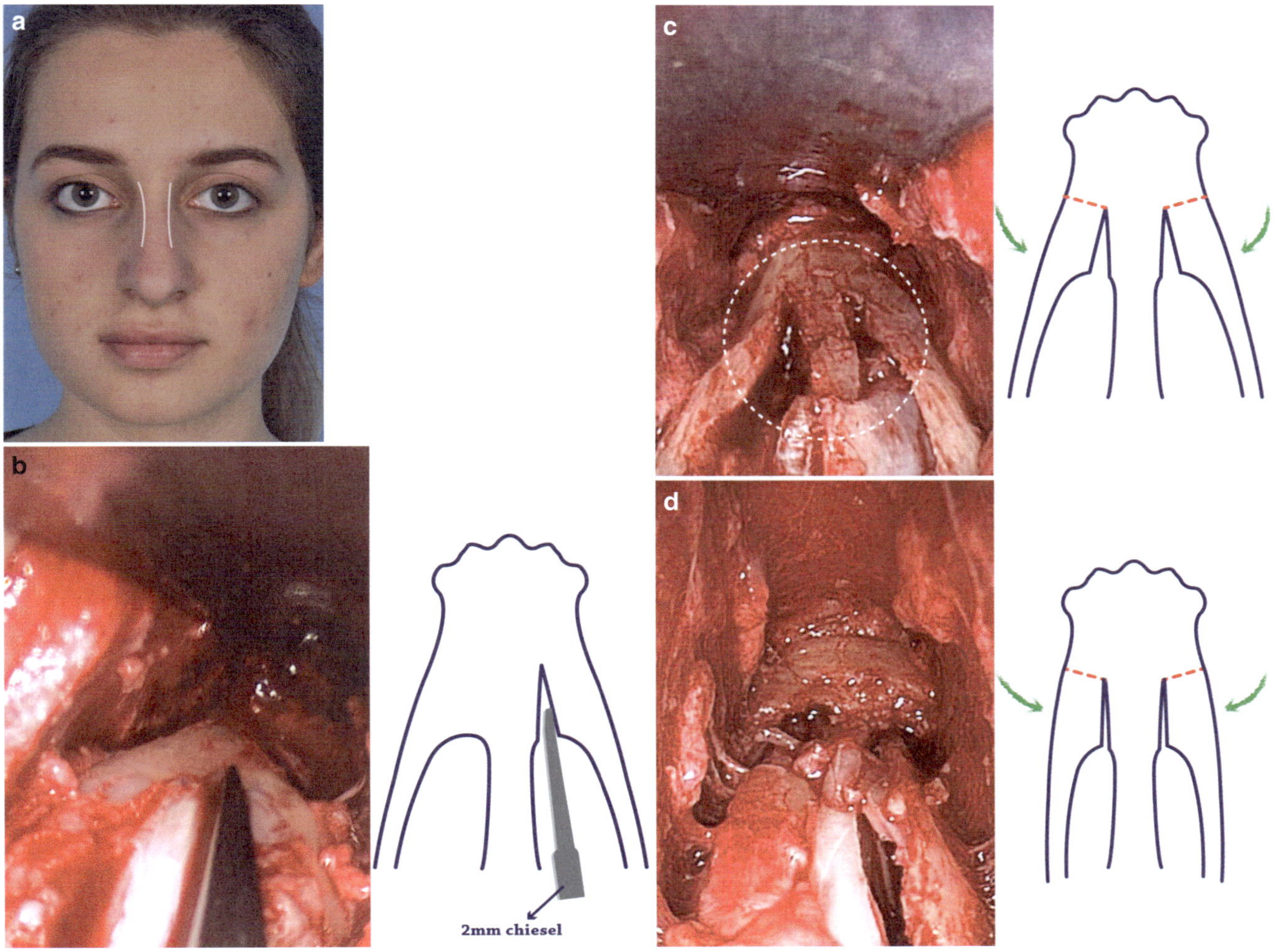

Fig. 7.24 (**a**) Preoperative photograph, wide nasal base is evident. (**b**) Chisel is placed from left side just near and parallel to septum. (**c**) Left medial osteotomy is performed. (**d**) Bilateral medial osteotomies are performed

7.3.6.3 Case 10

Approximately 10 years prior, the patient in this case underwent rhinoplasty surgery, performed by another surgeon. She had complaints about her wide nasal dorsum after surgery. Although osteotomy was performed, her nasal bones did not extend to the septum, which resulted in a wide dorsum (Fig. 7.38).

Revision surgery was performed by the author to correct these osteotomies. In dorsal endoscopic photos of the patient, the left nasal wall cannot be approximated to the midline, due to high septal deviation on the left side. Multiple longitudinal cuts were made to the septum; the deviation was corrected, and the septum was brought to the midline, which enabled nasal bone approximation to the midline after the osteotomies were performed (Fig. 7.39).

One-year postoperative photographs shown that the nasal pyramid is narrowed and open roof deformity is corrected (Fig. 7.40).

7.3.6.4 Case 11

In the photos of this representative case before primary surgery and immediately after osteotomy, the nasal bones approach each other in the midline, with the correct osteotomy (Fig. 7.41).

At 6 months postoperatively, however, there is an osteotomy opening, particularly on the left side. The bones tend to return to their former positions in time because neglected high septal deviation has pushed the lateral nasal wall (Fig. 7.42).

A revision surgery was performed. First, the left high septal deviation was corrected. Then osteotomies were reperformed (Fig. 7.43).

If the osteotomy is performed correctly, the long-term results will be satisfying.

7.3.6.5 Case 12

A 25-year-old woman requested a narrower appearance of her nose.

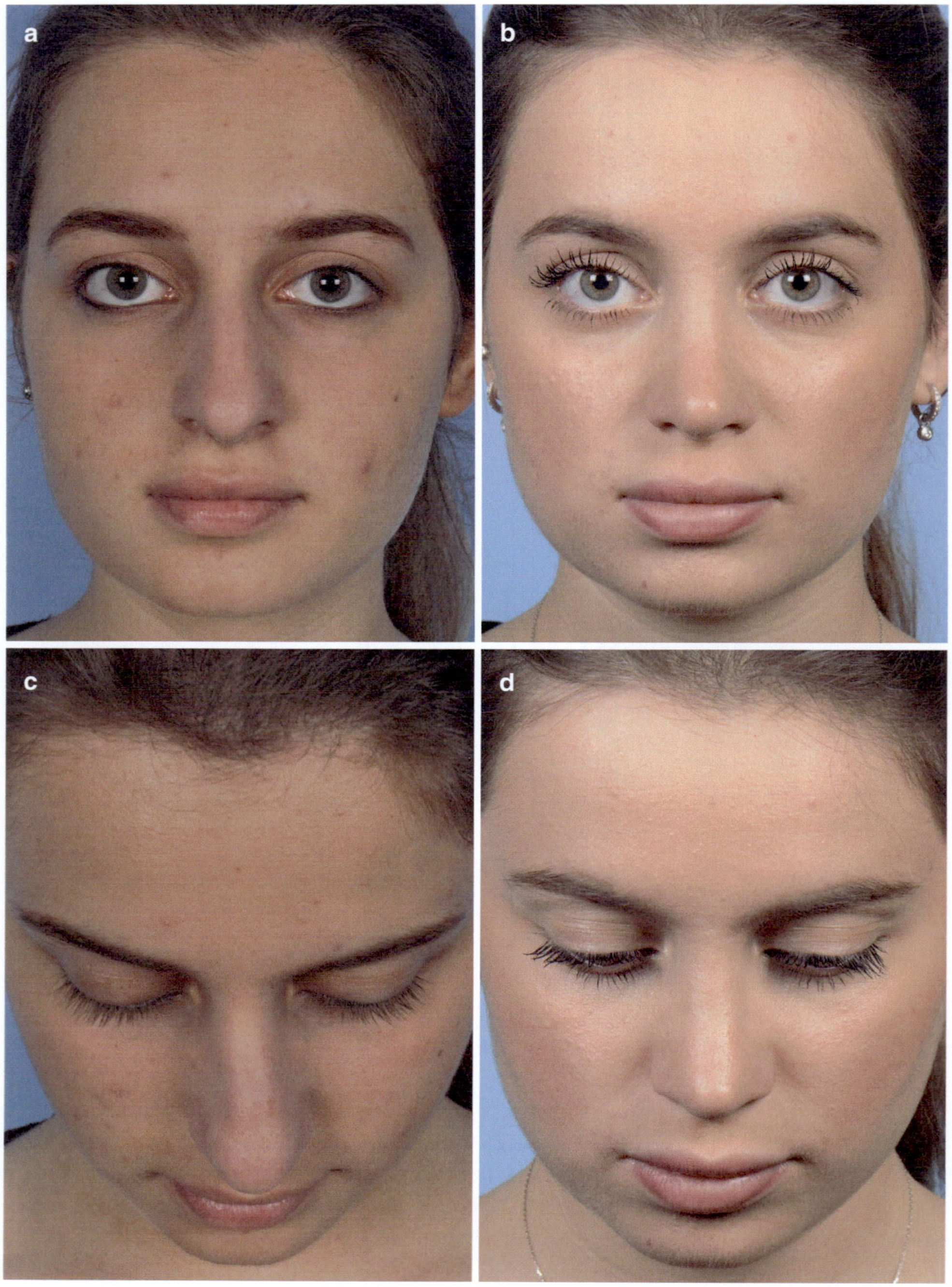

Fig. 7.25 (**a**) Preoperative photograph in frontal view. Wide nasal base, wide dorsum, and wide radix are evident. (**b**) 9-month postoperative photograph in frontal view. Both nasal base and dorsum are in their ideal positions. Narrowing of radix provides a more aesthetic transition for brow-tip aesthetic line. (**c**) Preoperative face-down photograph, wide bony dorsum is evident. (**d**) Postoperative face-down photograph, bilateral medial osteotomy was performed to narrow the dorsum

After hump removal, transverse and double lateral osteotomy were performed on the left side (more convex), and lateral and transverse osteotomy were performed on the contralateral side.

Preoperative and 15-year postoperative photographs show the result (Fig. 7.44).

7.3.7 Short Nasal Bone

Certain anatomic characteristics are relative contraindications to the use of osteotomies during rhinoplasty. It has been suggested that short nasal bone length may predispose patients to a greater risk of middle vault collapse after

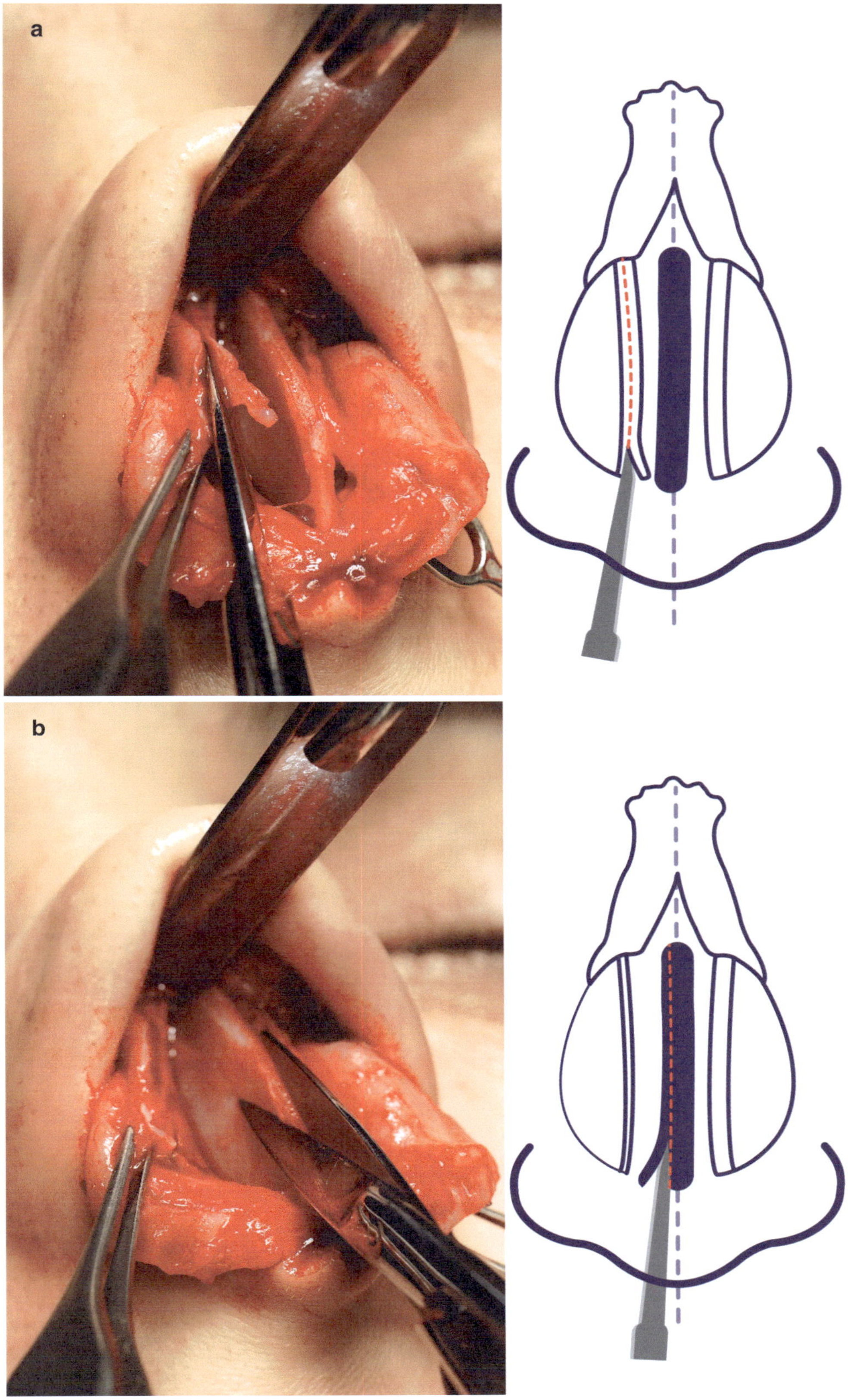

Fig. 7.26 (**a**) Upper lateral cartilage trimming via scissor or scalpel. (**b**) Septal cartilage trimming via scissor or scalpel

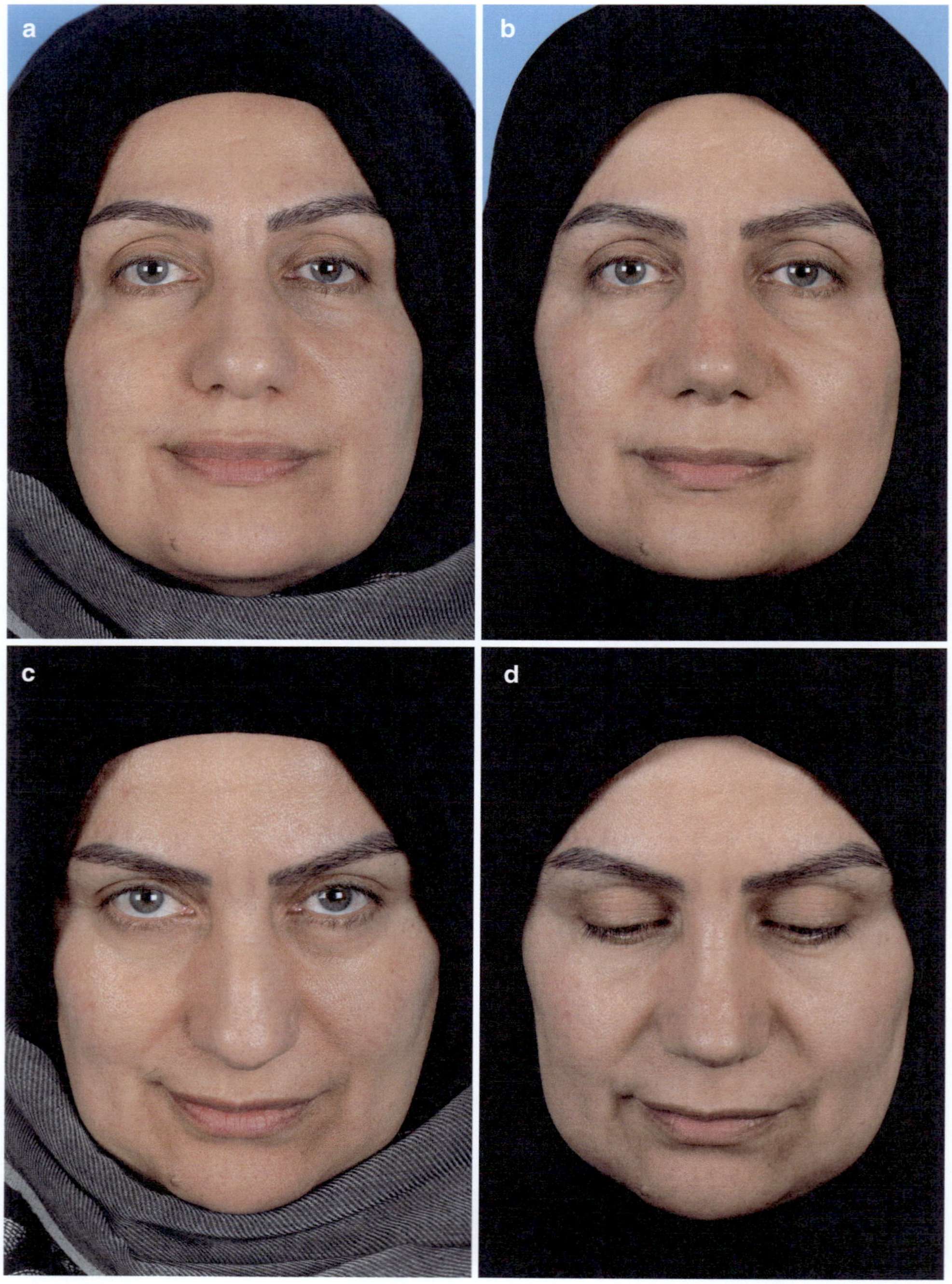

Fig. 7.27 (**a**, **c**) Preoperative and postoperative frontal and face-down photographs. (**b**, **d**) One-year postoperative photographs in frontal view, base–dorsum balance is ideal and brow-tip aesthetic line has a more aesthetic look. In this case, transdomal sutures, bilateral underlay lateral crural grafts, and columellar strut grafts are used for achieving the ideal nasal tip

osteotomy. Sheen and Sheen recommend against the use of osteotomies in patients with short nasal bones. In short nasal bones, the dorsal hump is almost entirely cartilaginous, and the resection of a cartilaginous roof and use of a spreader graft and camouflage graft constitute the main reconstruction method; osteotomy endangers the midvault and considerably reduces the support of the upper lateral cartilages. Therefore, there is a tendency for the upper lateral cartilages to collapse, causing nasal deformity and nasal valve obstruction.

To recognize a short nasal bone, its normal length must be known. Based on the findings of Setabutr's study, average external measurement of the nasal bone is 20.43 mm in normal cases; according to Sheen, 10 mm or less is regarded as a short nasal bone (distal border less than 1 cm beneath the intercanthal line) (Fig. 7.45).

In patients with a short nasal bone, a spreader graft can be used to close the open roof after hump removal.

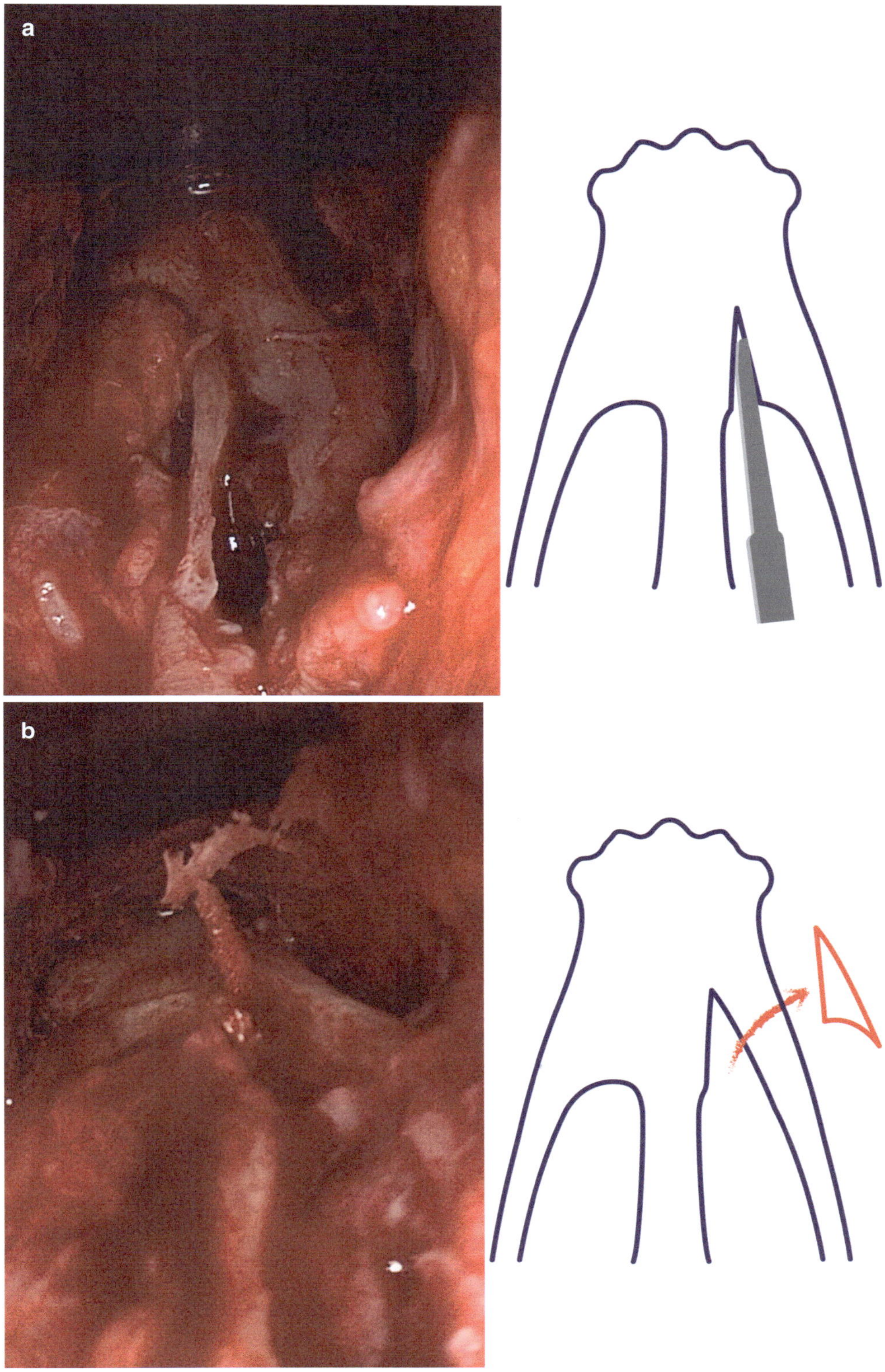

Fig. 7.28 (**a**–**c**) Left medial osteotomies and wedge-shaped bone removal

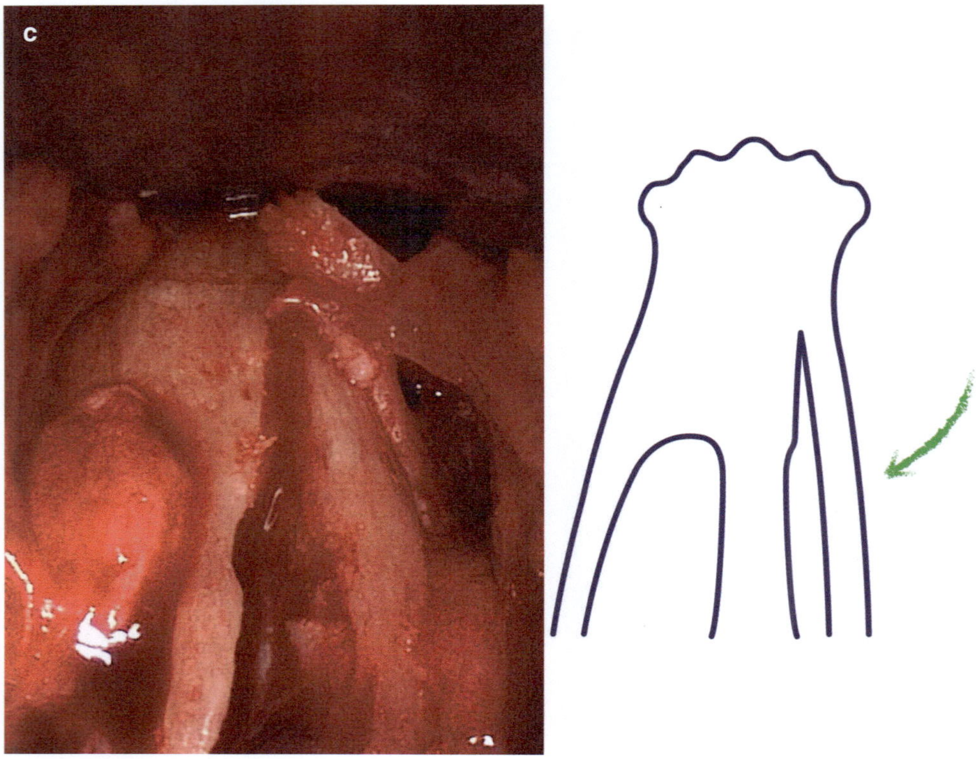

Fig. 7.28 (continued)

7.3.7.1 Case 13

In the representative case with a short nasal bone, after dorsal hump reduction, the open roof was closed with bilateral spreader grafts. No osteotomies or bone rasping were performed (Fig. 7.46).

If the nasal base is planned to be narrowed in the cases with a short nasal bone and wide bony base, the nasal bone base is rasped, and an osteotomy is not performed.

As in osteotomy, an incision is made with a scalpel immediately above the location where the inferior concha is attached. A very thin rasp is inserted through this incision, and the bone base is then rasped along the imaginary lateral osteotomy line. The operation is performed on both sides. Occasionally, the bony lateral nasal wall can also be rasped in cases where a short nasal bone is present with a good base width, but with convexity in the nasal walls.

7.3.7.2 Case 14

This patient desired a more elegant nose. Her dorsum and right bony base are wide with short nasal bones and the presence of a small dorsal hump (Fig. 7.47).

Osteotomy is not preferred in this case. Instead, the convexity in the right bony nasal wall is rasped. Bilateral spreader grafts were placed to close the open roof after humpectomy (Fig. 7.48).

Three years postoperative photographs show the outcome (Fig. 7.49).

7.3.8 Narrow Nasal Base

Although rarely observed, some patients exhibit a nasal hump along with a narrow or ideal bone base. In these patients, lateral osteotomy to close the open roof after hump removal may further narrow the already limited base, leading to undesirable aesthetic and functional problems. In such situations, spreader grafts may be used instead of osteotomy to close the open roof after hump removal.

7.3.8.1 Case 15

In this representative case, the basic problem is the nasal hump, while the bone base appears to be in an ideal location. It was possible to achieve an ideal dorsum view without performance of lateral osteotomy, by closing the open roof with a spreader that extended to the end point of the roof after the hump was removed (Fig. 7.50).

7.3.8.2 Case 16

In another case, the patient had a dorsal hump and droopy nasal tip, combined with a lack of too wide nasal bony base width. After hump removal, the open roof was constructed

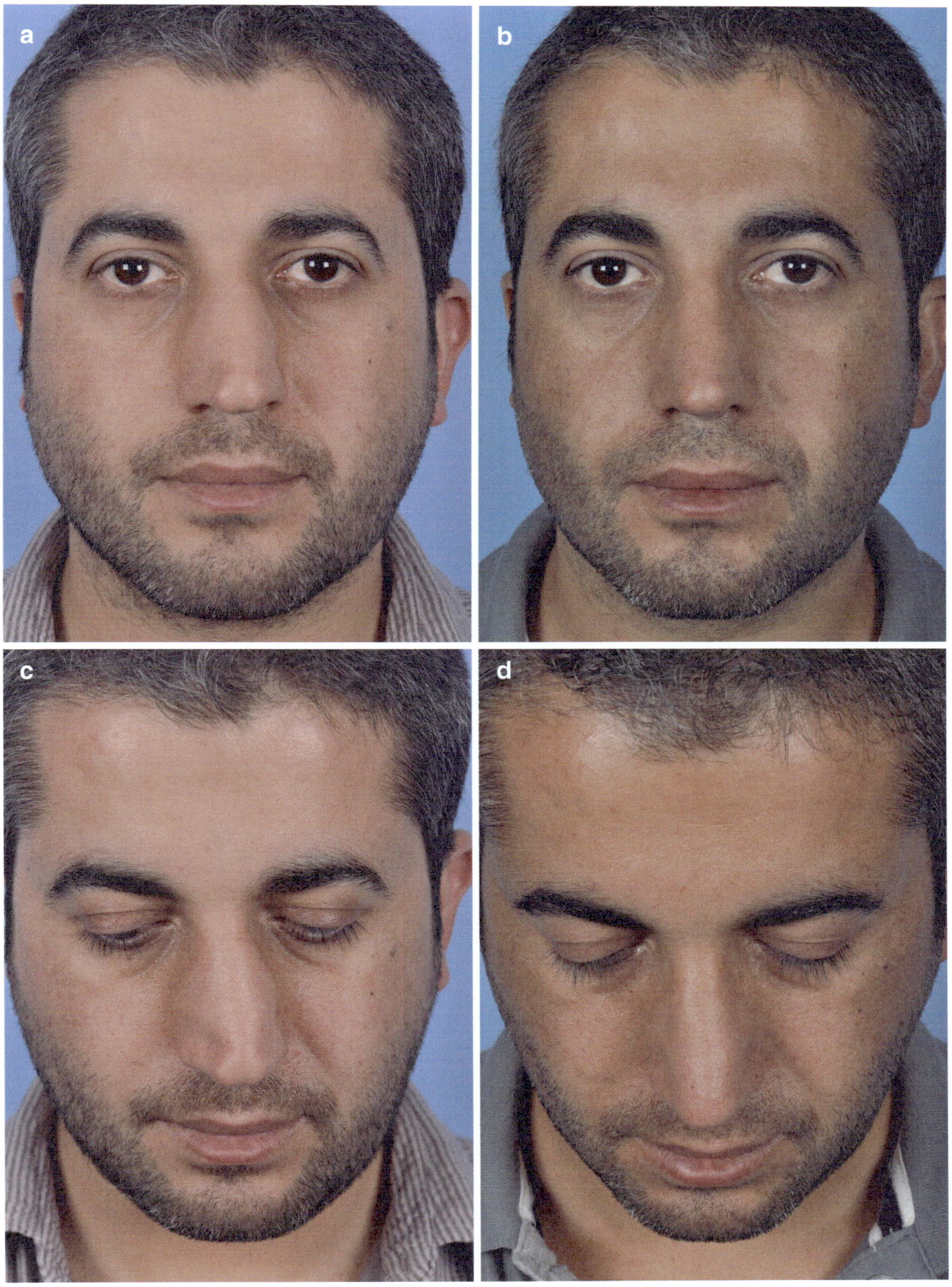

Fig. 7.29 (**a**–**c**) Preoperative frontal and face-down photographs. (**b**, **d**) One-year postoperative photographs in frontal view, base–dorsum balance is ideal and brow-tip aesthetic line has a more aesthetic look. In this case, transdomal sutures, bilateral underlay lateral crural grafts, and columellar strut grafts are used for achieving the ideal nasal tip

by spreader grafts and no osteotomy was performed (Fig. 7.51).

7.3.9 Narrow Nasal Root

In situations where the base of the nose narrows toward the radix, the imbalance between the nose root and middle of the nose continues because osteotomy narrows the nose base and nose root. To prevent this situation, it is necessary to exclude the root of the nose from the osteotomy. Transverse osteotomy, which begins from the open roof, should be extended in an oblique manner and meet with the lateral osteotomy more caudally than the level of the medial canthal ligament (Fig. 7.52).

7.3.10 Unique Situations

There are instances in which the nasal bone slant height is excessively short after hump removal, thus preventing sufficient narrowing to close the open roof deformity. When such

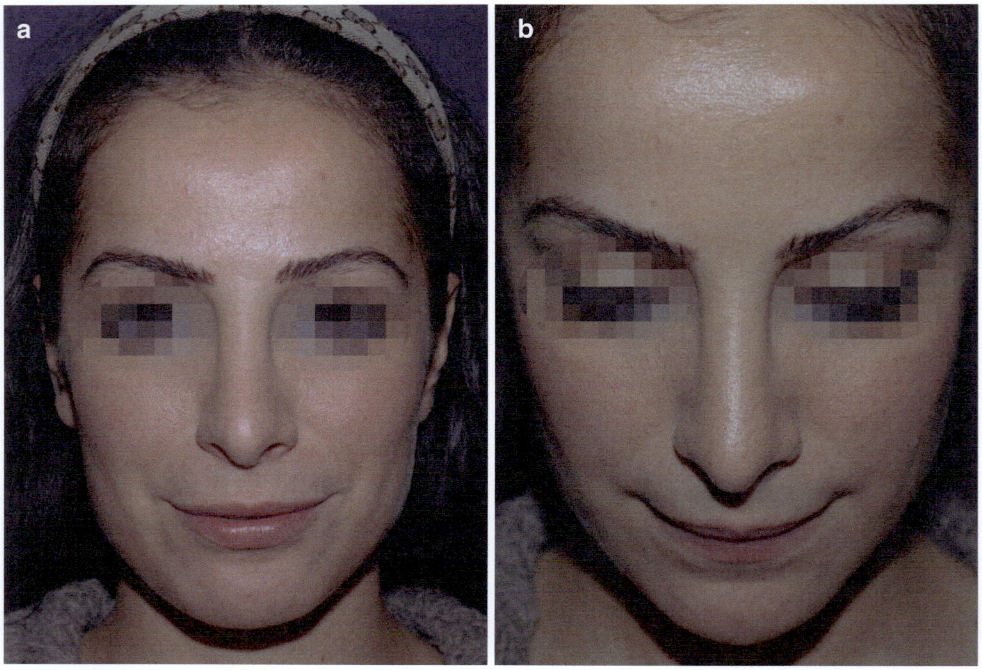

Fig. 7.30 (**a**, **b**) Sausage nose image

a situation is encountered during surgery, dorsal augmentation with cartilage grafting may be needed to close the open roof deformity. Otherwise, the dorsum remains fairly wide, despite the osteotomy. *While performing revision surgery in such a patient, augmentation of the dorsum along its length, rather than performance of recurrent osteotomy, enables the dorsum to appear narrower;* thus, an aesthetically ideal dorsum can be achieved (Fig. 7.53).

7.3.10.1 Case 17

In this representative case of a patient with a wide dorsum issue, the dorsum remains rather broad, although the nasal base is sufficiently narrowed. In this case, the problem is unrelated to insufficient osteotomy; an open roof deformity remains, and a narrower view is obtained when the dorsum is augmented (Fig. 7.54).

Another patient who is treated with a unique technique is shown below.

7.3.10.2 Case 18

Although there was no need for osteotomy in this representative case of a patient who underwent revision rhinoplasty, the inward collapse in the left nasal bone was corrected with soft tissues taken from above the nasal tip; a symmetrical appearance was subsequently achieved (Fig. 7.55).

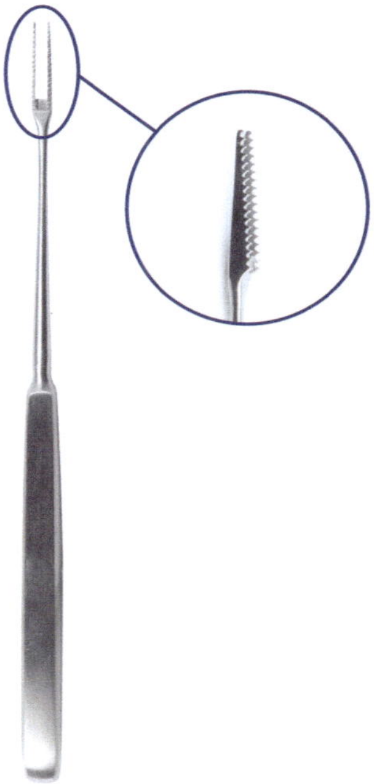

Fig. 7.32 Double saw

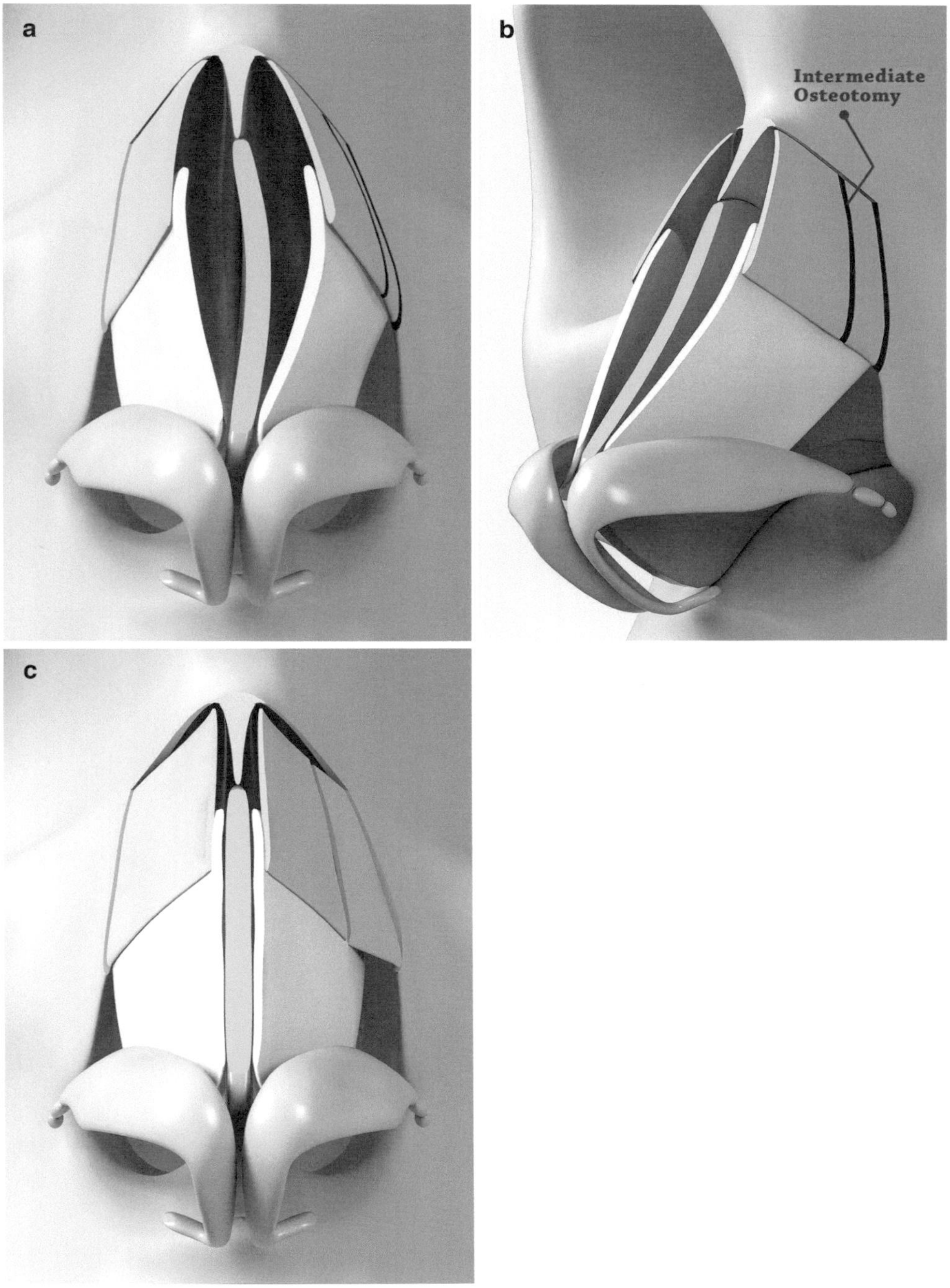

Fig. 7.31 (**a**) Asymmetric bone pyramid after hump removal. (**b**) Intermediate osteotomy line. (**c**) Symmetric bone pyramid after osteotomies

Preoperative planning is crucial in rhinoplasty, especially in osteotomy. Preoperative photos give an idea about osteotomy types and places that will be performed. **However, the surgeon must check the patient intraoperatively as they can change their decision based on surgical development.** Let us look at the example below.

7.3.10.3 Case 19

A patient was complaining about her deviated nose. Based on her preoperative photos, the right bony nasal wall seemed more long and convex. Therefore, performing double osteotomy on the right side was planned (Fig. 7.56).

After hump removal, it was seen that the left bony nasal wall was more convex than the right side. For this reason, the preoperative decision was changed. Double lateral osteotomy was performed on the left side (Fig. 7.57).

One year after the surgery, her deviation was corrected and ideal brow-tip aesthetic line was achieved (Fig. 7.58).

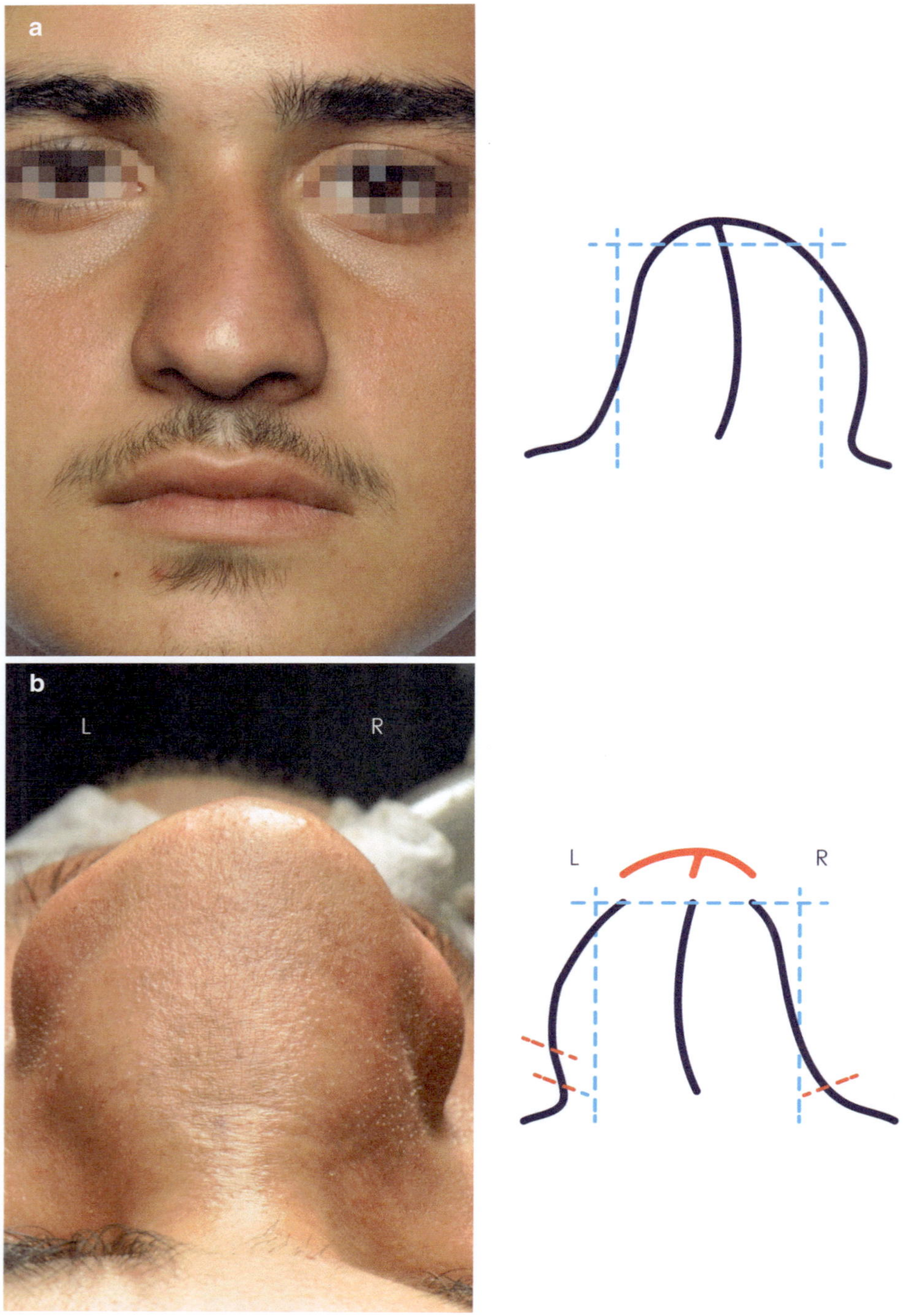

Fig. 7.33 (**a**) Deviation of the bony pyramid to the left. (**b**) The hump has been removed. (**c**) After transverse osteotomy, left double lateral osteotomy was done. (**d**) Symmetry achieved

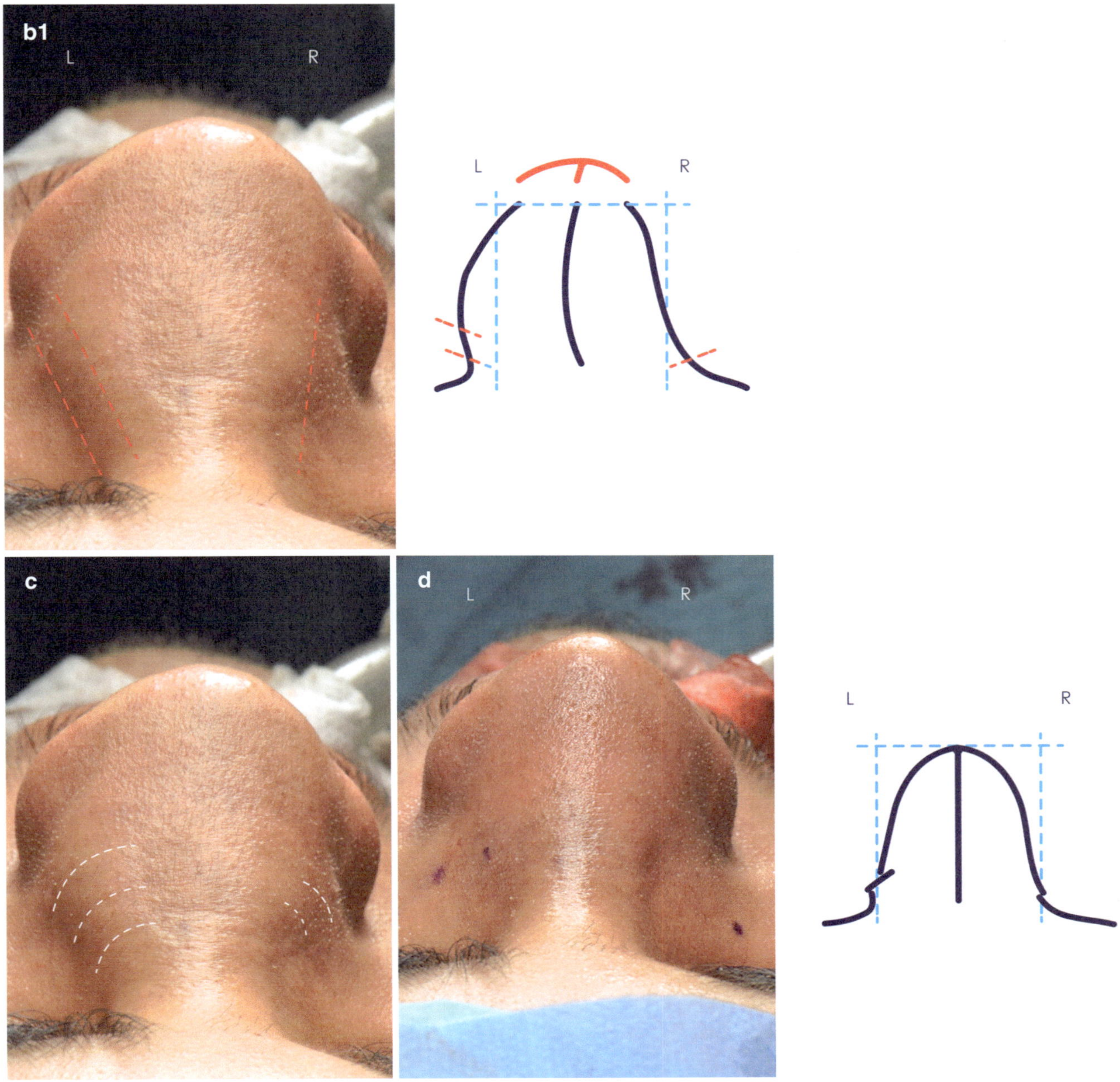

Fig. 7.33 (continued)

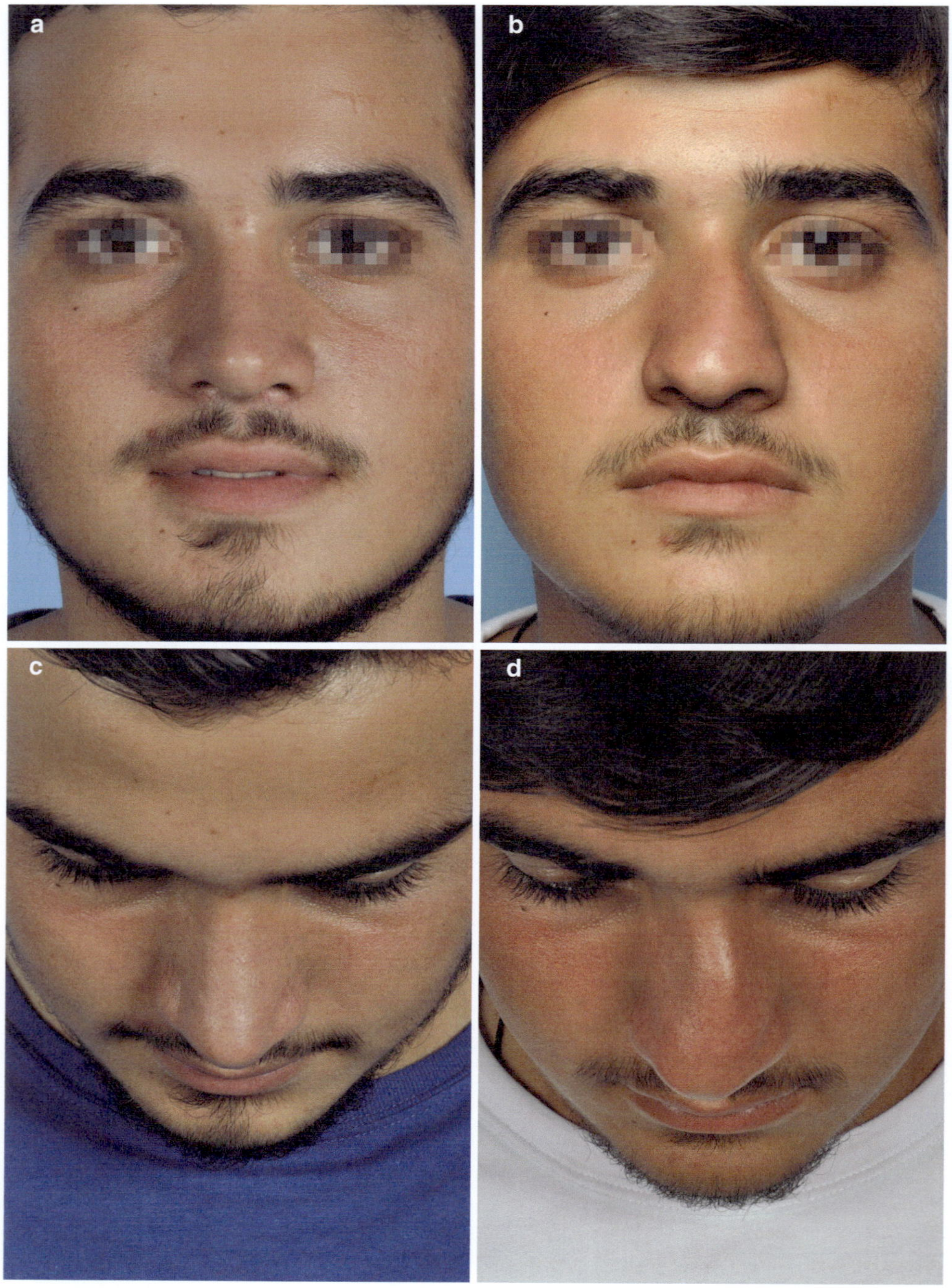

Fig. 7.34 (**a**, **c**) Preoperative frontal and face-down photos, convexity of left nasal bone is evident. (**b**, **d**) Two-year postoperative frontal and face-down photographs

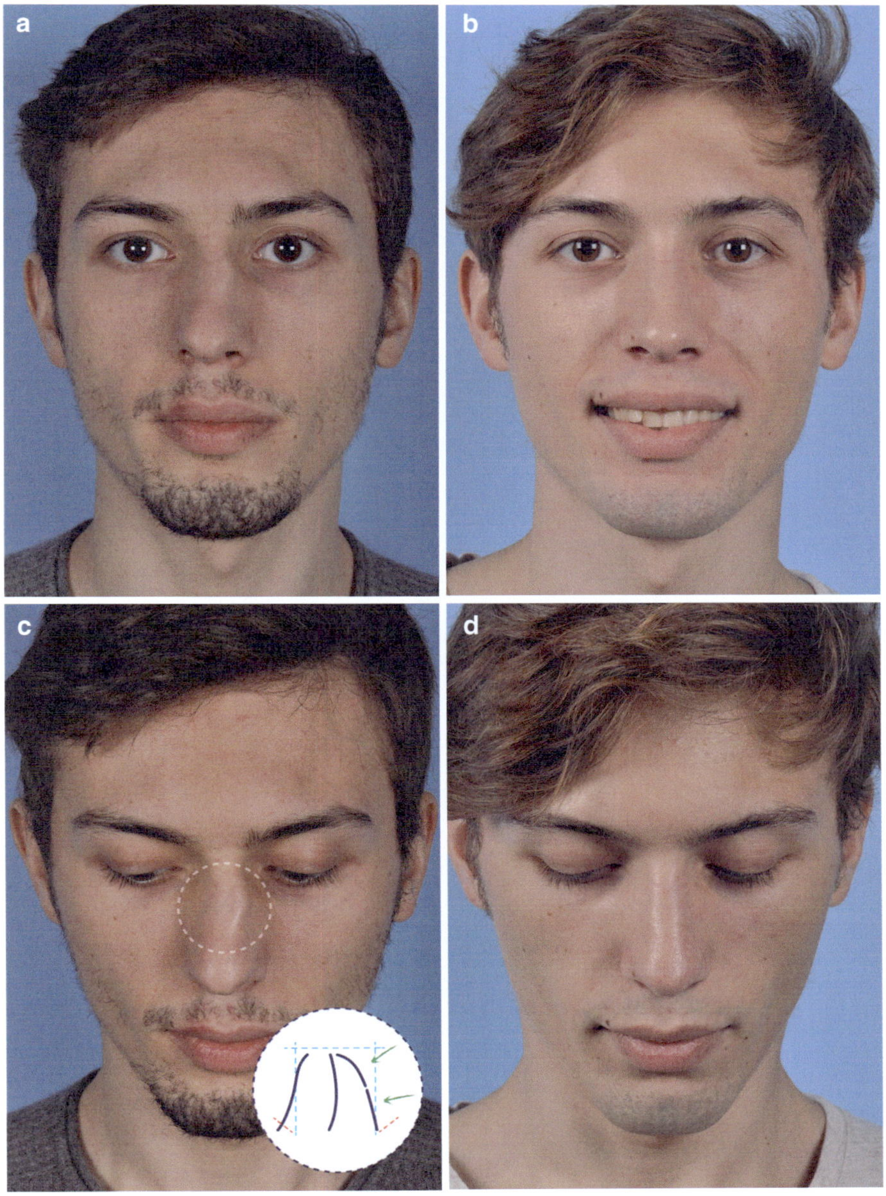

Fig. 7.35 (**a**, **c**) Preoperative frontal and face-down photographs, convexity of the left nasal bone is evident. (**b**, **d**) Four-year postoperative frontal and face-down photographs

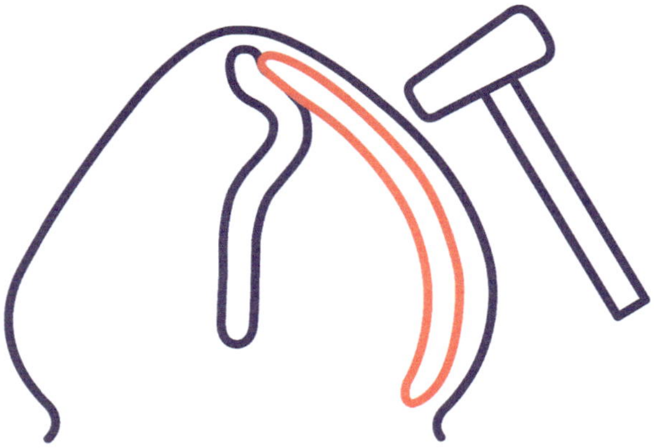

Fig. 7.36 Left high septal deviation limiting left nasal bone approximation to midline

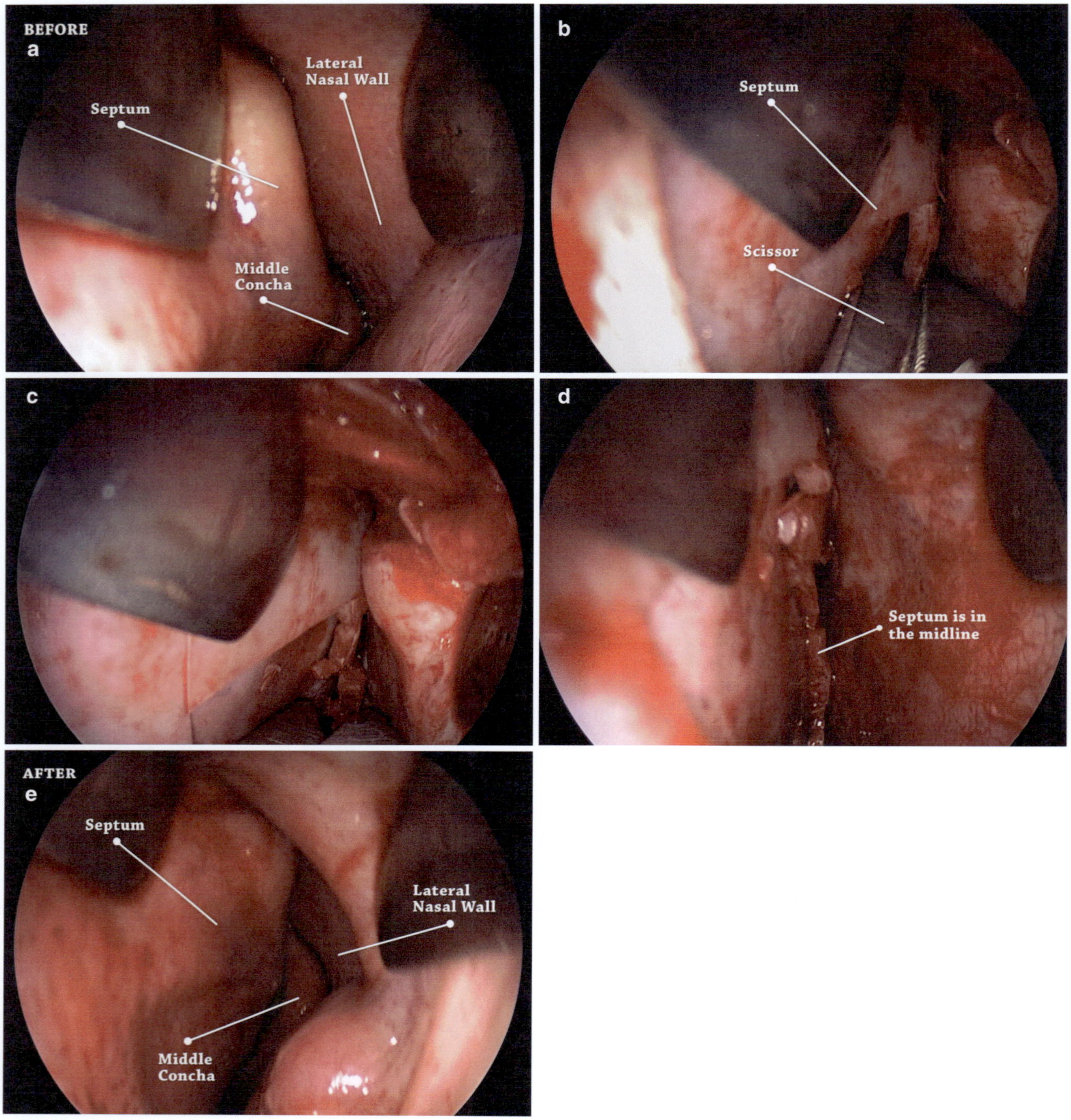

Fig. 7.37 (**a**) Intraoperative photograph, left nasal cavity. (**b**) Multiple incisions are made in septum with the help of scissors. (**c**) High septal deviation resistance is broken with these incisions. (**d**) Postoperative photograph, left nasal cavity

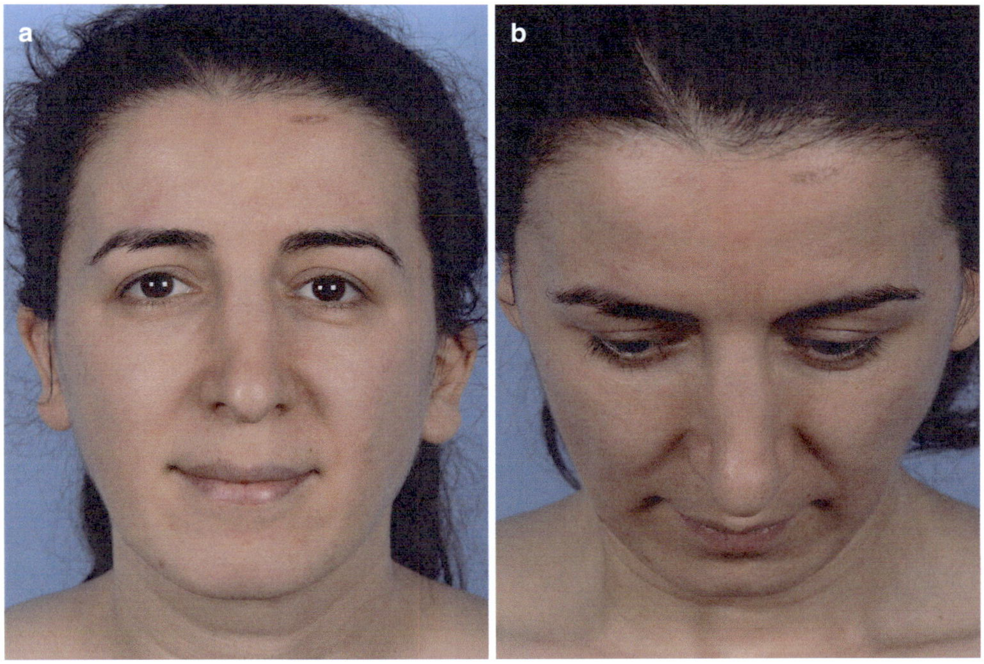

Fig. 7.38 (**a**, **b**) Preoperative frontal and face-down photos, open roof deformity is evident

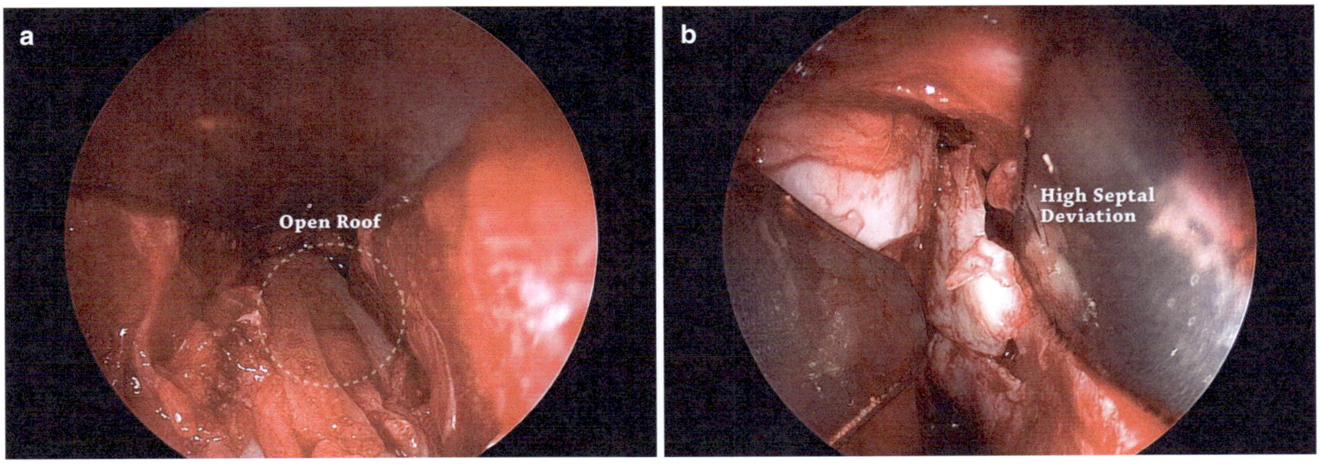

Fig. 7.39 (**a**) It is evident that left nasal bone is not in the midline due left high septal deviation (open roof deformity). (**b**) High septal deviation is seen

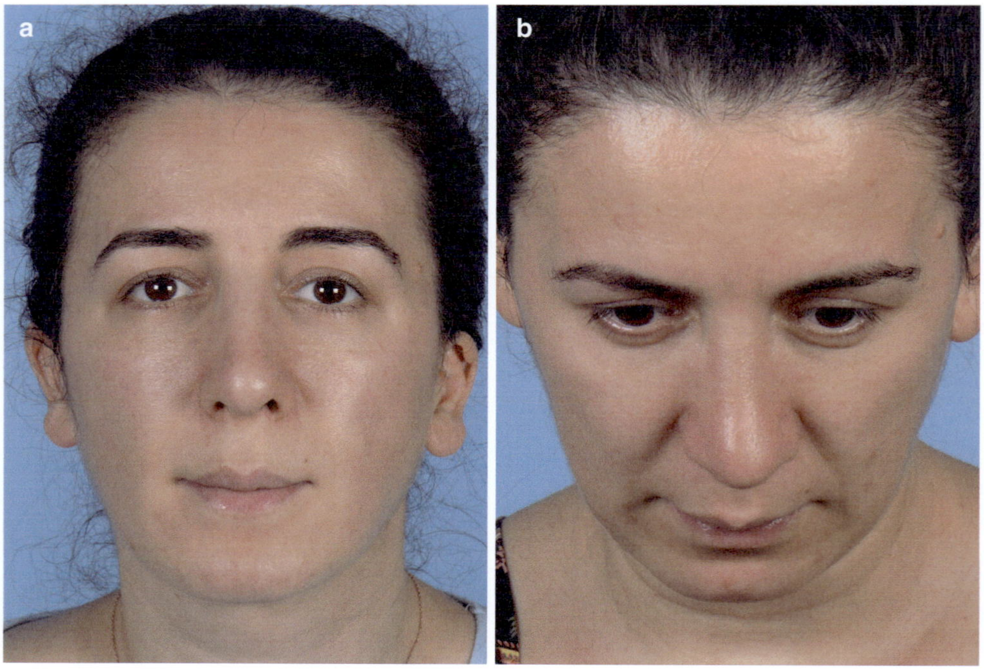

Fig. 7.40 (**a**, **b**) Postoperative frontal and face-down photos

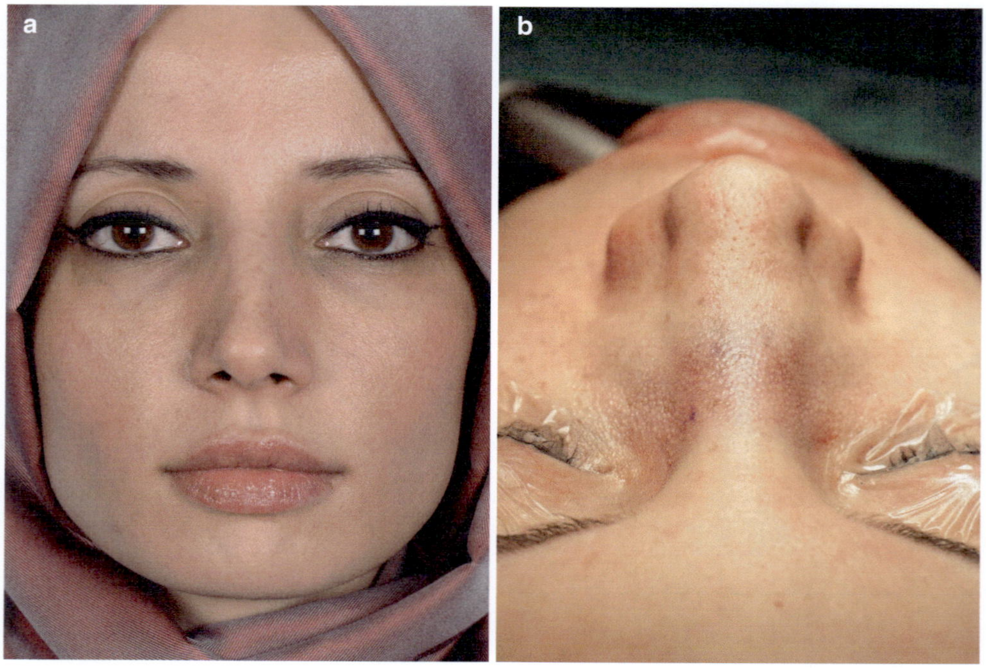

Fig. 7.41 (**a**) Preoperative frontal photograph. (**b**) Immediately after osteotomy

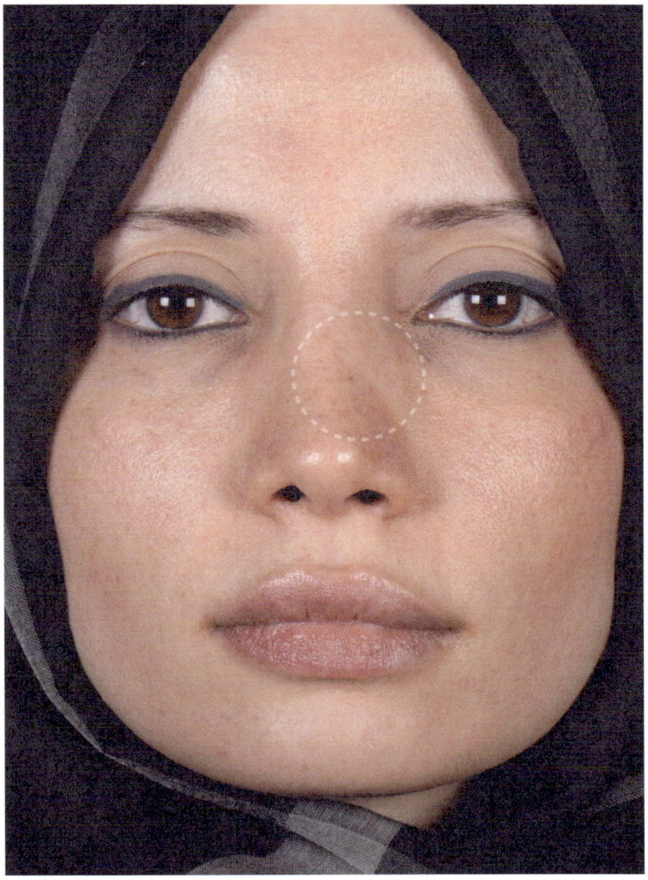

Fig. 7.42 There is a visible open roof deformity from previous rhinoplasty

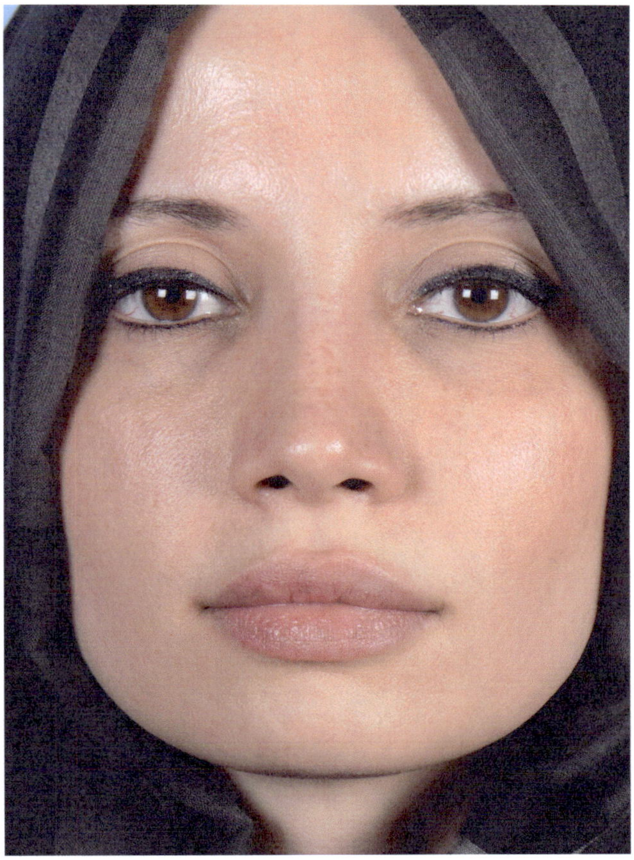

Fig. 7.43 After revision surgery the open roof is corrected

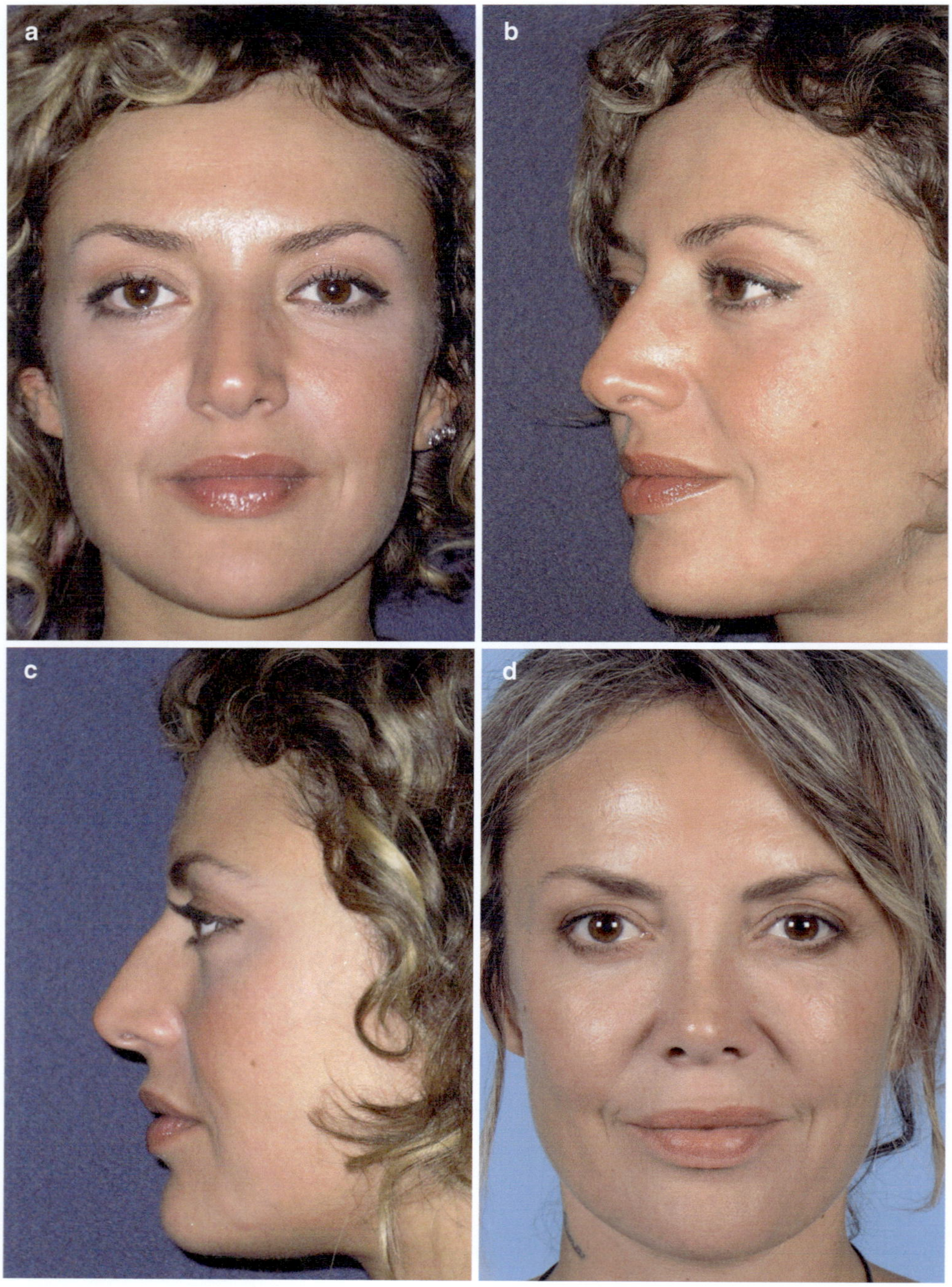

Fig. 7.44 (**a**–**c**) Preoperative photographs. The nose is slightly deviated to the right. The bony nasal pyramid is wide. (**d**–**f**) 15 years postoperative. The nose is straighter and the bony vault is narrower

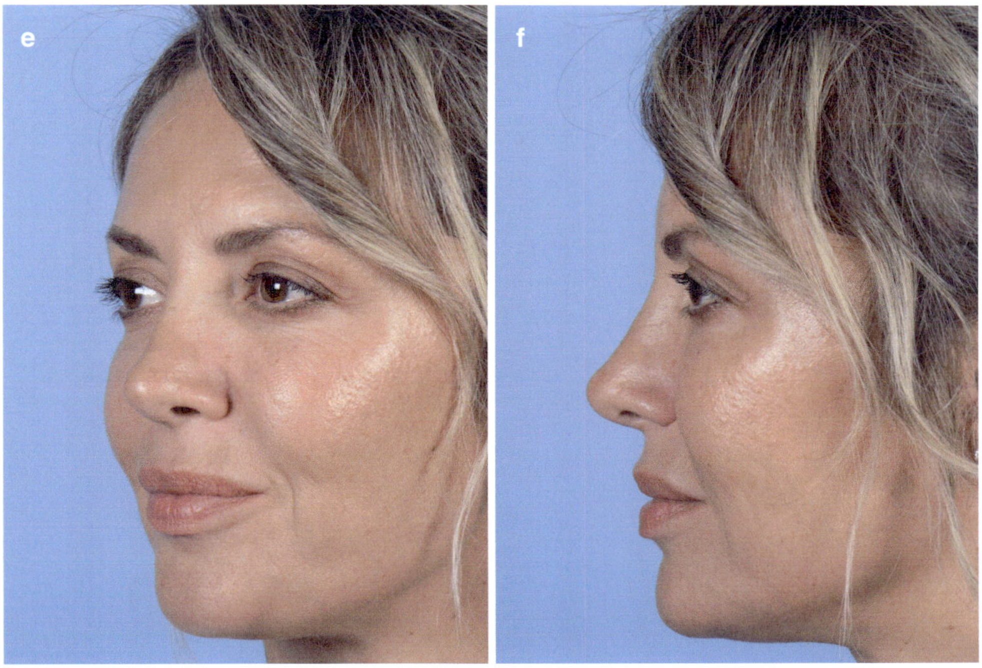

Fig. 7.44 (continued)

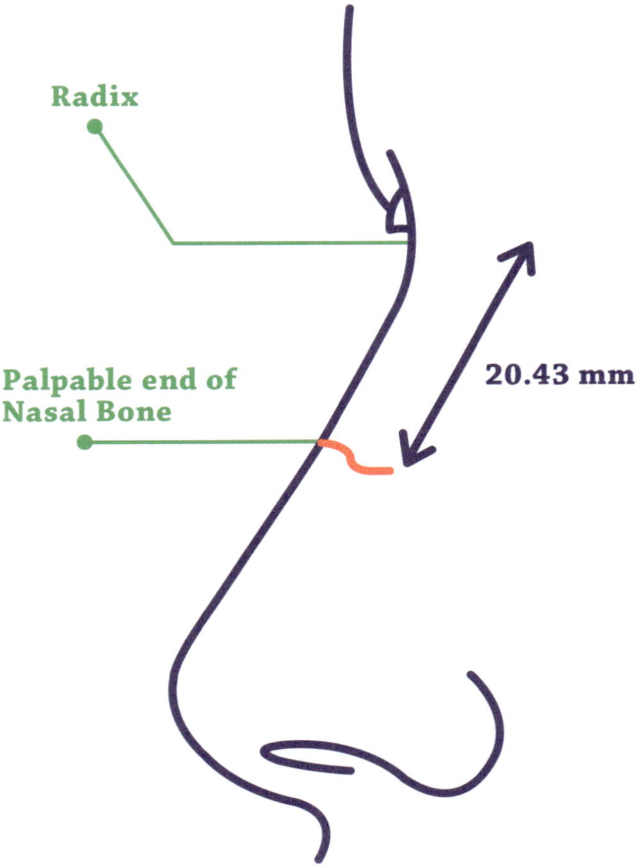

Fig. 7.45 Length of the nasal bone is measured from the lateral aspect of the radix to the palpable end of the nasal bone. The average length should be 20.43 mm

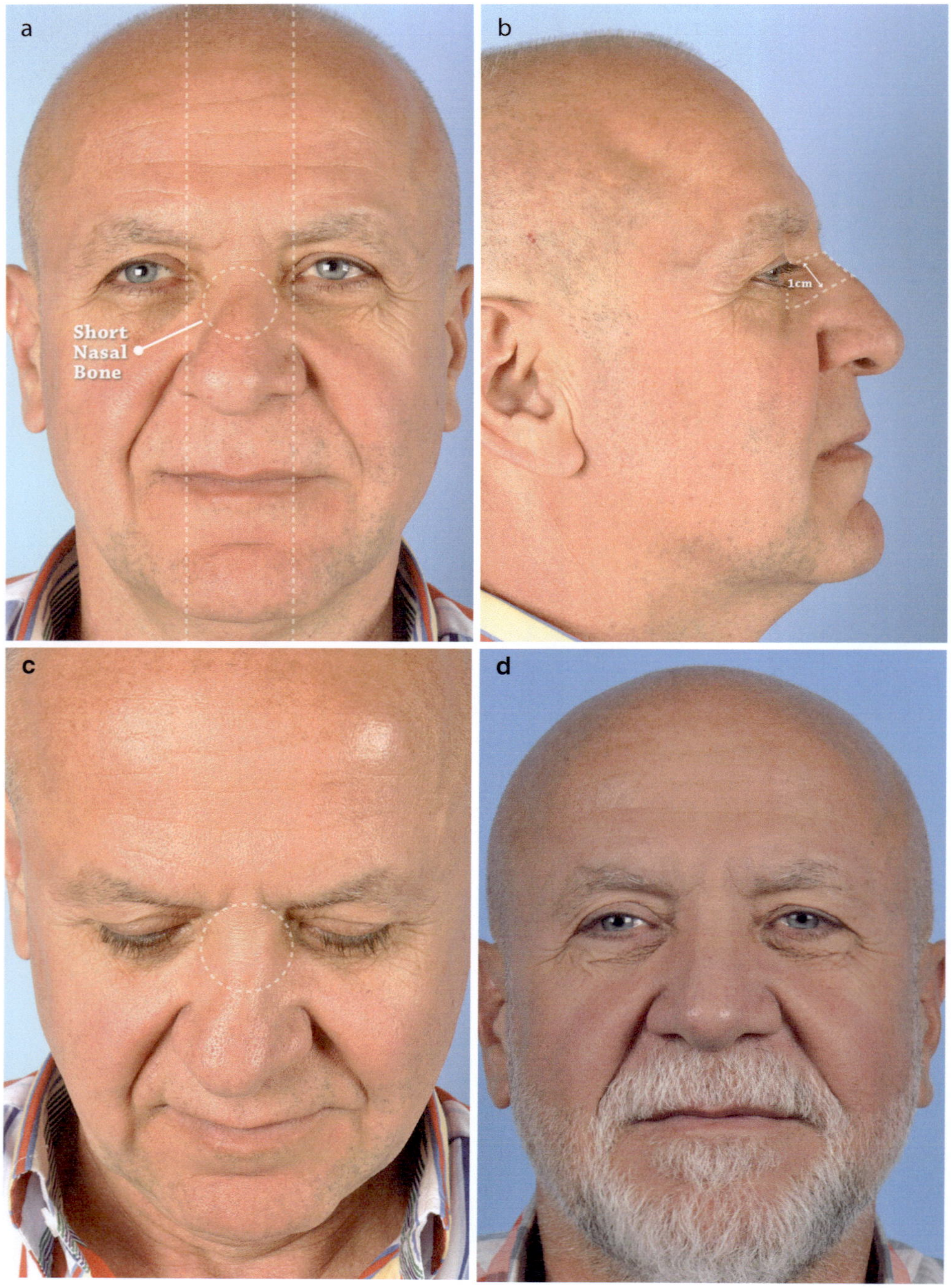

Fig. 7.46 (**a**) Preoperative frontal photograph, nasal axis is deviated to right side. The nasal base is not needed to be narrowed in this case. (**b**) Preoperative profile image shows the short nasal bones and presence of the small dorsal hump. (**c**) Nasal axis deviation to right side is evident. Brow-tip aesthetic line is disturbed due to deviation. (**d**) Five-year postoperative frontal photograph, nasal axis is in midline. The nose became midline with bilateral spreader grafts. (**e**) Five-year postoperative profile photograph, dorsal profile is smooth after hump removal. (**f**) The pyramid is straight and brow-tip aesthetic line is ideal

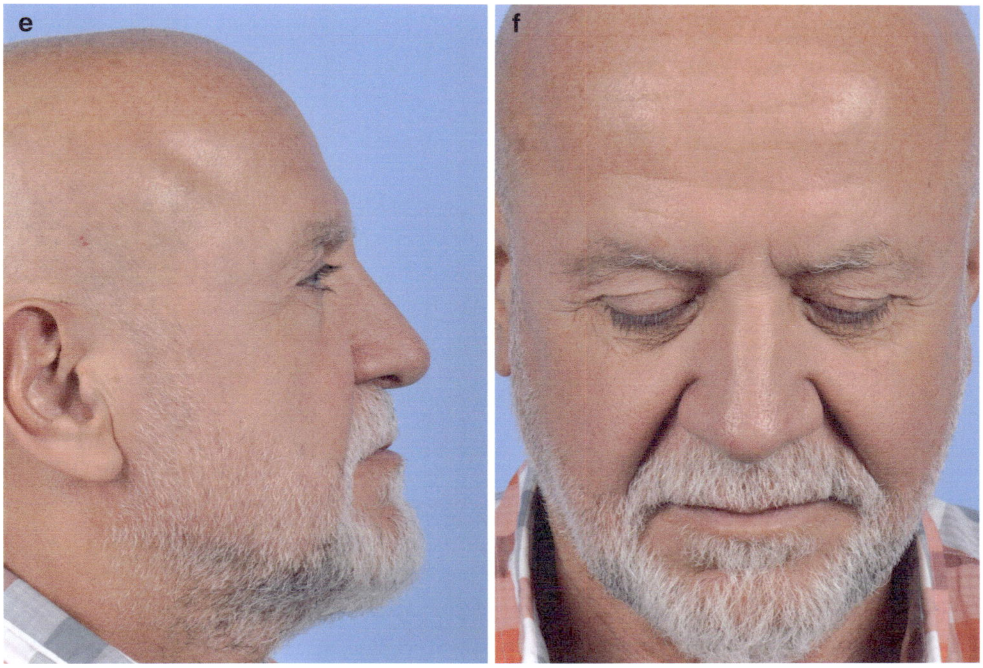

Fig. 7.46 (continued)

Fig. 7.47 (**a**–**c**) Right bony lateral nasal wall is more convex compared to left side

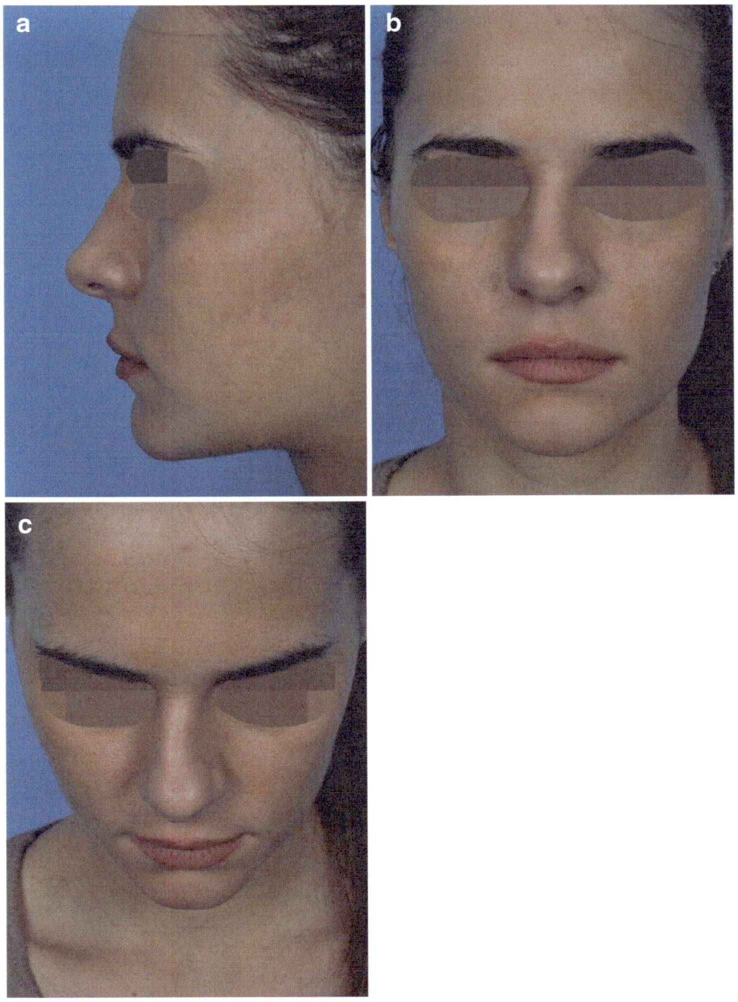

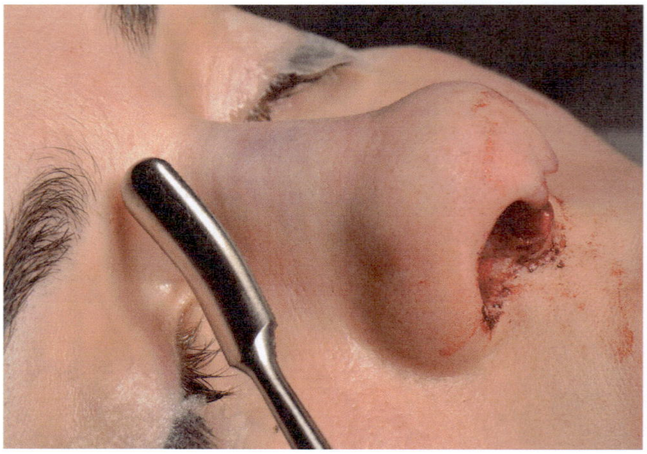

Fig. 7.48 After hump removal, the right bony wall was rasped and bilateral spreader grafts were placed

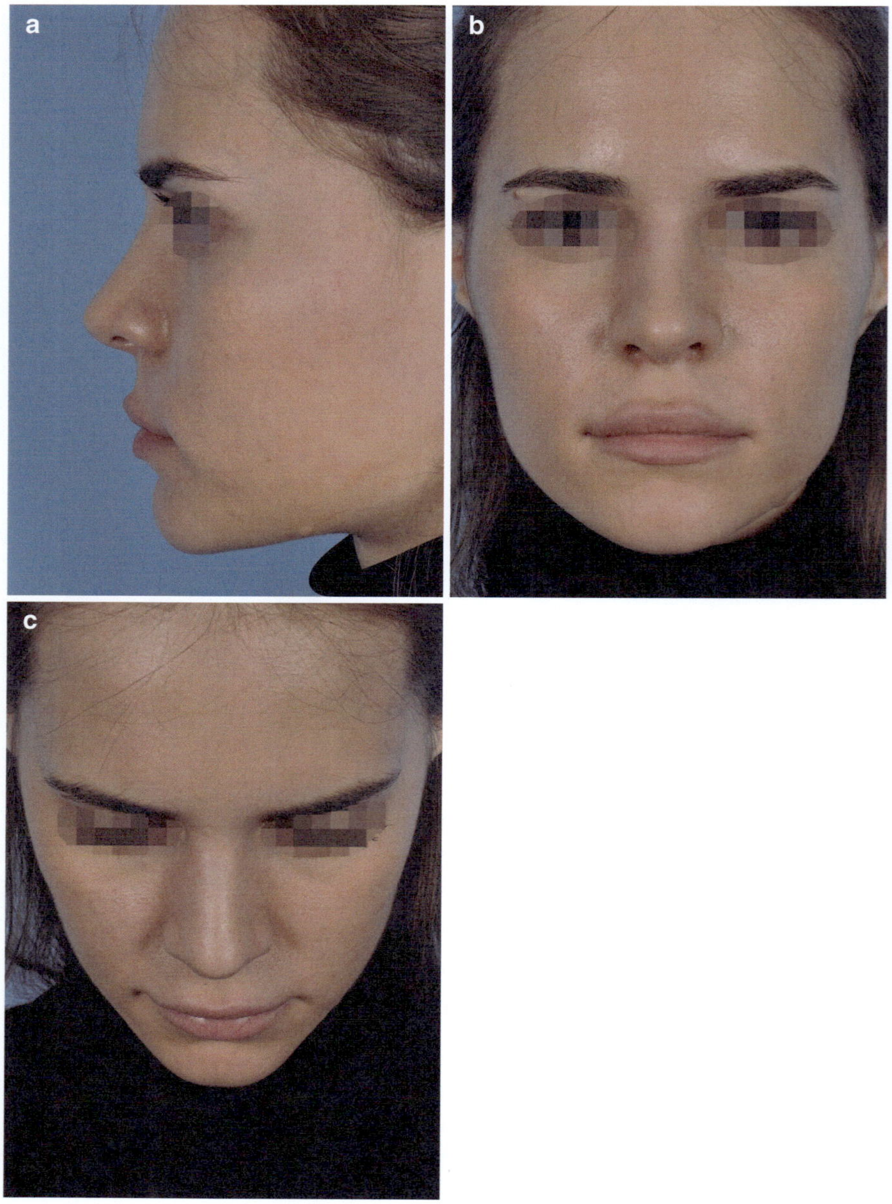

Fig. 7.49 (a–c) Postoperatively the patient showed improved nose appearance

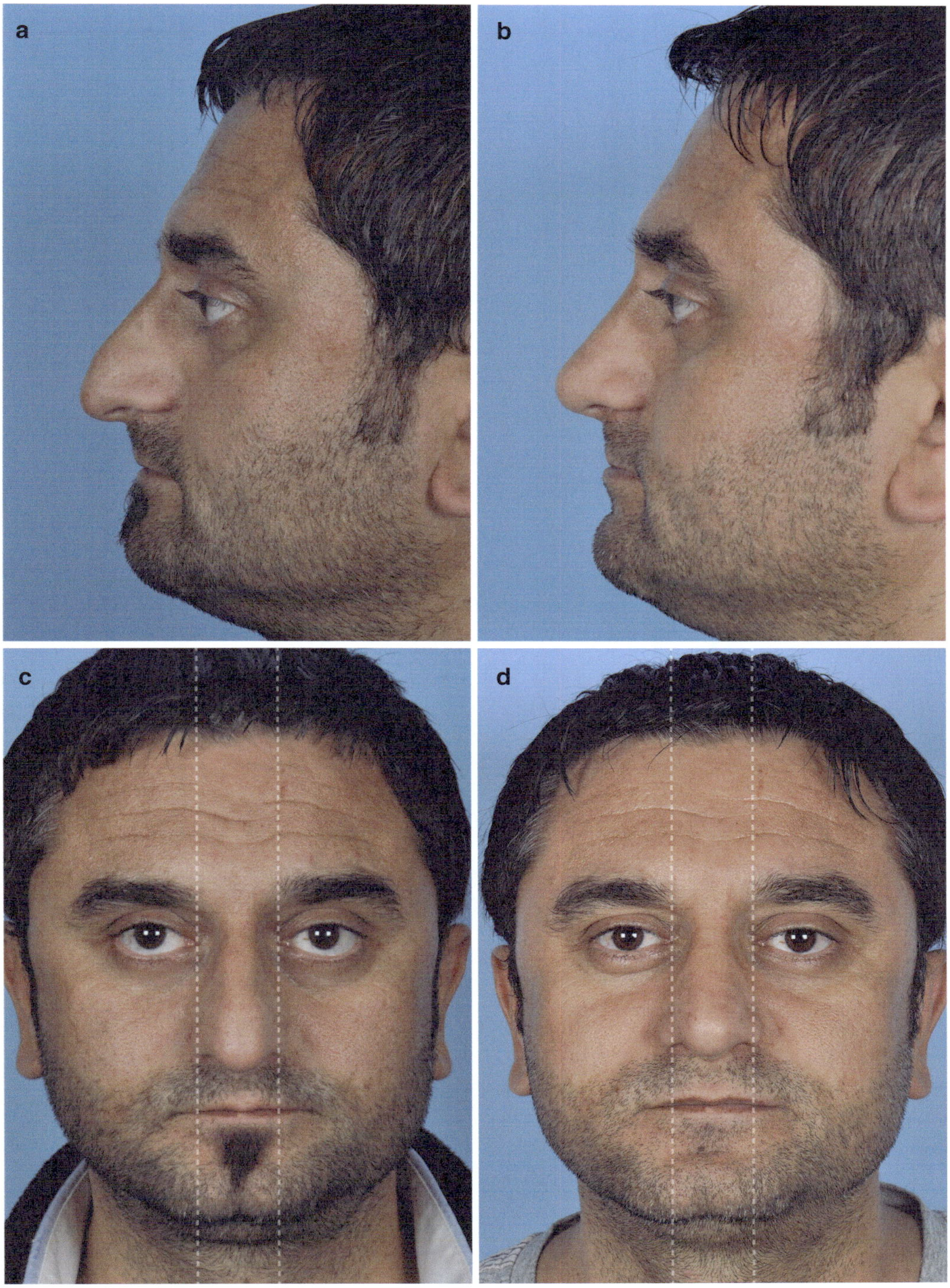

Fig. 7.50 (**a**) Preoperative profile photograph, dorsal hump, and droopy tip is clearly seen. (**b**) One-year postoperative profile photograph, dorsal profile is smooth and tip rotation is ideal. (**c**) Preoperative frontal photograph, nasal base is between medial canthus lines as if osteotomies were performed. (**d**) One-year postoperative frontal photo, no osteotomy was performed. (**e**) Preoperative face-down photograph, brow-tip aesthetic line is disturbed. (**f**) One-year postoperative face-down photograph, brow-tip aesthetic line is ideal

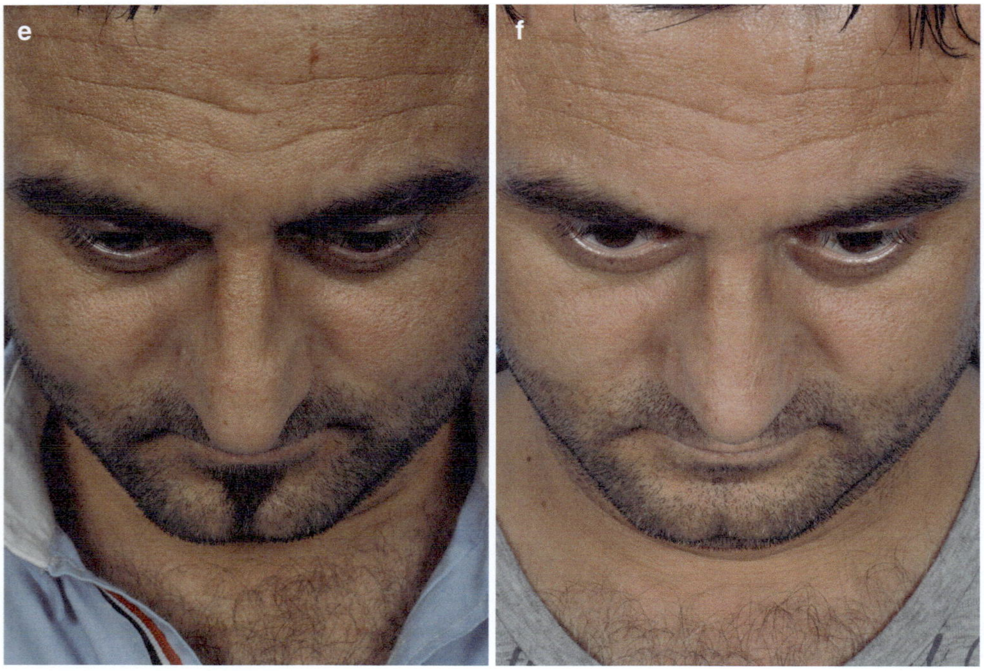

Fig. 7.50 (continued)

Fig. 7.51 (**a**–**c**) Preoperative frontal, lateral and face-down photographs. (**d**, **e**) After the hump removal, right unilateral spreader graft was used. (**f**–**h**) One-year postoperative frontal, lateral, and face-down photographs

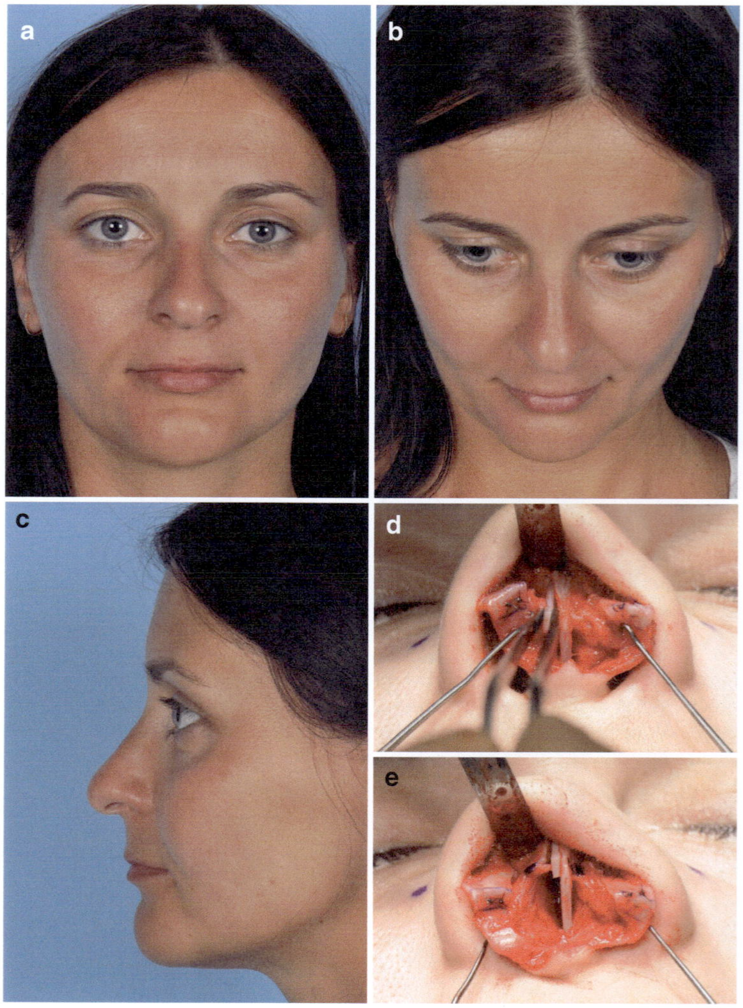

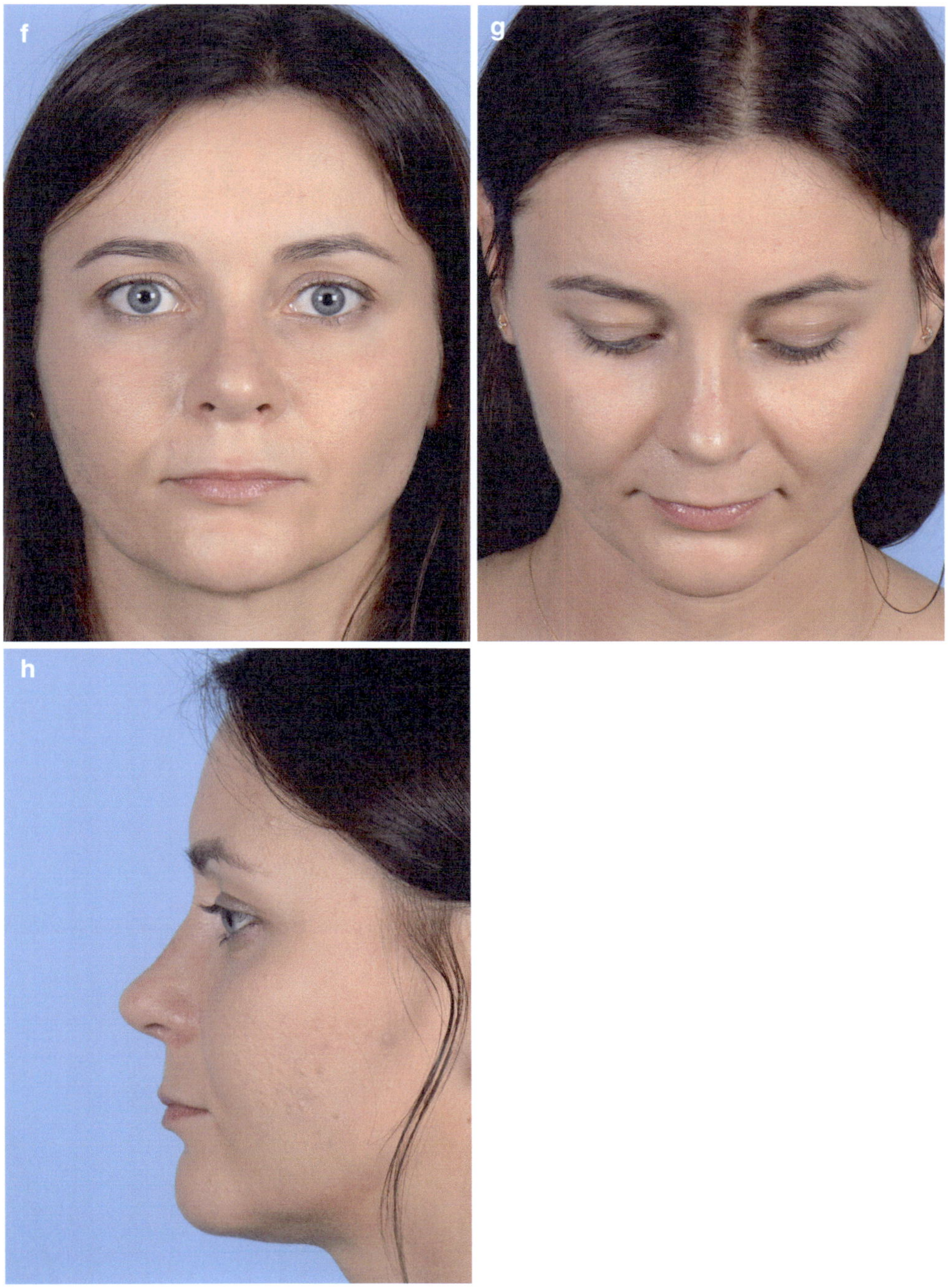

Fig. 7.51 (continued)

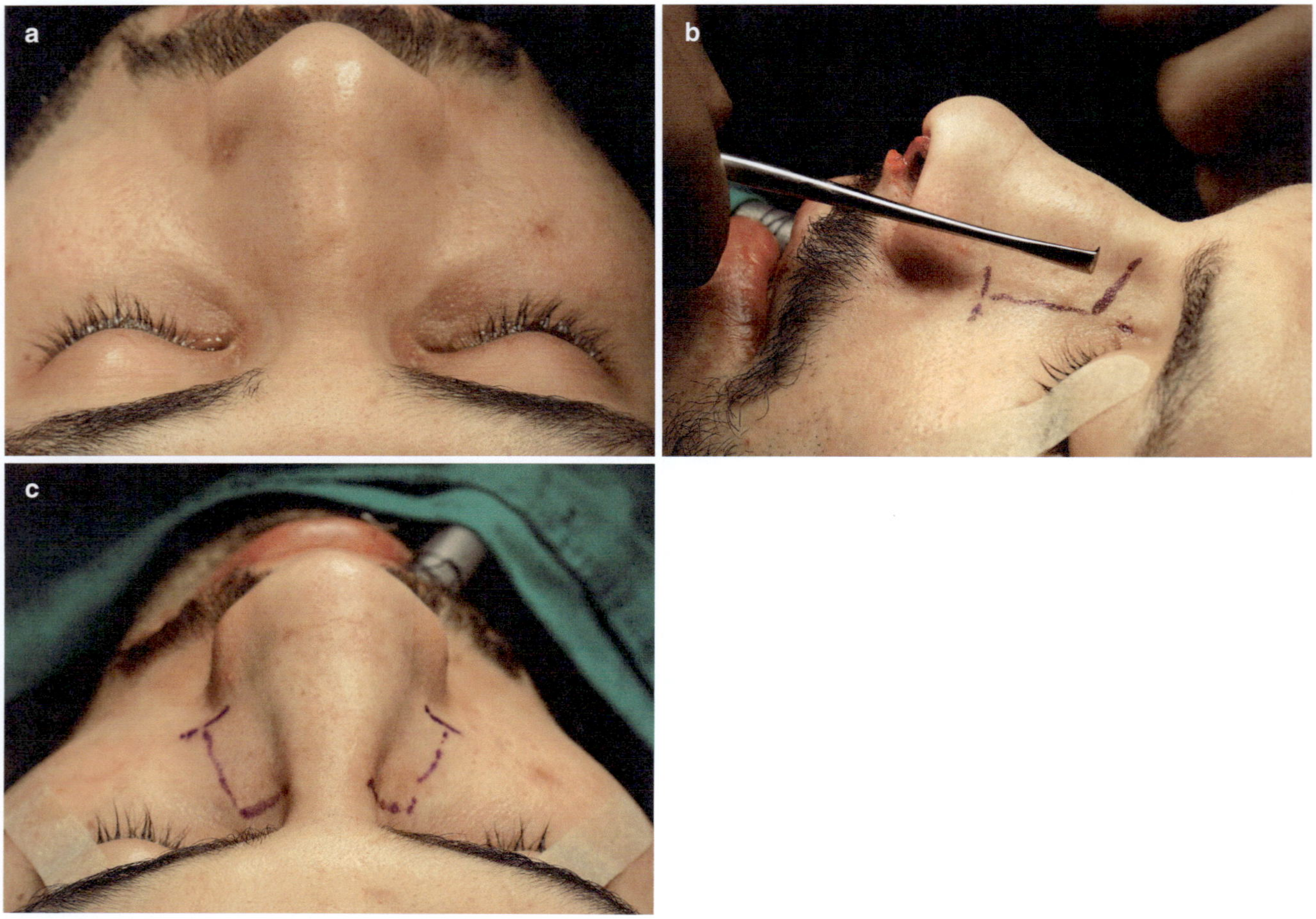

Fig. 7.52 (**a**) Intraoperative photograph, nasal root is narrow. (**b**) Intraoperative photograph, transverse osteotomy line is evident. (**c**) Intraoperative photograph, osteotomies are performed and nasal root is not included

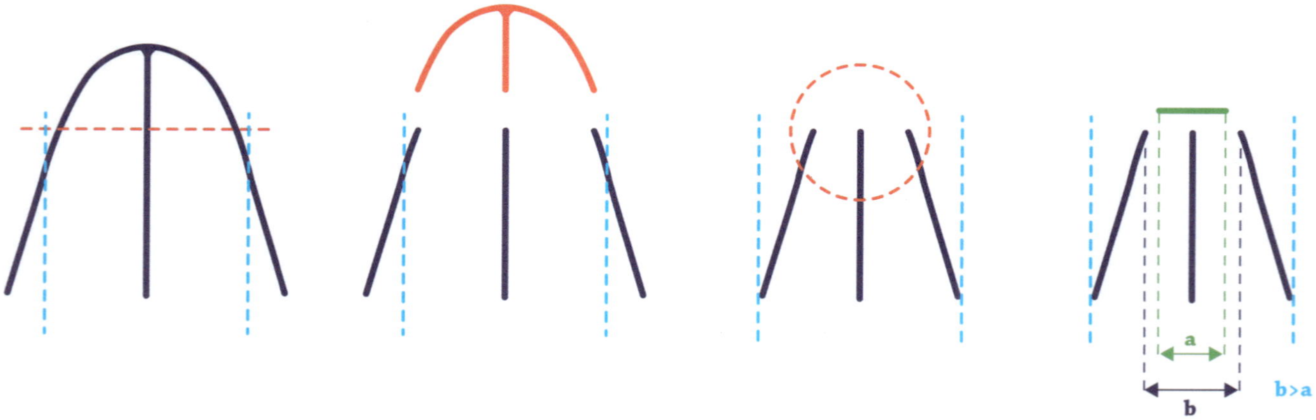

Fig. 7.53 In some cases with a huge hump, osteotomy is not enough to close the open roof. Onlay dorsal graft is kept in mind to close open roof deformity

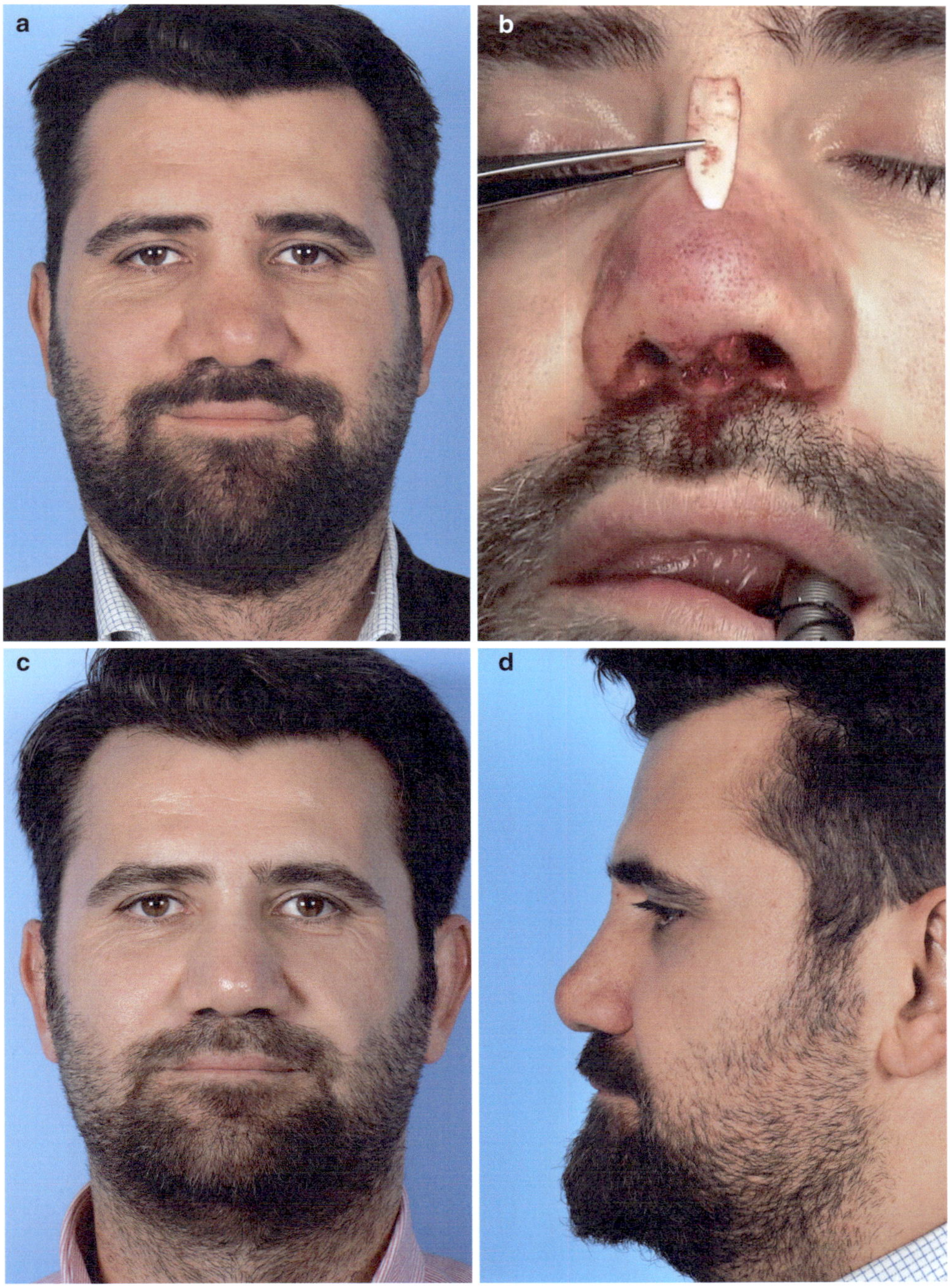

Fig. 7.54 (**a**) Revision case, preoperative photograph, the nasal dorsum is too wide (**b**) Intraoperative photograph; dorsal only graft (**c**) Postoperative photographs; nose looks narrower without osteotomy (**d**) Preoperative profile (**e**) Postoperative profile; the height of the dorsum is more uniform, and the tip position improved from the more ptotic position

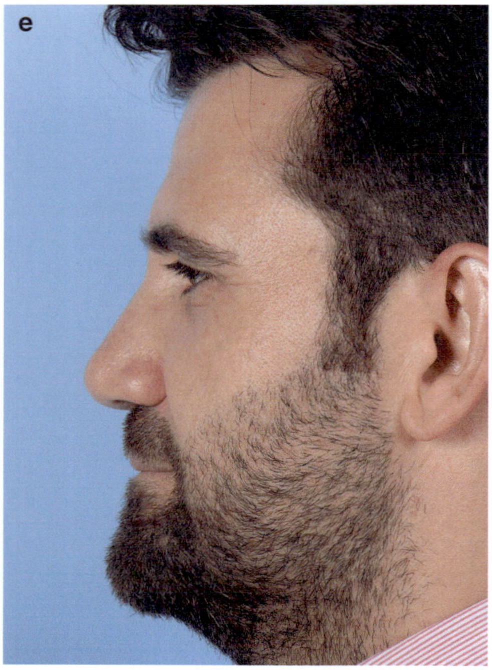

Fig. 7.54 (continued)

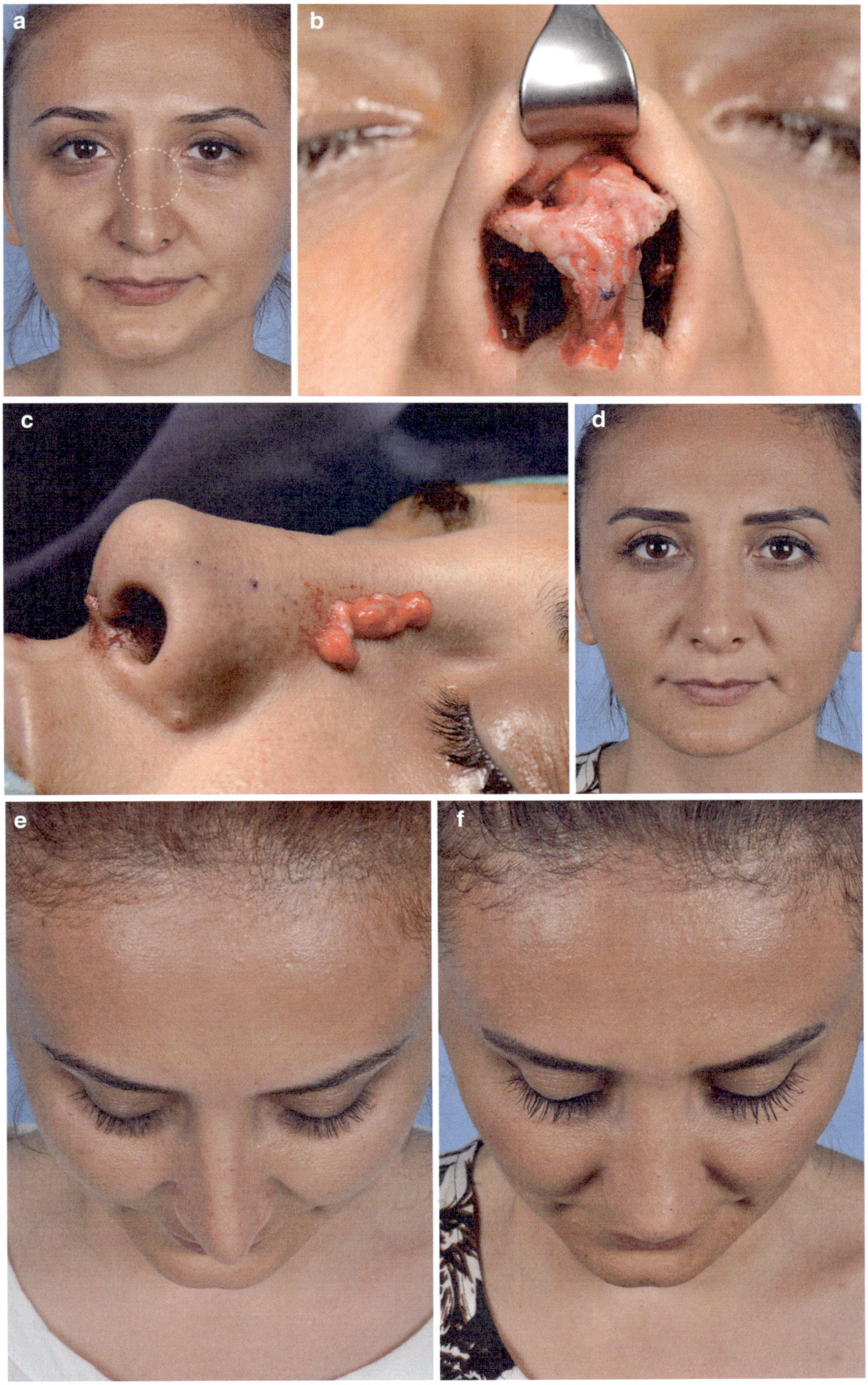

Fig. 7.55 (**a**) Preoperative frontal photograph, nasal tip asymmetry and collapse of left nasal bone are evident. (**b**) Intraoperative photograph, soft tissues on alar cartilages are evident. (**c**) Intraoperative photograph, soft tissues were put to the left nasal bone. (**d**) One-year postoperative frontal photograph, both tip asymmetry and left nasal bone collapse are corrected. (**e**) Preoperative face-down photograph. (**f**) Postoperative face-down photograph. (**g**) Preoperative base photograph, alar rim and nostril asymmetry are present. (**h**) One-year postoperative base photograph, both alar rim and nostril asymmetry are corrected

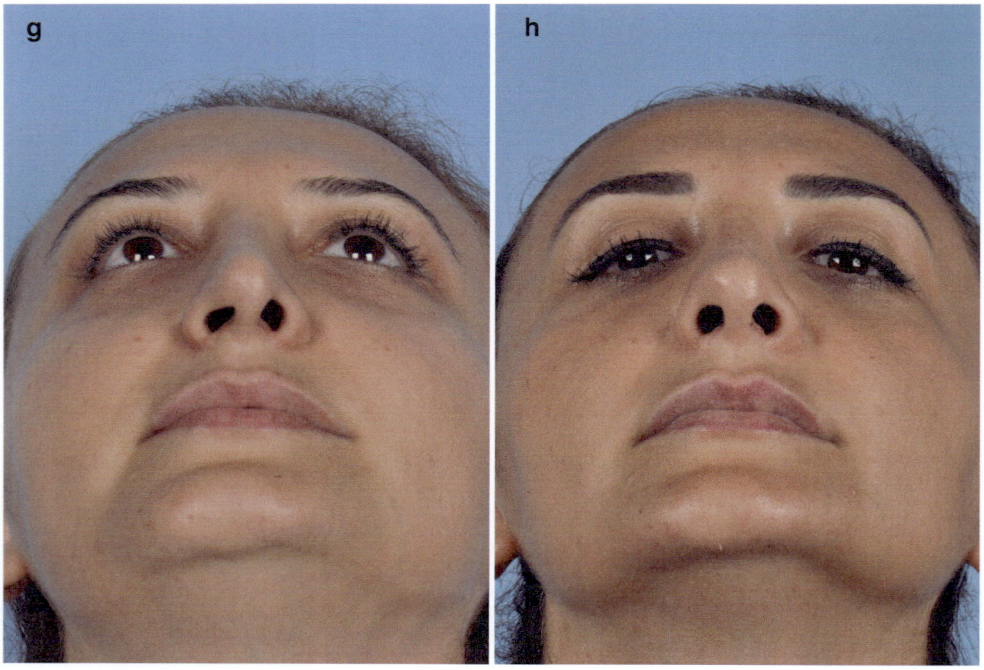

Fig. 7.55 (continued)

Fig. 7.56 (**a**, **b**) Preoperative photographs show that the right nasal bone is more concave than left

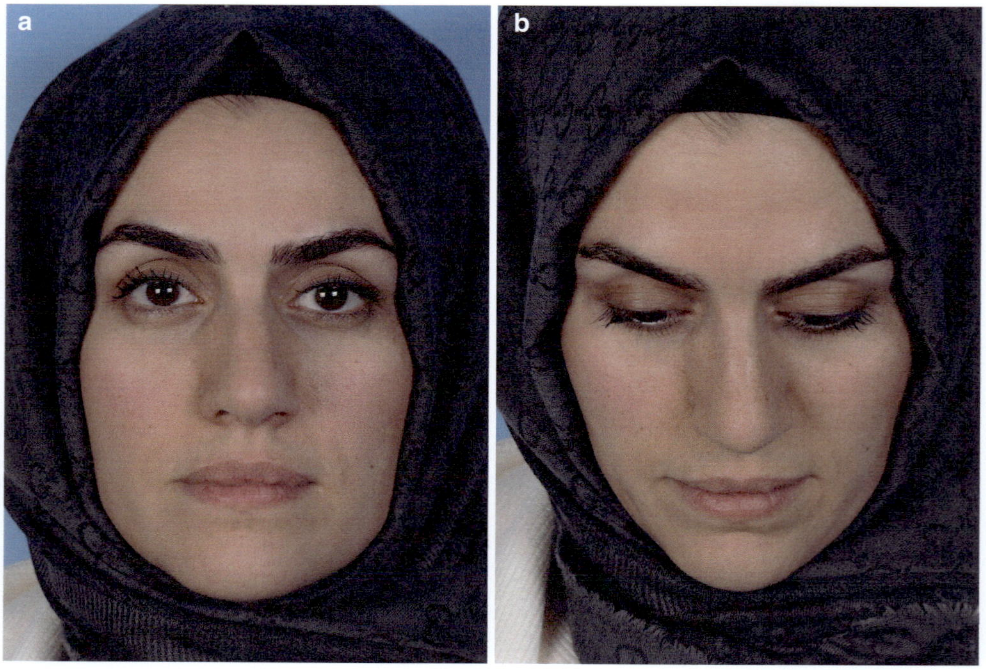

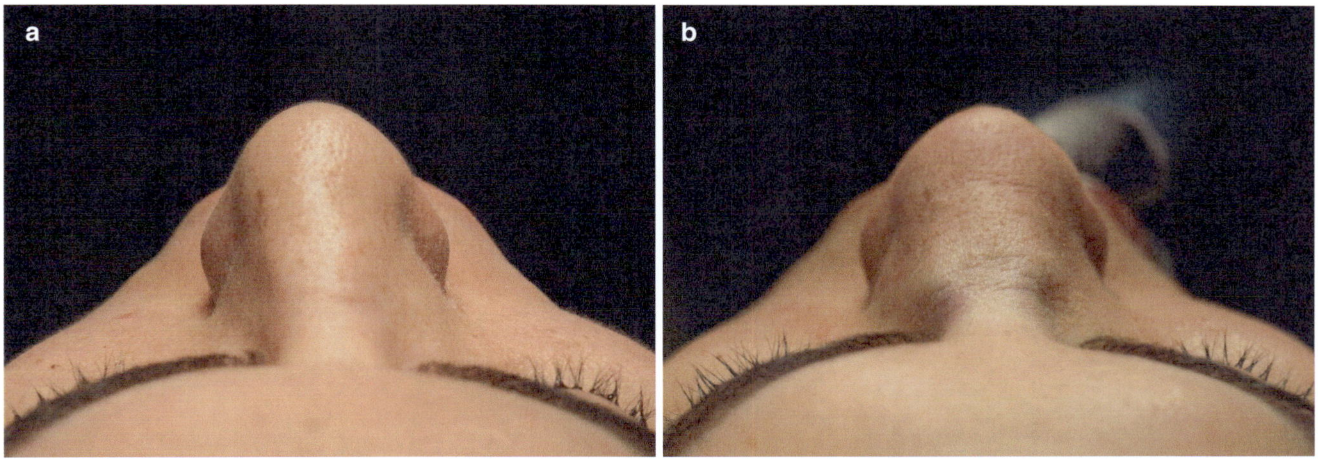

Fig. 7.57 (**a**) Before hump removal. (**b**) After hump removal, left nasal bone is more convex than the right one when compared to before removal

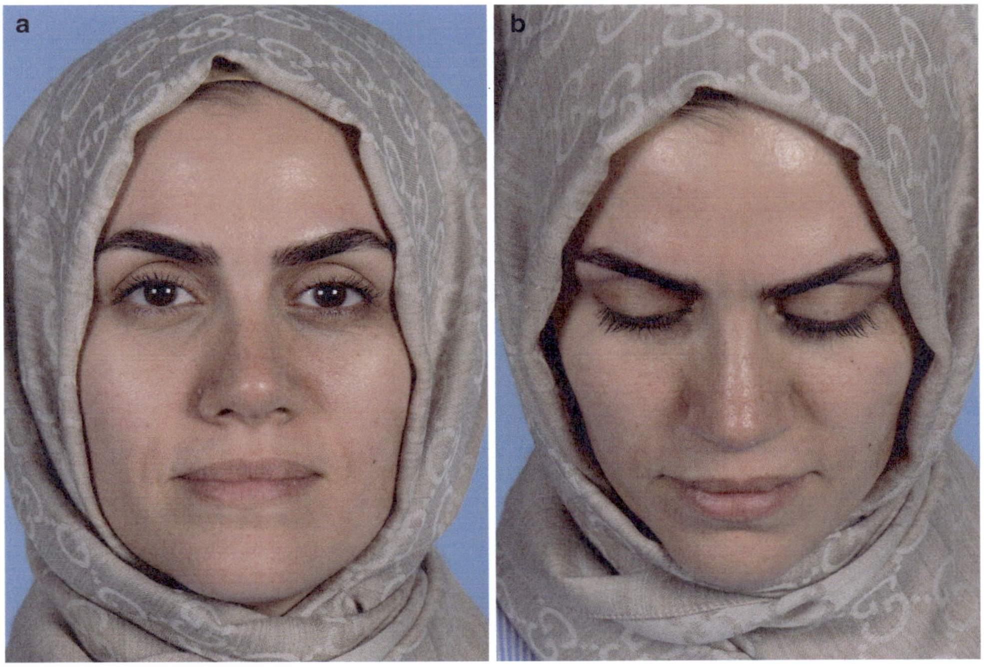

Fig. 7.58 (**a**, **b**) The bony base symmetry has been improved. Osteocartilaginous dorsum looks narrower and more defined

7.4 Conclusion

Osteotomy is an important component of rhinoplasty operations because it provides mobilization of the nasal bones and reshaping of the nose. Although it has these important effects, it also involves risks because it is primarily performed in a tactile manner without direct vision, and its effects are difficult to reverse. After hump removal is completed, the remaining nasal bones may be symmetrical or asymmetrical. Therefore, osteotomy approaches will differ depending upon the relationships among the nasal bones. Regardless of the osteotomy technique, the aim always remains closure of the open roof deformity caused by hump removal and achievement of an aesthetically natural nose by modifying the nasal base and dorsum to reach their ideal limits.

Figure 7.59 shows osteotomy performed on a cadaver.

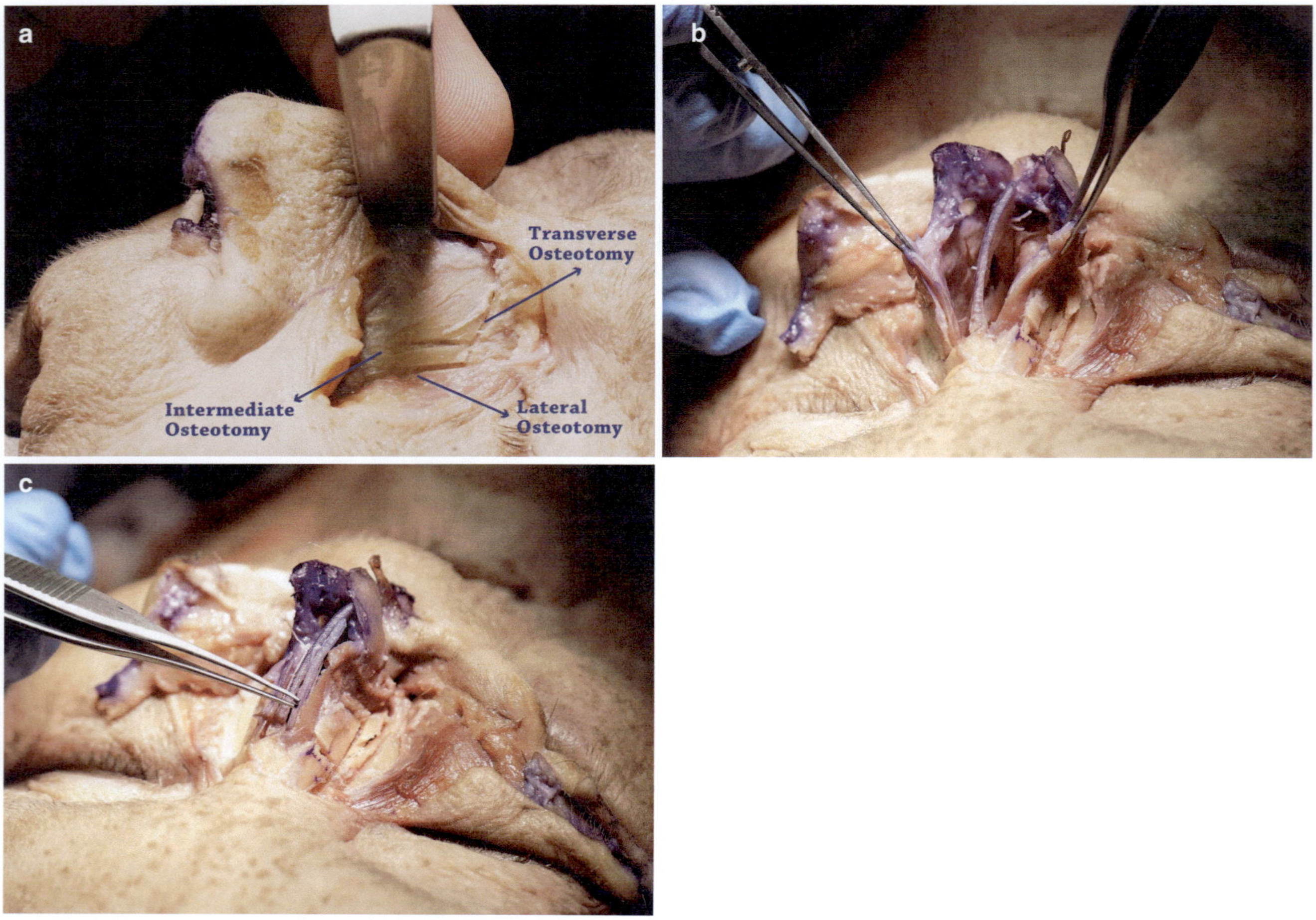

Fig. 7.59 (**a**) Osteotomy lines, the skin was removed. (**b**) Open roof after hump removal. (**c**) Open roof was closed with bilateral osteotomies

Disclosures The author reports no conflicts of interest or funding requiring disclosure.

Further Reading

Avsar Y. The oscillating micro-saw: a safe and pliable instrument for transverse osteotomy in rhinoplasty. Aesthet Surg J. 2012;32(6):700–8.

Azizzadeh B, Reilly M. Dorsal hump reduction and osteotomies. Clin Plast Surg. 2016;43(1):47–58.

Bohluli B, Moharamnejad N, Bayat M. Dorsal hump surgery and lateral osteotomy. Oral Maxillofac Surg Clin North Am. 2012;24(1):75–86.

Bracaglia R, Fortunato R, Gentileschi S. Double lateral osteotomy in aesthetic rhinoplasty. Br J Plast Surg. 2004;57(2):156–9.

Broadbent TR, Woolf RM. Anatomy of a rhinoplasty—saw technique. Ann Plast Surg. 1984;13(1):67–75.

Castro A, Jackson IT, Rademaker B. Rhinoplasty saw: a modified design. Ann Plast Surg. 1991;26(6):600–1.

Cerkes N. The crooked nose: principles of treatment. Aesthet Surg J. 2011;31(2):241–57.

Davis RE, Foulad AI. Treating the deviated or wide nasal dorsum. Facial Plast Surg. 2017;33(2):139–56.

Ghanaatpisheh M, Sajjadian A, Daniel RK. Superior rhinoplasty outcomes with precise nasal osteotomy: an individualized approach for maintaining function and achieving aesthetic goals. Aesthet Surg J. 2015;35(1):28–39.

Giampapa VC, DiBernardo BE. Nasal osteotomy—utilizing dual plane reciprocating nasal saw blades: a 6-year follow-up. Ann Plast Surg. 1993;30(6):500–2.

Gruber RP, Garza RM, Cho GJ. Nasal bone osteotomies with nonpowered tools. Clin Plast Surg. 2016;43(1):73–83.

Harshbarger RJ, Sullivan PK. Lateral nasal osteotomies: implications of bony thickness on fracture patterns. Ann Plast Surg. 1999;42(4):365–70; discussion 370–1

Harshbarger RJ, Sullivan PK. The optimal medial osteotomy: a study of nasal bone thickness and fracture patterns. Plast Reconstr Surg. 2001;108(7):2114–9; discussion 2120–1

Jang YJ, Wang JH, Lee BJ. Classification of the deviated nose and its treatment. Arch Otolaryngol Head Neck Surg. 2008;134(3):311–5.

Koçak I, Doğan R, Gökler O. A comparison of piezosurgery with conventional techniques for internal osteotomy. Eur Arch Otorrinolaringol. 2017;274(6):2483–91.

Kortbus MJ, Ham J, Fechner F, Constantinides M. Quantitative analysis of lateral osteotomies in rhinoplasty. Arch Facial Plast Surg. 2006;8(6):369–73.

Krane NA, Markey JD, Moneta LB, Kim MM. Aesthetics of the nasal dorsum: proportions, light, and shadow. Facial Plast Surg. 2017;33(2):120–4.

Moubayed SP, Most SP. Revision of the nasal dorsum. Facial Plast Surg. 2017;33(2):202–6.

Ozucer B, Özturan O. Current updates in nasal bone reshaping. Curr Opin Otolaryngol Head Neck Surg. 2016;24(4):309–15.

Potter JK. Correction of the crooked nose. Oral Maxillofac Surg Clin North Am. 2012;24(1):95–107.

Rohrich RJ, Ahmad J. Secondary rhinoplasty by the global masters. Boca Raton, FL: CRC/Taylor and Francis Group; 2017. p. 209–42.

Rohrich RJ, Gunter JP, Deuber MA, Adams WP. The deviated nose: optimizing results using a simplified classification and algorithmic approach. Plast Reconstr Surg. 2002;110(6):1509–23; discussion 1524–5

Rohrich RJ, Krueger JK, Adams WP, Hollier LH. Achieving consistency in the lateral nasal osteotomy during rhinoplasty: an external perforated technique. Plast Reconstr Surg. 2001;108(7):2122–30; discussion 2131–2

VanKoevering KK, Rosko AJ, Moyer JS. Osteotomies demystified. Facial Plast Surg Clin North Am. 2017;25(2):201–10.

Vuyk HD. A review of practical guidelines for correction of the deviated, asymmetric nose. Rhinology. 2000;38(2):72–8.

8 Dorsum: Final Touch the Dorsum

8.1 Introduction

Rhinoplasty is a thinking-, seeing-, and feeling-person operation. The art of rhinoplasty involves the ability to visualize the outcome of surgery intraoperatively, before the swelling resolves. Surgeons must therefore be able to see with their hands, feel with their eyes, and use their minds to integrate the two.

Rhinoplasty is a complex procedure in which every move has an effect. Most of the surgical manipulations in rhinoplasty, including bony hump removal, osteotomy, and middle vault reconstruction, involve the nasal dorsum. For this reason, dorsal surgery is of paramount importance with respect to the aesthetics and function of the nose. Although these procedures account for the majority of operations and resolve most of the preoperative issues, problems that significantly affect the surgical success may arise or persist after surgery. The surgeon may be preoccupied with managing problems related to other areas of the nose during surgery and may not observe dorsum-related problems due to distraction or fatigue, which may lead to dissatisfaction for both the patient and surgeon after surgery. In this chapter, the importance of an orderly check of the dorsum to detect aesthetic and functional problems will be discussed.

Closely checking the dorsum during the surgery is essential. Residual problems can be identified by palpation after dorsal maneuvers have been performed. The author recommends using wet surgical gloves to increase sensation during palpation (Fig. 8.1).

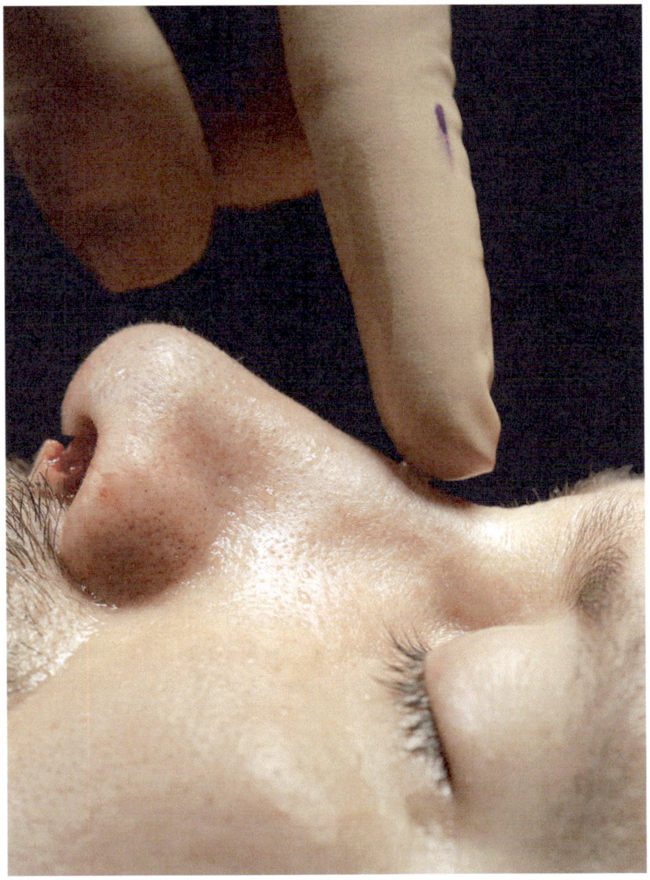

Fig. 8.1 The dorsum is palpated using wet gloves

Supplementary Information The online version contains supplementary material available at https://doi.org/10.1007/978-3-031-65619-4_8.

S. Şeneldir, *Photographic Atlas of Rhinoplasty*, https://doi.org/10.1007/978-3-031-65619-4_8

8.2 Treatment Strategy and Clinical Outcomes

First, palpate the bony dorsum starting from the radix to determine whether the bony vault is closed and the osteotomy line is smooth.

(a) If excess bone exists, rasping is necessary. Piezo, which allows the removal of bone spicules without applying much pressure, can be used as an alternative to the rasping at this point (Fig. 8.2).
(b) If a level difference exists due to concavity, cavities are filled. Bone dust is the most practical material for filling cavities on the bony dorsum. Bone dust acquired during rasping can be collected in a special bone dust collector and placed in cavities on the bony dorsum using bayonet forceps. Diced cartilage can be used when sufficient bone dust is not available (Figs. 8.3, 8.4, and 8.5).

After checking the bony dorsum, the point where the bony and cartilage vaults merge, known as the K-area, is palpated. Because the skin is the thinnest in this region, the K-area must be kept slightly higher than, or at the same level as, the supratip and radix to achieve the ideal dorsum. A low dorsum in the K-area may result in a curved appearance with thin skin postoperatively (Fig. 8.6).

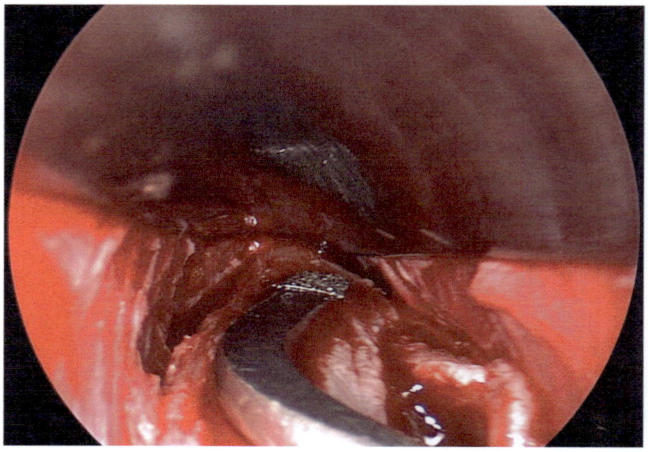

Fig. 8.2 Piezo device can be used to smooth irregularities after an osteotomy

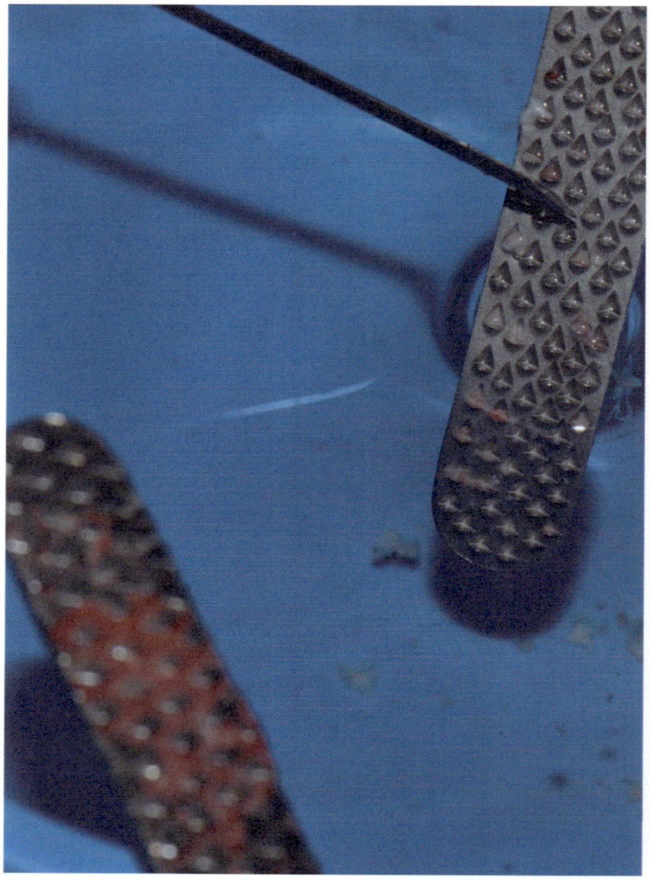

Fig. 8.3 Bone dust acquired during rasping can be collected

8.2.1 Case 1

A representative case of a minimal hump in which the K-area was lower than the supratip and radix caused by a small saddle nose deformity is shown here. The low K-area creates a problematic appearance on the profile view, as well as a split-nose appearance on the frontal view (Fig. 8.7).

Another important point that is necessary to focus on in the K-area is that, in cases in which a spreader graft is used, the cranial tip of the spreader graft may protrude toward the skin after osteotomies.

8.2.2 Case 2

Spreader grafts were used and, after performing osteotomies, the cranial tip of the spreader graft became visible. The excess part of the graft was removed, and the dorsal profile became ideal (Fig. 8.8).

Excess remaining after placement of the spreader graft may be overlooked by a surgeon who is fatigued toward the end of the surgery. The excess is invisible intraoperatively and can be visible in the postoperative mid-term period. Generally, excess in the K-area distorts the dorsum appearance and additional surgery is necessary to resolve the problem endonasally under local anesthesia.

In this representative case of a droopy nasal tip and minimal dorsal hump, the spreader graft excess in the K-area was missed intraoperatively. If the dorsum was palpated meticulously after osteotomy, the protrusion would have been noticed. Unfortunately, the cartilage excess appeared

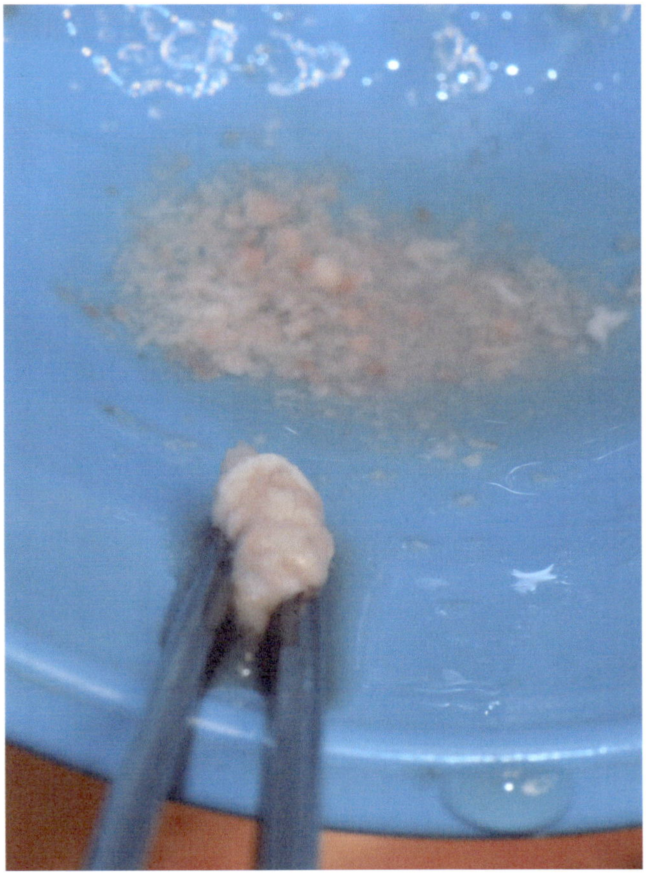

Fig. 8.4 Bone dust acquired during rasping can be collected

6 months after surgery, causing an irregular dorsum that was removed endonasally under local anesthesia (Fig. 8.9).

The supratip area is the last item to check on the dorsum. In most cases, patients want a straight dorsum with a small supratip break. Therefore, the surgeon must check to ensure a supratip break has been created. The tip–dorsum relationship must be checked repeatedly to avoid a Polly beak deformity.

The Polly beak deformity is a fullness in the supratip area caused by excessive soft tissue scarring (soft tissue poly beak) or excessive cartilage (cartilaginous poly beak) in that area. Soft tissue poly beak can result from excessive resection of the supra tip cartilaginous dorsum. The dead space under the skin can constitute scar tissue, leaving a soft tissue poly beak.

Cartilaginous poly beak deformity can be caused by:

(a) Excessive dorsal septal cartilage
(b) Loss of tip projection

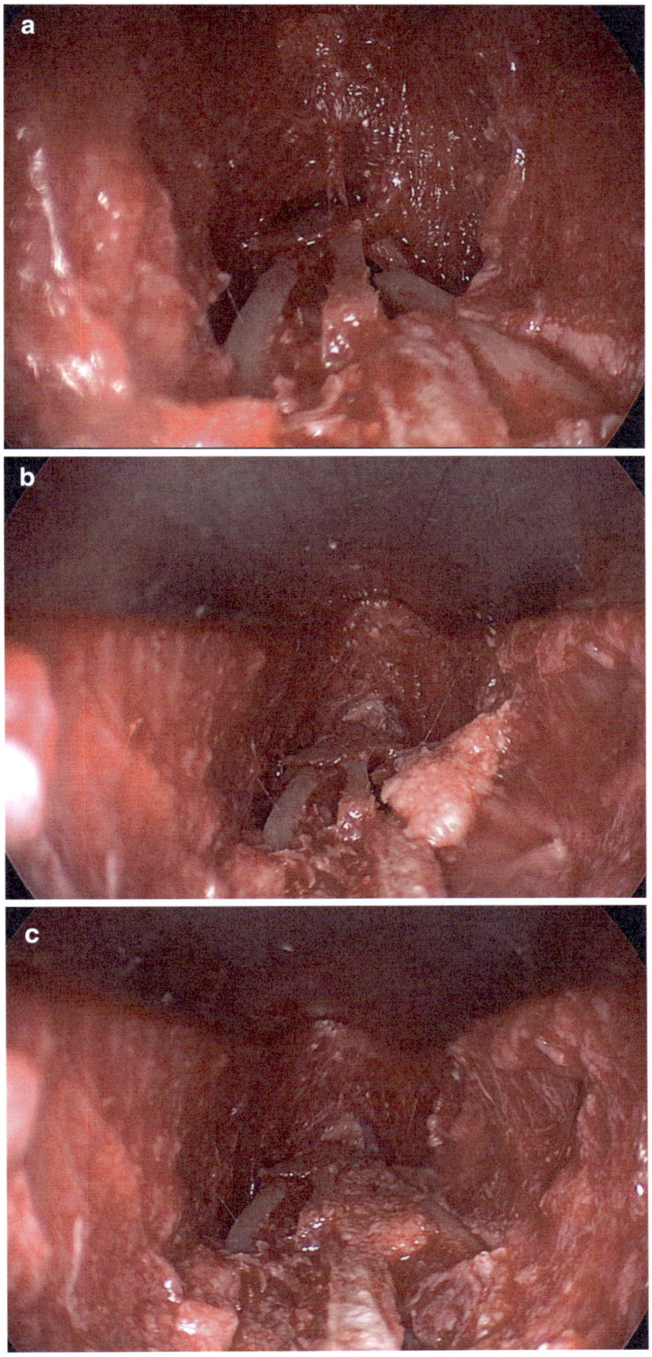

Fig. 8.5 (**a–c**) Bone dust can be used to fill the gap after nasal bone osteotomy

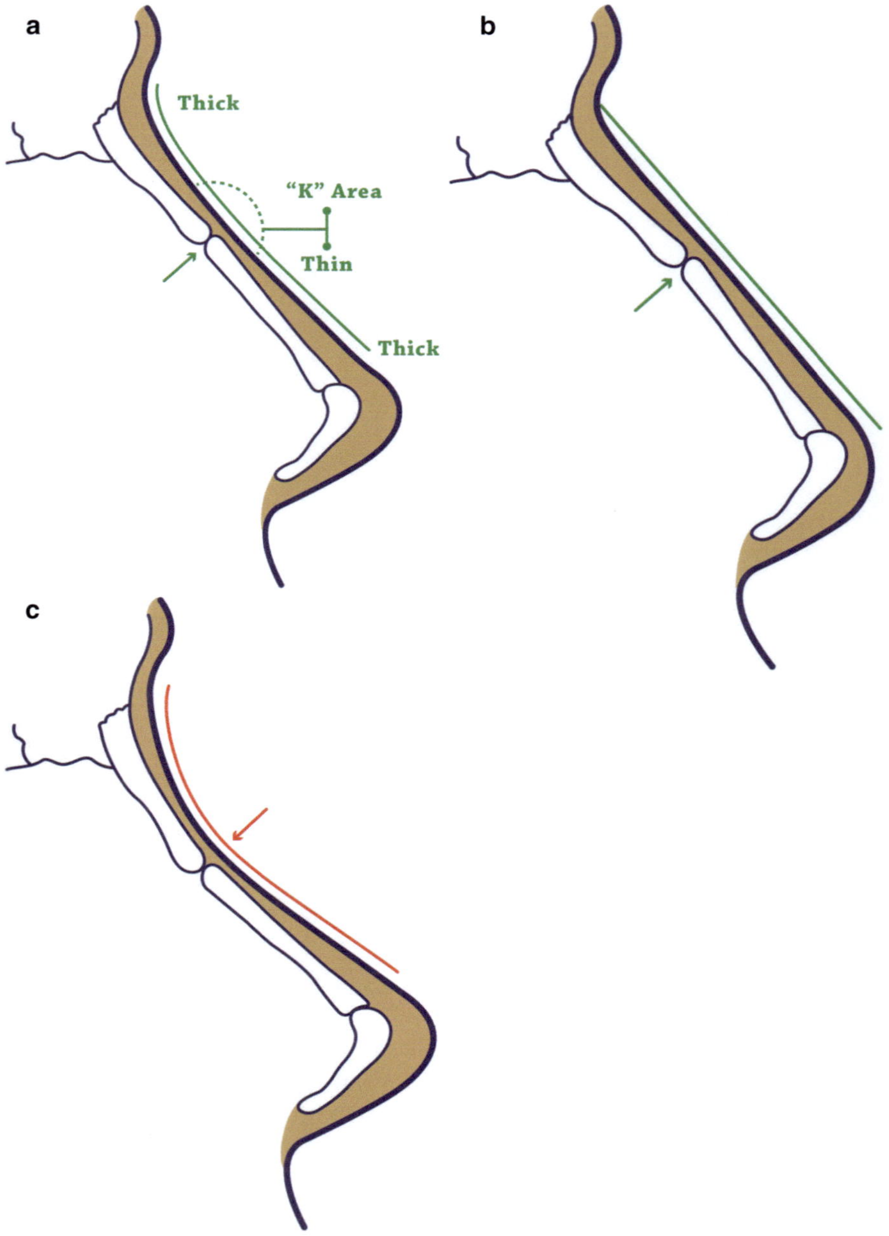

Fig. 8.6 (**a**–**c**) Illustrations of the ideal dorsum in a female (**a**), a male (**b**), and a curved dorsum caused by an over-reduction of the k-area (**c**)

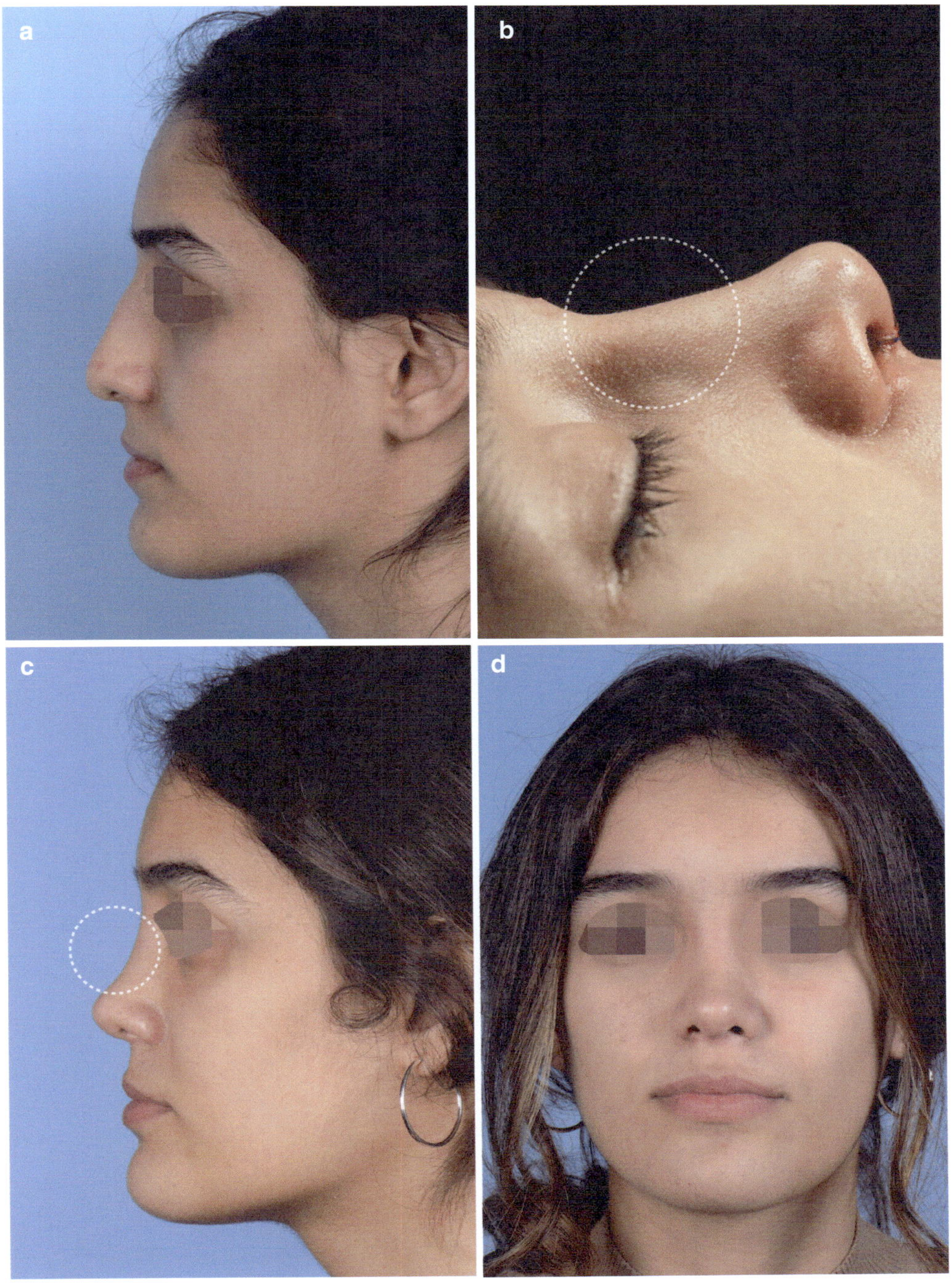

Fig. 8.7 (**a**) Profile-view photograph shows the preoperative slight nasal hump. (**b**) Well-formed dorsum during surgery. (**c**, **d**) One-year postoperative photograph shows a curved dorsum. Thus, despite a good intraoperative profile, failure to palpate the K-area sufficiently resulted in a curved dorsum postoperatively. In this case, the author was misled by using the eyes only. A frontal-view photograph at 1-year post-surgery shows a split appearance of the nose due to the curved dorsum

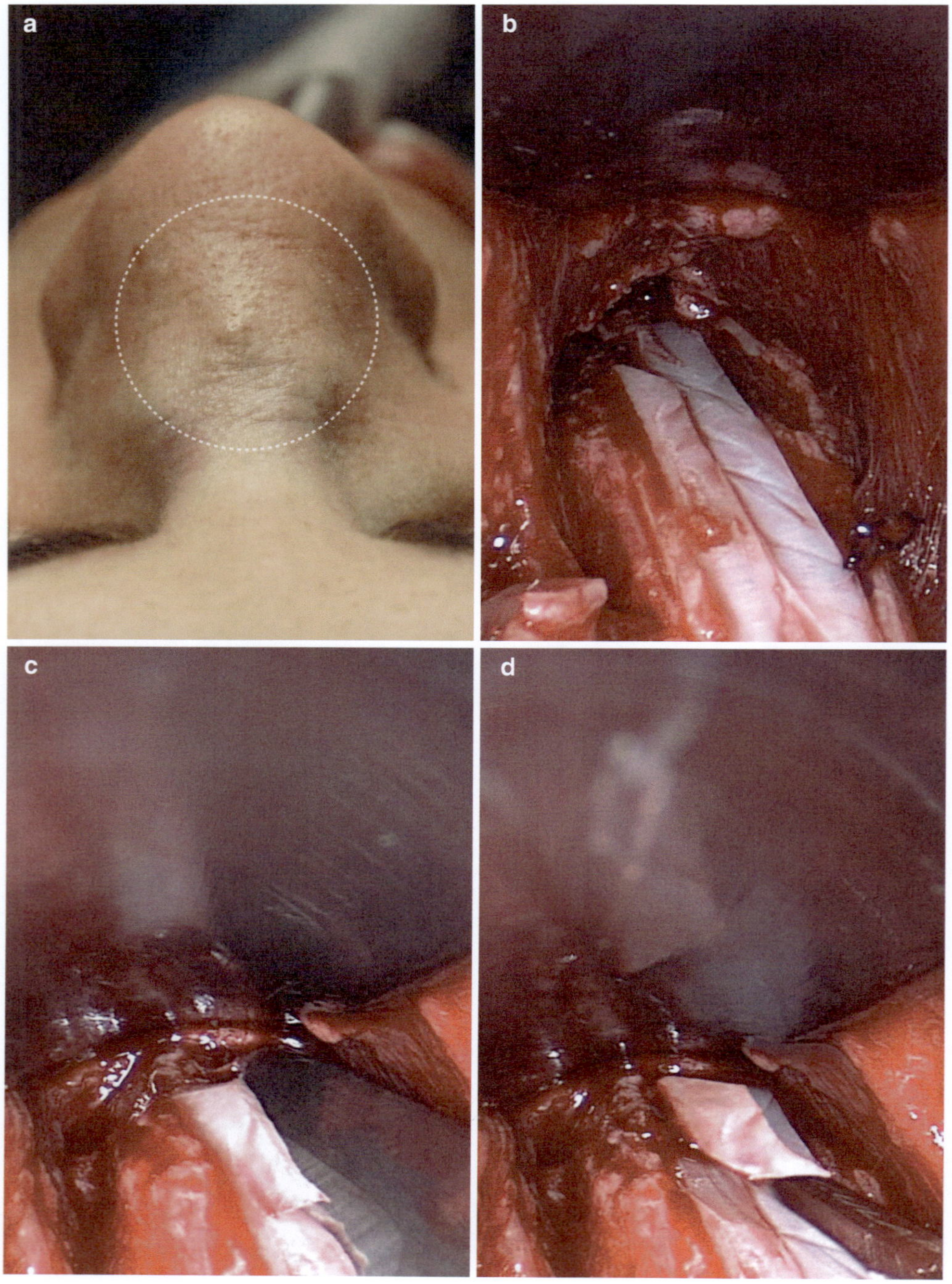

Fig. 8.8 (**a**) Intraoperative photograph shows the protrusion near the K-area. (**b**) Intraoperative endoscopic photograph shows the protrusion caused by the excess spreader graft. (**c**, **d**) Resection using a scalpel and removal of the excess graft material. (**e**) The right spreader graft after removal of the excess portion. (**f**) Intraoperative photograph shows a smooth dorsal profile after removal of the excess right spreader graft

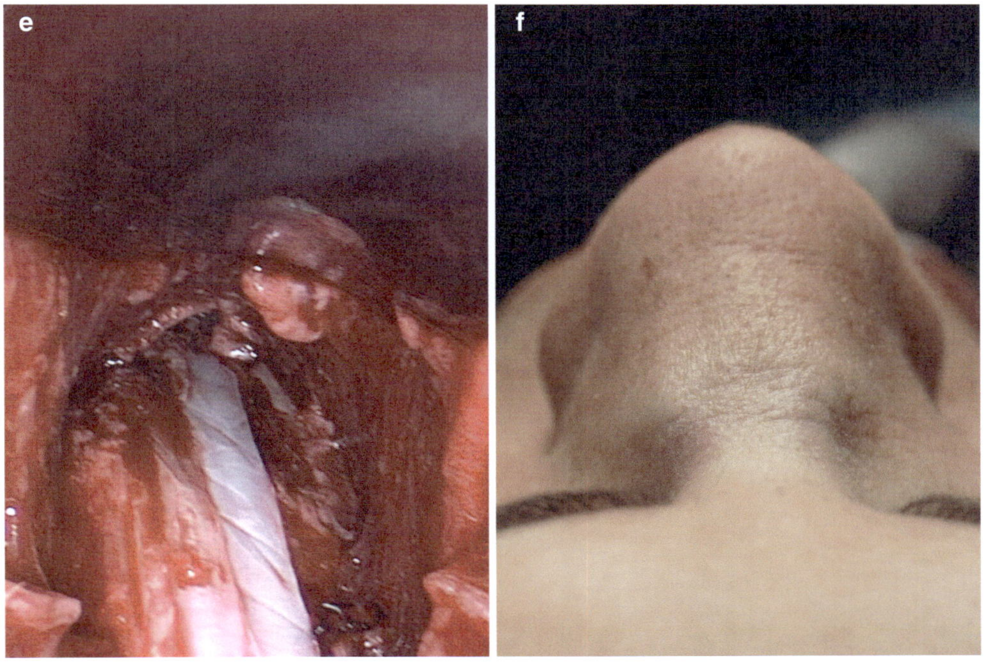

Fig. 8.8 (continued)

Fig. 8.9 (**a**) Preoperative profile-view of a patient with droopy tip and nasal hump. (**b**) Although intraoperative view shows the ideal dorsal profile, if the dorsum had been palpated, dorsal irregularity would have been revealed. (**c**) 6-month postoperative image showing an irregularity in the K-area caused by the cranial tip of the spreader graft. (**d**) An intraoperative image showing resection of the cartilage excess under local anesthesia during a second surgery performed by the author. (**e**) 6-months after revision surgery, an ideal dorsal profile is achieved

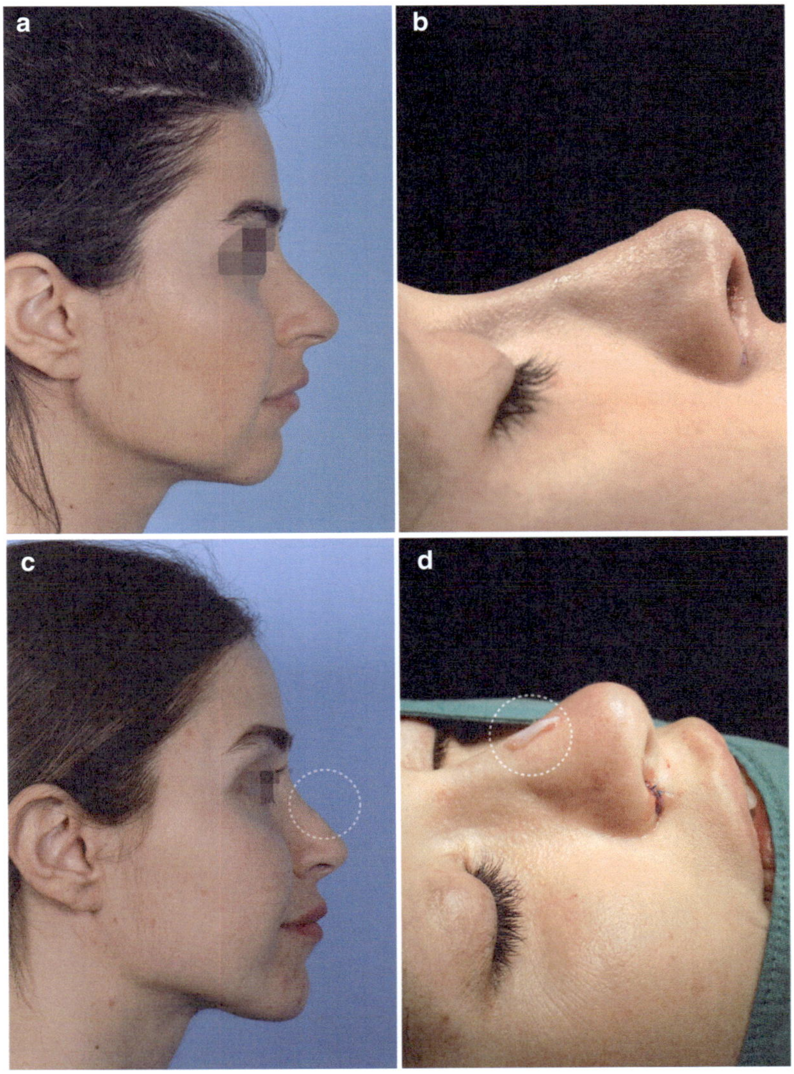

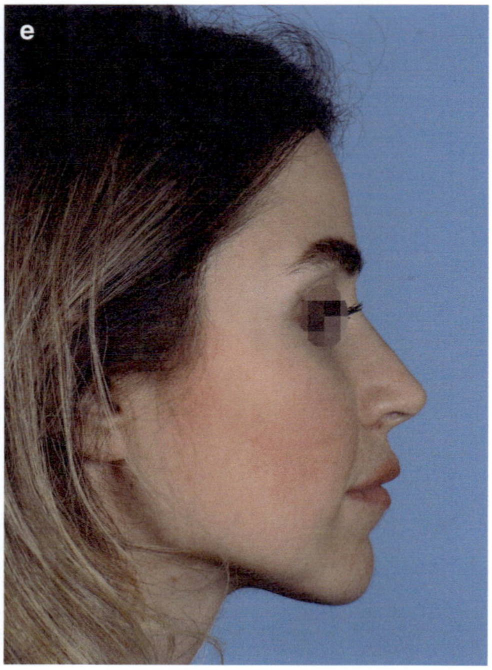

Fig. 8.9 (continued)

8.3 Excessive Septal Cartilage in the Dorsum

Overlooking septal excess in the supratip area may be caused by errors in planning the steps of the dorsal resection, or it may be missed in patients with a large dorsal hump. The importance of palpating the supratip with wet gloves and resecting excess cartilage to prevent these complications cannot be overstated. Furthermore, Polly beak deformity caused by excess septal cartilage can be readily corrected by exposing the supratip area via the endonasal or external approach and resecting the excess cartilage.

8.3.1 Case 4

A representative case of Polly beak deformity is shown here. The patient had undergone rhinoplasty 10 years earlier; however, nasal hump persisted, and she elected to undergo a second operation. The intraoperative photographs show that the Polly beak deformity was caused by excessive septal cartilage (Fig. 8.10).

8.3.2 Case 5

A second example of Polly beak deformity caused by excess septal cartilage in the dorsum is shown here. In this case, the supratip fullness stemmed from dorsal septal excess and the hanging columella was caused by caudal septal excess (Fig. 8.11).

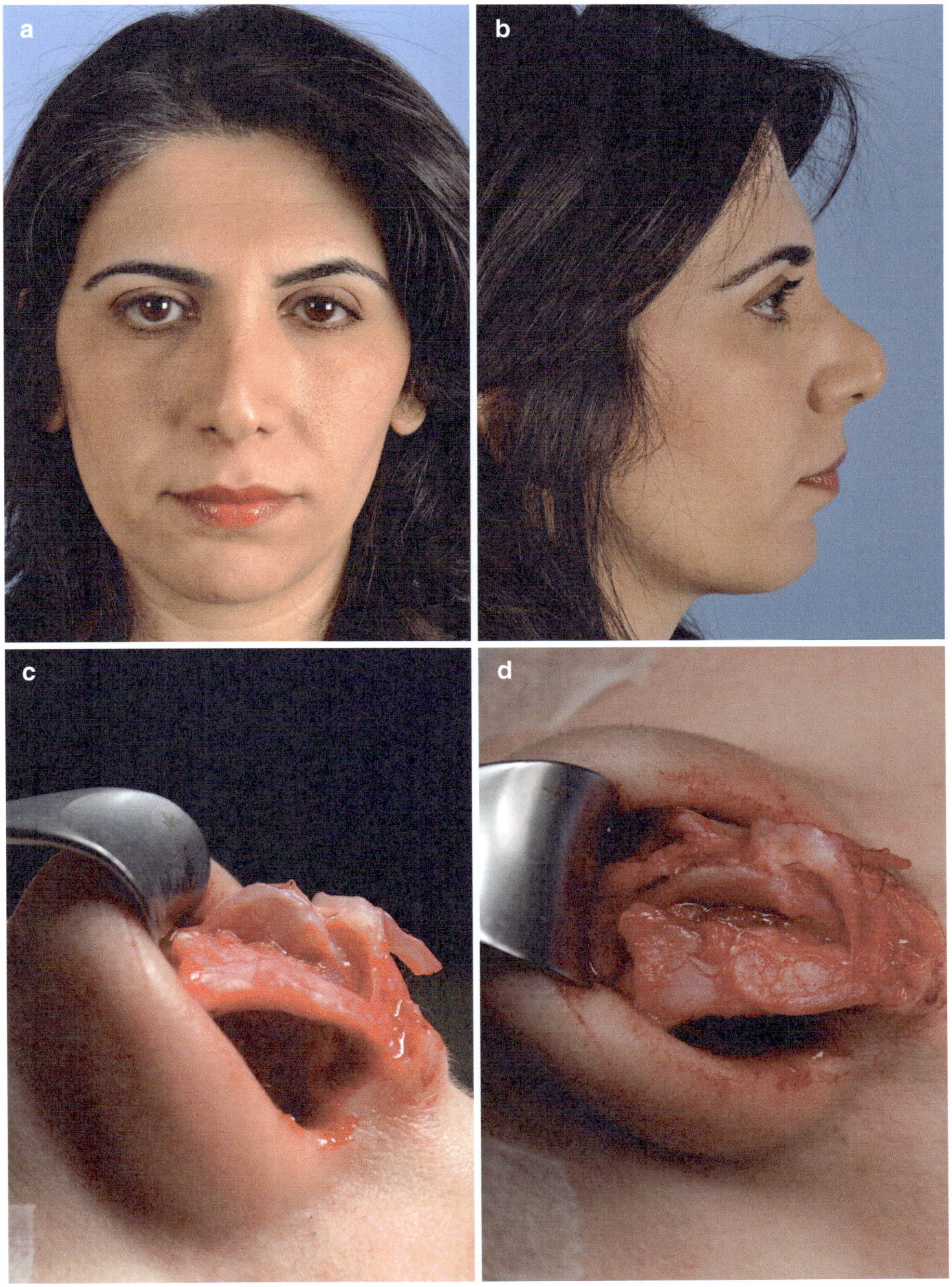

Fig. 8.10 (**a**, **b**) Preoperative photographs show Polly beak deformity in a revision case. (**c**, **d**) Intraoperative photographs showing cartilage excess in the septum. Excess cartilage was resected. (**e**, **f**) Frontal and profile photographs 3 years after revision surgery

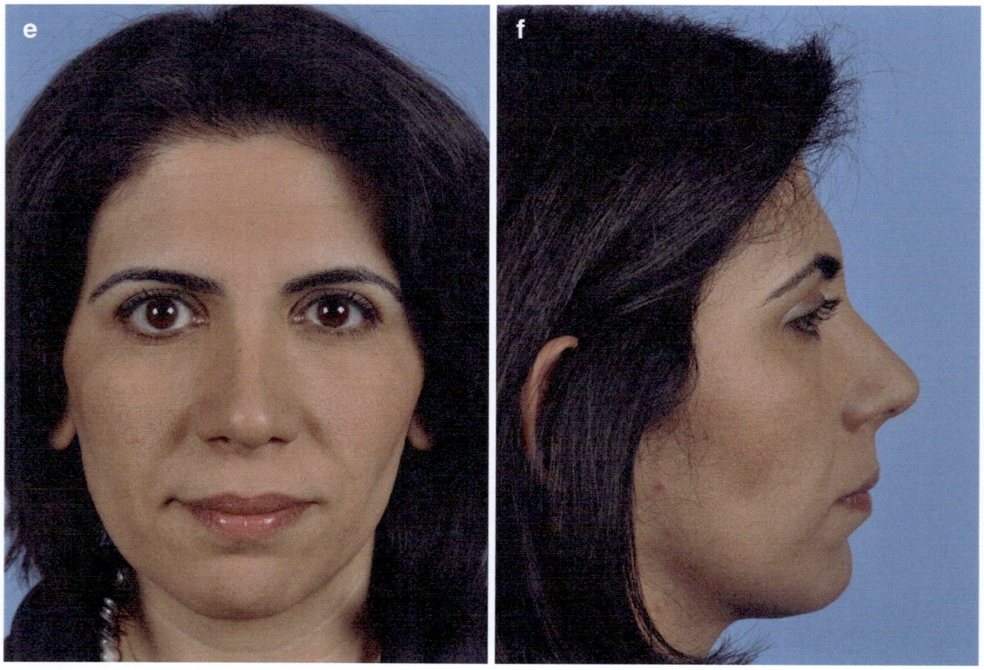

Fig. 8.10 (continued)

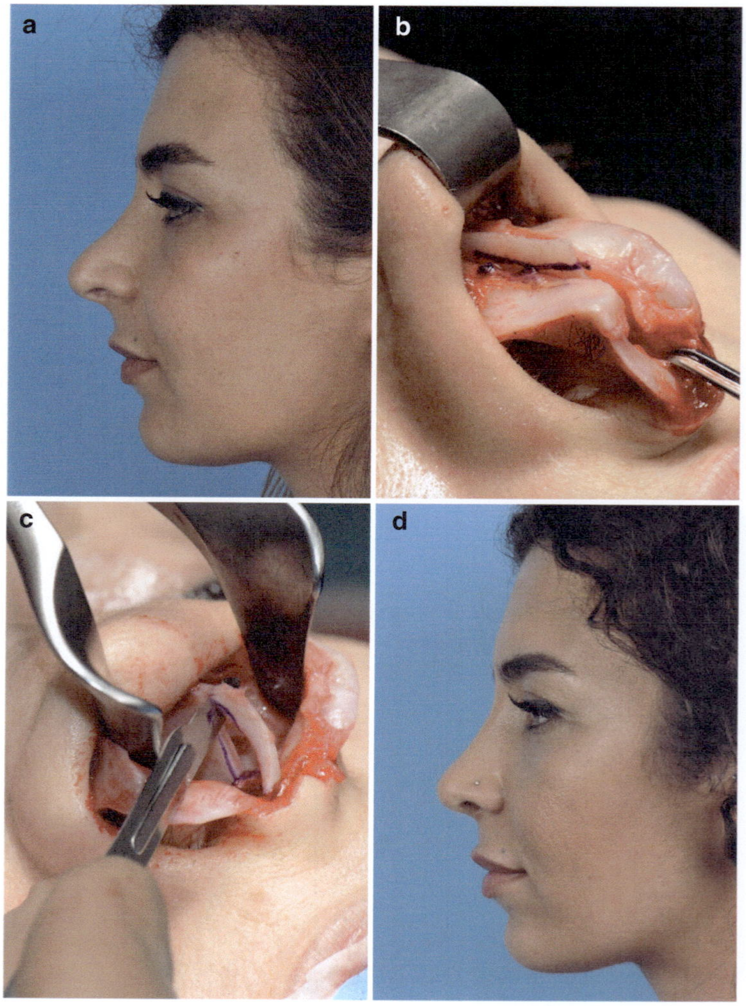

Fig. 8.11 (**a**) Patient with a Polly beak deformity caused by excess septal cartilage in the dorsum. Profile photograph showing supratip fullness and the hanging columella. (**b**, **c**) Marked areas indicating excess cartilage in the septum. (**d**) Photograph 2 years after resection of the excess cartilage

8.4 Polly Beak Deformity Caused by Lateral Crus

Lateral crura may cause Polly beak deformity. When unrecognized, persistent excess volume in the supratip area may occur as a result of the lateral crura overriding the dorsum. The problem is solved with the resection of the excess part of lateral crura (Fig. 8.12).

8.4.1 Case 6

This patient had a prior rhinoplasty in which the bony dorsum was resected and the cartilaginous dorsum was not touched (see Fig. 8.12).

Technical Pearl: If the hump caused by the lateral crura persists after cephalic resection, repositioning is necessary. Repositioning of the lateral crura moves the excess volume

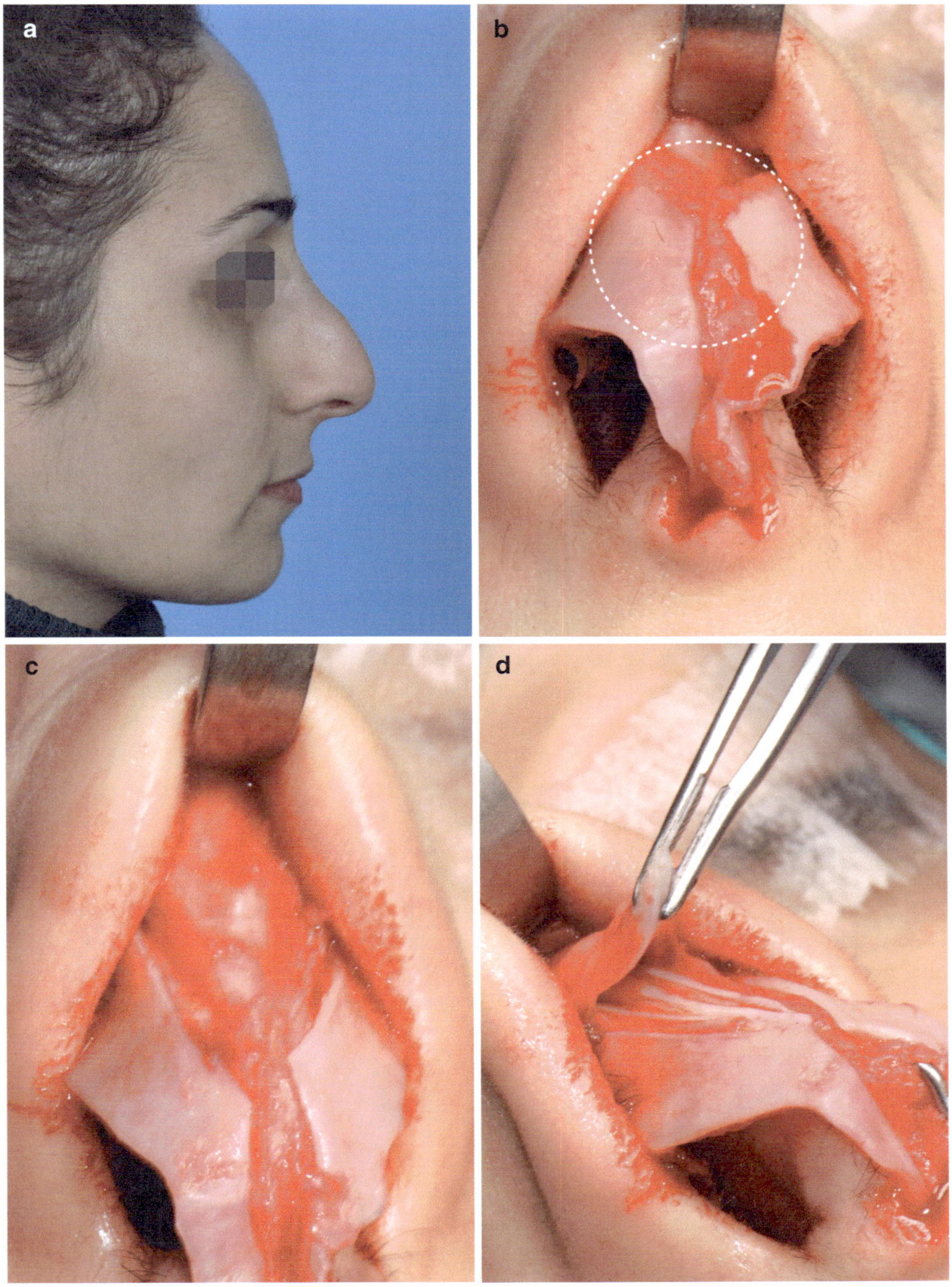

Fig. 8.12 (**a**) Preoperative profile view. (**b**) Intraoperative photograph showing the lateral crura overriding the dorsum The cartilaginous dorsal hump was caused by residual middle vault and the cephalic portion of the lateral crus. (**c**, **d**) Cephalic resection and removal of the excess cartilaginous dorsum. (**e**) One year after revision surgery; the dorsal profile was satisfactory

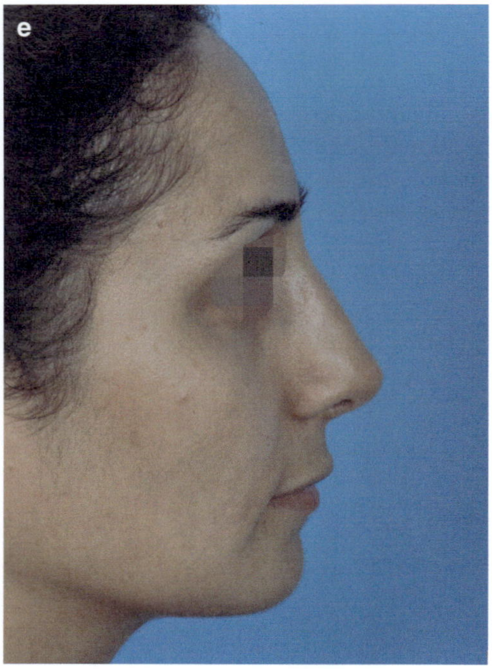

Fig. 8.12 (continued)

from the supratip to the lateral nasal wall, resolving the Polly beak deformity.

8.5 Loss of Tip Projection

The Polly beak deformity caused by excess septal cartilage and malpositioning of the lateral crura can be foreseen, although they are rare. Polly beak deformities caused by the loss of projection during the healing period may be unpredictable. Unless the tip is stabilized at the end of surgery, the projection may be lost, and the supratip will be higher than the tip. In fact, the main problem is not excess in the supratip, but insufficiency of the tip projection. Thus, it is crucial to ensure the tip is stabilized during surgery; if needed, the tip should be connected to the septum via the septocolumellar suture or septocolumellar strut (Fig. 8.13).

8.5.1 Case 7

Polly beak deformity caused by projection loss can be readily detected in the preoperative examination; when the tip is lifted slightly the fullness in the supratip disappears (Fig. 8.14).

The tip projection is regained following revision surgery, and the Polly beak deformity is resolved (Fig. 8.15).

After examination of the dorsal surface of the middle vault, the lateral nasal wall is palpated. Cavities in the lateral nasal wall should be checked carefully and filled with grafts if necessary. Cartilage is the most practical graft material for this purpose. Diced or *gently crushed cartilage* is placed in cavities using forceps. Grafts remain in place and do not resorb for a long period of time, which is why overgrafting must be avoided.

Technical Pearl: The nose must be assessed carefully before surgery to identify existing or potential cavities to achieve the ideal brow-tip aesthetic line. Thus, preoperative photographs are important. Frontal images made using single paraflash photography clearly reveal potential cavities (Fig. 8.16).

8.5.2 Case 8

In Fig. 8.16, the concavity on the right side still persists after hump removal, osteotomy, and the placement of bilateral spreader grafts. The intraoperative photographs in Case 8 show that the concavity was filled with diced cartilage (Fig. 8.17).

Two years later, an ideal brow-tip aesthetic line was achieved via both spreader grafts and diced cartilages (Fig. 8.18).

8.5.3 Case 9

Another patient had a concavity on the right nasal wall causing a break in the brow-tip aesthetic line. It was necessary to fill this concavity with crushed cartilage despite spreader grafting (Fig. 8.19).

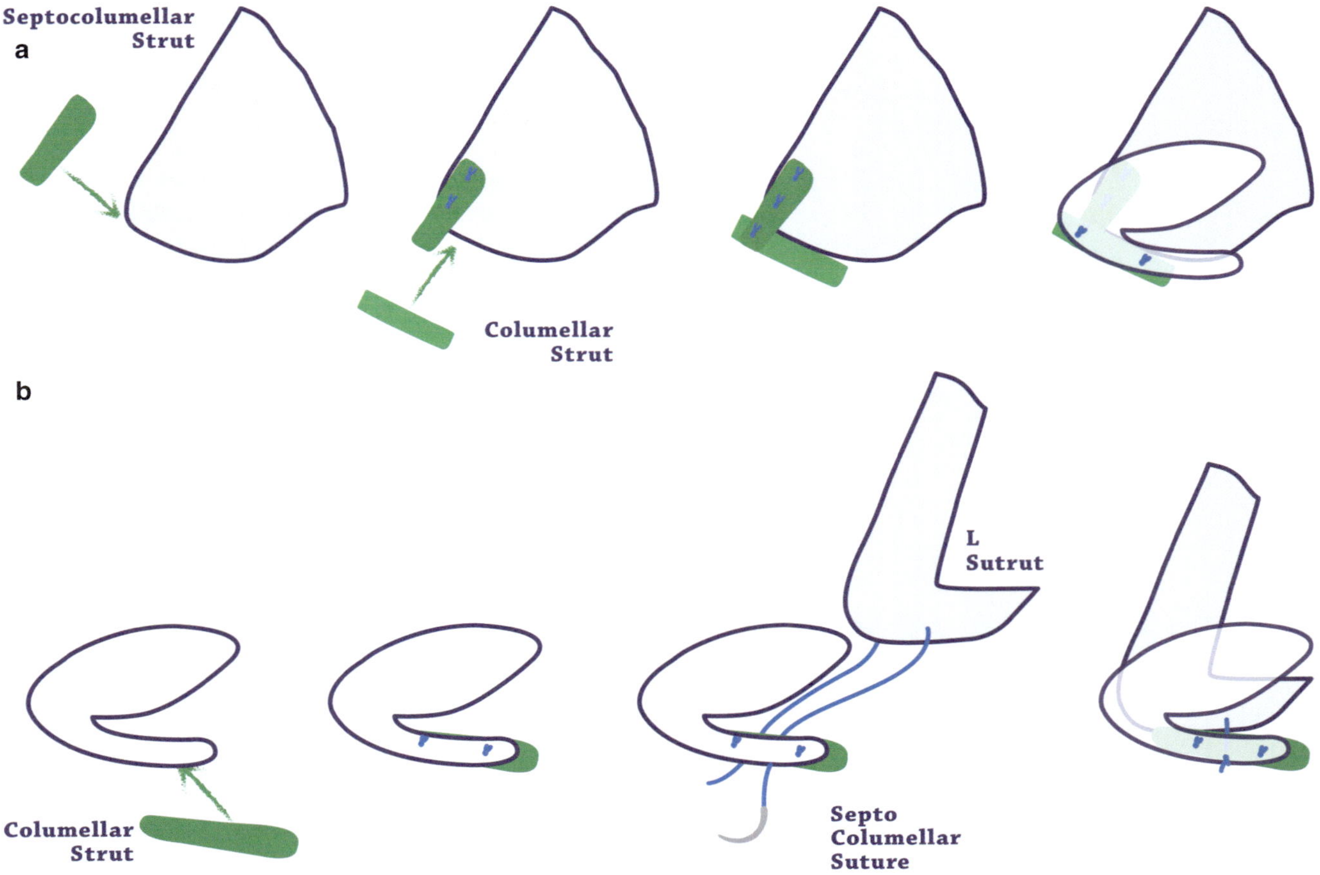

Fig. 8.13 (**a**) Columella septal graft: the tip and the columella are connected by suturing the graft in-between. It provides long-term tip stability. Septocolumellar graft is believed to provide the most support for nasal tip projection. Because the septum is extended by using this graft, it is much easier to protect the projection of the nasal tip. (**b**) Columella septal suture. A needle is passed between the leaves of the middle crura and then passed through the septum, which is usually at a same level to the columella septal entry. The suture provides tip stabilization and can correct any existing hanging columella. The septocolumellar suture effect is less than septocolumellar strut

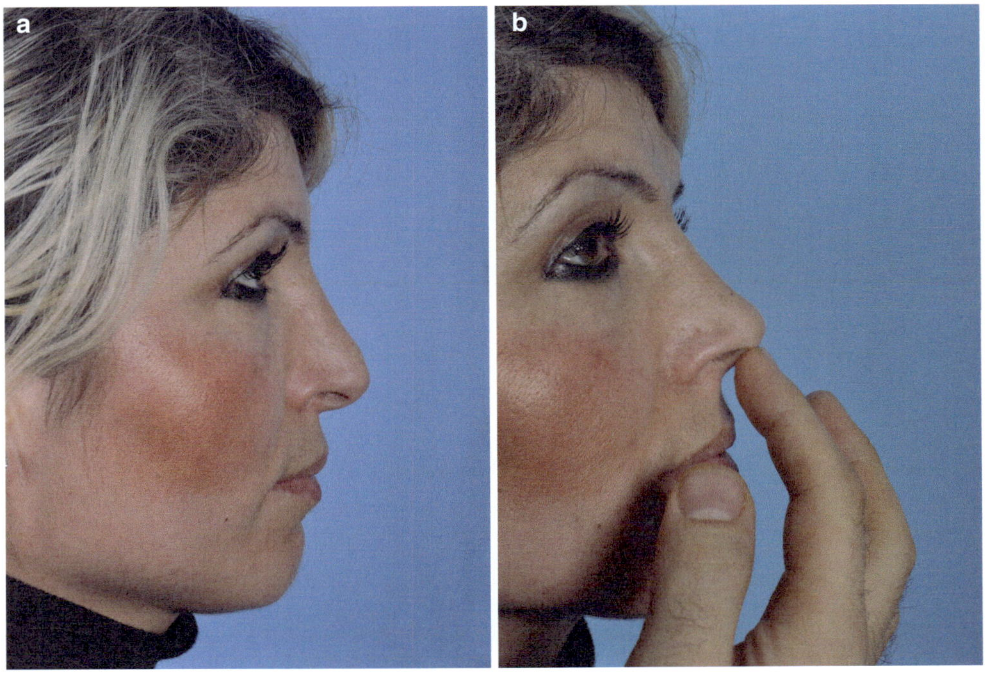

Fig. 8.14 (**a**) Patient with a Polly beak deformity caused by projection loss following rhinoplasty 5-years previously performed by another surgeon. The supratip fullness is readily visible. (**b**) After replacement of the lost projection, the supratip fullness disappears. This maneuver is a beneficial test to understand the reason of a poly beak

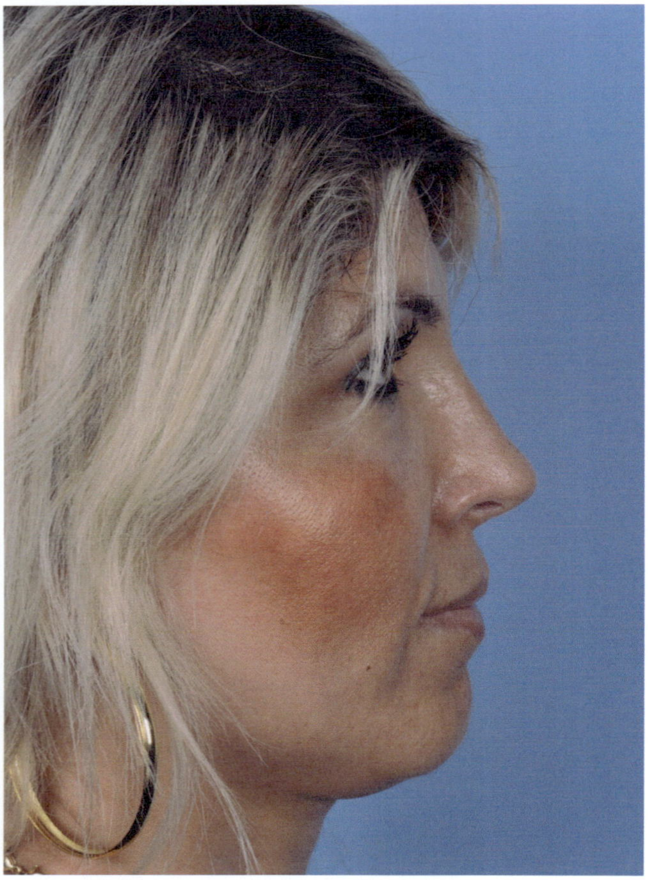

Fig. 8.15 The tip was supported and the projection is improved. The poly beak deformity is eliminated

Photographs taken 2 years after surgery from the frontal and face-down views show that the use of bilateral spreader graft and crushed cartilage filler achieved an ideal brow-tip aesthetic line (Fig. 8.20).

Camouflage grafts, whether crushed or diced cartilages, can be safely used to restore middle vault symmetry. Moving the septum to the midline position using a spreader graft or total septal reconstruction may not be sufficient to achieve middle vault symmetry. In such cases, camouflage grafts are effective.

8.5.4 Case 10

In this case, after septoplasty and bilateral spreader grafting, filling the right nasal wall concavity with crushed cartilage achieved bilateral middle vault symmetry (Fig. 8.21).

Technical Pearl: Fixing the crushed cartilage to the skin or the lateral nasal wall is not recommended because it can change the position of the cartilage. It is unlikely that carefully placed crushed cartilage will move.

8.5.5 Case 11

Preoperative photographs show two-sided concavity in a patient with middle vault asymmetry. Diced cartilage was used to fill the concavities to achieve bilateral middle vault symmetry (Fig. 8.22).

In contrast to concavity, convexity of the lateral nasal wall can create additional problems. Generally, the convexity stems from caudal excess of the upper lateral cartilages.

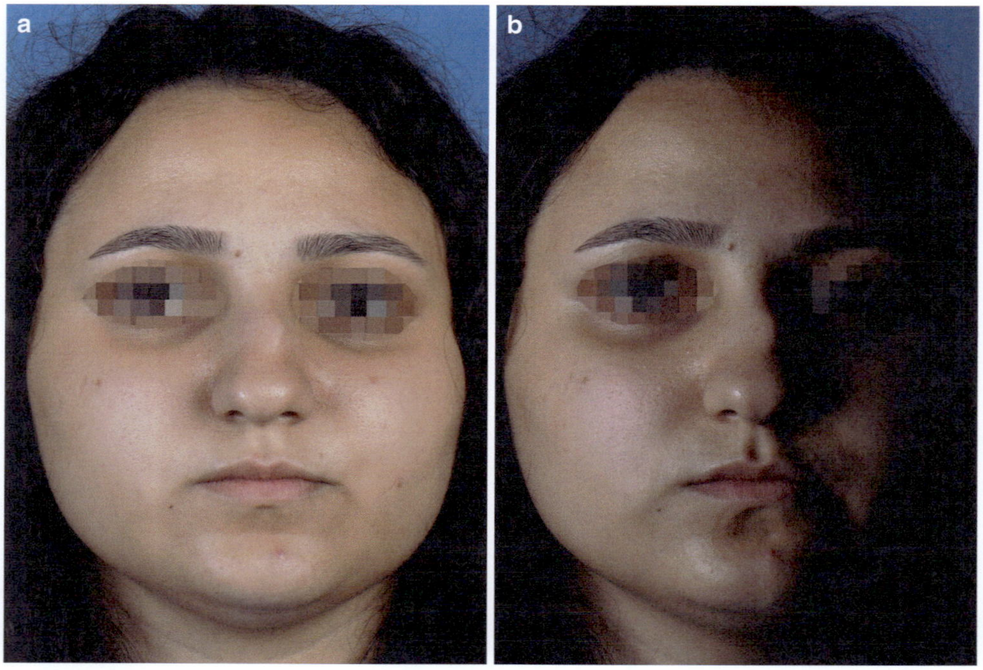

Fig. 8.16 (a, b) A comparison of images using single- (a) and dual-paraflash (b) photography. Concavities in the lateral nasal wall are clearly visible in the images using single-paraflash photography

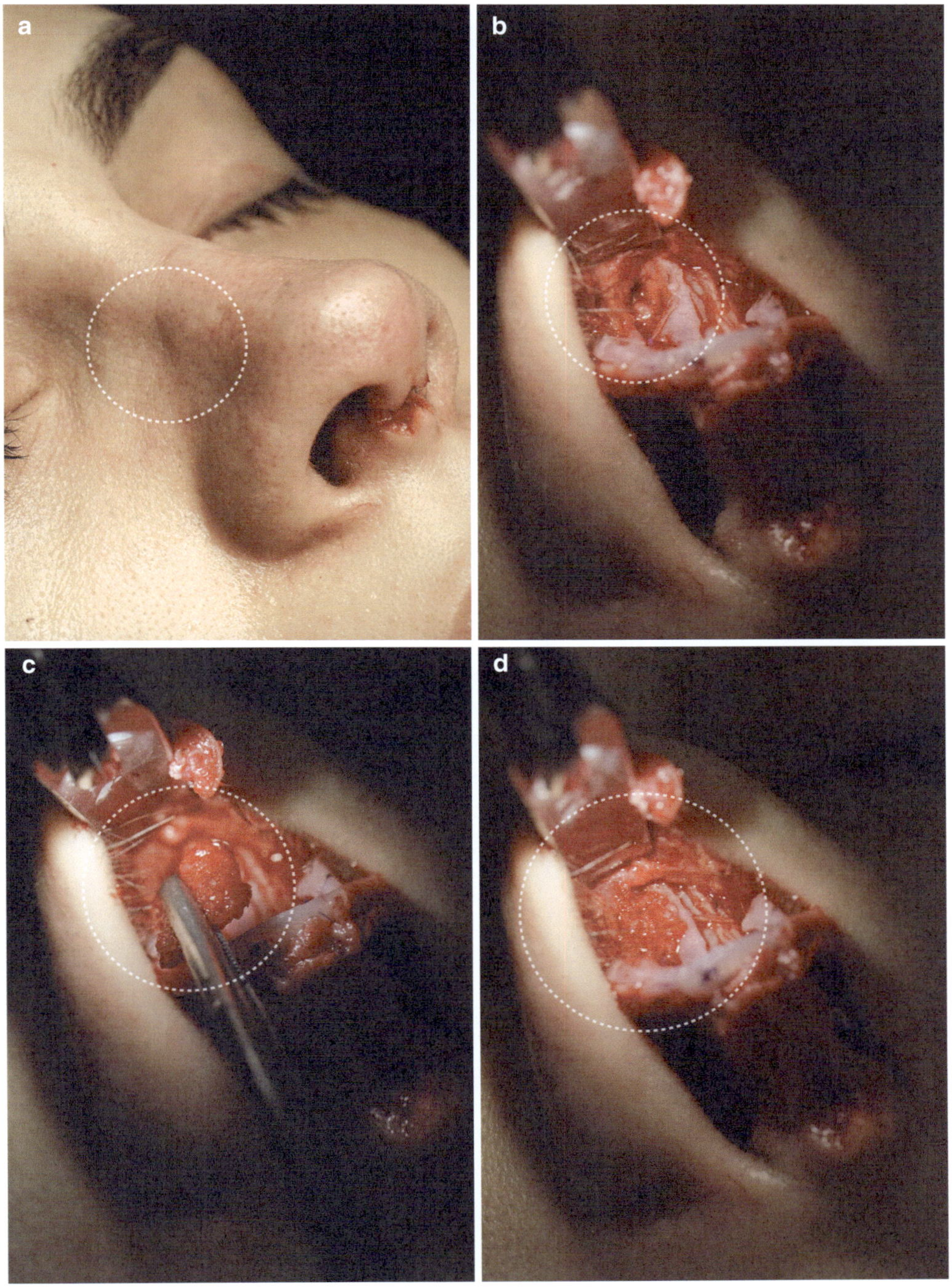

Fig. 8.17 (**a**) Shadow at the skin corresponding to concavity in the right nasal wall. (**b**) Concavity of the right upper lateral cartilage. (**c**, **d**) The concavity was filled with diced cartilage. (**e**) After filling the cavity, the shadow corresponding to the concavity disappeared

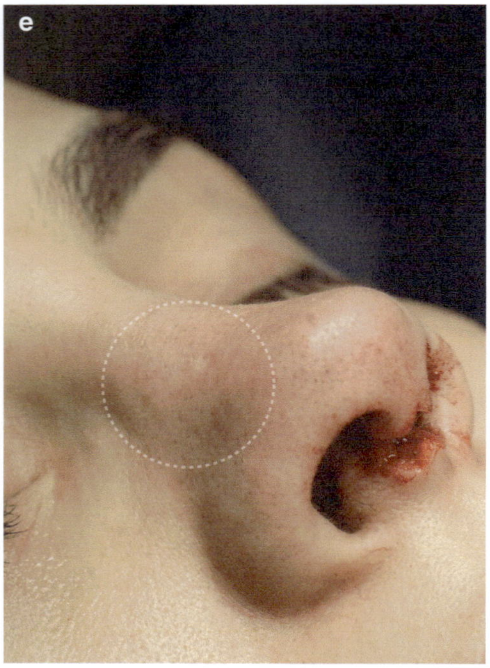

Fig. 8.17 (continued)

Fig. 8.18 (**a**, **b**) Dorsal aesthetic lines are improved

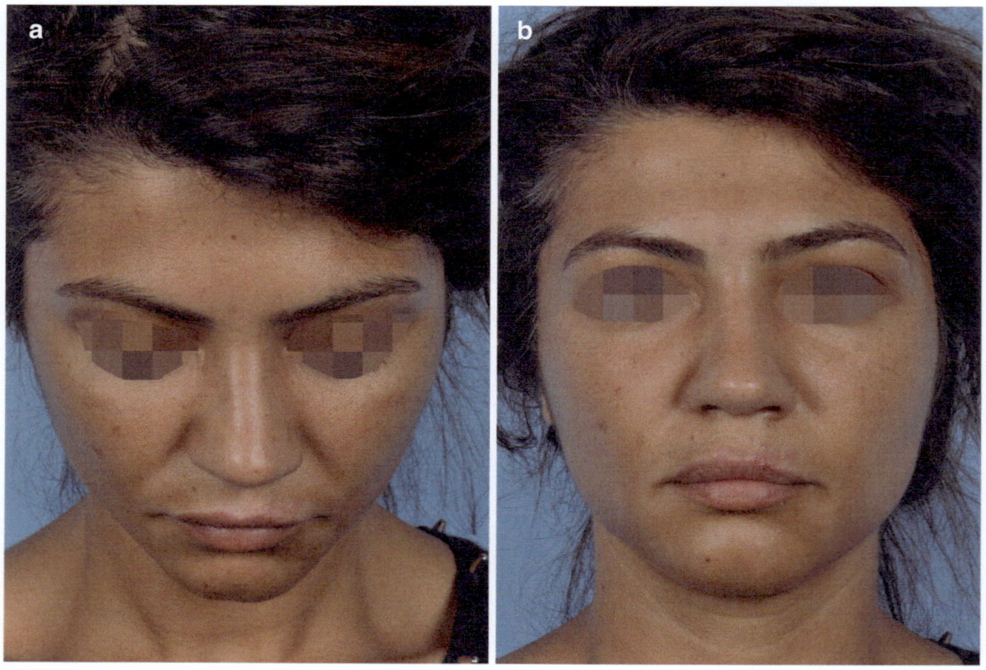

The convexity mostly occurs during surgery of droopy nasal tip patients that require rotation.

8.5.6 Case 12

This is a representative case of right alar sidewall convexity (Fig. 8.23); after osteotomy, middle vault reconstruction and nasal tip plasty were performed, and the caudal portion of the right upper lateral cartilage causing the convexity was removed, solving the problem.

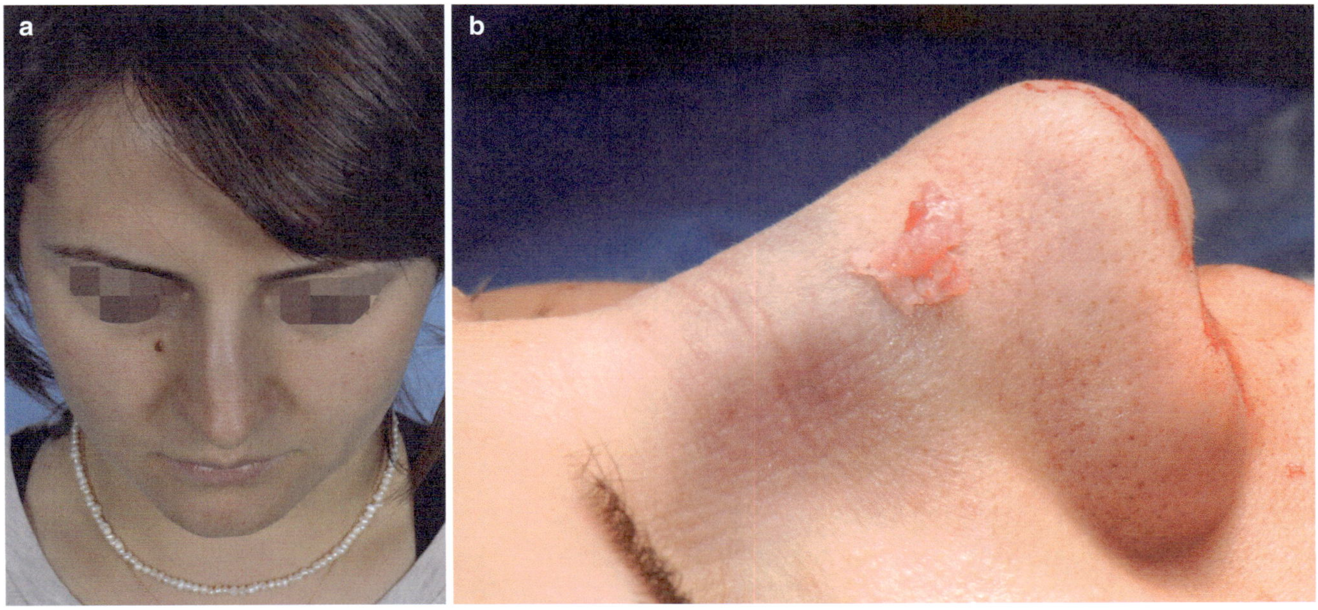

Fig. 8.19 (**a**) The preoperative face-down photograph clearly shows the concavity on the right nasal wall. (**b**) The concavity was filled with crushed cartilage

Fig. 8.20 (**a–d**) The crushed cartilage corrected the concavity and brow-tip aesthetic line break

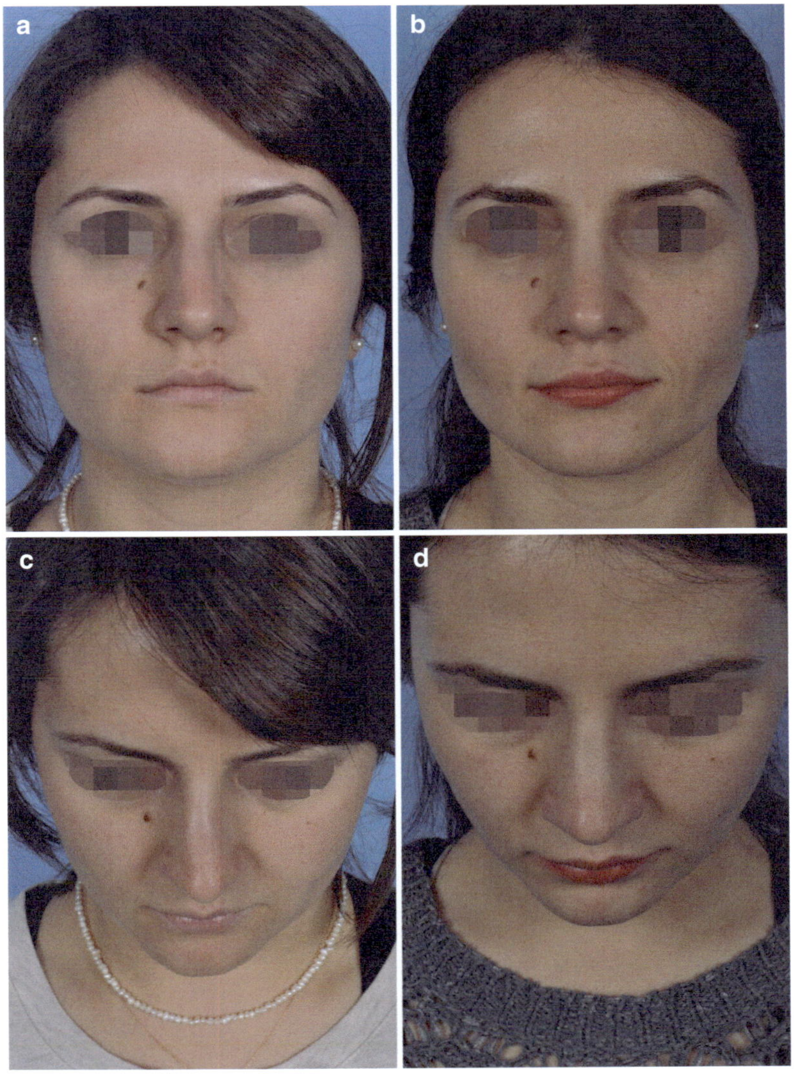

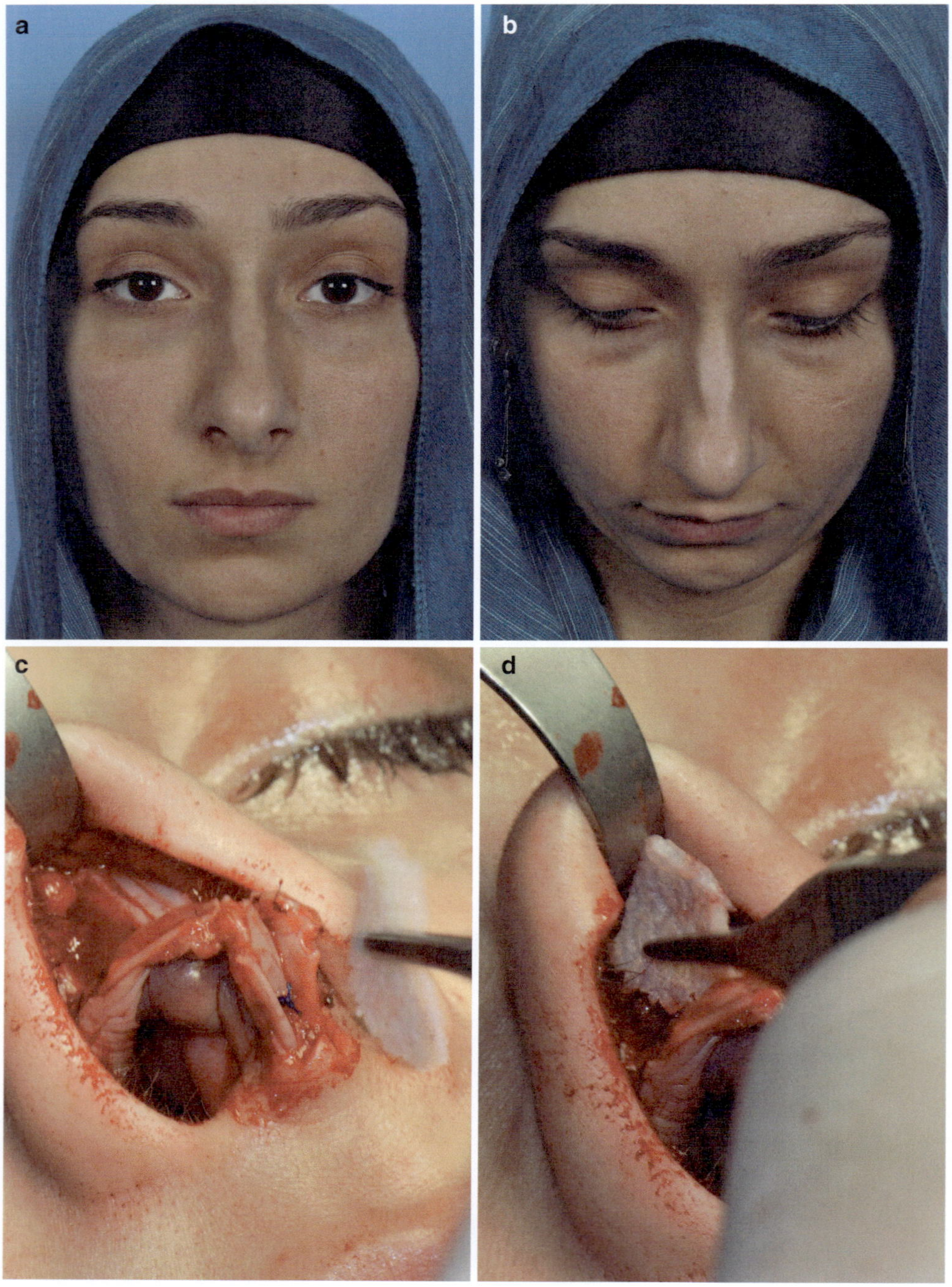

Fig. 8.21 (**a**, **b**) Preoperative photographs in the frontal and face-down views show middle vault asymmetries and weakness on the right side in particular. (**c**, **d**) Intraoperative photographs showing crushed cartilage placed in the right nasal wall. (**e**, **f**) Frontal and face-down photographs taken 1 year after surgery showing that bilateral middle vault symmetry was achieved

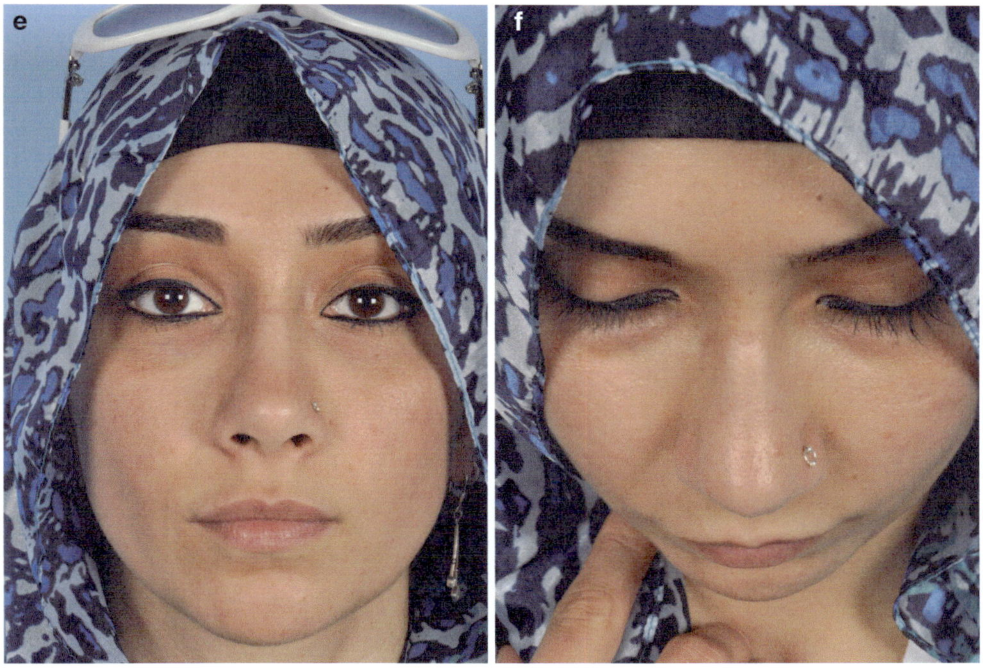

Fig. 8.21 (continued)

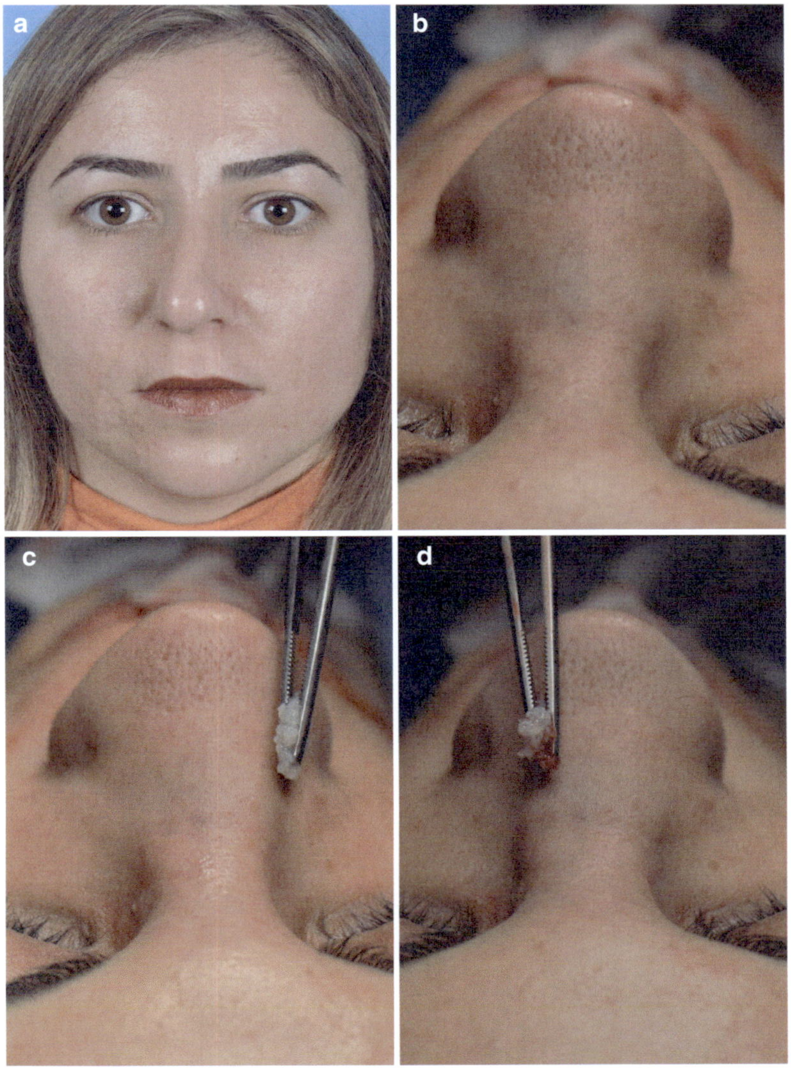

Fig. 8.22 (**a**) Preoperative frontal photograph showing severe asymmetry of the nasal dorsum and two-sided concavities on the lateral nasal walls. (**b**) Subtotal septal reconstruction achieved symmetry. (**c–e**) Final bilateral touch ups to the cavities using diced cartilage achieved excellent symmetry. (**f**) Two-year postoperative frontal photograph showing that the asymmetry was resolved, and the ideal brow-tip aesthetic line was achieved

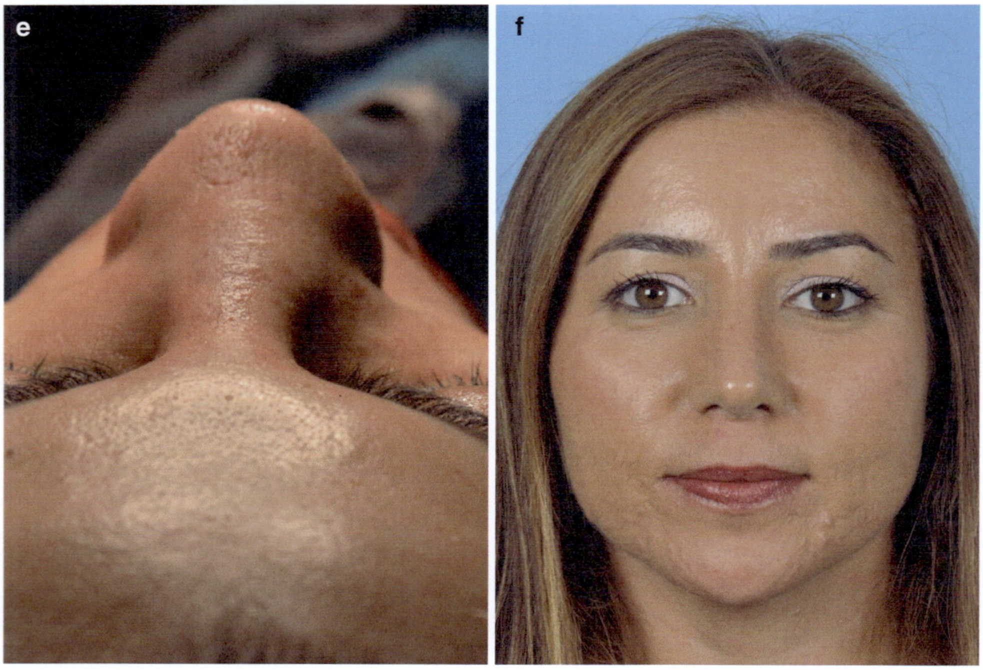

Fig. 8.22 (continued)

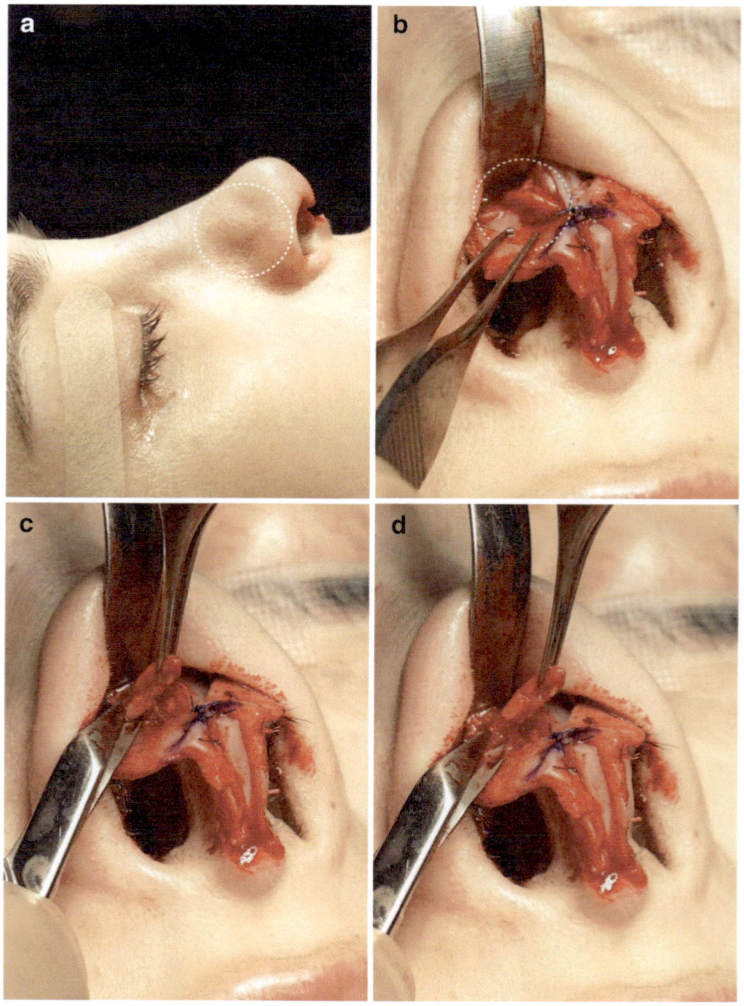

Fig. 8.23 (**a**) Intraoperative photograph of the patient with right alar sidewall convexity. (**b**) Source of convexity is the caudal excess part of the upper lateral cartilage. (**c**, **d**) Removal of the excess cartilage. (**e**) Convexity resolved on the alar side wall

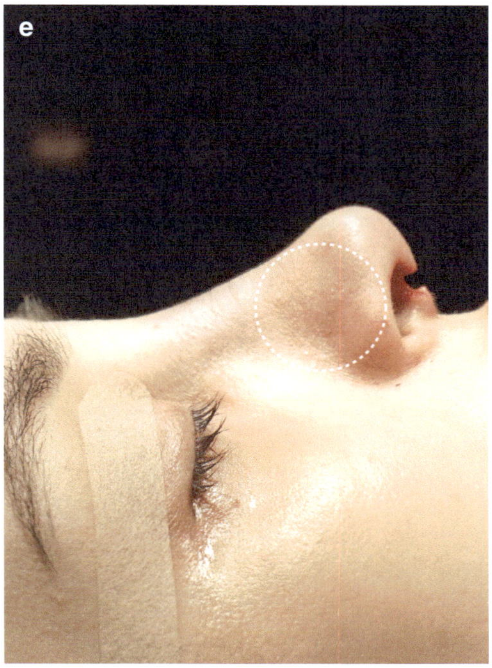

Fig. 8.23 (continued)

8.6 Conclusions

Surgeons generally tend to focus on the nasal tip and neglect the dorsum, which may cause them to overlook problems related to the dorsum as a result of long operating times and fatigue. In the final analysis, a straight dorsum is more important to patients than a fine tip. According to Kandathil et al. (2018), the reduction of dorsal height has a greater positive effect on social perception than the tip position. In this context, standard surgical steps may not be sufficient to achieve an ideal dorsum, making final touches to the dorsum crucial, which is why surgeons must be patient and carefully attend to potential problems.

In this chapter, we propose to meticulously inspect the osteocartilaginous vault at the end of the surgery to minimize errors related to the dorsum caused by surgeon's distraction during operation. Surgical outcomes can be improved by following the final touch and using diced or crushed cartilage and bone dust to camouflage the nasal dorsum.

Disclosures The author reports no conflicts of interest or funding requiring disclosure.

Further Reading

Hoehne J, Gubisch W, Kreutzer C, Haack S. Refining the nasal dorsum with free diced cartilage. Facial Plast Surg. 2016;32(4):345–50.

Kontis TC. The art of camouflage: when can a revision rhinoplasty be nonsurgical. Facial Plast Surg. 2018;34(3):270–7.

Robitschek J, Hilger P. The saddle deformity: camouflage and reconstruction. Facial Plast Surg Clin North Am. 2017;25(2):239–50.

Reference

Kandathil CK, Saltychev M, Moubayed SP, Most SP. Association of dorsal reduction and tip rotation with social perception. JAMA Facial Plast Surg. 2018;20(5):362–6.

9 Dorsum: Saddle Nose

9.1 Introduction

The principal cause of a saddle nose is weak (insufficient) septal support by the middle vault. A saddle nose is fundamentally a middle vault problem. However, in severe cases, the upper (bony) vault may also be affected.

An over-resected bony dorsum is often misdiagnosed as a saddle nose. Augmentation is the adequate treatment for over-resected bony dorsum, whereas this is not enough for the saddle nose treatment. Dorsal augmentation should be done after middle vault reconstruction, if necessary, in the saddle nose. For this reason, differential diagnosis of the saddle nose from over-resected bony dorsum is essential (Fig. 9.1).

The saddle nose deformity derives its name from the curved appearance of the nasal dorsum on a lateral view, resembling the depression of a horse's saddle. The curved appearance ranges from a slight supratip depression to total collapse of the dorsum because of the loss of septal cartilage and nasal bones that form the dorsal projection of the nose. A widened nasal dorsum is typically evident in a frontal view (Fig. 9.2).

The support structure most commonly affected in a patient with a saddle nose is the nasal septum. The key problem is serious structural compromise caused by loss of anterior septal cartilage between the keystone area (the "caudal septum") and the anterior nasal spine. If the nasal septum is weak or missing, the nasal vault collapses progressively over months or years because the nose is poorly supported, often accompanied by lateral compartment splaying. A saddle nose deformity affects not only the middle vault and nasal dorsum; all of tip deprojection, loss of tip definition, columellar retraction, alar collapse, and alar base widening may be evident. Apart from the poor aesthetic appearance, narrowing of the nasal airway affects nasal breathing and causes functional problems. A saddle nose deformity can arise after destruction of the septal vault, as follows:

A. On prior septal surgery, the following errors may have been made:
   - Dislocation of the septum from the nasal spine.
   - Excessive resection of the caudal septum.
   - Complete disruption or separation of the cartilaginous septum from the bony septum.

B. If rhinoplasty featuring septal surgery is planned, the above errors must not be made. Also, over-resection of the cartilaginous hump may cause the deformity. After execution of (recently popularized) dorsum preservation techniques, a supratip saddle nose is often encountered. If such techniques are employed, the amount of cartilage removed from the supratip must be minimized.

C. Nasal trauma can cause a saddle nose by directly disrupting septal integrity. Also, a post-traumatic septal hematoma or abscess can trigger saddling attributable to cartilaginous necrosis.

Supplementary Information The online version contains supplementary material available at https://doi.org/10.1007/978-3-031-65619-4_9.

S. Şeneldir, *Photographic Atlas of Rhinoplasty*, https://doi.org/10.1007/978-3-031-65619-4_9

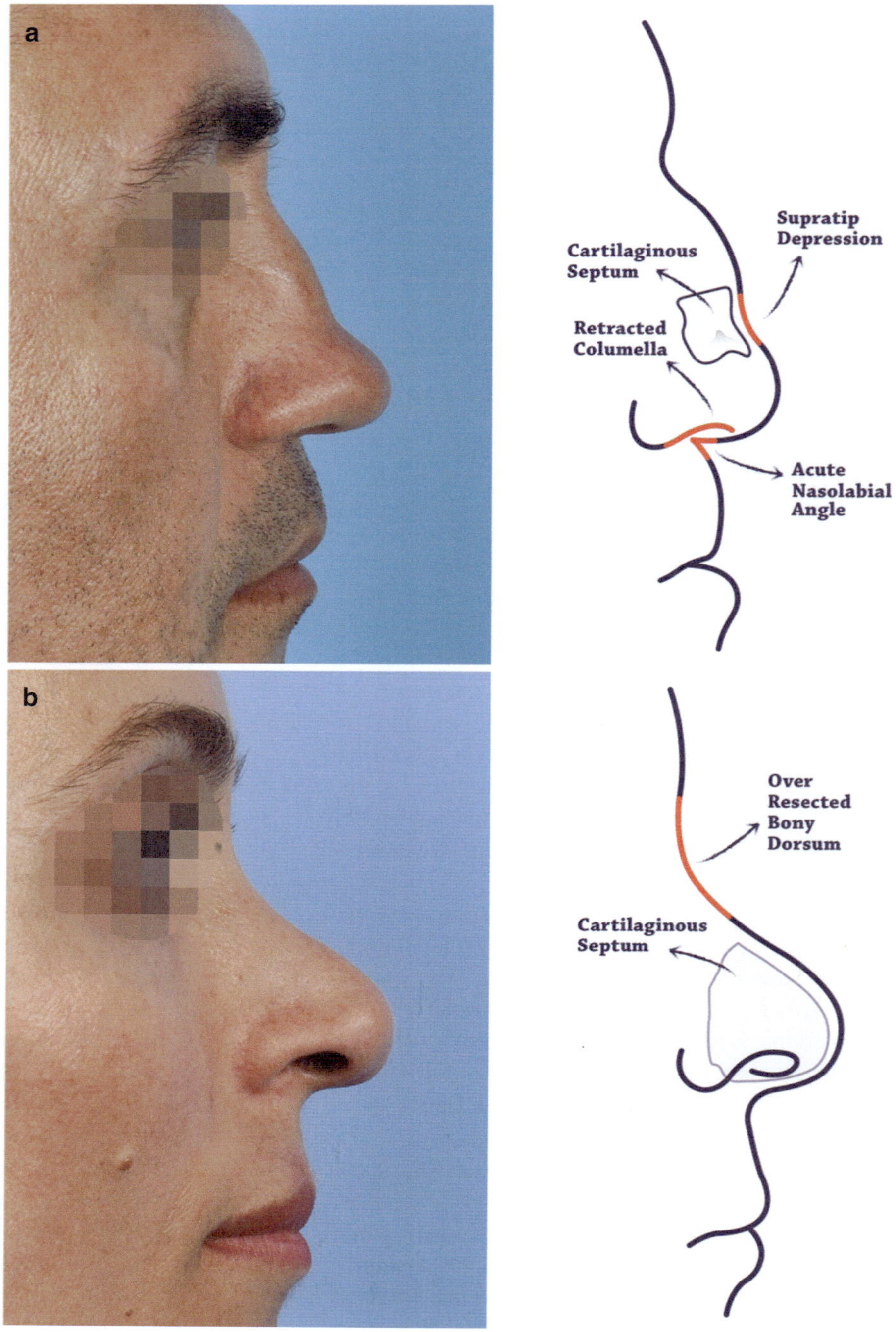

Fig. 9.1 (**a**) Saddle nose deformities in lateral view. Apart from the saddle-like appearance of the nose; the retracted columella, the acute subnasal angle, and the inadequate projection and rotation are other essential signs of septal deficiency. (**b**) However, an over-resected bony dorsum does not exhibit a specific nasal tip sign. The cases are different

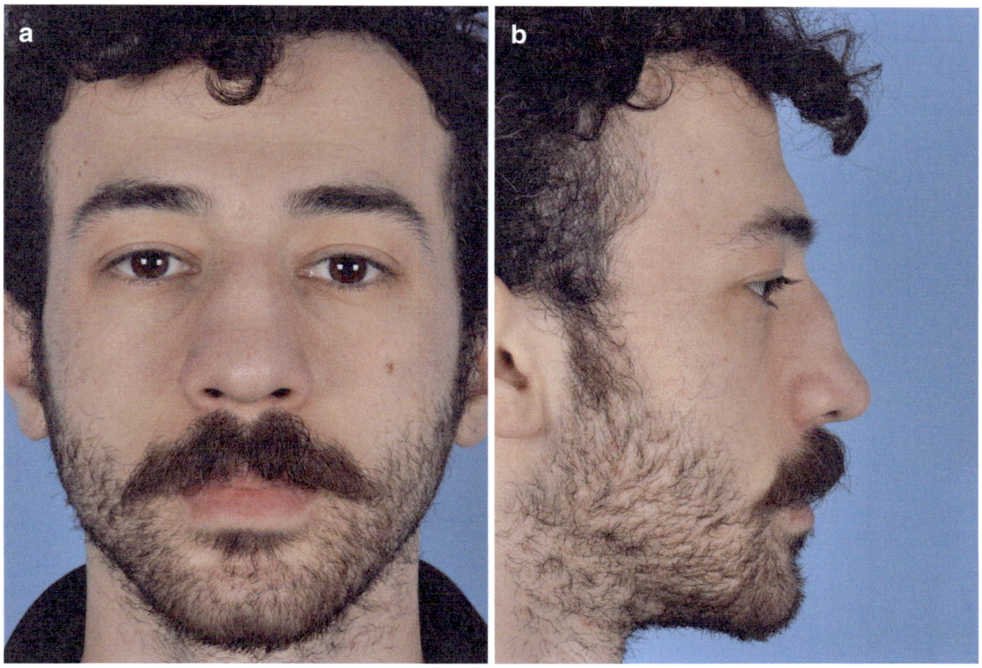

Fig. 9.2 (**a**, **b**) Frontal and profile photographs; the saddle nose deformity is evident

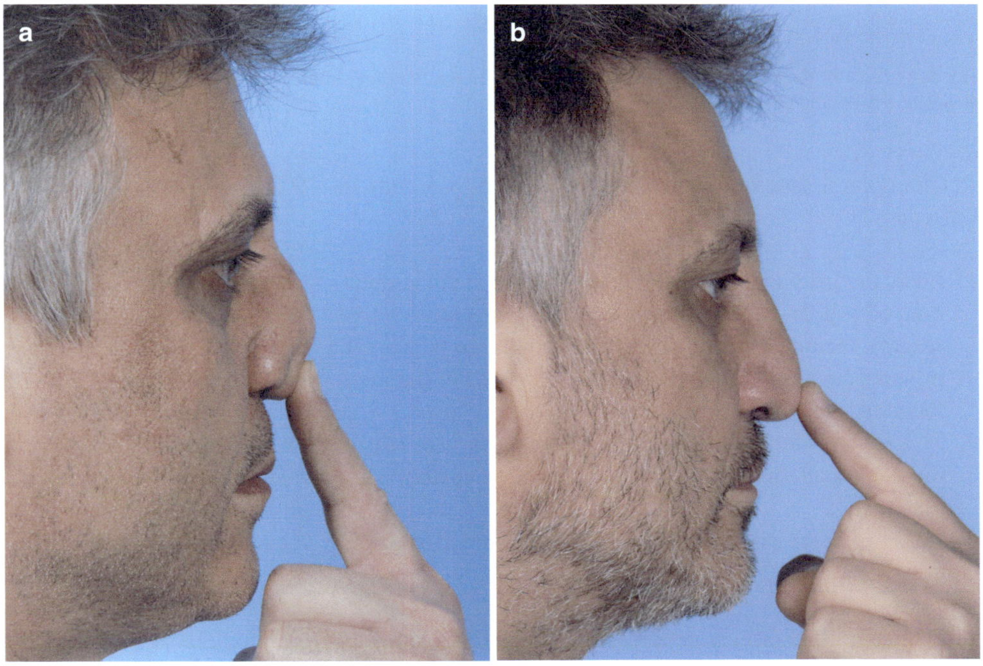

Fig. 9.3 (**a**) A typical sign of poor septal support. (**b**) Septal support is reestablished

9.2 Treatment Strategy

Several saddle nose classifications have been proposed by Seltzer et al., Vartanian, Tardy et al., and Daniel and Brenner; these seek to facilitate preoperative decision-making and prognostic predictions. However, our objective here was not to classify saddle deformities. We first focus on the septum; this is key. A comprehensive examination including photography of internal nasal structures (especially the septum) prior to surgery is essential. A septal perforation indicates either minimal or no septal support. The cartilaginous support can be checked by palpating the frontal septum with the thumb and forefinger. Also, if the nasal tip sticks to the face when the tip is pressed, septal support is lacking. This simple test emphasizes the etiological role played by the septum and the need to reconstruct septal support, especially in cases exhibiting progressive saddling (Fig. 9.3).

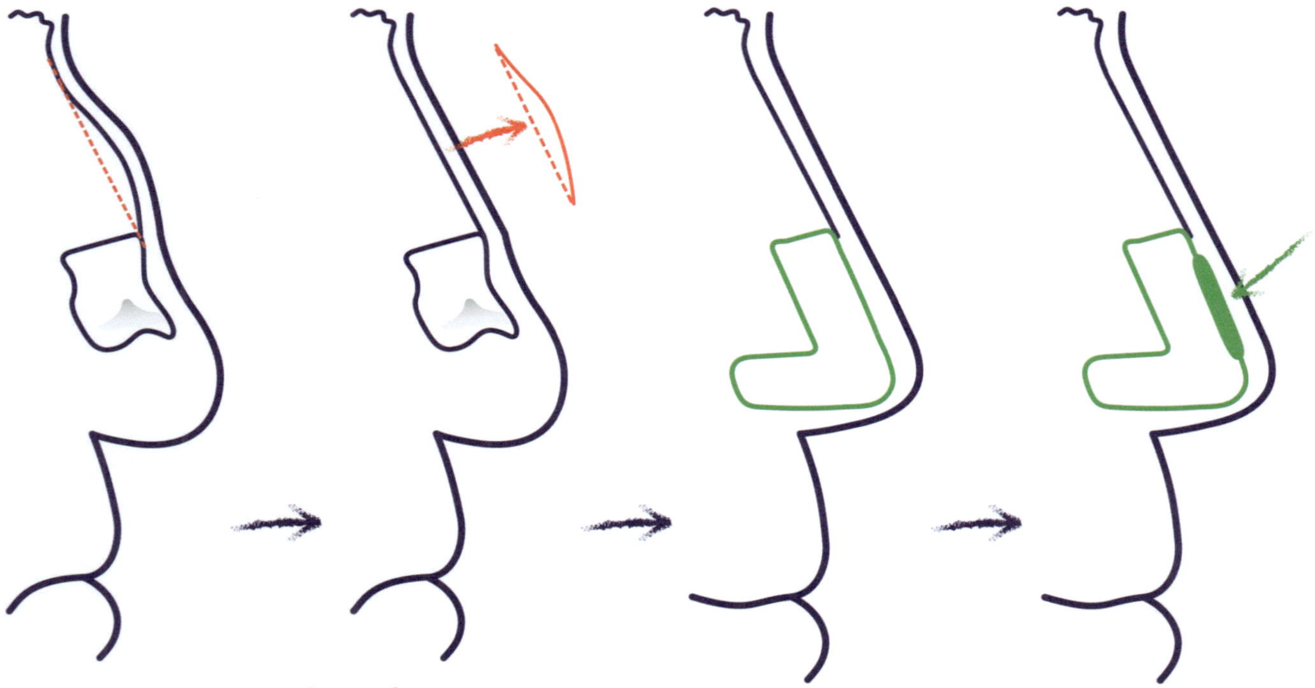

Fig. 9.4 Most of the saddle noses have a minor bony hump. Surgery should start resection of this bony hump, and then the middle vault is reconstructed; finally, the dorsum is augmented

Changing a saddle nose to an ideal dorsum proceeds in three steps:

1. First, the primary dorsum is addressed. A small proportion of saddle nose deformities developing after septal surgery include a bony hump. If such a hump is present, it is resected, and the bony dorsum is moved to the ideal location.
2. The septal vault is then reconstructed. The key step is major septal reconstruction; a solid foundation is essential.
3. If required, the dorsum is augmented to achieve aesthetic goals.

Thus, the aim is to create a reasonable dorsal height that is in balance with radix and tip proportions (Fig. 9.4).

Saddle nose surgery is not difficult. The idea is to reconstruct structures (especially the septum) that are missing or weak. Cartilage is the principal source of reconstructive tissue. Both otologic costal and cadaver cartilage can be used if the septum is not available. Auricular cartilage should be the last resort; the rigidity thereof is inadequate. We prefer to use cadaver costal cartilage because this behaves as otologic cartilage in the long term; no extra incision or surgery is required.

The need for cartilage must be discussed with the patient and a decision on cartilage source made via consensus.

9.3 Clinical Outcomes

We will proceed step-by-step through some cases.

9.3.1 Case 1

The first case is a male with trauma anamnesis; he claimed that he had never been operated upon. On the profile view, a minimal supratip depression, a minimal nasal hump, and an unsupported/under-projected nasal tip are evident. Initially, the radix needs attention to attain an ideal nasal profile. The radix exhibits ideal projection and location. It is possible to create an ideal dorsum by resecting the bony hump and augmenting the supratip concavity. It is essential to support and strengthen the septal cartilage (Fig. 9.5).

Thus, first, the minimal bony hump is removed (Fig. 9.6).

The second and the most important surgical step is the construction of a strong vault, focusing on the septum. Septoplasty had earlier been performed with placement of an L-strut; the caudal part of the strut gradually assumed a C-shape. It was thus weak and required strengthening. A batten graft was used to both correct the inclination and construct a strong septum. After removal of a reverse triangle of tissue from the convex part of the septum and suturing of a batten graft to the concave part, the septum became

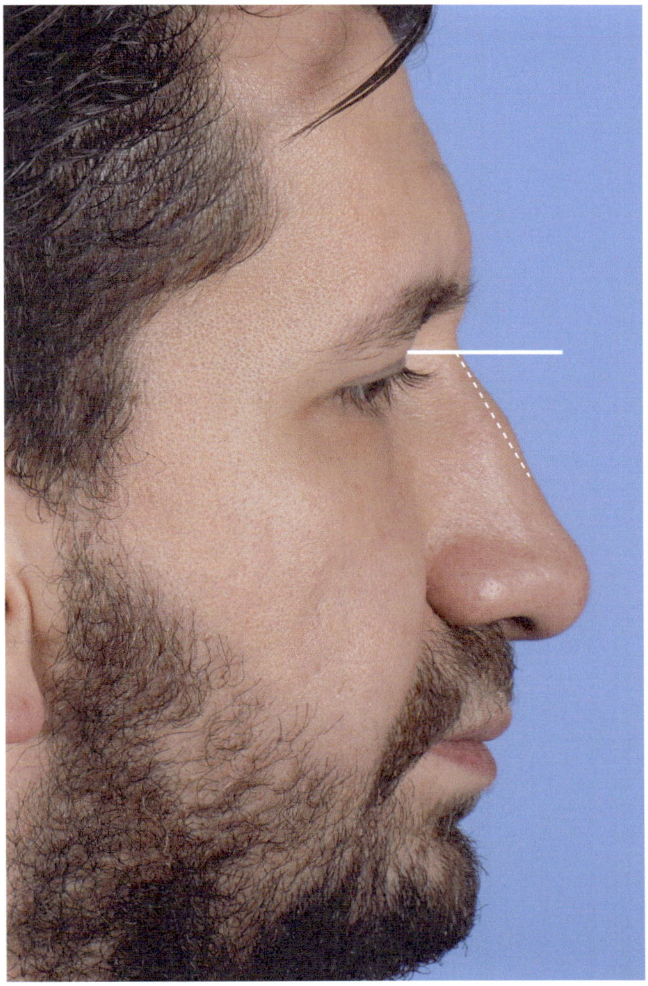

Fig. 9.5 Radix is an ideal position, minimal bony hump. Minor supra tip depression

both stabilized and flattened (septal vault reconstruction) (Fig. 9.7; Video 9.1).

The final step is augmentation of the supratip area to attain the final dorsum. Immediately after septal repair, the supratip area was palpated to assess the required augmentation volume. In this case, a cartilaginous supratip (prepared from the septum) 2 mm in thickness, 7 mm in width, and 7 mm in length, was appropriate. When engaging in segmental augmentation, the graft must be fixed to the dorsum via a suture. When the graft is ideally placed, it is initially fixed using an insulin injector and then more permanently fixed by placing absorbable sutures at various points (Fig. 9.8).

In this case, a steal suture, a columellar strut, a lateral crural graft, and a cup graft were used to form the tip. The results are shown in the photographs that comprise Fig. 9.9.

A more complicated case is shown next.

9.3.2 Case 2

In this case, which had septal surgery, a prominent supratip depression is evident in the profile view. Also, it is clear that a lack of septal support has caused the observed tip problems (Fig. 9.10).

The key step is septal reconstruction, which will achieve these results:

1. An increased dorsal projection.
2. Improved nasal breathing.
3. Resolution of the caudal septum-related tip problems.

The steps of saddle nose surgery are also appropriate here:

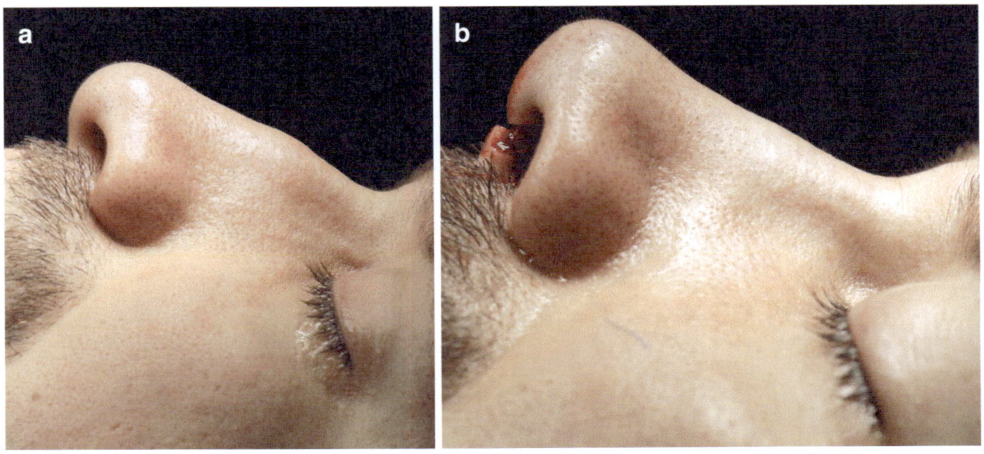

Fig. 9.6 (**a**) A photograph taken prior to work on the primary dorsum. (**b**) A photograph taken after primary dorsum work was completed

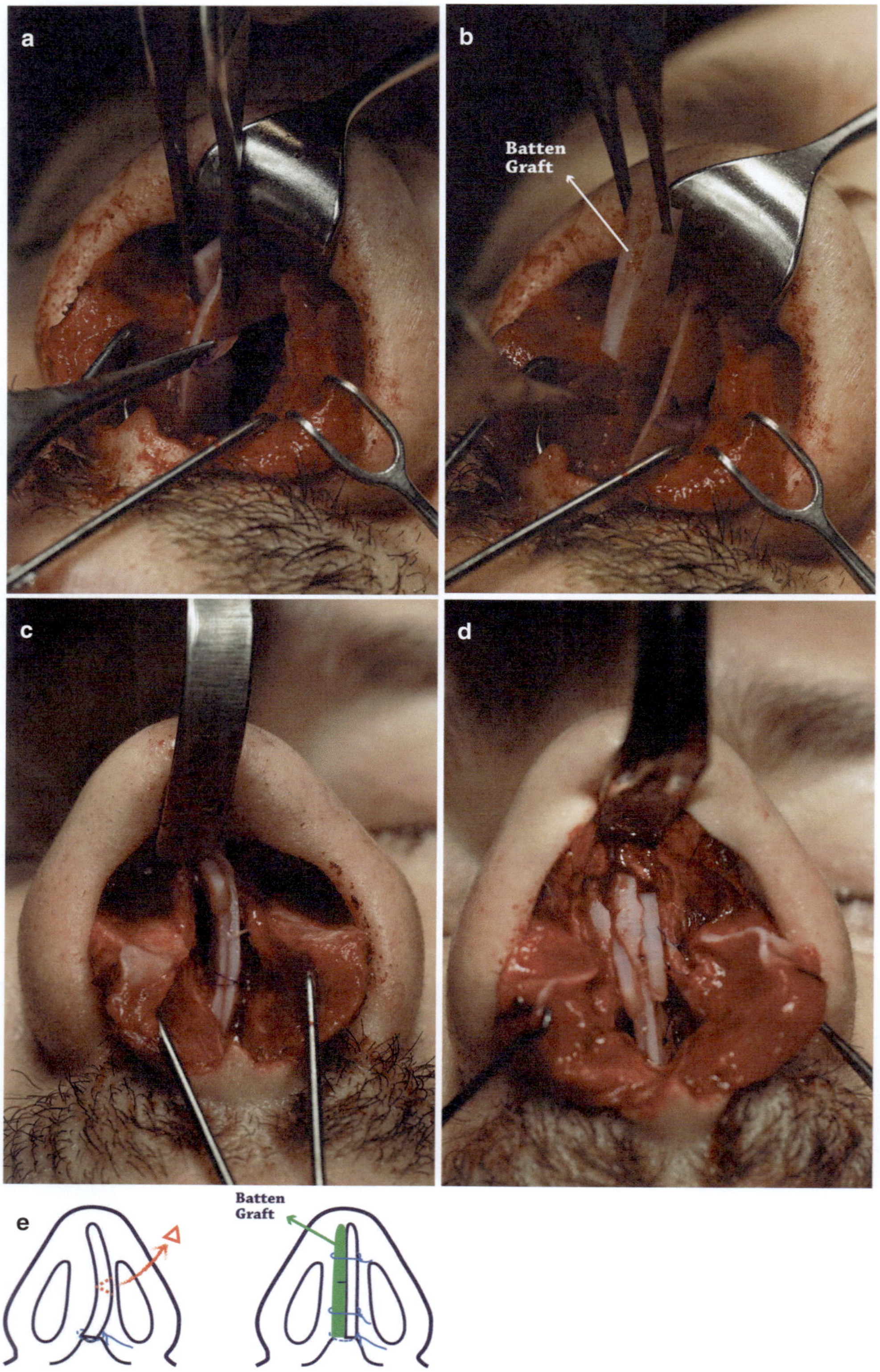

Fig. 9.7 (**a**) The reverse triangular area excised from the convex side of the caudal septum. (**b**, **c**) A batten graft placed and fixed on the concave side of the septal vault. (**d**) The entire dorsal septum was reconstructed using a bilateral spreader graft. (**e**) The batten graft clearly strengthened the septum

- First, during primary dorsum work, the bony hump is removed.
- As mentioned above, the critical step is always septal reconstruction. Thus, the septum is now reconstructed. If the septum is in focus, a caudal deficiency can be readily seen. In such cases, placement of extended spreader and caudal septal replacement grafts is optimal when reconstructing the septum. The extended and caudal septal

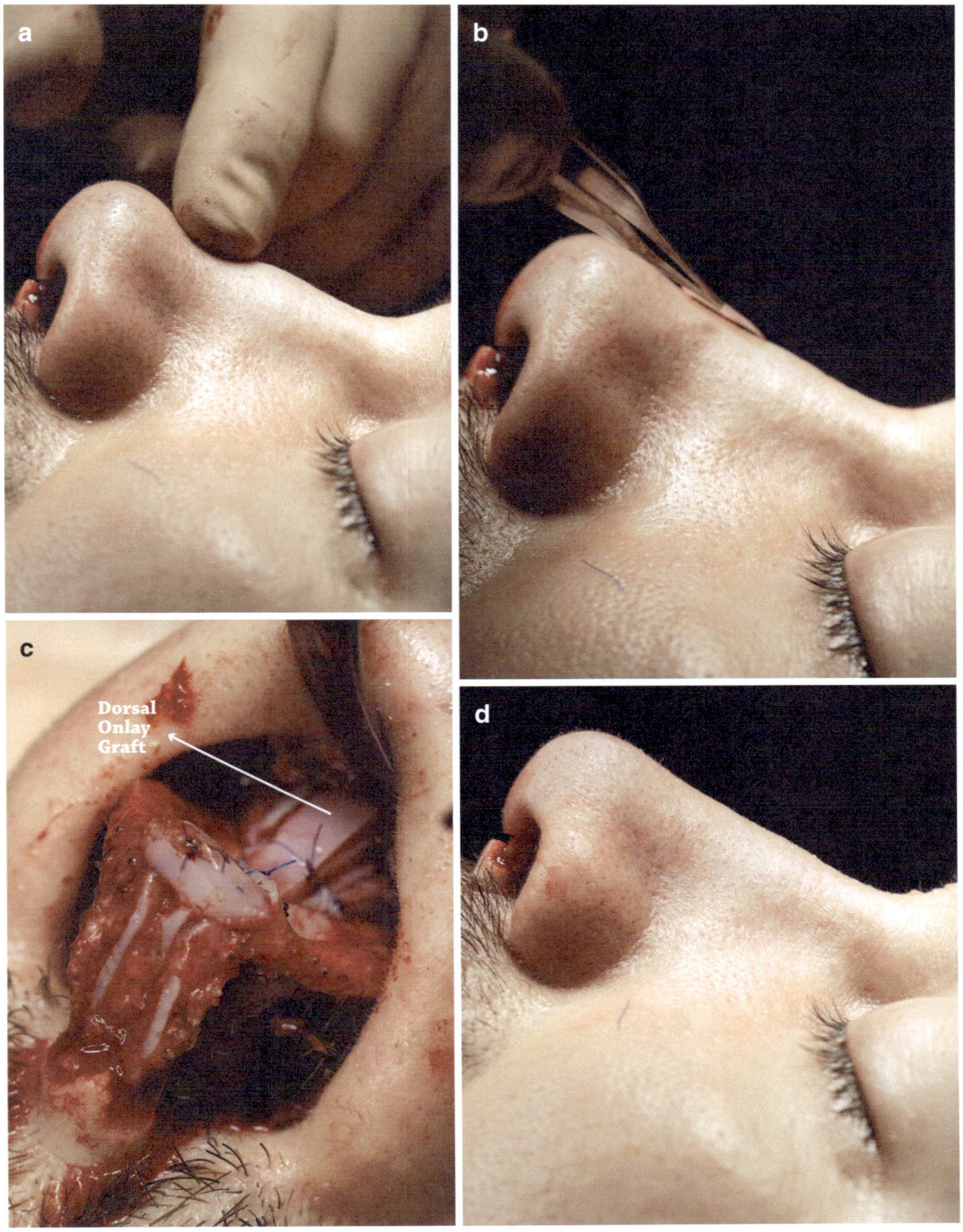

Fig. 9.8 (**a**) The dorsum is checked for proper sizing as a supra tip onlay graft. (**b**) Septal cartilage dorsal onlay graft. The graft is shaped, the edges are beveled, and it is ready for placement. (**c**) The graft secured with absorbable sutures. The around anterior septal angle is a comfortable spot to place a stabilizing suture. (**d**) Immediately after dorsal augmentation

replacement grafts are sutured, in turn, to the two sides of the septum. This method is appropriate when a remnant septum is available and its relationship with the ethmoid bone is intact (Fig. 9.11).

This approach requires strong, wide costal cartilages (Fig. 9.12).

Intraoperatively the remnant septum is evident (Fig. 9.13).

A caudal septal replacement graft is placed on the contralateral septal side and meets the extended spreader graft at an angle as close to 90° as possible (Fig. 9.14).

The extended spreader graft is sutured beside the nasal septum, at the concave aspect of the dorsal L-strut, using 5–0 polydioxanone (Fig. 9.15).

The caudal septal replacement graft is then suture-fixed to the extended spreader graft, the septum, and soft tissues around the anterior nasal spine (Fig. 9.16).

To elevate the cartilaginous nasal dorsum, the dorsal margin of the extended spreader graft can be extended beyond the existing dorsal height. Such modified positioning of extended spreader grafts readily elevates the dorsal height without any need for augmentation. An extended spreader graft should be placed more dorsally in the caudal end, and less dorsally in

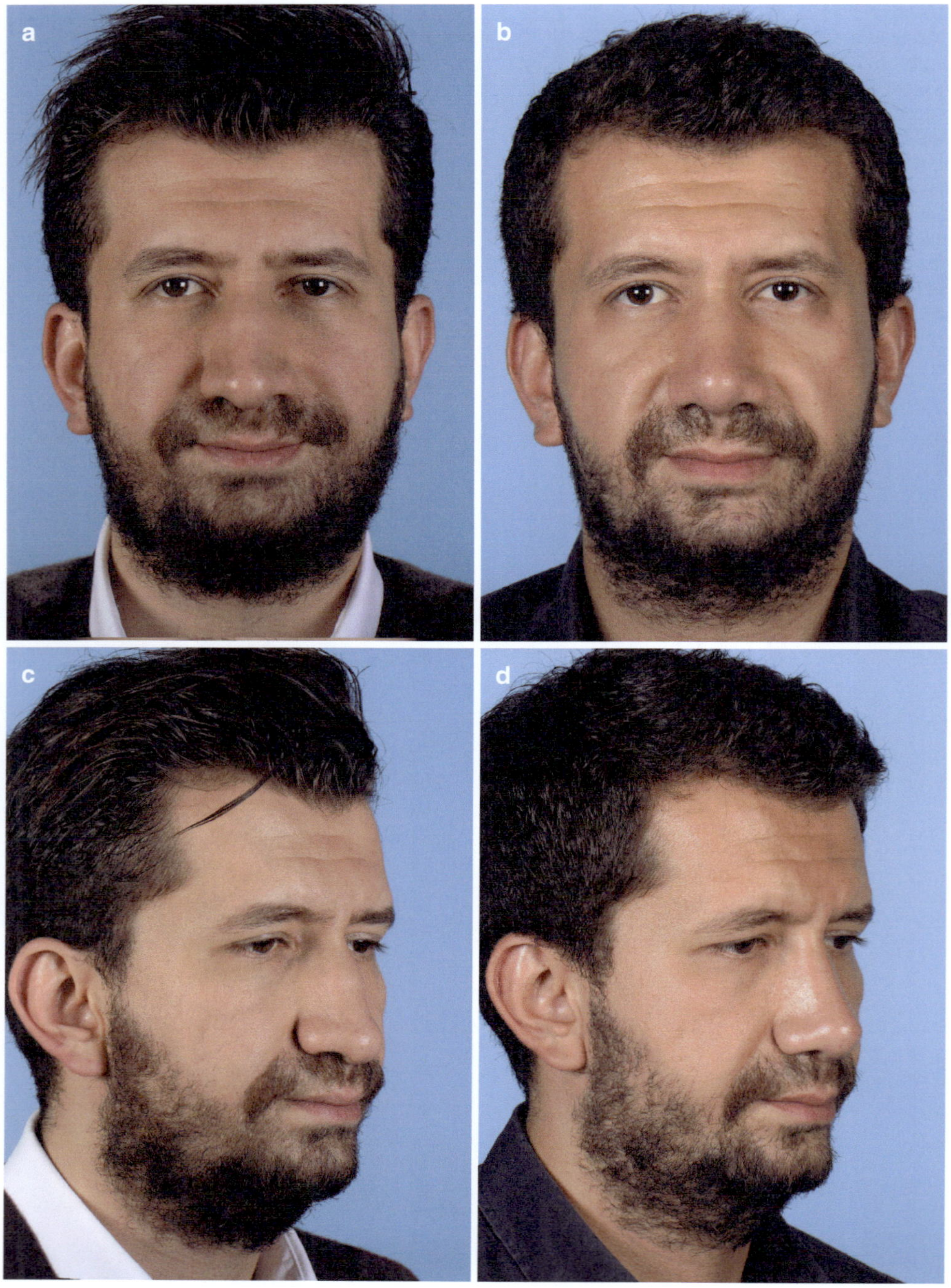

Fig. 9.9 (**a**, **b**) Before and after frontal photographs; dorsum is narrower with stronger middle vault and more defined tip, giving an overall frontal view of the nose a more pleasing appearance. (**c**, **d**) Before and after oblique photographs. Tip has gained rotation and projection. (**e–h**) Before and after profile: minor saddle deformity is restored. Dorsal profile alignment is improved. (**i**, **j**) Harmonious curves of dorsal aesthetic lines are achieved

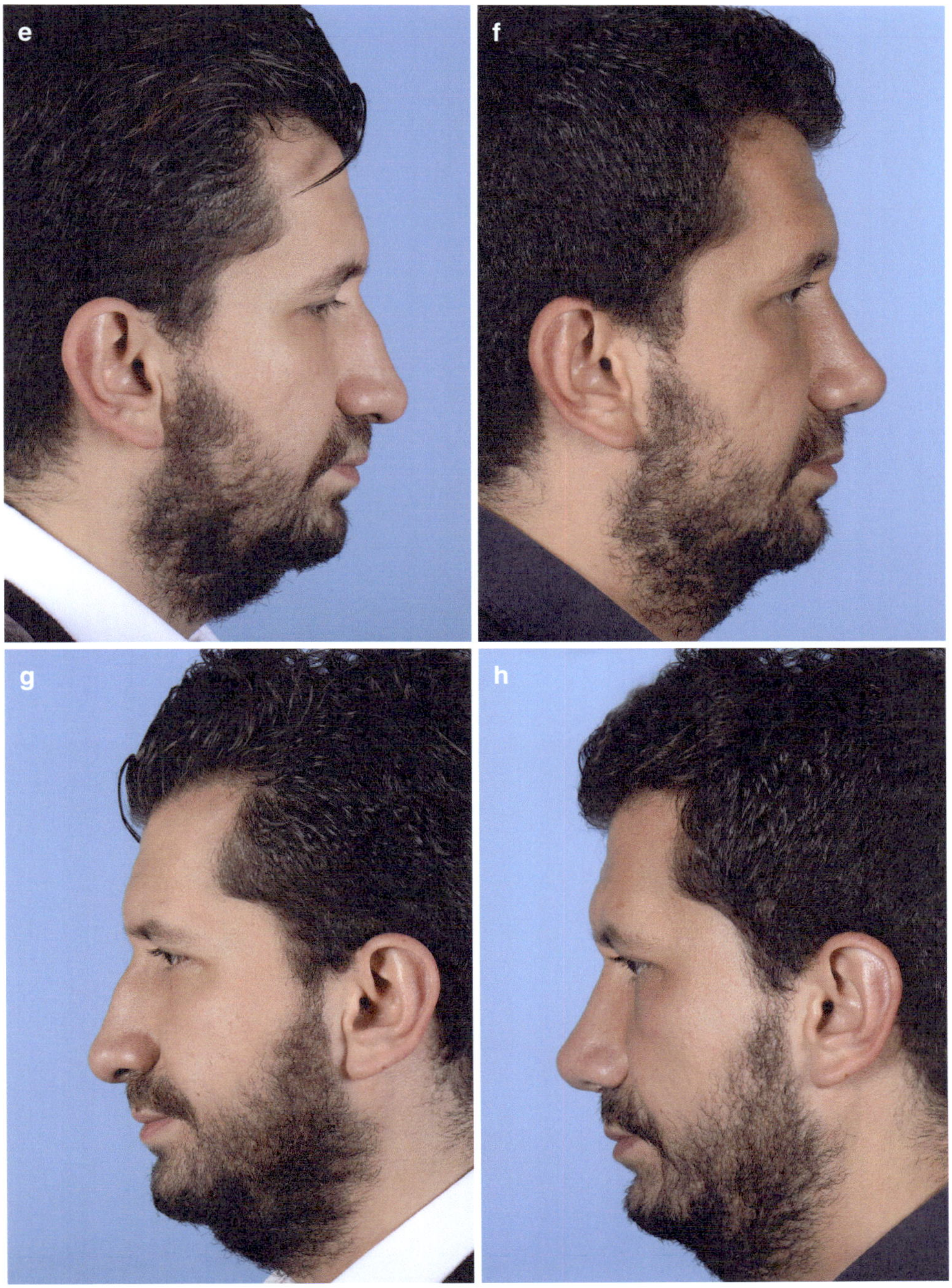

Fig. 9.9 (continued)

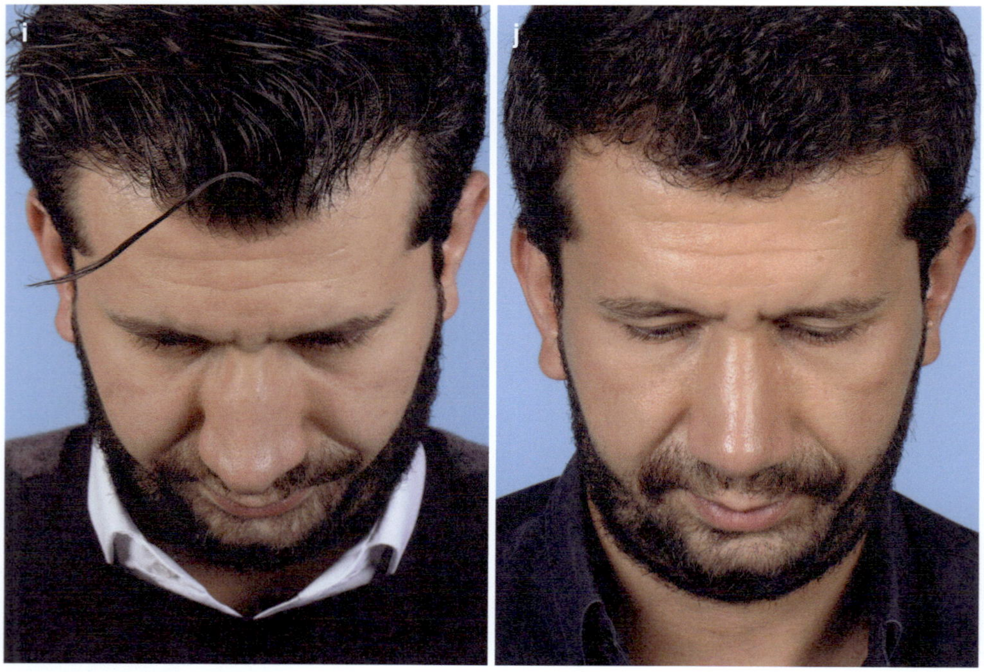

Fig. 9.9 (continued)

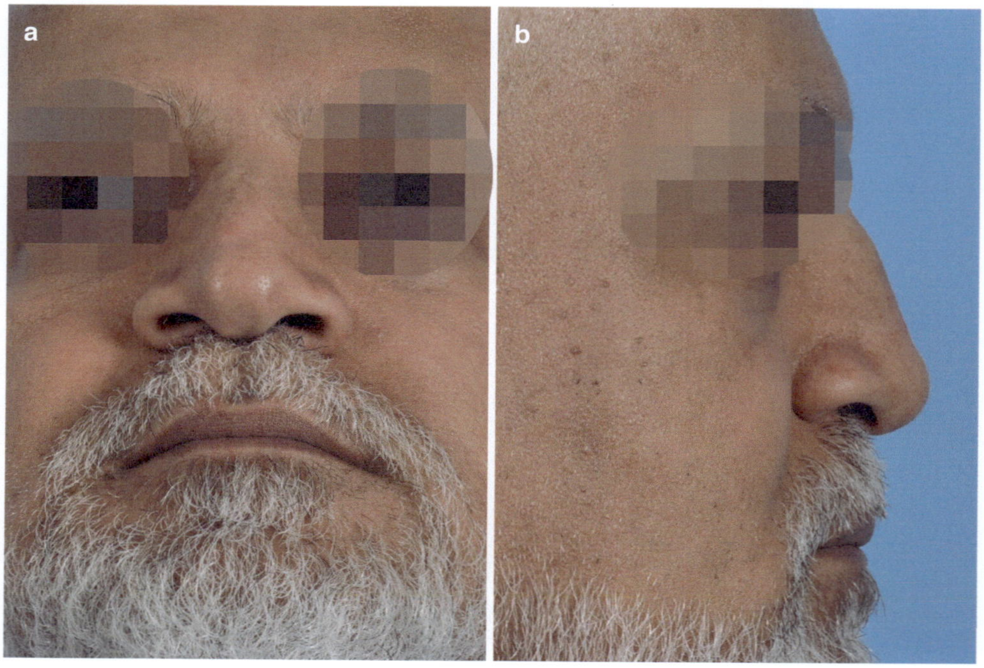

Fig. 9.10 (**a**, **b**) Loss of septal integrity results in a characteristic saddle nose deformity that is seen. Depression of the middle vault and dorsum, loss of nasal tip support, retraction of the columella, and widening of the nasal base. Functionally, the internal nasal valves are affected, leading to significant difficulties in breathing

the cephalic end. This creates a step deformity at the dorsal end of the remnant septum-spreader complex. To eliminate this, crushed cartilage can be added (Fig. 9.17).

Preoperative and 2-year postoperative photographs are shown in Fig. 9.18. The profile is improved without dorsal augmentation. Dorsal elevation corrected the saddle deformity and makes the dorsum appear narrower on frontal view. The caudal septum-related tip problem was solved. The nasal tip is also better defined. The nasolabial angle is more open and there is less alar flaring.

9.3.3 Case 3

Another case desired correction of saddle nose deformity that resulted from a nasal fracture. Prominent saddle deformity of cartilaginous dorsum causes flat appearance on the frontal view. A technique similar to that described above was used. Bony hump removal and septal reconstruction were enough to achieve straight nasal dorsum. Dorsal augmentation was not needed.

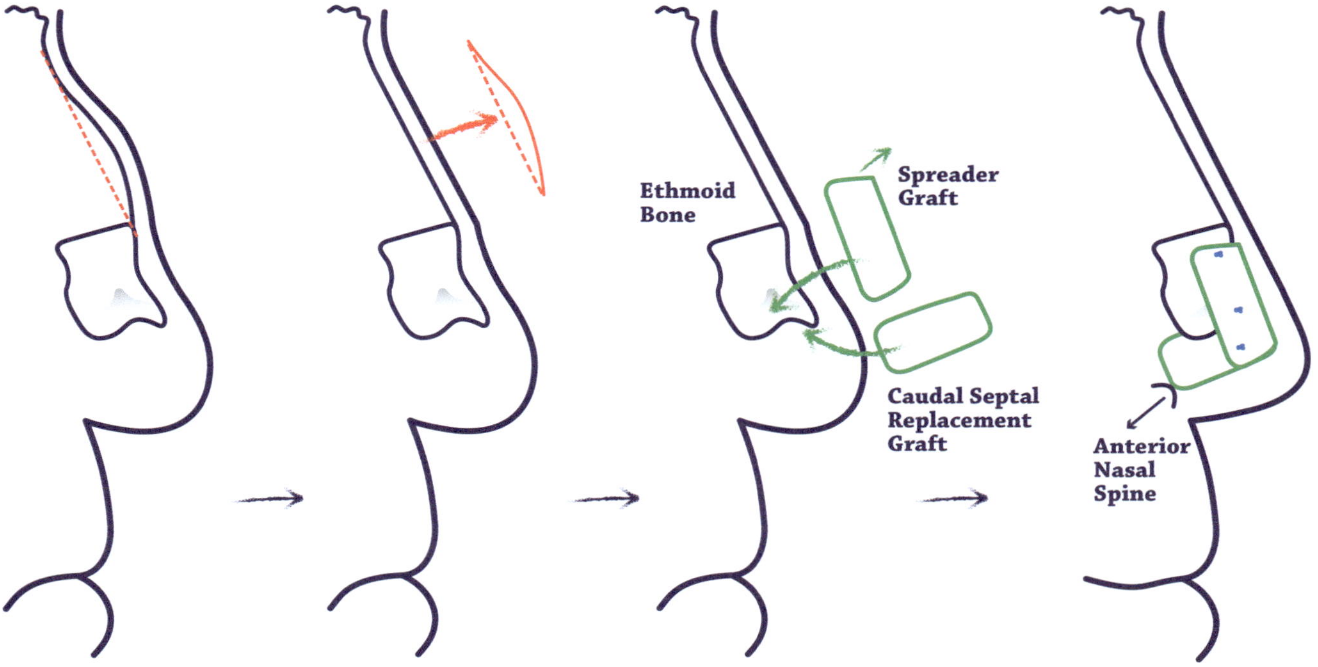

Fig. 9.11 When the caudal septum is absent or deficient, but the dorsal septum remnant is present and strong enough, caudal septal replacement graft, and a single spreader graft will be enough to reconstruct the middle vault

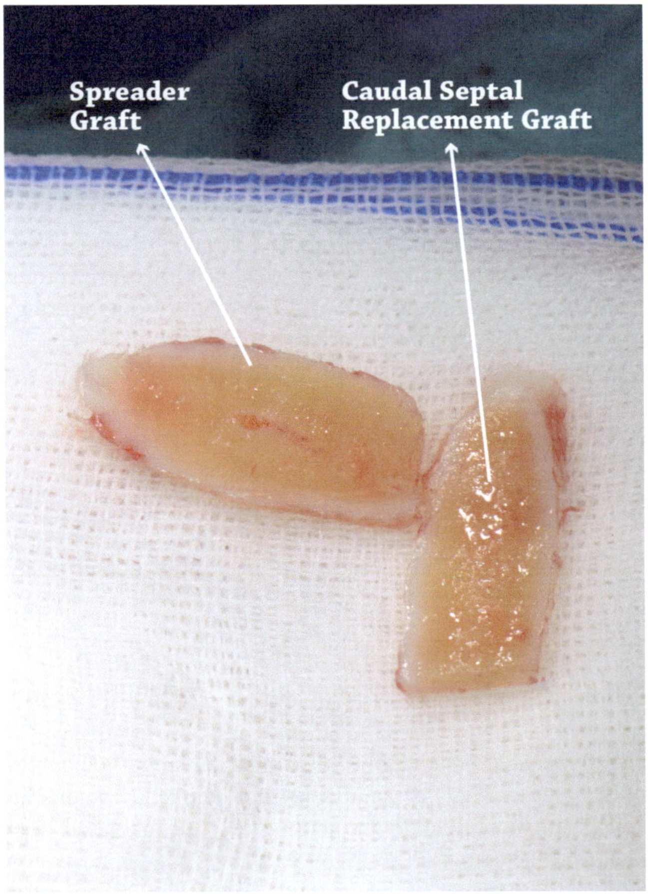

Fig. 9.12 Spreader graft size is larger than the standard size

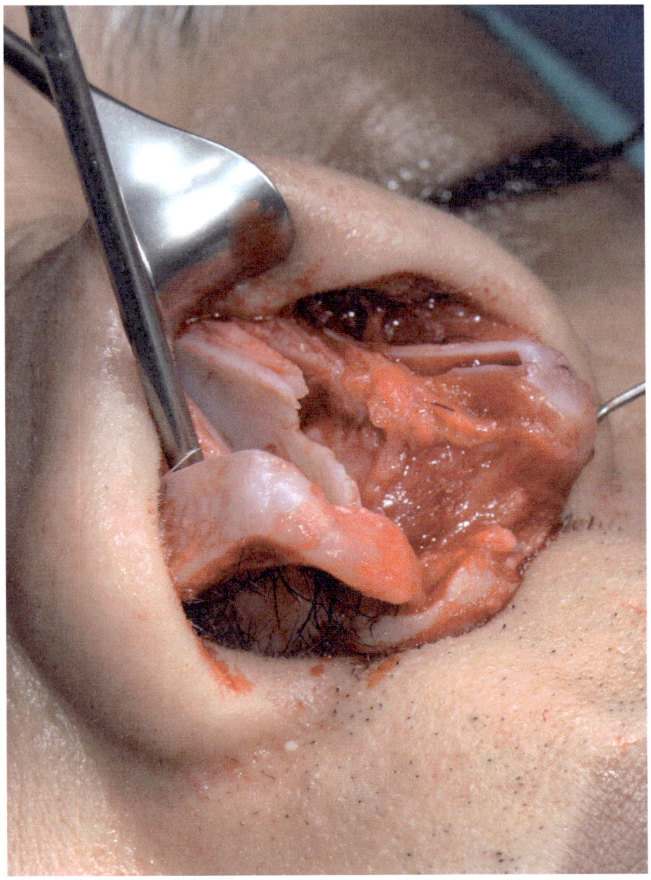

Fig. 9.13 Caudal septum is deficient

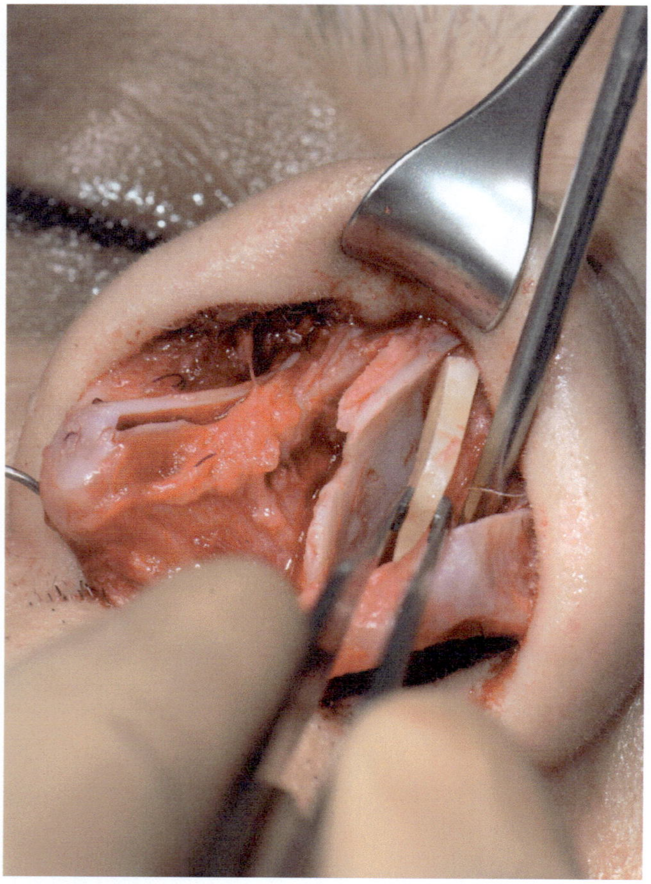

Fig. 9.14 Placement of septal replacement graft

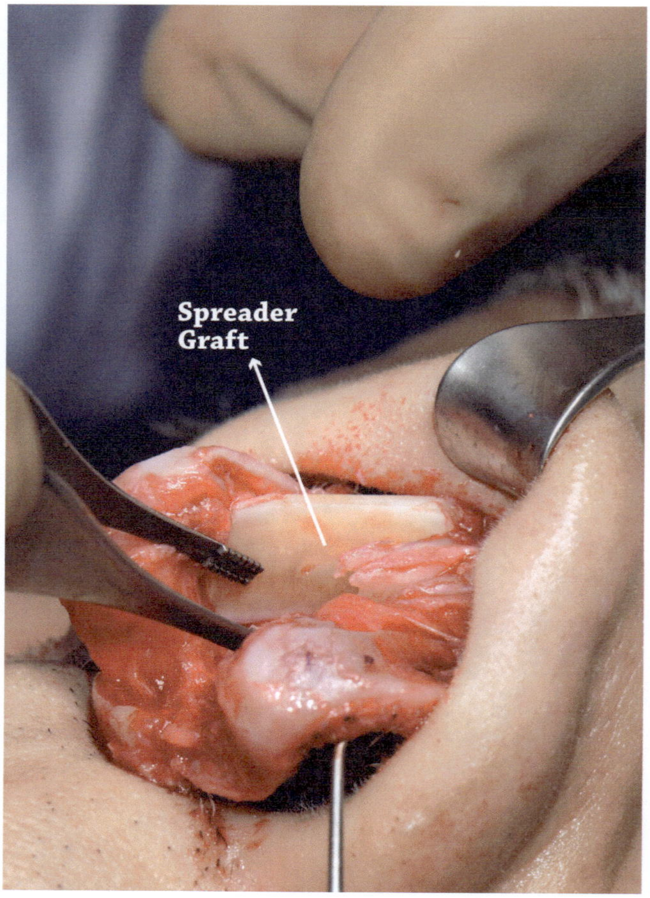

Fig. 9.15 Placement of spreader graft

Preoperative and 1-year postoperative photographs are shown in Fig. 9.19.

Technical Pearl: If the subnasal angle is acute and the columella is retracted, the surgeon should suspect a caudal septal deficiency and place a septal replacement graft.

Septal reconstruction may also feature placement of bilateral extended spreader and caudal septal replacement grafts. If the remnant septum is short, thin, and/or weak, either of these grafts alone will not be adequate. Both bilateral extended spreader and caudal septal replacement grafts should be placed.

9.3.4 Case 4

In the saddle nose deformity case shown here, bilateral extended spreader grafts were sutured to both sides of the dorsal strut, and a caudal replacement graft was sandwiched between these grafts (Figs. 9.20 and 9.21; Video 9.2).

This case's preoperative and 2-year postoperative photographs are shown in Fig. 9.22a–d.

In the cases reviewed, moving to the third treatment step (dorsum augmentation [as defined by the author]) was unnecessary because the dorsum was elevated when the middle vault was septically reconstructed. However, certain patients with advanced saddle noses require dorsum augmentation after septal reconstruction.

We use three types of grafts to this end:

- En bloc cadaver cartilage.
- Diced cartilage.
- Resected bony hump.

The following three cases explore how a dorsal onlay graft is placed.

9.3.5 Case 5

Another saddle nose deformity with septal surgery anamnesis. There are signs of caudal septum deficiency: supra tip depression, columellar retraction, an under-rotated and under-projected nasal tip (Fig. 9.23a).

After en block hump removal, the first crucial step involved rebuilding the septum. For this purpose, unilateral

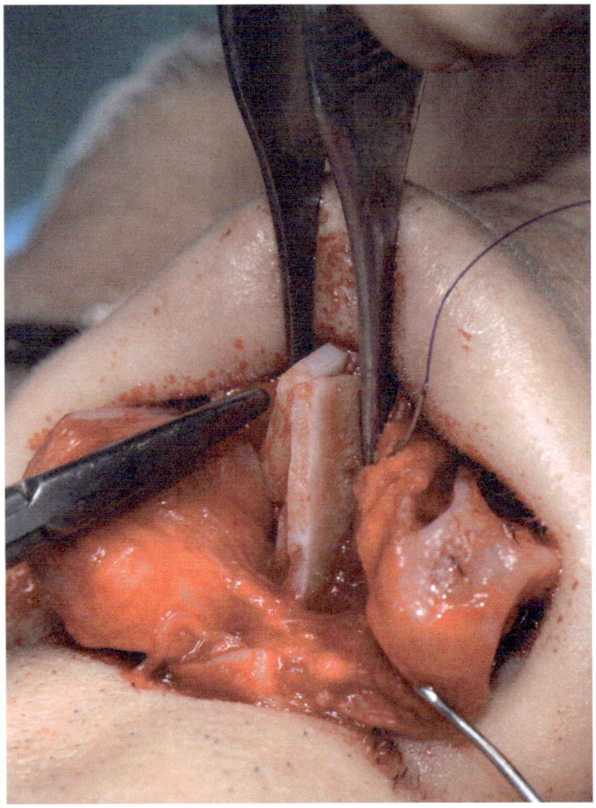

Fig. 9.16 Septal remnant, spreader, and replacement graft are sutured together with nonabsorbable suture material

spreader graft and septal replacement graft were used together (Fig. 9.23b–d). While this addressed many issues, it did not adequately elevate the supratip region on the nose bridge as in previous cases. Hence, additional volume was needed in the supratip area. The previously removed bone bump was placed back into the supratip region to achieve this. This adjustment reached the desired height, with prior contouring of the bump for shaping (Fig. 9.23e).

The 1-year postoperative photographs were obtained after caudal septal replacement and bilateral extended graft placement. No dorsal augmentation was needed (Fig. 9.23f).

When dorsal hump material is unavailable, we can utilize two alternative types of grafts.:

- *En bloc* cadaver cartilage.
- Diced cartilage.

The next two cases explore how a dorsal onlay graft is placed.

9.3.6 Case 6

The first patient evidenced a saddle nose deformity caused by prior septal surgery. Unlike the cases described above, no septal remnant was available for reconstruction. The septum required L-strut rebuilding. Cadaver cartilage was grafted within the tunnel to replace the dorsal septum; the tunnel opened into a septal mucoperichondrial flap under the bony dorsum. The cartilage was fixed to the nasal bones using non-absorbable sutures. The caudal tip of the cartilage was sutured to cartilage of the spine. Thus, the L-strut was reformed (Fig. 9.24).

A reconstructed L-strut acceptably raises the dorsum; this may also serve for augmentation. The author prefers to place diced cartilages freely, creating a dorsum projection of about 1–2 mm (Fig. 9.25).

Preoperative and 3-year postoperative photographs of the case are seen in Fig. 9.26.

The author prefers to use *en bloc* cartilage when dorsum projection is required more than 1–2 mm.

9.3.7 Case 7

In the case below, dorsal augmentation was necessary after bony hump rasping and septal reconstruction. En bloc costal cartilage was employed to this end (Fig. 9.27).

Preoperative and 7-year postoperative photographs of the case are shown in Fig. 9.28.

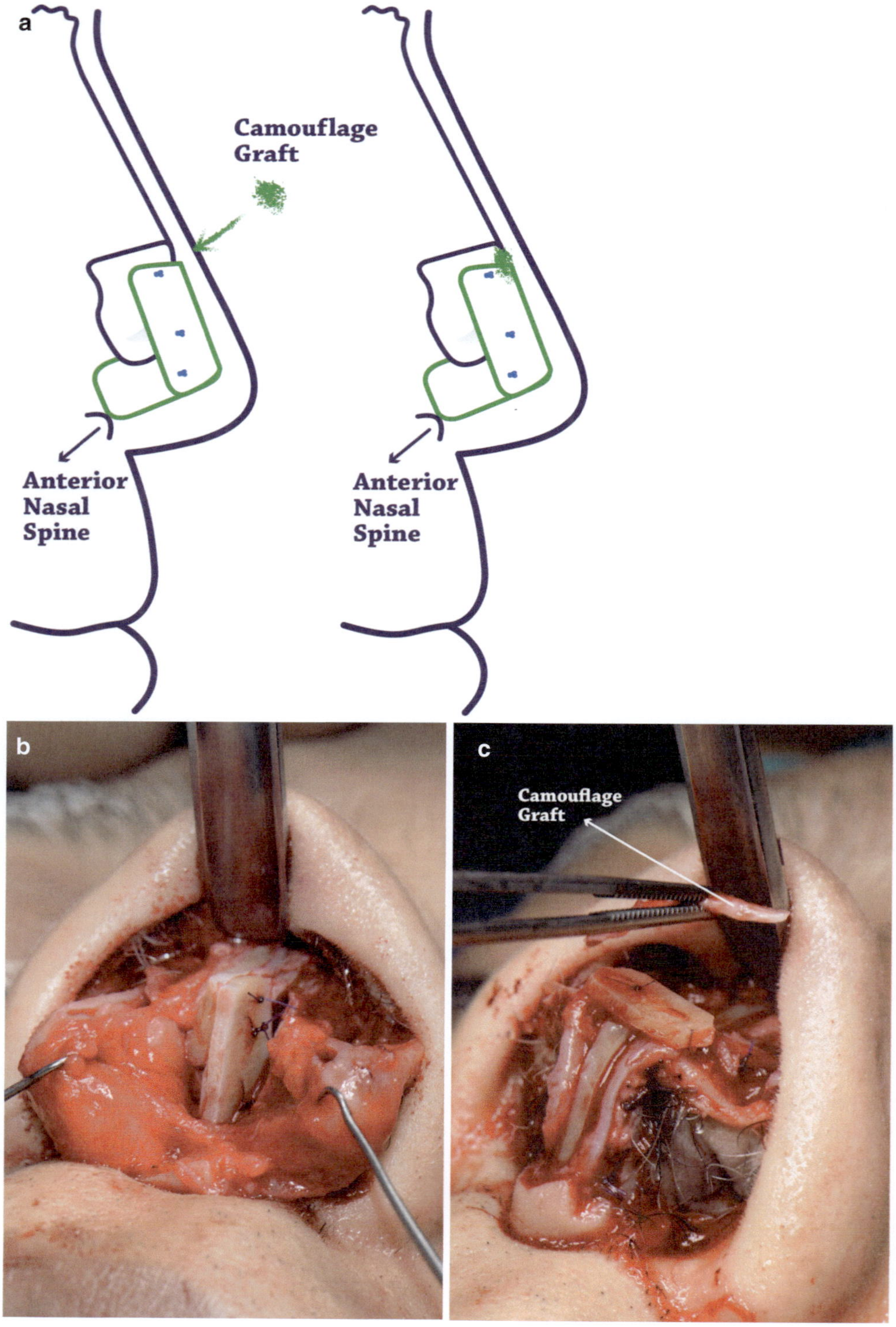

Fig. 9.17 (**a**) After replacing the grafts, their dorsal ends should be checked. In some cases, step deformity exists. Crushed cartilage as a camouflage graft might be needed to correct this. (**b**) There is a step in the marked area. (**c**) Crushed cartilage is placed

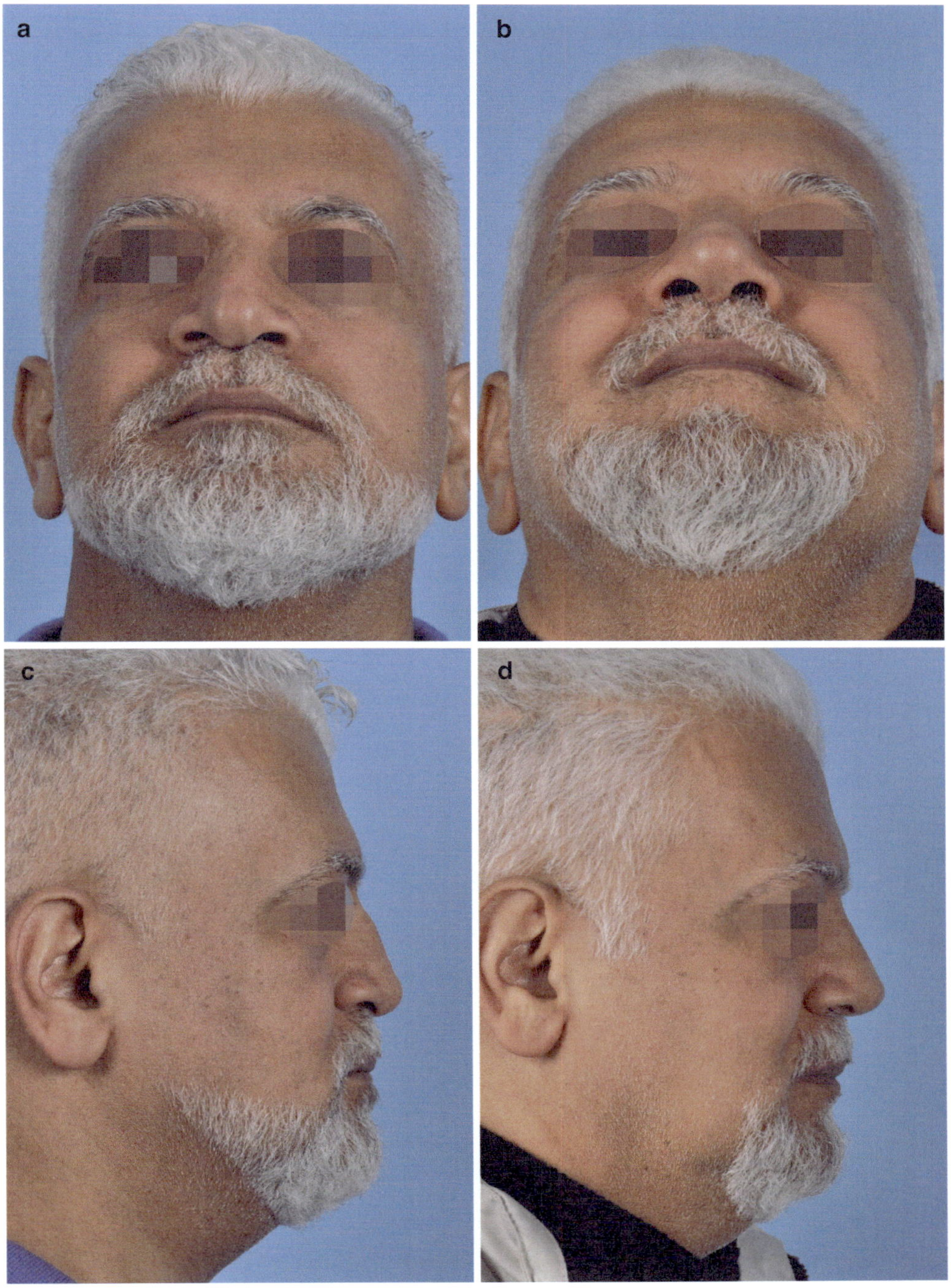

Fig. 9.18 (**a**, **b**) Before and after: the tip is more projected and rotated up. The nasal base is narrower. (**c**, **d**) Supratip depression has been eliminated. The dorsal line is straight. Nasal tip has gained projection and rotation. Nasalobial angle is more obtuse. (**e**, **f**) Osteocartilaginous dorsum looks narrower and more defined

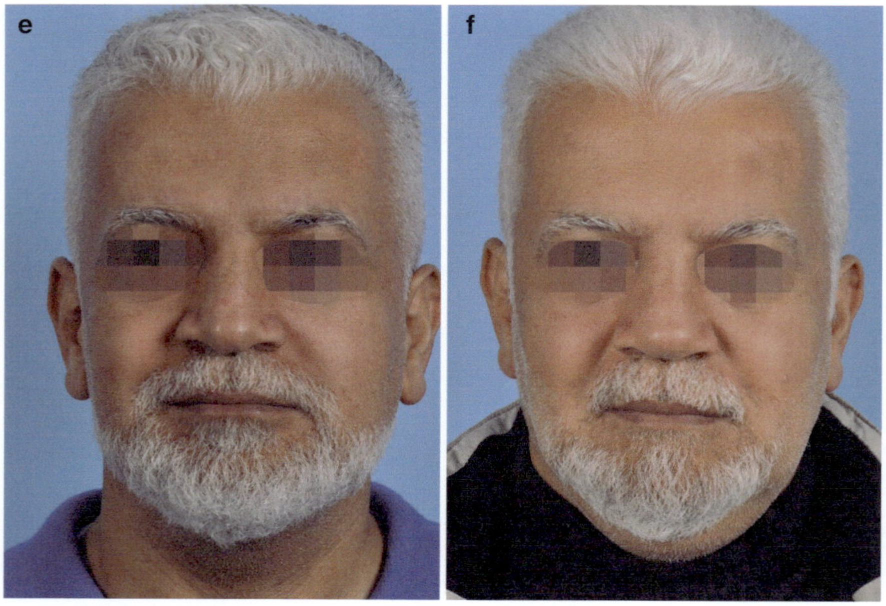

Fig. 9.18 (continued)

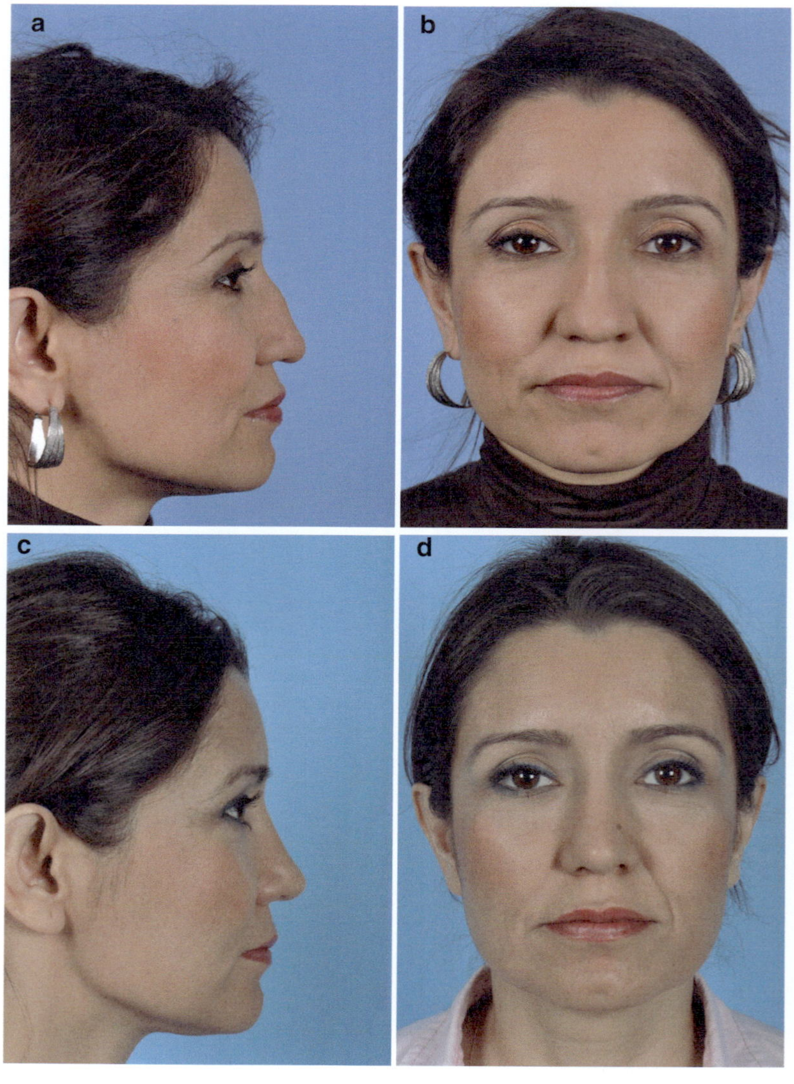

Fig. 9.19 (**a**, **b**) All of the typical tip and dorsum characteristics of a severe saddle nose deformity are apparent, as are an acute subnasal angle, a droopy under-projected tip, and a retracted columella. All of these features are attributable to the lack of a caudal septum. (**c**, **d**) The septal framework was reestablished using caudal replacement and extended spreader grafts

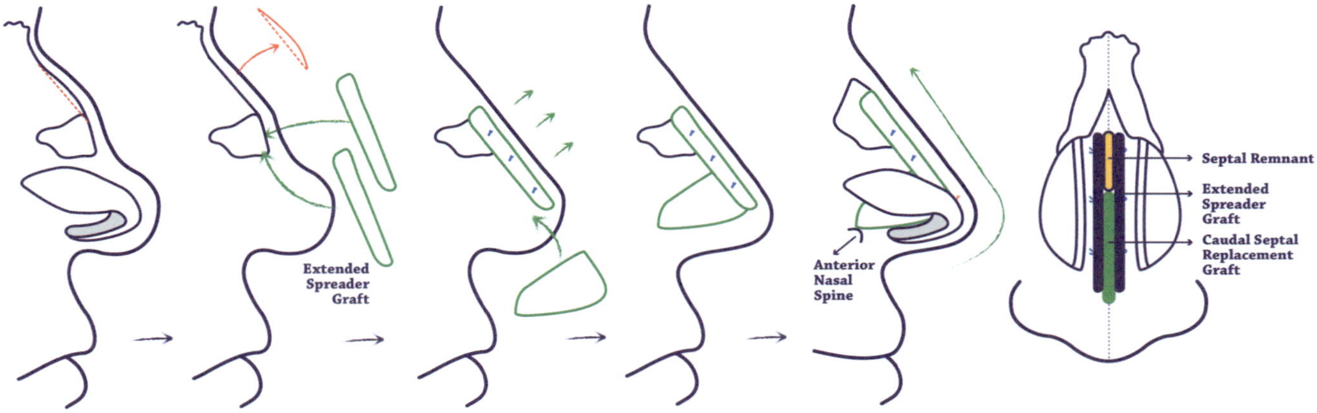

Fig. 9.20 When the caudal septum is absent and the dorsal septal remnant is not strong enough, bilateral extended spreader grafts and caudal septal replacement graft can be used for middle vault reconstruction

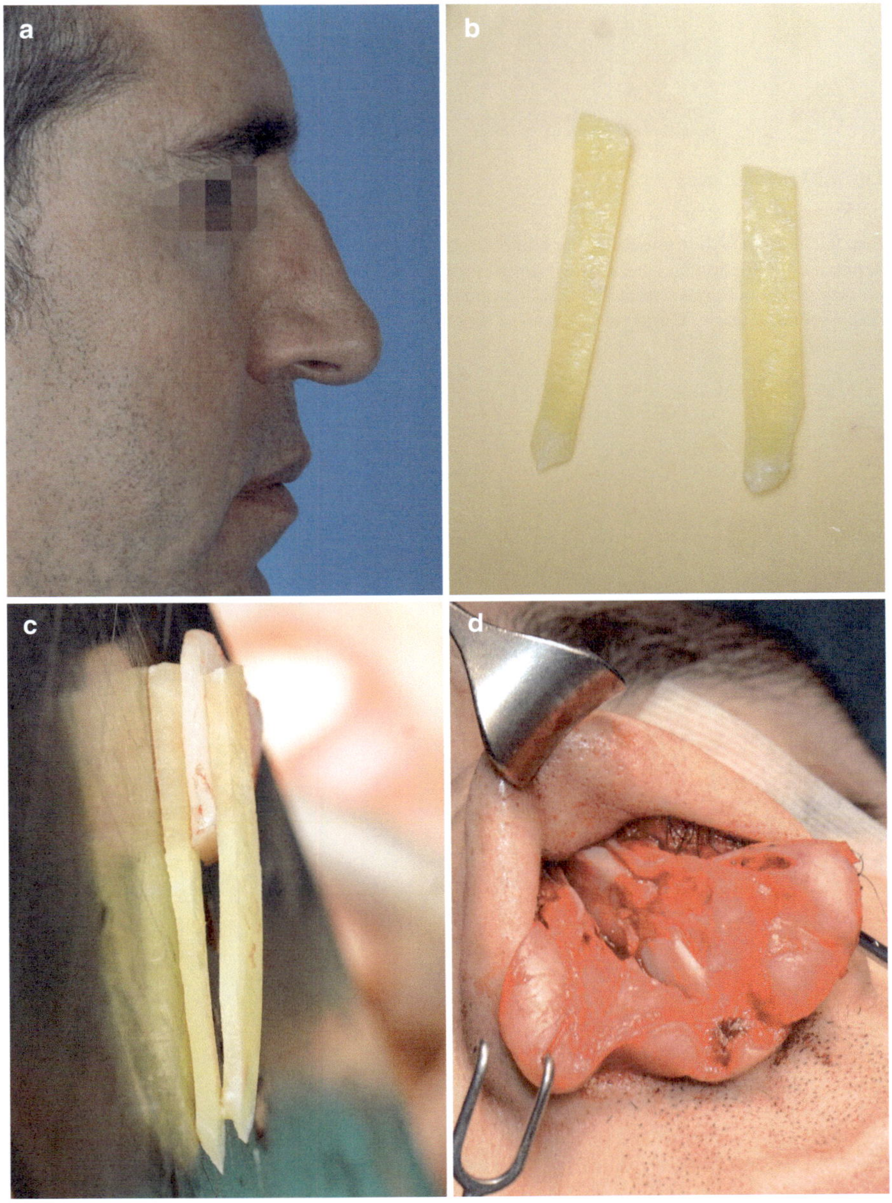

Fig. 9.21 (**a**) The preoperative profile photograph. (**b**) The extended spreader grafts. (**c**) The bilateral extended spreader graft and the sandwiched caudal replacement graft. (**d**) The dorsal septal remnant. (**e**, **f**) Intraoperative graft placement. The extended spreader grafts were sutured using 4–0 polydioxanone. The caudal replacement graft was placed between the extended spreader grafts and fixed with 5–0 polydioxanone sutures in an end-to-end manner relative to the native caudal septum and the anterior nasal spine

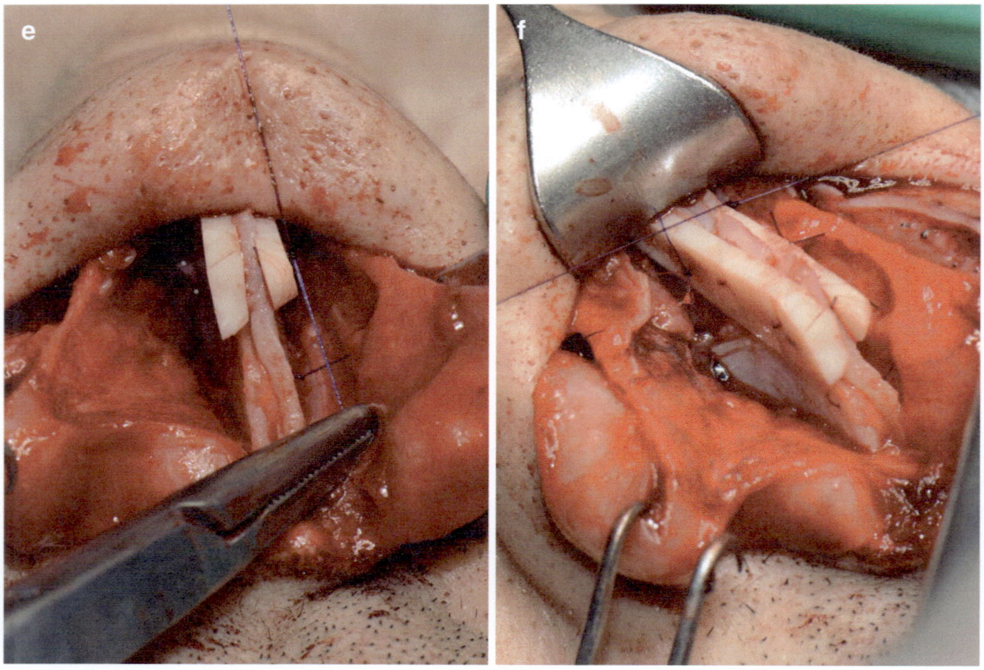

Fig. 9.21 (continued)

Fig. 9.22 (**a–d**) After removing the bony hump, septal reconstruction created an ideal dorsal profile and corrected both the retracted columella and the acute subnasal angle. Dorsal augmentation was not required

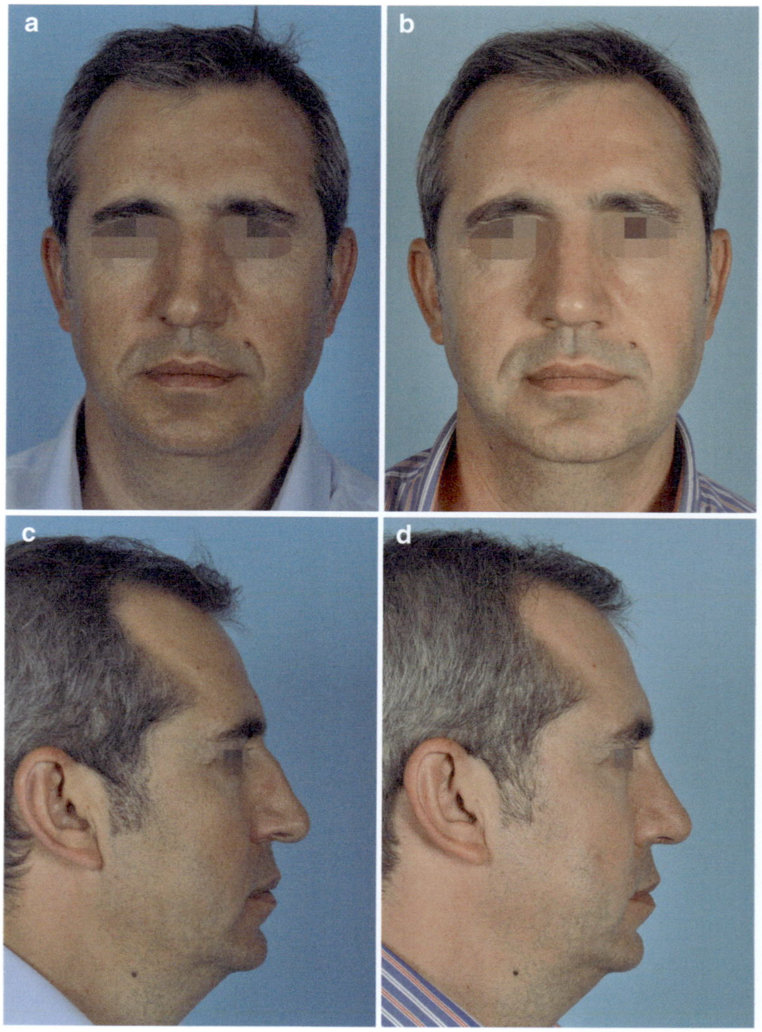

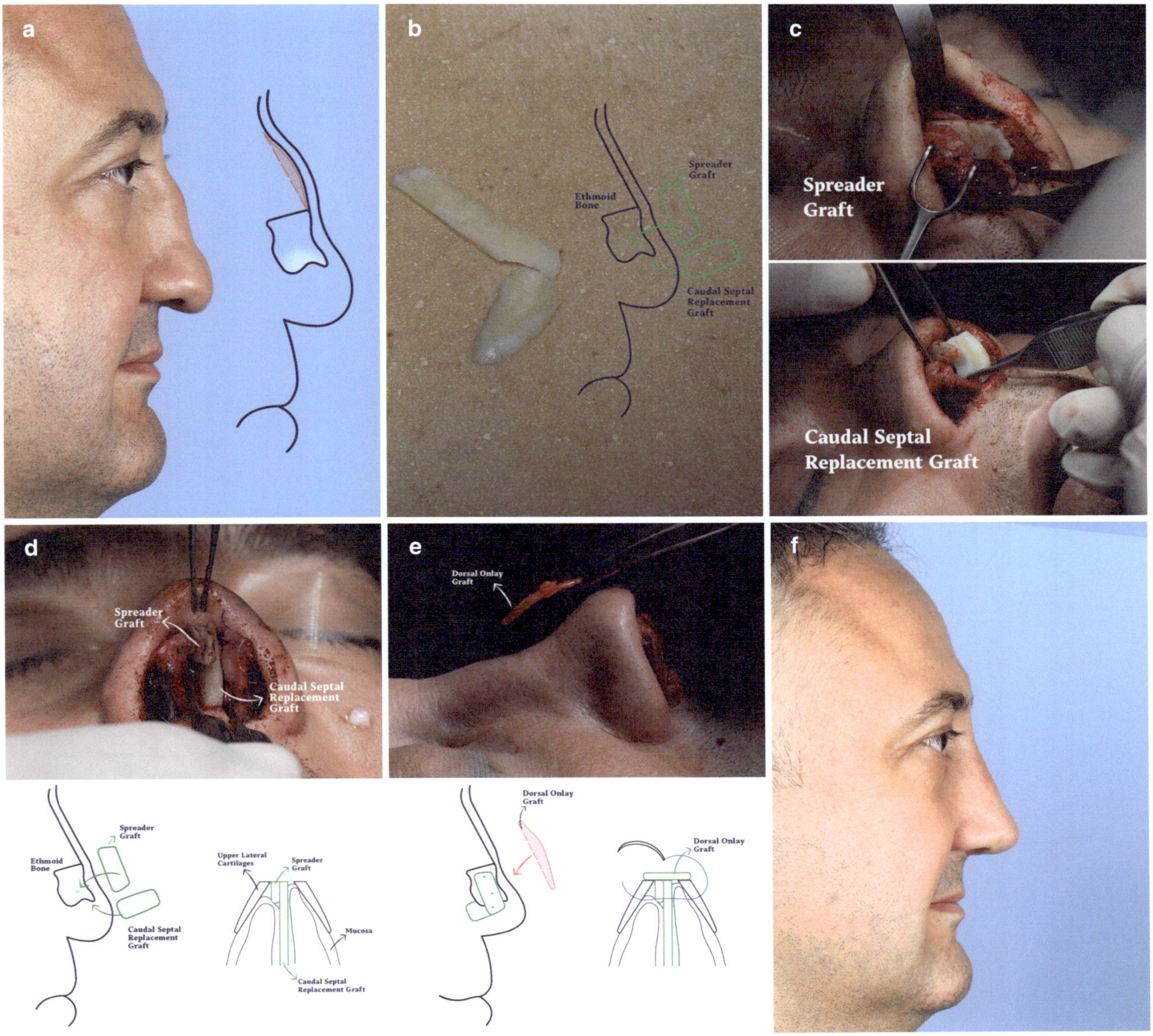

Fig. 9.23 (**a**) A typical saddle nose deformity due to caudal septum deficiencies. (**b–d**) To reconstruct the lower part of the septum, a unilateral spreader graft and a caudal septal replacement graft were used. Cadaveric cartilage was the graft material. The spreader graft was placed through a tunnel from the septal mucosa to the radix. As it fit well, the nasal bone was not secured, only fixed at a few points to the dorsal septal remnant. Then, the CSR graft was attached to the spreader graft and nasal spine, completing the septum reconstruction. (**e**) The excised bone hump was reshaped externally to achieve the required volume and contour for addressing the deficiency in the Supra tip. Subsequently, it was placed back over the deficient dorsal area. The dorsal onlay graft is secured onto the dorsum using a circular suture technique, beginning at the upper lateral aspect and passing through its corresponding opposite area. (**f**) After 1 year, the ideal appearance of the dorsal and tip was achieved. Reconstructing the septum resolved several issues in the tip. However, a steal suture was utilized, and bilateral medial crural strut graft was employed in the tip

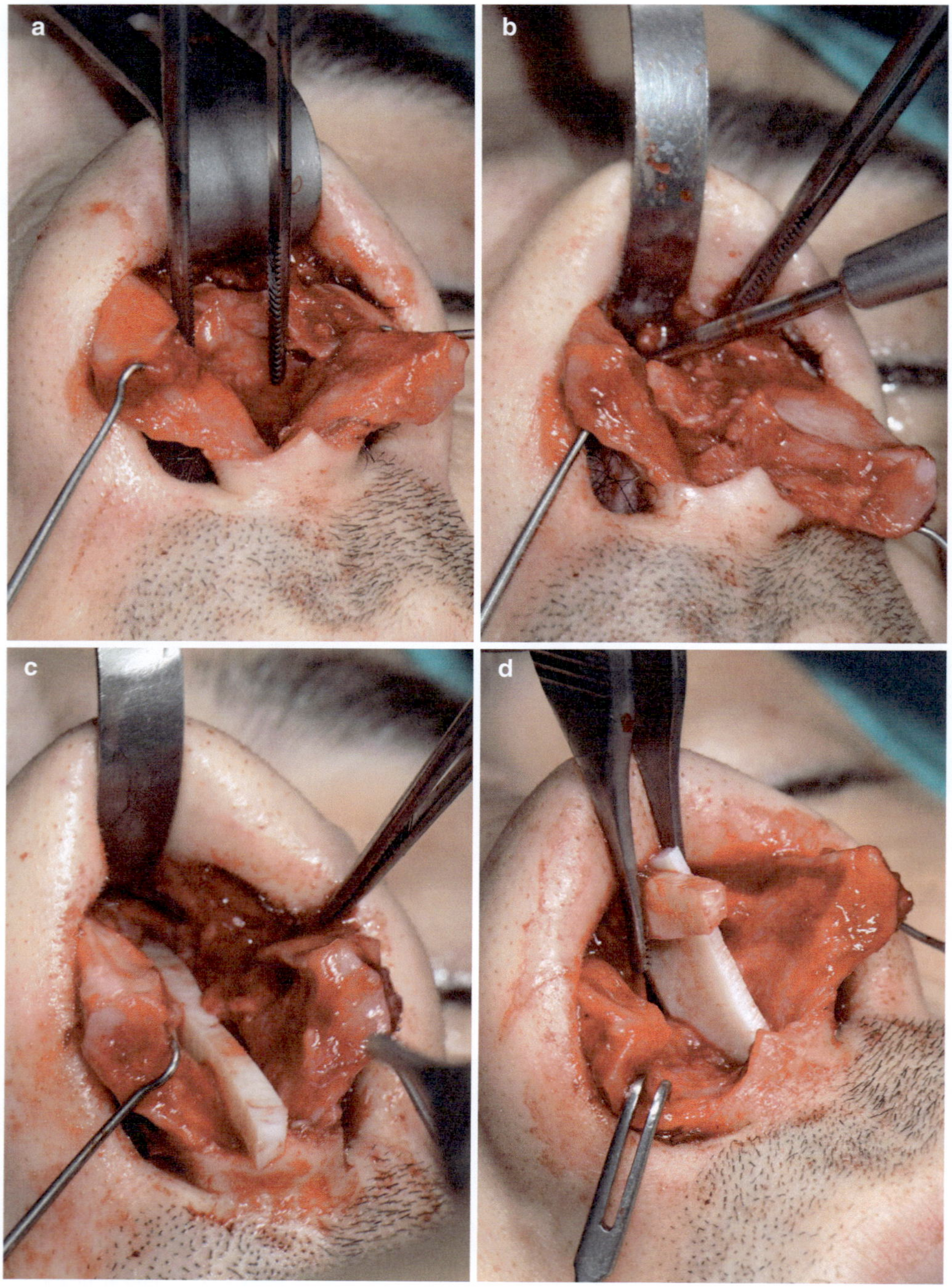

Fig. 9.24 (**a**) No septal cartilage is evident. (**b**) A septal mucoperichondrial tunnel is created under the nasal bones. (**c**) Cadaver cartilage serves as a dorsal septal replacement graft and is placed in the tunnel to create the dorsal part of the septum. (**d**) The caudal replacement graft is sutured to the dorsal septal replacement graft; this forms the caudal part of the septum. (**e**) The caudal replacement graft is sutured to the anterior nasal spine

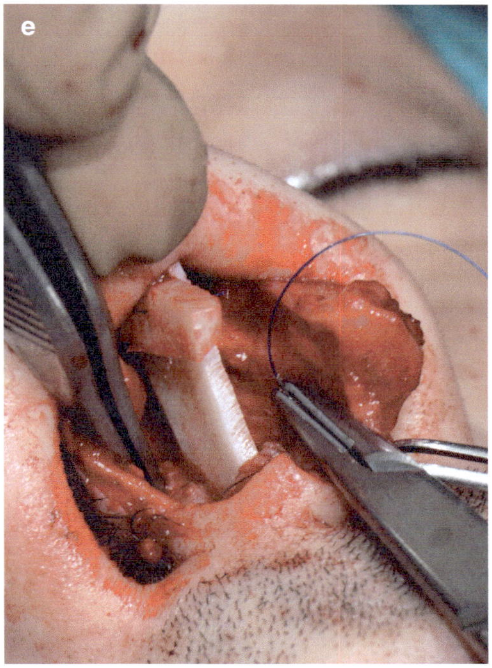

Fig. 9.24 (continued)

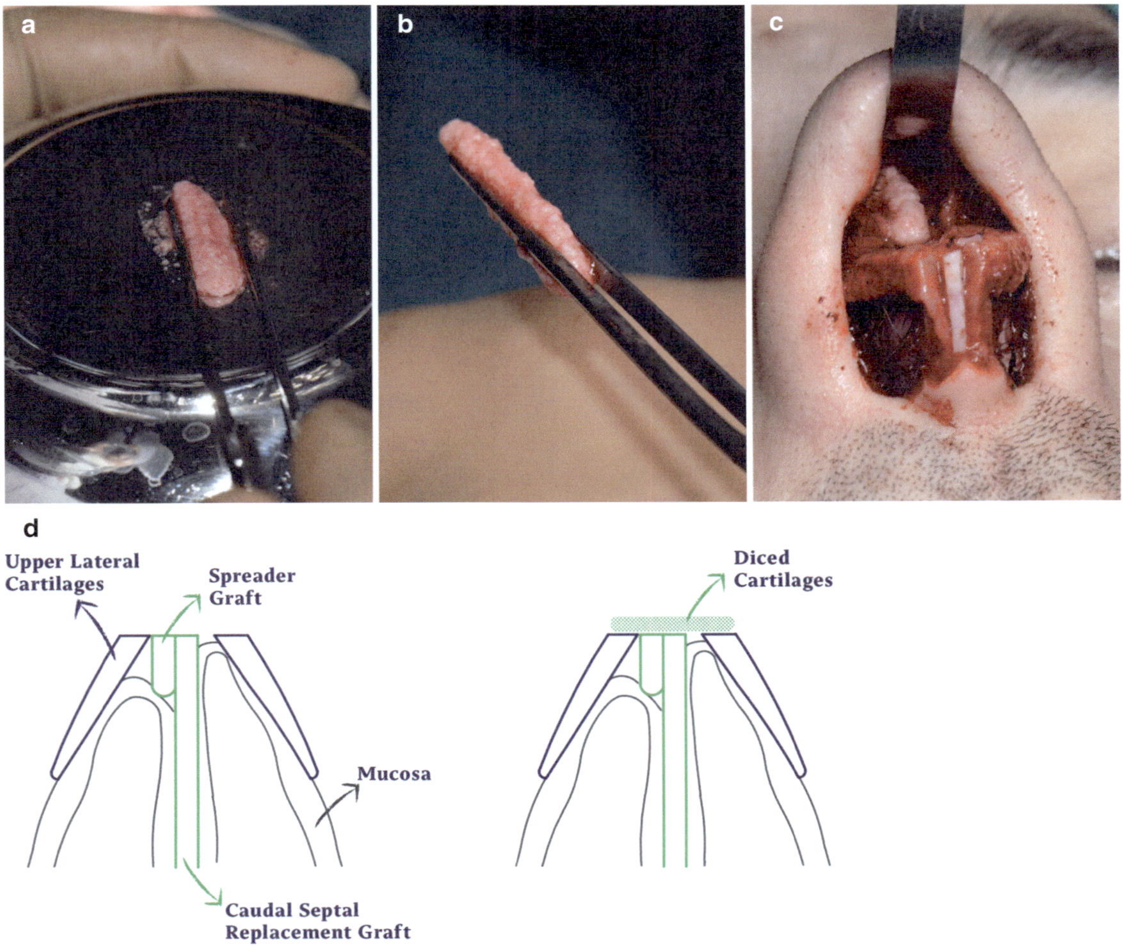

Fig. 9.25 (**a**–**h**) Diced cartilage was laid over the dorsum to gain projection

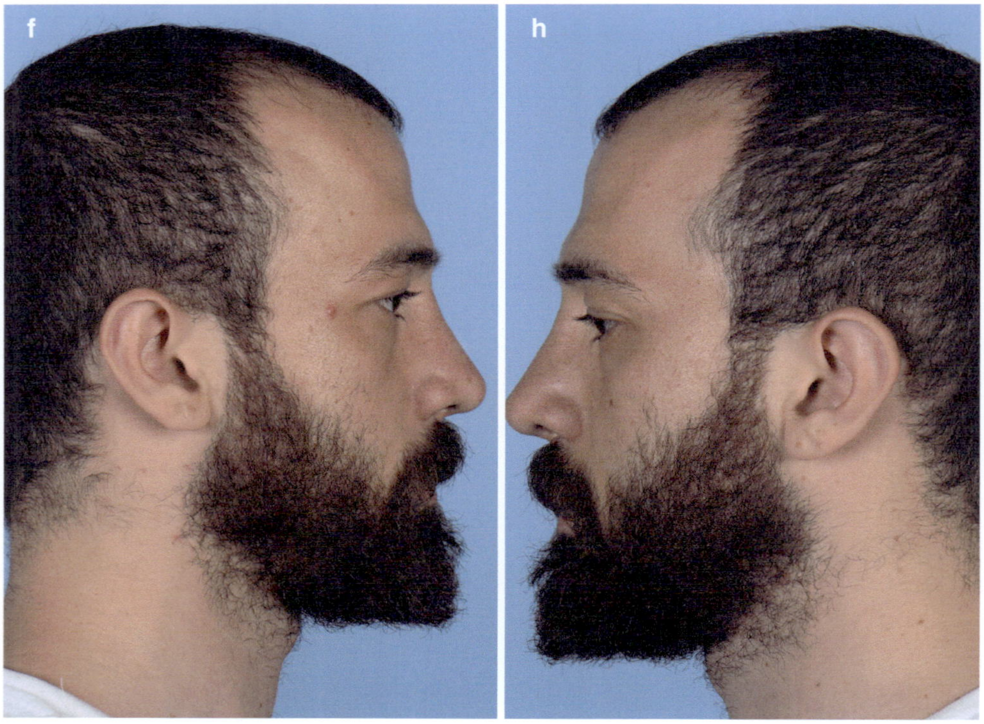

Fig. 9.25 (continued)

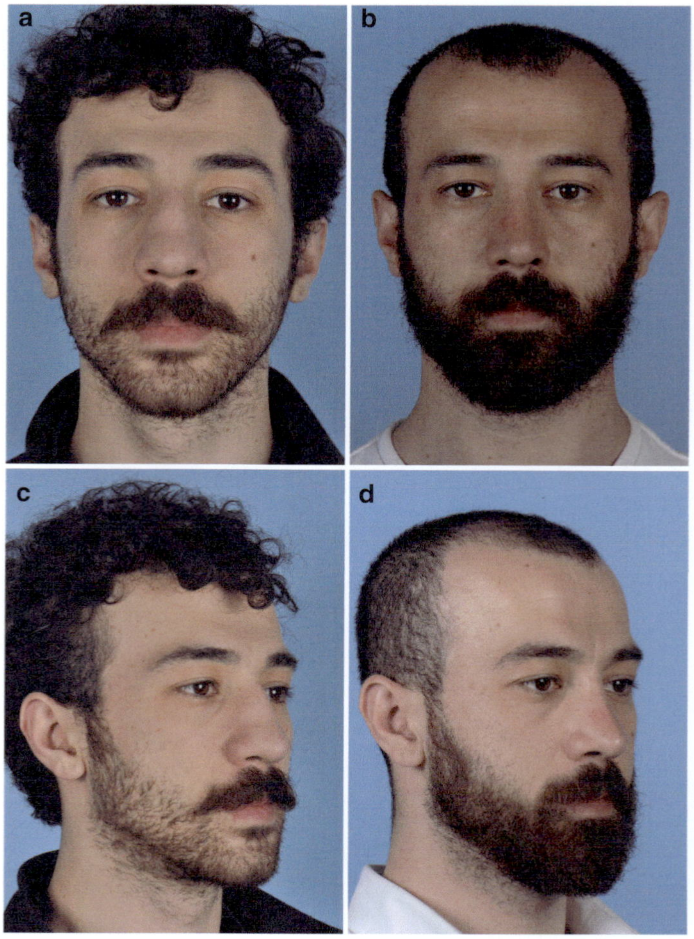

Fig. 9.26 (**a**, **b**) The width of the nose is normalized. (**c**, **d**) Bony dorsal hump has been eliminated. (**e–h**) Although the dorsal profile is improved, more dorsal projection is needed

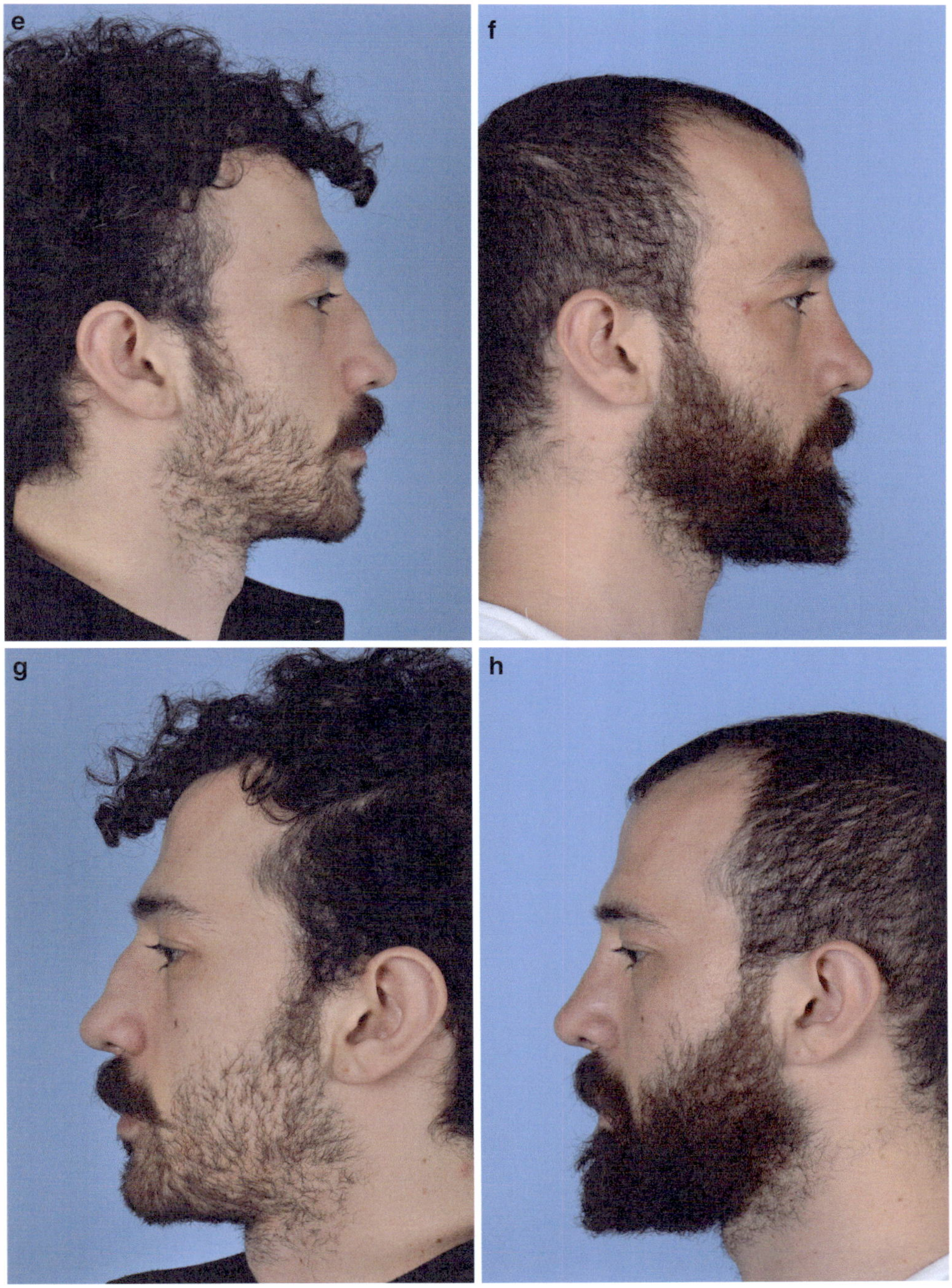

Fig. 9.26 (continued)

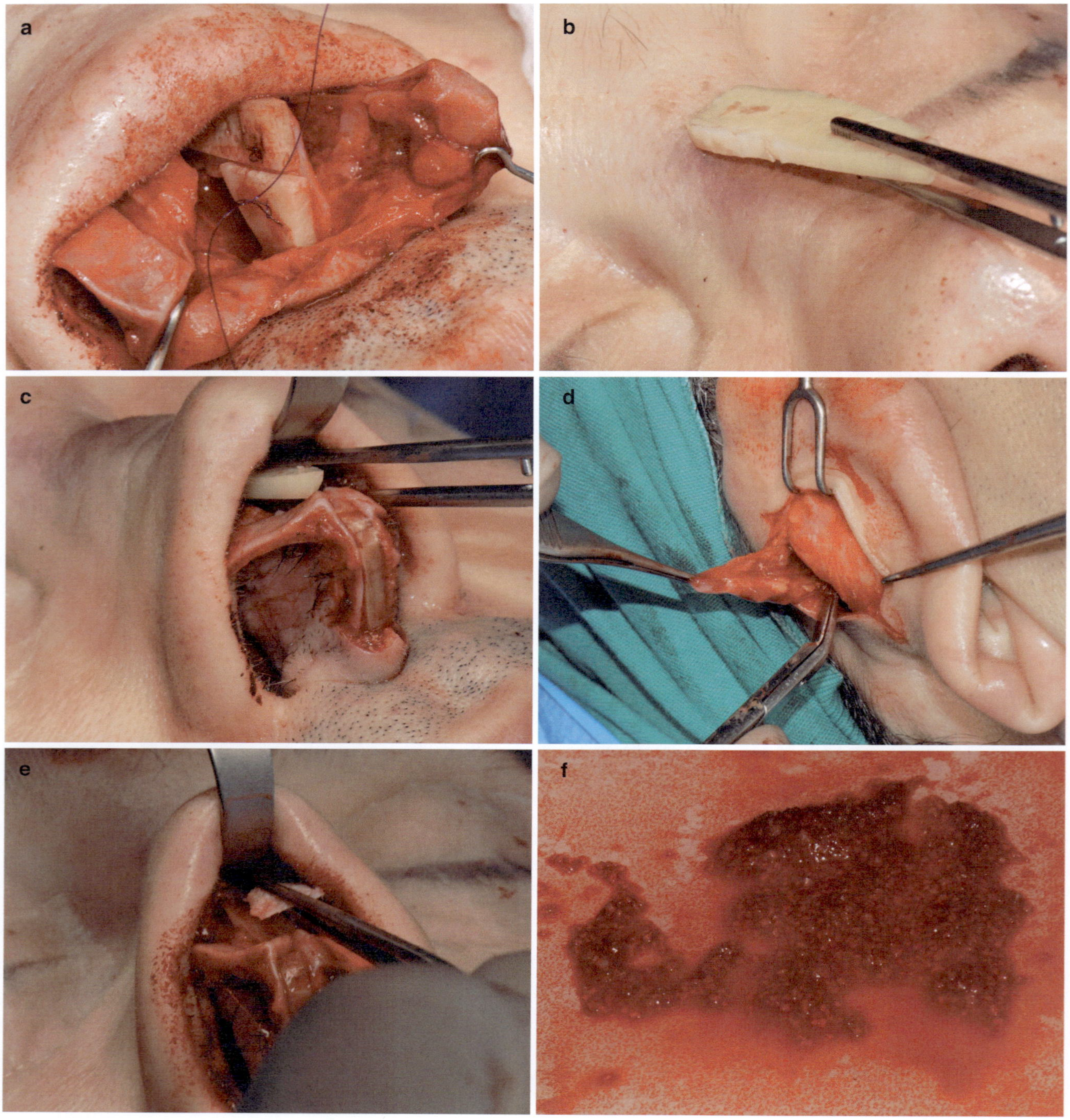

Fig. 9.27 (**a**) The septum is reconstructed with unilateral spreader graft and caudal septal button graft. (**b**, **c**) Previously prepared en bloc costal cartilage is placed on the newly formed L-strut to enhance dorsal projection. (**d**–**f**) Soft tissue (diced and crushed cartilage and post-auricular tissue) is placed near the costal cartilage to hide the graft

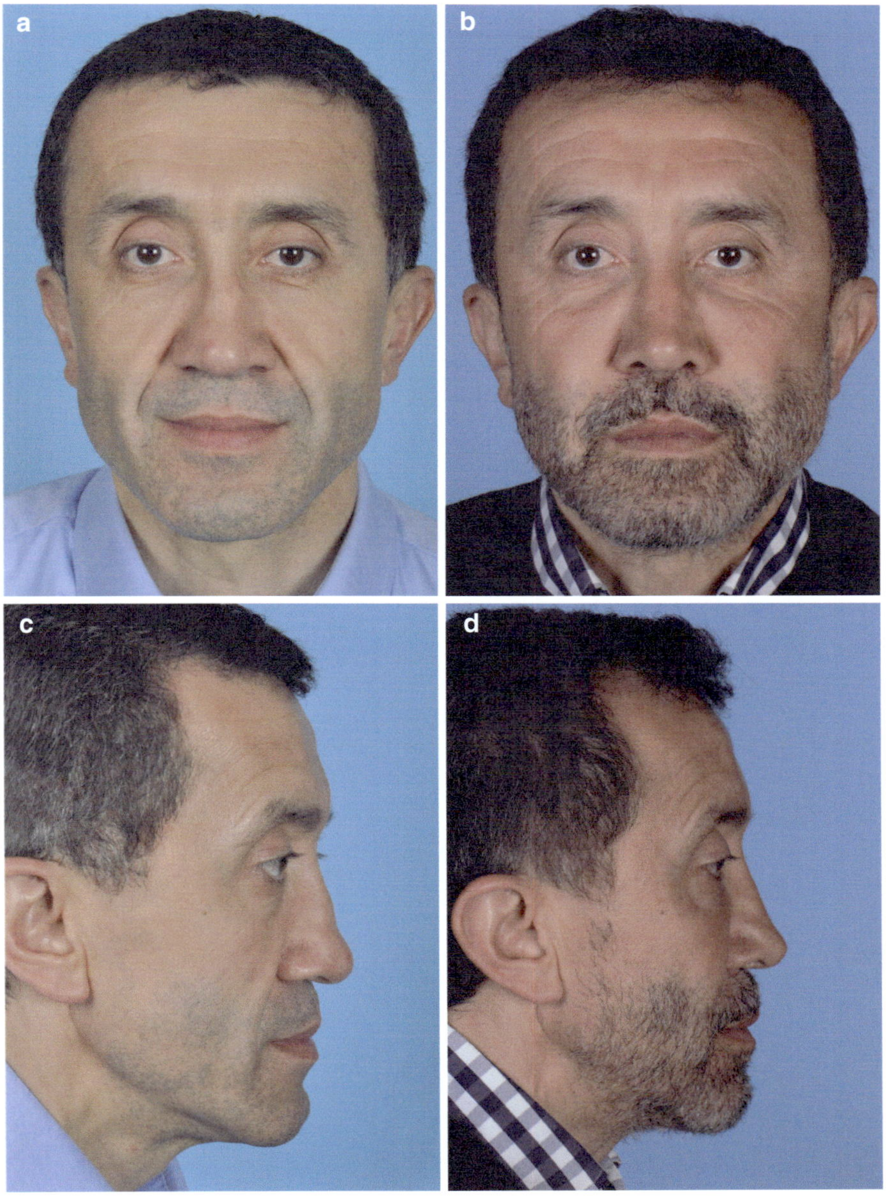

Fig. 9.28 (**a**–**n**) Before and after photographs: middle vault reconstruction and dorsal augmentation corrected the saddle nose deformity together and makes the dorsum appear narrower on frontal view. Retracted columella is improved and nasolabial angle is more obtuse

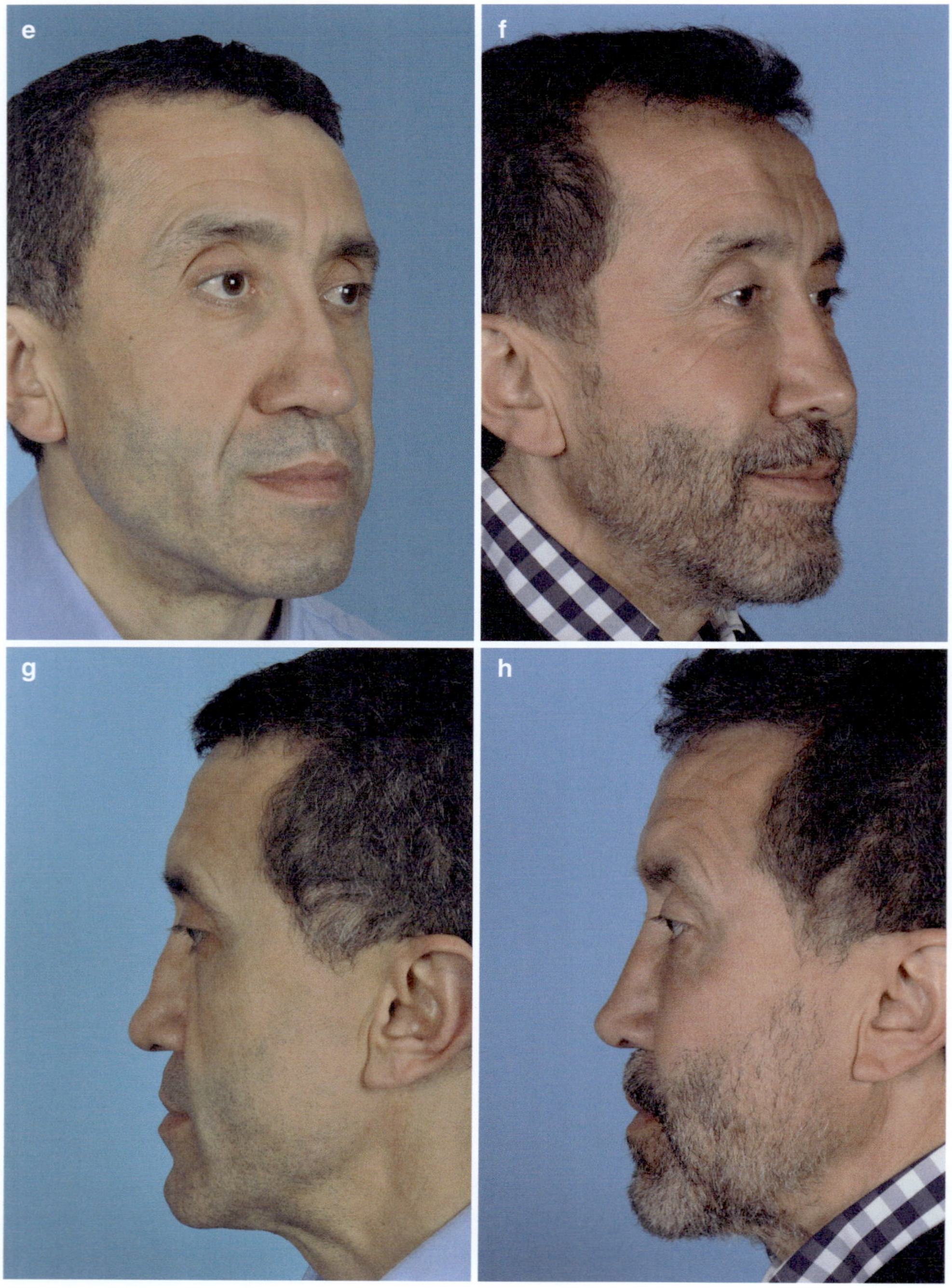

Fig. 9.28 (continued)

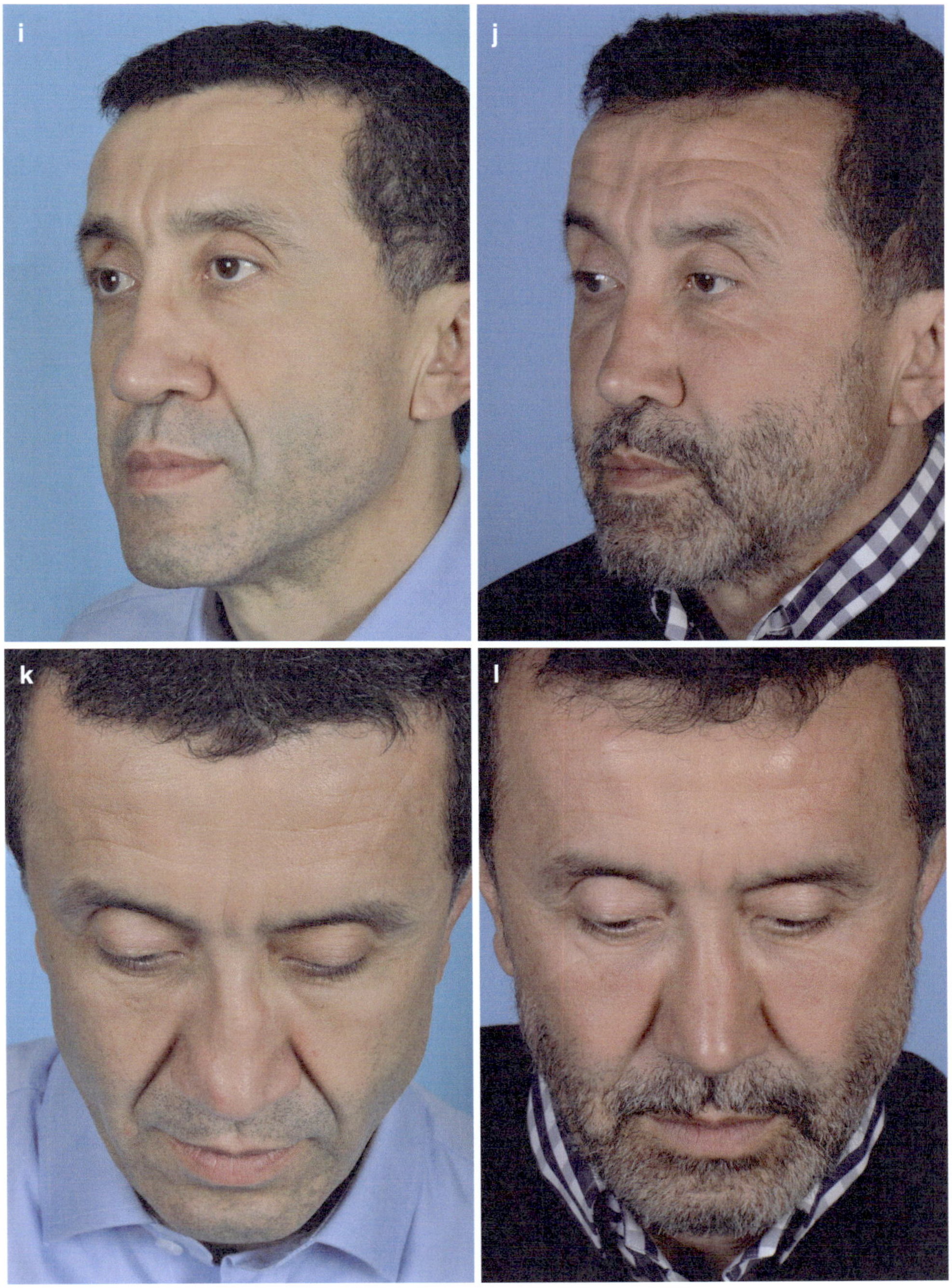

Fig. 9.28 (continued)

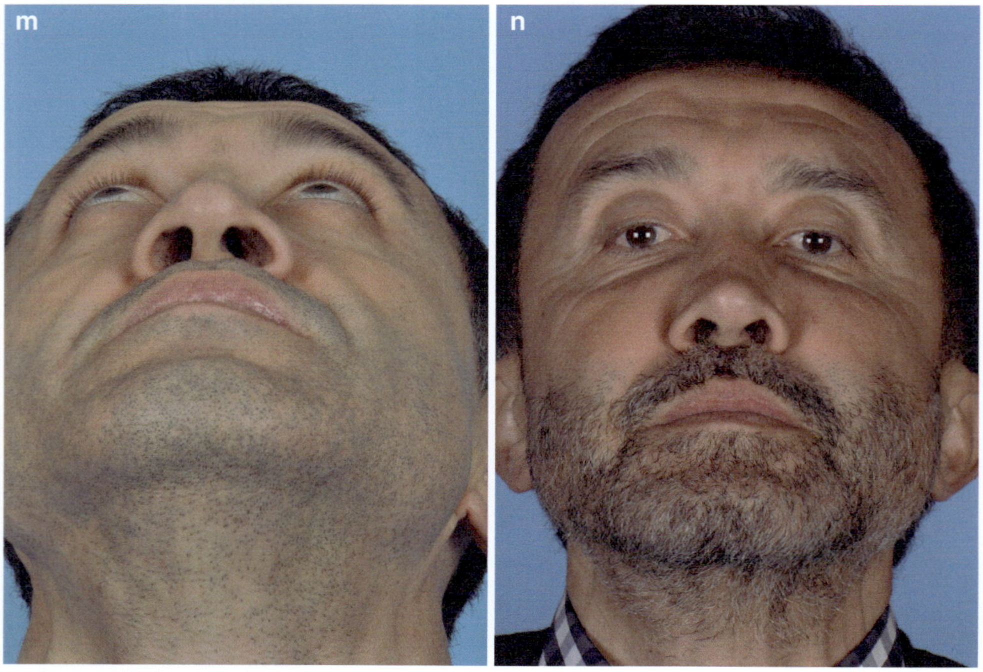

Fig. 9.28 (continued)

9.4 Conclusion

The nasal septum not only plays an important physiological role in terms of airflow maintenance but also supports the dorsum of the nose and contributes to nose height, length, tip, and position (optimally in the center of the face). When the structure is damaged, a saddle nose deformity develops. Dorsal augmentation should not be performed in the absence of septal reconstruction; the saddle nose will recur. However, an over-resected bony dorsum (often confused with a saddle nose deformity) can be treated via augmentation alone.

A typical example of an over-resected bony dorsum subjected to dorsal augmentation using costal cartilage is shown in Fig. 9.29.

Useful treatments for saddle nose deformity, one of the principal subjects of this chapter, are summarized in Fig. 9.30 (Video 9.3).

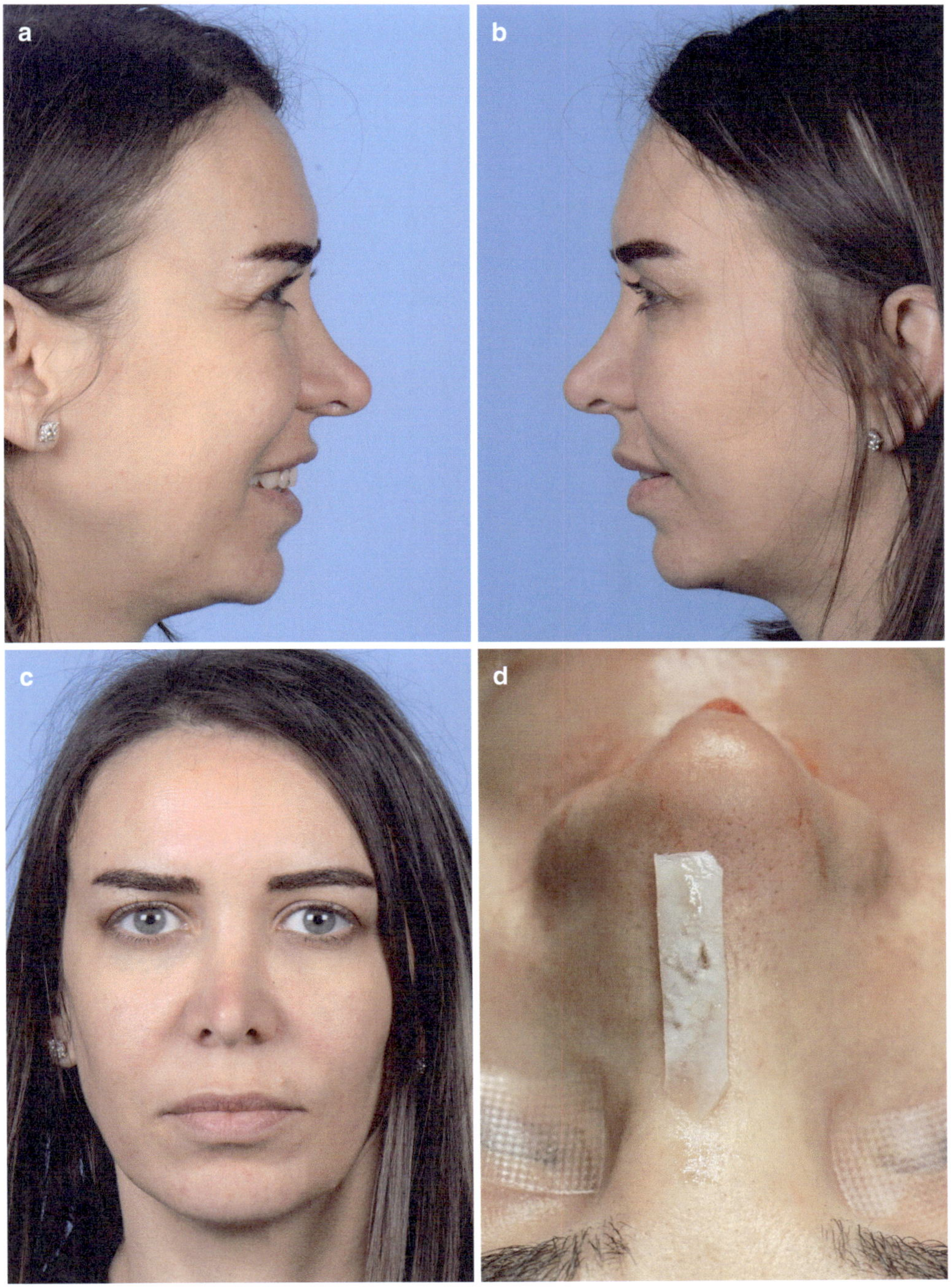

Fig. 9.29 (**a**–**c**) The dorsum had been over-resected previously. The tip projection was imbalanced with the dorsum. Septal support was looked strong enough, the main difference from the saddle nose. (**d**) Dorsal augmentation with costal cartilage was done. Septum was intact; therefore, septal reconstruction was not performed. (**e**–**g**) 1 year after. The nose appears straighter with more acceptable dorsal lines. The height of the dorsum is more uniform, and the tip position improved from the more ptotic position

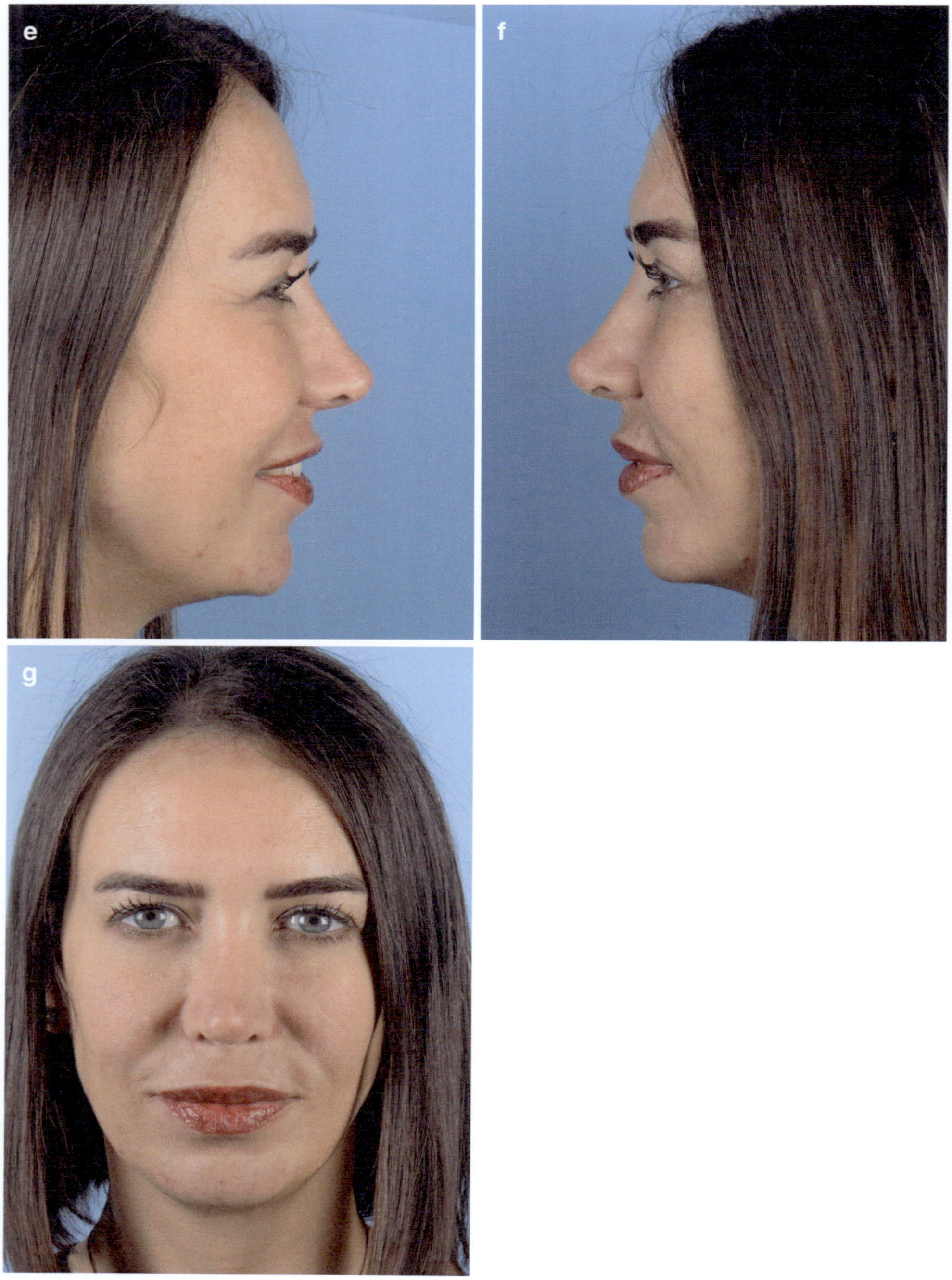

Fig. 9.29 (continued)

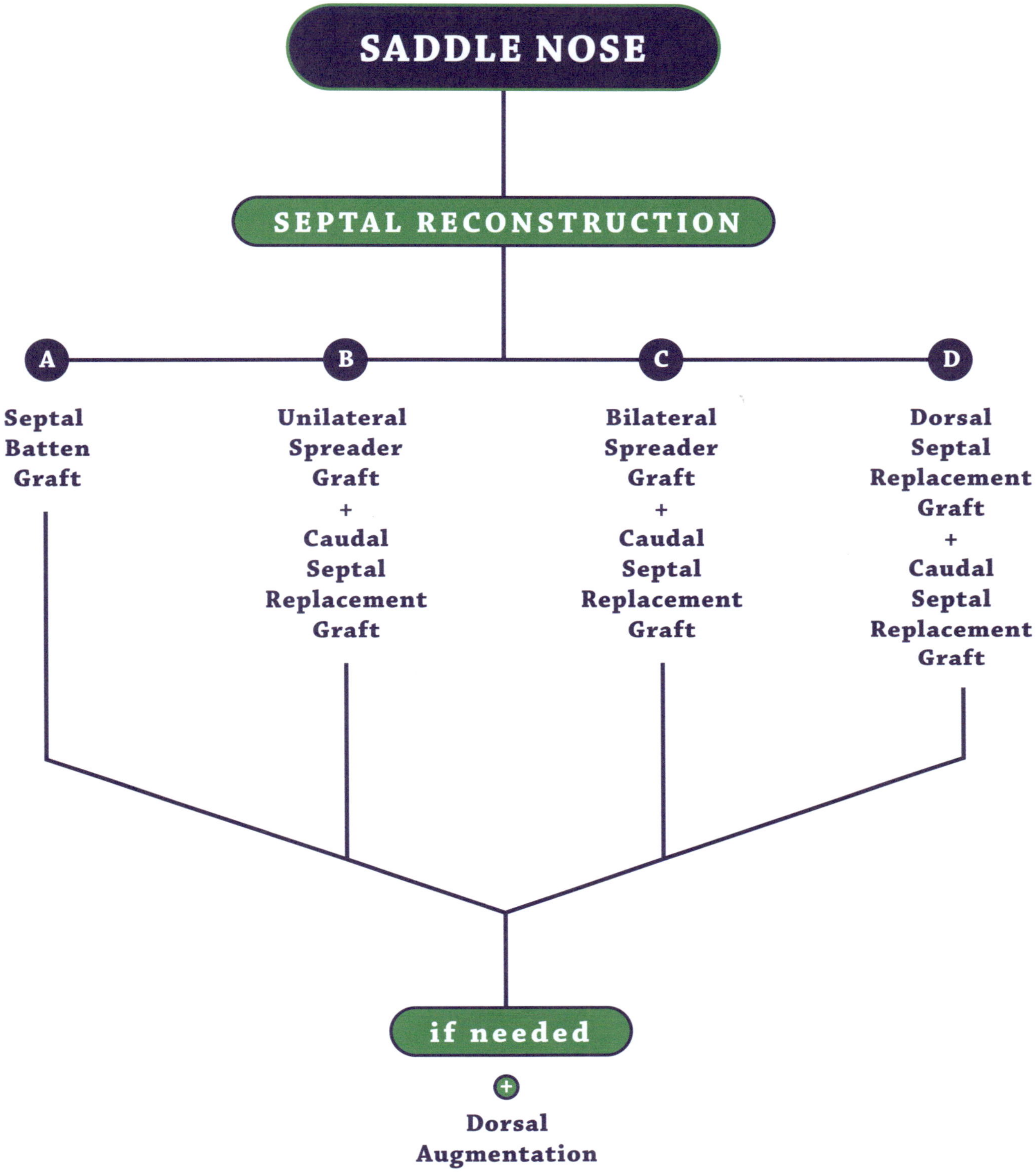

Fig. 9.30 The dorsal onlay graft has not only increased the height of the bridge on the lateral view but also improved the brow-tip aesthetic line on the frontal view

Disclosures The author reports no conflicts of interest or funding requiring disclosure.

Further Reading

Behrbohm H, Tardy ME. Essentials of septorhinoplasty: philosophy, approaches, techniques. New York, NY: Thieme; 2017. p. 210–24.
Boenisch M, Nolst Trenité GJ. Reconstructive septal surgery. Facial Plast Surg. 2006;22(4):249–54.
Chen YY, Jang YJ. Refinements in saddle nose reconstruction. Facial Plast Surg. 2018;34(4):363–72.
Daniel RK. Rhinoplasty: septal saddle nose deformity and composite reconstruction. Plast Reconstr Surg. 2007;119(3):1029–43.
Hamilton GS. Dorsal failures: from saddle deformity to pollybeak. Facial Plast Surg. 2018;34(3):261–9.
Lee HJ, Jang YJ. Correction of saddle and short noses. Curr Opin Otolaryngol Head Neck Surg. 2016;24(4):294–9.
Menick FJ. The interface of cosmetic and reconstructive rhinoplasty: the crucified tip, the saddlenose and the continuum of reconstruction and cosmesis. Philadelphia, PA: Saunders Elsevier; 2009.
Ponsky DC, Harvey DJ, Khan SW, Guyuron B. Nose elongation: a review and description of the septal extension tongue-and-groove technique. Aesthet Surg J. 2010;30(3):335–46.
Pribitkin EA, Ezzat WH. Classification and treatment of the saddle nose deformity. Otolaryngol Clin N Am. 2009;42(3):437–61.
Robitschek J, Hilger P. The saddle deformity: camouflage and reconstruction. Facial Plast Surg Clin North Am. 2017;25(2):239–50.
Toriumi DM, Bared A. Revision of the surgically overshortened nose. Facial Plast Surg. 2012;28(4):407–16.
Young K, Rowe-Jones J. Current approaches to septal saddle nose reconstruction using autografts. Curr Opin Otolaryngol Head Neck Surg. 2011;19(4):276–82.

10 Tip Anatomy and Analysis

10.1 Tip Anatomy

A basic understanding of the nasal tip anatomy is insufficient for successful tip surgery. Acquiring assessment of the anatomic variations presented by a patient and knowing surgical maneuvers to treat each tip variation will lead to successful tip surgery. Therefore, this chapter presents a limited overview of tip anatomy and basic terminology. Detailed anatomic variations and pathologies will be discussed in the following chapters regarding the nasal tip.

10.2 Basic Anatomy

The nasal tip is mainly supported by the lower lateral crura, known as alar cartilages or alar arches. Each alar arch is anatomically divided into lateral, medial, and middle crus.

The lateral crus begins at the domal junction and ends at the lateral nasal wall, where it meets with accessory cartilage. The lateral crus is the most important component of the nasal tip and makes a large contribution to tip definition and shape. In addition, the lateral crus supports the alar sidewall, which is crucial for nasal airflow.

The middle crus begins at the domal junction and ends at the columellar-lobular junction. It has two subunits: the domal and lobular segments.

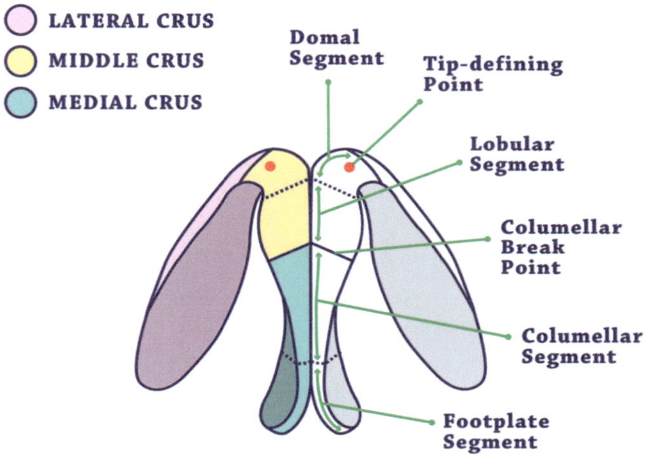

Fig. 10.1 Basal view of alar cartilages

The medial crus begins at the columellar lobular junction and ends at the footplates. It has two subunits: the columellar and footplate segments (Fig. 10.1).

To create an ideal tip, the cartilaginous septum should be stable, strong, and straight because the caudal septum supports the tip. The septal cartilage is a flat plate of irregular quadrilateral-shaped cartilage that varies in size. It is caudally continuous with the perpendicular plate of the ethmoids and inferiorly continuous with the vomer (Fig. 10.2).

S. Şeneldir, *Photographic Atlas of Rhinoplasty*, https://doi.org/10.1007/978-3-031-65619-4_10

Fig. 10.2 Nasal septum

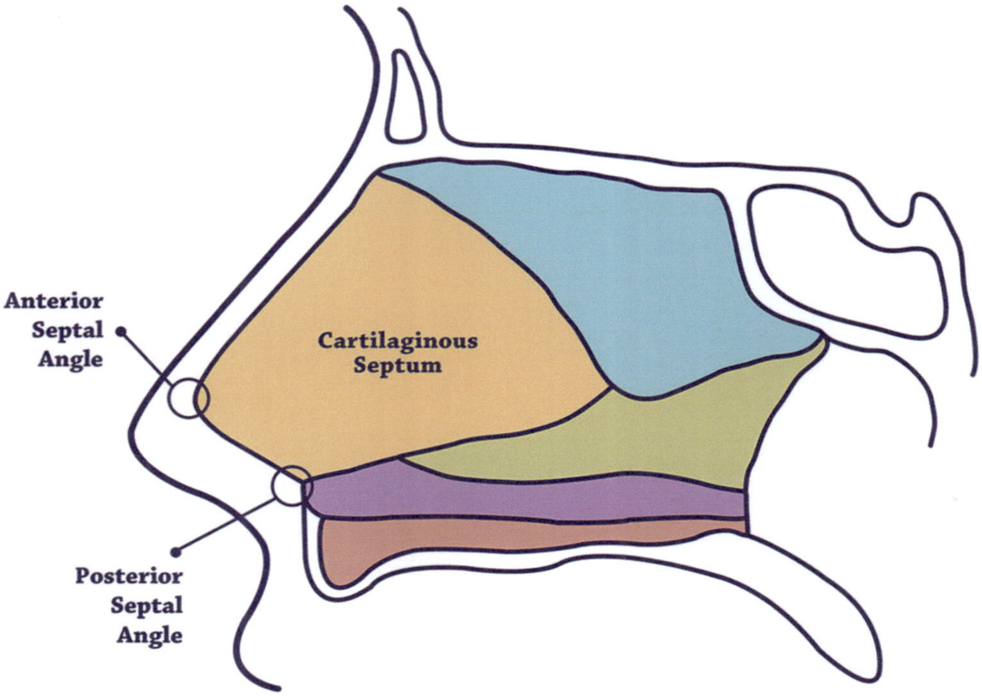

10.3 Directions

After these reminders regarding the basic nasal tip structure, it is necessary to identify directions to understand the subject (Fig. 10.3).

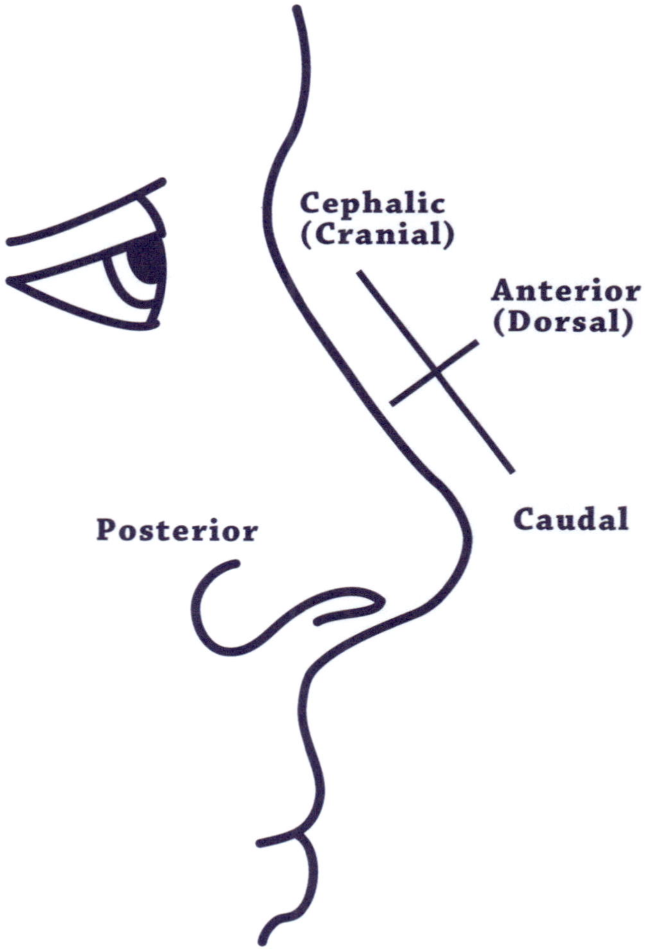

Fig. 10.3 Directions for the nose. Profile view

10.4 Terminology

The parameters of the nasal tip are as follows (Figs. 10.4, 10.5, 10.6, and 10.7):

1. **The tip rotation** is measured mainly by the *nasolabial angle*.

   The nasolabial angle is measured by a straight line through the most anterior and posterior edges of the nostril; this line creates the angle that transects a plump line.
2. **The tip projection** is measured mainly by the distance of the vertical plane passing through the alar crease to the nasal tip.
3. **The tip definition** points are located at the apex of the tip lobule and formed by the junction of the medial and lateral crura of each LLC. The cartilage in this area creates light reflection and affects perceived tip shape.
4. **The supratip** is the area immediately above the tip.
5. **The infratip lobule segment** is the area between the tip defining point and columellar break point.
6. **The columellar break point** is the point of transition between the columellar segment of the medial crus and the lobular segment of the middle crus. This transition point also creates an angle known as the columellar-lobular angle.

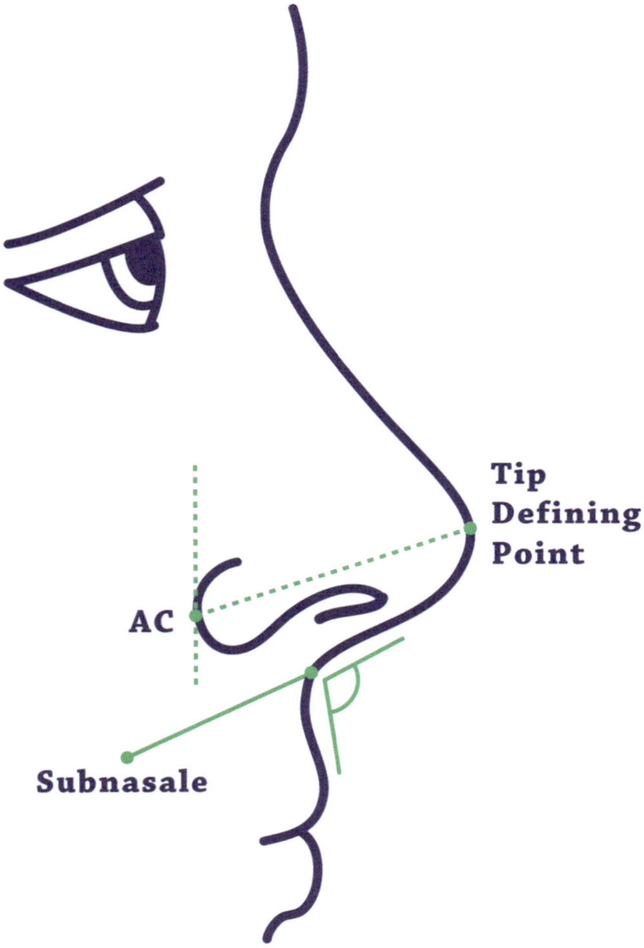

Fig. 10.4 The tip projection and rotation

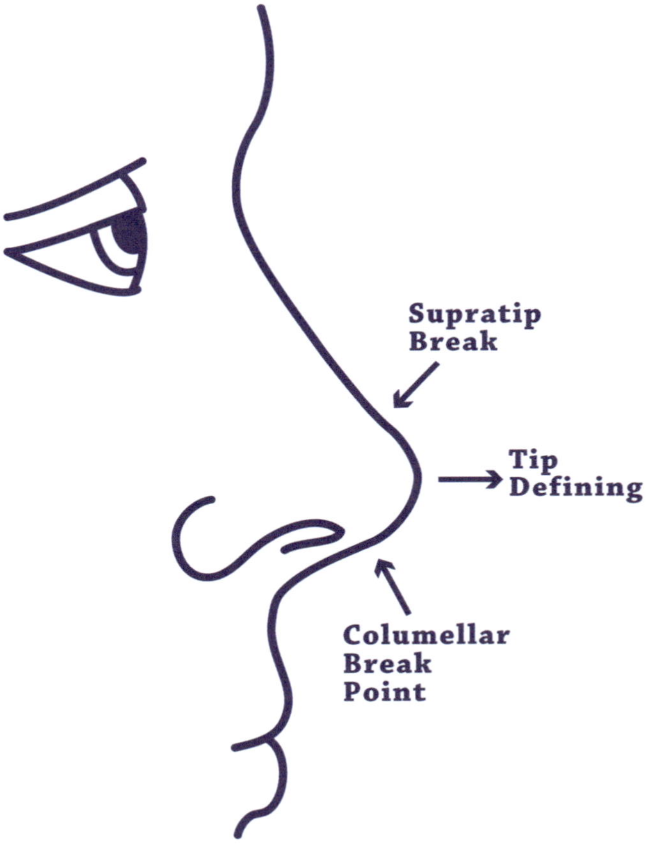

Fig. 10.5 Transition: points of the tip

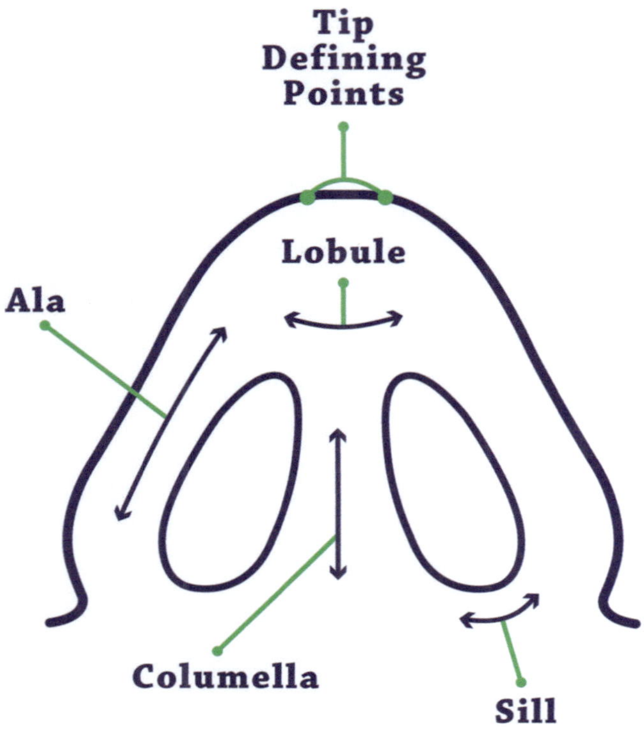

Fig. 10.6 Nasal base subunits

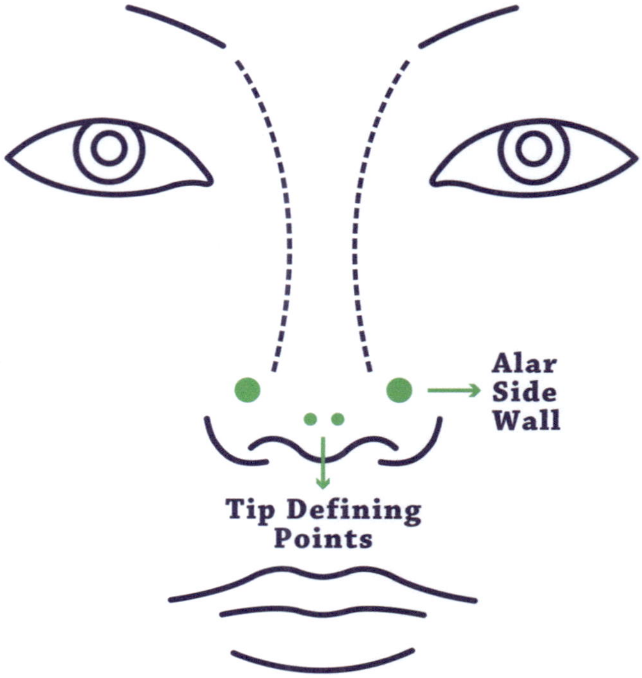

Fig. 10.7 Nasal subunits

Fig. 10.8 The main tip grafts

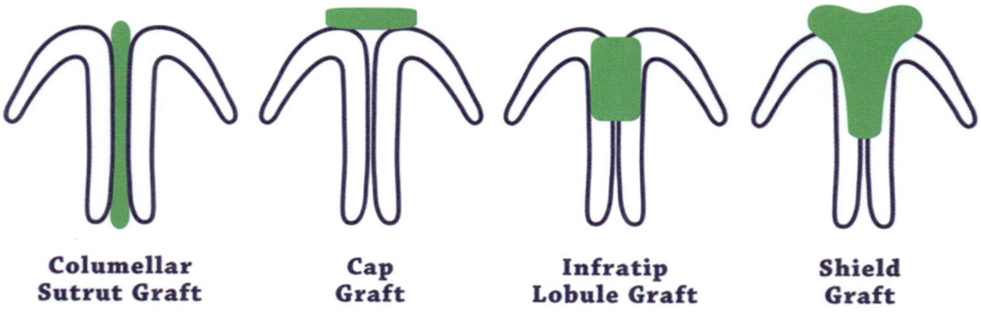

10.5 Grafts (Figs. 10.8, 10.9, and 10.10)

Onlay tip grafts constitute two types: cap graft and shield graft. These grafts facilitate tip projection and definition.

Lateral crural grafts are grafts placed on the lateral crus in an overlay/underlay fashion. These are used for lateral crus convexity and concavity or for strengthening the lateral crus.

Alar batten grafts are placed cephalically to the lateral crus. These are used for management of alar sidewall concavity.

Columellar strut grafts are used for reconstruction and strengthening of the middle/medial crus complex. These also enhance tip projection.

Columella lobular grafts are fixed to both middle and medial crura to form a stable tip.

Alar rim grafts are placed cranially to the lateral crus. These are used to treat alar rim retraction, to enhance tip lobule volume, and to camouflage and strengthen the alar wall when the cephalic border of the lateral crus is higher than its caudal border.

Infratip lobule grafts are used to treat infratip deficiency.

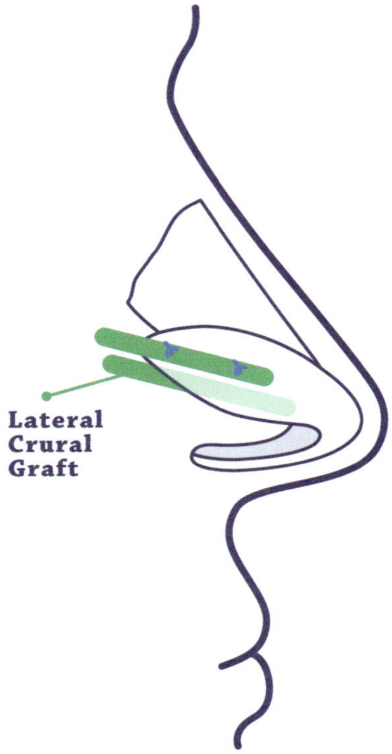

Fig. 10.9 Alar side wall grafts

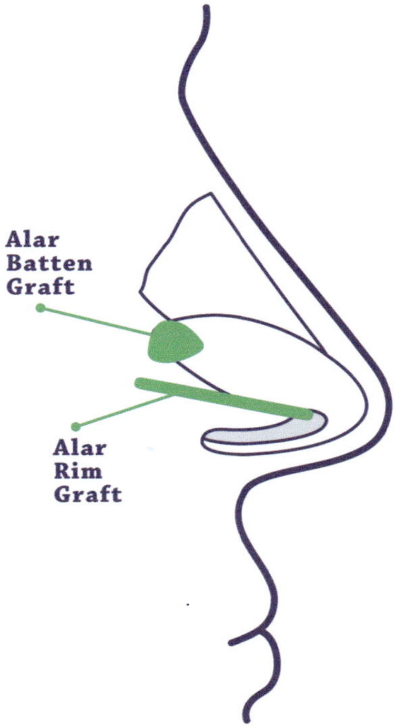

Fig. 10.10 Alar side wall grafts

Disclosures The author reports no conflicts of interest or funding requiring disclosure.

Further Reading

Daniel RK. The nasal tip: anatomy and aesthetics. Plast Reconstr Surg. 1992;89:216–24.

Gunter JP. Anatomical observations of the lower lateral cartilages. Arch Otolaryngol. 1969;89:599.

Janis JE, Ahmad J, Rohrich RJ. Rhinoplasty. In: Thorne CH, Chung KC, Gosain AK, Gurtner GC, Mehrara BJ, Rubin JP, et al., editors. Grabb and Smith's plastic surgery. 7th ed. Philadelphia, PA: Lippincott Williams and Wilkins; 2014. p. 512–29.

Pessa JE, Rohrich RJ. Nasal analysis and anatomy. Philadelphia, PA: Elsevier Saunders; 2013. p. 373–86.

Sheen JH, Sheen AP. Aesthetic rhinoplasty. 2nd ed. St. Louis, MO: Quality Medical; 1997. p. 50–92.

Tardy ME. Surgical anatomy of the nose. New York, NY: Raven Press; 1992. p. 36–72.

Toriumi DM. New concepts in nasal tip contouring. Arch Facial Plast Surg. 2006;8:156–85.

Zelnik J, Gingrass RP. Anatomy of the alar cartilage. Plast Reconstr Surg. 1979;64:650–3.

11 Plunging Nose, Under-Rotated Nasal Tip

11.1 Introduction and Brief Clinical History

Patients with a droopy nasal tip, which occurs when the tip of the nose is more caudal than its ideal configuration, appear older than their biological age. Following postsurgical recovery, patients may begin to receive compliments from their friends on how much younger they look, which makes them feel better and more attractive, and helps them appreciate how negatively their droopy nose affected their lives prior to surgery. This is a common motivation for rhinoplasty. The success of droopy nasal tip surgery is also important for the surgeon; when less-experienced surgeons succeed in correcting a droopy nasal tip, they receive positive feedback from the patient and their colleagues, increasing their motivation and prestige. The success of the surgery depends on the surgeon's anatomical knowledge, correct diagnosis of the underlying pathology, and selection of a surgical technique suitable for the patient. This chapter discusses droopy nasal tip, including the underlying pathology and treatment approaches (Fig. 11.1).

Rotation generally refers to the relationship between the nasal base and the rest of the face, in the profile view. It can be characterized from two angles:

1. Nasolabial angle
2. Columellar-lobular angle

These two angles provide information on deviations from the ideal in patients with an under-rotated nasal tip. Either one or both angles can show deviation, which may be the underlying cause of the droopy nasal tip appearance.

The columellar-labial angle, which is normally 90–95° in males and 95–105° in females, is lower in patients with an under-rotated nasal tip (acute columellar-labial angle), while the columellar-lobular angle is less than 45°. All maneuvers performed during droopy nasal tip surgery aim to bring these two angles as close to the ideal as possible (Fig. 11.2).

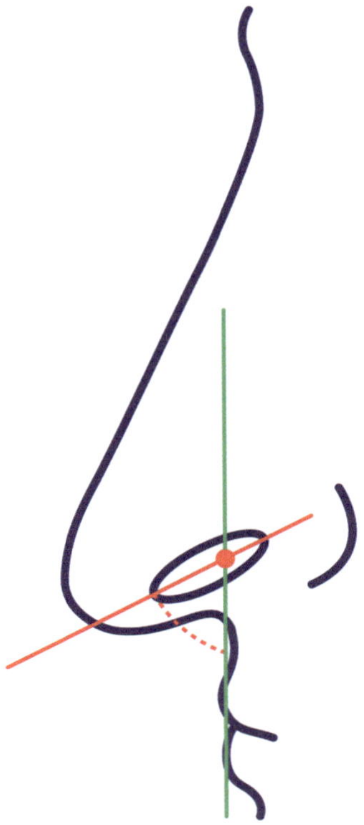

Fig. 11.1 Under-rotated nasal tip

Supplementary Information The online version contains supplementary material available at https://doi.org/10.1007/978-3-031-65619-4_11.

S. Şeneldir, *Photographic Atlas of Rhinoplasty*, https://doi.org/10.1007/978-3-031-65619-4_11

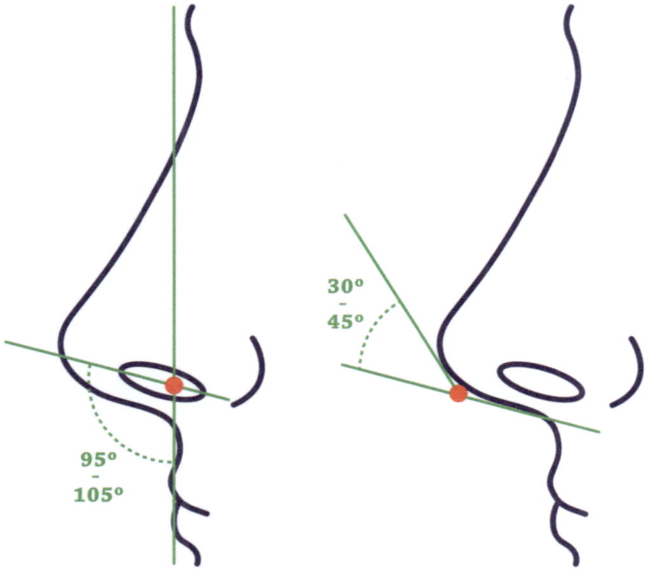

Fig. 11.2 Ideal nasolabial and columella-lobular angle in females

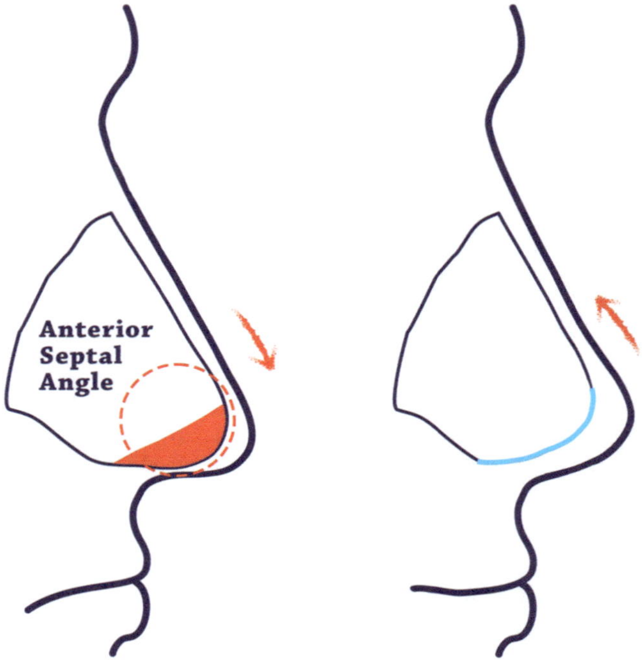

Fig. 11.3 (**a**) The red area shows excess caudal septum pushing the tip down. (**b**) Shortening the caudal septum via triangular resection gives rotation to the tip

11.2 Treatment Strategy

There are two main underlying causes of a droopy nasal tip:

1. Extrinsic factors, which are associated with the septum, the upper lateral cartilage, the skin, etc.
2. Intrinsic factors, which are associated with the alar cartilages.

11.2.1 Droopy Nasal Tip Associated with Extrinsic Factors

The first structure that should be addressed in all droopy nasal tip cases is the septum.

Two problems at the level of the septum can cause a droopy nasal tip:

1. Overdevelopment of the anterior septal angle
2. Deficiency of the posterior septal angle or nasal spine

11.2.1.1 Overdevelopment of the Anterior Septal Angle

In the case of overdevelopment of the anterior septal angle, an overdeveloped septal angle pushes the tip down. This condition is congenital. Droopy nasal tip associated only with anterior septal angle hypertrophy is rare and generally associated with intrinsic factors. In droopy tips associated only with septal hypertrophy, the septal segment pushing the tip down is resected. The resection is triangular, where the base of the resection must be in the dorsal septum (Fig. 11.3).

11.2.1.2 Case 1

The preoperative photograph shows an under-rotated nasal tip. The downward direction on the tip caused by the caudal septum is evident. The long lateral crura also contributes to the nasal tip's low positioning.

The initial step in achieving the ideal nasal tip rotation involves a conservative resection in the anterior septal angle area, considering tipples as the subsequent stage to complete perfect rotation (Fig. 11.4; Video 11.1).

Technical Pearl: Resection must proceed in a stepwise manner and an excessive amount of cartilage must not be resected at once.

11.2.1.3 Deficiency of the Posterior or Septal Angle or Nasal Spine

In the case of deficiency of the posterior septal angle or nasal spine, the tip drops down due to an absence of base support. These cases show all signs of caudal septal deficiency, such as columellar retraction, an acute nasolabial angle, long upper lip, under-projected tip, etc. This is especially common in patients with previous septal surgery (Fig. 11.5).

Droopy nasal tip, associated with deficiency of the posterior septal angle or nasal spine, generally develops after radical septal surgery. The primary surgeon may either over-resect the caudal septum or cause the deformity in some other way.

While the first step in treatment is reconstruction of the caudal septum on which the tip sits, the second step is reconstructing the alar cartilages. If the columellar-labial angle (subnasal)

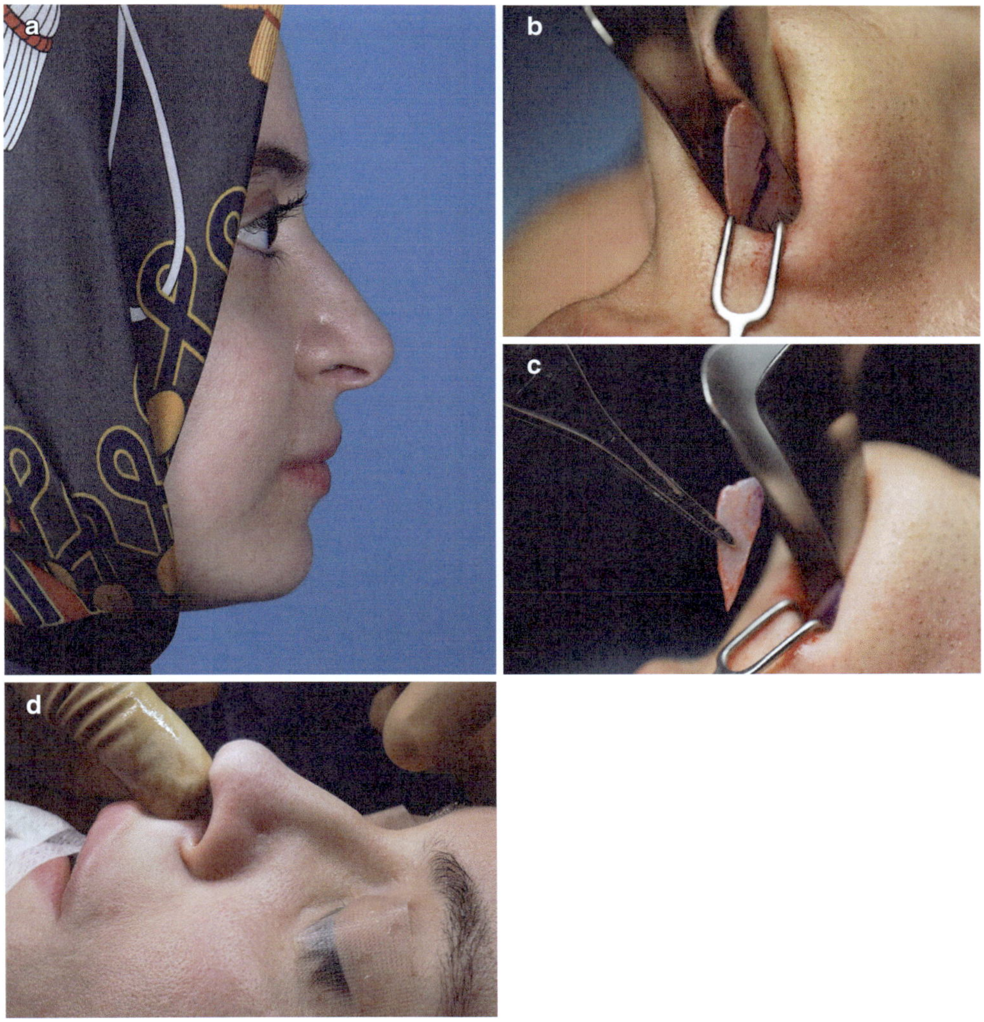

Fig. 11.4 (**a**) Mild degree drop nasal tip. (**b**, **c**) "V"shaped caudal septal resection. (**d**) Manual palpation can guide deciding what cartilage to remove. (**e**) Shows the effect of resection; note the difference between the photos before and after performing caudal resection about rotation. (**f**) Postoperative image. The ideally rotated nasal tip was attained through the implementation of the tip cost technique combined with caudal resection

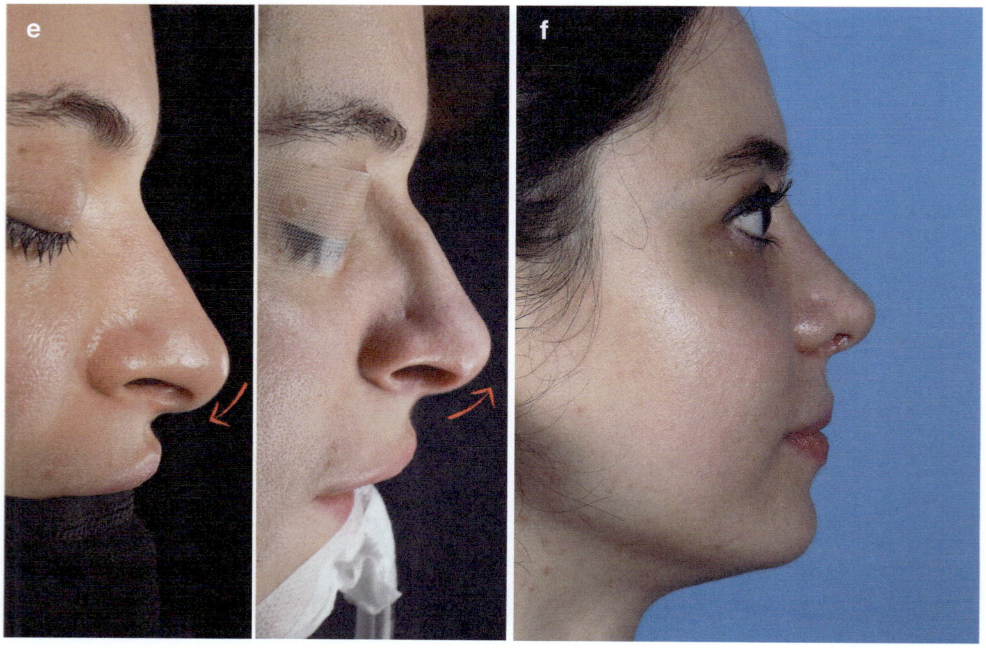

Fig. 11.4 (continued)

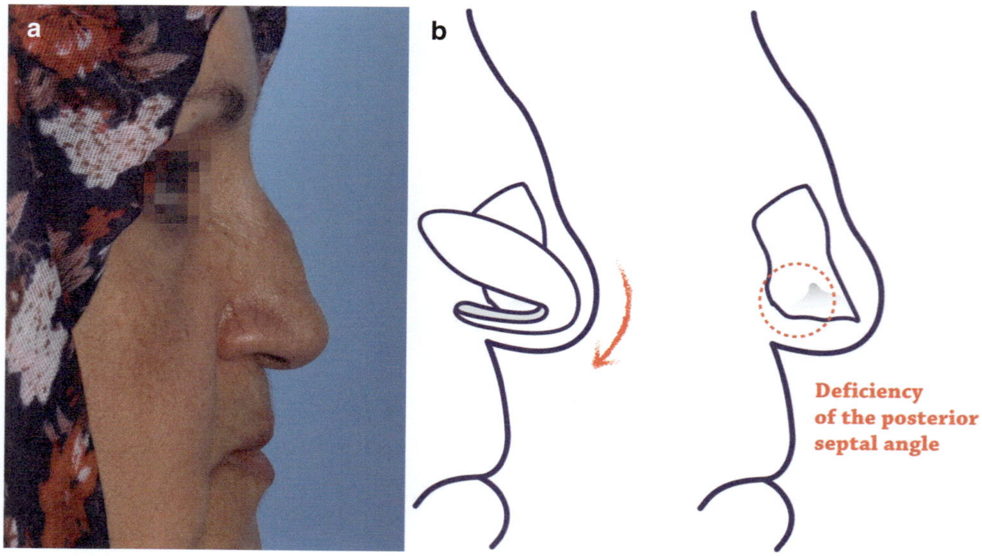

Fig. 11.5 (**a**, **b**) Droopy nasal tip due to deficiency of the caudal septum

is still deficient, a third step involving the use of a columellar plumping graft or pre-maxillary graft may be applied.

In such cases, a strong dorsal segment must first be constructed to achieve a strong caudal septum. While a spreader graft is used to reinforce the dorsal segment, a septal replacement graft or septal batten graft can be used for reconstruction of the caudal segment. If the dorsal segment of the septum is already sufficiently strong, the surgeon can directly reinforce the caudal segment.

In cases where there is an insufficient amount of dorsal septal remnant, the dorsal segment is first reconstructed with bilateral spreader grafts, and the septal replacement graft is then caudally fixed in between these two spreader grafts (Fig. 11.6).

In cases where there is a sufficient amount of, but a curved and deformed, dorsal segment, it is first reconstructed with a spreader graft; then, a caudal septal replacement graft or septal batten graft is used to reconstruct the caudal aspect of the septum (Fig. 11.7).

In cases where there is a sufficient amount of septum, but its caudal aspect is deformed, a septal replacement graft can be used alone for reconstruction (Fig. 11.8).

Columellar plumping and pre-maxillary grafts are useful in droopy nasal tip treatment by compensating for the inadequate nasolabial angle.

- Plumping grafts consist of crushed cartilage derived from the septum, auricle, costa, etc., and are inserted into a pocket opened between the footplate and the nasal spine (Fig. 11.9).
- ≥Pre-maxillary grafts are typically placed along the caudal edge of the apertura piriformis and correct retraction at the pre-maxilla. Although some surgeons prefer to use alloplastic graft material, any cartilage remaining unused at the end of the surgery can be employed as graft material (Fig. 11.10; Video 11.2).

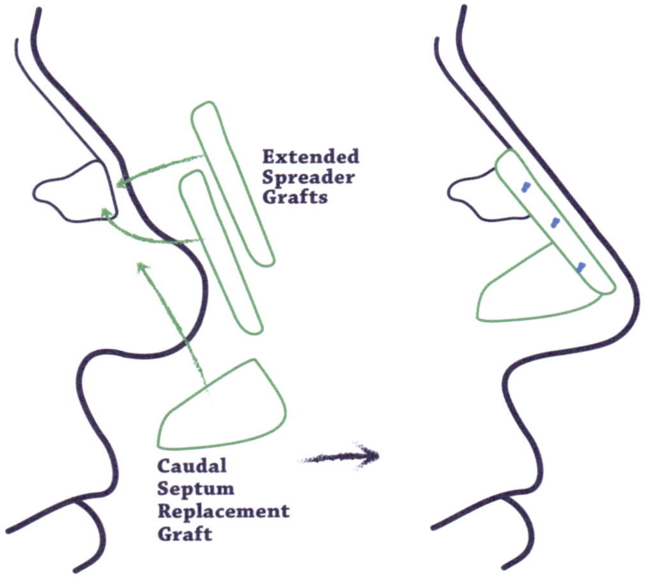

Fig. 11.6 Caudal and dorsal septal deficiency. Bilateral extended spreader grafts and caudal replacement graft can reconstruct the entire septum together

11.2.1.4 Case 2

Figure 11.11 shows a droopy nasal tip patient who underwent septal surgery 10 years ago. *This case shows all signs of caudal septal deficiency.*

Intraoperative photos showed severe nasal axis deviation at the dorsal septum. In addition, the caudal septum is deformed due to this deviation and the previous surgery, and therefore does not provide adequate support to the alar cartilage (Fig. 11.12).

First, the dorsal septum was reconstructed. A spreader graft was fixed to the concave plane; the graft was placed at the starting point of the concavity and extended through the anterior septal angle (Fig. 11.13).

Second, a septal batten graft was placed between the underside of the spreader and the nasal spine, and then sutured to the septum using nonabsorbable sutures to strengthen the caudal septum (Fig. 11.14).

After reconstruction to achieve a strong septal frame, the pre-maxillary graft was inserted freely within the

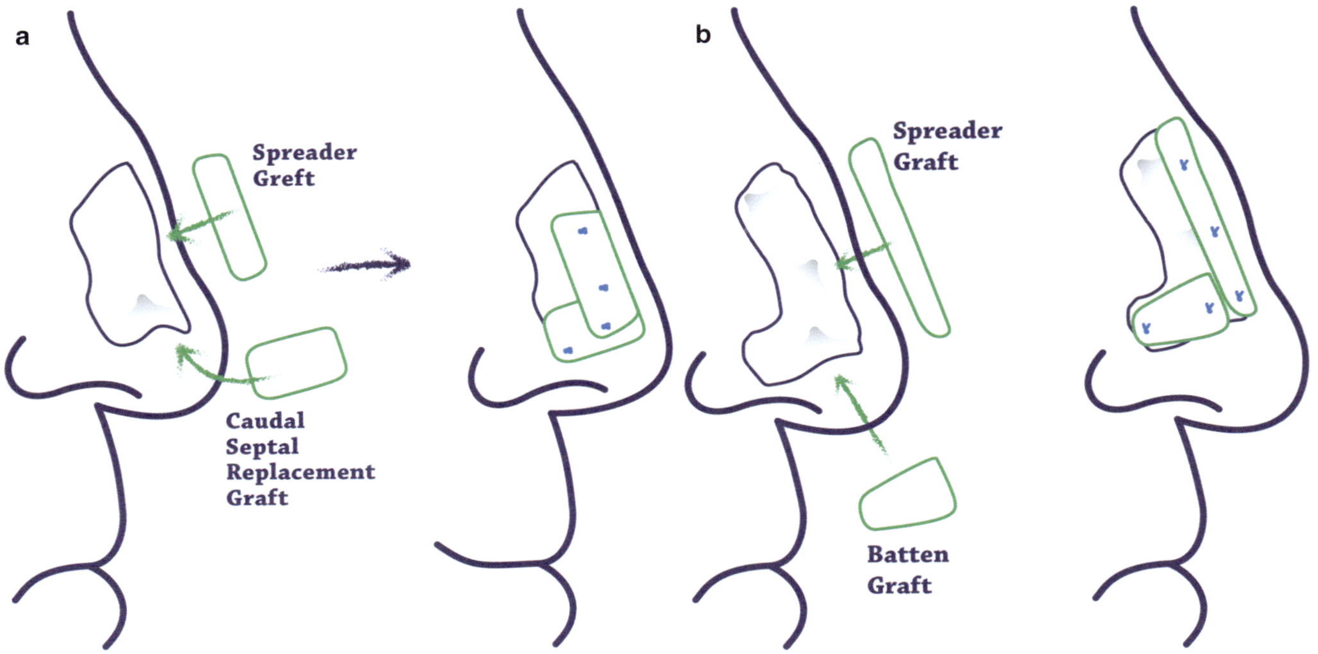

Fig. 11.7 (**a**) Caudal septal deficiency with deformed dorsal septum. Unilateral extended spreader grafts and caudal replacement graft can reconstruct the caudal septum together. (**b**) Deformed caudal and dorsal septum together. Spreader graft and septal batten graft can strengthen the entire septum

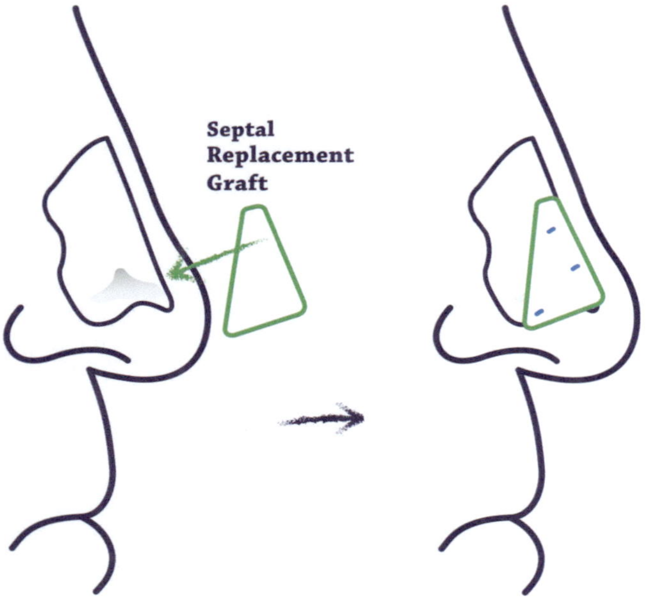

Fig. 11.8 There is a sufficient amount of septum but the caudal part is deformed and weak. Septal replacement graft can strengthen the entire septum alone

pocket, then opened from under and next to the columella to compensate for the pre-maxillary deficiency and improve tip rotation by increasing the columellar-labial angle.

The final step involved correction of the alar configuration. Sutures, a columellar strut, and a cap graft were used to reshape the tip (Fig. 11.15).

Preoperative and postoperative photographs of this case are seen in Fig. 11.16. The tip has been rotated and is well projected. More columellar shows.

Another case of droopy nasal tip due to the deficiency of the posterior septal angle is shown next.

11.2.1.5 Case 3

A 63-year-old patient with a history of septal surgery complained of nasal obstruction and droopy nasal tip. His under-rotated tip stems from a deficiency of caudal septum. The caudal septum was reconstructed. The nose is shorter with the correction of an under-rotated tip (Fig. 11.17).

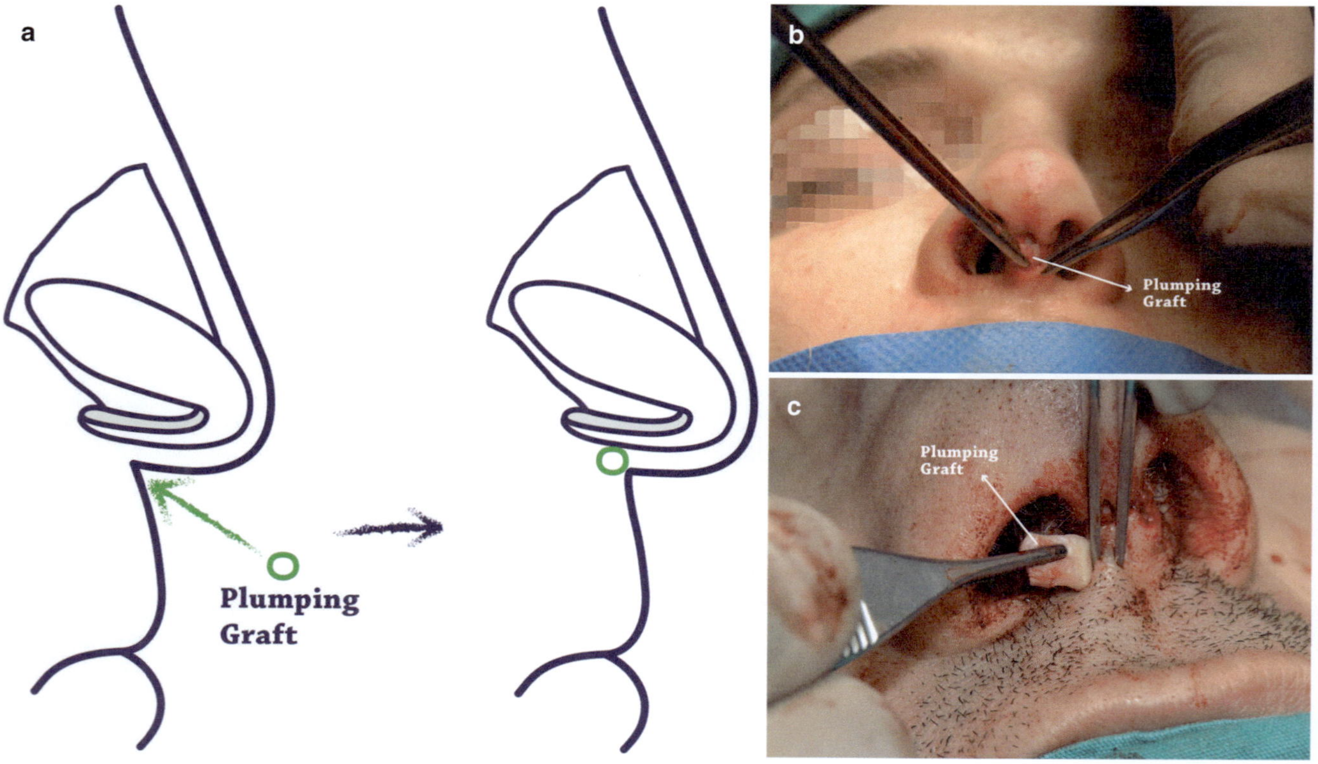

Fig. 11.9 (**a–c**) The graft can either be placed in front of the nasal spine between the two medial crura or within a separate incision made next to the nasal spine

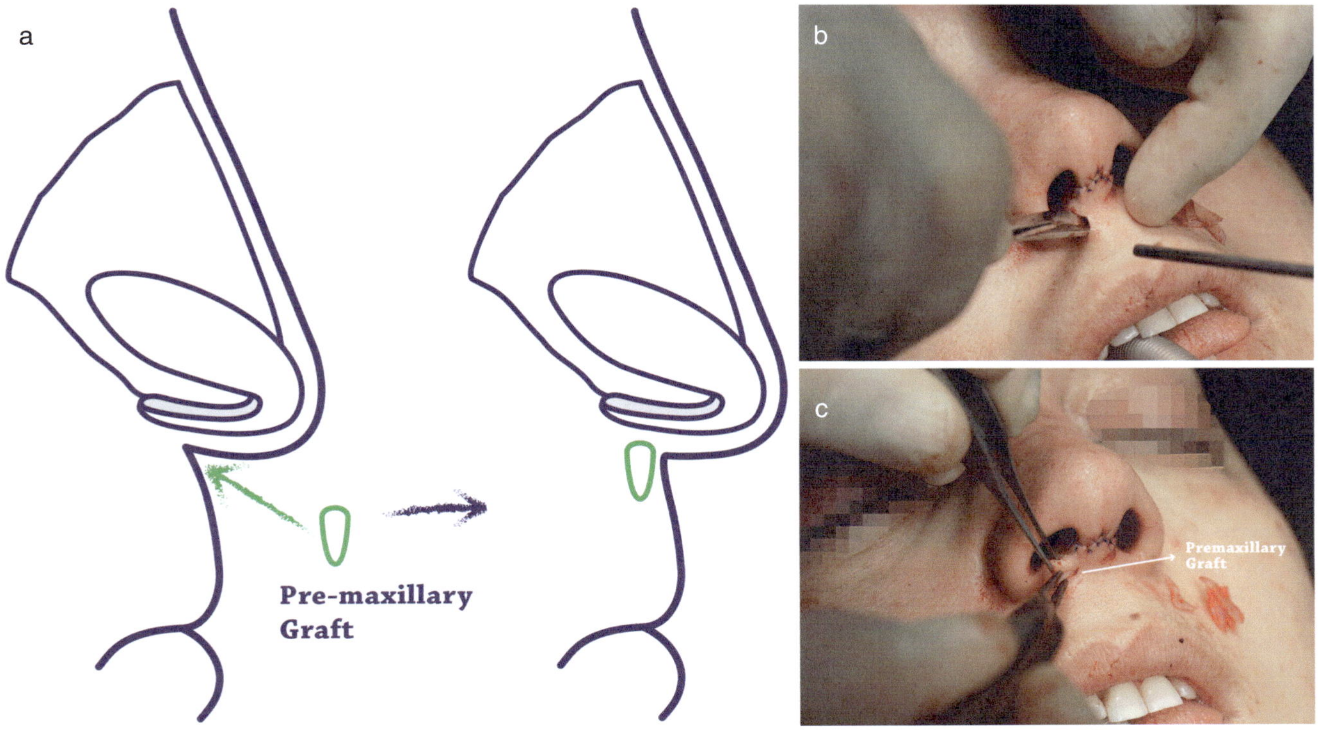

Fig. 11.10 (**a–c**) A pre-maxillary graft is inserted into a small incision made immediately in front of the nostril

Fig. 11.11 Right illustration shows typical findings of the droopy nasal tip due to deficiency of caudal septum

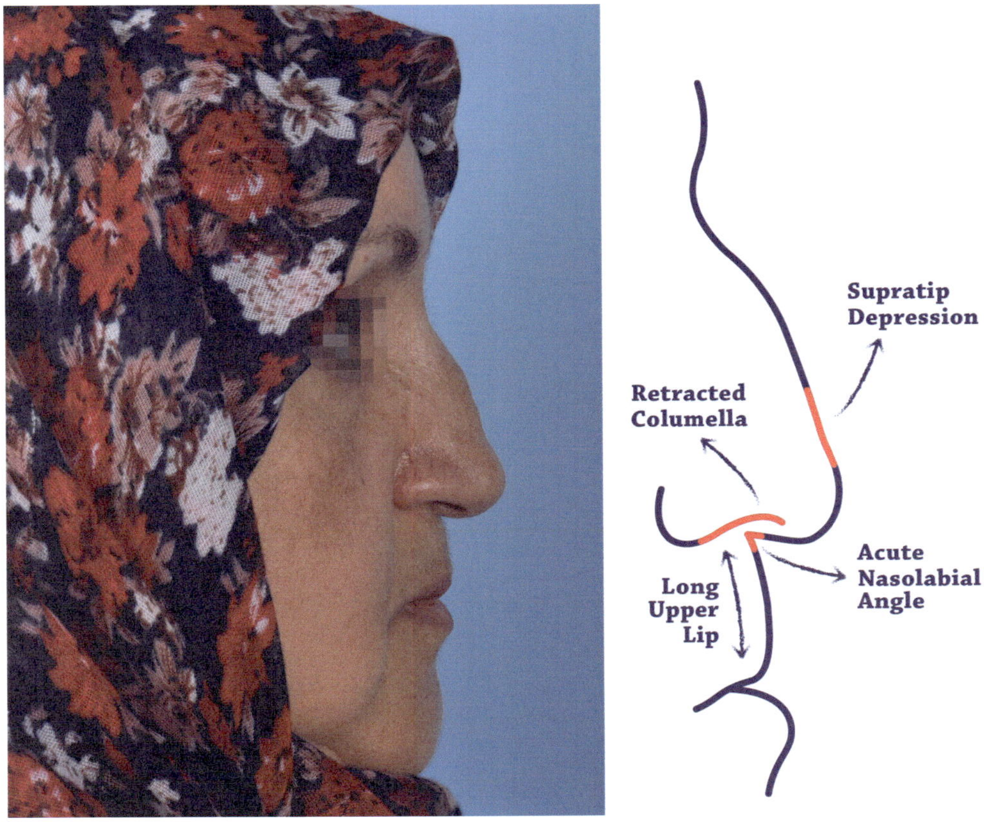

11.2.2 Droopy Nasal Tip Associated with Intrinsic Factors

Anatomical problems of the alar cartilages are among the main underlying causes of a droopy nasal tip (Fig. 11.18).

- Long lateral crura is the leading cause.
- Malposition of the lateral crura, which represents another alar cartilage abnormality, also results in a droopy nasal tip.

Any of the above problems associated with the lateral crus may be the underlying cause of a droopy nasal tip, and each is treated differently.

11.2.2.1 Treatment of Droopy Nasal Tip Associated with Long Lateral Crura

There are three main stages in the correction of a droopy nasal tip and reconstruction of a "delicate tip."

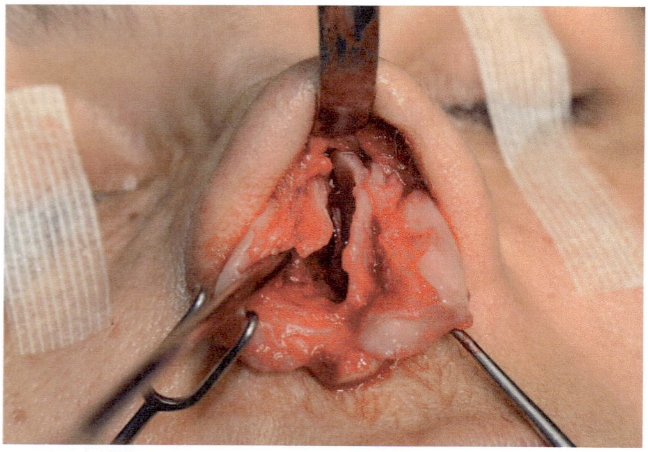

Fig. 11.12 Deformed caudal and dorsal septum

- **In the first stage, the lateral crus is shortened, deformities of the alar arch are corrected, and a new alar cartilage anatomy is created. The rotation is corrected during this stage. Three different techniques can be used for this purpose.**
  - Lateral crural steal suture: the lateral crus is shortened by 3–6 mm with this technique.
  - Concomitant overlap steal tip-plasty (COST): The lateral crus is shortened by 6–10 mm with this technique.
  - Vertical alar resection (VAR): the lateral crus is shortened by ≥10 mm with this technique.

The technique selected depends on how much shortening of the lateral crus is desired.

- **In the second stage, strong tip support is provided by construction of a satisfactory alar arch. Columellar strut placement and dome equalizing suture are essential during this stage.**

A columellar strut must be used during droopy tip surgery for the following reasons:

1. Stability: stabilizes the newly constructed alar arch.
2. Symmetry: symmetrically connects the two alar arches at the midline.
3. Preservation: preserves the projection gained via use of the steal suture.

"Dome-equalising suture" is used after placement of the columellar strut. This suture crosses the cranial edges of the new dome and connects the edges at the midline. Nonabsorbable polypropylene sutures are preferable.

The dome-equalizing suture serves the following three purposes:

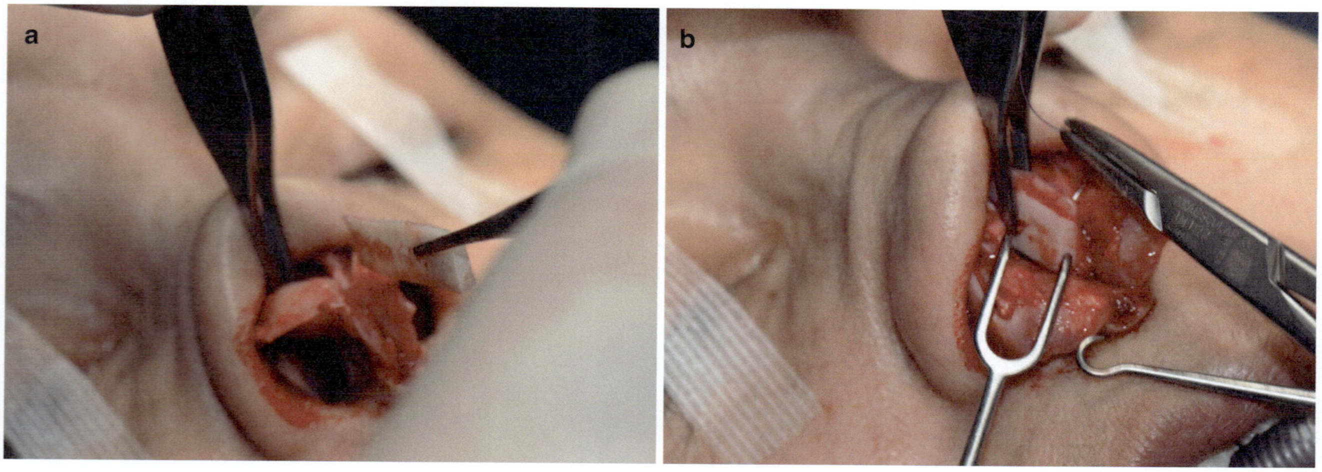

Fig. 11.13 (**a**, **b**) Unilateral costal cartilage spreader graft

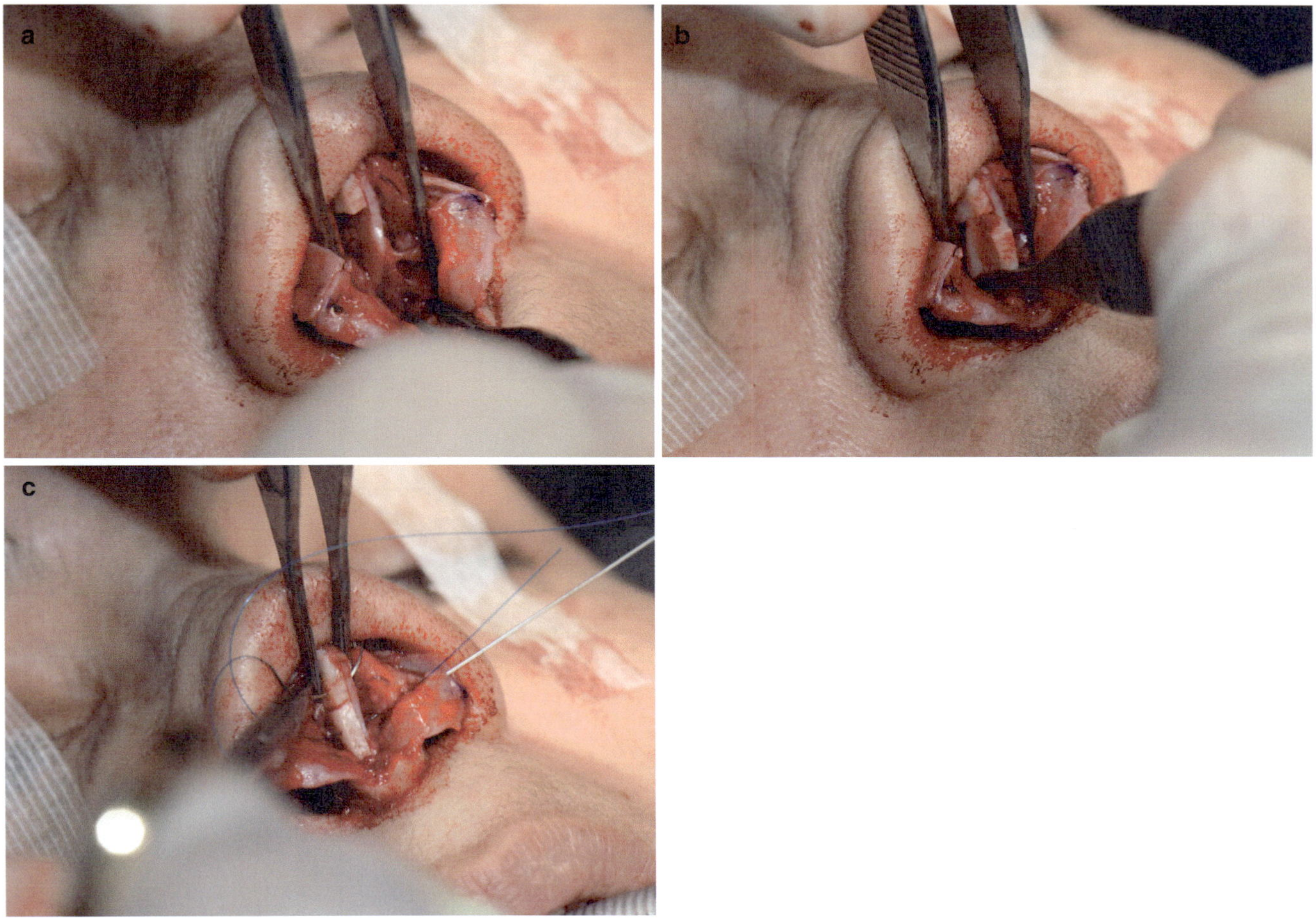

Fig. 11.14 (**a–c**) Placement of costal batten graft

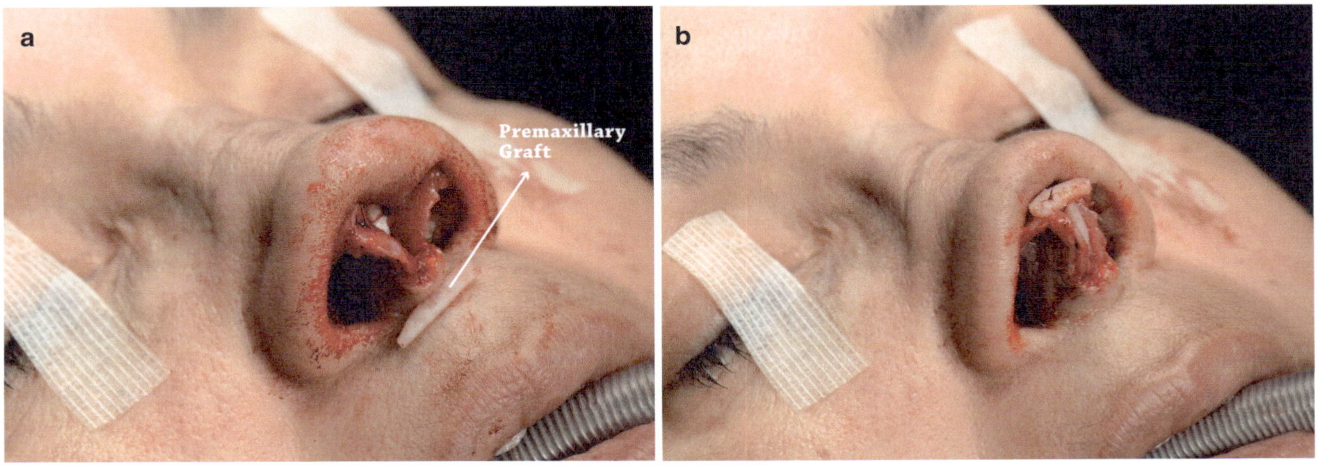

Fig. 11.15 (**a**) The premaxillary graft was used to contribute to tip projection and rotation. The graft of costal cartilage was inserted in a surgical pocket created at the base of the columella. (**b**) Bilateral transdomal suture, columellar strut, costal cap graft

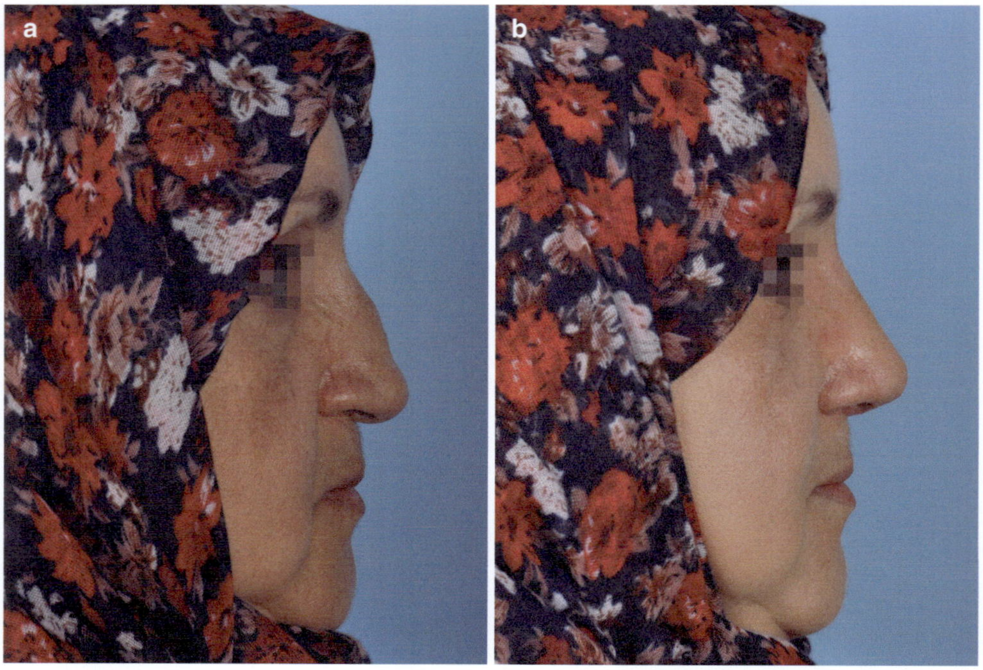

Fig. 11.16 (**a**, **b**) Results of the surgery described above. The drooping tip has been improved significantly, following mainly caudal septal reconstruction. The maxilla was filled with premaxillary graft and a prominent subnasale is achieved

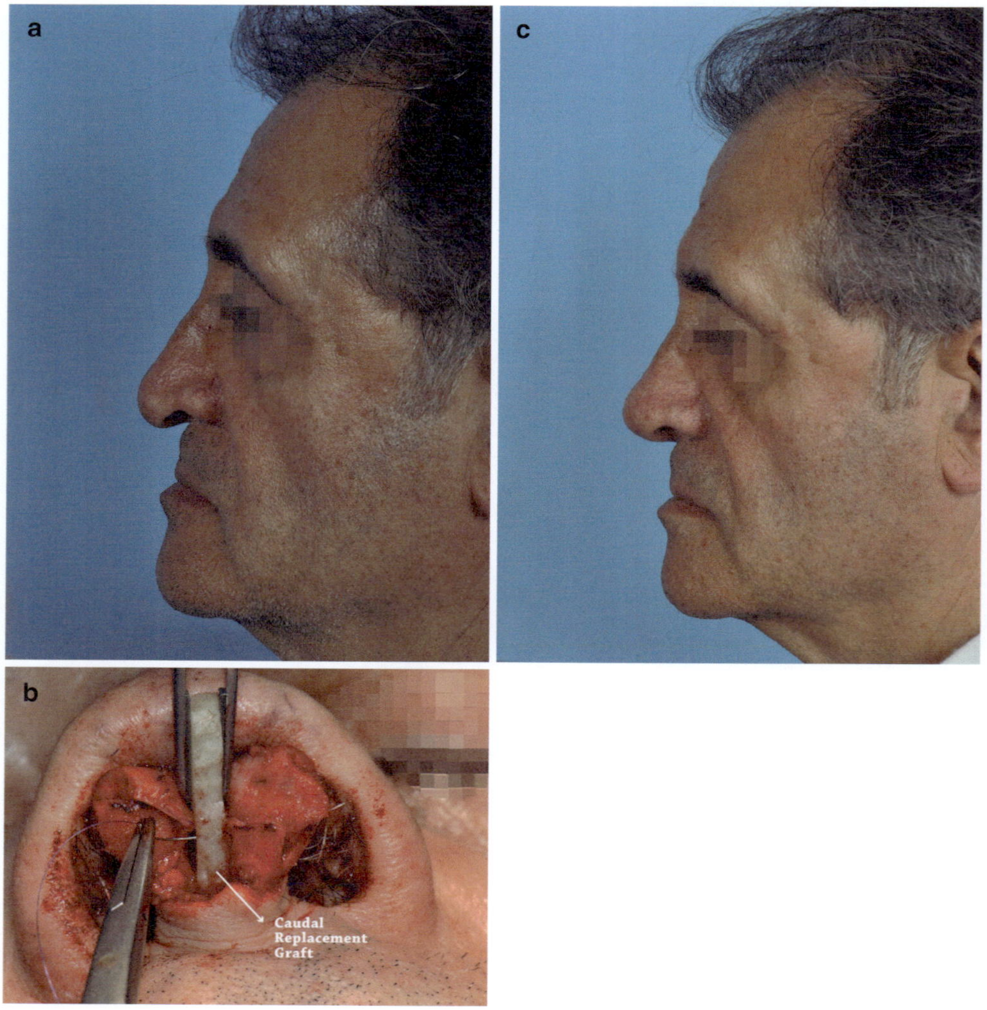

Fig. 11.17 (**a**) A preoperative photograph. (**b**) A caudal replacement graft and a unilateral spreader graft were used for caudal septal reconstruction. (**c**) A postoperative photograph

1. It eliminates any differences in level between the two domes and renders them symmetrical.
2. It elevates the cranial edge of the lateral crus and thus further stabilizes the ideal plane achieved using the transdomal suture.
3. It corrects any discrepancy in angulation between the two dome points.

Establishing an ideal angle between the domes (90°) allows the skin to rest on a wide plane, which in turn is advantageous for long-term tip stability (Fig. 11.19; Video 11.3).

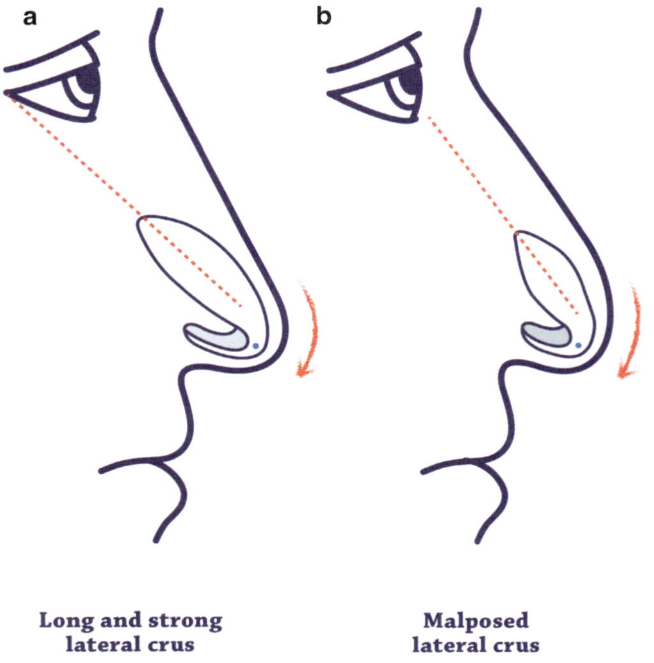

Fig. 11.18 (**a**) The long lateral crus pushes the tip down. (**b**) Although normal in length, the lateral crus pushes the tip down because it is directed toward the medial canthus

In patients with structurally weak alar cartilage or thick skin, if the use of columellar strut and dome equalizer suture is not considered sufficient for tip stabilization, the other alternative is the medial-middle crural strut. This graft can give more support than the columellar strut. If you feel this technique is insufficient for support, the reshaped alar arch must be fixed to the septum. A tip supported by a stable septum maintains its stability in the long term. A septocolumellar strut or septocolumellar suture can be used; the objective is not to gain additional projection and rotation, but rather to maintain the stability of the new structure (Figs. 11.20a, b and 11.21a, b; Videos 11.4 and 11.5).

- **In the third and final stage, the objective is to improve tip definition to achieve a natural and attractive tip appearance. Surgery is terminated when the definition of the newly constructed alar cartilage is satisfactory. Otherwise, an onlay tip graft can be used. A cap graft gives rise to a light reflection at the nasal tip.**

The following must be considered carefully when using a cap graft:

- The width of the cap graft should correspond to the distance between the final dome points and should be at the upper limit in thick-skinned patients, but not in excess of 10 mm.
- Especially in thin-skinned patients, cap grafts should always be camouflaged. For thick-skinned patients camouflaging may not be necessary.
- Cap grafts should be placed securely immediately over the dome created with sutures and should not shift toward the caudal or cranial aspect.

An onlay lateral crural graft can be used to accentuate the light reflection along the alar rim (Fig. 11.22).

Fig. 11.19 The dome-equalizing suture

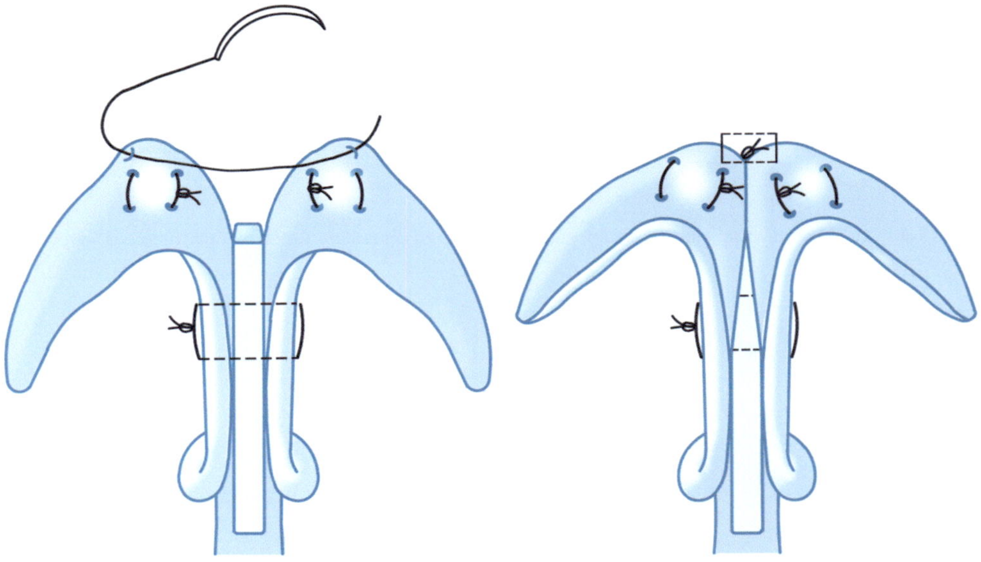

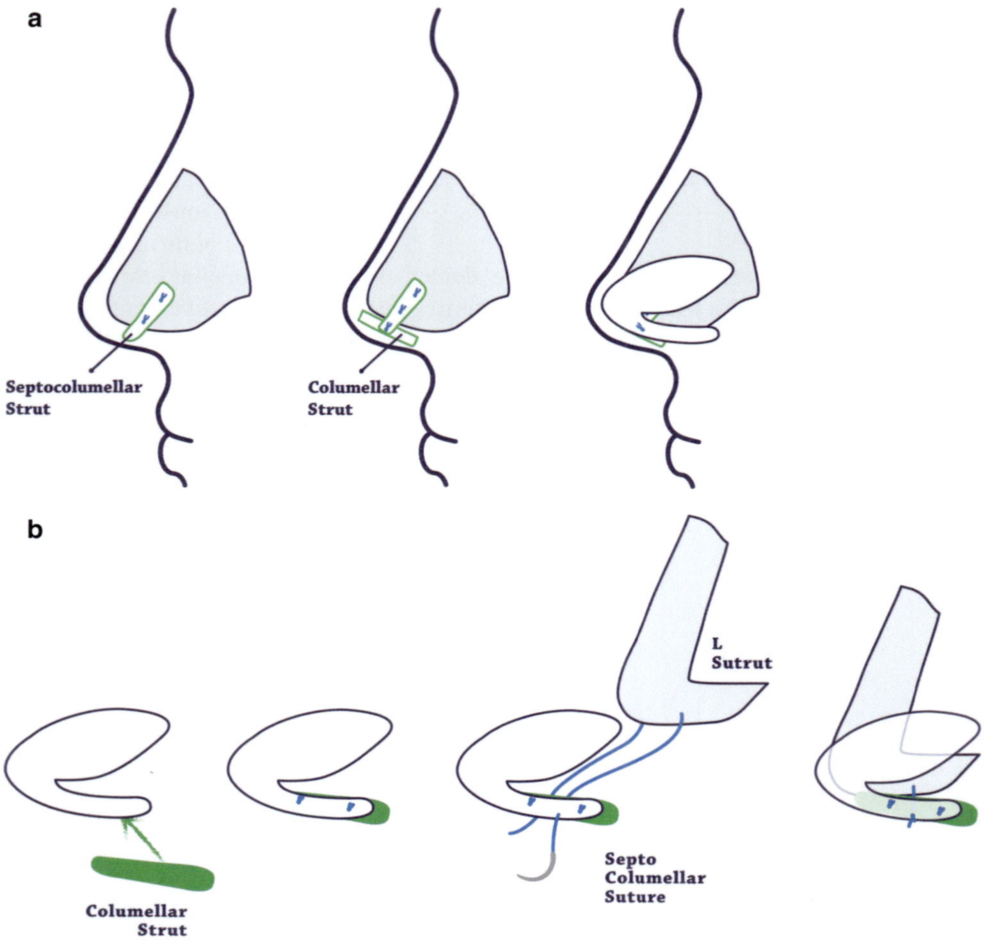

Fig. 11.20 (**a**) The septum and columella are connected via placement of a permanent suture or by using a piece of cartilage, the latter of which creates a stronger connection. (**b**) The septum and columella are connected via placement of a permanent suture or by using a piece of cartilage, the latter of which creates a stronger connection

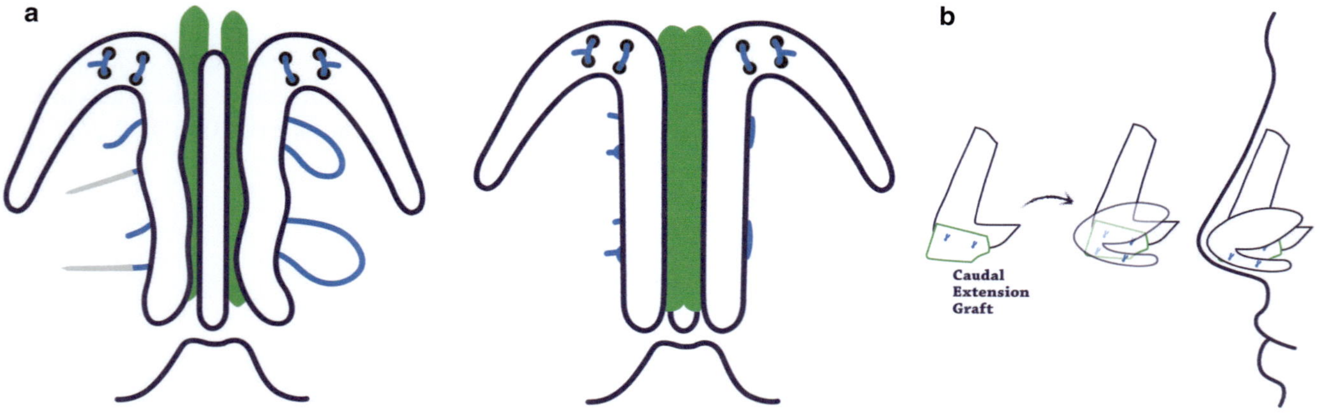

Fig.11.21 (**a**) Medial/Middle crural struts; each strut secured separately to the alar cartilage. (**b**) Septal extension graft

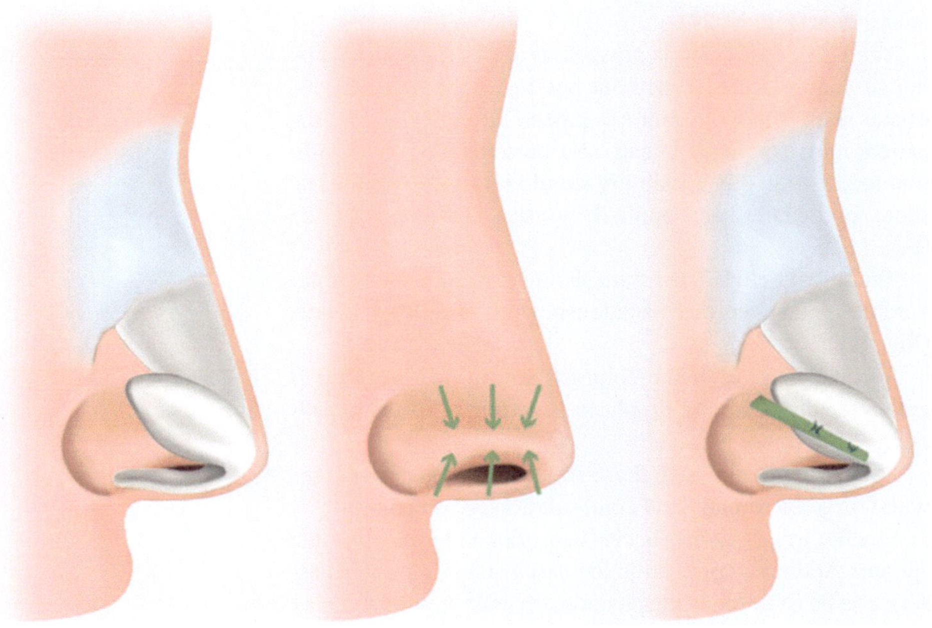

Fig. 11.22 (**a–c**) A lateral crural graft should start in the lateral part of the new dome and extend to the apertura piriformis along the alar rim. The graft is sutured to the crus at a number of locations to firmly secure it in place. The preferred suture material is 6–0 polydioxanone suture. Insertion of the graft into the pocket opened at the side of the graft would provide additional stability

11.3 Example Cases

Each technique introduced above will now be considered in detail via a number of example cases.

11.3.1 Correction of Tip Rotation with a Lateral Crural Steal Suture

The steal suture is essentially a transdomal mattress suture. The term "steal suture," in literal terms, refers to the "stealing" of an excess portion of the lateral crus and transferring it to the medial crus. A new dome point is created on the lateral crus using a transdomal mattress suture. While the lateral crus is shortened, the middle crus is elongated. This shortened lateral crus increases the tip rotation.

A schematic diagram (profile view) of nasal tip alteration following application of the lateral crural steal technique is seen in Fig. 11.23 and Video 11.7.

The lateral crural steal suture not only increases rotation, but also results in a more favorable shape of the lateral crus, with better dome definition and increased projection. Lateral crural steal suture is an efficient method for treating droopy nasal tip in patients with a long lateral crus and short middle crus, i.e., for patients with a droopy and under-projected nasal tip.

11.3.2 Technique of Lateral Crural Steal Suture

First, cephalic trimming of the alar cartilage is performed. Now the question is, how much should be trimmed? It varies from patient to patient. It is not a question of how much we remove but how much remains. The width of the remaining part should be 6–8 mm.

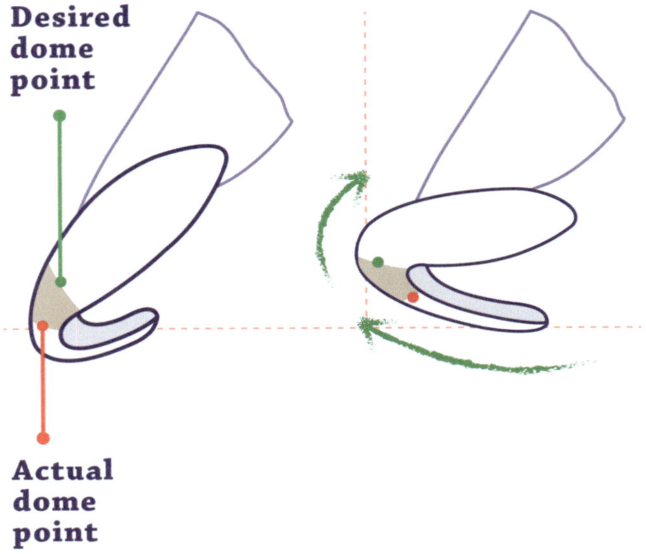

Fig. 11.23 How a suture can be used to provide rotation. Increasing the length of the medial crura by shortening the length of the lateral crura results in increased tip rotation. The dome is advanced laterally onto the lateral crus

Steal suture can be applied in both the open and closed approaches; the order of the seps and the logic underpinning the technique remain the same. Here, we will begin by discussing use of the steal suture in the open approach.

The actual dome point is marked. Then, the desired dome point is marked on the lateral crus. The distance between the two marked points is the segment to be "stolen" from the lateral crus (Fig. 11.24).

The new dome point is grasped with forceps and a transdomal suture is placed without passing it through the vestibular skin. When the suture is passed through the skin, the patient may experience a bad odor postoperatively; in addition to crusting, this possibility should be kept in mind. The same procedures are applied on the contralateral side (Fig. 11.25).

Technical Pearl: The suture should also correct any unfavorable caudal–cranial relationship of the lateral crus (Fig. 11.26).

Second, fixation of the columellar strut following bilateral symmetrical suture tip plasty is performed. Also, equalizing dome suture is used.

After completion of all these stages, stable alar cartilages with corrected rotation and configuration are obtained.

Finally, tip projection is checked prior to terminating the surgery. Additional projection increases of 1–2 mm, if necessary, can be achieved using an onlay tip graft. Use of an onlay graft also has the advantage of improving tip definition.

Technical Pearl: When the alar cartilage configuration is corrected, the tip is moved backward; however, the upper lat-

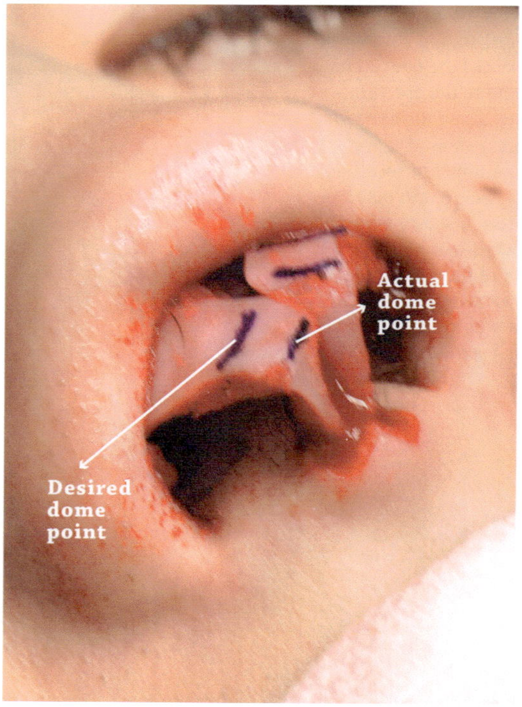

Fig. 11.24 Location of new dome creation

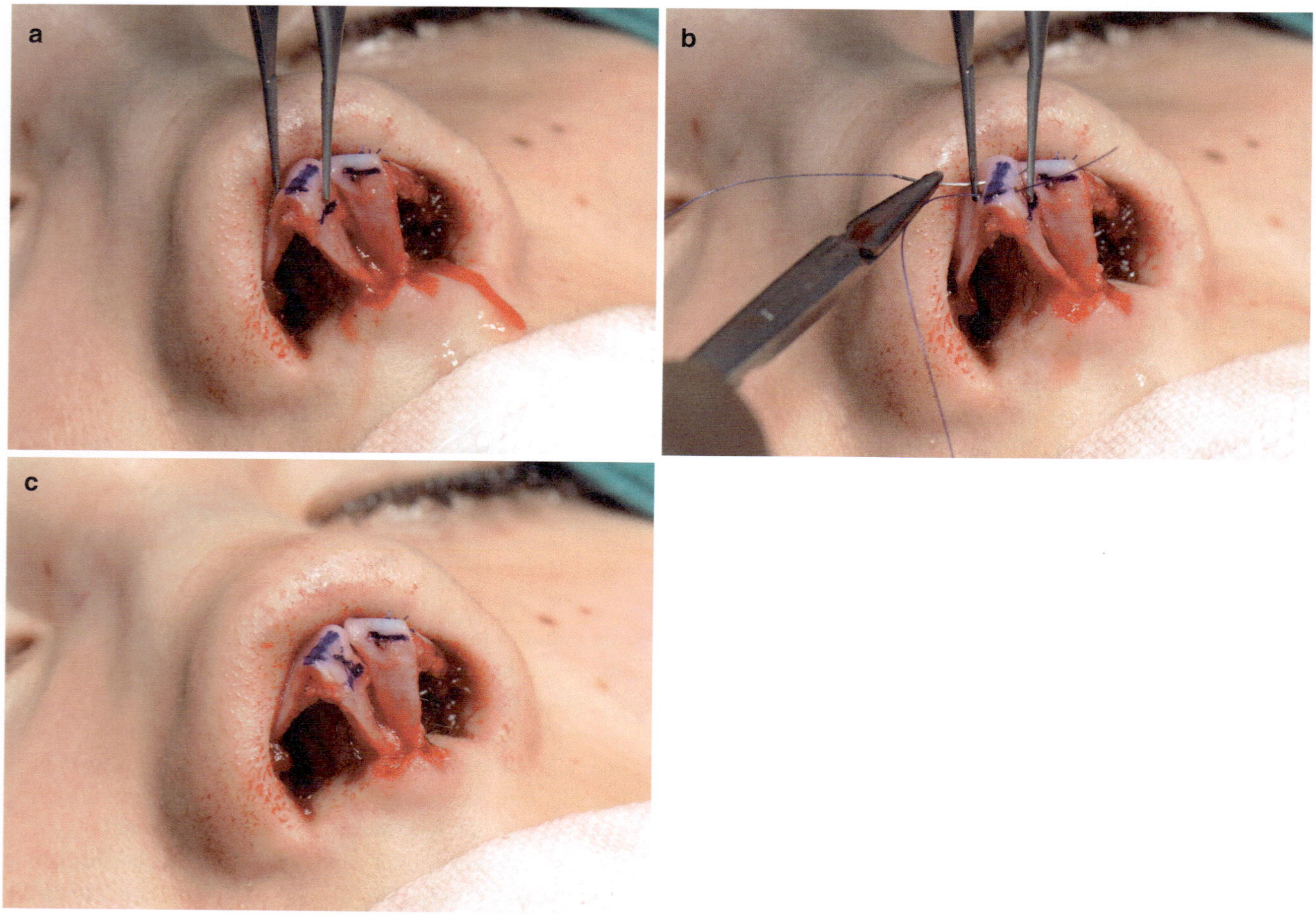

Fig. 11.25 (a–c) Nonabsorbable suture materials causing minimal tissue reaction, such as 5–0 polypropylene sutures, are preferable. Absorbable sutures may degrade even before the end of the surgery

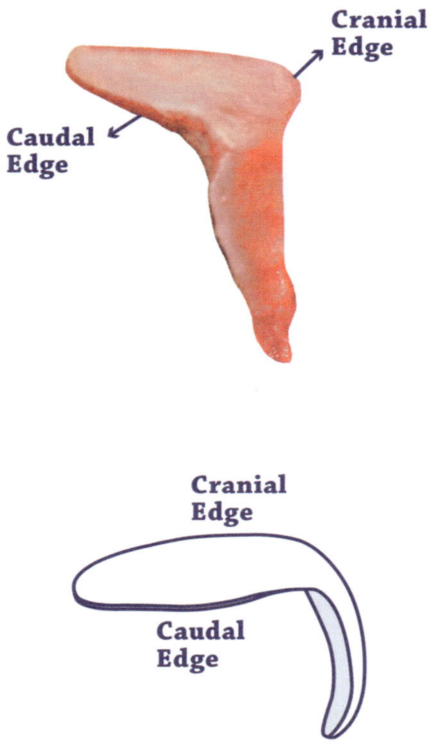

Fig. 11.26 The caudal and cranial edges of the ideal lateral crus are in the same plane

eral cartilage may prevent the tip from moving back. If this happens, the excess segment of the upper lateral cartilage must be resected, otherwise the excess segment may push the tip forward and later manifest as bulging at the lateral nasal wall during the recovery period (Fig. 11.27).

In conclusion, steal suture is an efficient technique for use in droopy nasal tip cases that also require projection gain.

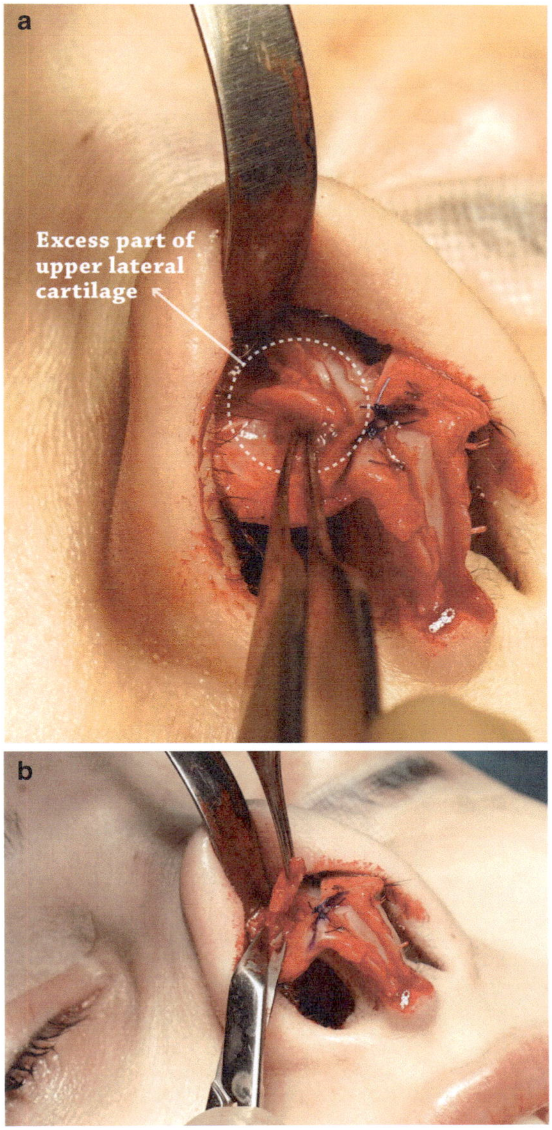

Fig. 11.27 (**a**, **b**) The excess segment of the upper lateral cartilage prevents setback of the lateral crus caudally. The excess segment is resected with scissors

11.3.3 Clinical Outcomes: Droopy Nasal Tip Corrected with the Steal Suture Technique

This section presents cases of droopy nasal tip corrected with the steal suture technique.

11.3.3.1 Case 4

Three main problems were identified in the lateral view of the first case: a droopy nasal tip, under-projection, and a short infratip lobule (Fig. 11.28).

The intraoperative lateral view showed the alar cartilage anatomy. While the long lateral crus positioned the tip down, the short middle crus was responsible for both under-projection and the short infratip lobule (Fig. 11.29).

Attention must be paid to the extent of shortening of the lateral crus and elongation of the middle crus. The alar arch, which was reconfigured using the steal suture technique, was stabilized by the columellar strut (Fig. 11.30).

Preoperative and 1-year postoperative photographs show correction of the droopy nasal tip and increased projection. The front view shows improved tip definition via the steal suture. All of the advantages of the steal suture technique were apparent in this case (Fig. 11.31).

11.3.3.2 Case 5

This is another droopy nasal tip case expected to respond to the steal suture technique. The lateral view photograph highlights the droopy nasal tip, under-projection, and short infratip lobule (Fig. 11.32).

The alar cartilage anatomy indicates that the long lateral crus and short middle crus were the underlying causes of the problems outlined above (Fig. 11.33).

Tip configuration was corrected with the suture, stealing from the lateral crus and elongating the middle crus. The suture also corrected the configuration of the lateral crus. While the caudal aspect of the lateral crus was below the cranial aspect before placing the suture, they were in the same plane after suture placement (Fig. 11.34; Video 11.8).

Preoperative and 2-year postoperative photographs show increased rotation and projection of the tip via suturing, and elongation of the short infratip lobule (Fig. 11.35).

11.3.3.3 Case 6

In this patient, the droopy nasal tip was accompanied by a short infratip lobule with resulting under-projection (Fig. 11.36; Video 11.9).

Attention should be paid to the intraoperative alar arch configuration before and after placing the suture. The steal suture shortened the lateral crus and elongated the middle crus, leading to tip rotation and projection. Additional stability was achieved in this thick-skinned patient using a septocolumellar suture. Lateral crural grafts were placed bilaterally to achieve light reflection from the oblique angle (Fig. 11.37).

In the 3-year postoperative period, tip rotation was corrected. There was elegant light reflection over the lateral crura and the alar rim was pronounced at an oblique angle (Fig. 11.38).

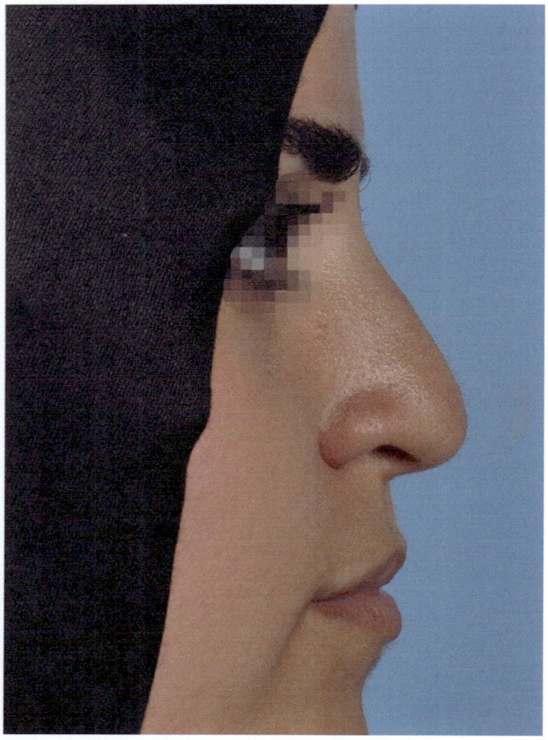

Fig. 11.28 Preoperative photograph

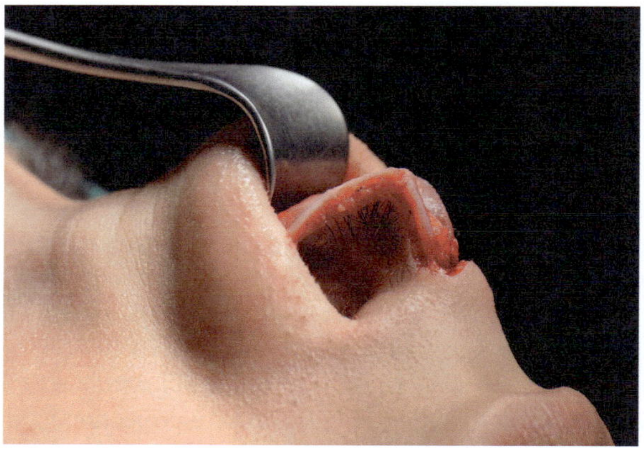

Fig. 11.29 Steal suture was an ideal solution in this case

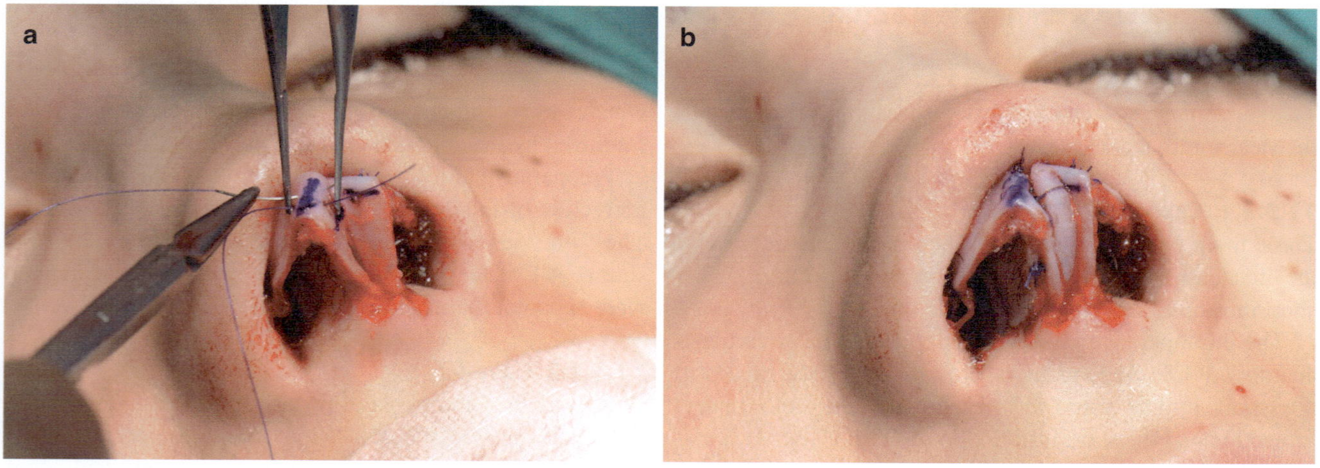

Fig. 11.30 (**a**, **b**) Bilateral crural steal suture has been applied and then columellar strut was fixed to stabilize the base of the tip

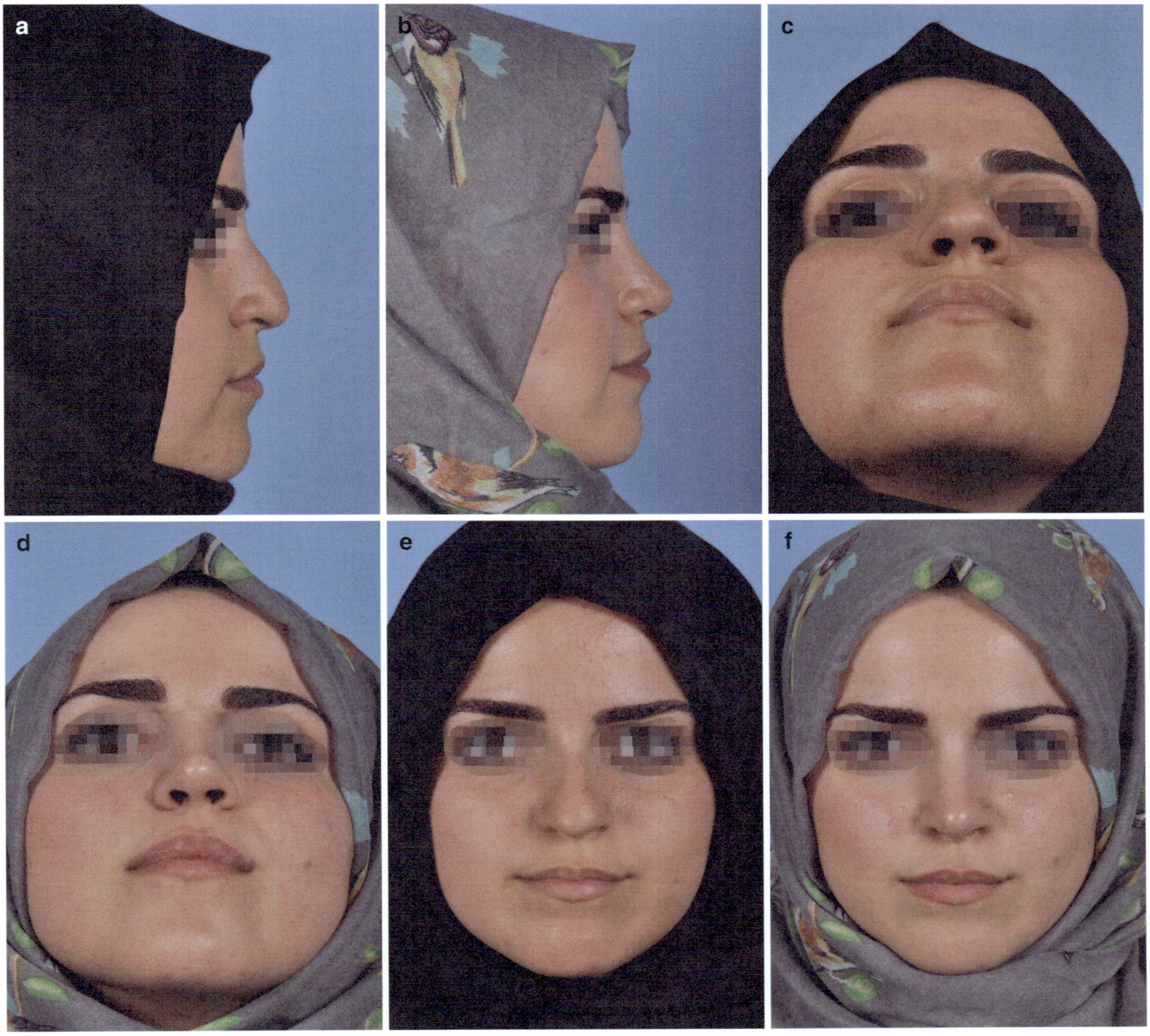

Fig. 11.31 (a–f) The preoperative and 12-month postoperative frontal, lateral, and basal views. Tip rotation, projection, and definition are improved

Technical Pearl: If shortening of the lateral crus by 3–6 mm is sufficient to correct a droopy nasal tip, the steal suture can be used alone.

When lateral crural steal suture is performed with appropriate indications, the nasal tip will not deteriorate, and will instead retain its anatomical integrity over the long term. Let us look at an example in Case 7.

11.3.3.4 Case 7

This young woman desired aesthetic improvement of her nose. The tip was under-rotated with long lateral crura and short medial crura. Steal suture was used to correct this problem (Fig. 11.39).

11.3.4 Droopy Nasal Tip Treatment with the COST Technique

The COST technique aims to add a medial crural division and overlap to the lateral crural steal suture. The steal suture serves to shorten the lateral crus. The segment that is stolen from the lateral crus and moved to the middle crus may disturb the configuration of the alar arch. This becomes more likely as the segment becomes longer. A segment 6–10 mm in length may impair the configuration of the middle crus, in which case the columellar strut would not suffice to correct the impaired configuration. Thus, the tension and distortion in the middle/medial crural complex must be relieved; this is

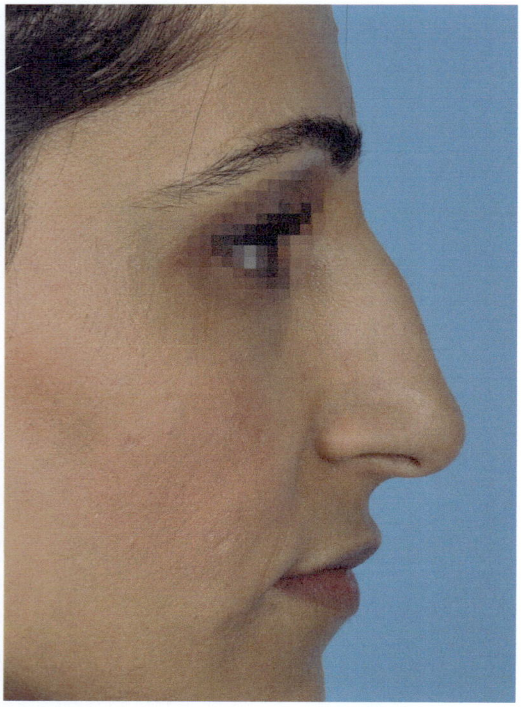

Fig. 11.32 Preoperative photograph

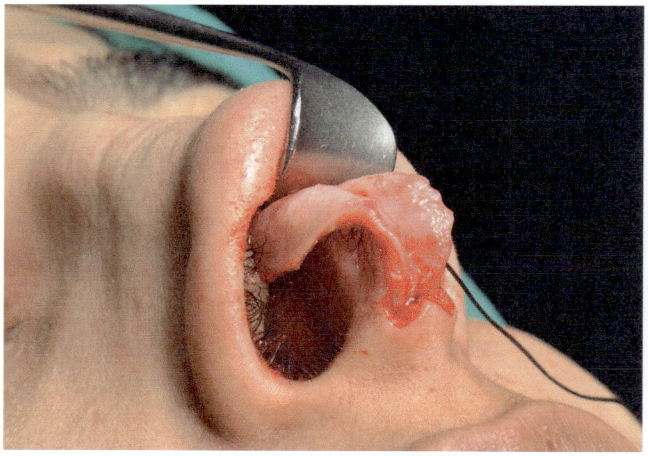

Fig. 11.33 Long lateral crura with unfavorable caudal–cranial relationship

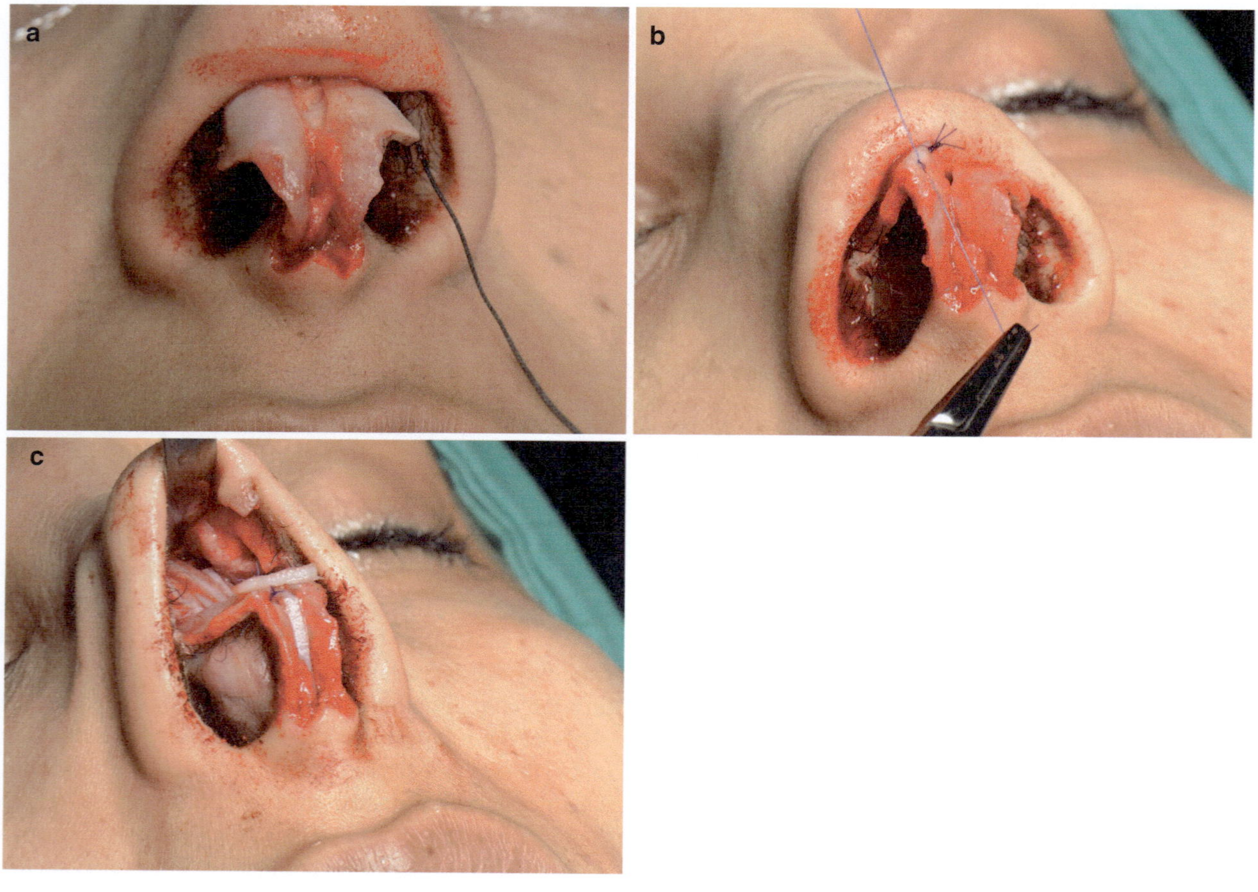

Fig. 11.34 (a–c) Placement of the columellar strut using the steal suture technique represents standard practice. A cap graft is additionally used to gain more projection

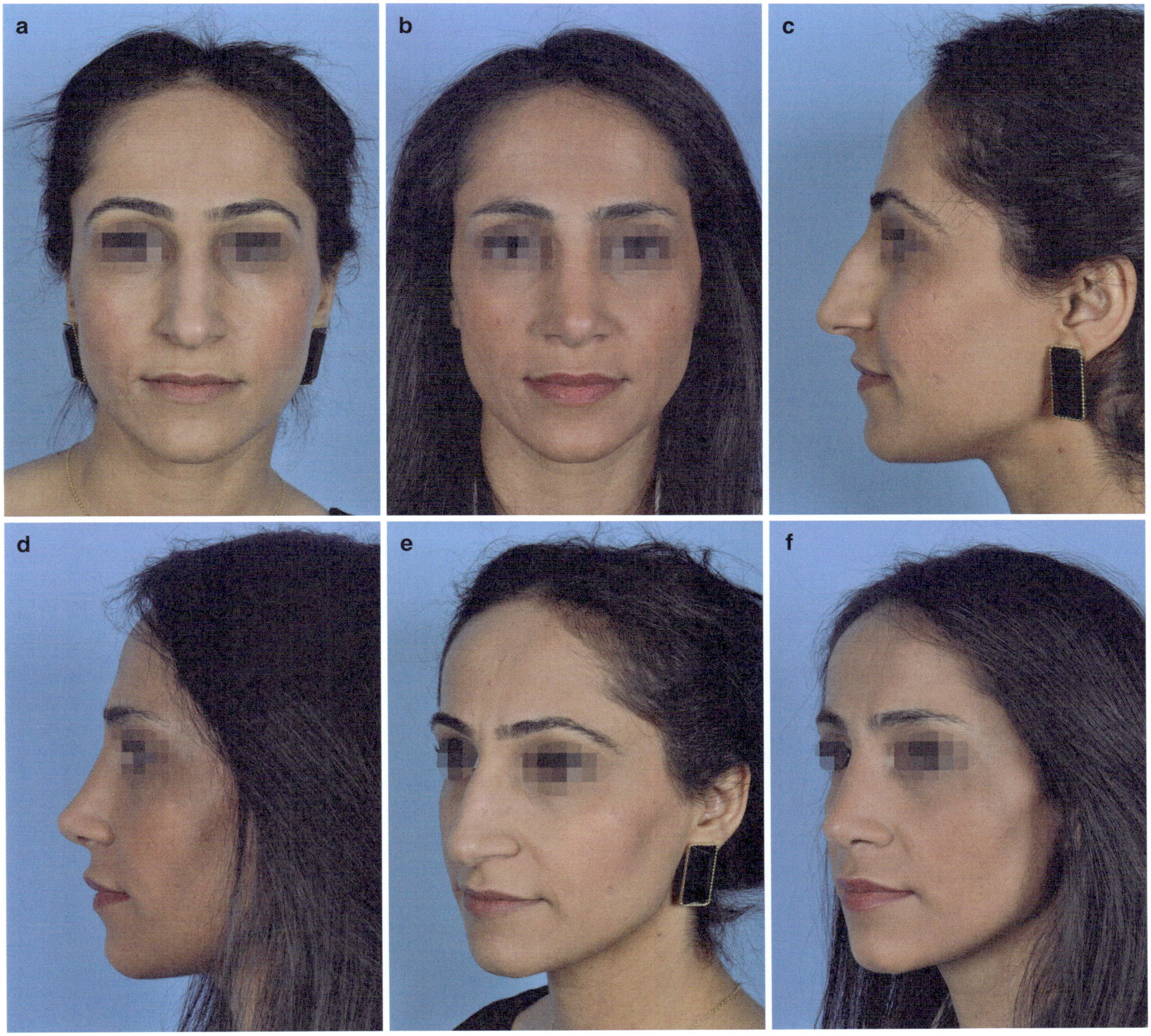

Fig. 11.35 (**a–f**) The preoperative and 2-year postoperative frontal, lateral, and oblique views. Tip rotation, projection, and definition are improved

where the medial-crural overlap will be effective. Postoperative deformities may emerge if the operation is terminated without relieving this tension.

An intraoperative example of the situation above is shown in Fig. 11.40: An approximately 7-mm segment is stolen from the crura to correct the droopy nasal tip. The 7-mm segment moved from the lateral crus to the medial crus corrects the droopy tip but lengthens the infratip lobule, pushing the columella anteriorly. The surgeon must avoid terminating surgery without correcting the configuration, as such a tip would not have a natural and attractive appearance. Therefore, medial crural overlap is performed to achieve the ideal appearance.

How should the COST technique be performed? Let us examine the COST technique by way of an example (Fig. 11.41).

11.3.4.1 Case 8

After applying the steal suture, overlap starts by dividing the medial crus at the point of maximum tension. The division creates two stumps; one above and the other below the point of maximum tension. The upper stump is dissected from the vestibule up to the dome and is slid over the lower stump until configuration irregularities are corrected; this is why the technique is termed *overlap*. As soon as the desired configuration is achieved, the proximal flap is sutured over the

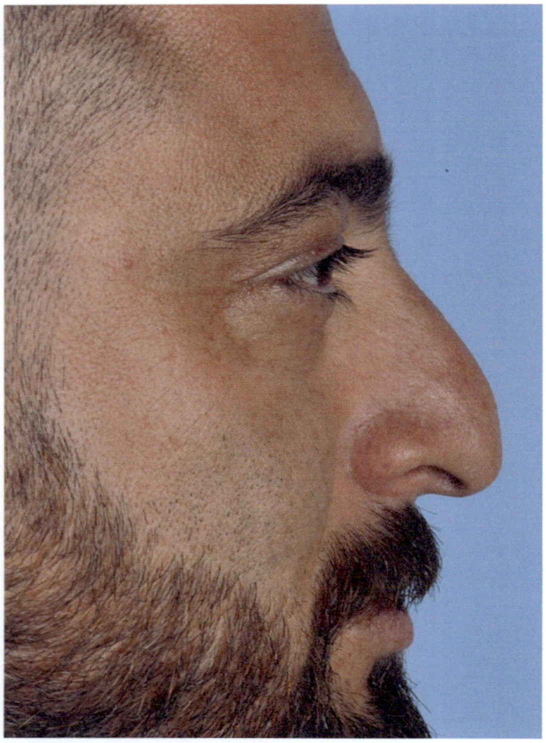

Fig. 11.36 Profile view. Tip position requires rotation and projection

distal stump. The overlap not only corrects the middle/medial crural configuration deformity, but also improves any asymmetries in the alar arch. Configuration of the alar arch improves once the COST technique is completed. Rotation resulting from shortening of the lateral crus increases and configuration deformity resulting from the overlap improves (Fig. 11.42).

Once bilateral overlap has been performed and the new configuration of the alar arch has been created, the next step is tip stabilization. While columellar strut and dome-equalizing suture are standard techniques for this purpose, it may be necessary to add a septocolumellar suture or septocolumellar strut in some cases.

In this patient, a septocolumellar suture was added to the columellar strut and the dome-equalizing suture (Fig. 11.43).

Dividing and overlapping the medial crus would shorten the segment moved to the medial crus by a steal suture, which would result in deprojection. In this case, onlay tip grafting may be necessary to improve projection (Fig. 11.44).

One-year postoperative photographs of the case on whom COST technique was performed are shown in Fig. 11.45.

In cases of droopy nasal tip presenting with asymmetric alar cartilage, the COST technique may be applied unilaterally as seen next, in Case 9.

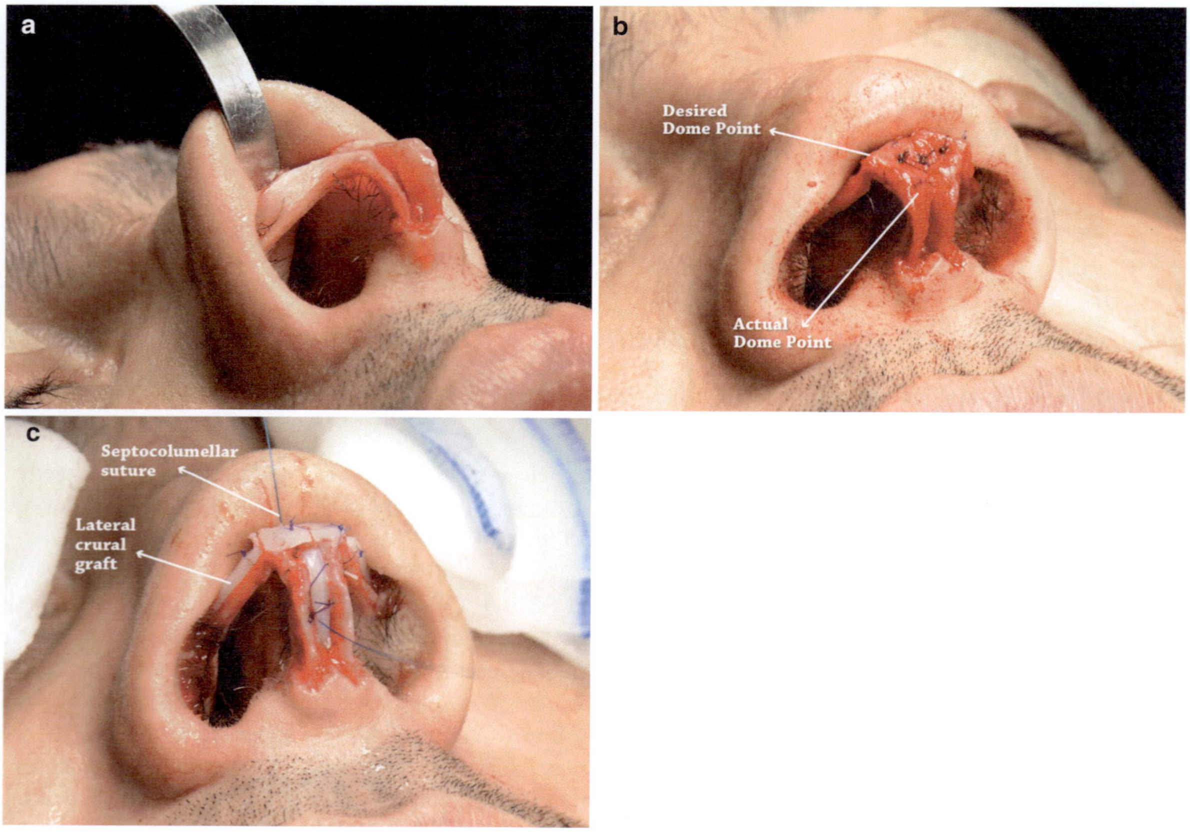

Fig. 11.37 (**a**) Before placing the steal suture. (**b**) After placing the steal suture, lateral crura are shortened while, on the contrary, infratip lobule is lengthened. (**c**) Final enhanced nasal tip anatomy. Columellar strut, cap graft, lateral crural graft, and septocolumellar suture

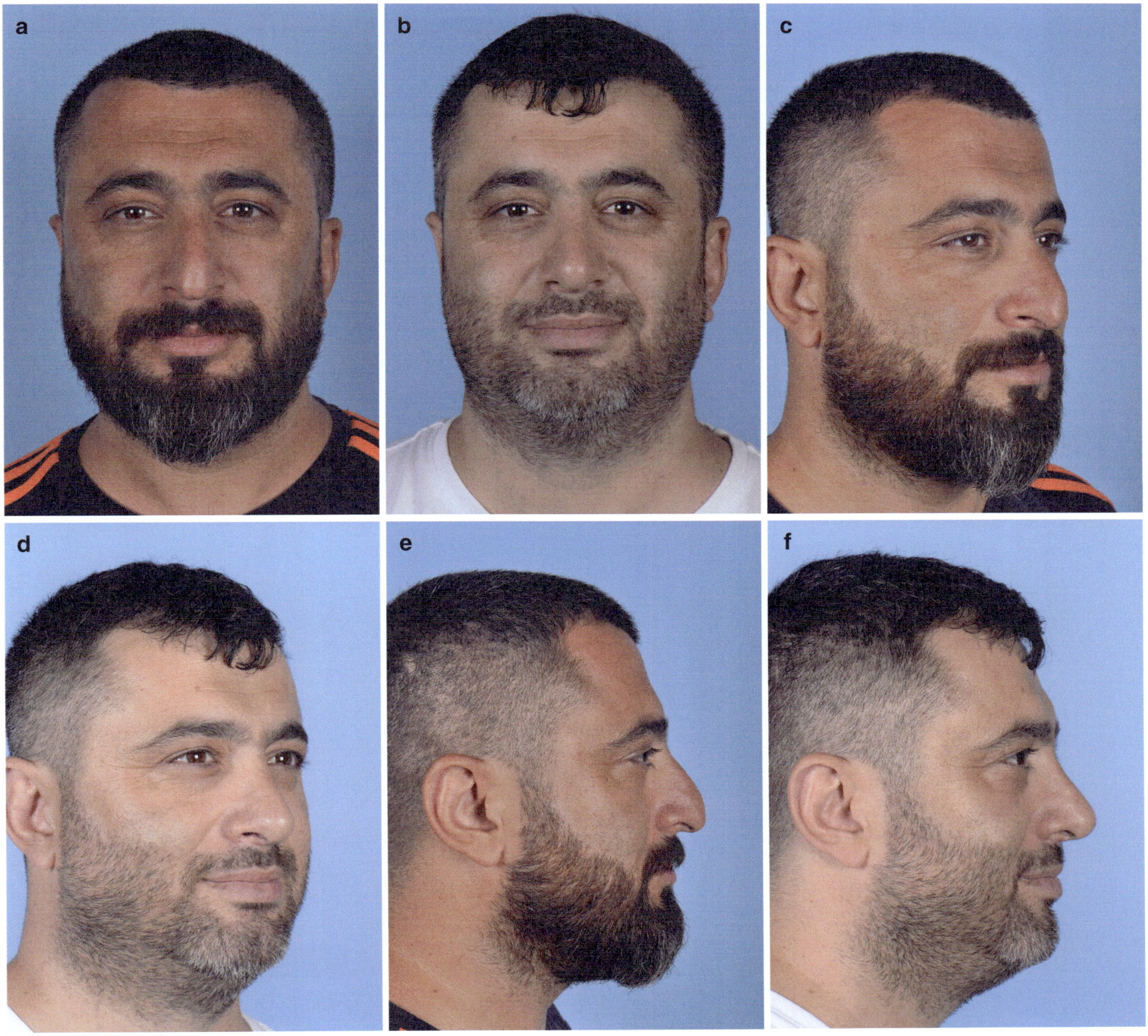

Fig. 11.38 (a–f) Postoperative photographs. Nasal tip is well projected and rotated, and infratip lobule is more aesthetic shaped

11.3.4.2 Case 9

An example is presented here. A thick-skinned male patient with a droopy nasal tip had a long lateral crus and overdeveloped septal cartilage, pushing the tip downward. At the same time, the configuration of the medial and middle crura is not ideal, leading to a narrow columella lobule angle. Moreover, both the columellar and lobular segments are elongated (Fig. 11.46).

An 8 mm shortening was contemplated to attain the ideal length of the lateral crus. Nevertheless, the existing medial crural incongruity increased further after the steal suture, resulting in the elongation of the leg portion of the alar arch (Fig. 11.47).

The misconfiguration of the medial/middle crura and their shortening were resolved through division and overlap (Fig. 11.48).

A septocolumellar strut and columellar were used together because the patient had thick skin. A cap graft was used for tip definition, whereas a lateral crural graft was preferred for alar rim definition. Dome-equalizing suture improved the tip definition (Fig. 11.49).

Photographs of the patient taken 1 year postoperatively are shown in Fig. 11.50.

Patients with droopy nasal tips and preoperative middle/medial crus deformities are potential candidates for the overlap technique. The steal suture would further

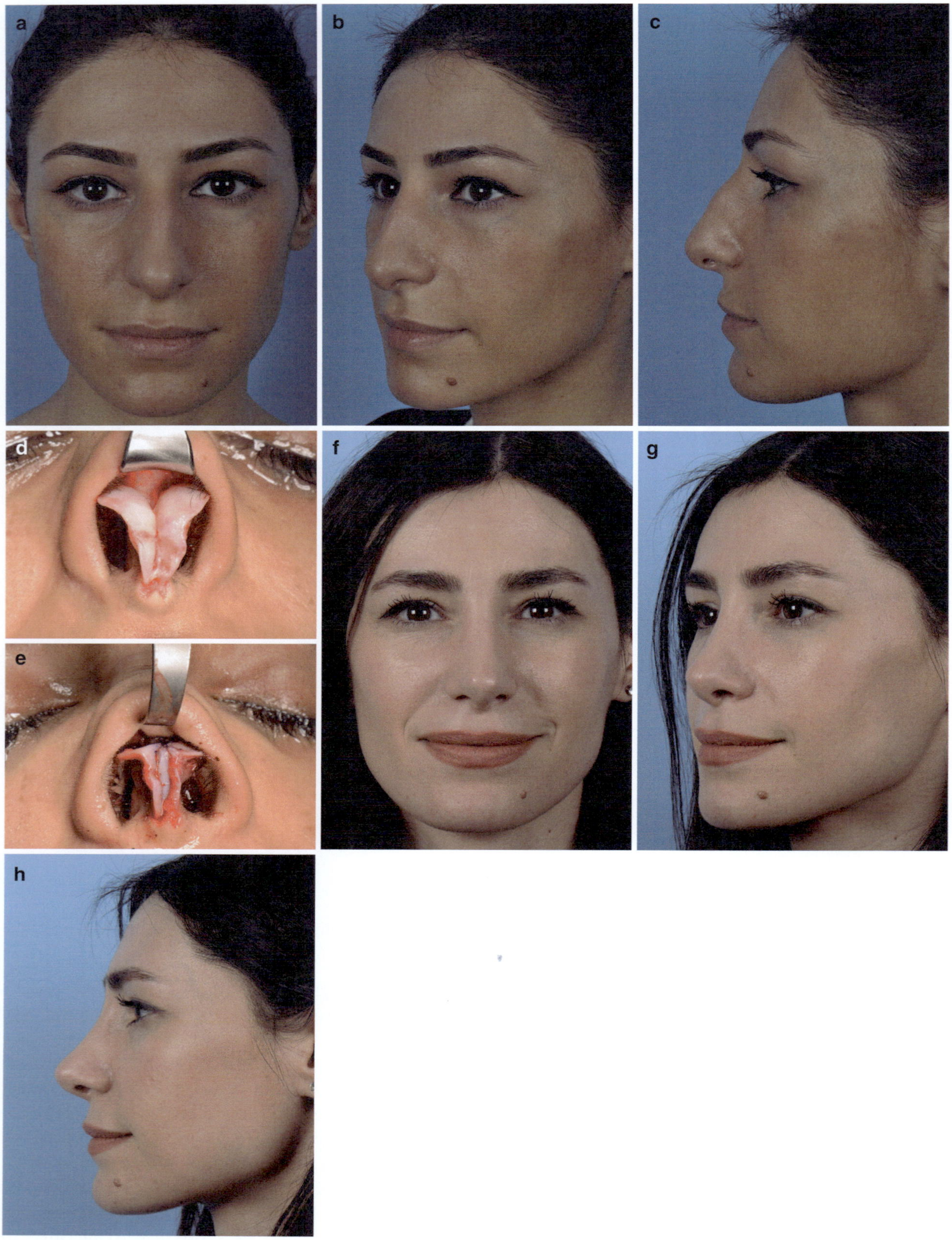

Fig. 11.39 (**a–c**) Preoperative photographs. (**d**, **e**) Lateral crural steal suture is performed. (**f–h**) Five-year postoperative photographs

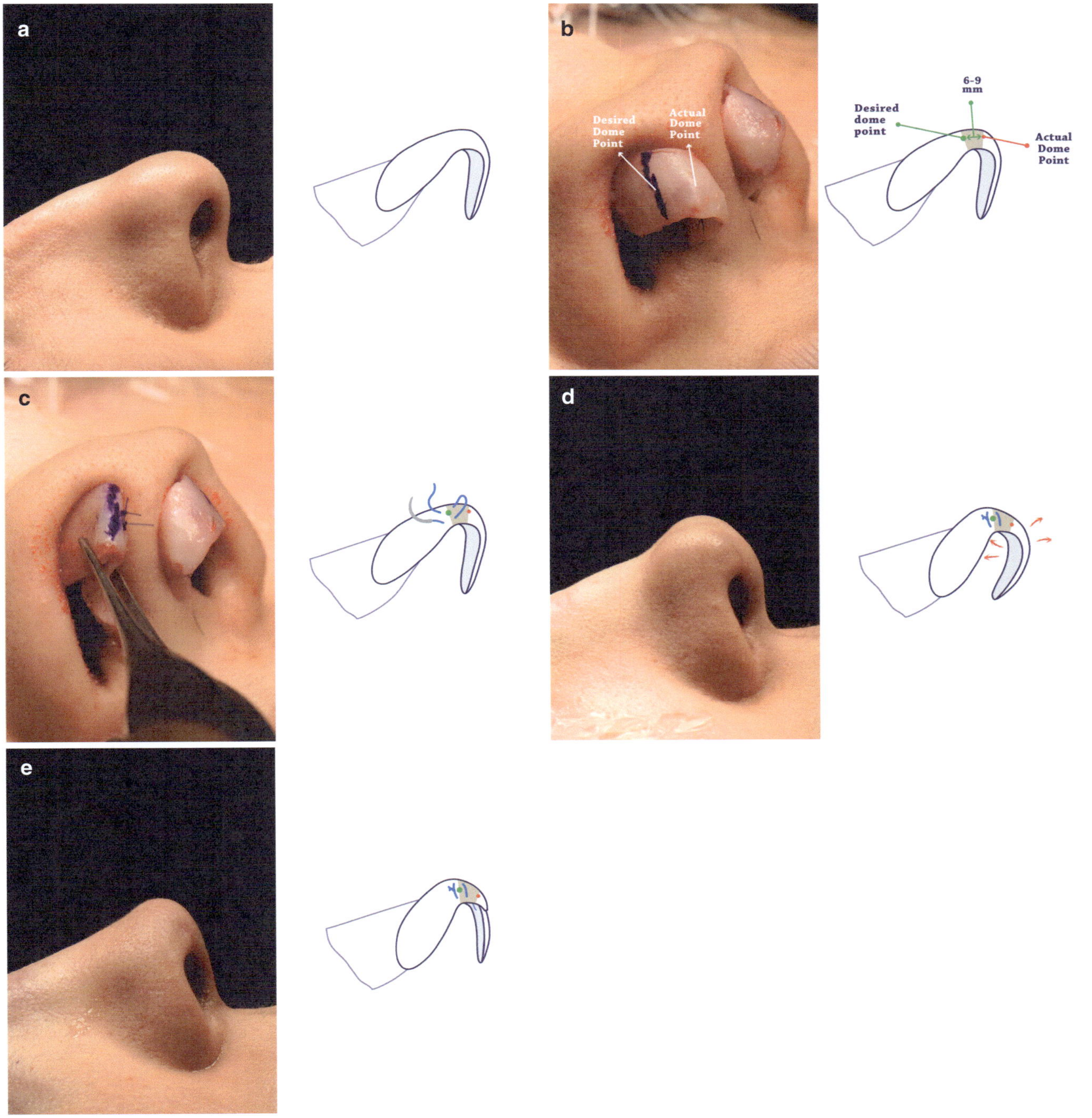

Fig. 11.40 (**a**) Intraoperative profile view. (**b**) Alar cartilage anatomy. The desired dome point is marked. (**c**) Bilateral steal sutures were placed and a columellar strut was applied. (**d**) Attention should be paid to the appearance following only steal suture and columellar strut placement. Many deformities were apparent in this case. Therefore, it was necessary to change the strategy. (**e**) The overlap technique was applied without touching the steal suture, and the configuration improved

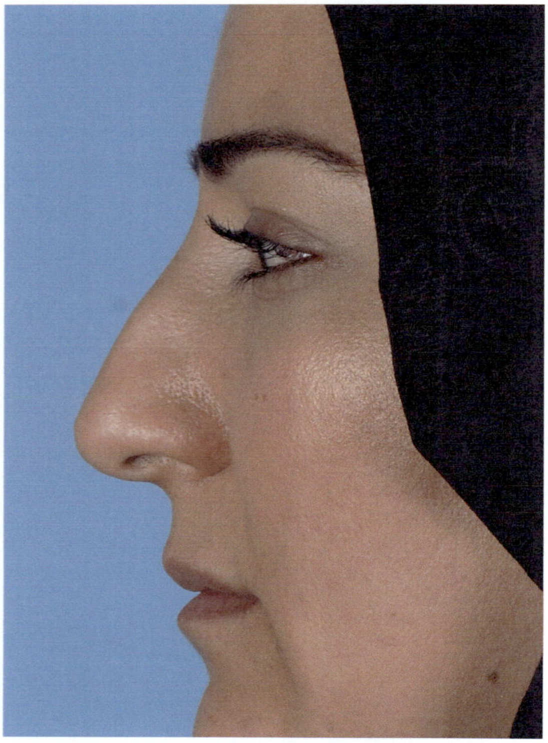

Fig. 11.41 Preoperative profile photograph

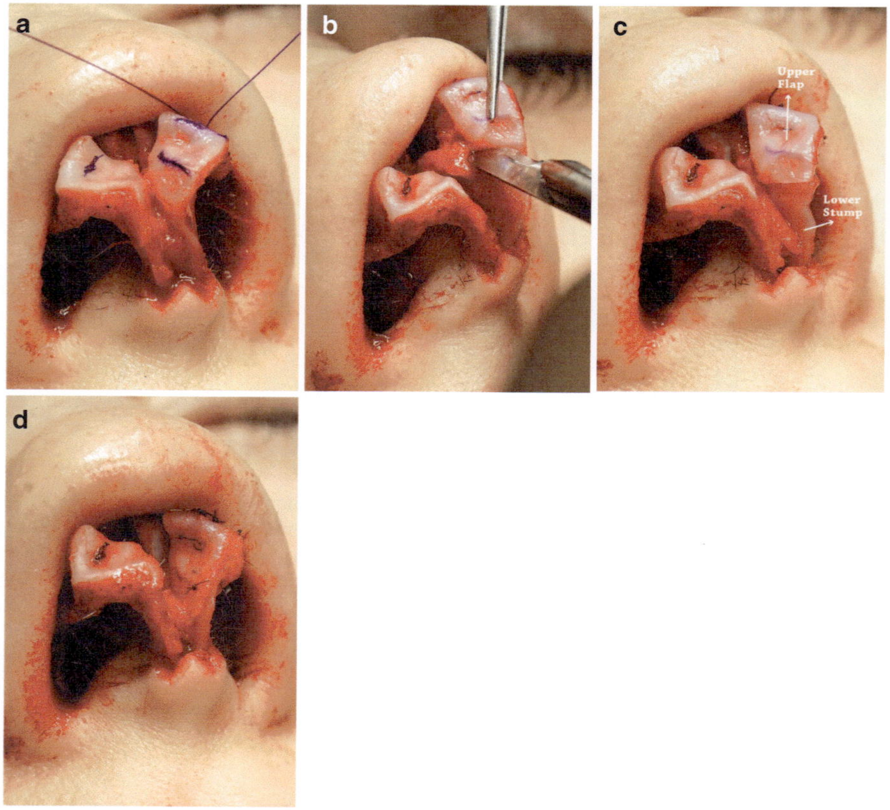

Fig. 11.42 (**a**) First, 8-mm lateral crus segments were moved bilaterally to the medial crus. The lateral crus was shortened but the configuration of the medial crus was disturbed. (**b**) Alar cartilage division was performed at the point of maximum tension. (**c**) The upper flap was elevated from the skin sliding over the lower stump to find its ideal location. (**d**) Compare the alar cartilage at the left side versus the right side, paying attention to the differences in configuration; the alar cartilage on the left appears completely corrected with the overlap whereas the cartilage on the right has a deformed appearance

disturb an already impaired intermediate/medial crural configuration (Fig. 11.51).

A typical example of the situation above is shown next, in Case 10.

11.3.4.3 Case 10

In this case, pay attention to the patient's droopy nasal tip and hanging columella due to middle/medial crus deformity (Fig. 11.52).

Intraoperative alar configuration shows long lateral and middle/medial crus deformities (Fig. 11.53).

The bilateral crural steal suture was performed to shorten the lateral crura (Fig. 11.54).

The overlap was performed (Fig. 11.55).

The septocolumellar strut was used for extra tip stability because of the thick skin (Fig. 11.56).

The operation was finished by using cap and lateral crural grafts in order to gain projection and definition (Fig. 11.57).

Preoperative and postoperative photographs are shown in Fig. 11.58. Tip rotation has been a more aesthetic level. Hanging infratip lobule is improved.

11.3.4.4 Case 11

Another example related to the COST technique, long-term results of the case below (Fig. 11.59).

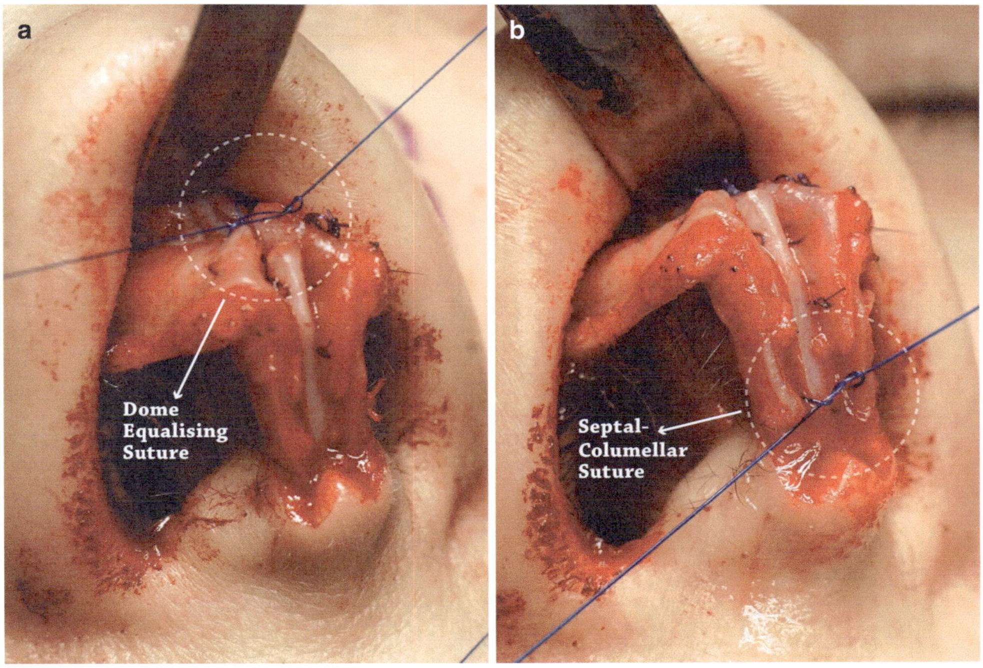

Fig. 11.43 (**a**) Dome equalizing suture and columellar strut are standard for stabilizing of the tip**.** (**b**) Due to thick nasal skin, the newly formed alar arch should receive extra support by using septocolumellar suture

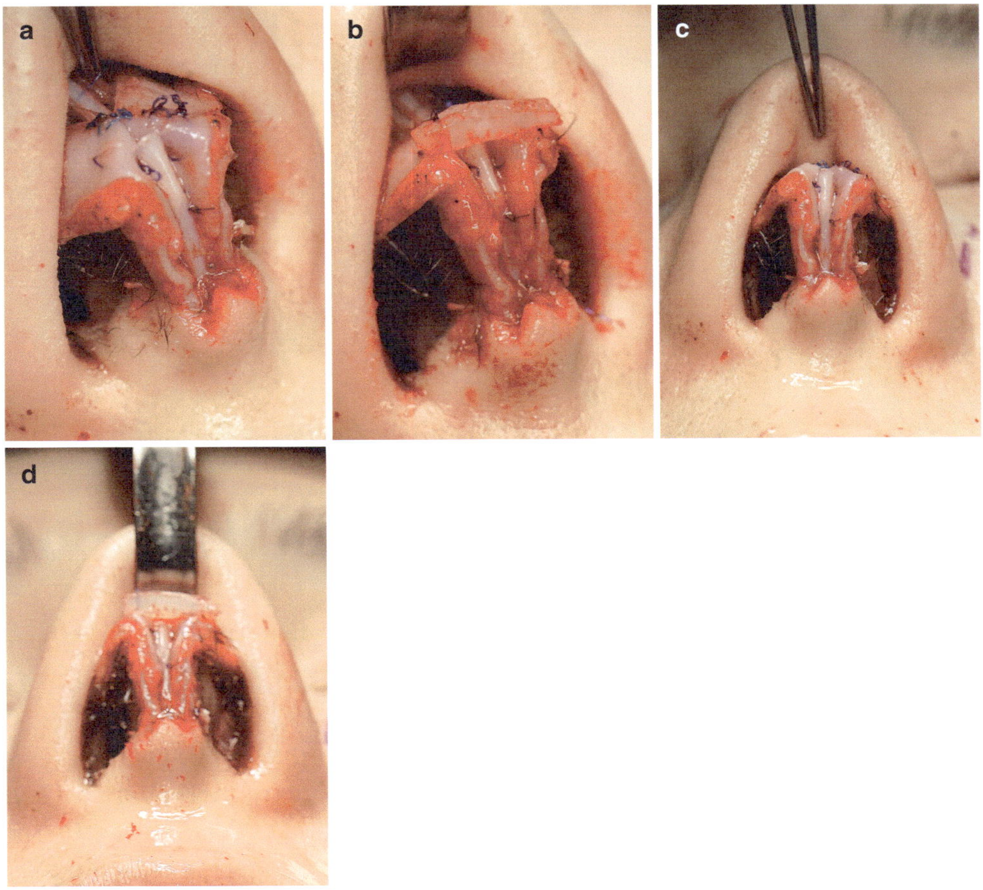

Fig. 11.44 (**a–d**) Attention should be paid to the relationship between the dorsum and the tip. The distance between the tip-defining point and the dorsum is around 6 mm. The surgeon should not finish the surgery without increasing the projection. An additional 3 mm of tip projection is needed to achieve the ideal tip–dorsum relationship. A thick cap graft is suitable for this purpose. Attention should be paid to the projection before and after the cap graft, and to the distance between the tip and the dorsum. In this case, the distance, which was 9 mm preoperatively, is appropriate for an ideal postoperative tip–dorsum transition

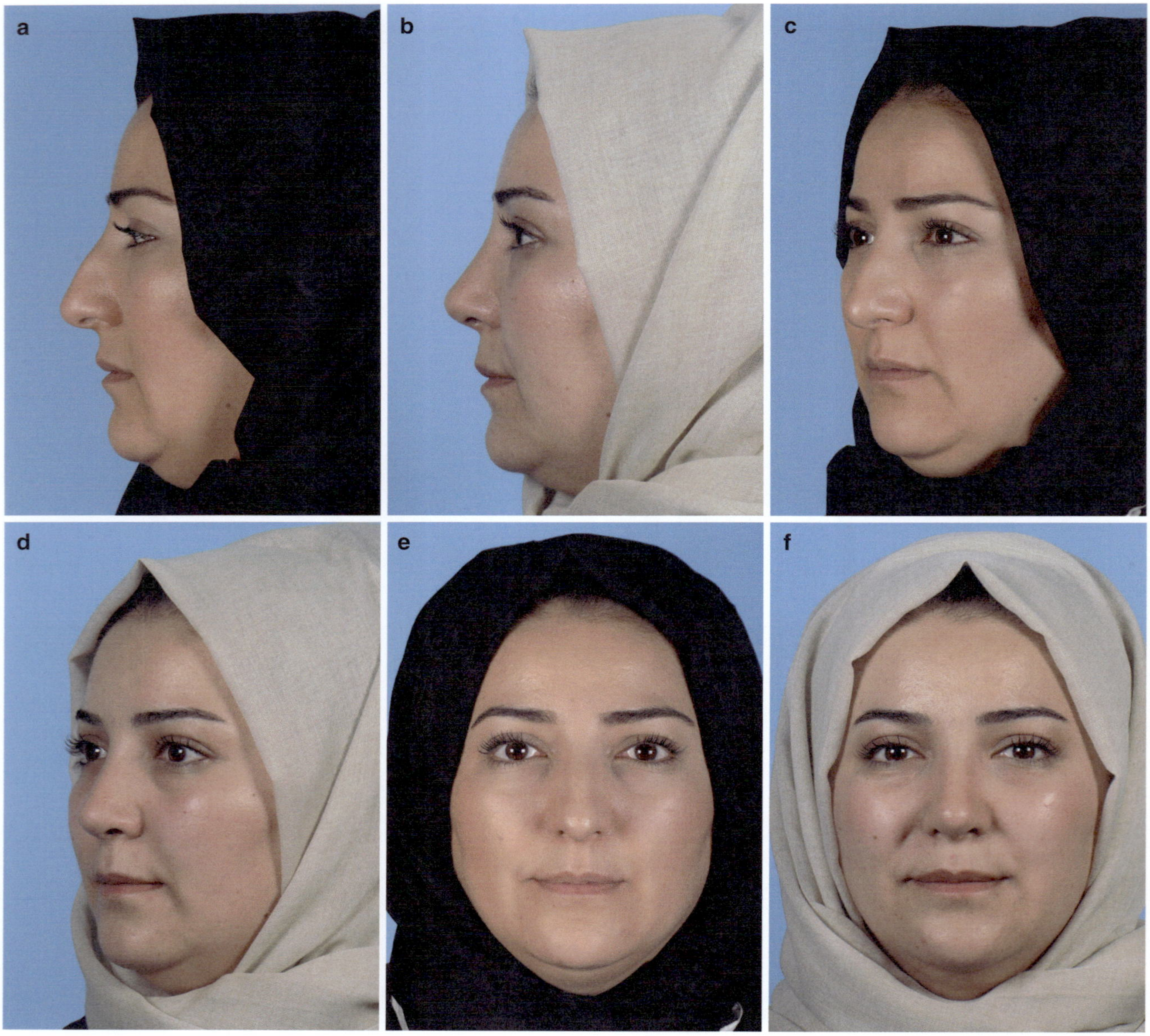

Fig. 11.45 (**a–f**) Preoperative and postoperative images. The tip has gained rotation. More pleasing, feminine, nasolabial angle. The favorable relation between dorsum and tip projection

Preoperative photographs indicated a long lateral crura in the oblique view. The configuration deformity in the middle/medial crural complex was remarkable in the profile view. The surgical technique involved application of suturing to shorten the long lateral crus and overlap to correct the configuration deformity at the middle/medial crural complex, as this deformity would become more pronounced after suturing.

As discussed above, treatment of droopy nasal tip gives the face a younger appearance, as in the following example.

11.3.4.5 Case 12

Droopy nasal tip caused by a long lateral crus can be seen in the preoperative oblique view (Fig. 11.60). Also, the preoperative lateral view shows middle/medial crus configuration disorder. The COST technique was applied in this case and yielded satisfactorily.

11.3.5 Droopy Nasal Tip Treatment with Vertical Alar Resection (VAR Technique)

If the lateral crus requires shortening by more than 10 mm to correct the droopy nasal tip, the VAR technique should be used rather than the steal suture. The VAR technique involves excision of the excess portion of the lateral crus by a vertical cut just lateral to the dome. In the presence of any deformity of the lateral crus, this technique has several advantages.

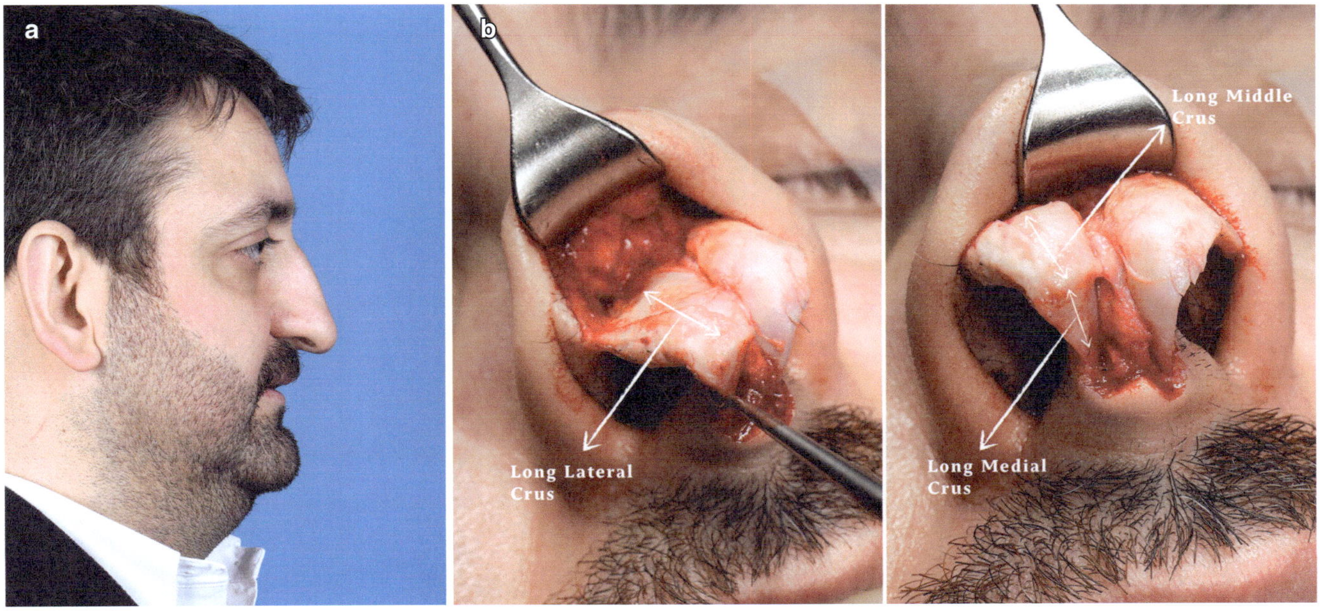

Fig. 11.46 (**a**) Bottom-heavy nose, the profile view of the nose showing an under-rotated nasal tip with a nasolabial angle of less than 90 degrees, while the columellar-lobular angle is less than 45°. (**b**) The anatomy of alar cartilages seen from the oblique view; lateral crus is too long, the caudal septum is over-developed, and long middle-medial crura

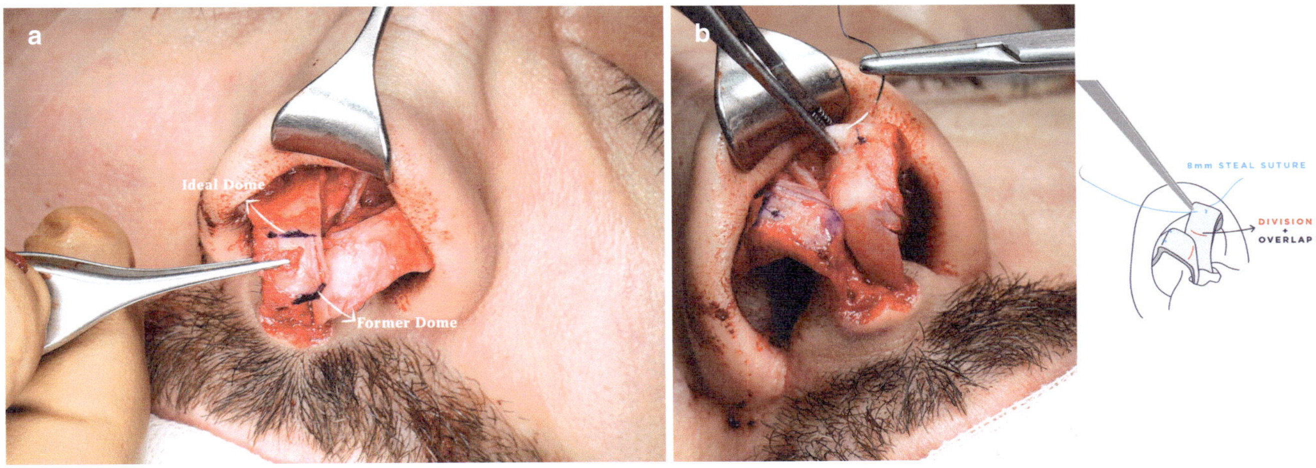

Fig. 11.47 (**a**) The ideal dome point was marked. This is approximately 8 mm lateral to the former dome. (**b**) After the steal suture, the already long medial, middle crura became even longer, necessitating division and overlapped at this stage

Resection can also correct such deformities. The long lateral crus mostly presents with additional configurational deformities, such as excessive convexity or concavity. Another advantage of the VAR technique is that it provides access to both the lateral crus and the middle crus.

How can we perform VAR technique? VAR technique is shown in the illustrations in Fig. 11.61 and Video 11.11.

Patients requiring VAR often present with a hypertrophic and alar solid arch. In such cases, the columellar strut would suffice for tip stabilization following VAR.

Patients requiring VAR often present with a weak alar arch and heavy skin. A septocolumellar strut, bilateral medial-middle crural strut, or SEG would be needed in such cases.

Technical Pearl: When removing the cartilage, an angled resection must be performed, in such a way that the short edge lies caudally, and the longer edge remains cranially directed.

A columellar strut graft creates a stable, symmetric, and strong nasal base. The columellar strut graft can be either straight or angled. Care must be taken to avoid the columellar strut graft touching the nasal spine or the septum. Fixation must be performed in at least two different points using 4–0 rapid Vicryl sutures. The suture is passed through the vestibular skin, medial crus, columellar strut, and medial crus, and turned back to make a knot.

Technical Pearl: The lateral nasal wall must constantly be reinforced during VAR. The excess portion removed from

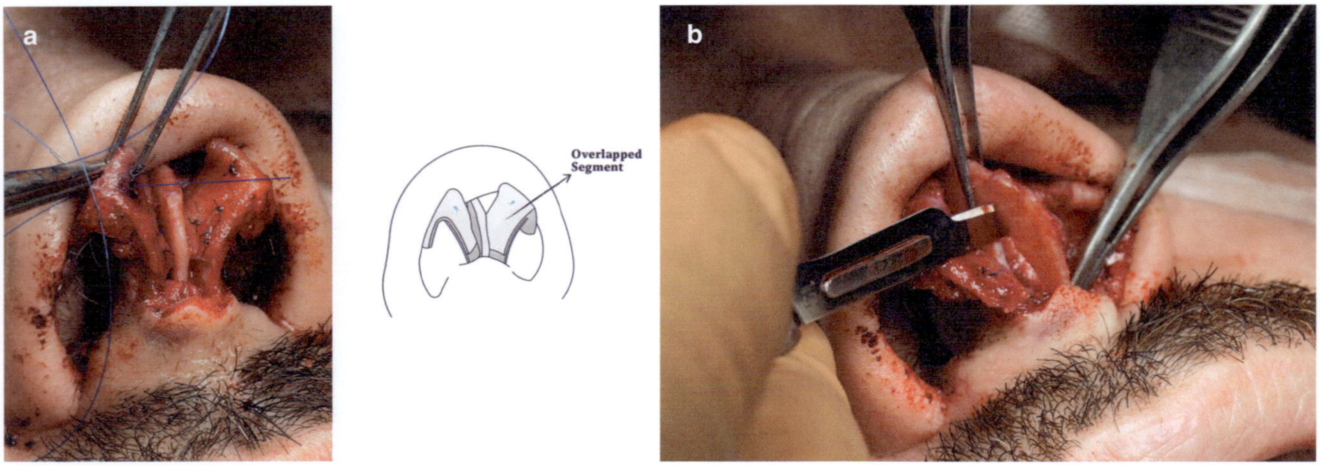

Fig. 11.48 (**a**) Bilaterally, the distal parts were slid over the proximal parts and secured with a 6/0 absorbable suture until the configuration disorder was corrected, resulting in an achieved fixed alar configuration. (**b**) The excess caudal septum, which was pushing down the nasal tip, was resected

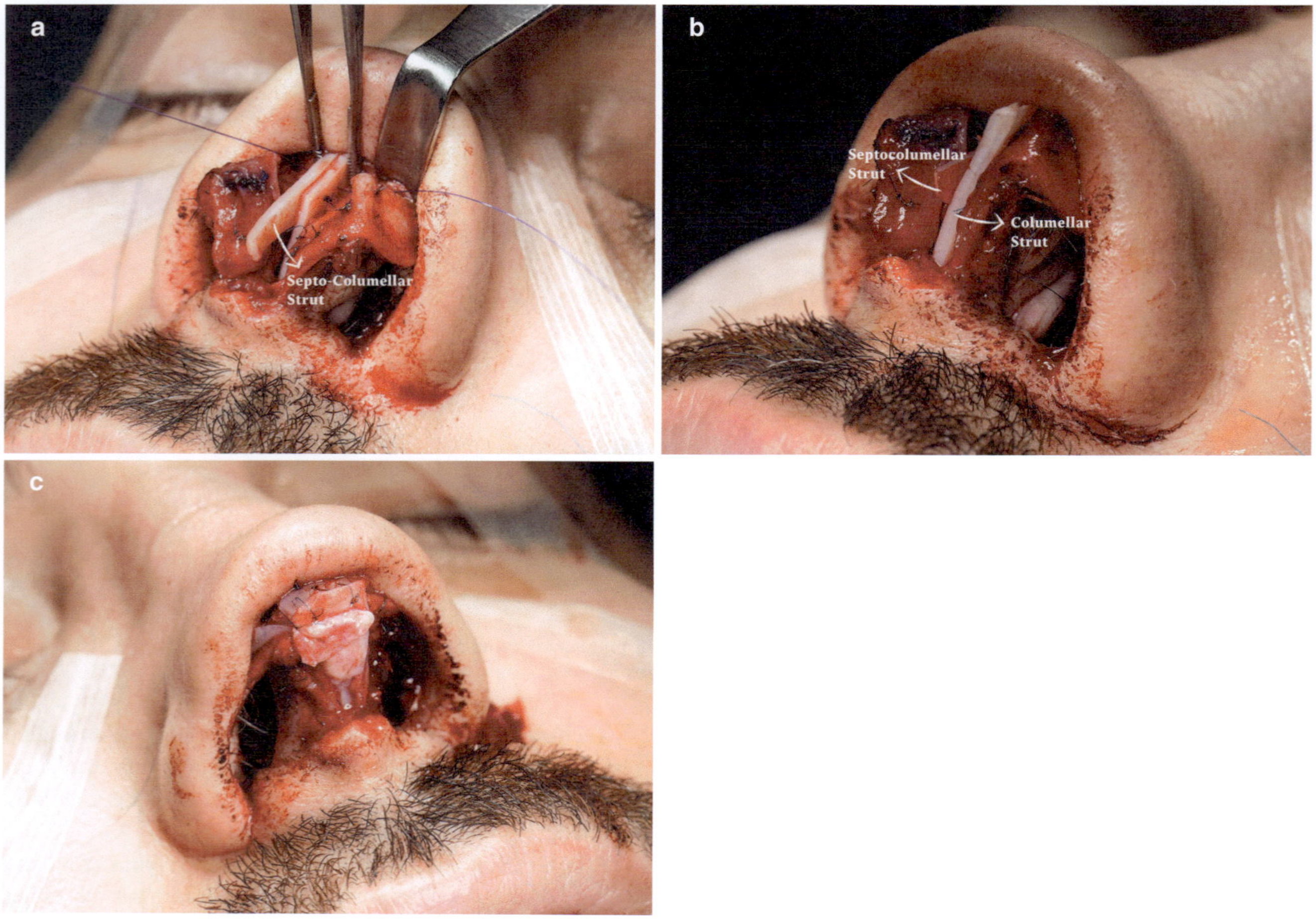

Fig. 11.49 (**a**) Septoculumellar graft placement. (**b**) Columellar strut placed and secured with septocolumellar strut. (**c**) The overlap aimed at correcting the misconfiguration of the mid-medial crura resulted in a loss of projection. To optimize the projection, a 3 mm cap graft was utilized

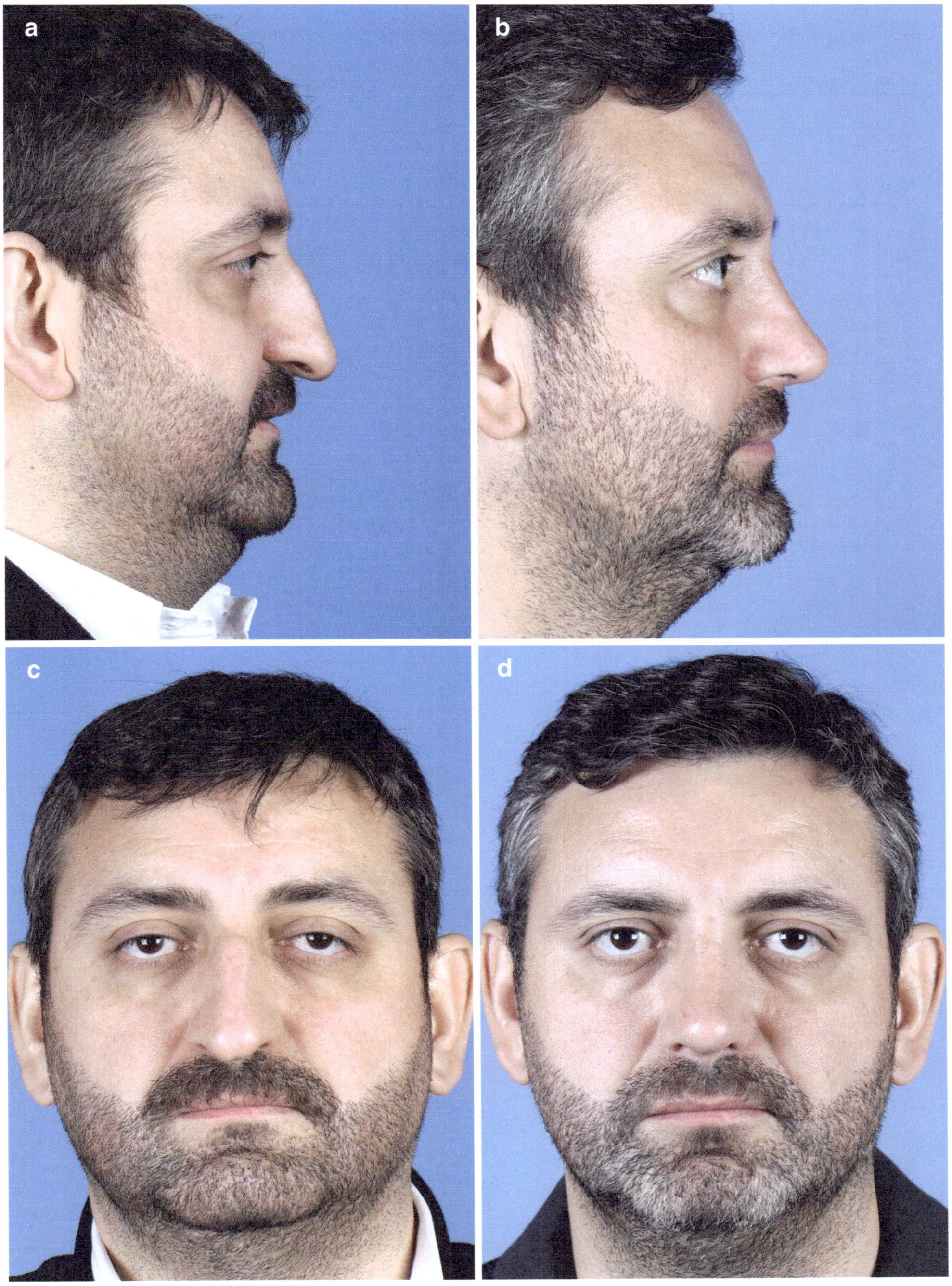

Fig. 11.50 (**a–f**) Preoperative and postoperative photographs, despite having thick skin correction of a ptotic, asymmetrical tip was achieved with a COST technique and septocolumellar strut

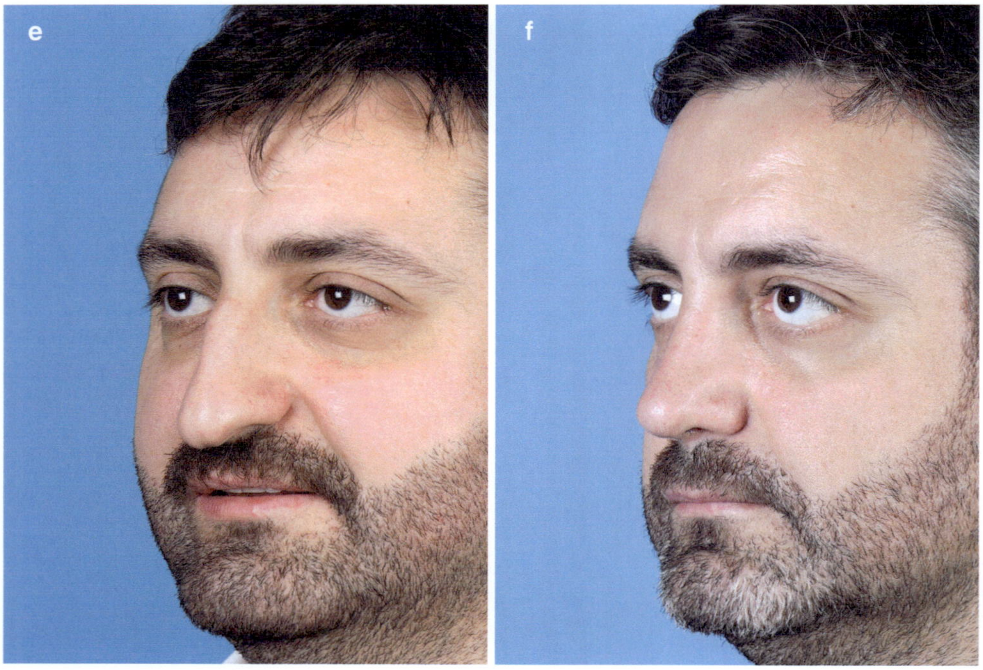

Fig. 11.50 (continued)

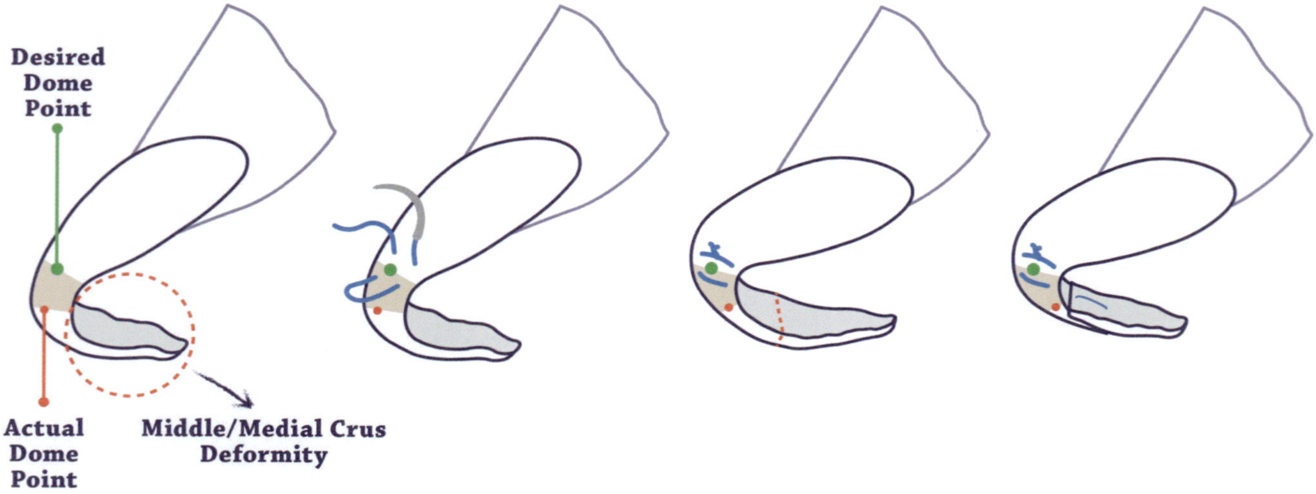

Fig. 11.51 The suture may aggravate an already existing deformity, as shown in the illustration (Video 11.10)

the lateral crus is used as an alar batten graft. A pocket is opened immediately beneath the caudal border of the lateral crus toward the apertura piriformis, where the graft is inserted. If the graft is shaped to fit precisely into the pocket, there would be no need for fixation. The lateral crural graft can also be used for this purpose.

A lateral crural graft should also be considered an alternative to an Alar button graft to strengthen the lateral nasal wall. The lateral crural graft should also be considered an alternative to an Alar button graft to enhance the lateral nasal wall.

11.3.5.1 Case 13

The VAR technique is discussed here with reference to a case of droopy nasal tip. Attention should be paid to the length of the lateral crus; shortening a 10-mm lateral crus would only correct the tip configuration (Fig. 11.62; Video 11.12).

The alar arch was divided immediately next to the dome, creating two stumps. The lateral stump was elevated from the vestibular skin. The excess portion of the lateral crural flap was resected. This was followed by end-to-end suturing of the flap with the distal stump, such that the crural segments reached the ideal length (Fig. 11.63).

A columellar strut was used as a stable base, a dome-equalizing suture was applied for definition, and a cap graft and camouflage graft were used for projection. The resected part from the lateral crus was used as an alar batten graft to reinforce the lateral nasal wall. The lateral crural graft created light reflection at the alar rim (Fig. 11.64).

Preoperative and postoperative photographs are shown in Fig. 11.65.

The most common question asked about the VAR technique is how much cartilage should be removed. Excessive cartilage is always exposed once the dome is cut and the lateral crus elevated. However, on average, it may be necessary to remove about 10 mm of cartilage tissue.

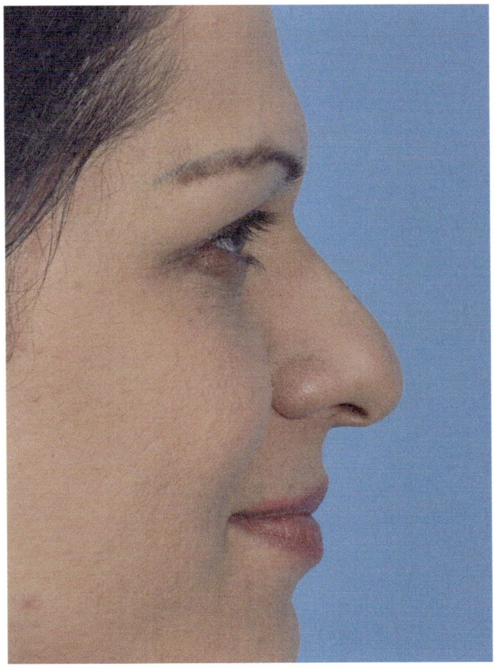

Fig. 11.52 Droopy nasal tip with hanging columella

11.3.5.2 Case 14

The VAR technique can also be applied with the delivery approach; the surgical steps are the same. Here, we show a case of droopy nasal tip corrected with the delivery technique (Fig. 11.66; Video 11.13).

Symmetrical resection may appear challenging with the endonasal approach. However, with good intraoperative analysis and correct marking, it is not difficult to achieve symmetry. The VAR technique starts with marking of the actual dome points; suspending the two domes when marking provides good exposure. In this way, dome points can be marked symmetrically. Then, an incision is made lateral to the marked dome, excising the excess portion of the crus. Following bilateral excision, end-to-end anastomosis is completed using 6–0 absorbable sutures. A columellar strut and cap graft are then fixed to the alar cartilages exposed through either of the nostrils and a dome-equalizing suture is applied (Fig. 11.67).

Photographs of the patient taken 1 year postoperatively showed correction of the droopy tip (Fig. 11.68).

11.3.5.3 Case 15

Figure 11.69 shows another case of droopy nasal tip (Video 11.14). The preoperative lateral view indicated an advanced, hypertrophic, and long lateral crus.

The length of the lateral crus must be analyzed intraoperatively. Such a long lateral crus can only be shortened by resection (Fig. 11.70).

Photographs taken 1 year postoperatively showed complete correction of the droopy nasal tip (Fig. 11.71).

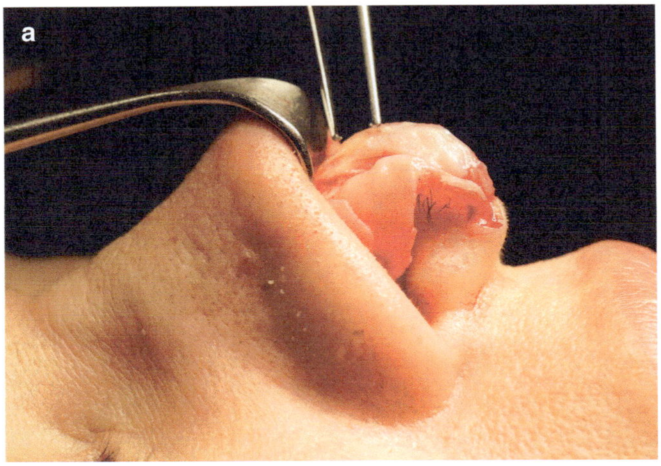

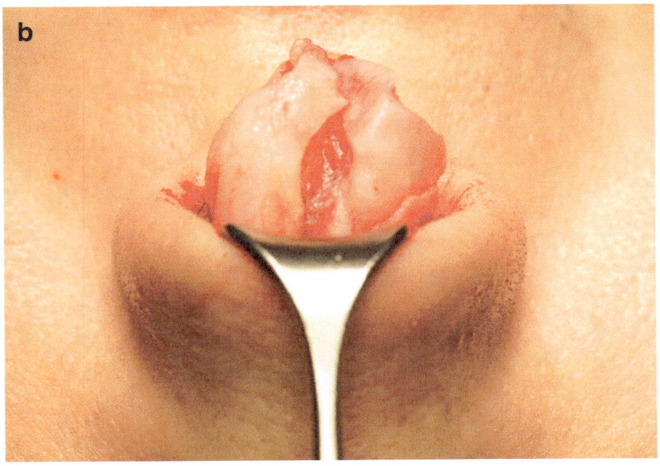

Fig. 11.53 (**a**) Disfigured middle/medial crus. (**b**) Too long lateral crura

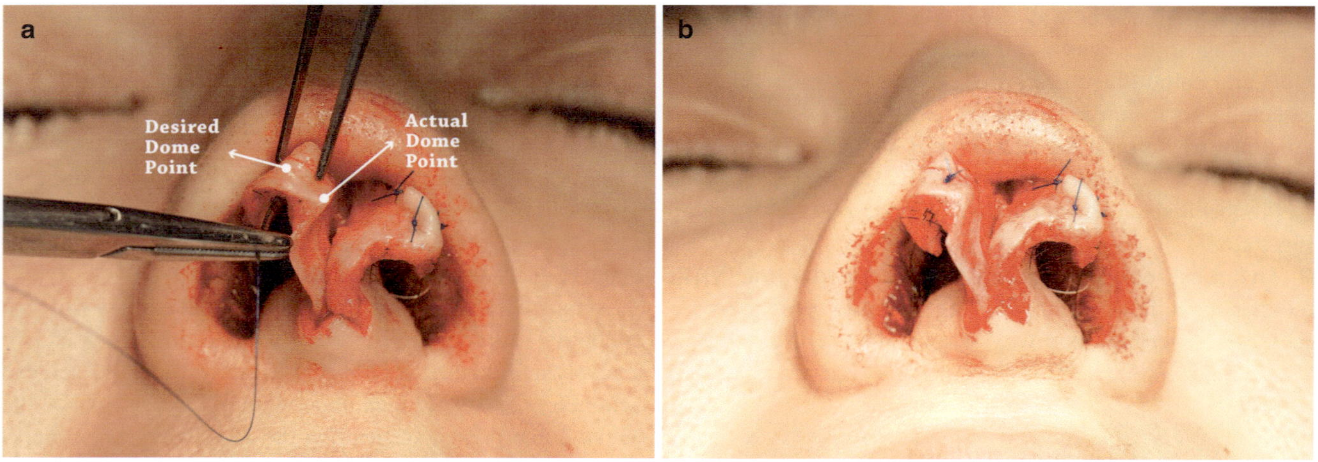

Fig. 11.54 (**a**, **b**) Lateral crural steal suture has provided an increase in tip projection and rotation at the expense of lateral crura

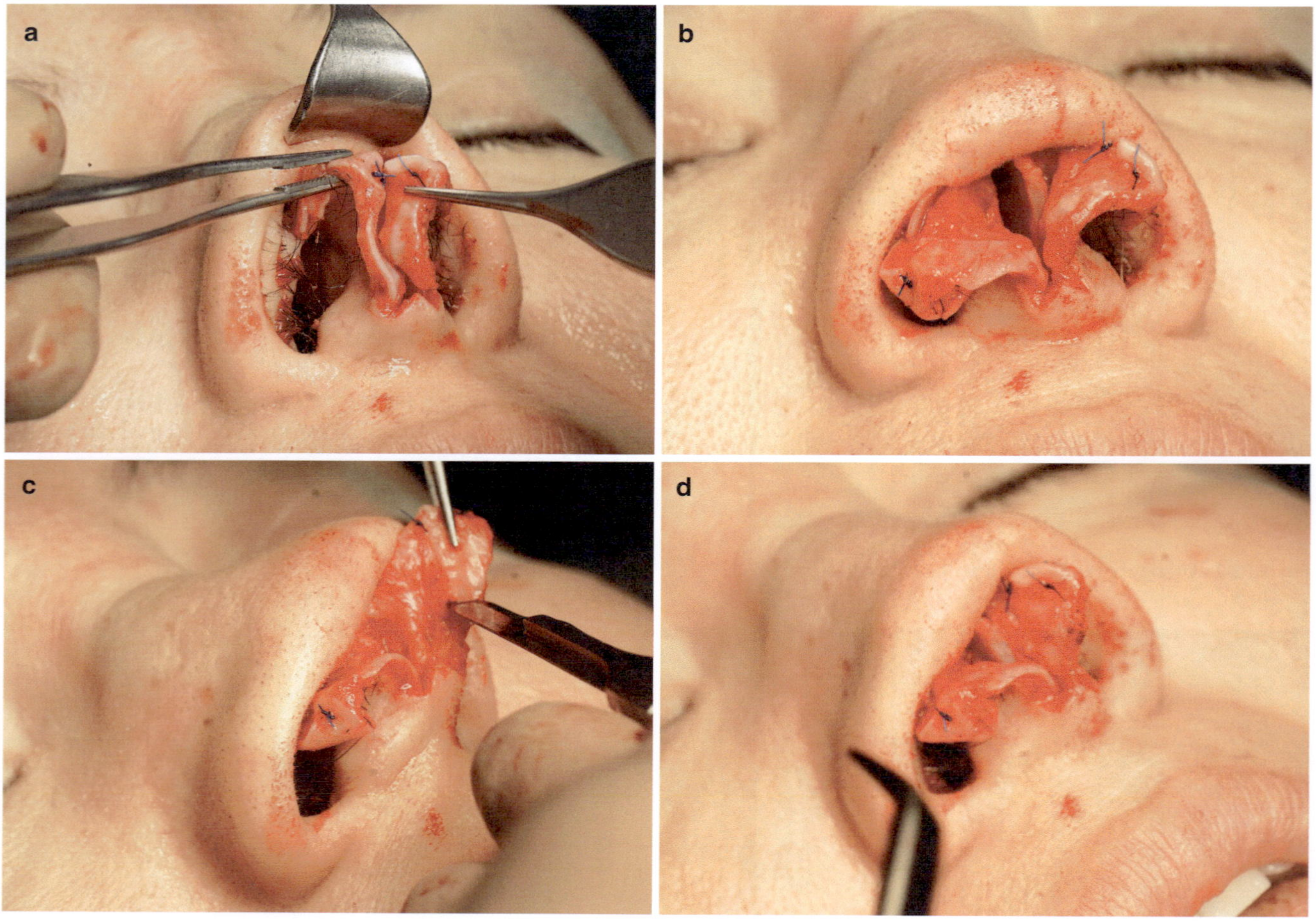

Fig. 11.55 (**a**, **b**) Lateral crura and the dome points look symmetrical while middle/medial crura are asymmetric and deformed. (**c**, **d**) Unilateral dividing and overlap were finished, and then the same process would be performed for the contralateral side

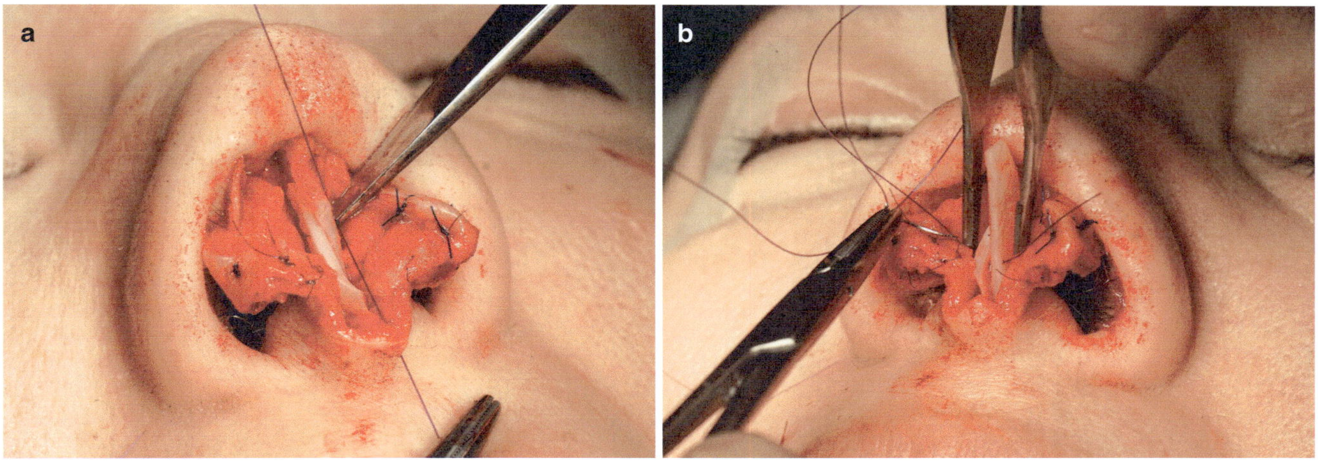

Fig. 11.56 Septocolumellar strut anchors the caudal septum to the intercrural columellar strut. (**a**) It should be fixed to the concave side of the septum, preferably with nonabsorbent suture. (**b**) Distal part of the graft is sutured to the columellar strut

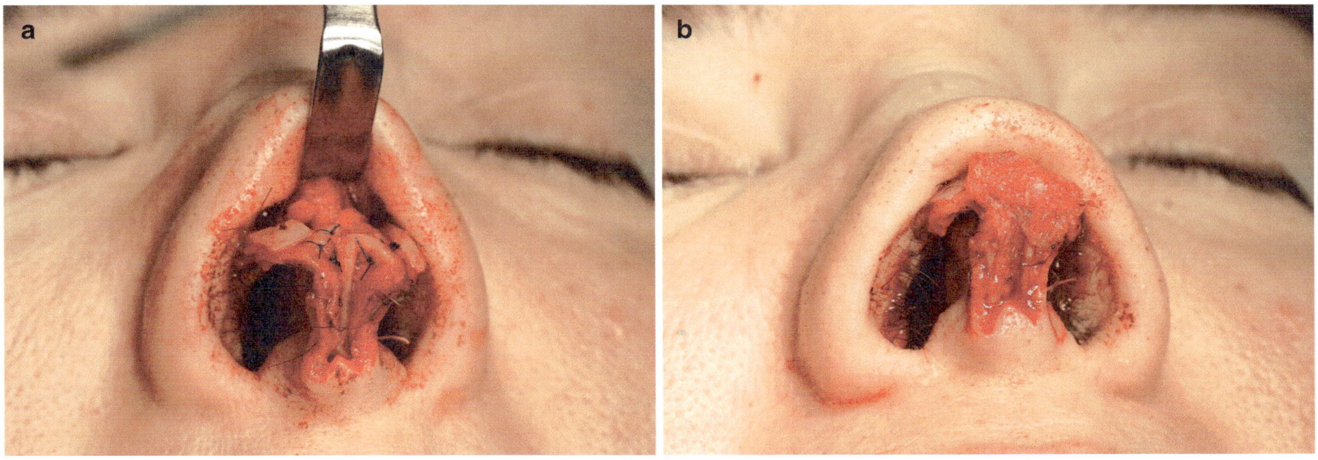

Fig. 11.57 (**a**) The columellar strut is sutured to the medial crura. (**b**) Cap graft, bilateral lateral crural graft, and camouflage graft

11.3.5.4 Case 16

The VAR technique can also be used in a droopy nasal tip with a thin-skinned patient. It would be sufficient to camouflage the graft when using an onlay tip graft. Three years after the operation, this thin-skinned patient did not show any tip irregularity due to the treatment (Fig. 11.72a–d; Video 11.15).

11.3.5.5 Case 16

This technique is safe, reliable, effective, simple, and easily applicable by surgeons at all levels of experience. When applied with correct indications, the long-term results of the VAR technique are pleasing. The VAR technique was applied in this patient due to the droopy nasal tip. The tip remained stable and no deformities were seen in the 5-year postoperative photographs (Fig. 11.73).

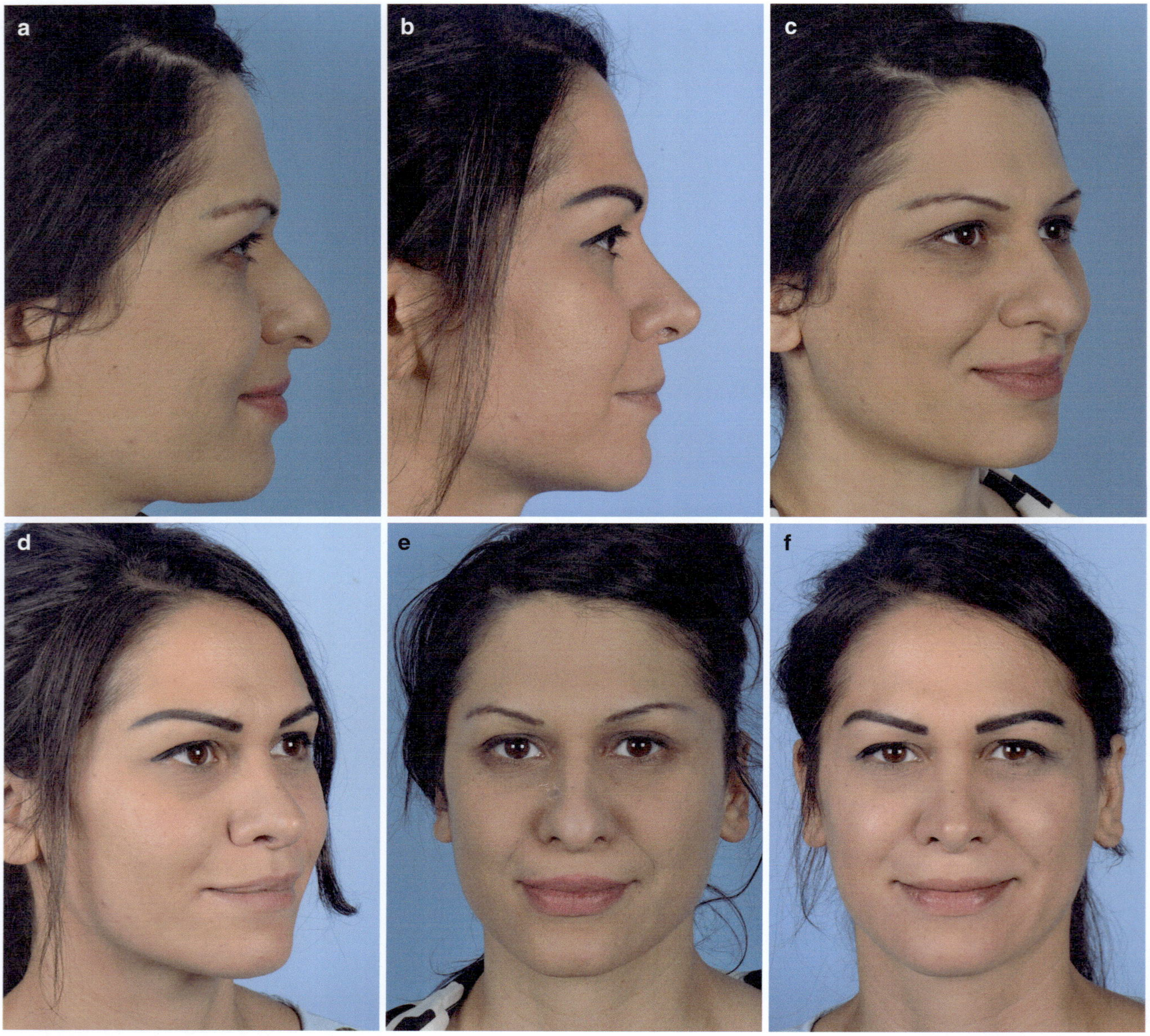

Fig. 11.58 (**a–f**) Preoperative and 8-year postoperative photographs, the patient underwent COST to correct a hanging columella and droopy tip together

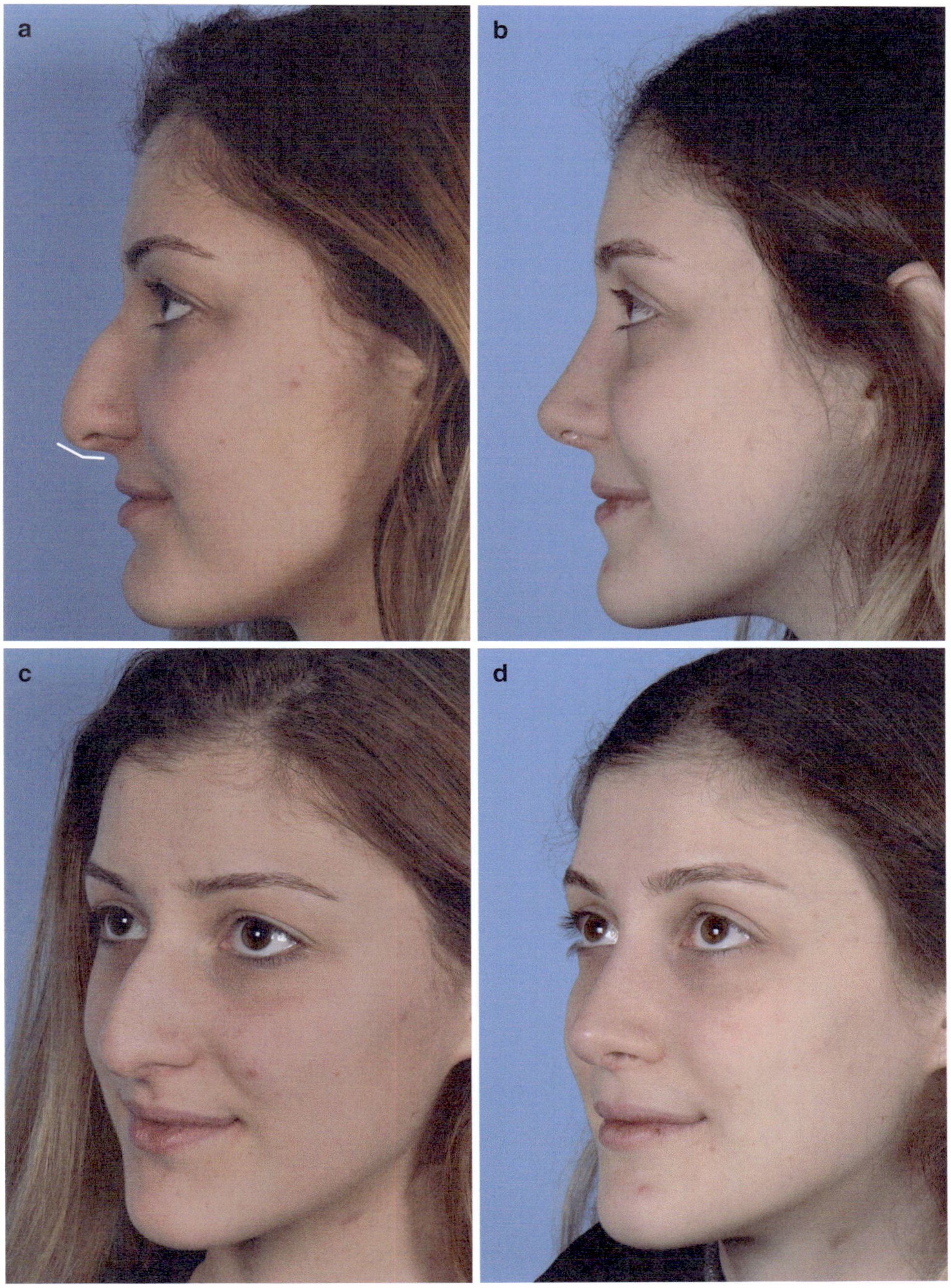

Fig. 11.59 (**a–d**) Analysis of 4-year postoperative photographs confirmed that the appropriate surgical technique, i.e., COST technique, was chosen in this case

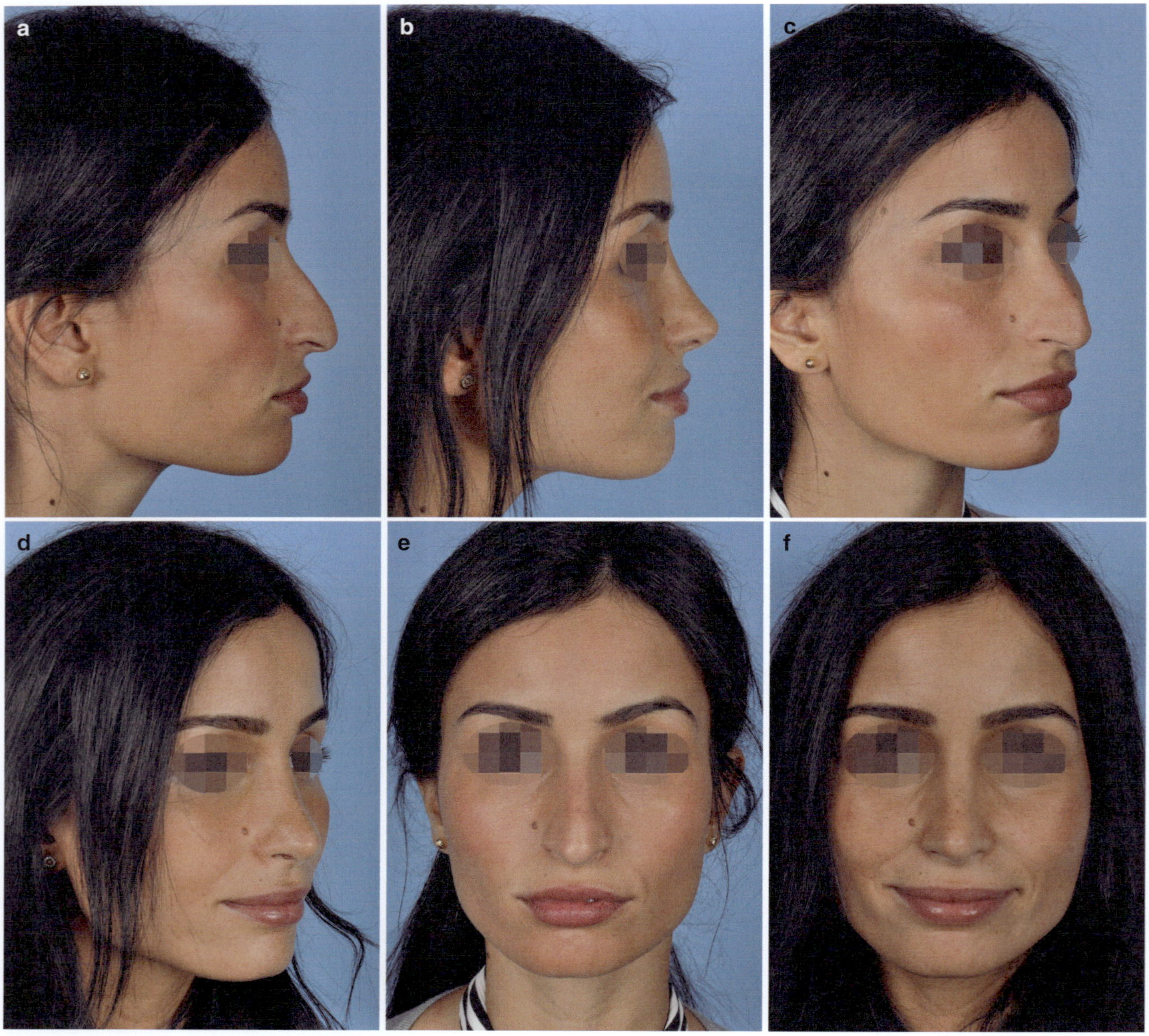

Fig. 11.60 (**a–f**) Preoperative and postoperative photographs. COST technique was applied while medial crural overlap corrected the disfiguration of middle/medial crural complex, steal suture increased the tip rotation

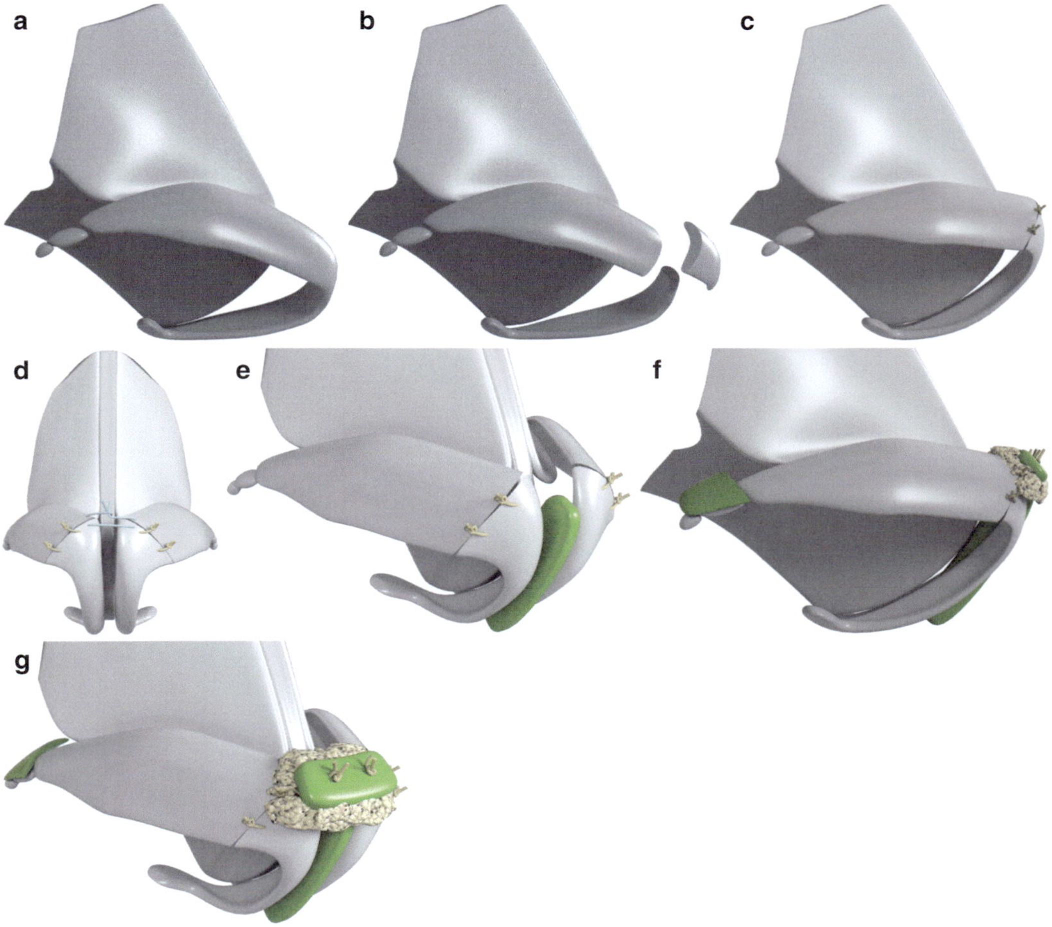

Fig. 11.61 (**a**) The illustration shows a droopy nasal tip resulting from a long lateral crus. (**b, c**) Vertical resection of the excess part of lateral crura: end-to-end suture (reestablishment of alar arch). (**d–f**) Columellar strut dome-equalizing suture and, alar batten graft (stabilization of alar arch). (**g**) Definition provided by the cap and camouflage graft

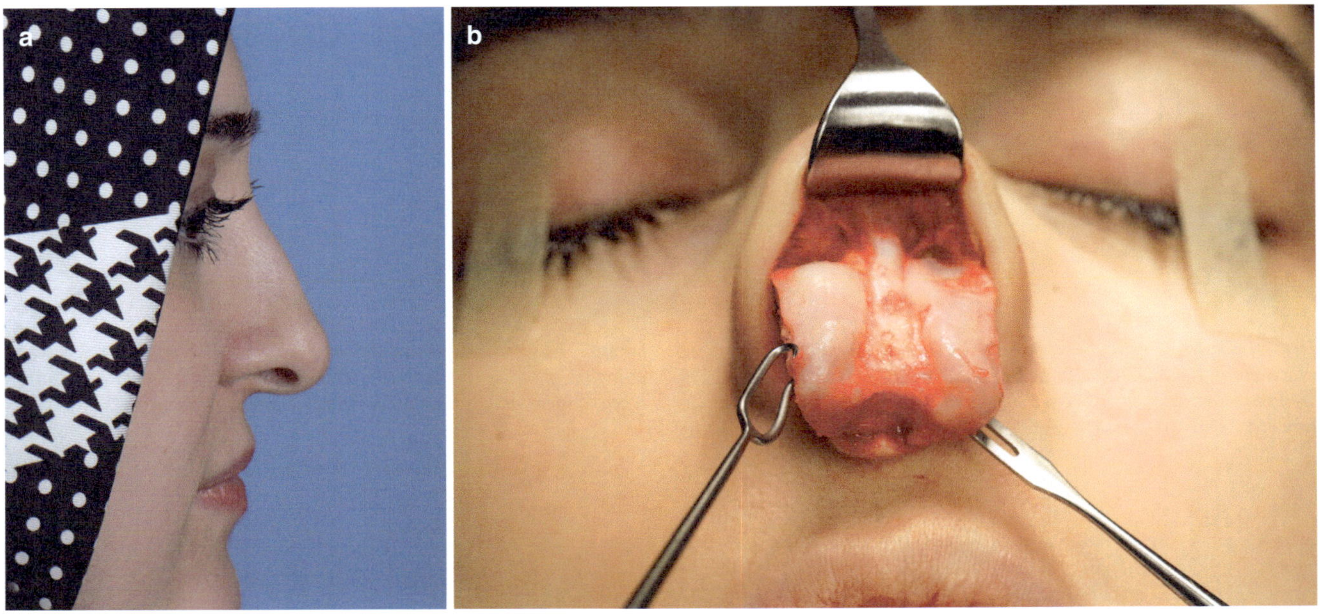

Fig. 11.62 (**a**, **b**) The lateral crura are both too long, causing a droopy tip, and too convex, resulting in a wide tip

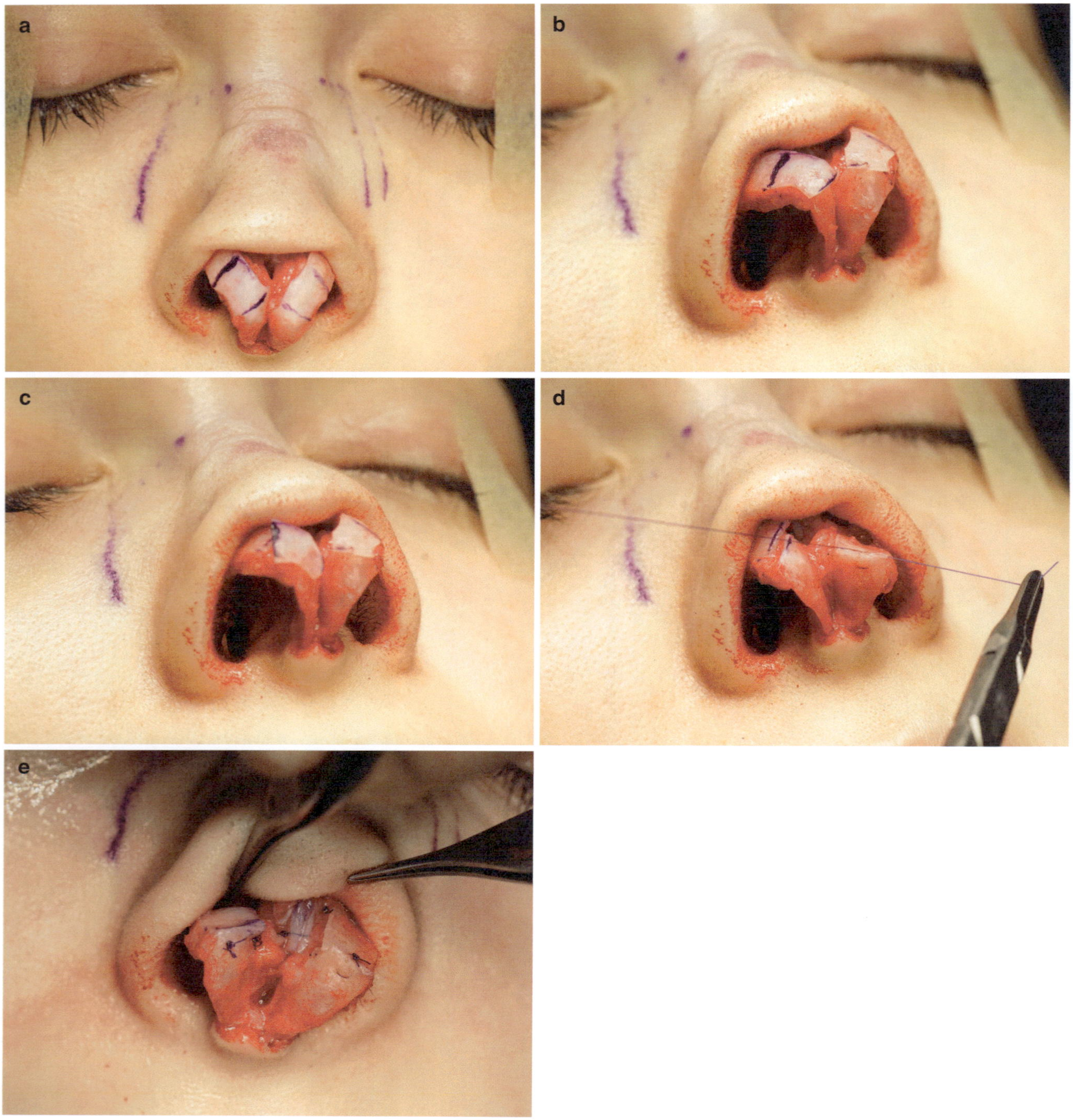

Fig. 11.63 (**a**) The segment to be excised was marked on the lateral crura. (**b**, **c**) An incision was made immediately next to the dome. The lateral crus was detached from the skin with resection of the excess portion. (**d**) The two stumps were approximated end-to-end by matrix suture. The caudal aspect of the lateral crus was averted upward when applying the matrix suture. (**e**) After bilateral suturing, the lateral crura were of ideal length relative to the alar cartilages

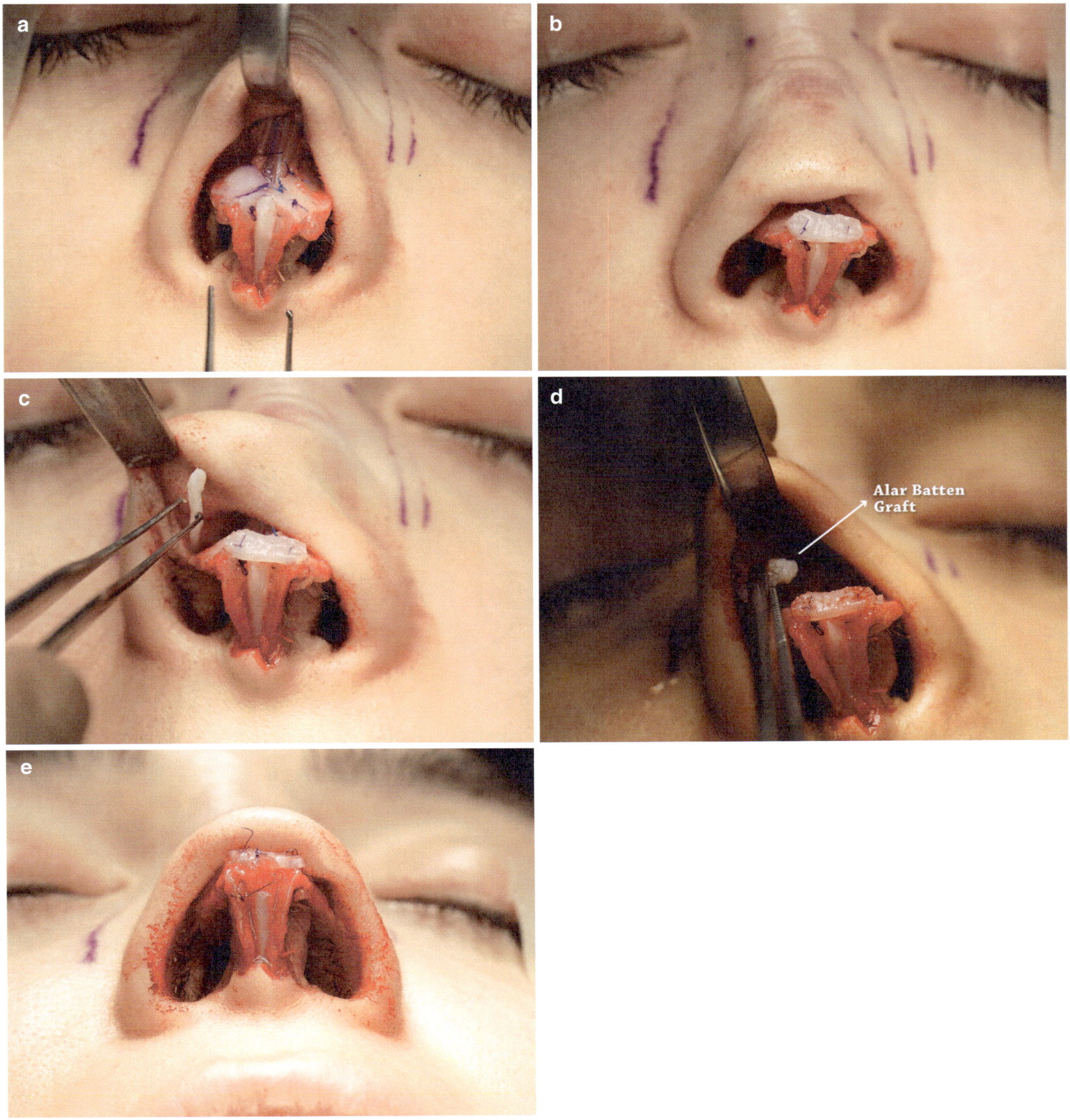

Fig. 11.64 (**a**) A stable tip was achieved using a columellar strut and dome-equalizing suture. (**b**) A cap graft provided both projection and definition. (**c**) The lateral crural graft was fixed bilaterally. (**d**) The excess portion of the cartilage trimmed from the lateral crus was used as an alar batten graft to support the lateral nasal wall. (**e**) The cap graft was camouflaged with crushed cartilage. The final enhanced tip anatomy can be seen in the photograph

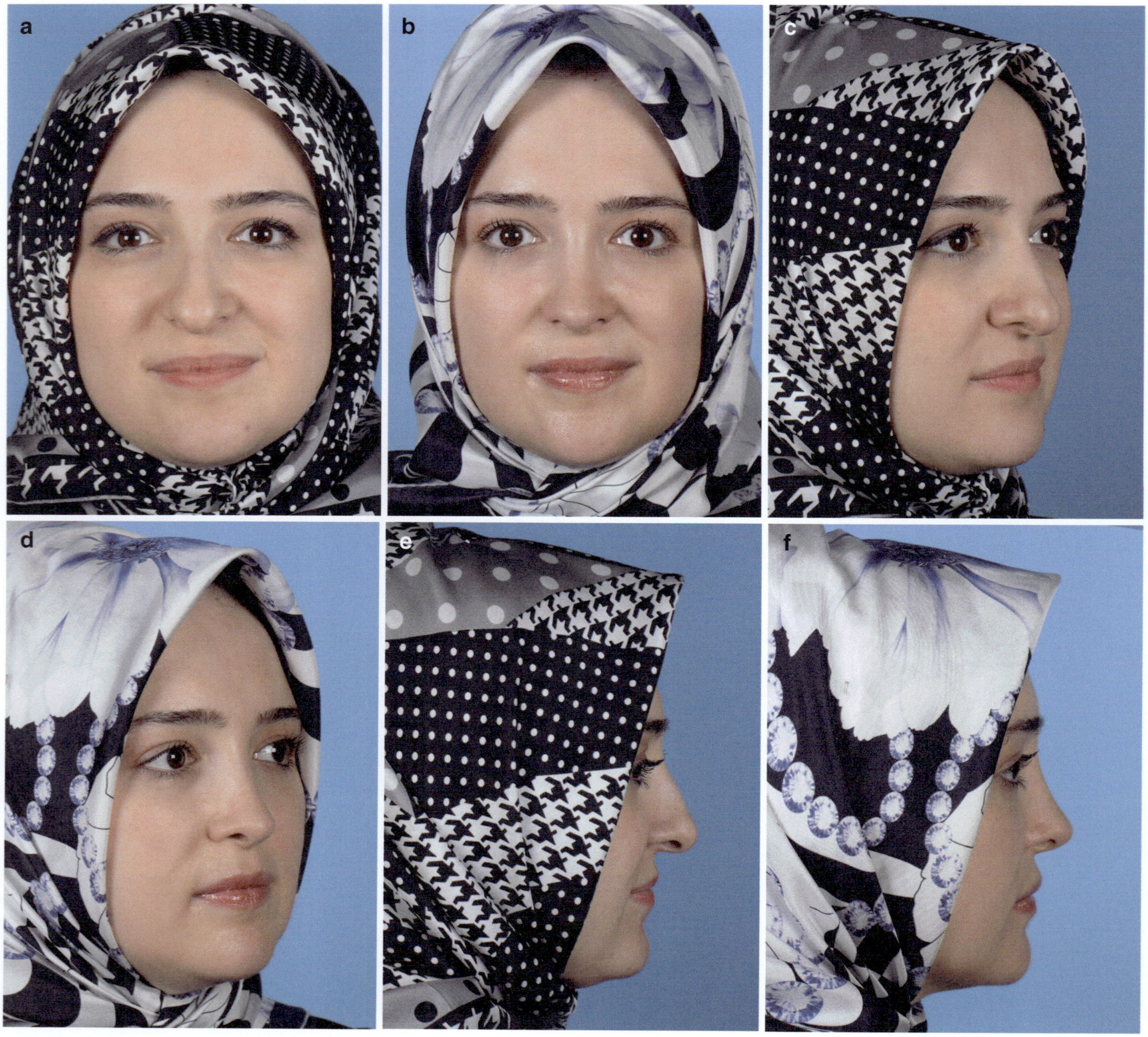

Fig. 11.65 (**a–f**) The VAR technique simultaneously provides solutions to the droopy nasal tip, wide tip, and tip asymmetry problems

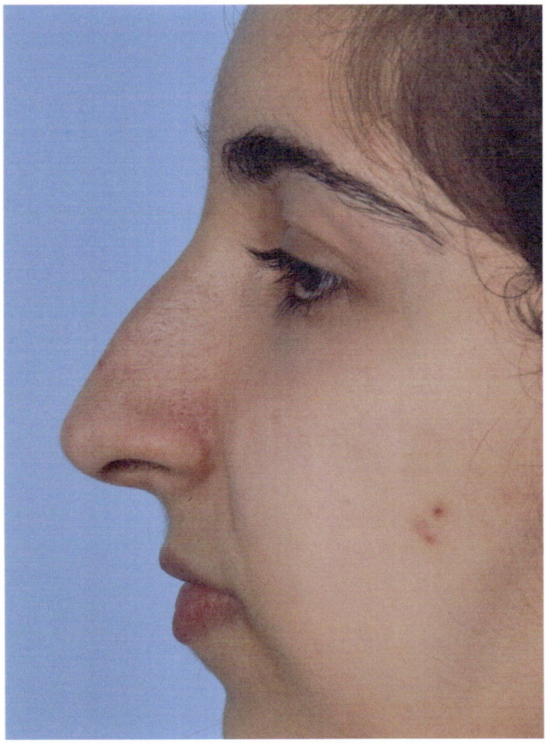

Fig. 11.66 Lateral view, droopy nasal tip

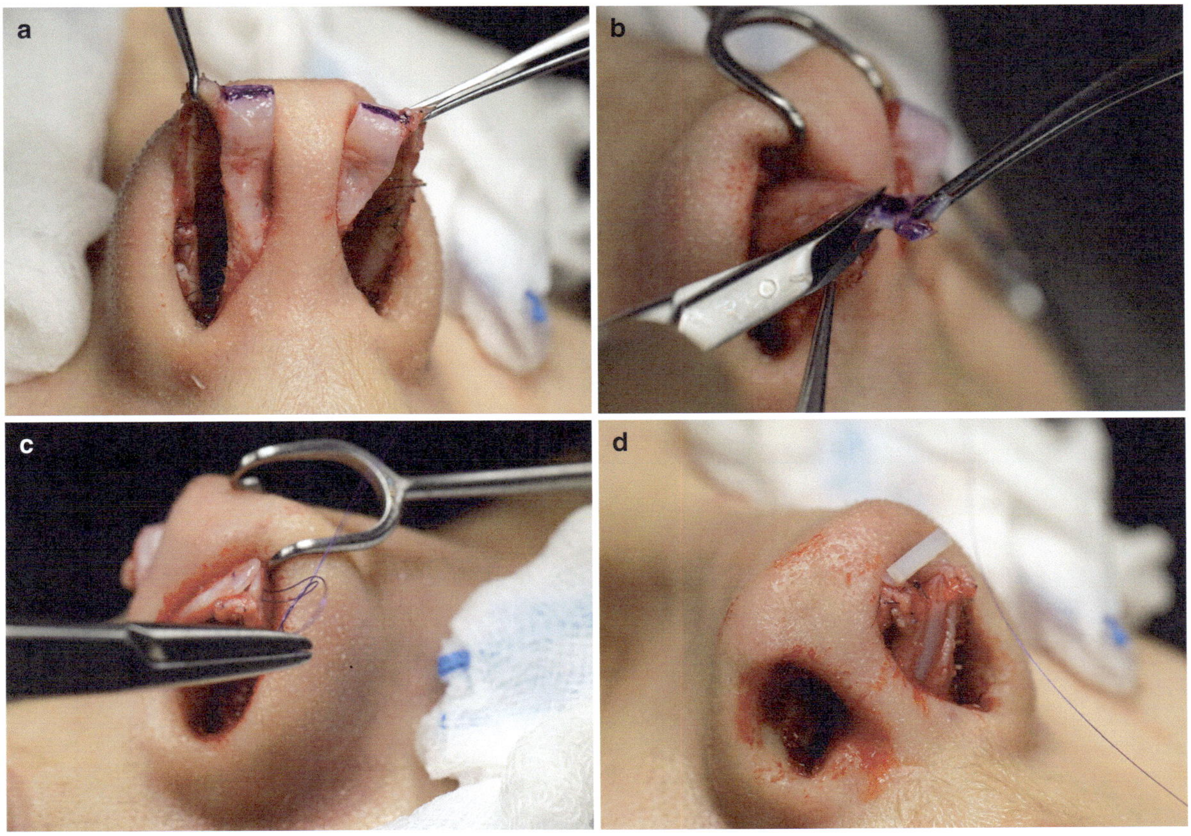

Fig. 11.67 (**a–d**) In the closed technique, the key to symmetrical resection is correct initial marking of the dome point. It is useful to suspend the alar arch simultaneously from each of the nostrils. To achieve the ideal lateral crural length, a resection of approximately 12 mm was performed in this case

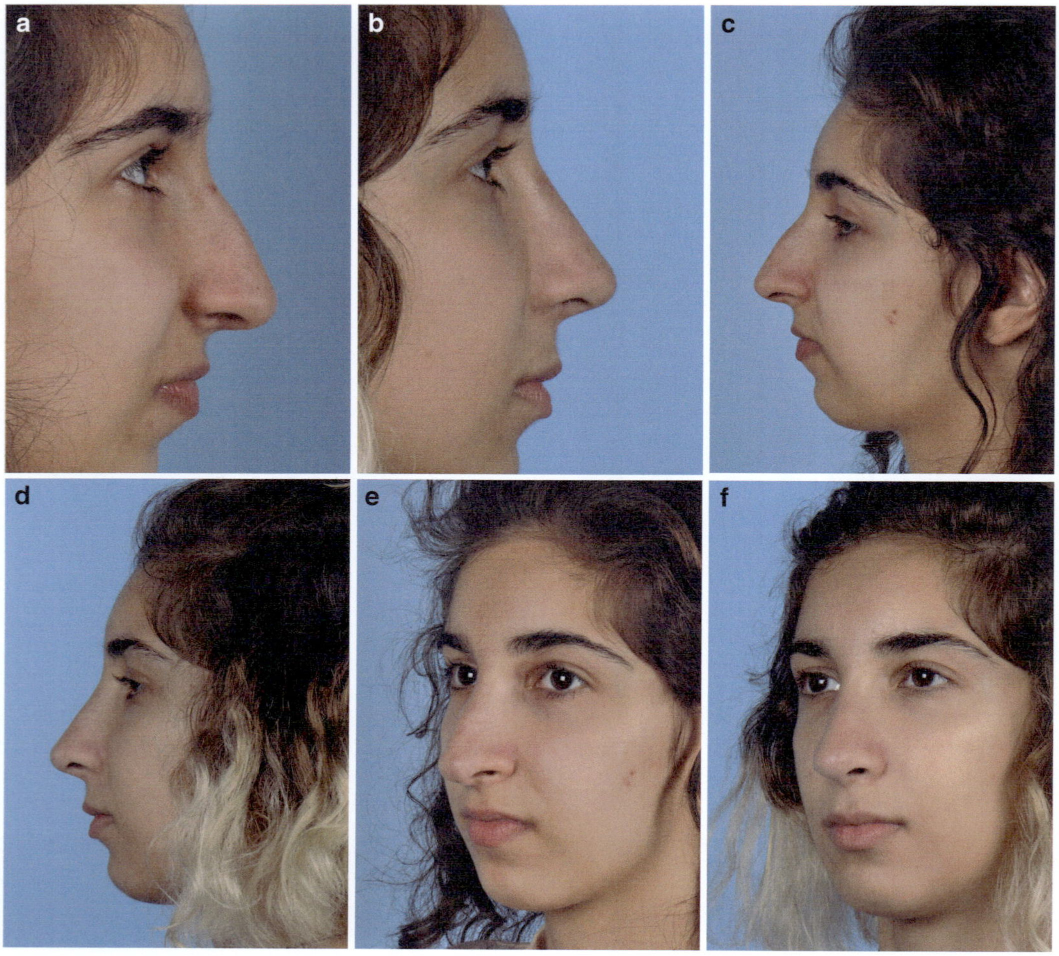

Fig. 11.68 (**a–f**) Comparison photographs of preoperative and 1-year appearance demonstrate correction of the droopy nasal tip, appropriate projection, and refinement of the tip

Fig. 11.69 The tip, evidently counter-rotated and over-projected, reveals excessive nostril, overdeveloped caudal septum, and thin skin

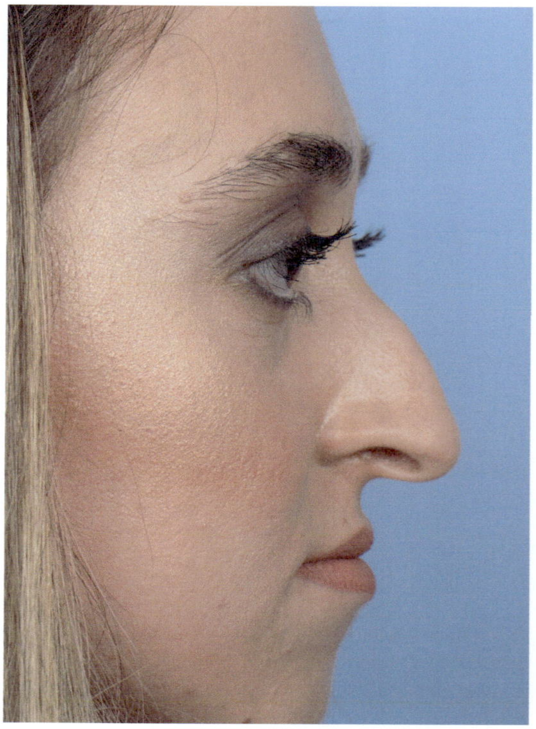

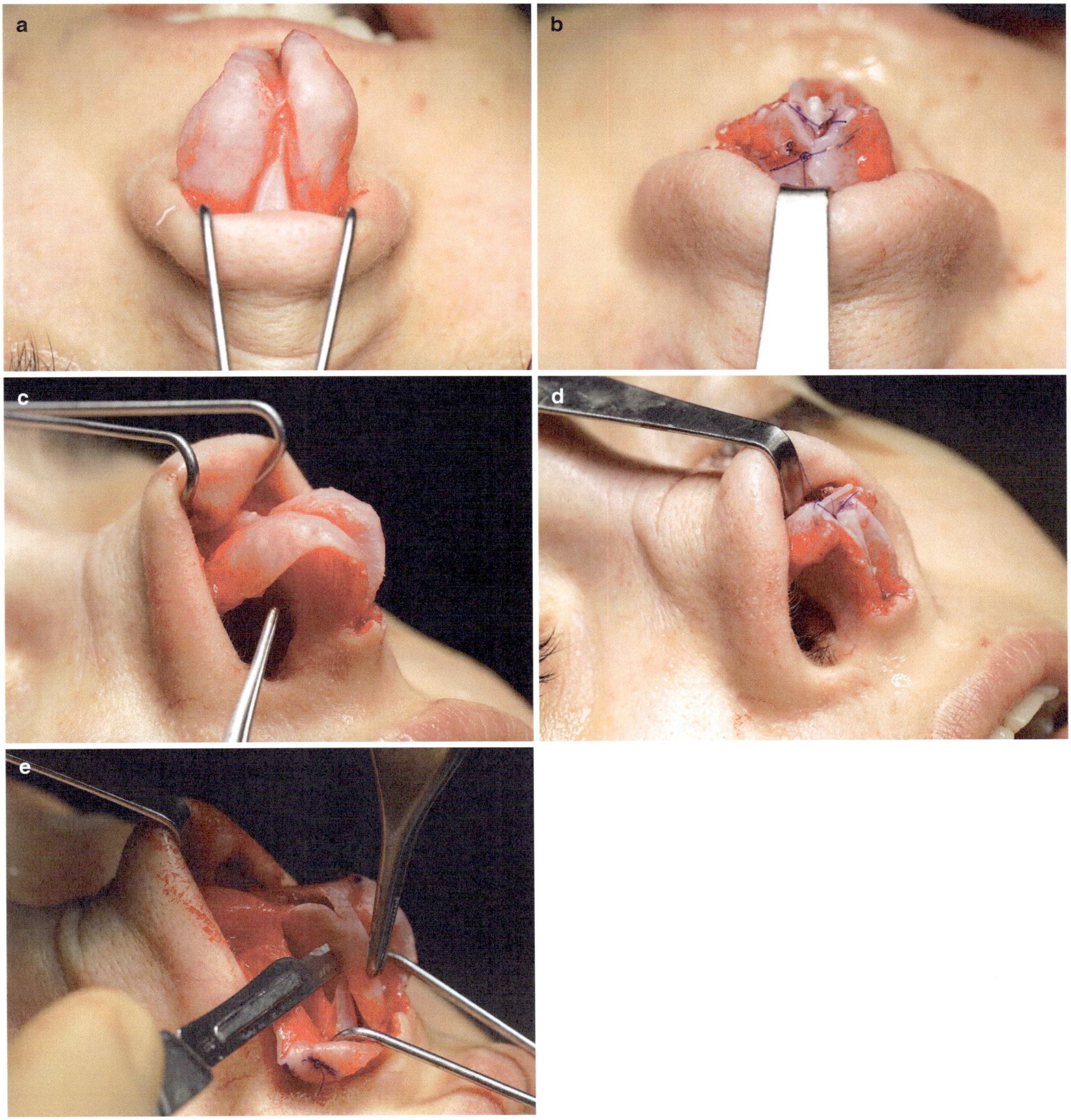

Fig. 11.70 (**a–e**) Following resection, the lateral crus was remarkably shortened. To restore the alar arch configuration, a resection of almost 15 mm was performed. Excess part of caudal septum that pushes the tip down was also resected

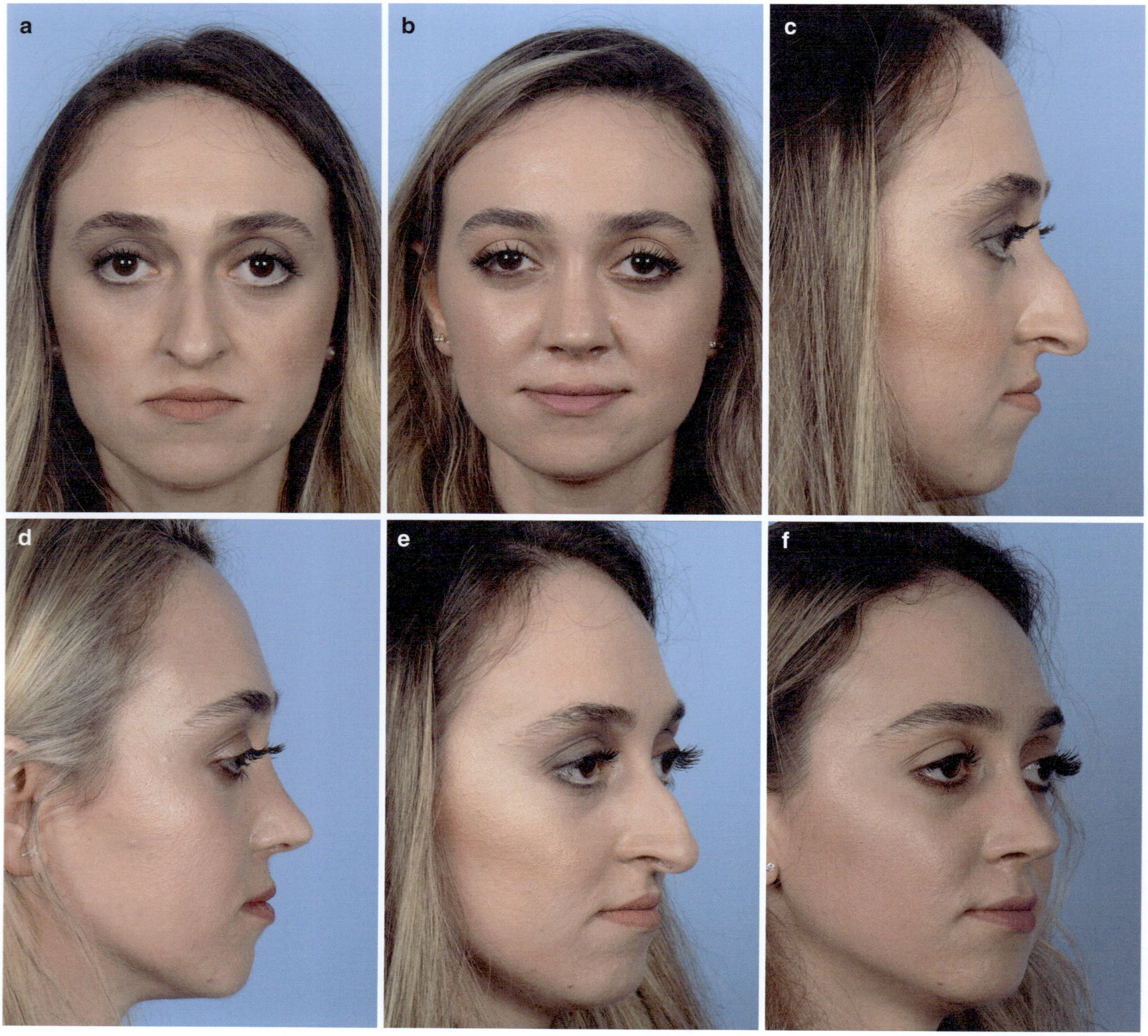

Fig. 11.71 (**a–f**) Postoperative photographs show increased tip rotation as well as deprojection of her tip to create a more balanced nose. Note the improvement of the nostril appearance and alar–columellar relationship

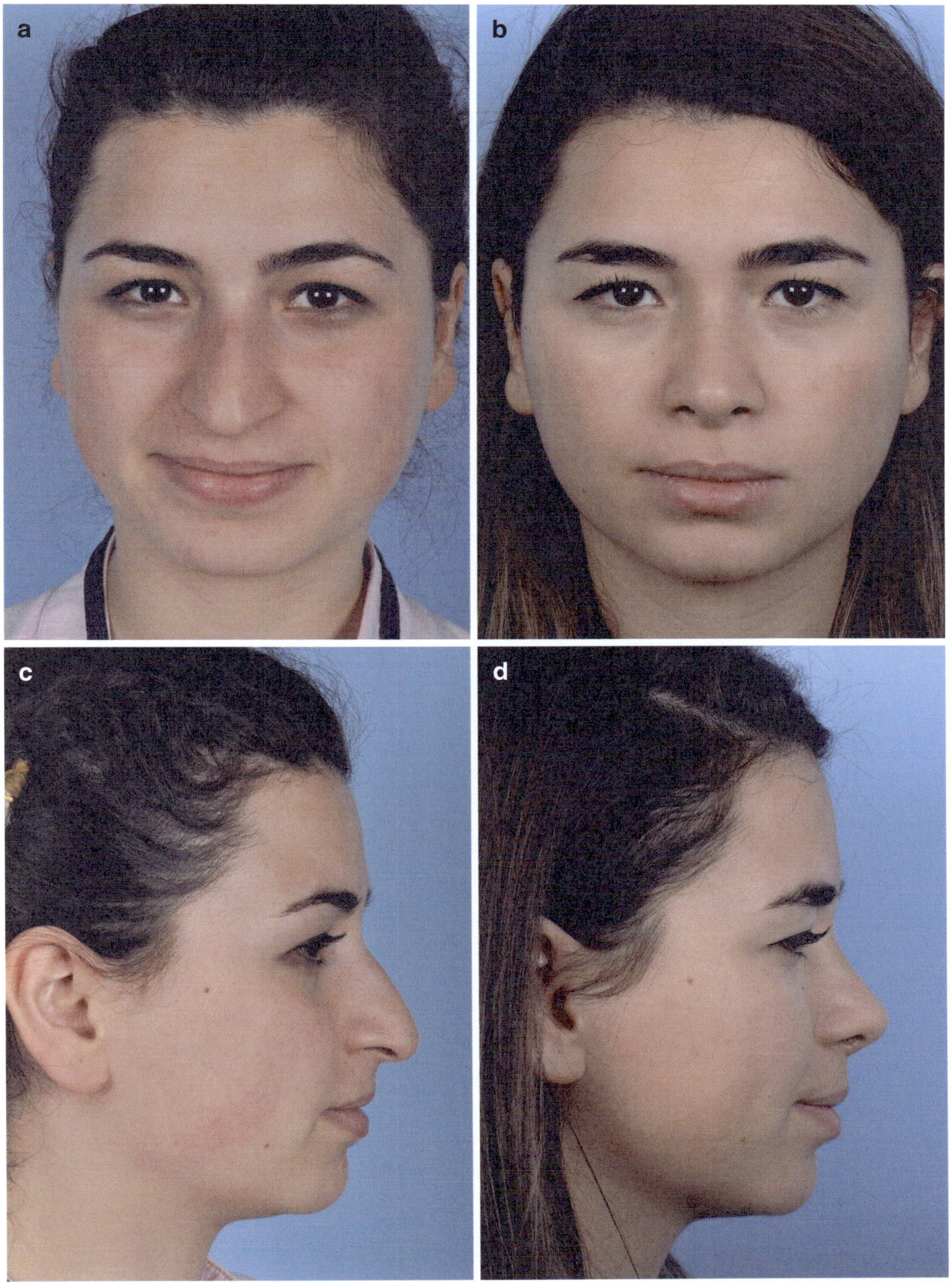

Fig. 11.72 (**a–d**) Open approach was done. Anterior septal angle was reduced. Lateral crura were shortened with vertical alar resection. A columellar strut, dome equalizing suture, cap graft, camouflage graft, alar batten graft, and septocolumellar suture were placed

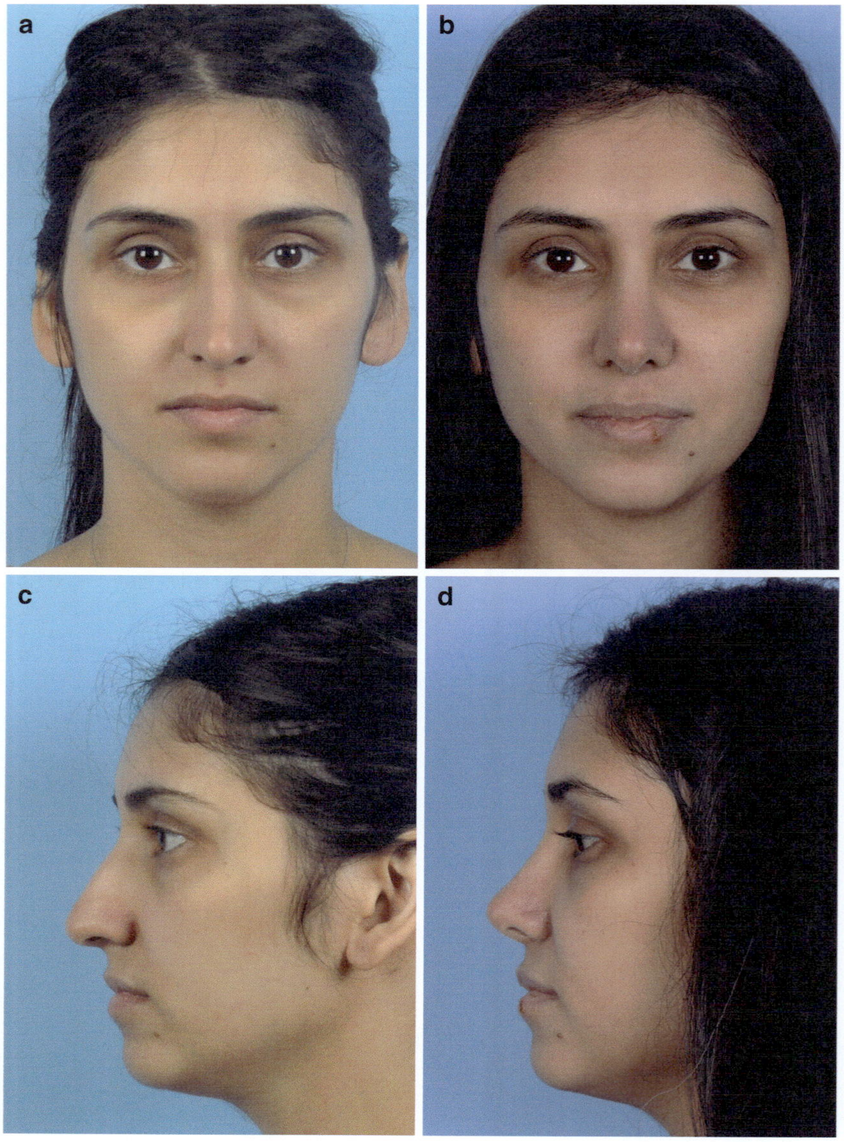

Fig. 11.73 (**a–d**) Patient with droopy nasal tip is shown pre- and 5-years postoperatively. She is pleased with the aesthetic result. Long-term result is very satisfactory

11.4 Malpositioned/Cephalically Oriented Lateral Crus

The axis of the ideal lateral crus must point the outer canthus toward the same side. Any deviation from the ideal position would be in the cephalic direction, causing different types of deformity depending on the degree of deviation. In the most advanced cases, the axis points toward the medial canthus, which is termed as a malpositioned or cephalically oriented lateral crus (Fig. 11.74).

A cephalically oriented lateral crus creates a propulsive force, pushing the tip inferiorly. If the weak medial crus cannot resist this force effectively, the tip will droop down. Droopy nasal tip resulting from a malpositioned lateral crus can be accompanied by weakness in the alar side wall, as well as alar retraction (Fig. 11.75).

11.4.1 Treatment of Malpositioned Lateral Crus

The key to treatment of a malpositioned crus is removal of and ideal repositioning of the cartilage. To perform this surgery successfully, the surgeon should ensure that the direction of the lateral crus is truly toward the medial canthus. If positioned between the medial canthus and the lateral canthus, there would be no need to change its position because other techniques, such as suture plasty, alar batten graft, and so on, would suffice.

A malpositioned lateral crus can be corrected by completely dissecting the crus from its original position, for placement into the pocket opened in its ideal position after separation from the attached tissues.

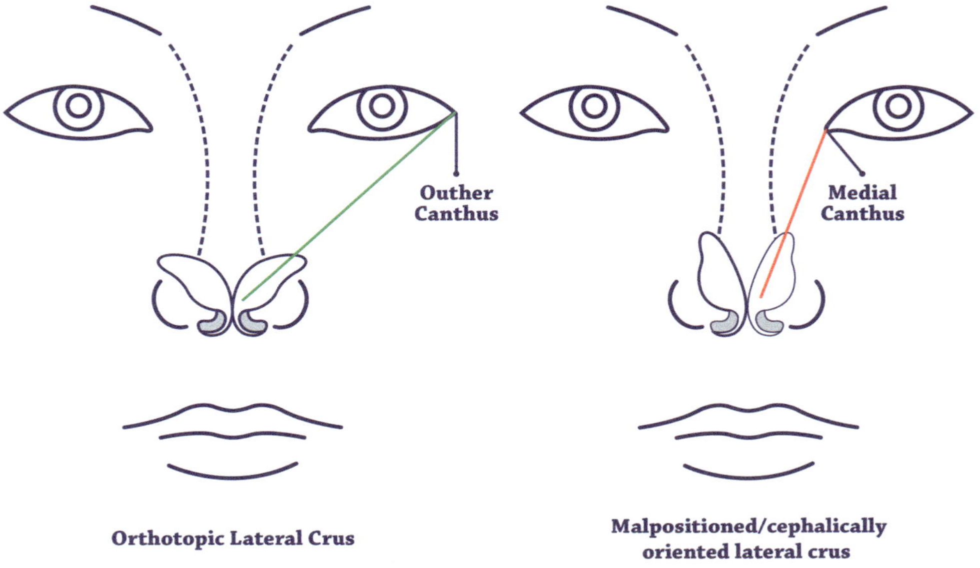

Fig. 11.74 Note the contrast between the normal lateral crus on the left and malpositioned one on the right

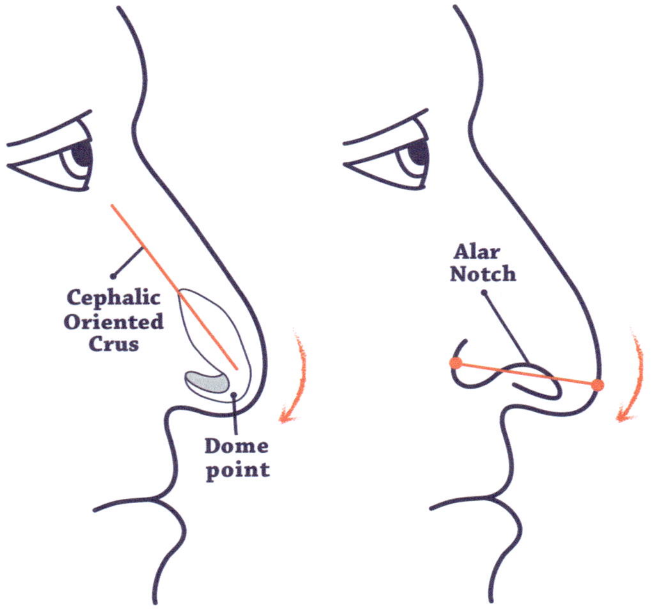

Fig. 11.75 The malpositioned lateral crura can move the domes caudally, thus the tip is positioned counter-rotated. Cephalic positioning of the lateral crus does not parallel the alar rim. Alar retraction and notch caused by a lack of support to the lateral position of the nostril

Before repositioning, the lateral crus must be reinforced by adding a straight cartilage beneath, or by lateral crural turn-in. In this way, the lateral crus becomes more resistant and surface issues, such as convexity or concavity, are resolved (lateral crural graft) (Fig. 11.76).

Technical Pearl: Auricular cartilage is not recommended to be used as a lateral crural graft.

How can we perform lateral crural repositioning? Let us examine the repositioning technique by way of an example.

11.4.1.1 Case 17

This patient has droopy nasal tip that stems from malpositioned lateral crura (Fig. 11.77).

A simple intraoperative test can be performed to check if there is true malposition. Both domes were pulled downward at the dome point by a double hook, creating a concavity at the lateral nasal wall pointing toward the medial canthus. Simultaneously, the cephalic edges of the lateral crura must appear parallel to each other from above (Fig. 11.78; Video 11.16).

The first step of surgery is to completely separate the lateral crus from the vestibular skin. Although some surgeons suggest performing an injection between the crus and the skin in advance to facilitate dissection, we feel that there is no need for such an injection. Also, starting dissection from the caudal aspect facilitates the procedure (Fig. 11.79).

Technical Pearl: The surgeon should not start the malpositioned cartilage surgery operation via cephalic resection.

The dissection must start at the dome point, and then progress to the point where the lateral crus extends to the apertura piriformis, followed by complete removal of the crus. The surgeon must then check whether the lateral crus has sufficient strength and length before the operation proceeds to the second step.

In the second step, the lateral crus is cut with a scalpel from its midpoint all the way through, avoiding a full-fold cut, and then turned-in and fixed at four points with absorbable sutures. The portion remaining under the fold behaved like a lateral crural graft. We thus achieve a strong lateral crus, with no superficial problems, ready for placement in its new position (Fig. 11.80).

The third step is to identify the dome point, which should not be in its previous position but rather on the lateral crus, because the medial crus was short in this case. The columella

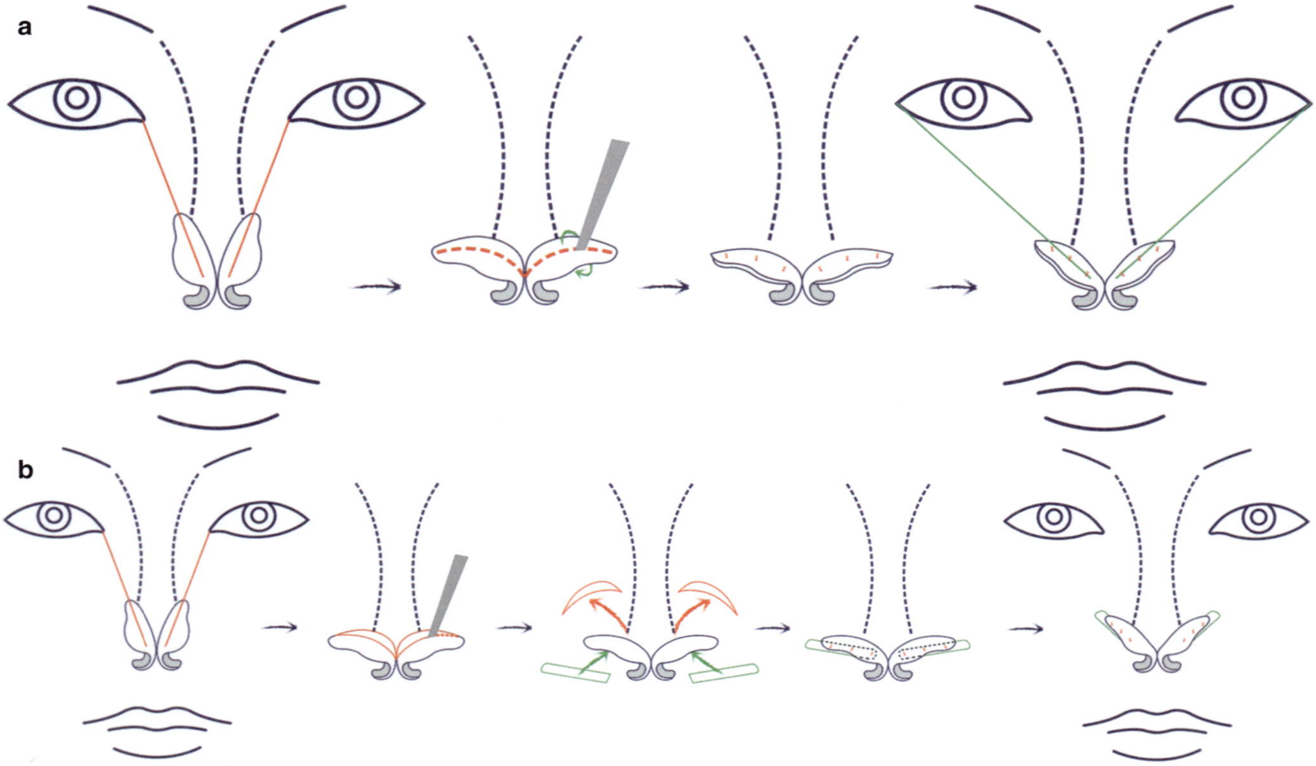

Fig. 11.76 (**a**) In primary cases, lateral crural turn-in would mostly serve this purpose. (**b**) In revision cases, septum or costal cartilage graft would be the appropriate choice (lateral crural graft)

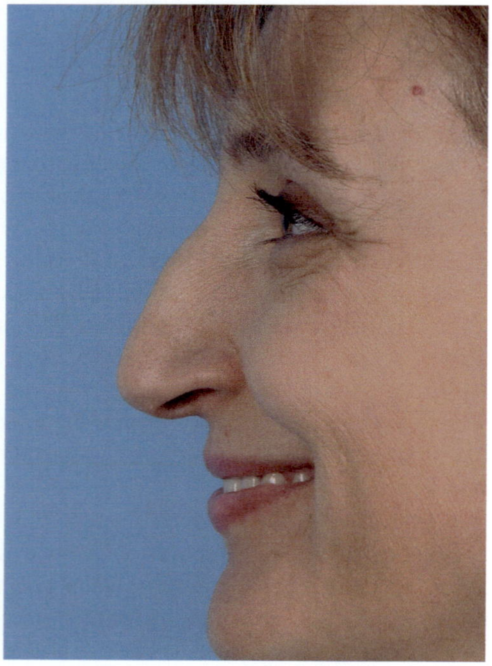

Fig. 11.77 Droopy nasal tip with thick skin

was lengthened by creating a new dome on, and stealing from, the lateral crus. This increased the rotation and projection of the tip. The suture was a standard matrix dome suture (Fig. 11.81).

In the fourth step, the new position of the lateral crus was identified. Using dissection scissors, a small pocket was opened on the footprint of the outer canthus, and the crus was inserted inside (Fig. 11.82).

Technical Pearl: The pocket should not be too large, and should be fashioned in such a way that the crus can be well-accommodated.

The fifth step was to apply the septocolumellar suture, providing stability and symmetry at the nasal base.

In every case undergoing repositioning surgery, the newly created tip should be fixed at the septum to ensure that it does not lose projection or rotation in the long term.

Septocolumellar suture would suffice in the majority of cases. The suture may be ineffective in thick-skinned or older patients, where it may be necessary to use a septocolumellar strut or septal extension graft.

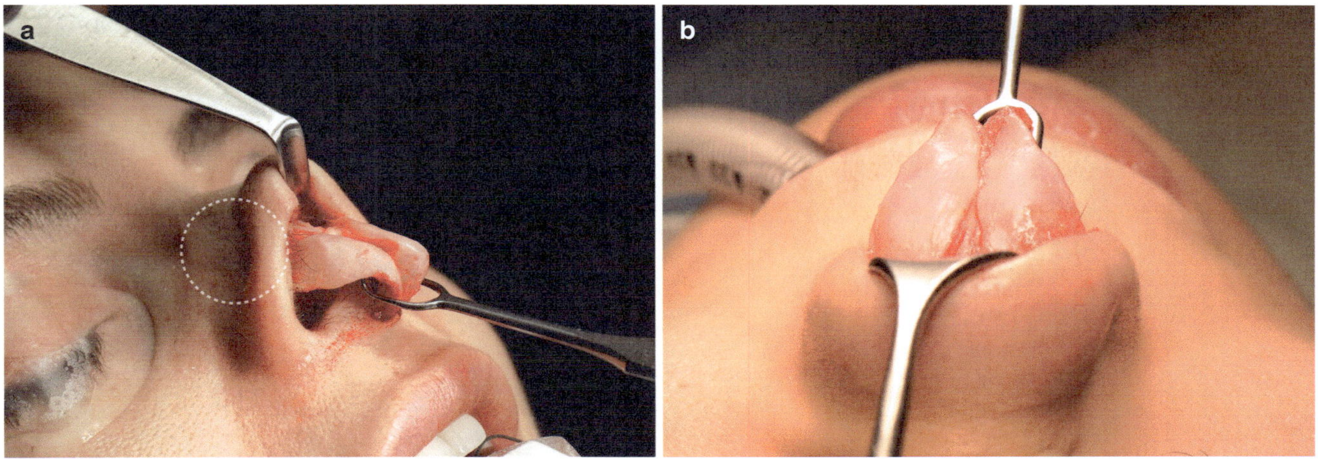

Fig. 11.78 (**a**, **b**) Typical intraoperative findings of malposed lateral crura

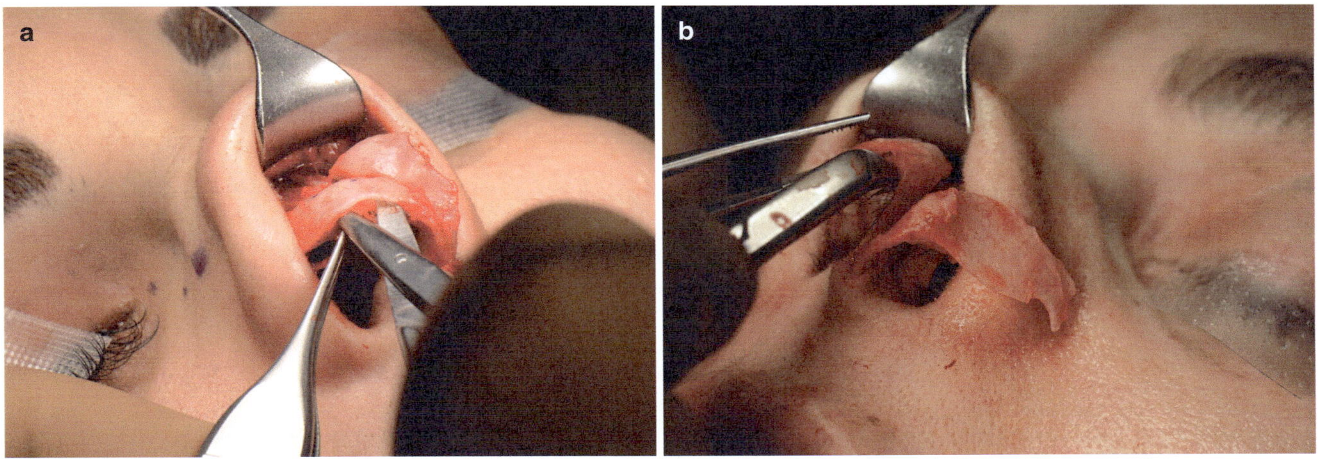

Fig. 11.79 (**a**, **b**) Lateral crura dissected from vestibular skin

Finally, if there is any need for extra projection and/or definition, a cap graft may be added (Fig. 11.83).

Two-year postoperative photographs show that correcting the position of the lateral crus solved not only the droopy tip, but also the wide tip (Fig. 11.84).

11.4.1.2 Case 18

Figure 11.85 shows lateral and intraoperative views of another patient with a droopy nasal tip (Video 11.17). Observation of the lateral crura parallel to each other sufficed for diagnosis of a malpositioned crus. Repositioning corrected both the droopy nasal tip and the disturbed alar–columellar relationship.

Two years after the repositioning surgery, the nasal tip had a completely restored appearance and excessive columellar show had improved (Fig. 11.86).

A septal extension graft can also be considered for long-term tip stability in very thick-skinned patients, and in those with an extremely droopy nasal tip. Although septal extension grafts are rarely preferred in our practice, they can still be used in selected patients. The graft prepared from the septum in a rectangular shape was sutured onto the caudal septum, overlapping three-fourths of the graft size. It was then sutured by bringing its free edge and the two media crura together, creating a strong connection between the tip and the septum (Fig. 11.87).

11.4.1.3 Case 19

Here, we analyze a thick-skinned patient with malpositioned lateral crus. The lateral crura appeared parallel in the intraoperative view, leading to a typical malpositioned appearance (Fig. 11.88).

The main maneuver was lateral crural repositioning, but due to skin thickness another technique was needed for more stabilization. Three quarters of the septal extension graft was fixed at the caudal aspect of the septum, whereas the free edge was fixed at the middle medial crus complex (Fig. 11.89).

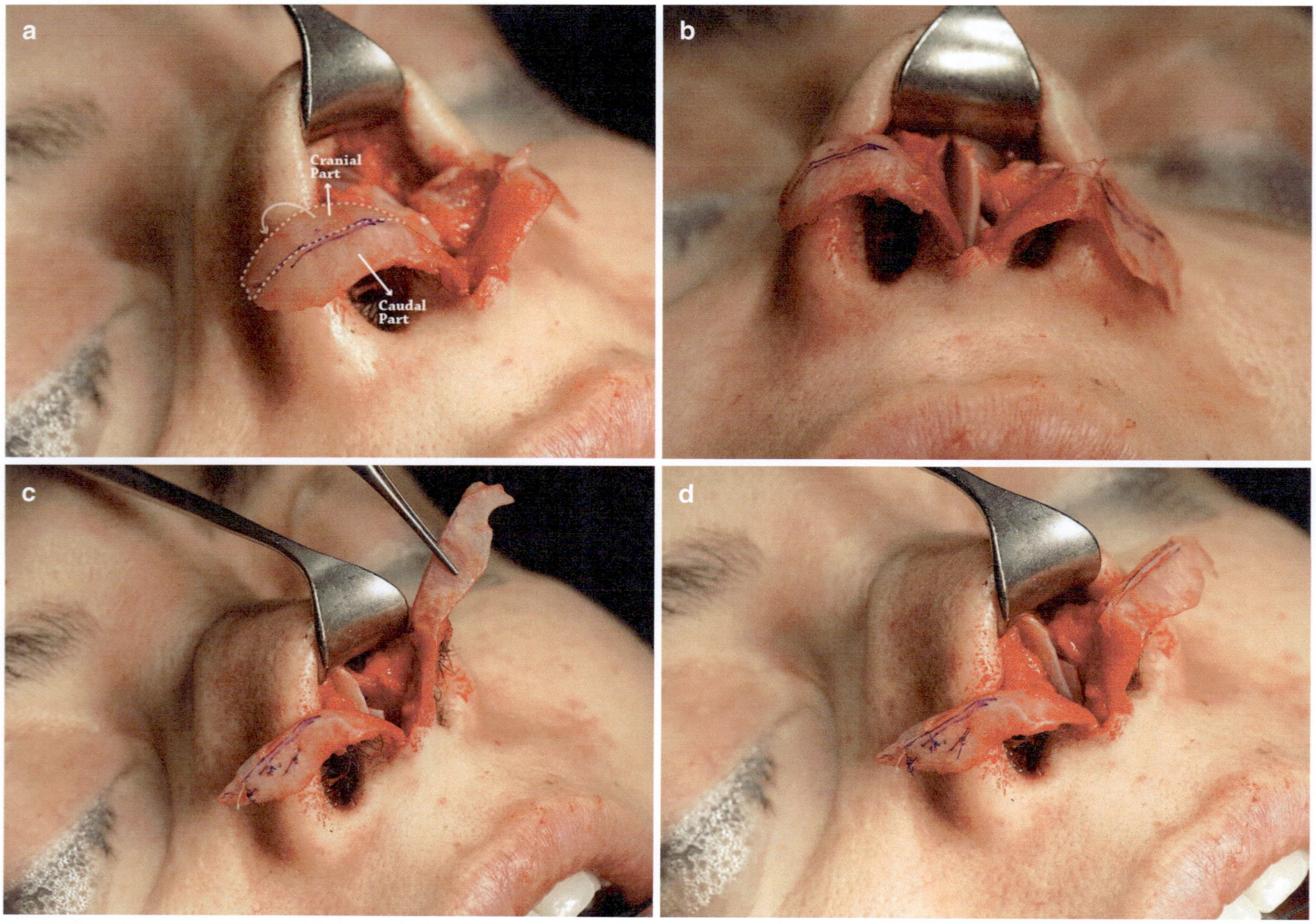

Fig. 11.80 (**a–d**) The lateral crus of the lower lateral cartilage is subdivided into two segments, a caudal and a cranial. The caudal should be the main component of the lateral crus, and its width must be around 6–8 mm. The cranial turn-in flap is created. Then the flap is secured with two to three 5–0 absorbable sutures, with the knot placed above the surface of the caudal part

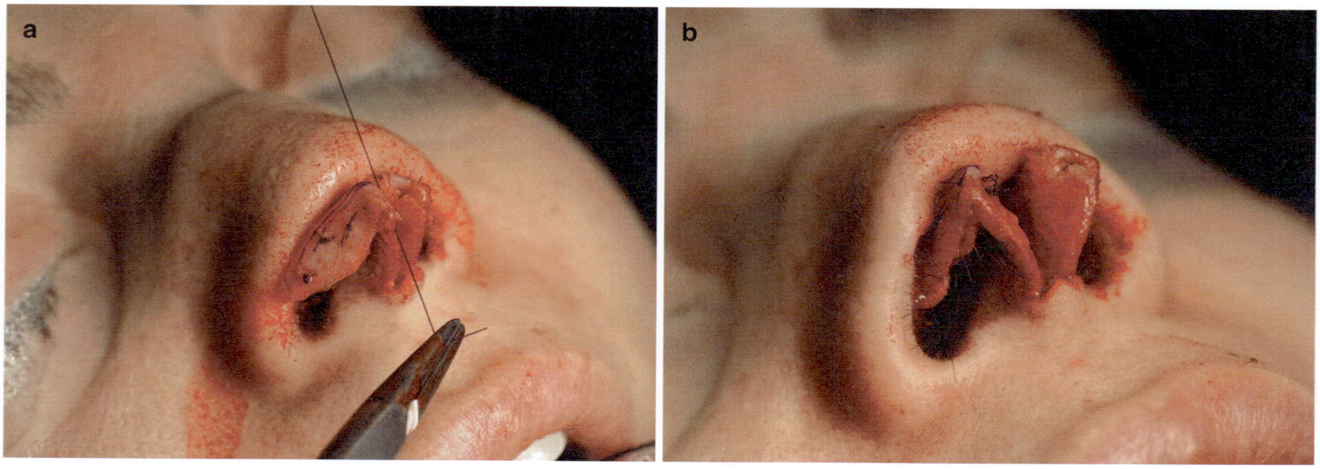

Fig. 11.81 (**a**, **b**) The new domes are formed by transdomal suture

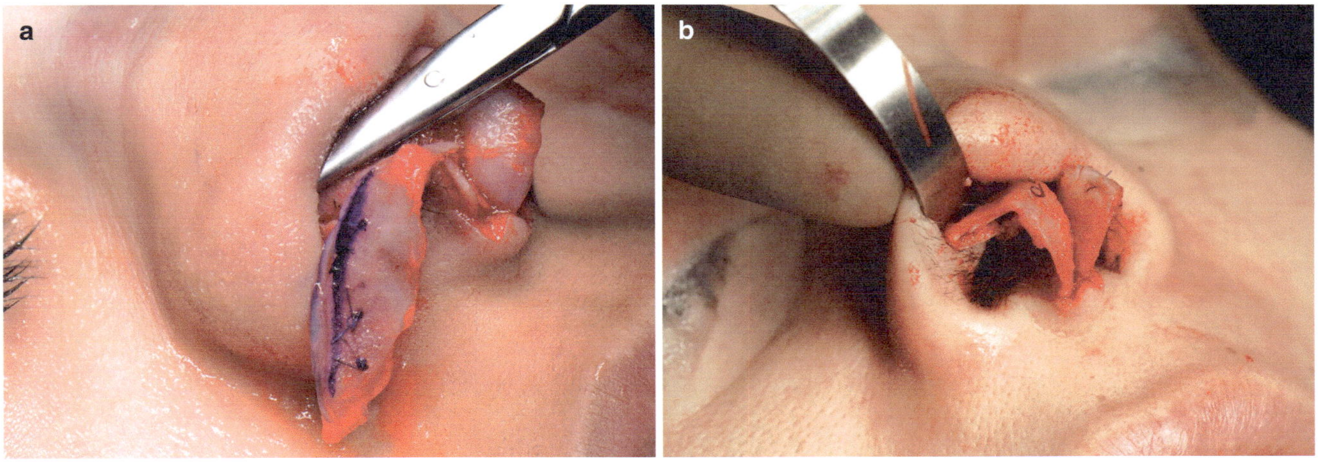

Fig. 11.82 (**a**, **b**) Placement of lateral crura into caudally dissected pockets

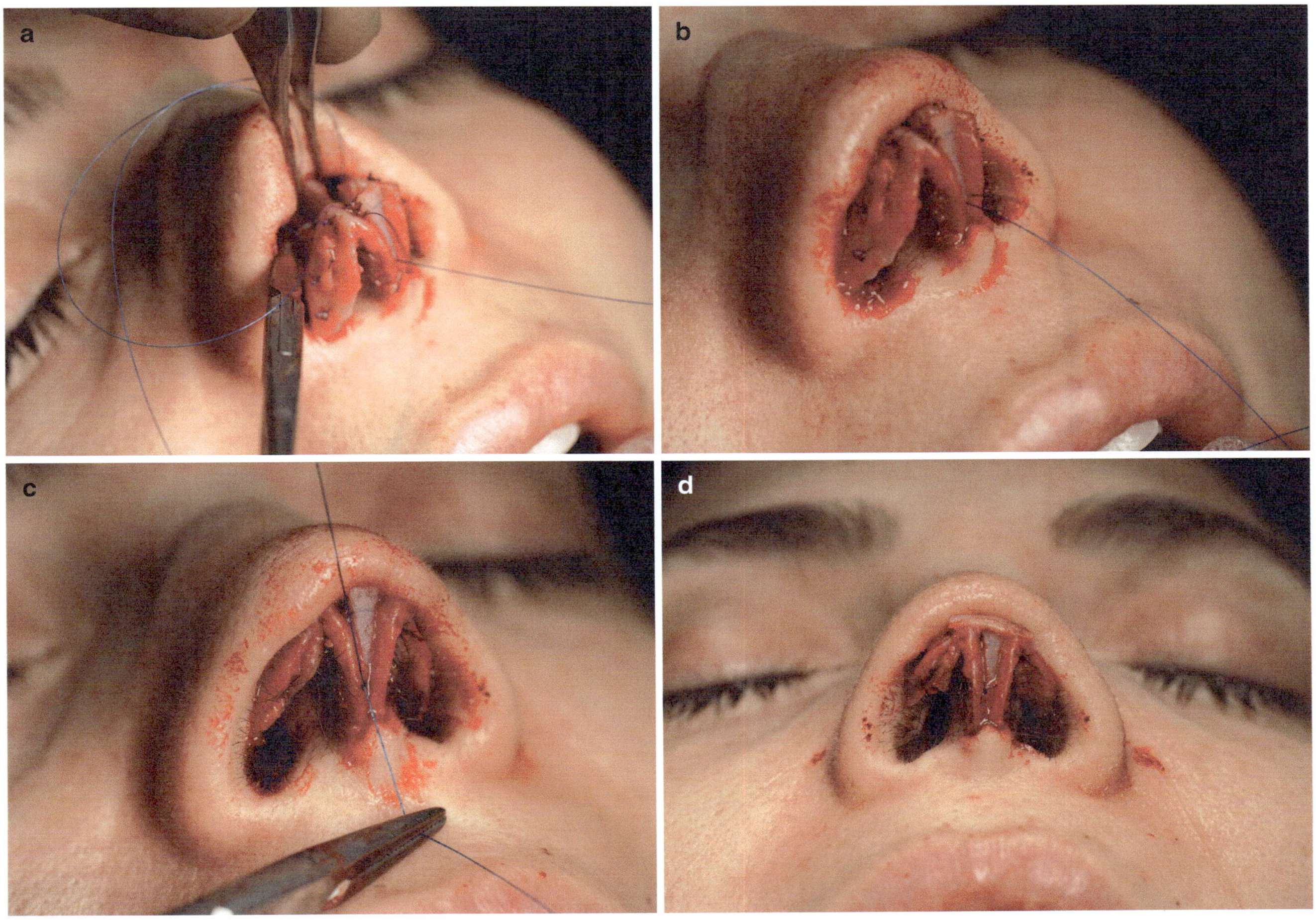

Fig. 11.83 (**a–d**) Placement of septocolumellar suture. Onlay tip graft placed horizontally over dome

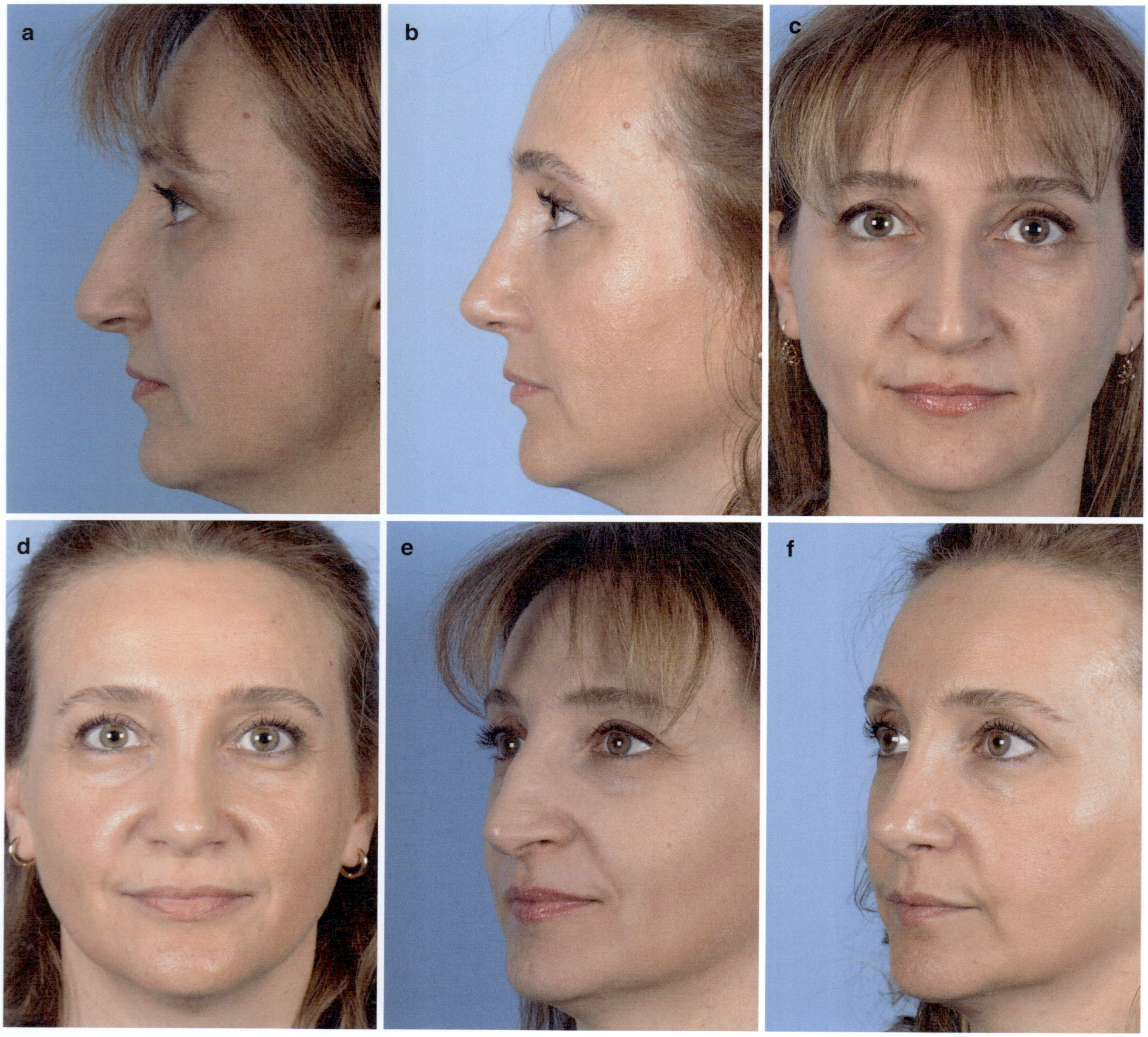

Fig. 11.84 (**a**, **b**) In profile, the tip rotation has been improved, the dorsum is refined, and there is some persistent supra tip fullness. (**c**, **d**) Postoperatively, the nose appears shorter because of the rotation of the nasal tip. (**e**, **f**) Postoperatively, the change in location of the lateral crus has provided a more aesthetic appearance of the alar sidewall and alar rim

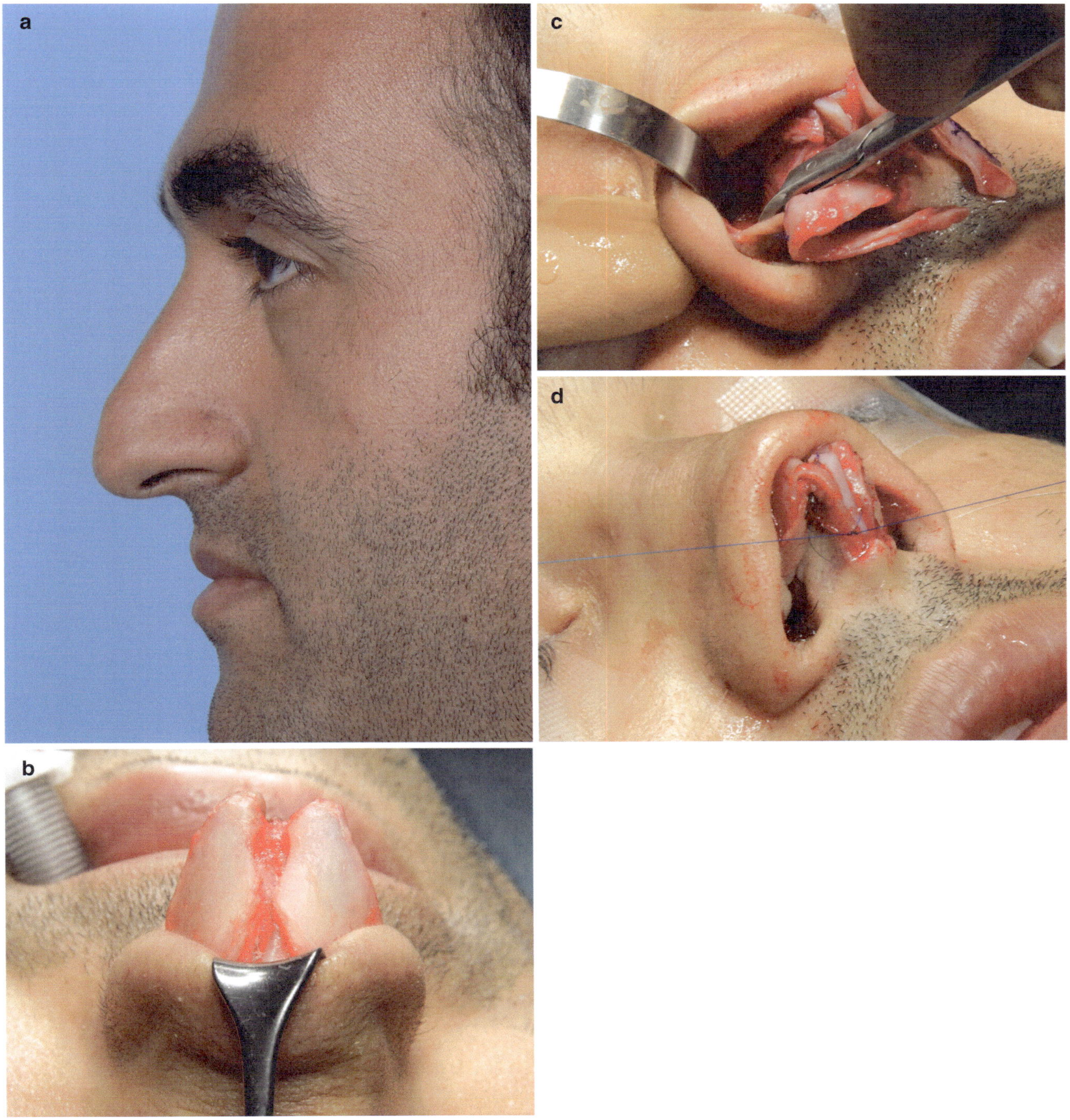

Fig. 11.85 (**a**) Preoperative lateral view, demarcating the borders of the alar cartilage is seen. This boundary is referred to as a malpositioned lateral crus and is associated with a droopy tip deformity. (**b**) Typical intraoperative finding of cephalically oriented lateral crura, each lateral crus almost parallel the other. (**c**, **d**) Creation of a caudally positioned pocket and placement of newly formed lateral crus into the pocket. Septocolumellar suture for extra stabilization of the tip

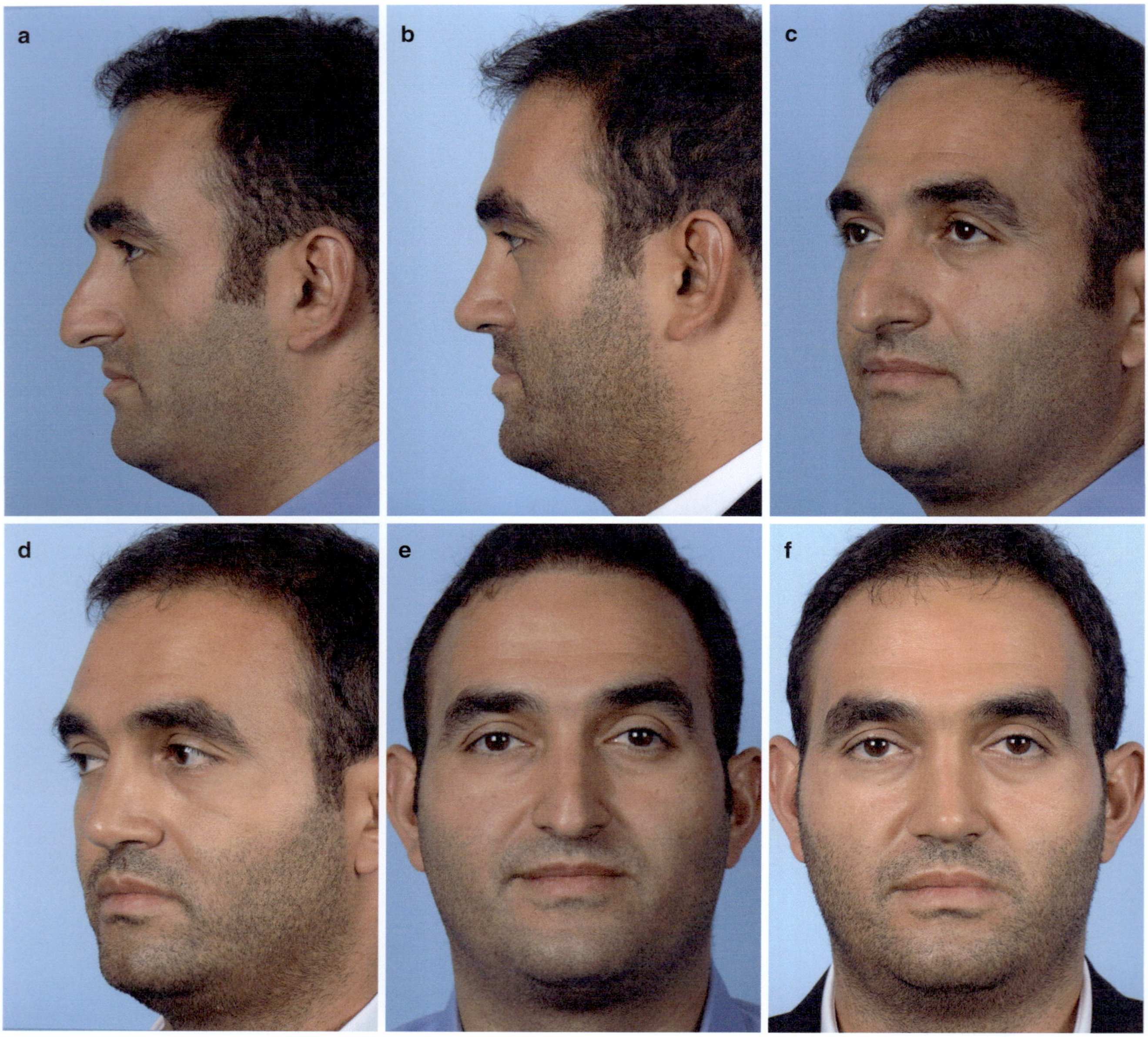

Fig. 11.86 (a–f) The droopy tip was improved with reposition surgery

Any deficiency in the pre-maxillary area may cause the tip to appear droopy, as discussed earlier in this chapter. This case presented with pre-maxillary deficiency. A pre-maxillary graft was used to resolve the problem. A graft prepared from the septum was used to fill the pre-maxilla (Fig. 11.90).

Photographs taken 2 years postoperatively showed improvement of the droopy tip (Fig. 11.91).

In previously operated patients, a persistent droopy tip may result from a malpositioned lateral crus. In addition, the lateral crus may become deformed due to surgery. In such cases, either septum or costal cartilage could be used for lateral crural grafting.

In the next case, we will look at the typical one.

11.4.1.4 Case 20

Here, we examine the profile view of this patient, who was previously operated by another surgeon. A retracted alar accompanying the droopy nasal tip allowed the malpositioned lateral crus pathology to be pinpointed (Fig. 11.92).

Repositioning surgery was applied in this patient with a malpositioned crus (Fig. 11.93).

Photographs of this patient at 1 year after repositioning surgery of the septal cartilage showed improvement at the droopy nasal tip (Fig. 11.94).

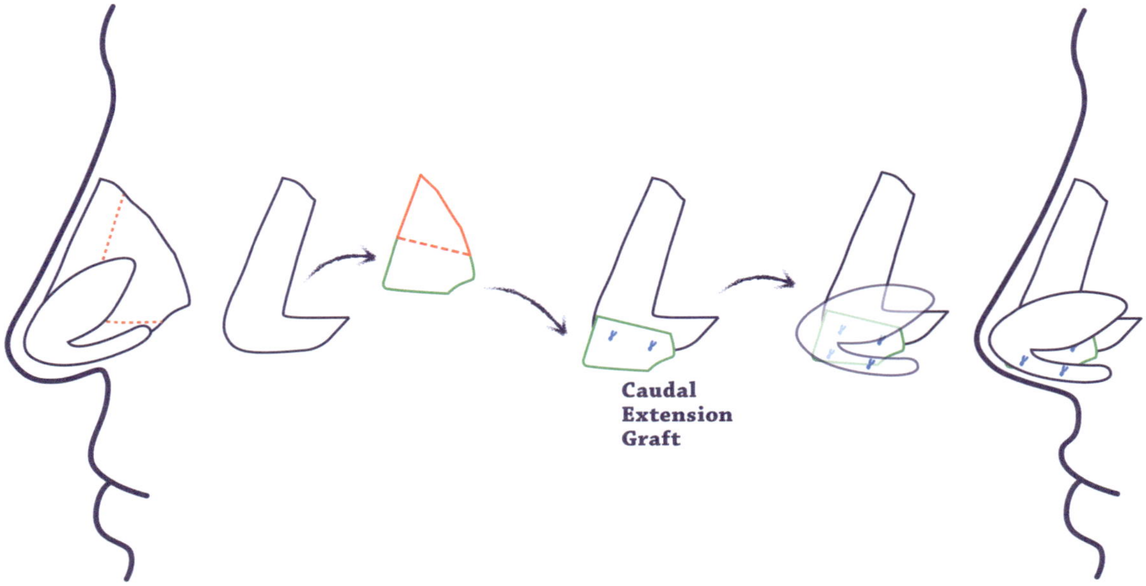

Fig. 11.87 The septal extension graft is harvested from the septum and then affixed to the caudal septum and the medial crura with adequate force to maintain nasal tip support

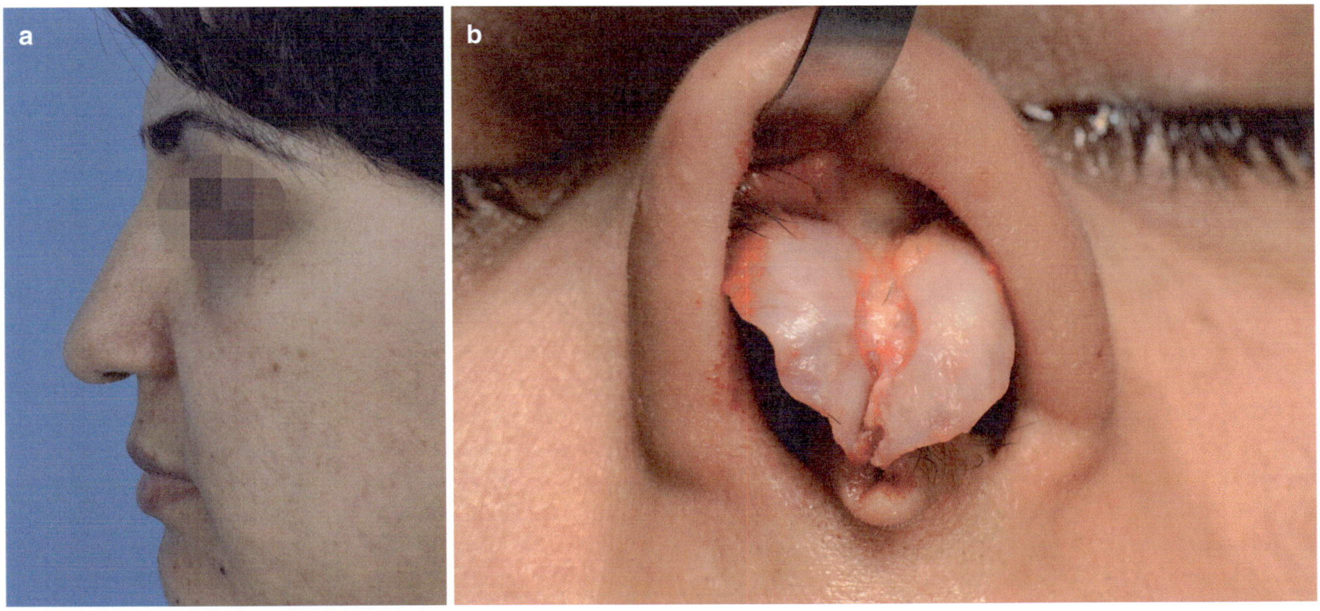

Fig. 11.88 (**a**, **b**) Droopy nasal tip with heavy skin. Droopy appearance is mostly caused by malpositioned lateral crura with a lack of supporting caudal septal structure. Premaxillary deficiency also contributes

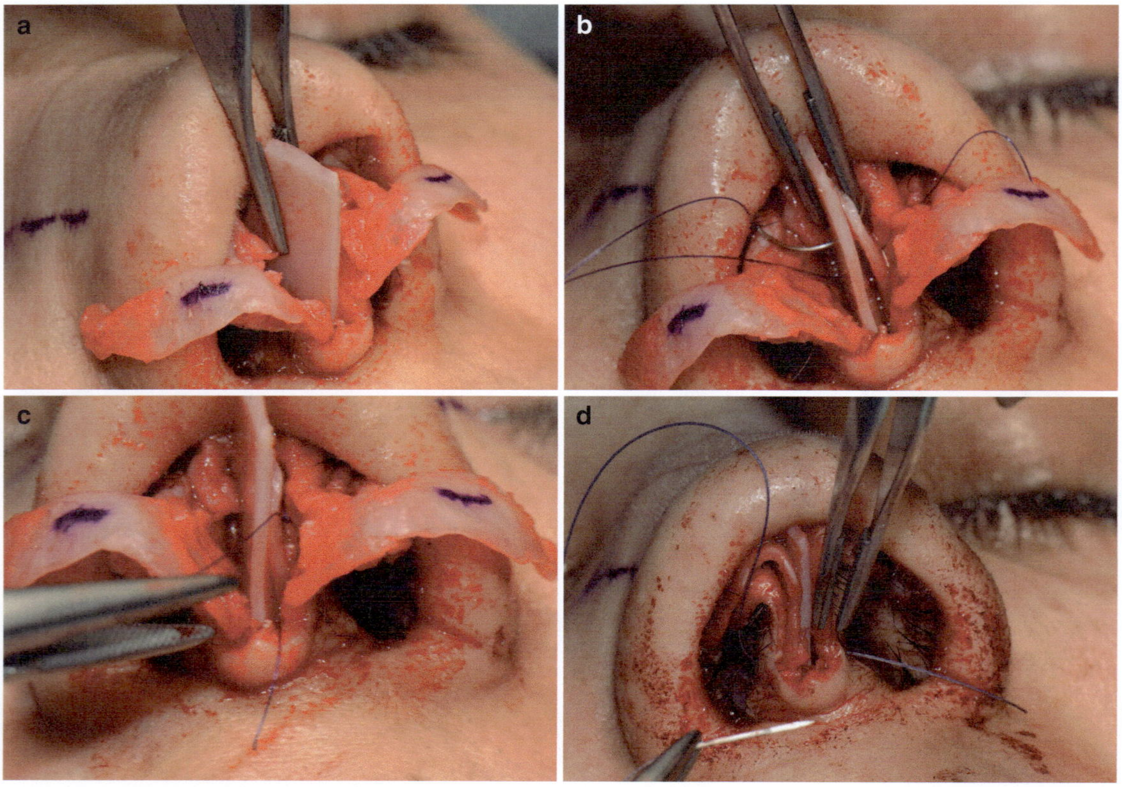

Fig. 11.89 (**a–d**) The graft is overlapped and sutured to the caudal septum for maximal support, and then the medial crura are sutured to the caudal part of the graft

Repositioning surgery applied to the droopy nasal tip provides successful outcomes in the long term when applied with proper indications and correct technique.

In the next case we will look at an example long-term result.

11.4.1.5 Case 20

This patient with droopy nasal tip had undergone repositioning surgery due to malpositioned lateral crus, and had a stable tip 6 years after surgery (Fig. 11.95).

Technical Pearl: What lends stability to a lateral crus moved to a new and ideal position?

- A septum connected to the tip (via septocolumellar suture, septal extension graft, etc.).
- A pocket fashioned such that the lateral crus fits inside (avoiding too large a space in the pocket).
- A lateral nasal wall splint, which must be done before placing the external nasal splint, i.e., before completing all surgical steps. A silicon splint the size of a coin is placed at the outer and inner sides of the lateral nasal wall. The two splints are sutured with 4–0 polydioxanone sutures, which are removed after 7 days. The splint provides stability as it remains in place, facilitating settlement of tissues (Fig. 11.96).

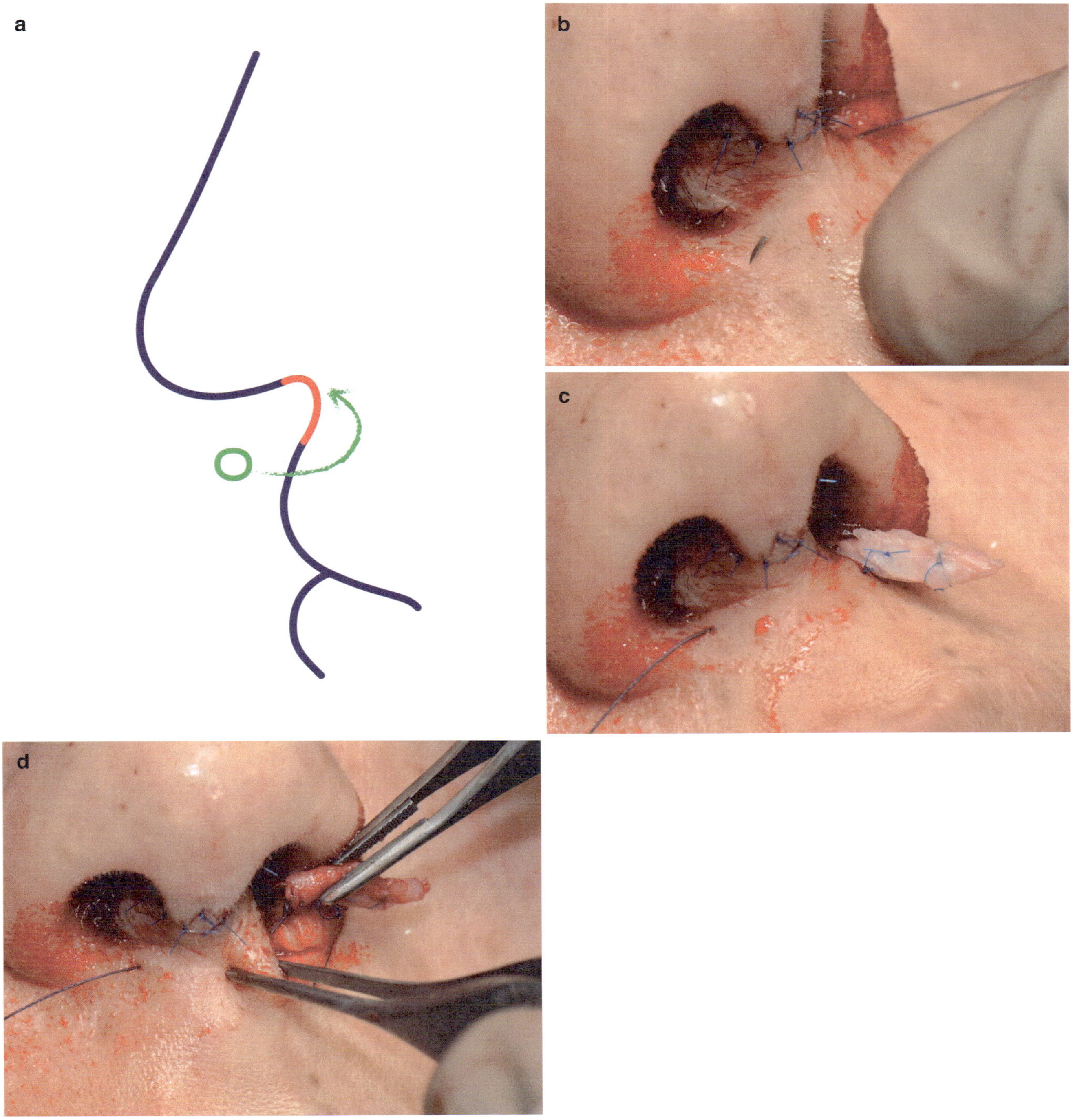

Fig. 11.90 (**a**) The nasal spine and septum are not altered in a patient with a short caudal septum and a closed columellar-labial angle. A premaxillary or plumping graft is usually necessary to help open the angle. (**b**) Stab incision, create a pocket above the premaxilla, then insert the plumping graft with suture guide. (**c**, **d**) A separate incision was made immediately next to the columella, opening a pocket into which the graft was inserted

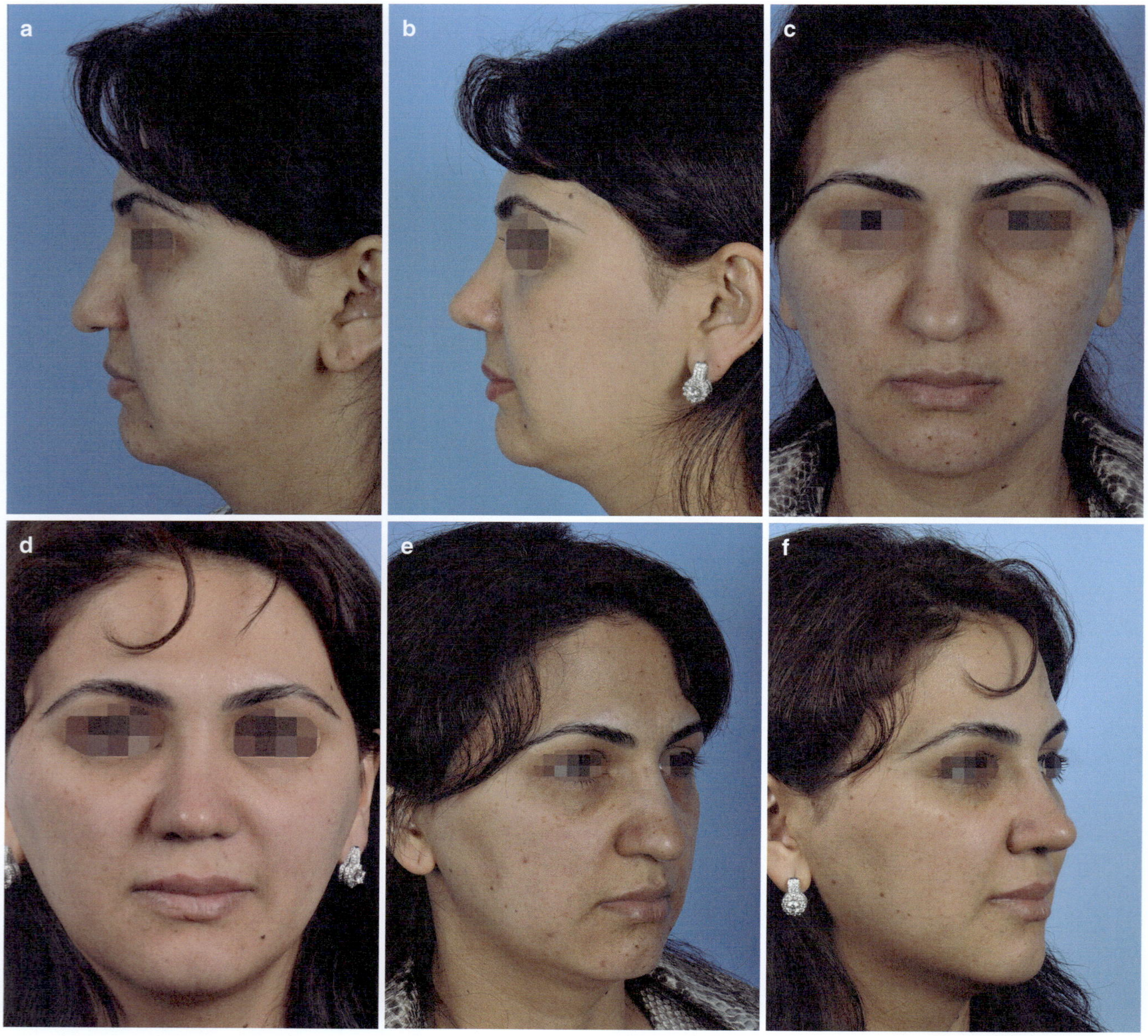

Fig. 11.91 (**a–f**) Postoperative images demonstrate increased tip rotation, projection, and refinement. Caudal septal extension graft ensured stability for the newly formed tip after reposition surgery. The inadequate columellar-labial angle was corrected by premaxillary and caudal septal extension graft, which contributed to the increased rotation

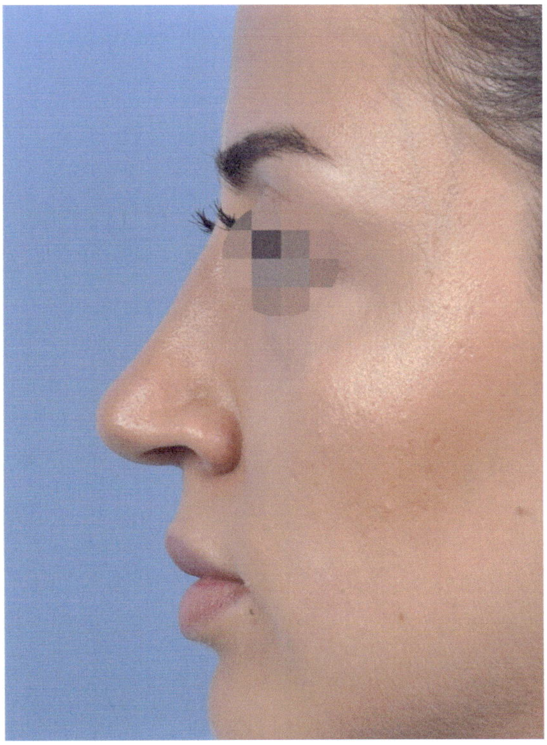

Fig. 11.92 This patient had bilaterally deformed malpositioned lateral crura and inadequate tip rotation

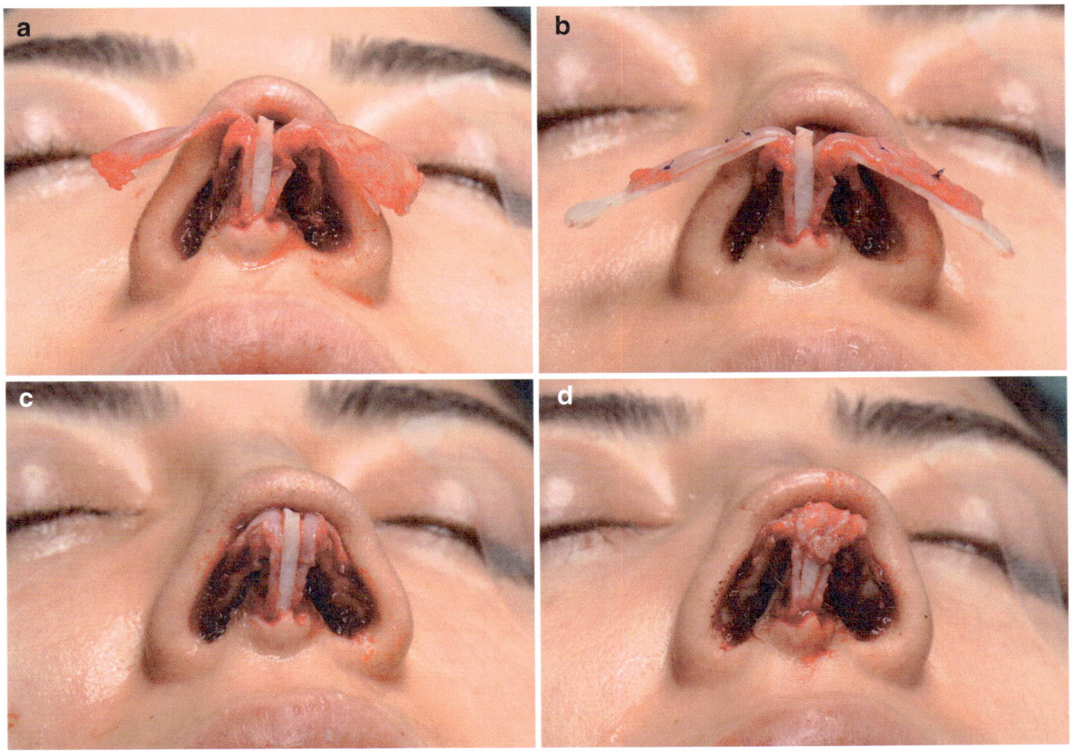

Fig. 11.93 (**a–d**) Septal cartilage was used to reinforce the lateral crus. A 5–6-mm-wide and 1–2-mm-thick septal graft must extend from the dome to the apertura piriformis. The prepared graft was sutured under the deformed lateral crus at three separate points. The newly created strong lateral crus was then moved to its ideal position

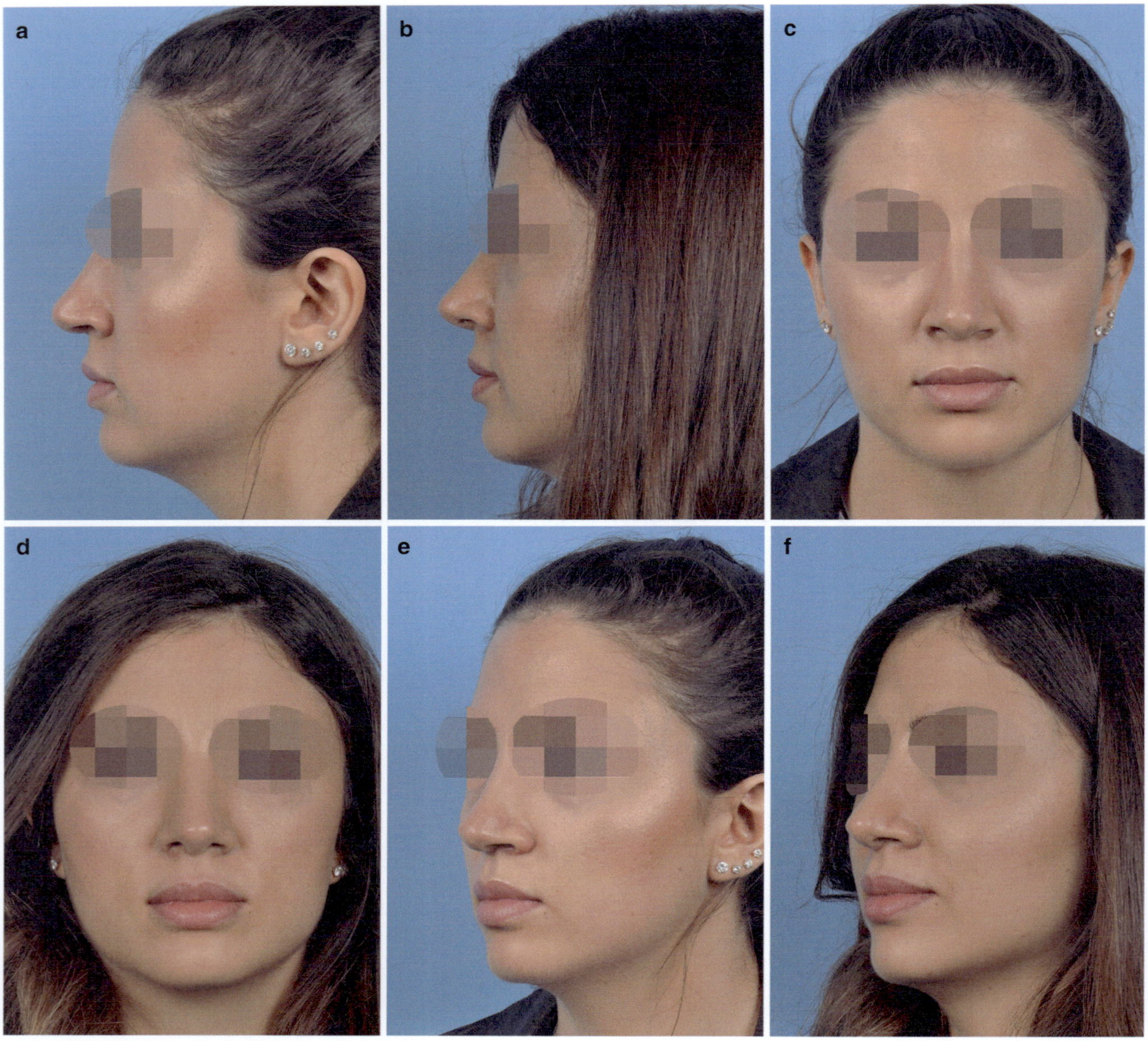

Fig. 11.94 (**a–f**) Patient is shown before and 12 months after repositioning of the lateral crura, tip grafts, and septocolumellar suture. There is increased tip rotation with a more balanced infratip lobule and increased the columellar-lobular angle. Note the ablation of the alar wall hollows and the alteration in alar rim contour after lateral crural repositioning

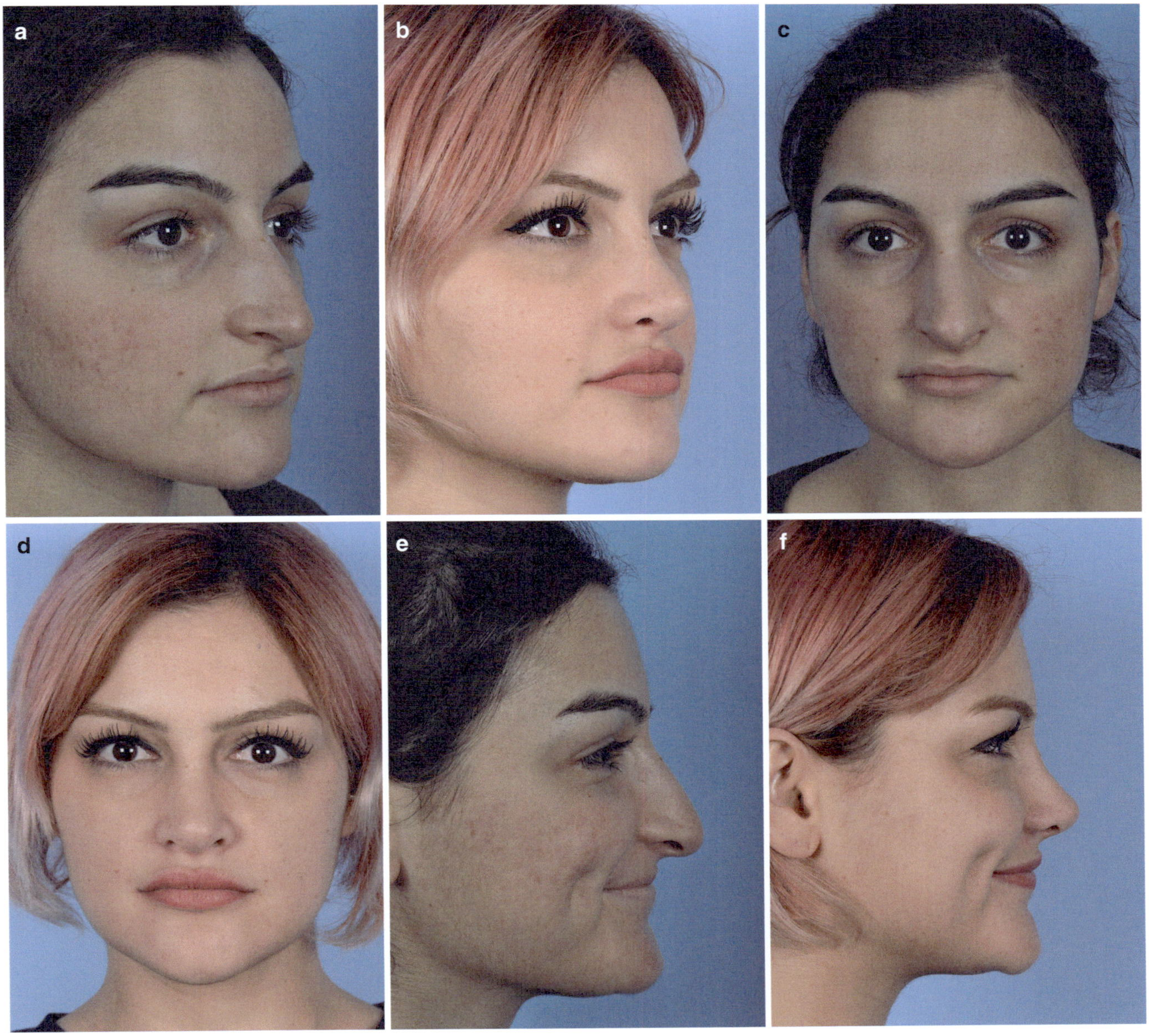

Fig. 11.95 (**a–f**) Patient has an acute columella-lobular angle and a noticeable ptotic nasal tip. Lateral crural reposition surgery was performed to correct the acute columellar-lobular angle and rotate tip. Patient is shown 5 years postoperatively

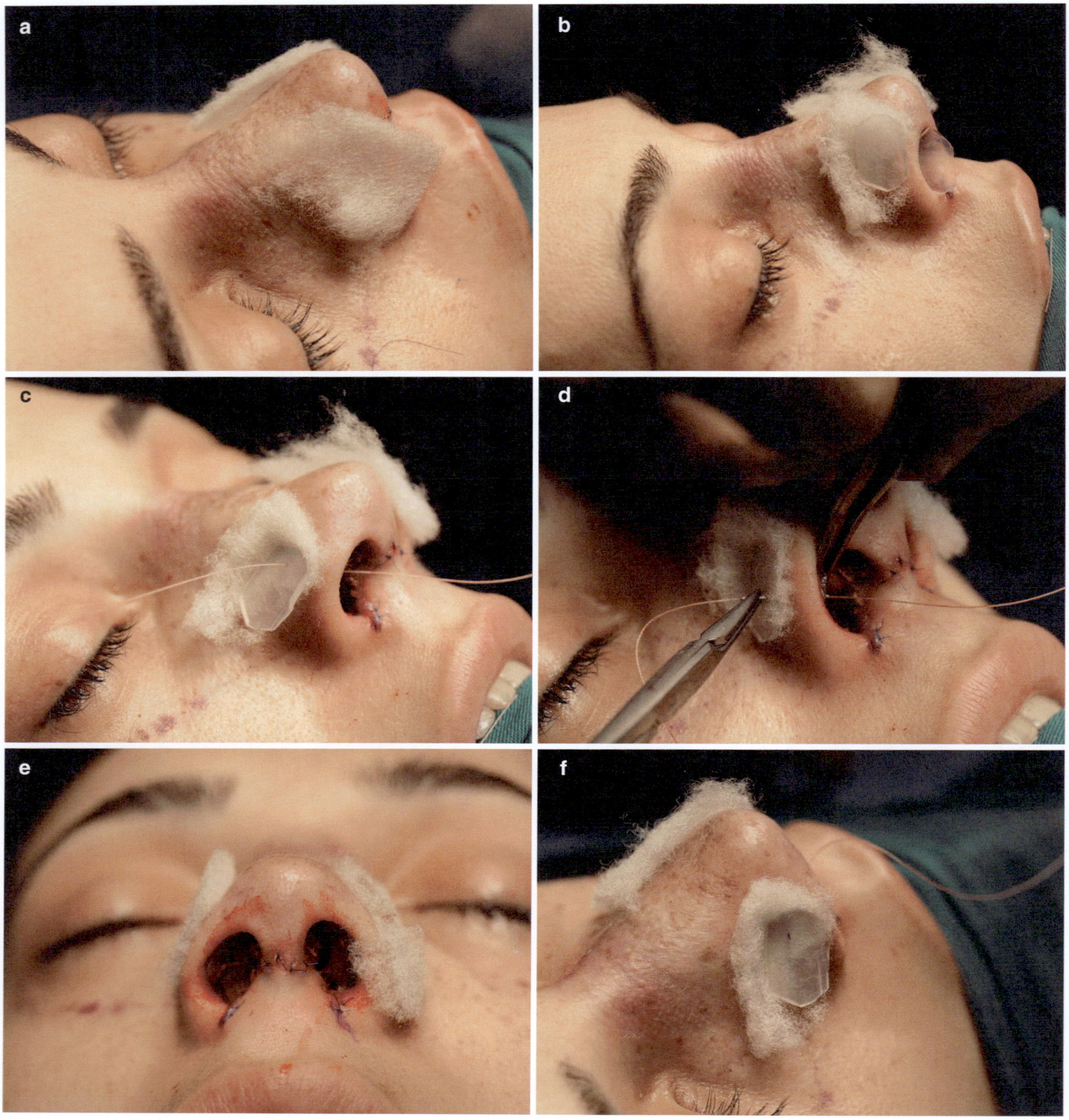

Fig. 11.96 (**a–f**) A suture connecting the splints together that is not knotted too tightly

11.5 Conclusion

A step-by-step approach is used for rotation of the tip. Evaluation of the caudal septum is performed first. If this is not deficient, then the excess anterior septal cartilage may be excised. Then, the position and length of the lateral crus are checked, because the main reason for a droopy nasal tip is a long or malposed lateral crus.

- Repositioning surgery should be performed if the lateral crus is malposed; if the lateral crus is long, three different techniques can be used for this purpose (Fig. 11.97).

We present three different droopy nasal tip cases due to long lateral crus, treated with three different techniques.

1. In this case, the nasal tip was slightly under-rotated; therefore, 3–6 mm shortening of the lateral crus was sufficient. Lateral crural steal suture should be preferred (Fig. 11.98; Video 11.18).
2. In the second case, droopy nasal tip was accompanied by hanging columella. COST technique was performed where 6–10 mm shortening was needed. Postoperatively, tip rotation was increased and hanging columella is absent (Fig. 11.99; Video 11.19).
3. In the last case with a severely under-rotated tip, vertical alar resection (VAR) was performed. Lateral crus was shortened more than 10 mm. Postoperatively, the tip was well defined and rotated (Fig. 11.100; Video 11.20).

In conclusion, crural steal suture is preferred if 3–6 mm shortening is sufficient, while the COST technique allows for 6–10 mm of shortening. For cases of droopy nasal tip in which more than 10 mm of shortening is necessary, VAR technique should be chosen.

The nasal tip is repositioned to achieve the necessary upward position. The next step is to stabilize the nasal tip, which can be achieved with three different procedures, i.e., use of a columellar strut, septocolumellar strut, or septocolumellar suture. After stabilizing the tip, the lateral nasal wall must be strengthened. An alar batten graft or lateral crural strut is commonly used for this purpose. Finally, an onlay tip graft can sometimes be used for tip definition.

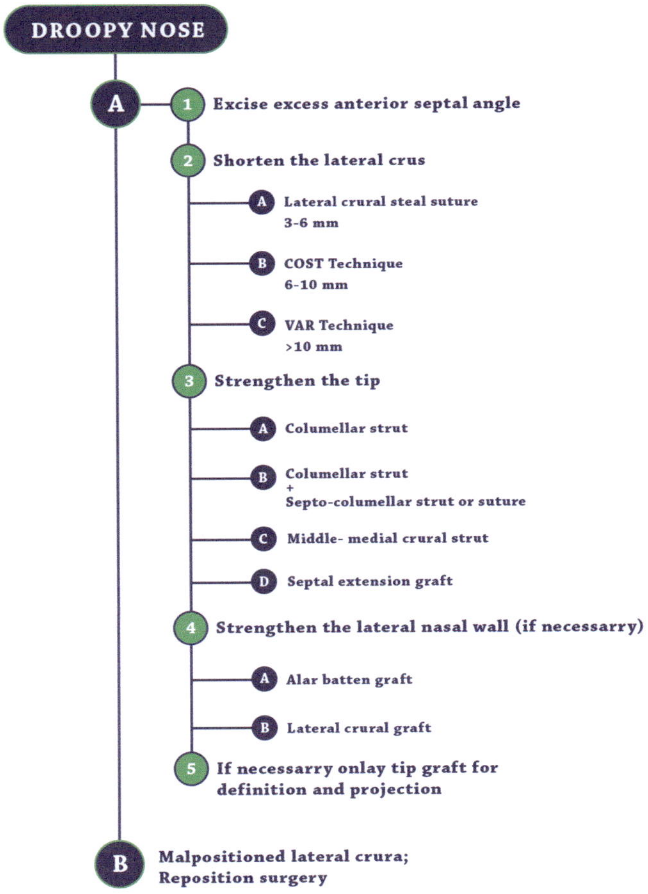

Fig. 11.97 Summary of the droopy nasal tip treatment

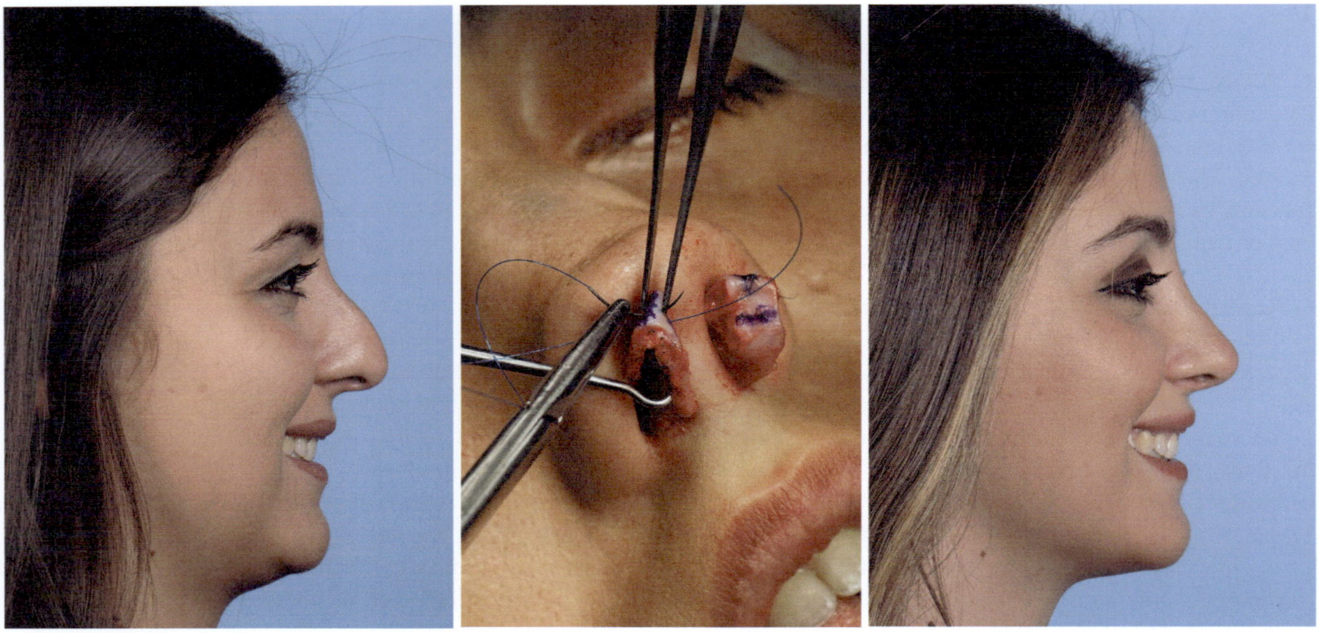

Fig. 11.98 Mild droopy nasal tip. Steal suture should be the primary maneuver to correct mild. The anterior septal angle can be resected if it needed

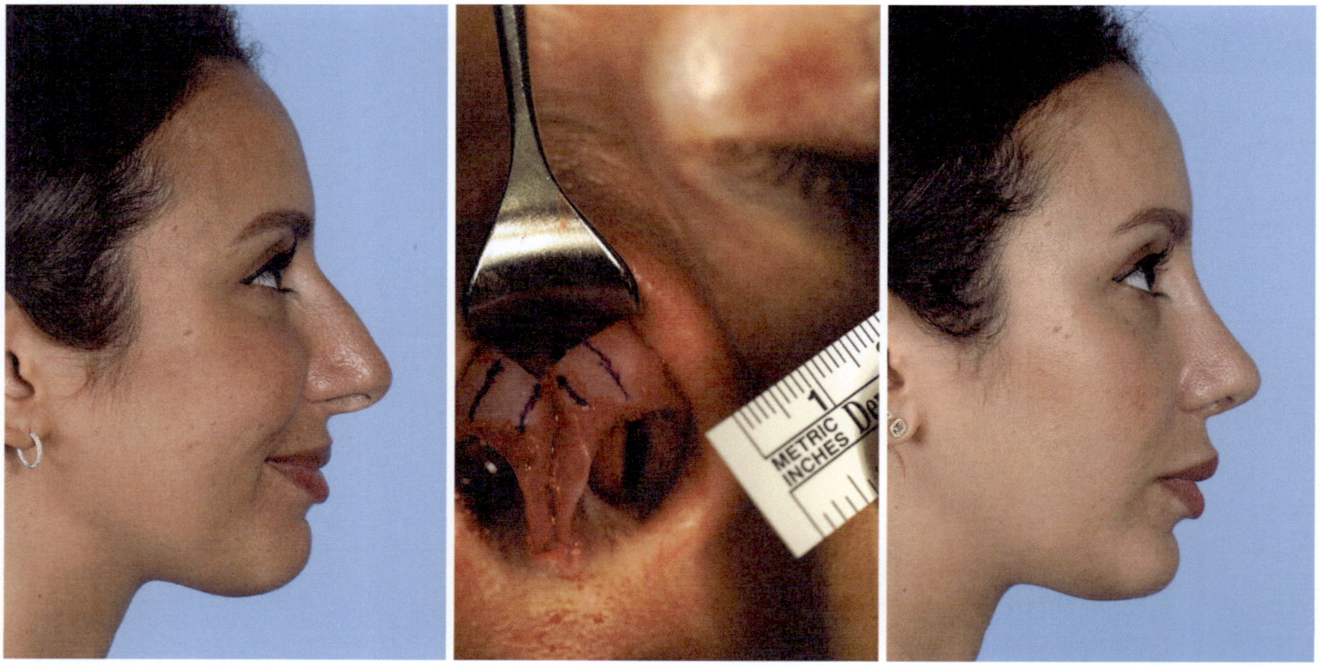

Fig. 11.99 Moderate droopy nasal tip. COST technique should be a useful maneuver to correct moderate. This technique also can correct alar-columellar discrepancy at the same time if it exists. Septal work can contribute if needed

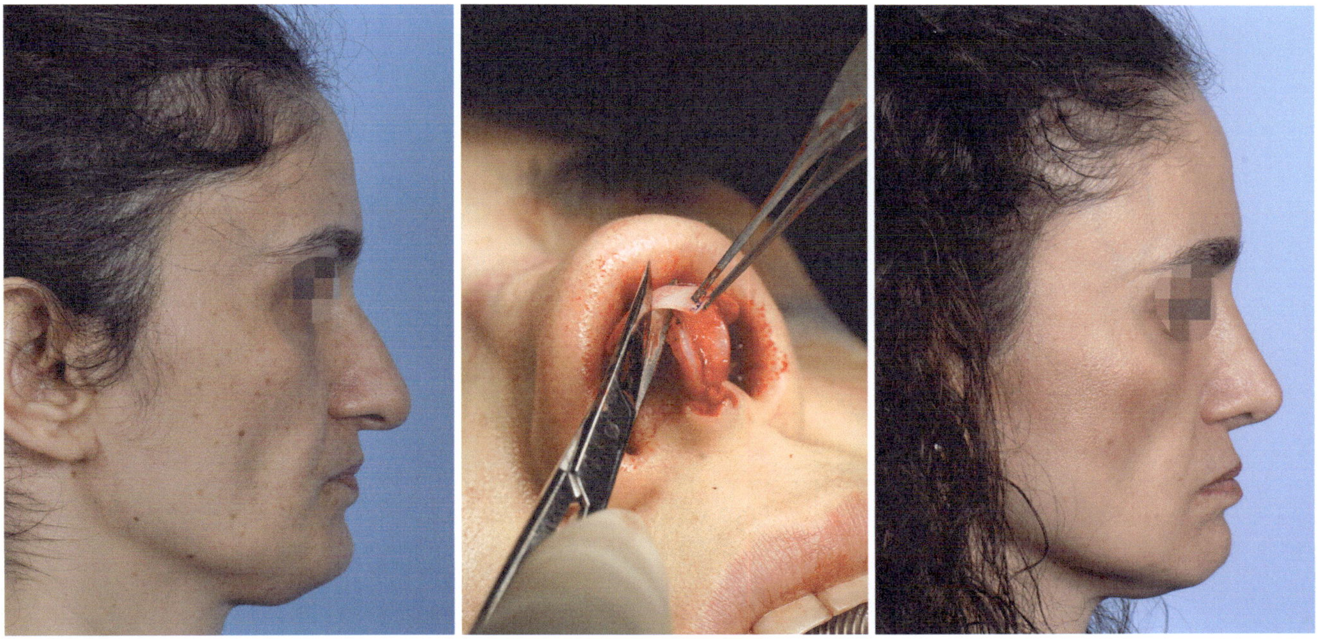

Fig. 11.100 Severe droopy nasal tip. In some cases, suture techniques do not work and should not be forced. An alternative strategy can be required. Vertical alar resection provides an opportunity for this purpose

Disclosures The author reports no conflicts of interest or funding requiring disclosure.

Further Reading

Ahmed O, Dhinsa A, Popenko N, Osann K, Crumley RL, Wong BJ. Population-based assessment of currently proposed ideals of nasal tip projection and rotation in young women. JAMA Facial Plast Surg. 2014;16(5):310–8.

Apaydin F. Projection and deprojection techniques in rhinoplasty. Clin Plast Surg. 2016;43(1):151–68.

Bitik O, Uzun H, Kamburoğlu HO, Dadaci M. Nasal tip suspending transfixion suture. Aesth Plast Surg. 2014;38(2):309–15.

Cerkes N. Nasal tip deficiency. Clin Plast Surg. 2016;43(1):135–50.

Davis RE. Lateral crural tensioning for refinement of the wide and underprojected nasal tip: rethinking the lateral crural steal. Facial Plast Surg Clin North Am. 2015;23(1):23–53.

Foda HM. Management of the droopy tip: a comparison of three alar cartilage-modifying techniques. Plast Reconstr Surg. 2003;112(5):1408–17; discussion 1418–21

Ha RY, Byrd HS. Septal extension grafts revisited: 6-year experience in controlling nasal tip projection and shape. Plast Reconstr Surg. 2003;112(7):1929–35.

Ingels K, Orhan KS. Measurement of preoperative and postoperative nasal tip projection and rotation. Arch Facial Plast Surg. 2006;8(6):411–5.

Kuran I, Öreroğlu AR, Efendioğlu K. The lateral crural rein flap: a novel technique for management of tip rotation in primary rhinoplasty. Aesthet Surg J. 2014;34(7):1008–17.

Rohrich RJ, Hoxworth RE, Kurkjian TJ. The role of the columellar strut in rhinoplasty: indications and rationale. Plast Reconstr Surg. 2012;129(1):118e–25e.

Rohrich RJ, Kurkjian TJ, Hoxworth RE, Stephan PJ, Mojallal A. The effect of the columellar strut graft on nasal tip position in primary rhinoplasty. Plast Reconstr Surg. 2012;130(4):926–32.

Şeneldir S, Altundağ A, Dizdar D. Cutting the holy dome: the evolution of vertical alar resection. Aesth Plast Surg. 2018;42(1):275–87.

Şirinoğlu H. The effect of the short and floating columellar strut graft and septocolumellar suture on nasal tip projection and rotation in primary open approach rhinoplasty. Aesth Plast Surg. 2017;41(1):146–52.

Sood VP. Surgery of the nasal tip. Indian J Otolaryngol Head Neck Surg. 1999;51(1):1–5.

Toriumi DM. New concepts in nasal tip contouring. Arch Facial Plast Surg. 2006;8(3):156–85.

Xavier R. Nasal tip plasty: the delivery approach revisited. Aesth Plast Surg. 2013;37(1):16–21.

Yeşiloğlu N, Sarici M, Temiz G, Yildiz K, Mersa B, Filinte GT. Hezarfen wings: a lower lateral cartilage-based cartilage suspension technique for the adjustment of nasal tip rotation and projection and the correction of supratip deformity. J Craniofac Surg. 2014;25(3):983–7.

12 Over-Rotated Nasal Tip

12.1 Introduction

Deflection at either or both the nasolabial and columella-lobular angles can result in an over-rotated nasal tip and is the main cause of excessive upward rotation. The normal nasolabial angle is between 90° and 95° in men and 95° and 105° in women, while the columella-lobular angle is between 30° and 45°. An increase in these angles results in upward deflection of the tip, in turn causing an over-rotated nasal tip. Surgery for an over-rotated nasal tip aims to achieve the ideal normal nasolabial and columella-lobular angles (Fig. 12.1).

An over-rotated nasal tip is rarely congenital, but can be caused by certain conditions; however, it is mostly due to nasal surgery. An over-rotated nasal tip mainly stems from the caudal septum and alar cartilages.

The original version of this chapter was revised. The original (print and online) version of the book was inadvertently published with the faces masked in a few images. The correction to this chapter is available at https://doi.org/10.1007/978-3-030-44325-2_22

Supplementary Information The online version contains supplementary material available at https://doi.org/10.1007/978-3-031-65619-4_12.

S. Şeneldir, *Photographic Atlas of Rhinoplasty*, https://doi.org/10.1007/978-3-031-65619-4_12

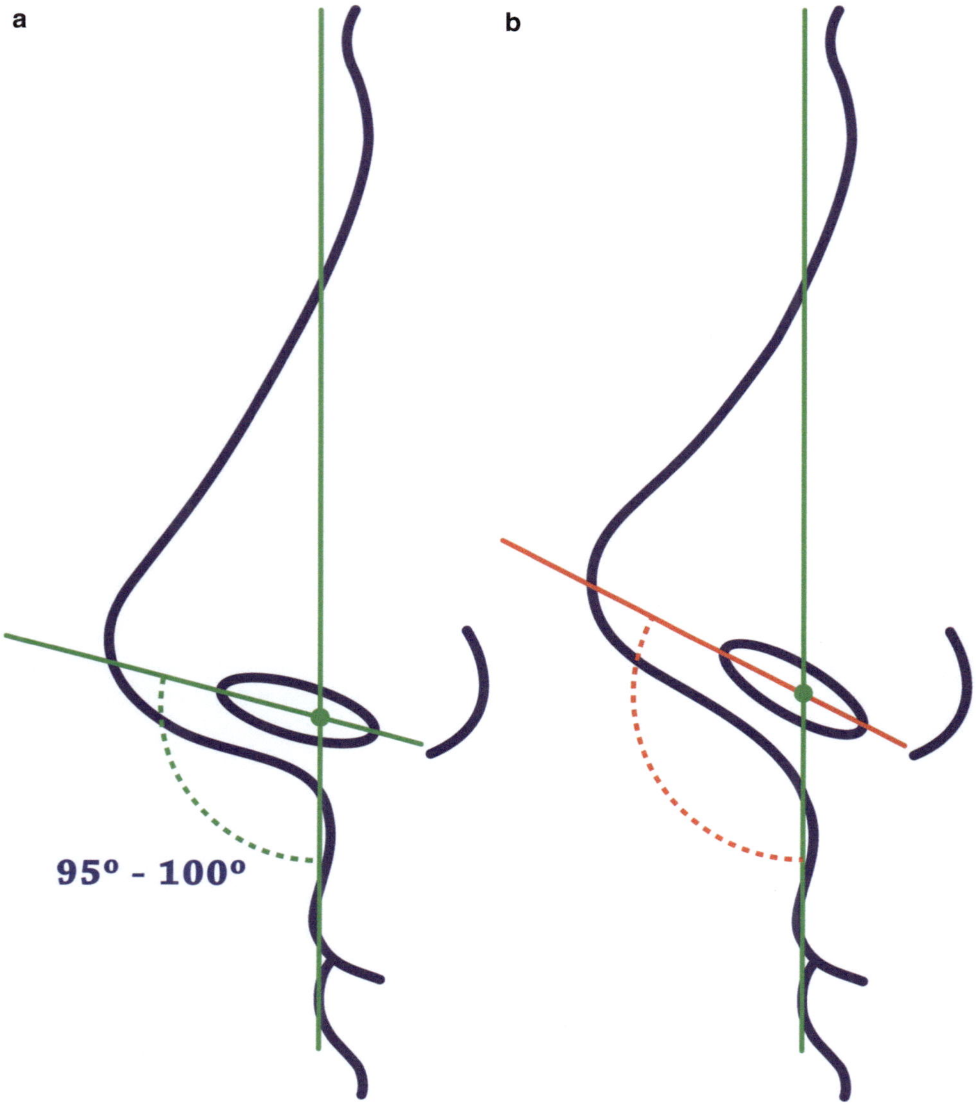

Fig. 12.1 (**a**, **b**) Nasolabial angle. The degree of tip rotation is determined by reference to a straight line through the most anterior and posterior edges of the nostril. The nasolabial angle is the angle at which this line transects a plumb line. (**c**, **d**) Illustration of the columella-lobular angle; a 45° angle is considered normal

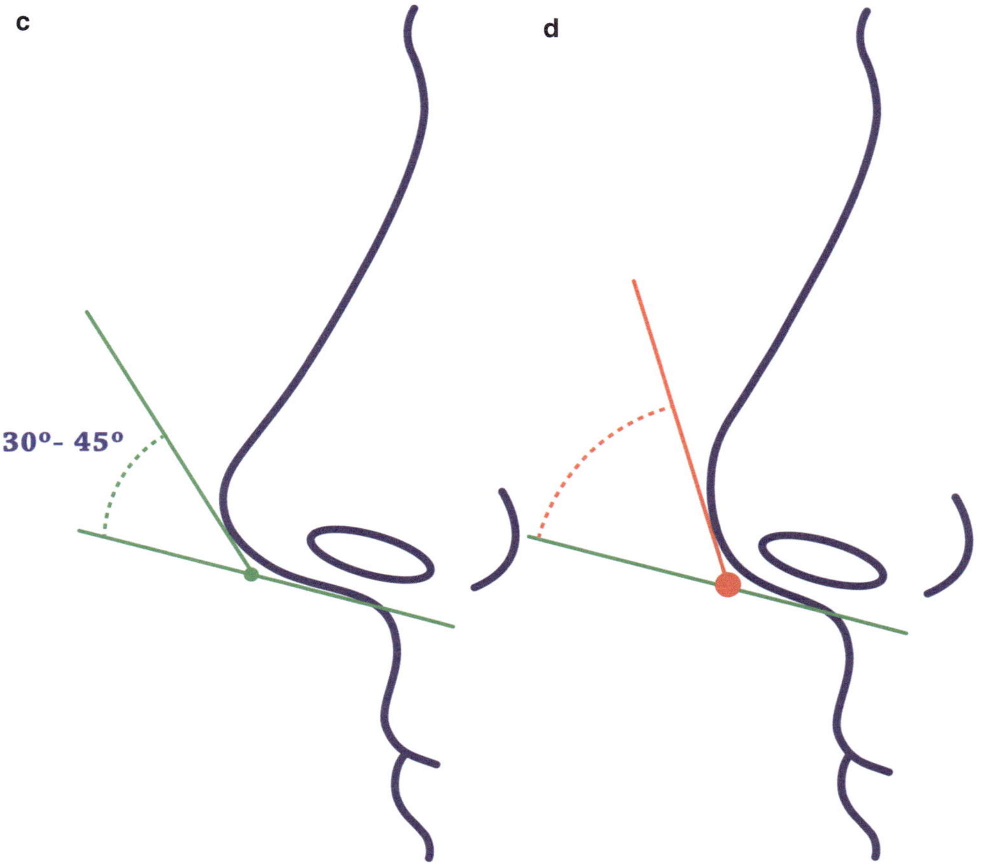

Fig. 12.1 (continued)

12.2 Caudal Septum-Based Over-Rotated Nasal Tip

(a) Excessive resection of the caudal septum without tip stabilization leads to over-rotation. In this representative case, the tip rotation is ideal preoperatively, but aggressive septal resection to shorten the nose by the initial surgeon resulted in an over-rotated tip (Fig. 12.2a, b).

There are no other tip over-rotation problems caused only by the septum, as shown in Fig. 12.2. Examining the case photos, the tip does not have any major negative aspects, except a bulbous appearance. There are no serious problems in the lateral nasal wall or alar rim, because the lateral crus is intact (Fig. 12.3).

Technical Tip: If a surgeon wants to shorten the nose in the case of an ideally rotated tip, the caudal septum must be resected parallel to the caudal border of the septum. Note that resection of the dorsal part of the caudal septum is important for adjusting the degree of tip rotation. If the point of resection is located cephalically in the dorsal part of the septum, the tip rotation increases such that the tip inclines backward (Fig. 12.4).

(b) Overgrowth of the posterior septal angle and nasal spin pushes the tip upward. Dorsal septal deficiency is one reason for an over-rotated nasal tip, but an excessive ventral septum can cause the same problem.

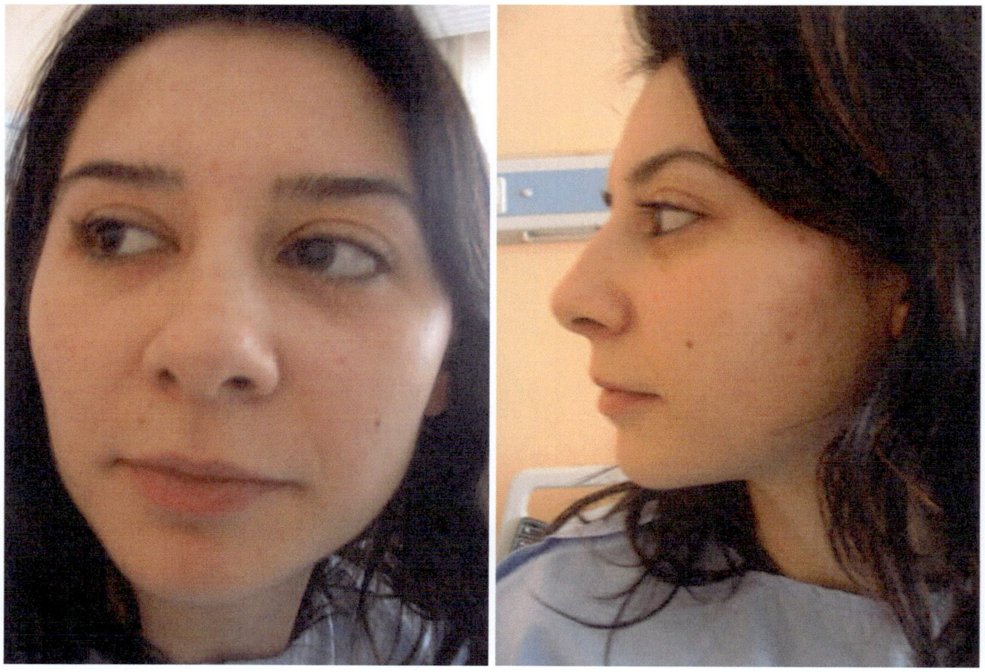

Fig. 12.2 (**a**, **b**) Before first rhinoplasty, there was no need for excessive septal trimming

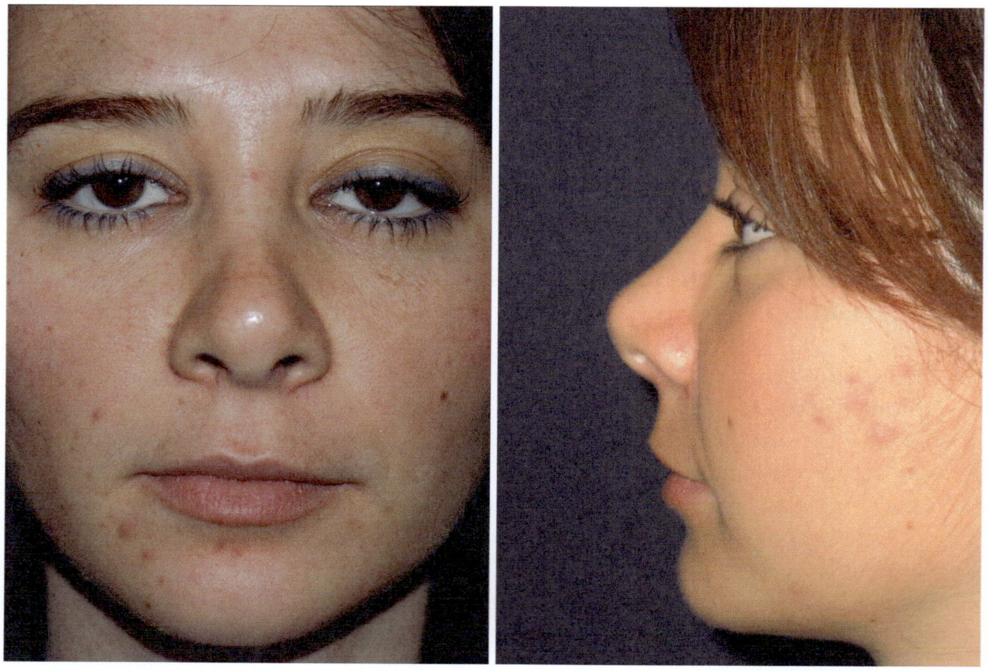

Fig. 12.3 (**a**, **b**) After first rhinoplasty, there is no sign about alar cartilage deformity. Over-rotated nasal tip comes from a deficiency of the anterior septal area

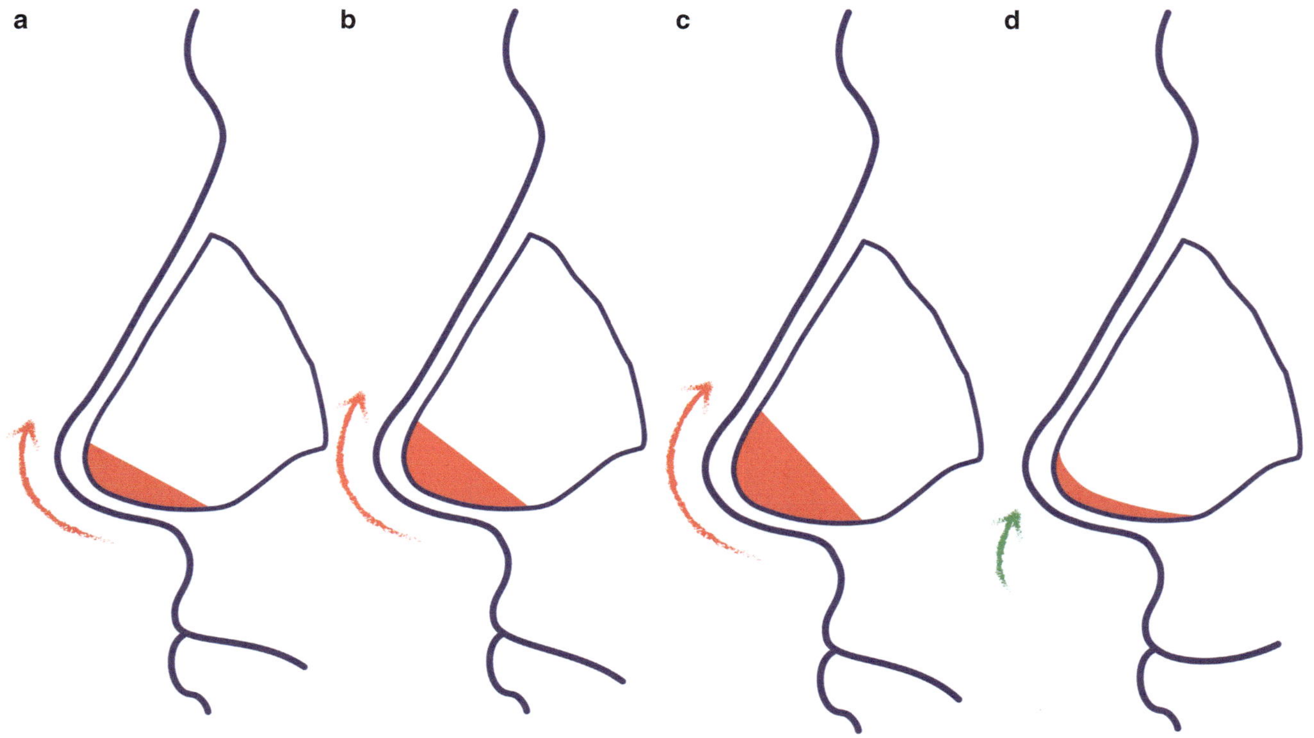

Fig. 12.4 (**a**–**c**) Caudal septal resections causing over-rotated nasal tips. (**d**) An ideal caudal septal resection with tip rotation in the normal range

12.3 Alar Cartilage-Based Over-Rotated Nasal Tip

(a) Overzealous resection of the lateral crura may result in over-rotation and retraction. In the past, surgeons believed that the only way to narrow the nasal tip was through cephalic resection of the lateral crus, which was resected aggressively. However, with greater resection, the lateral crus becomes weaker. Moreover, if the middle-medial crus complex is long and strong, it tends to lie cranially; this type of over-rotation can shorten and weaken the lateral crus, which may in turn cause retraction and a pinched nasal tip (Fig. 12.5).

(b) Overdeveloped or strong middle/medial crus complex. When long and strong middle/medial crura accompany a short and weak lateral crus, the tip will over-rotate.

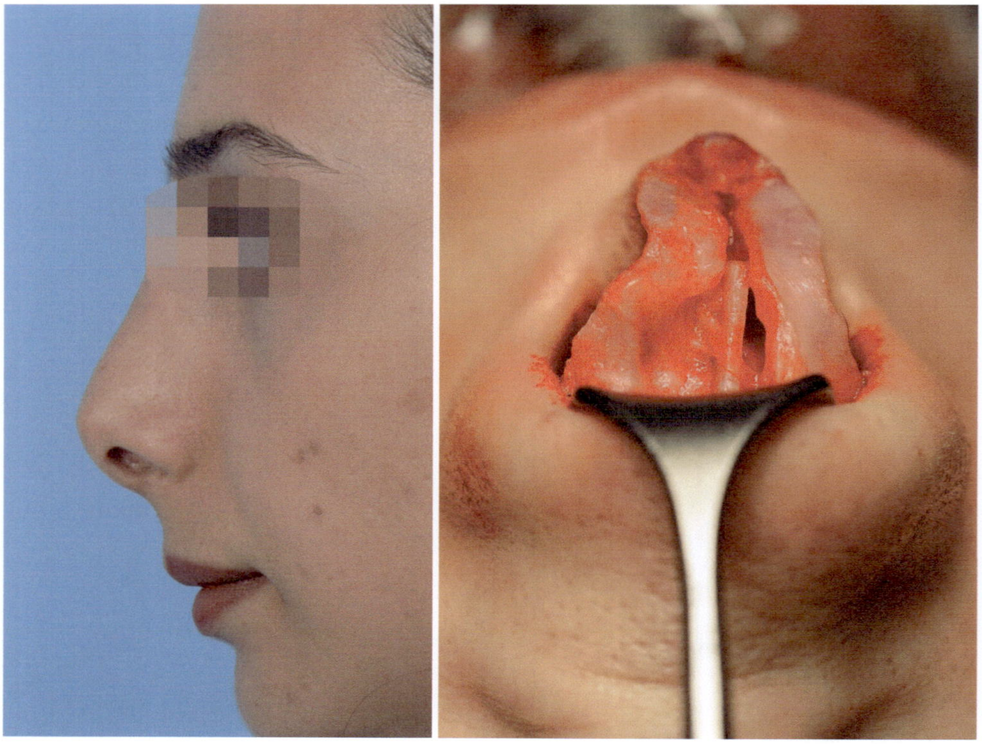

Fig. 12.5 (**a**) Preoperative profile image shows an over-rotated nasal tip. (**b**) Intraoperative image shows that the over-rotation was caused by overzealous cephalic resection of the lateral crura

12.4 Treatment Strategy

After a detailed history-taking and preoperative examination, the restrictive effects of the skin on the surgical outcome must be discussed with the patient. Where possible, it is beneficial to show the patient possible consequences of surgery using computer imaging to ensure realistic expectations. The patient should be informed that if septum extension is needed, costal cartilage may be harvested and, if alar retraction occurs, composite grafts from the ear may be needed. The timing is crucial for revision cases and surgical procedures must be postponed until the skin becomes sufficiently elastic to perform surgery.

An over-rotated nasal tip can be treated by operating **in three different areas,** separately or simultaneously, depending on the case.

1. **Septum:** If the anterior septal angle area is deficient, the septum may be extended caudally from the anterior septal angle. The most likely cause of an over-rotated nasal tip is deficiency of the anterior part of the caudal septum.

   If the deficient part of the septum is augmented, the tip will de-rotate and affect the columella-lobular angle, which will become obtuse instead of acute.

   To perform the augmentation, three grafts are needed: two extended spreader grafts and a septal extension graft. These grafts are used to move the tip from an anterior septal angle to a more caudal position (Fig. 12.6).

   If there is overgrowth of the posterior septal angle, the excess should be resected. Over-rotation of the nasal tip occurs when anterior nasal spin and caudal septal hypertrophy cause fullness of the subnasale. Increased fullness in this area is caused by a prominent caudal septum and gives the illusion of increased rotation, although the nasolabial angle is within normal limits. If posterior septal angle hypertrophy exists, the tip will be pushed upward. A triangular strip, with its base located dorsally, is resected to de-rotate the nasal tip (Fig. 12.7).
2. **Alar cartilage:** If the lateral crura are short, weak, and malformed, they should be strengthened and lengthened. If the middle-medial crus complex is longer than ideal, it should be shortened (Fig. 12.8).
3. **Infratip lobule:** Filling the infratip lobule is beneficial for lengthening the tip and making it appear less rotated (Fig. 12.9).

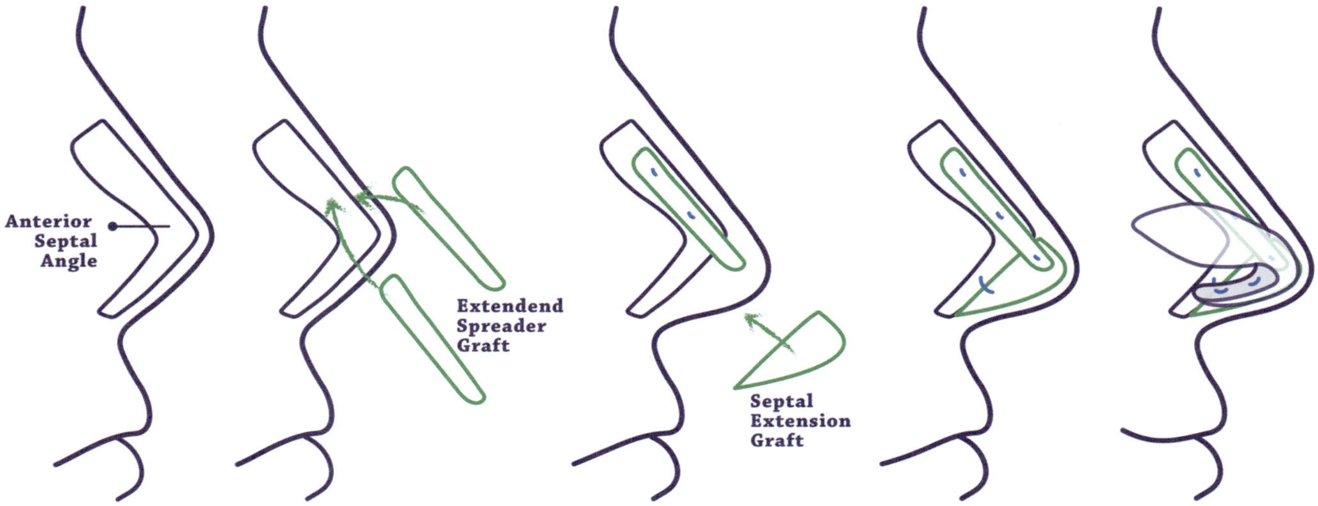

Fig. 12.6 Generally, two extended spreader grafts and a caudal replacement graft are sufficient for lengthening the nose

Fig. 12.7 Posterior caudal septal hypertrophy resection

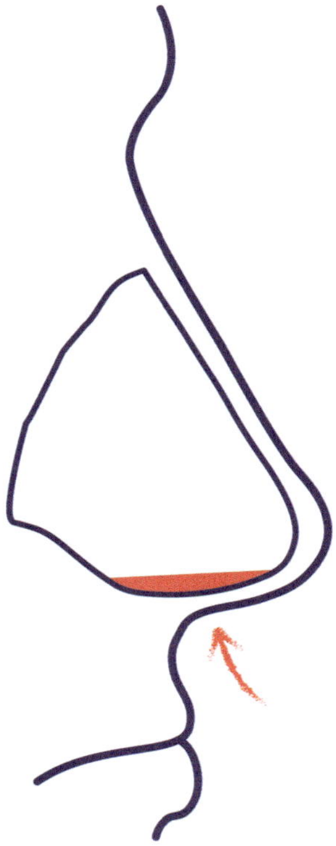

Fig. 12.8 Medial crural steal suture moves the dome defining points more caudal in position

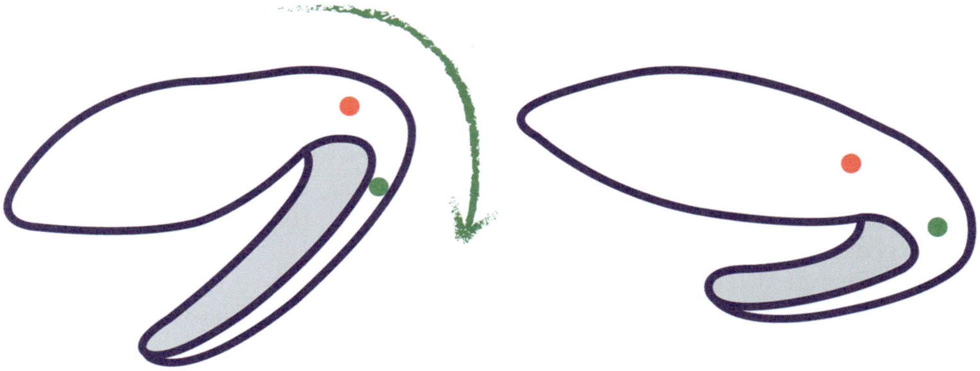

Fig. 12.9 Double layer tip graft to add length to the nose

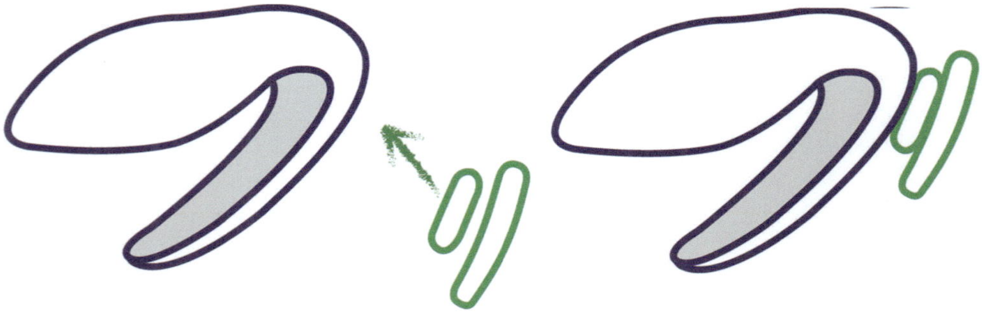

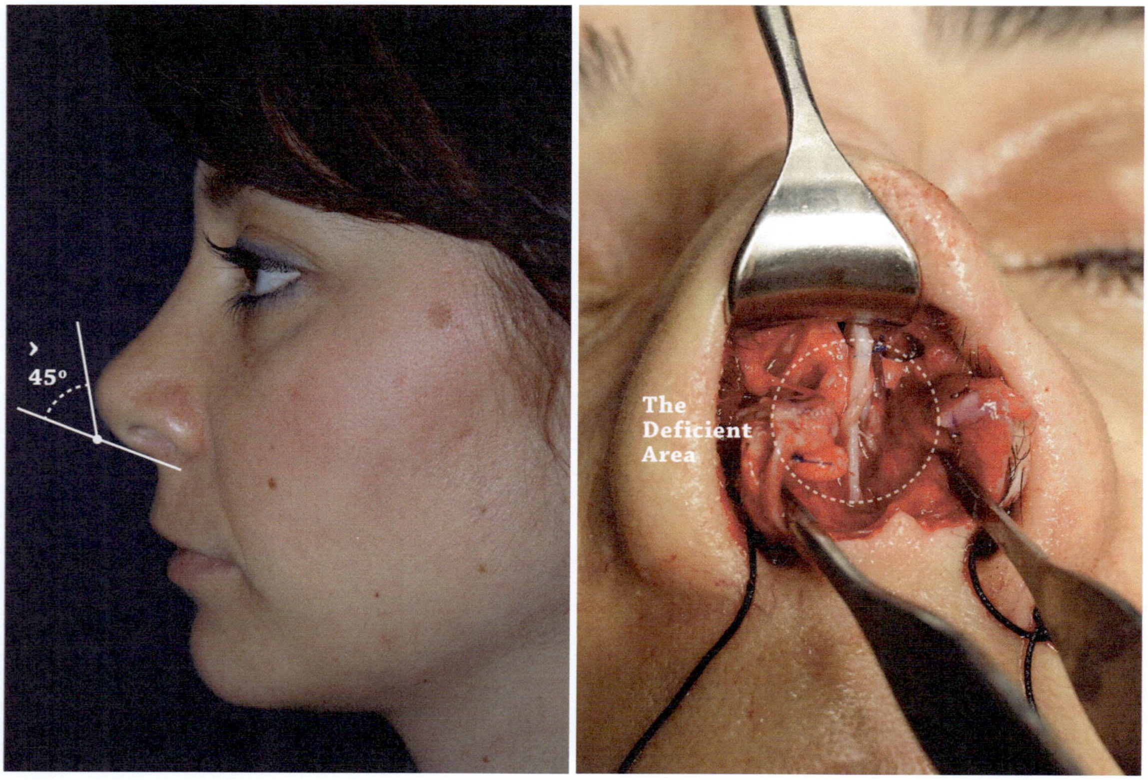

Fig. 12.10 (**a**) Over-rotated nasal tip, preoperative profile view. (**b**) Deficiency of the anterior septal angle area is evident

12.5 Clinical Outcomes

12.5.1 Case 1

A 25-year-old presented for evaluation of a cosmetic deformity of her nose caused by a previous rhinoplasty. Her tip is over-rotated and, overall, the nose is short (Fig. 12.10). Her nasal tip was analyzed in Fig. 12.3. The reason for over-rotation is a deficiency of anterior septal area of the caudal septum. If the nose appears short and the tip over-rotated because of a deficient caudal septum, reconstruction of the septum will provide an elongated appearance.

To counter-rotate, the tip, two extended spreaders, and caudal septal extension graft should be used. The spreaders start from beneath the nasal bones and lie beyond the caudal septum. Normally, a spreader graft terminates in the anterior septal angle, but the extended spreader graft in this case exceeds the anterior septal angle. The nose elongates caudally by the same amount as it exceeds the anterior septal angle.

An extended spreader graft is placed precisely in a subperichondrial pocket between the septum and upper lateral cartilages. Once its position is confirmed, the spreader grafts are fixed directly to the septum using two polydioxanone mattress sutures and the caudal extent of the spreader graft is then fixed to the caudal extension graft. The bottom of the septal extension graft must be fixed to the anterior nasal spin (Fig. 12.11).

Photographs taken 6 years postoperatively are shown in Fig. 12.12. The nasal tip has been counter-rotated, increasing the length of the nose.

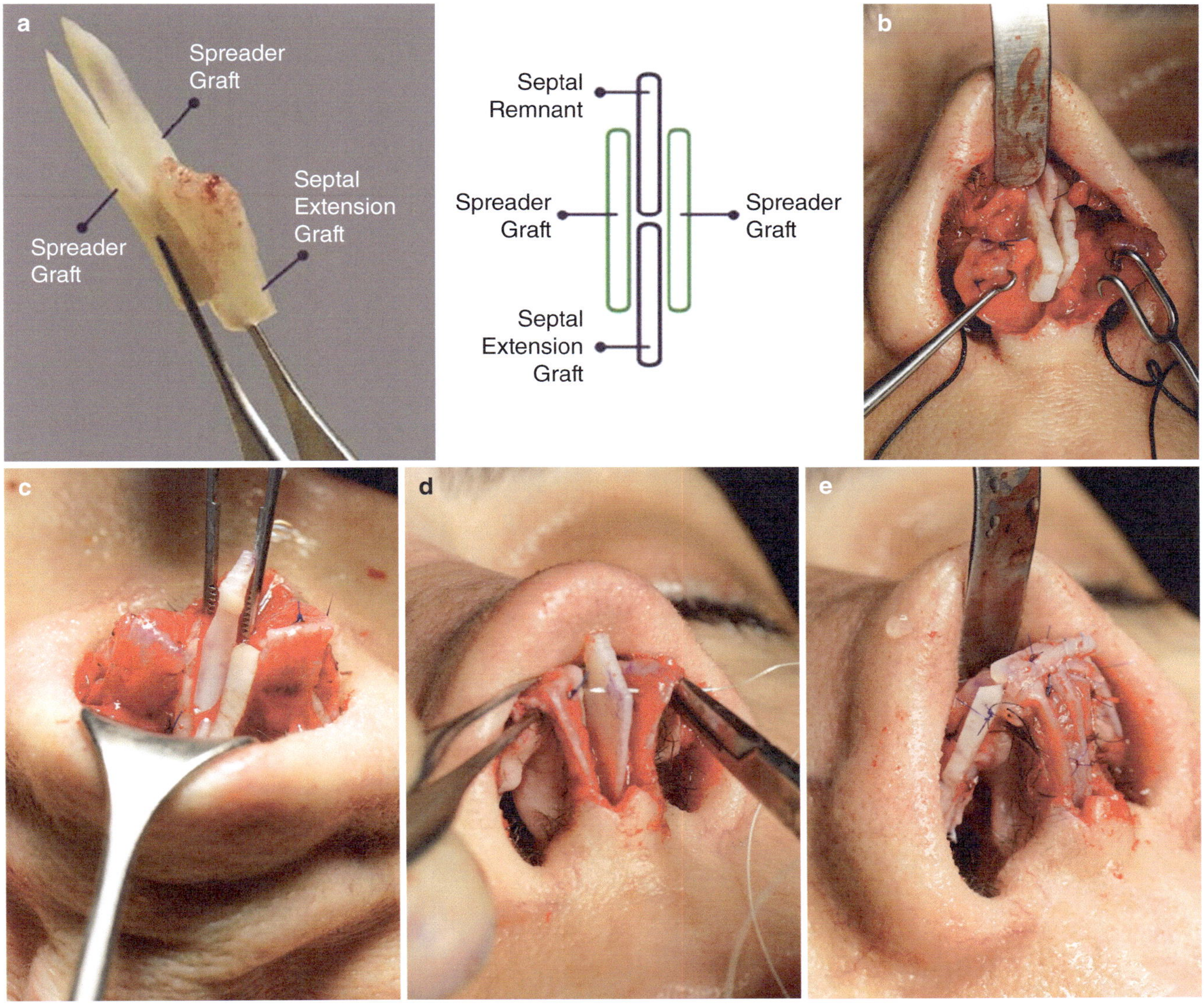

Fig. 12.11 (**a**) The bilateral spreader grafts and extended septal extension graft are seen extra-corporally. (**b**) The spreader grafts were sutured on both sides of the septum using permanent sutures. (**c**) The septal extension graft was sutured with permanent sutures between the spreader grafts and nasal spin. (**d**) The medial and middle crus were fixed to the septal extension grafts caudally. (**e**) While the lateral crura were strengthened via the lateral crural grafts, the cap graft increased the definition

If the lateral crura are short and weak, and the middle medial crus is long and strong relative to the lateral crura, the tip will appear over-rotated. To de-rotate the tip while also strengthening and elongating the lateral cartilage, the middle medial crus should be shortened. Two techniques can be used to de-rotate the tip:

- *Medial crural steal suture*: A steal suture steals a segment from the middle crus and gives it to the lateral crus. Consequently, the lateral crus is elongated, while the middle crus shortens, which causes tip de-rotation. The main disadvantage of this suture is that it decreases the projection.
- *Medial crural overlap*: The overlap not only shortens the medial crus but also corrects any configuration problems. However, it does not affect the length of the lateral crus.

Both of these techniques should be combined with the lateral crural graft, because lateral crural grafts are very useful for:

- Strengthening the lateral nasal crura.
- Pushing the tip forward.
- Repairing any minor alar retraction.

Technical Tip: The medial crural overlap technique is an alternative to a medial crural steal suture if the configuration of

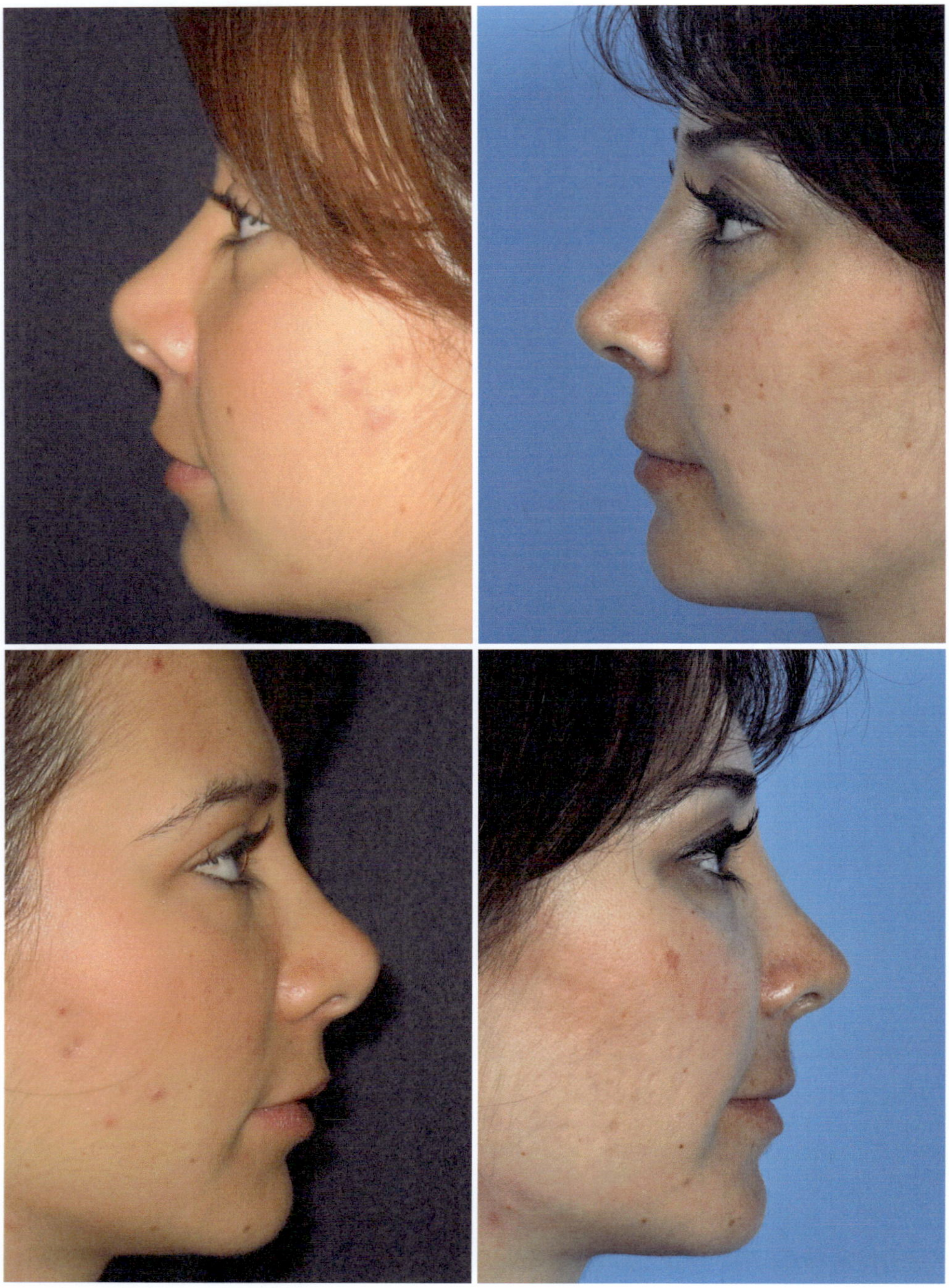

Fig. 12.12 (**a–h**) Before and after views. The nose is longer, with corrected over-rotated tip

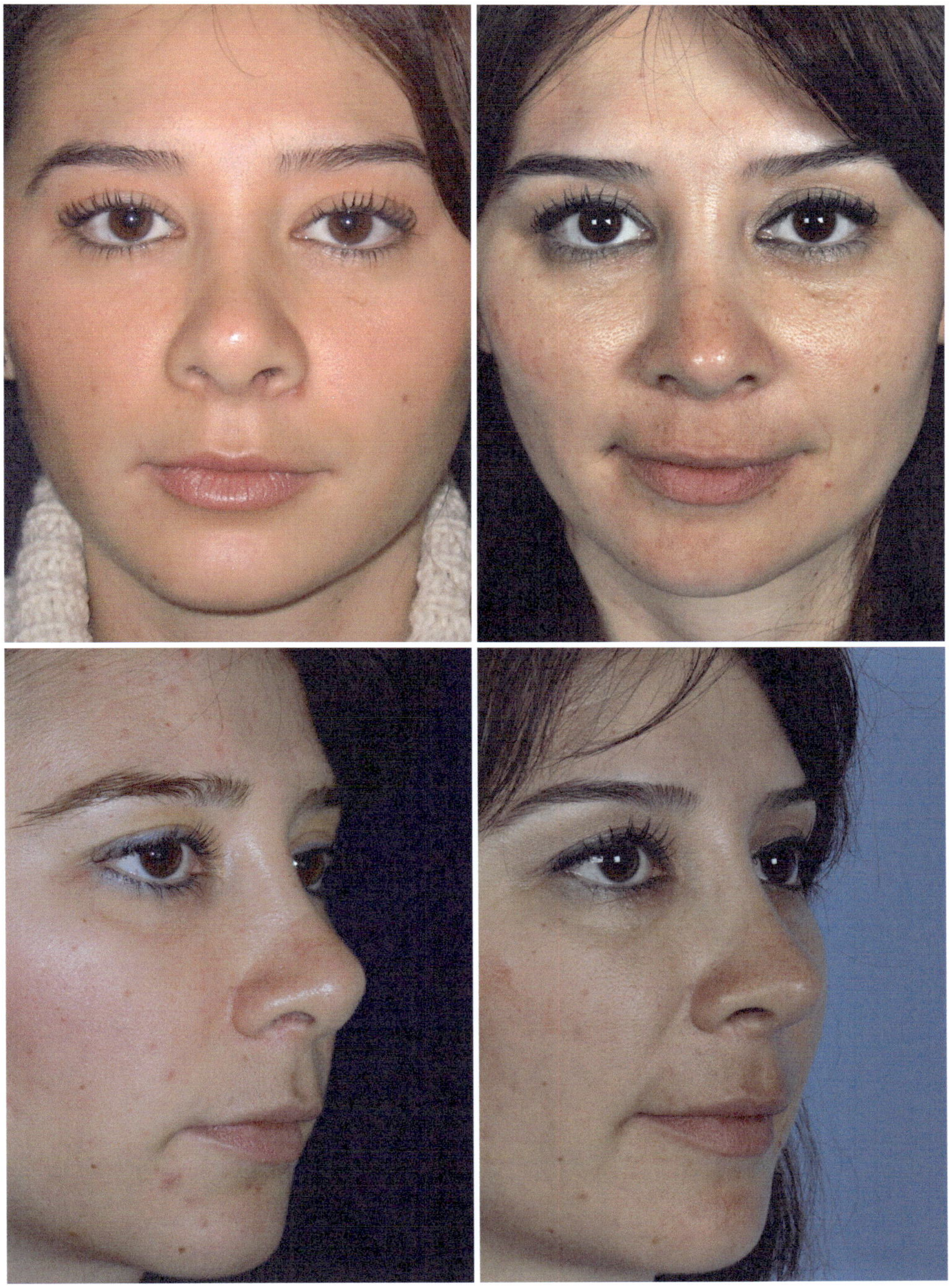

Fig. 12.12 (continued)

the medial crus is distorted. In both techniques, the lateral crura must be strengthened with lateral crural grafts (Fig. 12.13).

12.5.2 Case 2

Now we consider a revision case with over-rotation. This patient underwent rhinoplasty 5 years earlier. Her nasolabial and columella–lobular angles are greater than ideal. The lateral crura appear short and weak, while the medial/middle crura are long and strong. The nasal spin and posterior septal angle are clearly hypertrophic (Fig. 12.14).

The surgical steps used in this case are shown in intraoperative photographs. Over-rotation is evident due to the excessive columella-lobular angle (Fig. 12.15).

The caudal septum is trimmed because the overdeveloped posterior part of the caudal septum pushes the tip upward (Fig. 12.16).

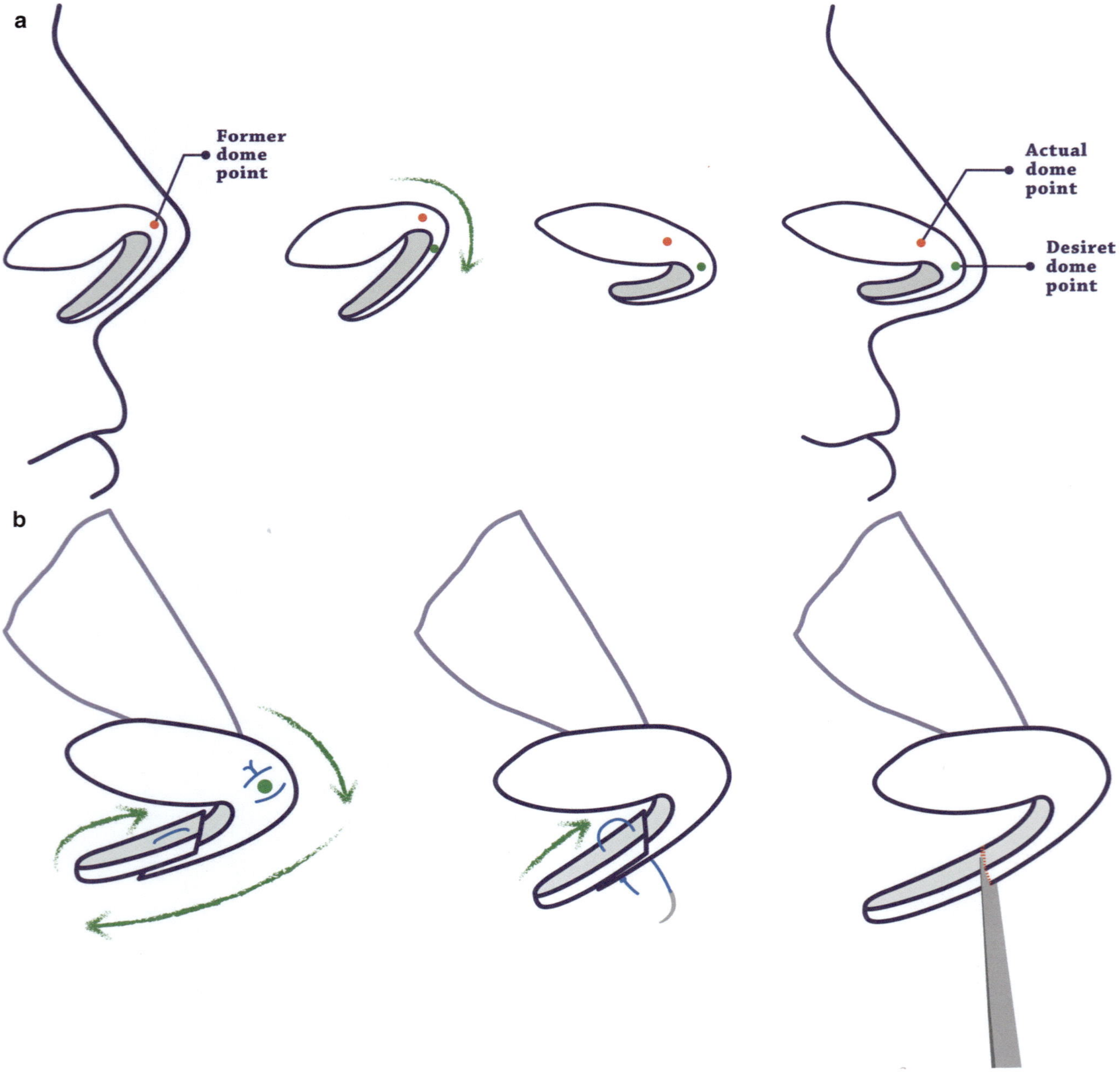

Fig. 12.13 (**a**) The medial crural steal suture should be positioned caudal to the anatomical dome. Using this de-rotation suture, the lateral crus elongates and the middle crus shortens. This suture also corrects the columella-lobular angle. (**b**) The medial crural overlap de-rotates the tip because it shortens the columella

Tip suturing techniques that reposition the nasal tip complex are the mainstay of providing a finer tip. For this purpose, medial crural steal suture can be used in over-rotated nasal tip cases.

Using a medial crural steal suture, the new dome-defining point was moved more caudally, thereby shortening the medial crura while lengthening the lateral crus (Fig. 12.17).

The suture decreased the tip projection that was regained with a cap graft camouflaged with fibrous soft tissues. Lateral crural grafts were placed bilaterally to strengthen the lateral crura (Fig. 12.18).

The degree of tip rotation was rendered more favorable by using a medial crural steal suture and caudal septal trimming (Fig. 12.19).

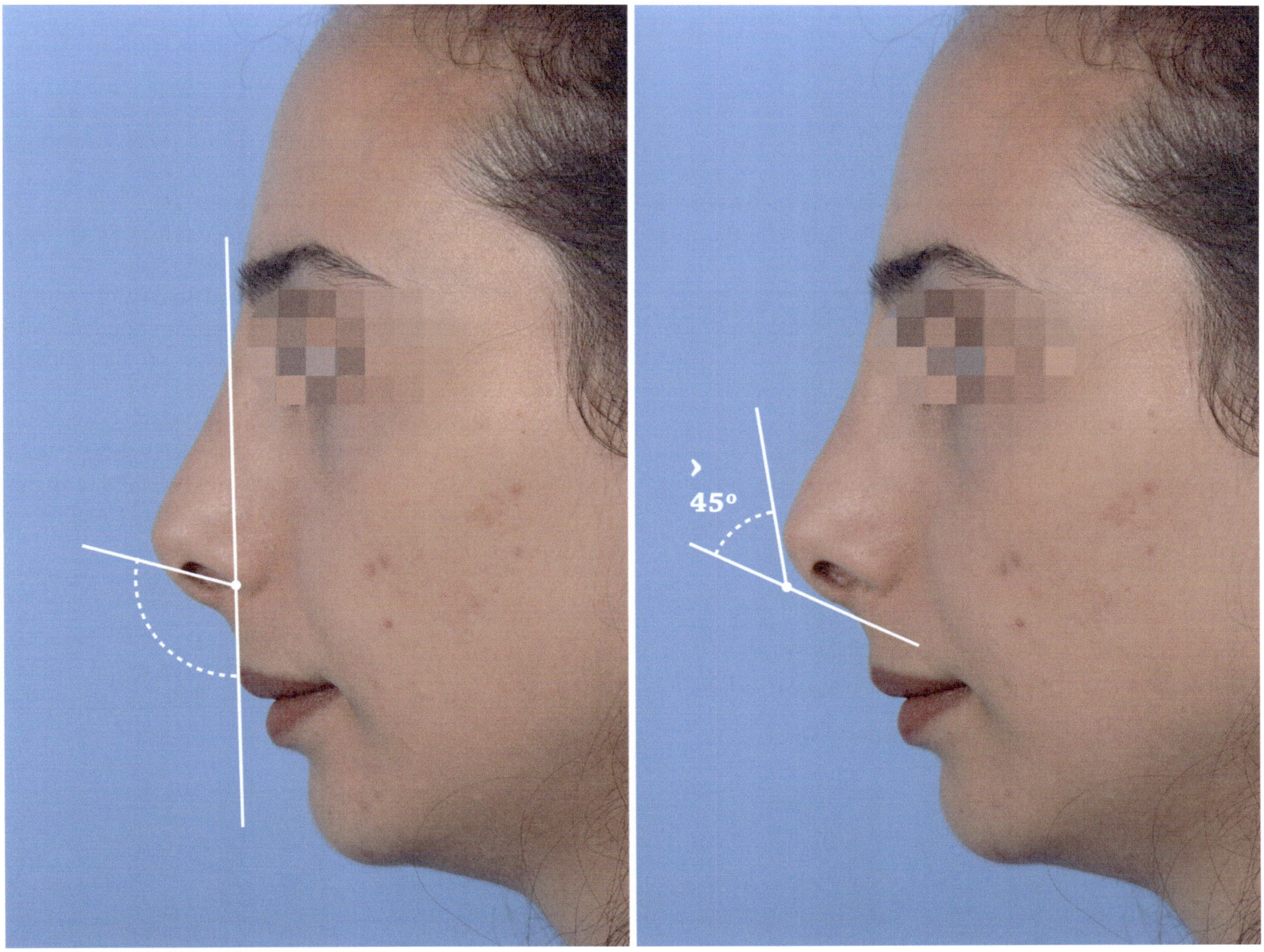

Fig. 12.14 (**a**) The nasolabial angle. (**b**) The columella–lobular angle

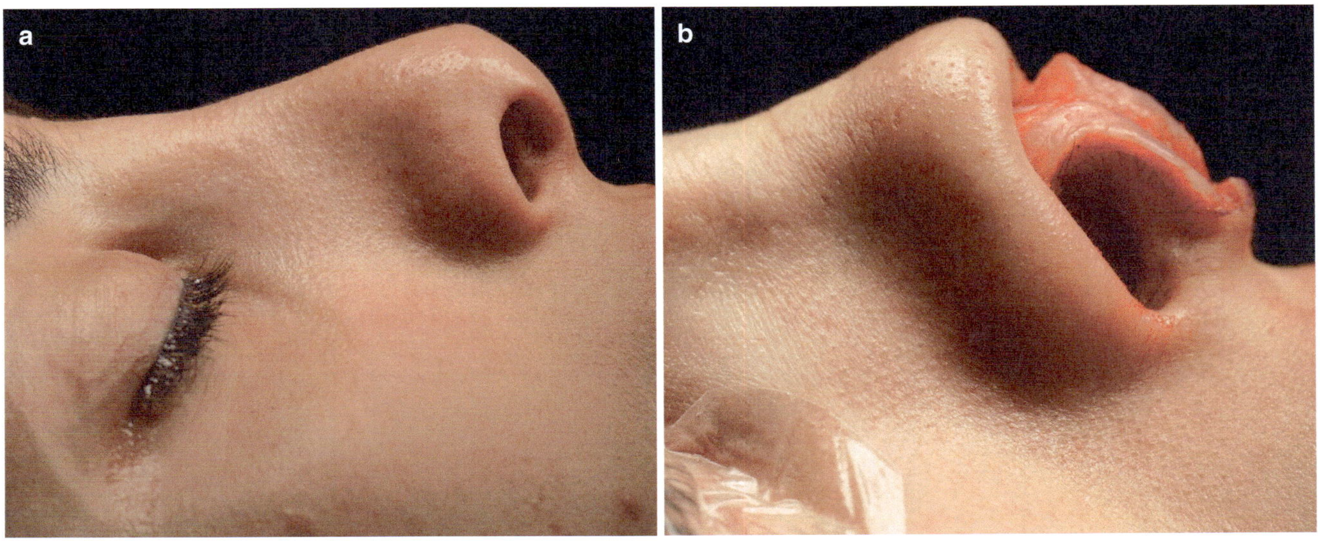

Fig. 12.15 (**a**, **b**) Long and flat middle/medial crura, not noticeable columella-lobular angle

Preoperative and 1-year postoperative photographs are shown in Fig. 12.20.

12.5.3 Case 3

Another case with an over-rotated nasal tip is shown here. In this case, the medial crural steal technique was the main maneuver. The intraoperative lateral view shows that the medial crus was long; a steal suture would be effective in this situation (Fig. 12.21).

The desired dome-defining points were marked under the actual ones and a transdomal suture was performed (Fig. 12.22).

Weak lateral crura are evident (Fig. 12.23).

Bilateral lateral crural grafts were placed to strengthen the lateral crura (Fig. 12.24).

A cap graft was used to project and define the tip, and an infratip lobular graft was used to improve the columella–lobular angle by increasing the fullness of the infratip (Fig. 12.25).

The alar rim retraction may continue despite the overlay lateral crural graft. Severe alar retraction deformities can be treated with a composite graft harvested from the ear. In this case, an ear composite graft was used for alar retraction on the right side (Fig. 12.26).

Photographs taken 1 year postoperatively are shown in Fig. 12.27.

In cases with an over-rotated, over-projected nasal tip with alar-columellar disharmony, the medial crural overlap technique is suitable. Division and overlap at the medial

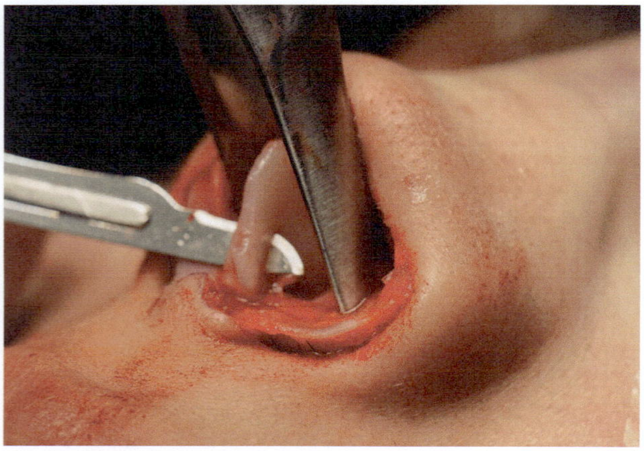

Fig. 12.16 Resect the posterior part of the caudal septum

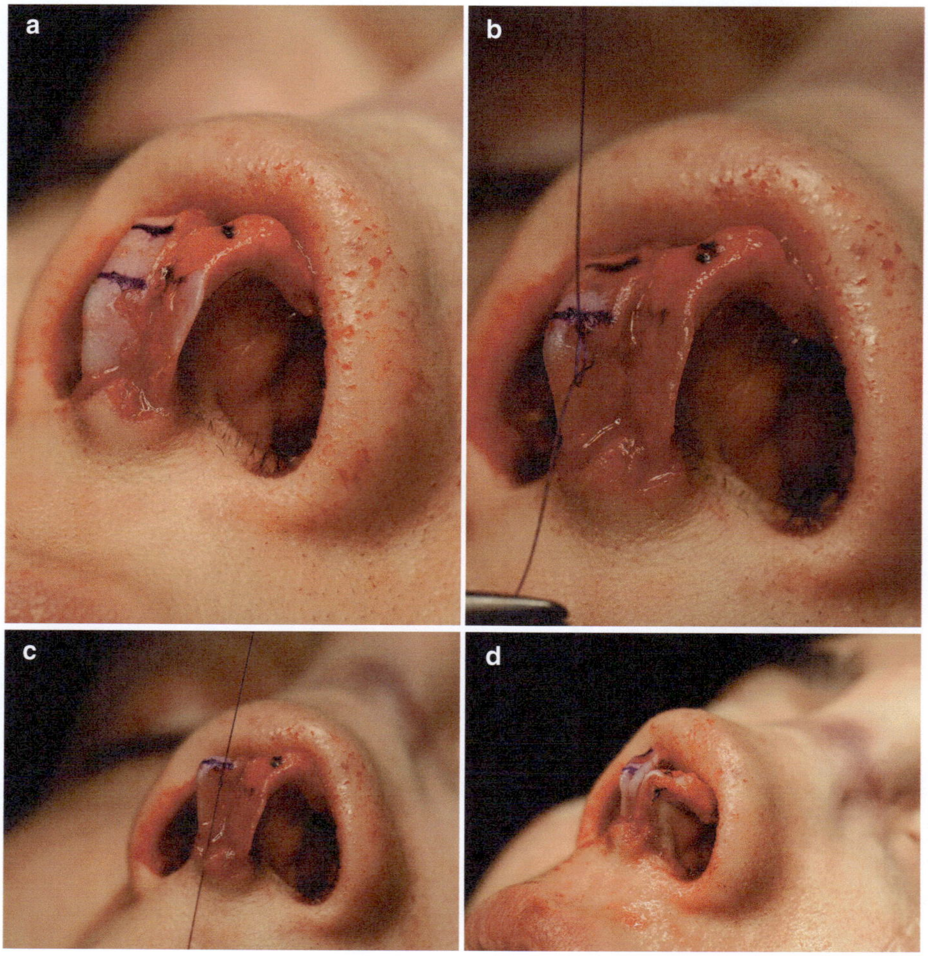

Fig. 12.17 (**a–d**) The medial crus is advanced laterally onto the lateral crus and fixed in its new positioning using a 5–0 nonabsorbable mattress suture just below the newly established dome

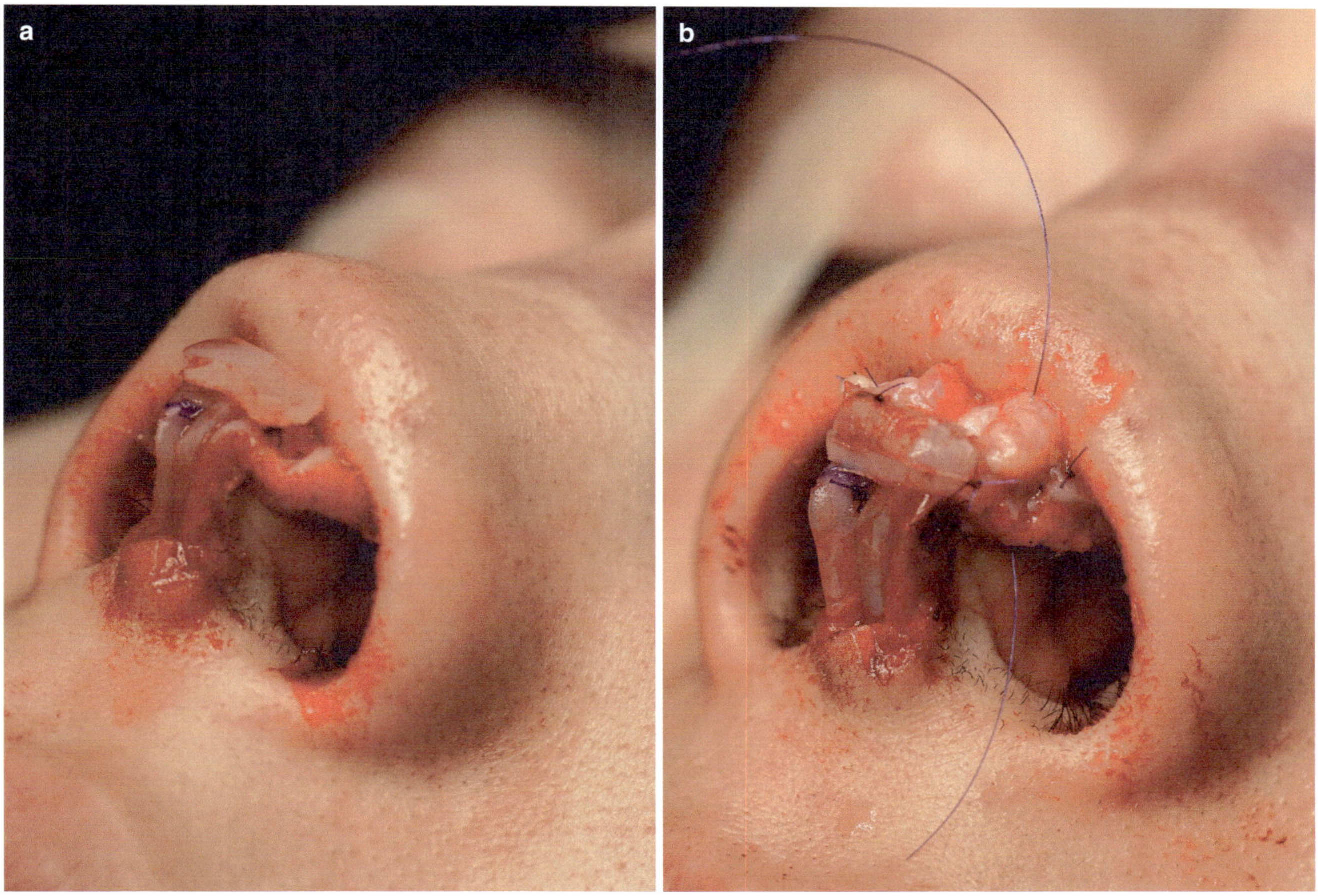

Fig. 12.18 (**a**, **b**) Following independent creation and fixation of the right and left domes, columellar strut, caudally positioned tip graft, lateral crural grafts, and camouflage graft are placed

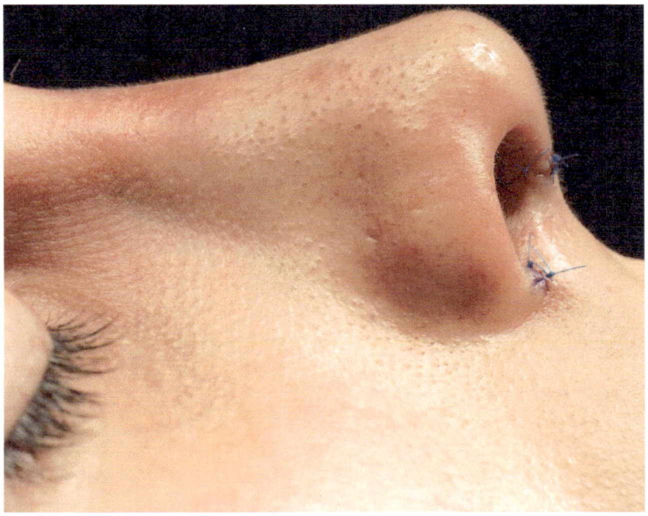

Fig. 12.19 Immediately after surgery

crura will achieve moderate deprojection and rotation. Let us examine a typical example.

12.5.4 Case 4

A 28-year-old woman previously underwent rhinoplasty; the tip was over-rotated and over-projected with a long medial crura and short lateral crura. Excessive nostril show and a hanging infra tip lobule were also present (Fig. 12.28).

The photographs in Fig. 12.29 show the intraoperative clinical findings.

A caudal septal replacement graft harvested from homologous costal cartilage was used to strengthen and lengthen the caudal septum (Fig. 12.30).

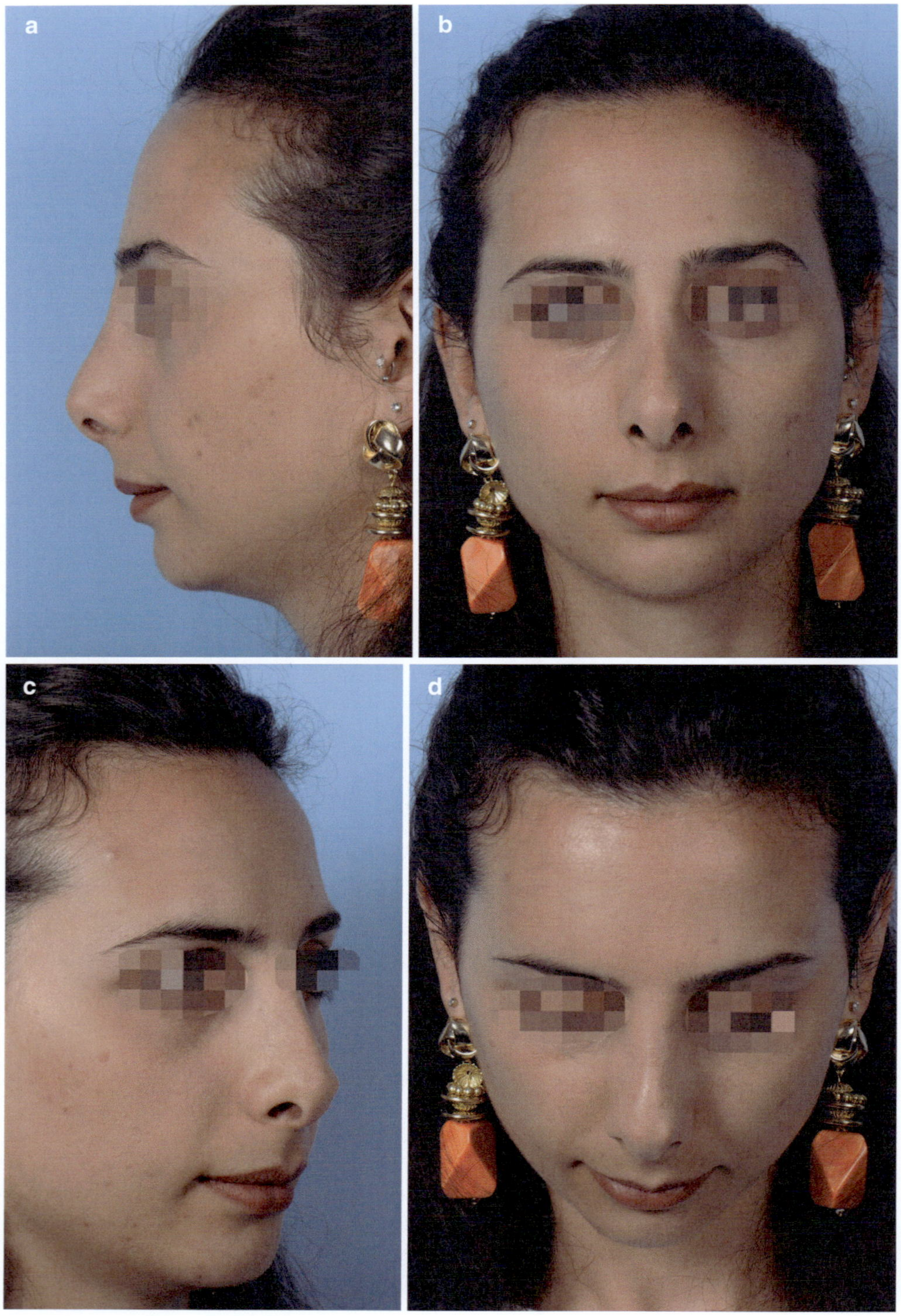

Fig. 12.20 The patient before (**a–d**) and 12 months after (**e–h**) elongation of a secondary short nose using medial crural steal suture and posterior caudal septal resection

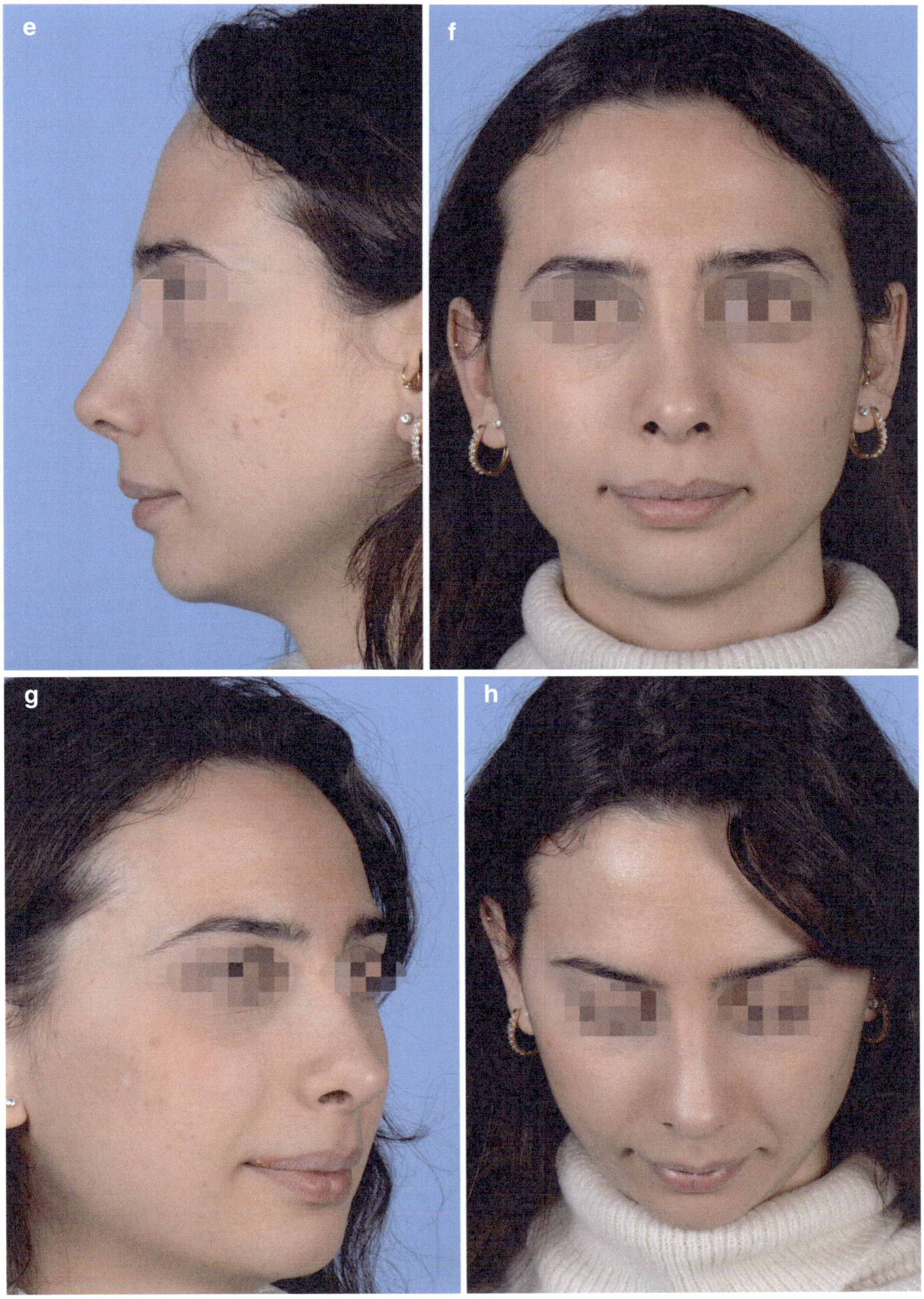

Fig. 12.20 (continued)

Then, the lateral crura were detached from the vestibular skin. To strengthen and lengthen the lateral crus, a lateral crural graft was placed under the lateral crus. Grafts were harvested from homologous costal cartilage. Then, the newly formed lateral crura were placed in their previous positions (Fig. 12.31).

The medial crural overlap is indicated in patient who has severe over-rotation associated with over-projection. After lateral crural reconstruction, the medial crura were cut and overlapped each other. Tip grafts are necessary to achieve the proper tip definition, rotation, and projection. Finally, a columellar strut, cap graft, and crushed cartilage used as an infratip lobular graft were secured with absorbable sutures (Fig. 12.32).

Preoperative and 2-year postoperative photographs are shown in Fig. 12.33.

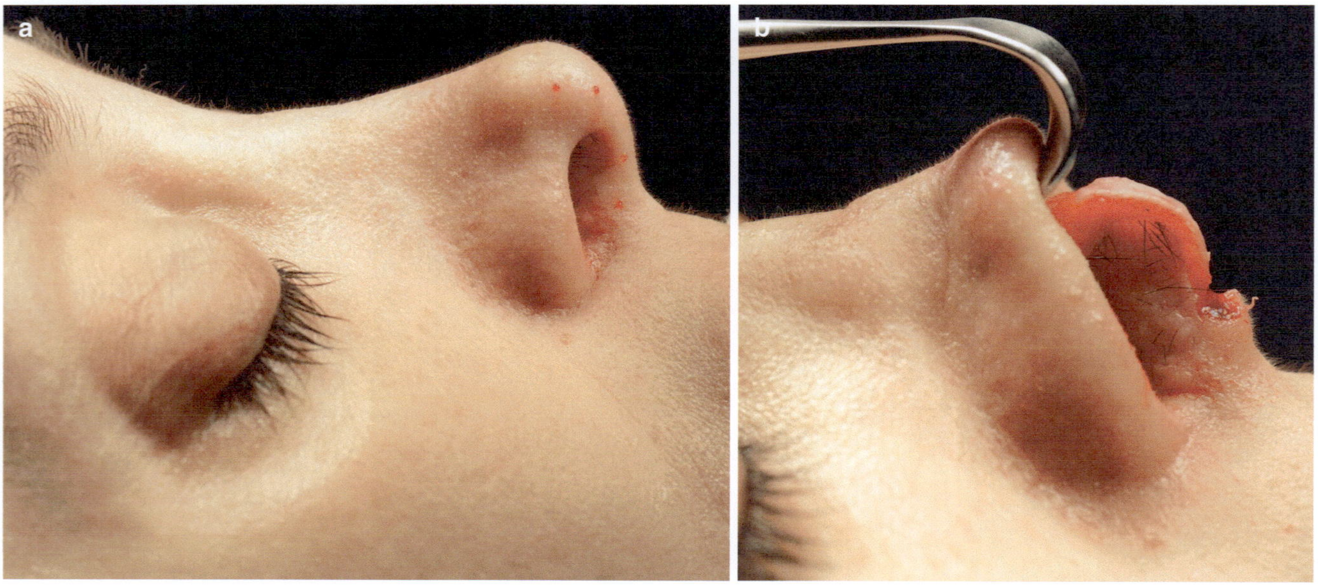

Fig. 12.21 (**a**, **b**) This patient had undergone two prior rhinoplasties. Cephalic over-rotation stems from weak lateral crura and long and strong middle crura

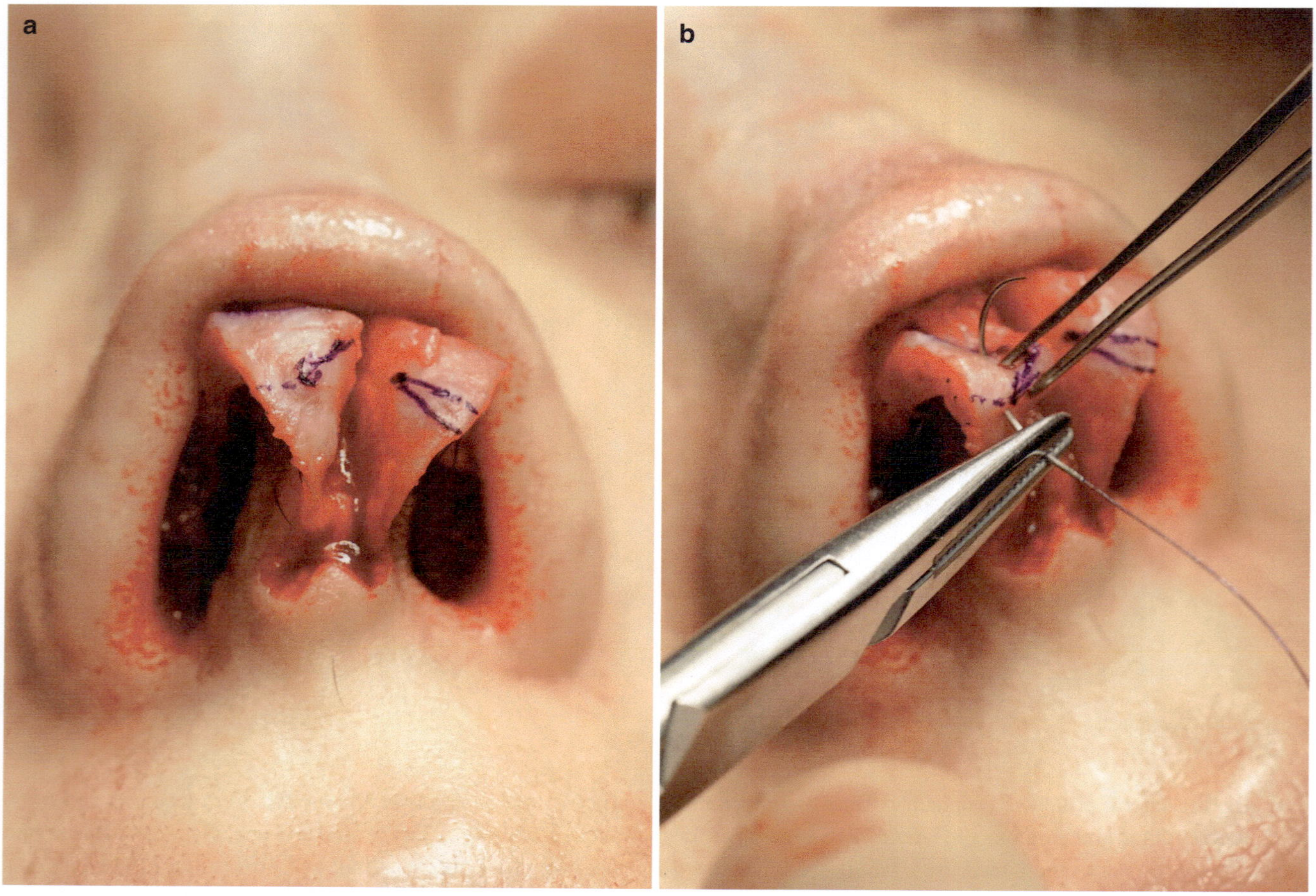

Fig. 12.22 (**a**, **b**) The new dome points created in a more caudal position

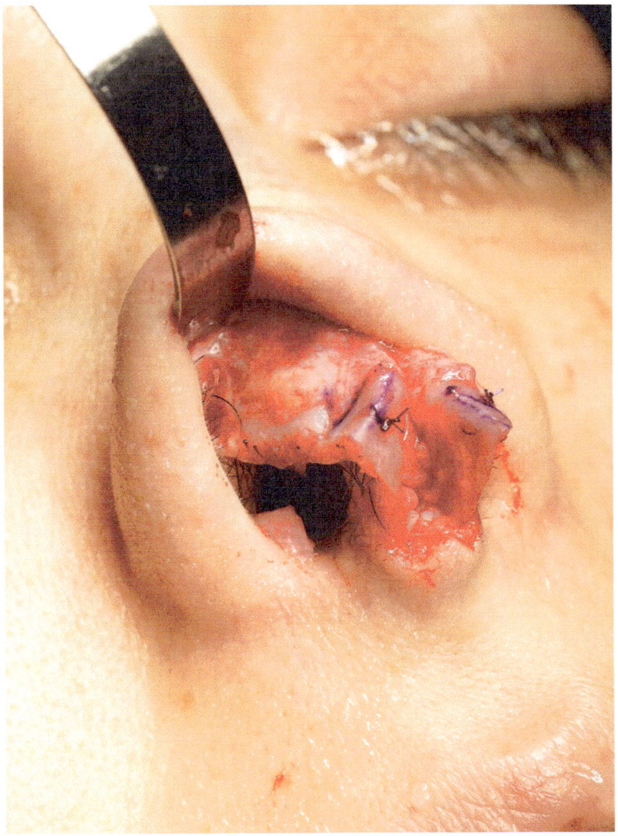

Fig. 12.23 In the MCS technique, the medial crura are advanced onto the lateral crura, resulting in an increase in the length of the lateral crura at the expense of the medial crura

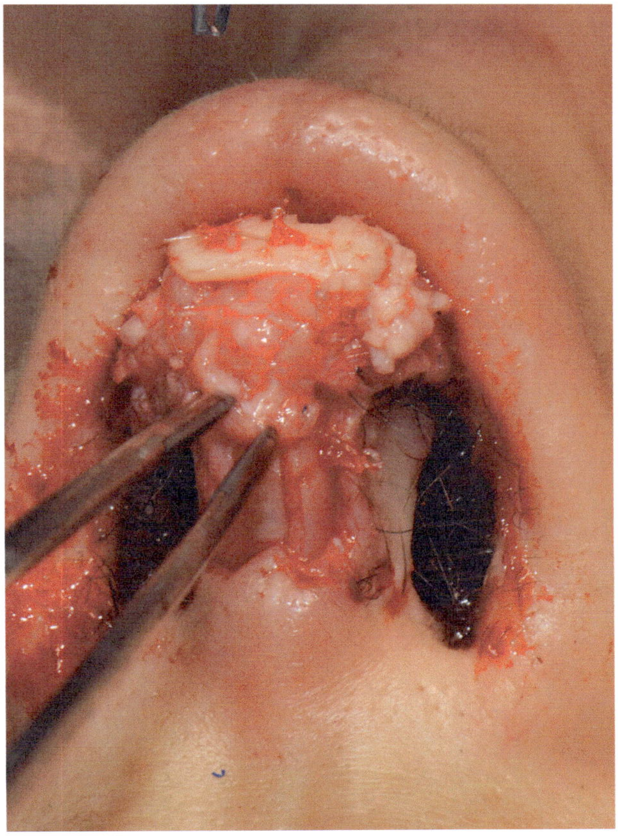

Fig. 12.25 A combination of onlay and infratip grafts further elongates the nasal tip complex more caudally

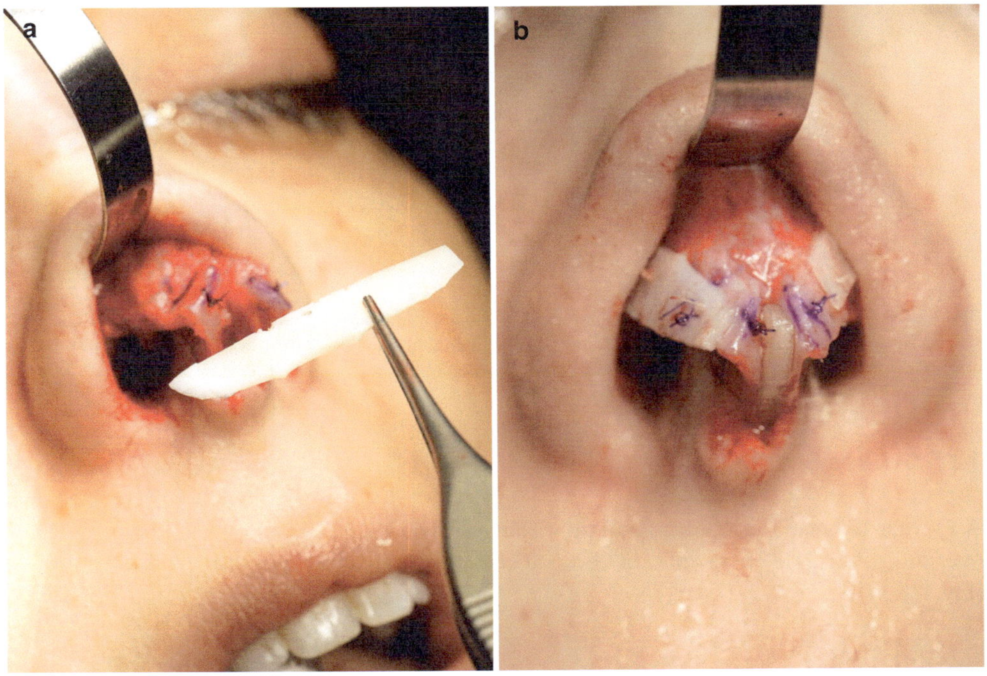

Fig. 12.24 (**a**, **b**) The lateral crural weakness was corrected with lateral crural grafts after creating new domes

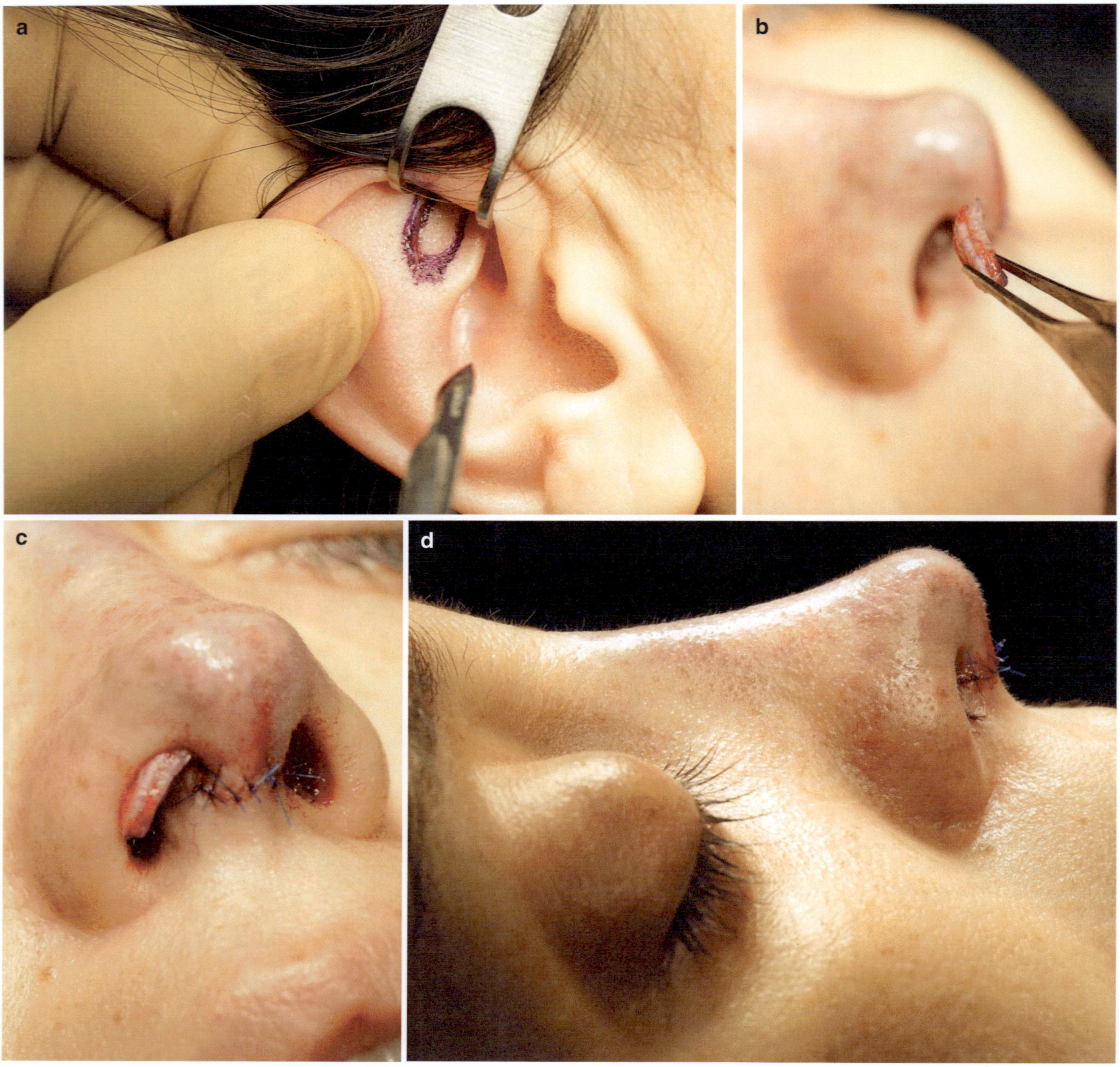

Fig. 12.26 (**a**) The composite graft was harvested from the right triangular fossa. (**b**) The ear composite graft. (**c**, **d**) The graft was placed in a marginal rim incision. Note that the size of the graft depends on the degree of alar retraction. The graft should fit the defect precisely and be at the point of maximum retraction. The graft in this case was sutured

12.5.5 Case 5

A 24-year-old man felt that his nasal tip was over-rotated and over-projected. He also has a history of rhinoplasty (Fig. 12.34).

Division and overlap of the medial crura shortened the leg of the nasal tip. The overlap helped to achieve the ideal nasal tip rotation, projection, and symmetry. Lateral crural grafts were used for lateral crural reconstruction (Fig. 12.35).

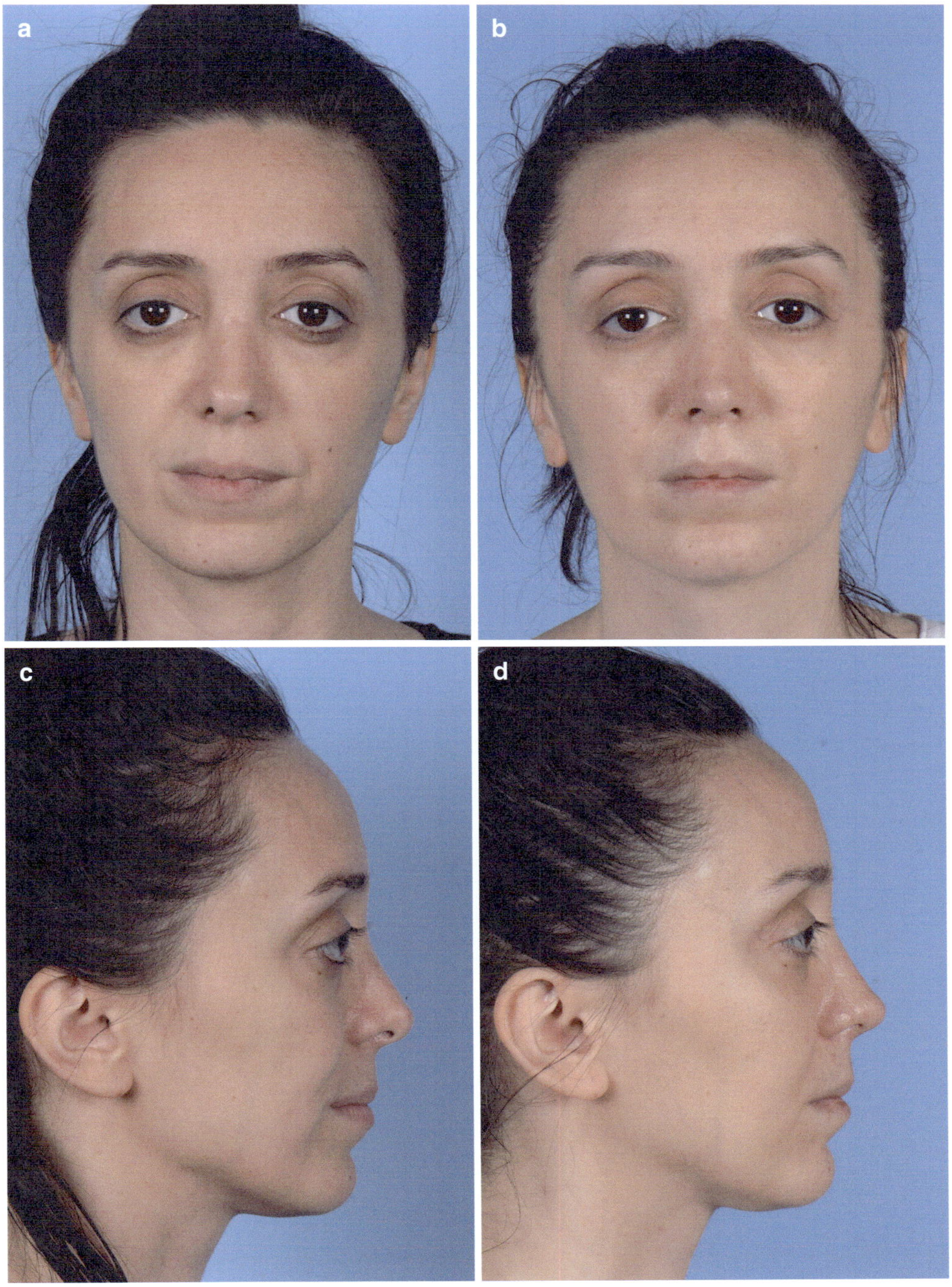

Fig. 12.27 (**a**–**f**) Before and after views. (**a**, **b**) A balanced nasal tip as seen from the frontal view. (**c**, **d**) The lateral view demonstrates an improved columella-lobular angle and alar columellar relationship. (**e**, **f**) Composite graft and lateral crural graft corrected the depressed alar grooves and the pinched appearance of the nasal tip

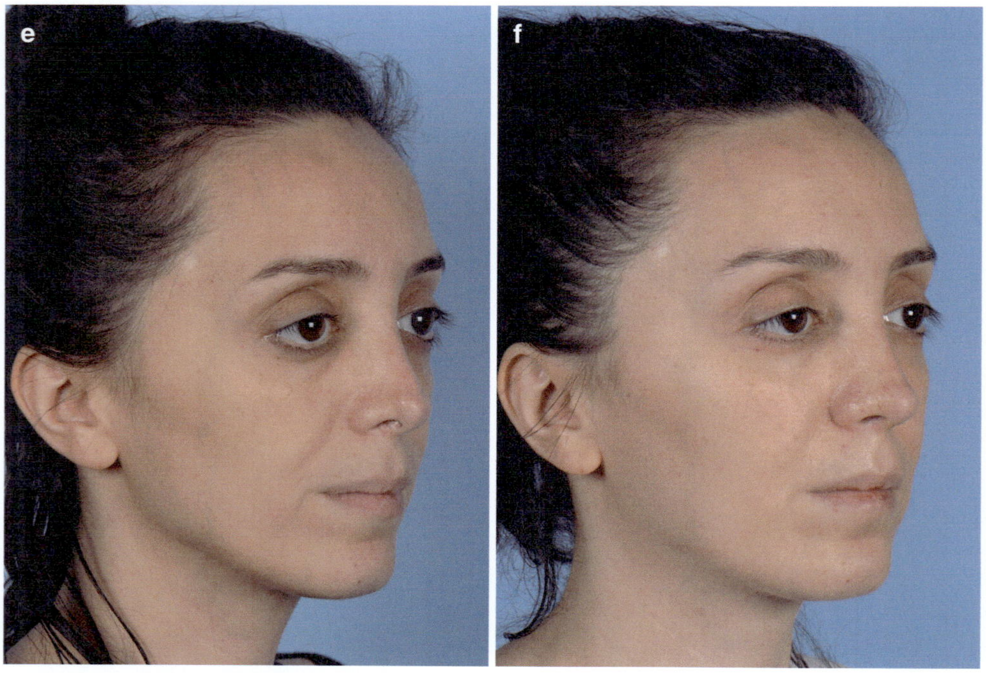

Fig. 12.27 (continued)

Fig. 12.28 (**a**, **b**) The alar–columellar disharmony was due to medial crural misconfiguration; the overlap technique is suitable in such a situation

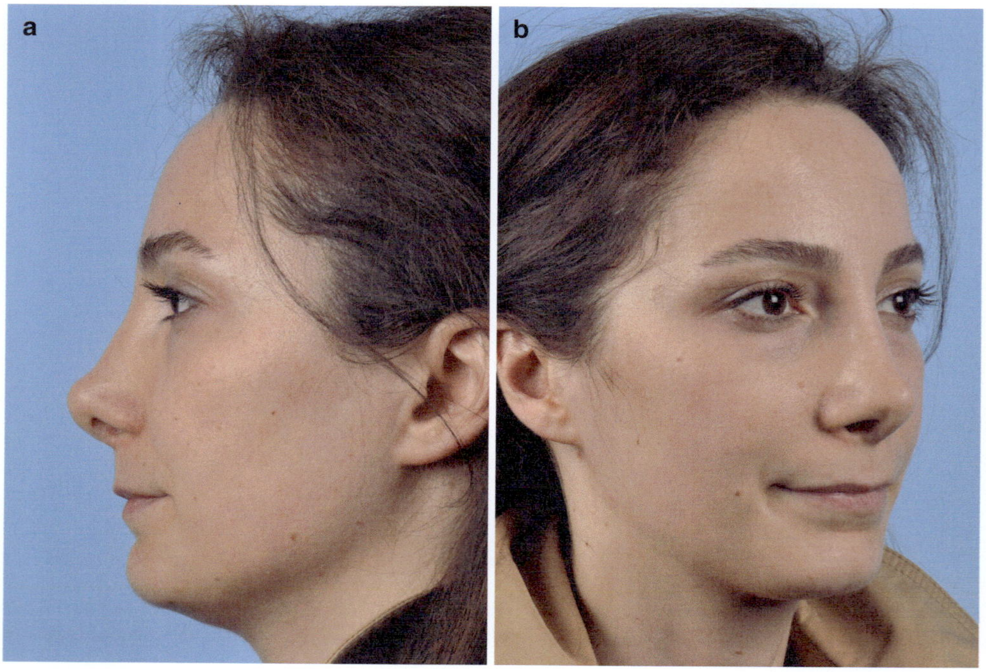

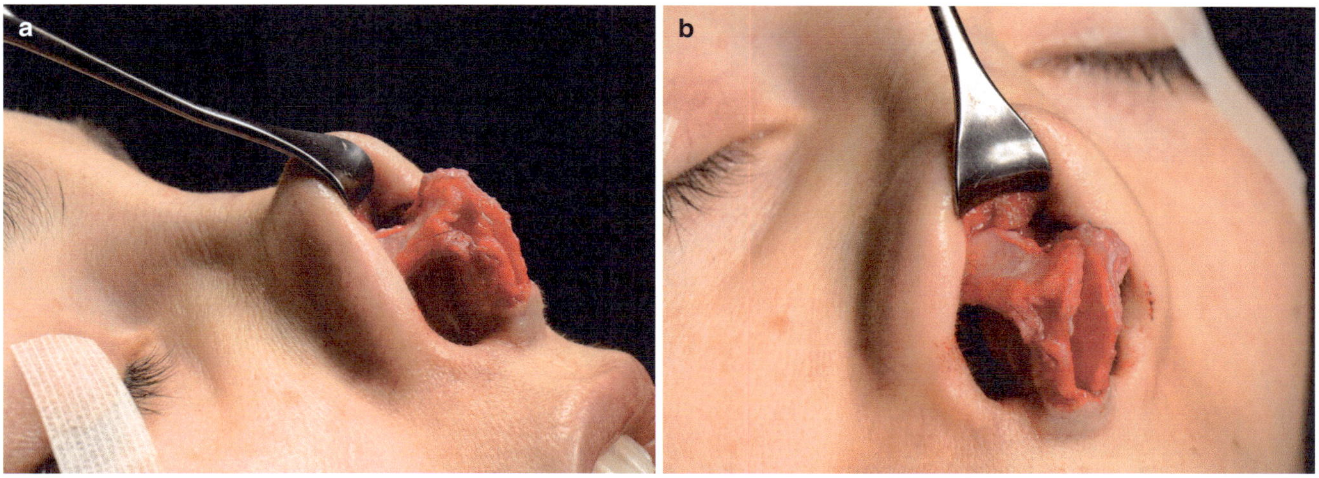

Fig. 12.29 (a, b) Severely deformed lower lateral cartilage complexes

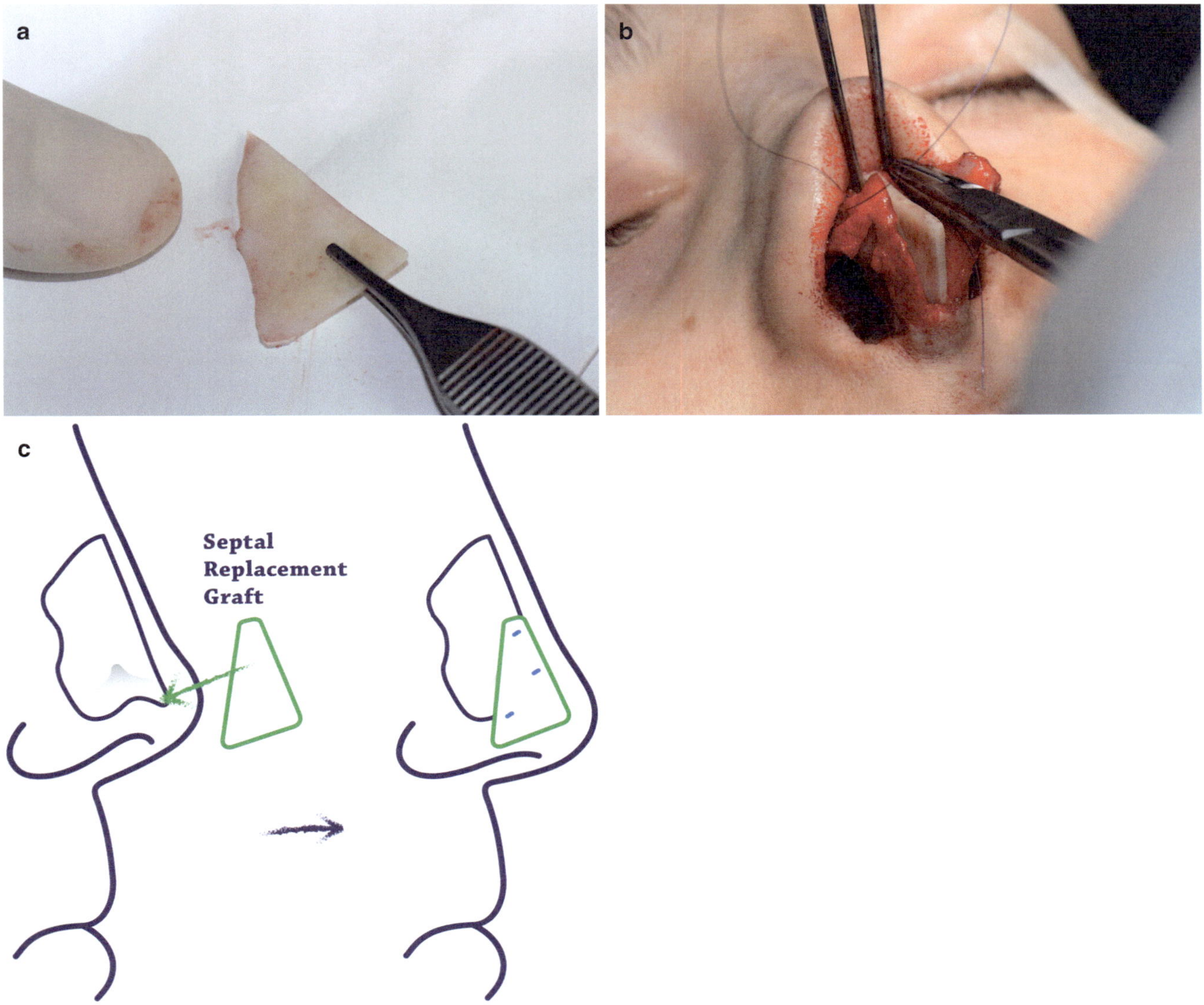

Fig. 12.30 (a–c) Septal replacement graft was added on the concave side beyond the anterocaudal septum proportional to the elongation necessary and fixed to the septum

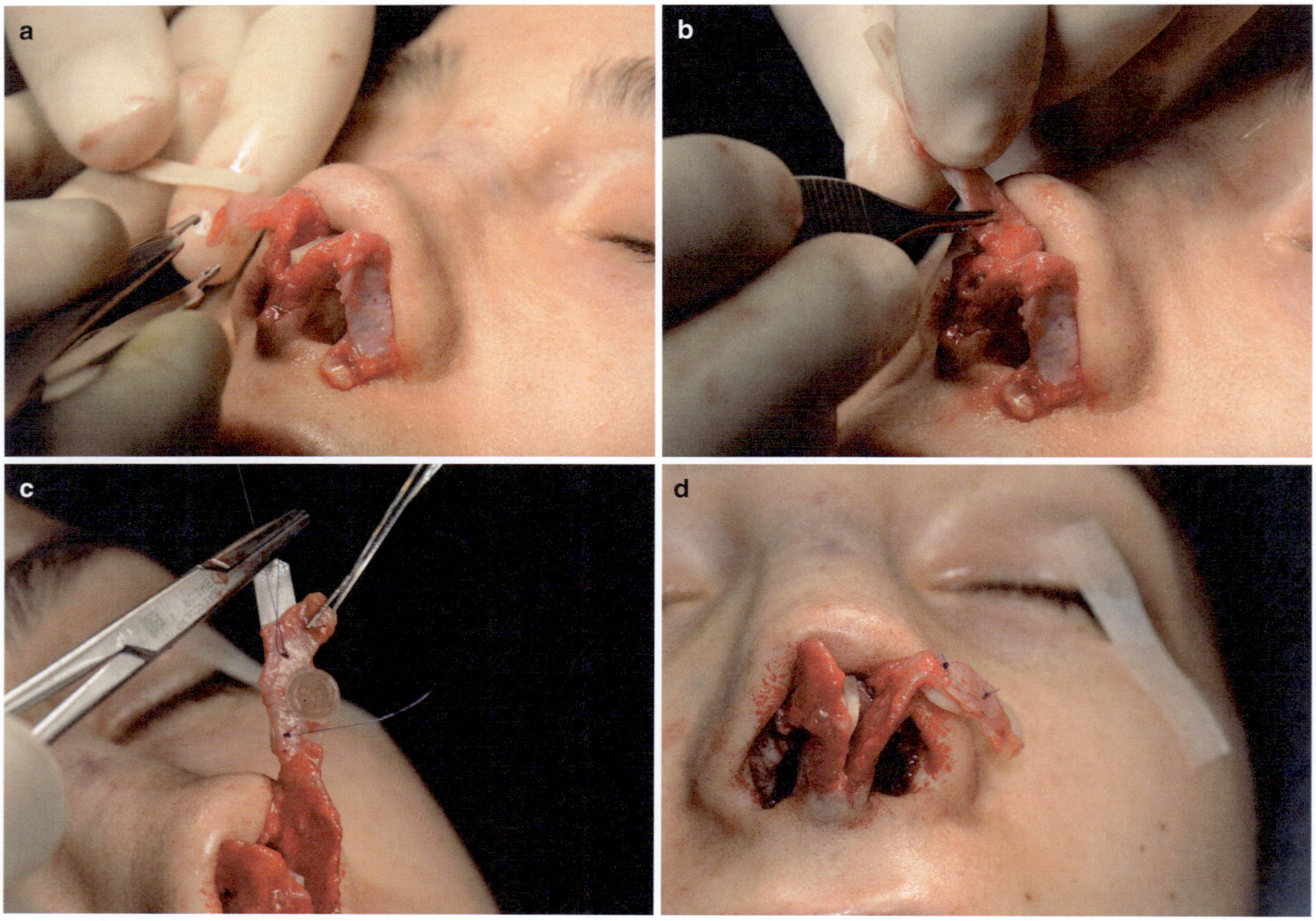

Fig. 12.31 (**a–d**) In this case, lateral crura were dissected from the underlying vestibular skin and the lateral crural graft was sutured to the undersurface of the crus, providing additional support and length for weak and short lateral crural cartilage

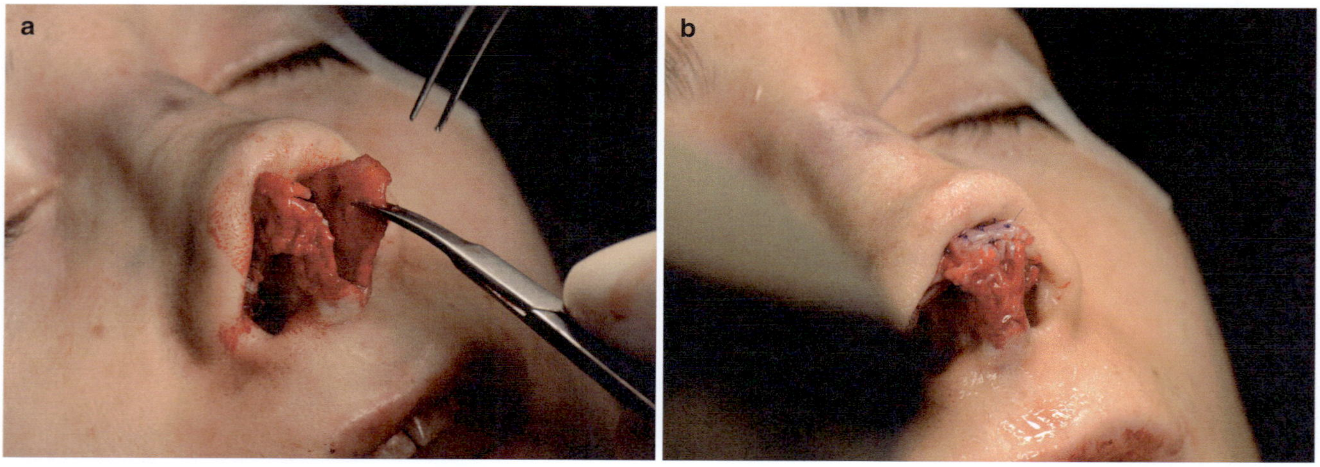

Fig. 12.32 (**a**) With the medial crural overlap technique, the medial crus is shortened by vertically transecting it and overlapping the cut edges. An incision is planned so as to cross the midportion of the medial crus on each side. The cartilage is then cut. The free proximal and distal ends of the transected medial crus are then overlapped and fixed with a 5–0 permanent, transcartilaginous, horizontal, mattress-type stitch. (**b**) Tip grafts set tip projection, hide tip asymmetries, and improve tip rotation

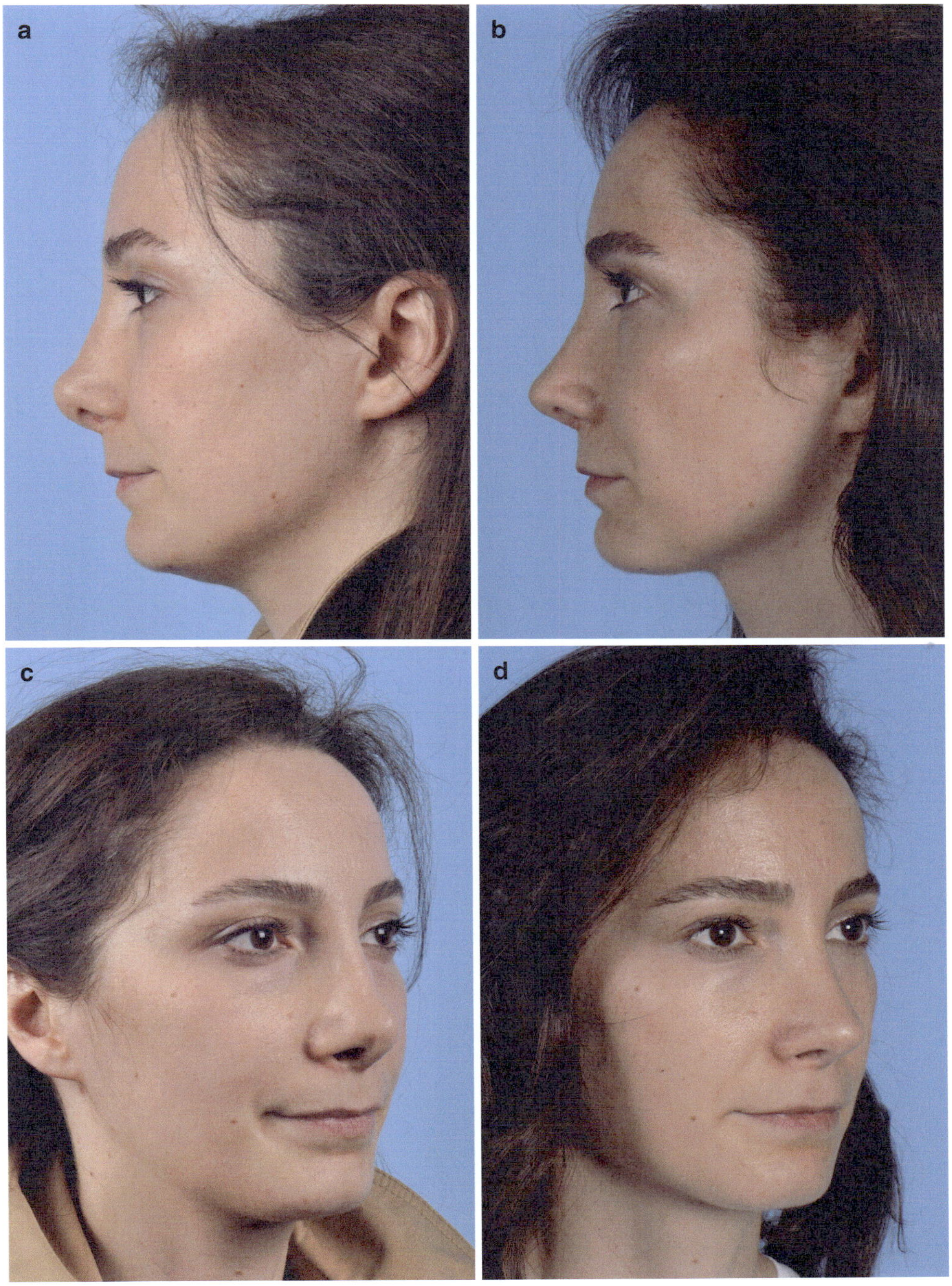

Fig. 12.33 (**a**–**h**) Pre- and postoperative views. The nasal tip is well projected. The tip has been counter-rotated. There is decreased show of the columella. The alar–columellar relationship has been significantly improved

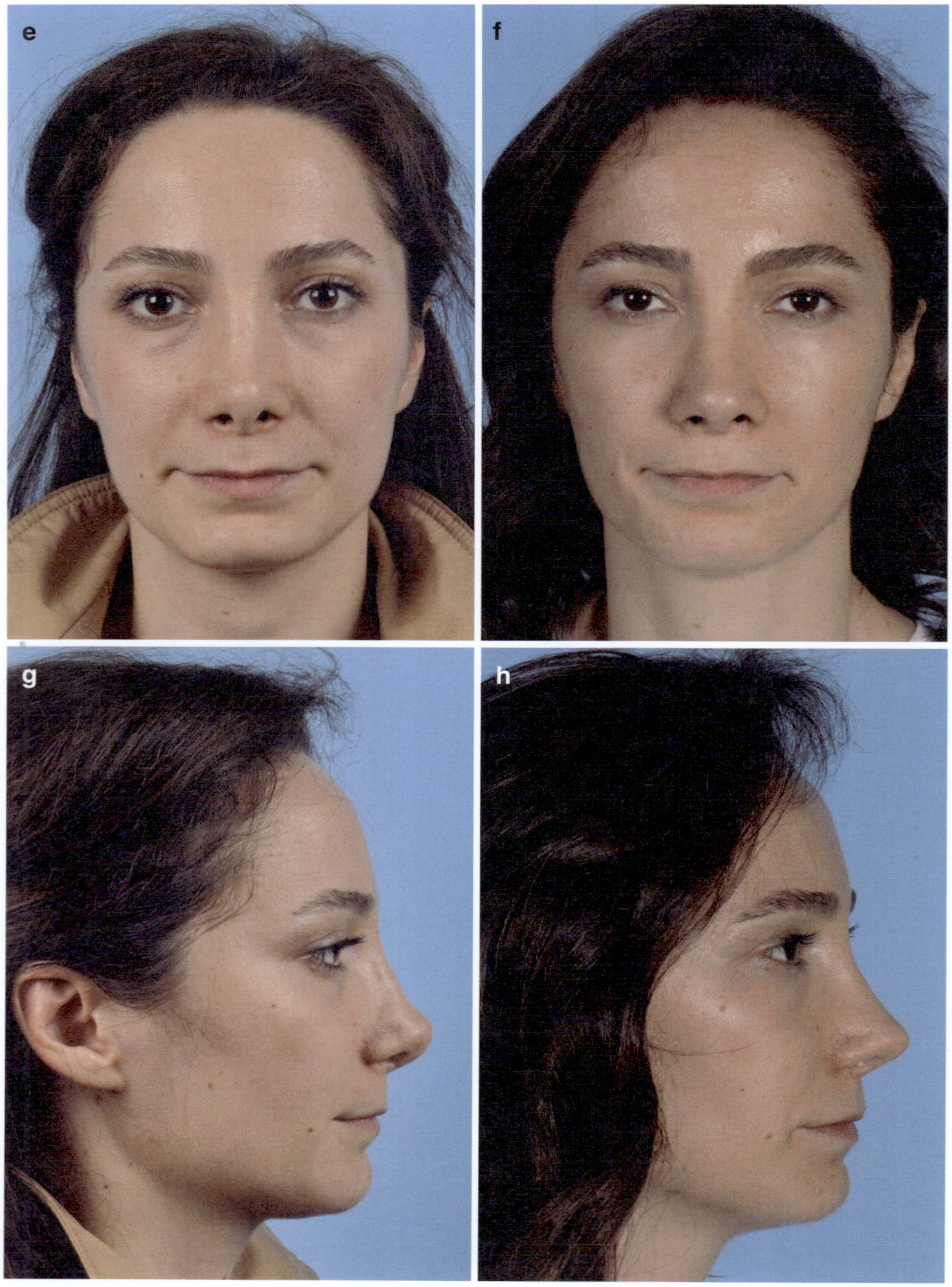

Fig. 12.33 (continued)

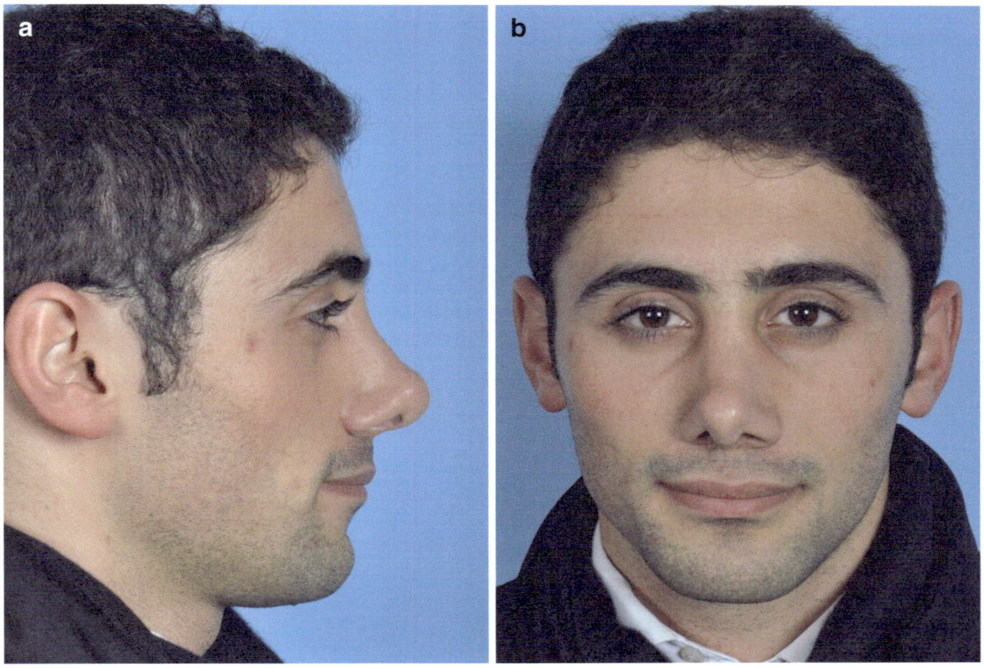

Fig. 12.34 (**a**, **b**) The nose is over-rotated and over-projected and the tip is asymmetric

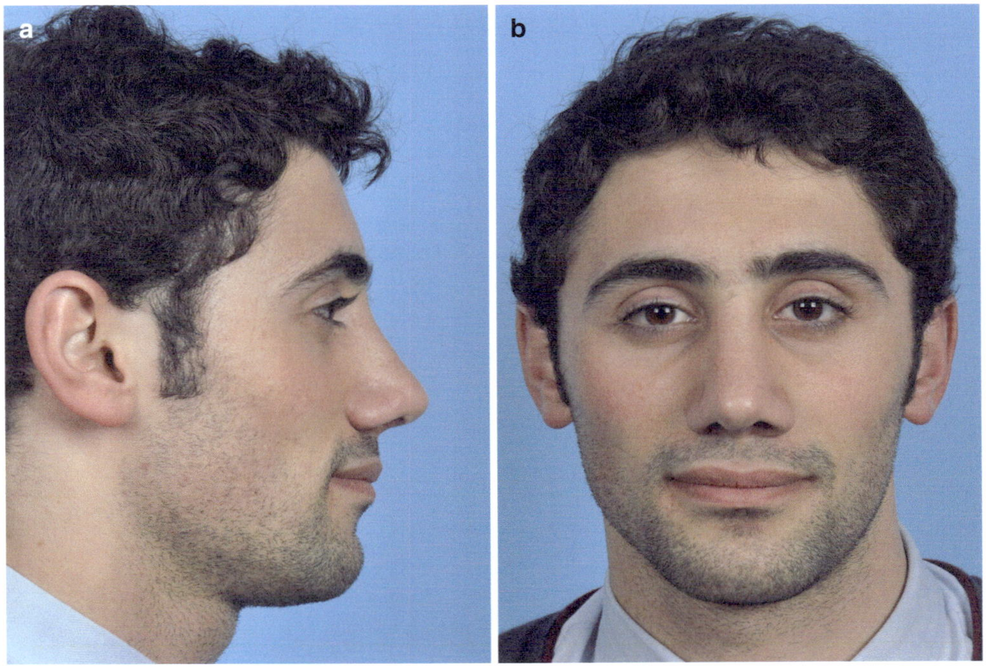

Fig. 12.35 (**a**, **b**) Photographs 1-year postoperatively. The nasal tip has been de-projected and under-rotated. The tip asymmetry has been eliminated, and alar side walls are stronger

12.6 Conclusion

In over-rotated tip surgery, strong tip support is essential to maintain the achieved ideal tip projection and rotation; in other words, the long-term result of any tip technique depends mainly on the amount of available tip support. One of the major tip support structures is the caudal septum. If the septum was previously excised or is congenitally deficient, it should be reconstructed. Another important factor is the status of the alar cartilages. The alar cartilages and their subunits should be examined separately. Depending on the problem, some parts should be strengthened (e.g., the lateral crus), while others should be shortened (e.g., the middle/medial crus) to bring the alar cartilage anatomy into ideal alignment.

Remember that the skin limits both alar cartilage and septal maneuvers; this should be discussed with the patients and their expectations should be realistic.

Disclosures The author reports no conflicts of interest or funding requiring disclosure.

Further Reading

Akkus AM, Eryilmaz E, Guneren E. Comparison of the effects of columellar strut and septal extension grafts for tip support in rhinoplasty. Aesth Plast Surg. 2013;37(4):666–73.

André RF, Vuyk HD. Reconstruction of dorsal and/or caudal nasal septum deformities with septal battens or by septal replacement: an overview and comparison of techniques. Laryngoscope. 2006;116(9):1668–73.

Byrd HS, Andochick S, Copit S, Walton KG. Septal extension grafts: a method of controlling tip projection shape. Plast Reconstr Surg. 1997;100(4):999–1010.

Cone JD, Hobar PC. The short nose. Clin Plast Surg. 2016;43(1):169–76.

Foda HM. The caudal septum replacement graft. Arch Facial Plast Surg. 2008;10(3):152–7.

Gruber RP. Surgical correction of the short nose. Aesth Plast Surg. 2002;26(Suppl 1):S6.

Gunter JP, Rohrich RJ. Lengthening the aesthetically short nose. Plast Reconstr Surg. 1989;83(5):793–800.

Hobar PC, Adams WP, Mitchell CA. Lengthening the short nose. Clin Plast Surg. 2010;37(2):327–33.

Huang J, Liu Y. A modified technique of septal extension using a septal cartilage graft for short-nose rhinoplasty in Asians. Aesth Plast Surg. 2012;36(5):1028–38.

Jung DH, Jin SG, Hyun SM. Correction of short nose. Facial Plast Surg Clin North Am. 2018;26(3):377–88.

Kim MH, Choi JH, Kim MS, Kim SK, Lee KC. An introduction to the septal extension graft. Arch Plast Surg. 2014;41(1):29–34.

Naficy S, Baker SR. Lengthening the short nose. Arch Otolaryngol Head Neck Surg. 1998;124(7):809–13.

Park JH, Mangoba DC, Mun SJ, Kim DW, Jin HR. Lengthening the short nose in Asians: key maneuvers and surgical results. JAMA Facial Plast Surg. 2013;15(6):439–47.

Ponsky DC, Harvey DJ, Khan SW, Guyuron B. Nose elongation: a review and description of the septal extension tongue-and-groove technique. Aesthet Surg J. 2010;30(3):335–46.

Rikimaru H, Kiyokawa K, Watanabe K, Koga N, Nishi Y. A new therapeutic strategy for lengthening severe short nose. J Craniofac Surg. 2010;21(2):495–8.

Şeneldir S, Kırgezen T. Vertical alar folding (VAF): a useful technique for correction of long and concave lateral crura in rhinoplasty. Aesth Plast Surg. 2019;43(5):1269–78.

Şeneldir S, Altundağ A, Dizdar D. Cutting the holy dome: the evolution of vertical alar resection. Aesth Plast Surg. 2018;42(1):275–87.

Senyuva C, Yücel A, Aydin Y, Okur I, Güzel Z. Extracorporeal septoplasty combined with open rhinoplasty. Aesth Plast Surg. 1997;21(4):233–9.

Seyhan A, Ozden S, Ozaslan U, Sir E. A simplified use of septal extension graft to control nasal tip location. Aesth Plast Surg. 2007;31(5):506–11; discussion 512–3

Suh MK, Ahn ES, Kim HR, Dhong ES. A 2-year follow-up of irradiated homologous costal cartilage used as a septal extension graft for the correction of contracted nose in Asians. Ann Plast Surg. 2013;71(1):45–9.

Suh YC, Jeong WS, Choi JW. Septum-based nasal tip plasty: a comparative study between septal extension graft and double-layered Conchal cartilage extension graft. Plast Reconstr Surg. 2018;141(1):49–56.

Toriumi DM. Subtotal septal reconstruction: an update. Facial Plast Surg. 2013;29(6):492–501.

Toriumi DM, Bared A. Revision of the surgically overshortened nose. Facial Plast Surg. 2012;28(4):407–16.

Toriumi DM, Patel AB, DeRosa J. Correcting the short nose in revision rhinoplasty. Facial Plast Surg Clin North Am. 2006;14(4):343–55. vi

Woo JS, Dung NP, Suh MK. A novel technique for short nose correction: hybrid septal extension graft. J Craniofac Surg. 2016;27(1):e44–8.

Wu PS, Hamilton GS. Extracorporeal septoplasty: external and endonasal techniques. Facial Plast Surg. 2016;32(1):22–8.

13 Wide Nasal Tip

13.1 Introduction

Alar cartilage abnormalities are the principal cause of wide nasal tips, although thick skin may also widen the nasal tip. To ensure successful surgery, the surgeon must have a good knowledge of the ideal cartilage anatomy and variations thereof. Seven anatomical features of the alar cartilage that influence tip shape are as follows:

1. **The domal separation angle**: The between-dome angle should be about 90°. The nasal tip widens and increases in size as the angle increases (Fig. 13.1).
2. **The domal definition angle**: This angle should be acute; the greater the angle, the wider the tip. In other words, the length of the domal arch should be approximately 4 mm. The tip widens as the arch lengthens (Fig. 13.2).
3. **The crural surface:** The ideal lateral crural surface is smooth or mildly convex. The tip widens as convexity increases. Excessive lateral crural convexity is the most common cause of alar cartilage deformities (Fig. 13.3).
4. **The surface area of the lateral crus**: The tip volume is proportional to this area. As the crural surface widens caudally, tip volume increases, and the tip becomes more prominent (Fig. 13.4).
5. **The positions of the caudal and cranial margins of the lateral crus**, which must lie in the same plane (Fig. 13.5; Video 13.1). If the caudal margins of the lateral crura lie below the cephalic margins, the tip appears wide (Fig. 13.6).
6. **The positions of the lateral crura**: Ideally, each lateral crus points toward the outer canthus. As the tip moves toward the inner canthus, the lateral crus assumes a cephalic position. Patients presenting with such positioning typically exhibit a parenthesis-shaped tip deformity or a wide nasal tip. On an oblique view, the line of demarcation between the nasal subunits (tip/dorsum/lateral sidewall) is highly visible. If the orientation is favorable, the caudal margins of the lateral crura of the lower lateral cartilages (LLCs) can be measured from the midline, and are ideally at least 30° (Fig. 13.7). A cephalically malpositioned lateral crus presents with a parenthesis-like deformity, shadows lateral to the nasal tip, a wide tip, notched alar rims, and a nose that is almost square when viewed from below. In addition, such patients exhibit the Polly beak deformity; the lateral crura fill the supra-tip area and the external nasal valve collapses because of a lack of caudal cartilage in the lateral nasal wall. The severity of such malpositioning varies; all of these factors may be involved to some extent.
7. The lateral crural length determines tip bulbosity. A long lateral crus widens the tip laterally. A long and overdeveloped lateral crus not only creates a wide nasal tip but also may make the tip droopy and/or over-projected (Fig. 13.8).

Supplementary Information The online version contains supplementary material available at https://doi.org/10.1007/978-3-031-65619-4_13.

S. Şeneldir, *Photographic Atlas of Rhinoplasty*, https://doi.org/10.1007/978-3-031-65619-4_13

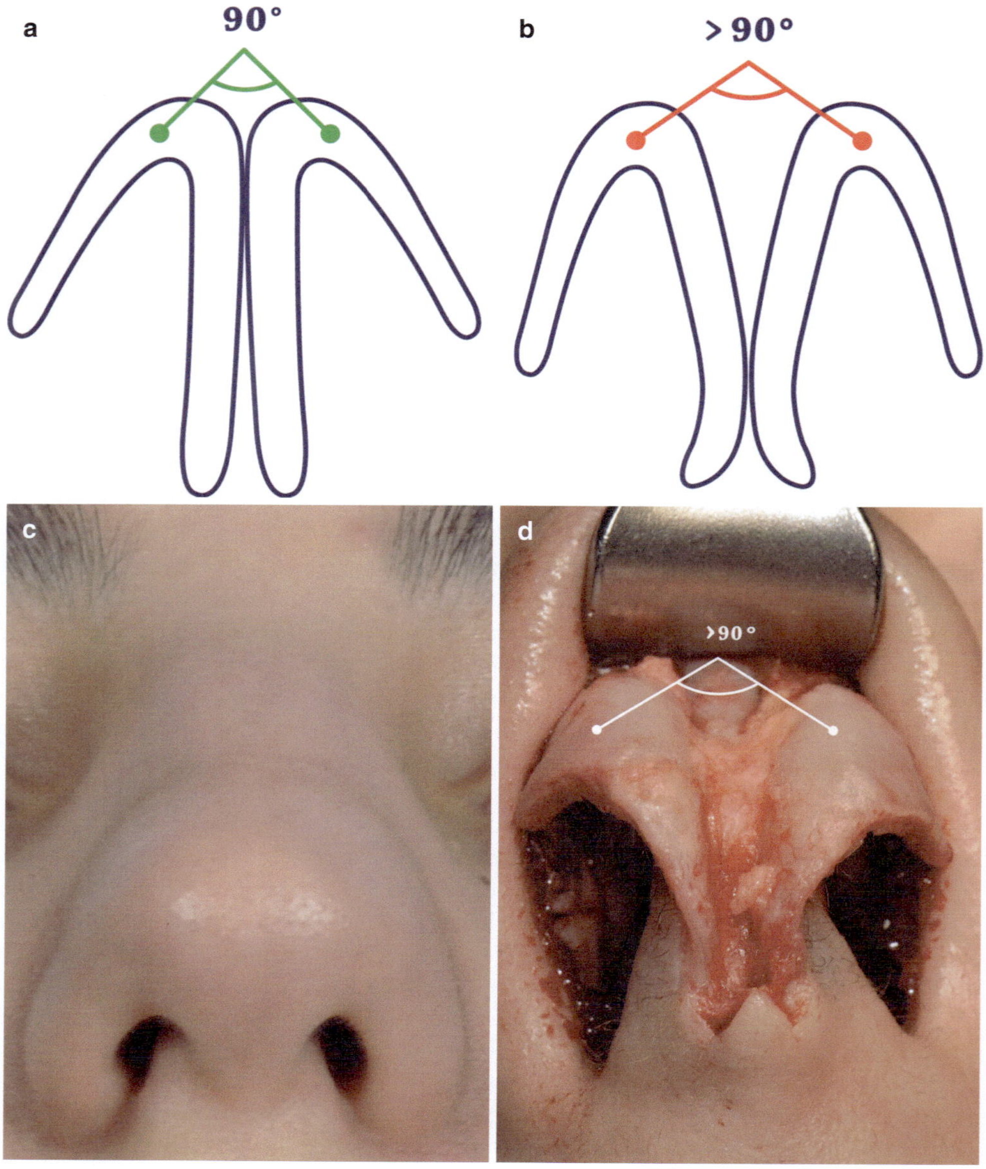

Fig. 13.1 (**a**) The ideal domal separation angle. (**b–d**) Larger angle

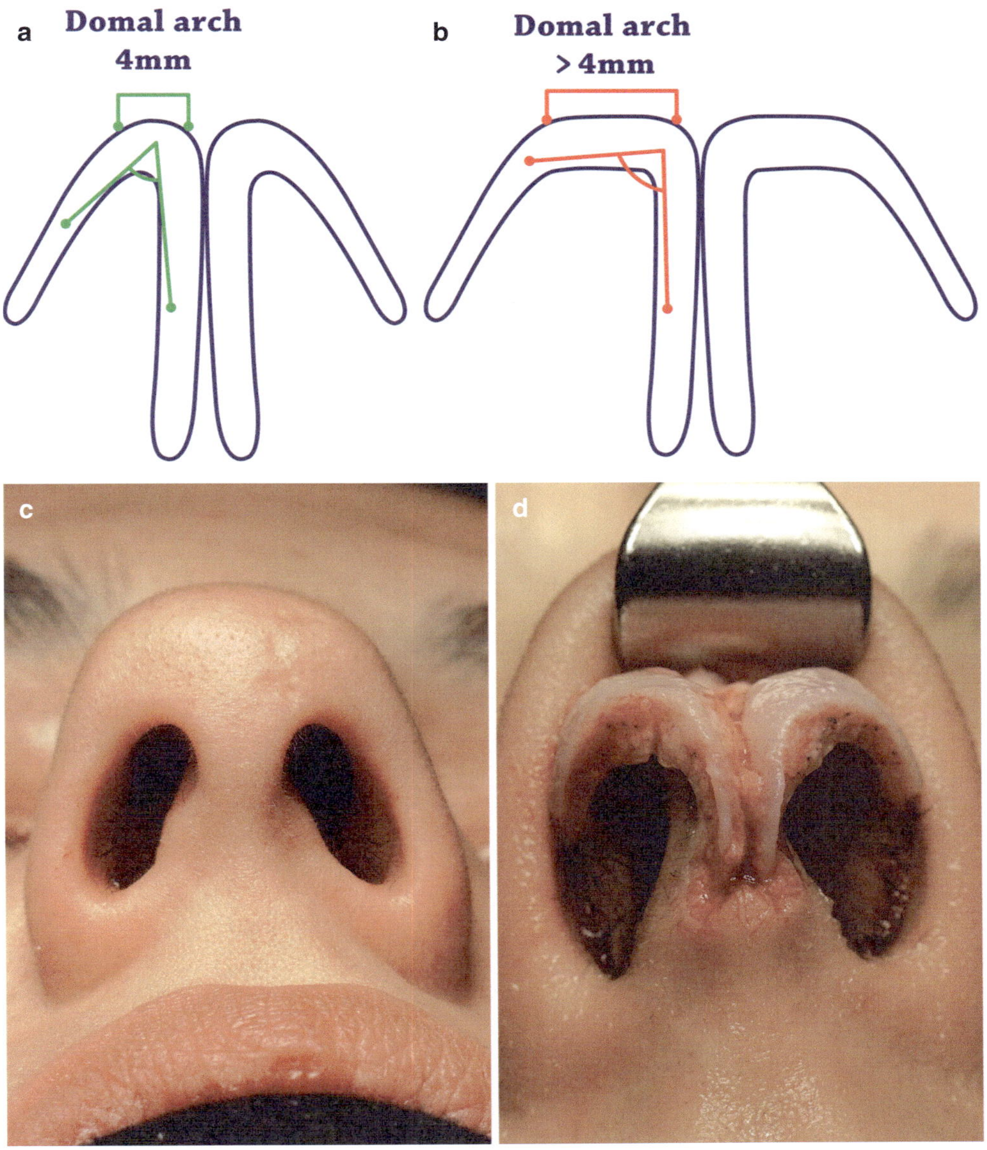

Fig. 13.2 (**a**) The ideal domal definition angle and length of domal arch. (**b–d**) Longer domal arches

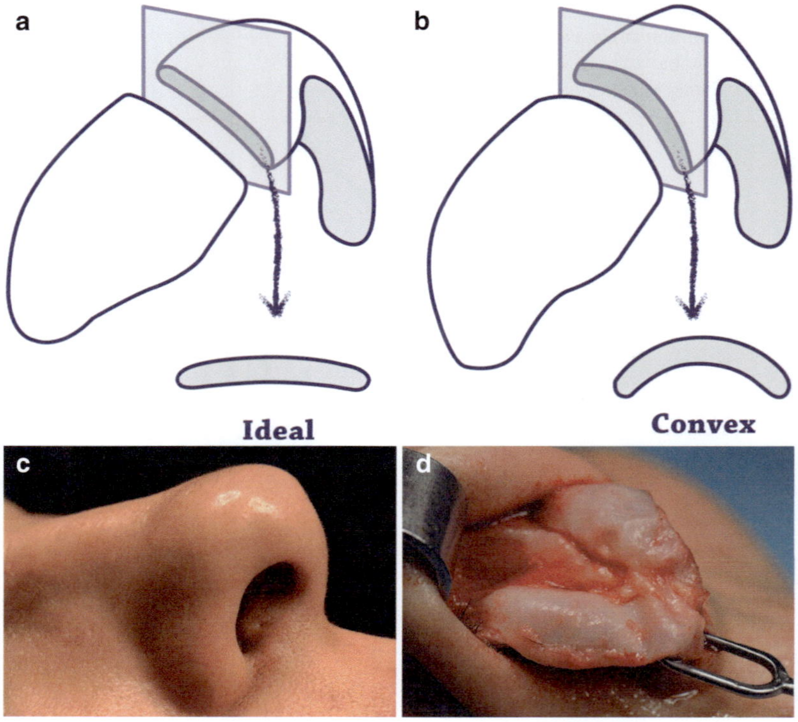

Fig. 13.3 (**a**) The ideal lateral crural surface. (**b–d**) Excessive lateral crural convexity

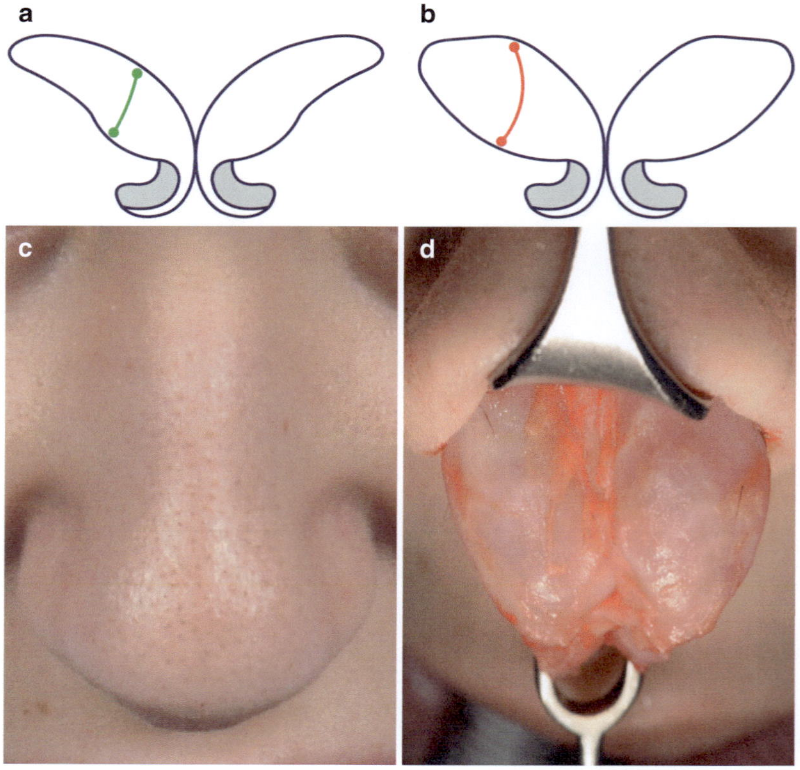

Fig. 13.4 (**a**) The ideal lateral crural surface. (**b–d**) A caudally wide crural surface

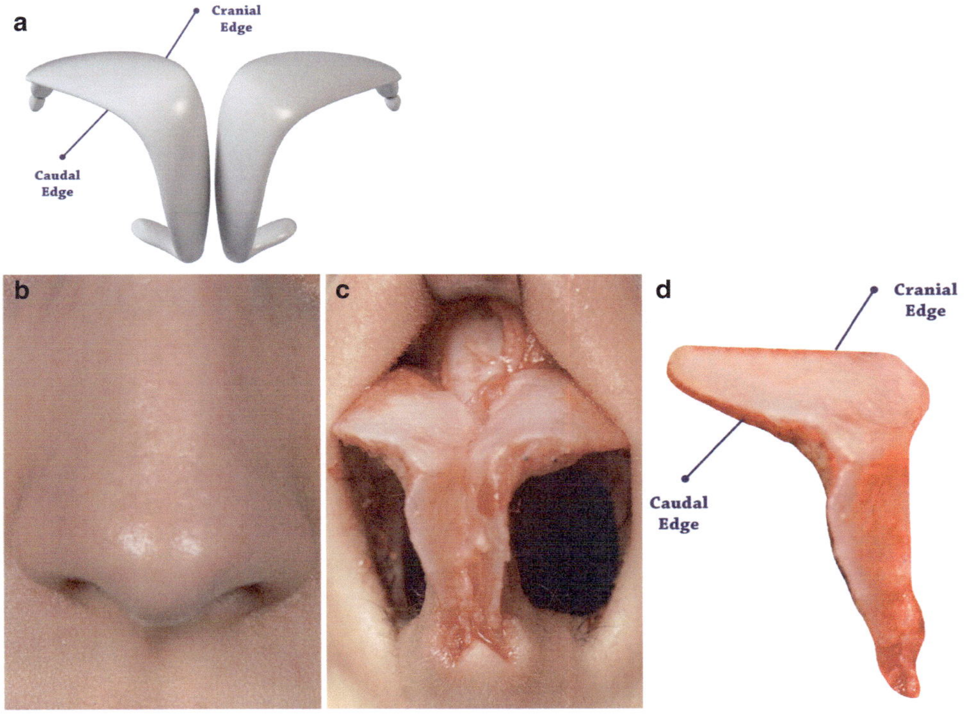

Fig. 13.5 (**a**) The ideal caudal–cranial relationship at the lateral crus. (**b**) The ideal nasal tip. (**c**) An anatomical view of the patient featured in (**b**). (**d**) Relevant relationships

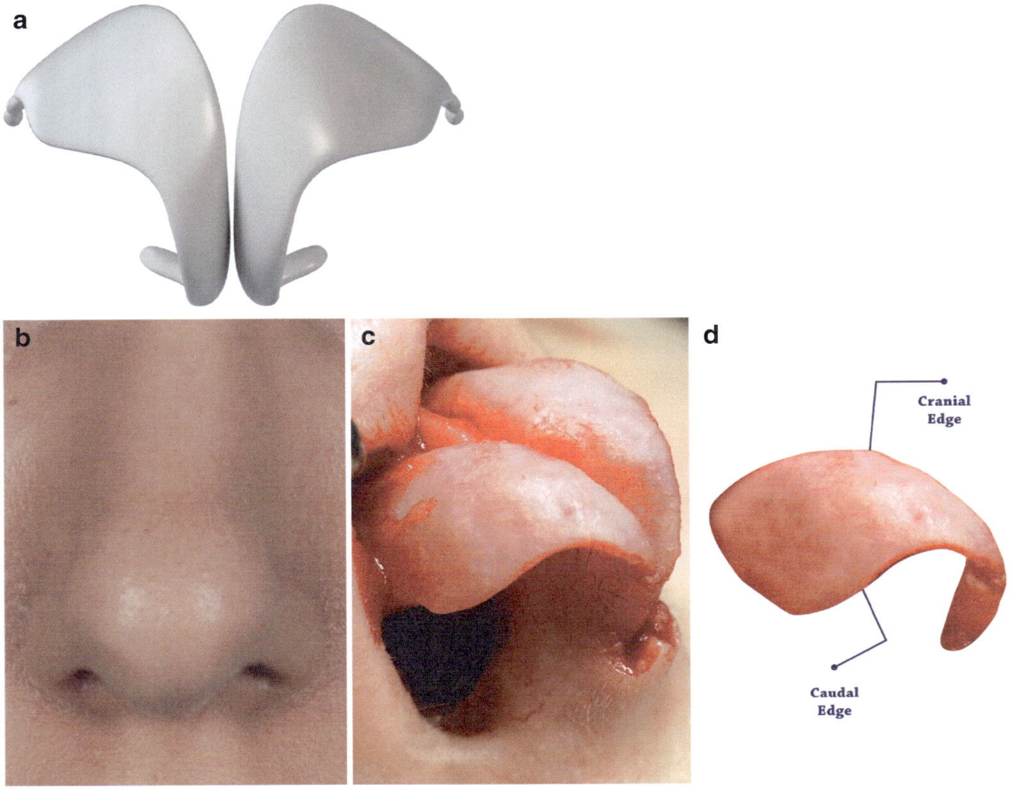

Fig. 13.6 (**a**) An unfavorable caudal–cranial relationship at the lateral crus. (**b**) A wide nasal tip. (**c**) Tip wideness is attributable to the inappropriate caudal–cranial relationship at the lateral crus. (**d**) Relevant relationships

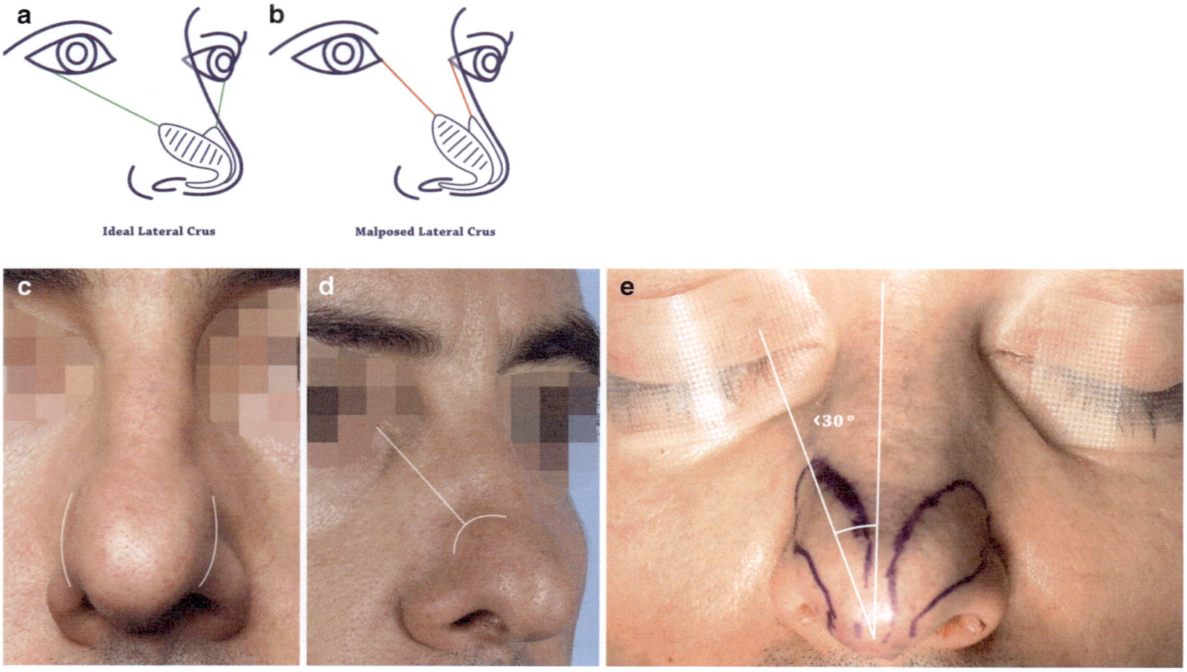

Fig. 13.7 (**a**) The ideal position of the lateral crus. (**b**) A malpositioned lateral crus. (**c**, **d**) The clinical appearance of a malpositioned lateral crus. (**e**) A narrower crural angle

Fig. 13.8 (**a**) The green line indicates the length of the lateral crus. (**b**) The red line indicates the length of a long lateral crus. (**c**, **d**) The clinical appearance of a long lateral crus

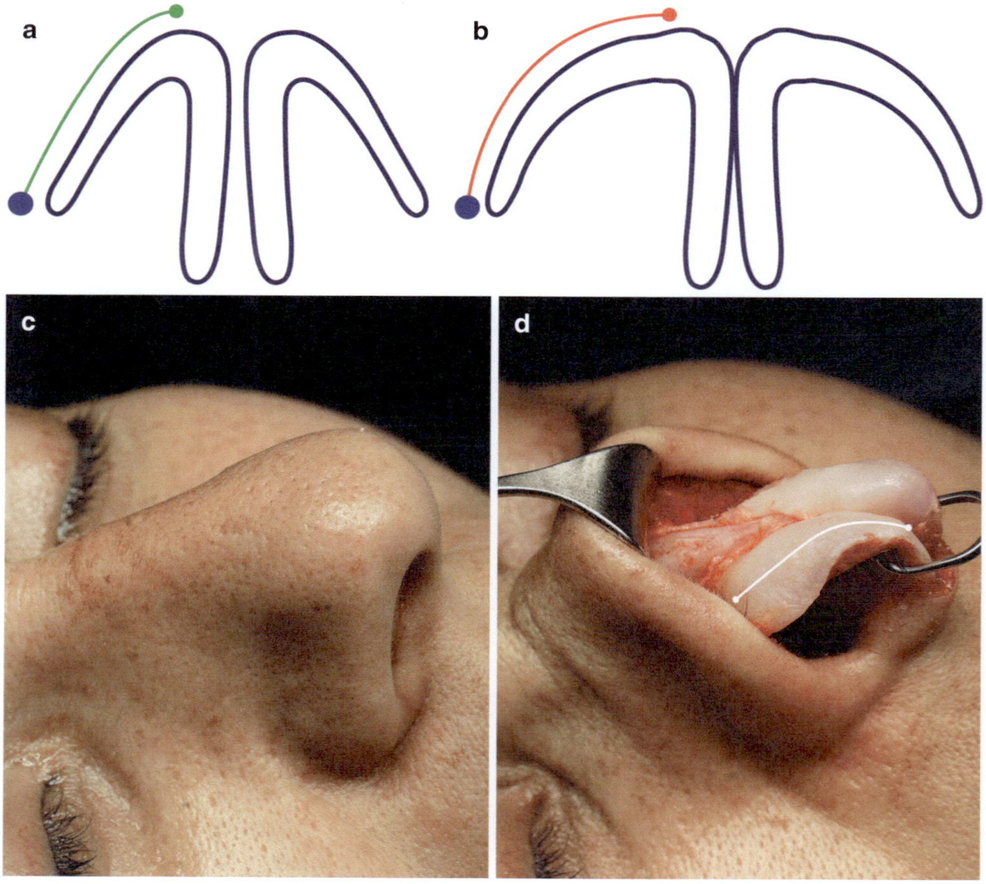

13.2 Treatment Strategy

The key to successful wide tip surgery is recognition of the problems mentioned above, correction of anatomical and configurational deformities of the alar cartilages, and adequate tip stabilization and definition.

The treatment features three principal suites of techniques:

- Basic techniques.
- Intermediate techniques.
- Advanced techniques.

13.2.1 Basic Techniques

Five approaches are valuable when narrowing a somewhat wide nasal tip.

1. Cephalic trimming of the alar cartilages.
2. Transdomal suturing.
3. Placement of dome-equalizing sutures.
4. Columellar strut placement.
5. Cap grafting.

For most wide nasal tips, these tools suffice.

Surgery may involve either a closed or open approach and all available tools can be used during either approach. The degree of mastery of a given technique will dictate the approach of choice. This chapter discusses both approaches to wide nasal tip surgery.

13.2.1.1 Cephalic Trimming of Alar Cartilages

After the alar cartilages are dissected and exposed, attention should turn to the lateral crura. Firstly, the crural surfaces should be reduced. Cephalic resection proceeds over the entire caudocranial axis until an average of 5–7 mm of transverse cartilage remains. Cephalic resection reduces the cephalic width of the lateral crus and the surface area, such that tip volume is decreased. Over-resection should be avoided because it weakens the alar side wall and, in the mid- to-long term, may trigger complications such as a pinched nasal tip or alar retraction (Fig. 13.9).

Resection should commence at precisely the point where the domal arch ends, and should end when the line parallel to the caudal edge of the lateral crus is reached; also, the incision should not be straight. This treatment transforms a large spherical tip into an oval tip that may appear equally bulbous to the patient (Fig. 13.10).

Meticulous dissection/resection is critical; if removed intact, the cartilage is a good source of graft material that can be placed in many different regions of the nose. Four grafts can be produced using the cephalic excess:

- A lateral crural graft can be sutured onto or under the lateral crus to correct any configurational deformity.

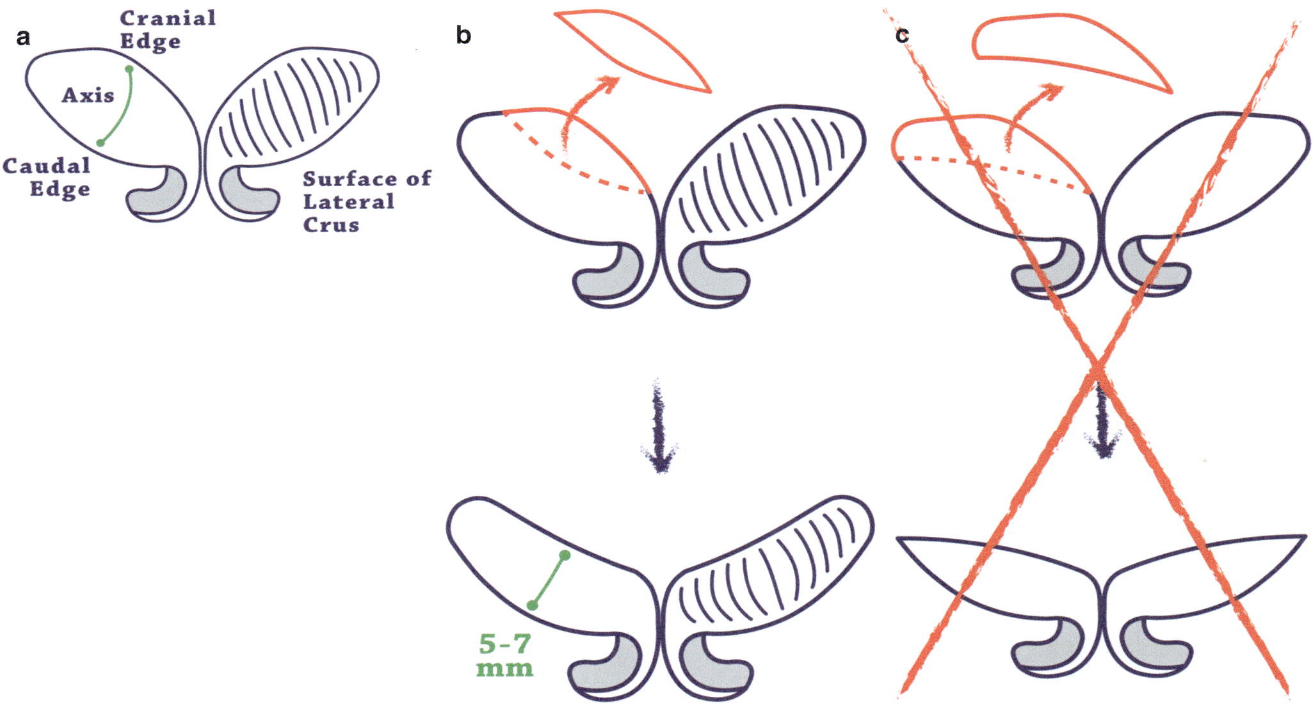

Fig. 13.9 (**a**) The surface of the lateral crus. (**b**) Correct resection. (**c**) Incorrect resection

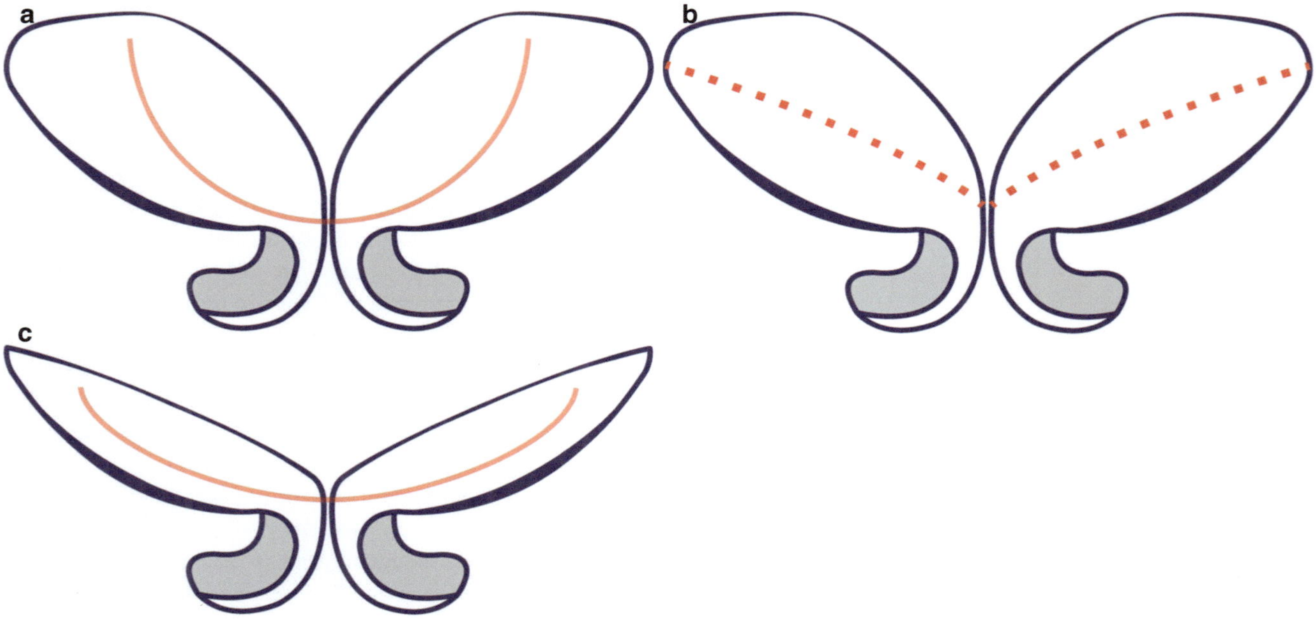

Fig. 13.10 (**a**) A wide, spherical nasal tip. (**b**) Incorrect resection. (**c**) A wide, oval nasal tip

- An onlay tip graft.
- A radix graft.
- A camouflage graft.

Cephalic resection is simple but important when reducing the nasal tip (Figs. 13.11 and 13.12; Videos 13.2 and 13.3).

13.2.1.2 Horizontal Transdomal Mattress Suturing

Next, a small permanent mattress suture involving the cartilage just medial and lateral to the dome should be placed. It is helpful to perform initial dome penetration in the medial-to-lateral direction, followed by a needle pass back through the dome (i.e., laterally to medially). The suture ends exit the cartilage deep within the interdomal area, which is the ideal site in which to safely bury the suture knot.

This suture essentially

- Shapes the alar cartilages.
- Narrows the domal arch.
- Reduces the convexity of the lateral crus.
- Corrects its caudocranial relationship of the lateral crus.
- Slightly increases projection.

In this way, most of the anatomical problems that arise when alar cartilages cause a wide nasal tip are resolved. The suture renders a disorganized/loose dome both straighter and narrower, and stabilizes the alar cartilage (Fig. 13.13).

Although the transdomal suture may appear simple, it is in fact very complex; the surgeon must pay attention to many aspects of suture placement. Incorrect suturing may exacerbate existing problems or even cause new ones. It is critical that the relationship between the caudal and cranial edges of the lateral crus is appropriate, as discussed above. When the caudal margin of the lateral crus is lower than the cephalic margin, marginal alar support may be lacking, and a shadow could form between the nasal tip and the alar lobules, thus isolating the tip and creating the appearance of a boxy ball. The caudal and cranial edges are thus ideally apposed and the transdomal suture is then placed. Thus, it is helpful if an assistant uses a hook to elevate the caudal edge. Alternatively, the forceps should be placed in a position that moves the caudal edge upward; only then is the transdomal suture placed. Random suturing must be avoided (Fig. 13.14; Video 13.4).

The caudal edge will move downward if the relationship between the caudal and cranial edges is ignored, such that revision will be required. If performed inappropriately, domal suturing will create an abnormal relationship between the caudal and cephalic margins of the lateral crura (Fig. 13.15).

Technical Pearl: Another critical point requiring attention when placing a transdermal suture is where to position the new dome. Do not position the dome laterally in broad noses exhibiting ideal rotation and projection. Otherwise, over-projection or over-rotation may create a highly undesirable narrow tip.

When utilizing the Transdomal suture, the objective is to juxtapose the rising domal convexity with the concurrently increasing lateral crura concavity.

How is Transdomal Suturing Performed Using the Open Approach? Fig. 13.16 illustrates this technique (Video 13.5).

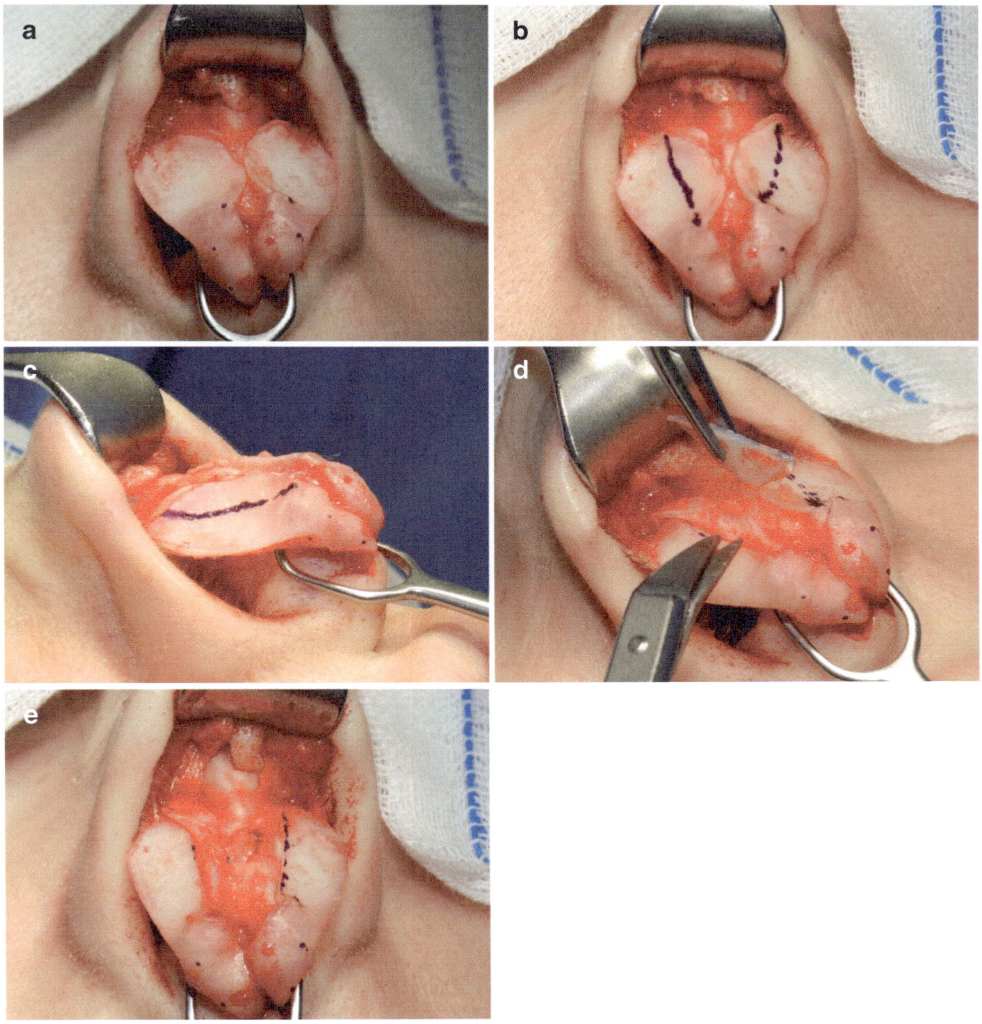

Fig. 13.11 (**a–e**) Cephalic excision of the crus using an open approach

How is Transdomal Suturing Performed Using the Closed Approach? While an open (external) approach affords good access to the alar cartilages, a closed approach also provides exposure adequate for suture repair (Fig. 13.17; Video 13.6).

After conservative alar cartilage volume reduction, the points defining the dome are marked. The assistant surgeon elevates the caudal edge of the lateral crus, using a hook, to neutralize the propulsive force of the lateral crus skin envelope. The caudal margin of the lateral crus moves superiorly (closer to the skin envelope) and the cephalic margin moves inferiorly (away from the envelope). Thus, the same-side lobule and alar do not compromise the lateral crural plane. The caudal edge is placed parallel to the cranial edge. The new dome is squeezed between the two ends of the forceps and the transdomal mattress suture is placed. Both alar cartilages are exposed from the same vestibule to check symmetry. A 5–0 polypropylene horizontal mattress transdomal suture is placed to narrow and reorient the alar cartilage dome.

13.2.1.3 Dome-Equalizing Suturing

This type of suturing creates the ideal interdomal angle and brings the lateral crus to the ideal plane at the same time. Polypropylene suture materials should be used. The two domes are sutured together just cranial to the newly formed dome-defining points. The suture commences at the lateral aspect of one dome and is passed through the medial aspect. The suture then enters the medial aspect of the other dome and exits from the lateral aspect. The suture is then tied, and the knot is left in the midline (Fig. 13.18; Video 13.7).

13.2.1.4 The Columellar Strut

This strut increases nasal base stability and contributes to nasal tip projection; the tip now seems narrower.

Ideally, the columellar strut graft should be straight and prepared from rigid cartilage. The graft should be placed between the newly formed dome-defining point and the point where the medial crus ends. Recall that an overlarge strut may touch the anterior nasal spine; this is undesirable.

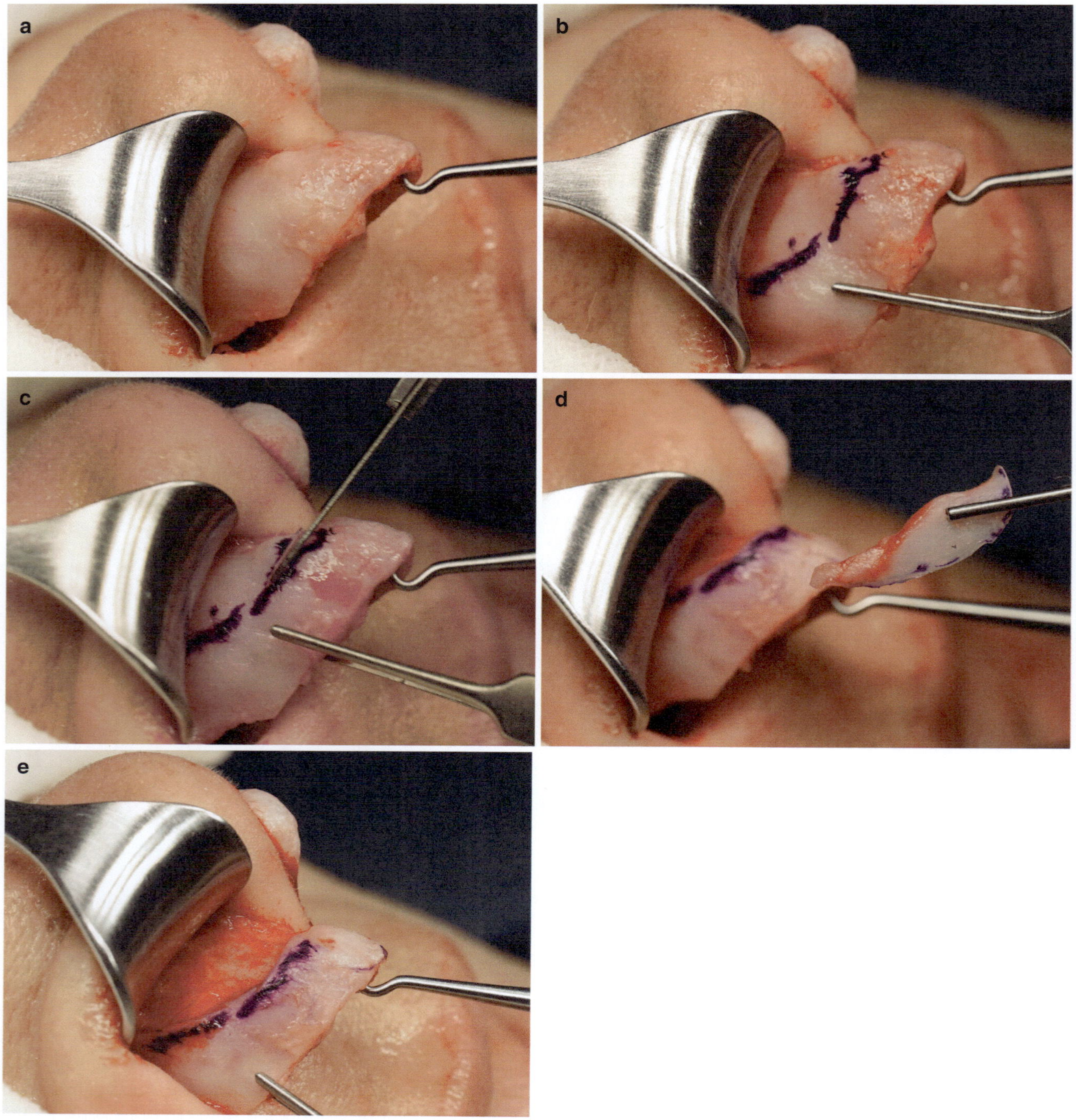

Fig. 13.12 (**a–e**) Cephalic excision of the crus using a closed approach

An absorbable 4.0 suture should be placed using a straight needle. The suture commences in the vestibular skin of either side, and the knot is left on the skin. The suture will dissolve in 3–4 weeks (Fig. 13.19; Video 13.8).

13.2.1.5 The Cap Graft

A small graft placed on the dome narrows the tip (Fig. 13.20; Video 13.9).

13.2.2 Clinical Outcomes

The cases in this section show the surgical steps of wide nasal tip correction with basic techniques.

13.2.2.1 Case 1

A 22-year-old woman requested better tip definition and narrowing of the nasal tip (Fig. 13.21). Basic tip techniques

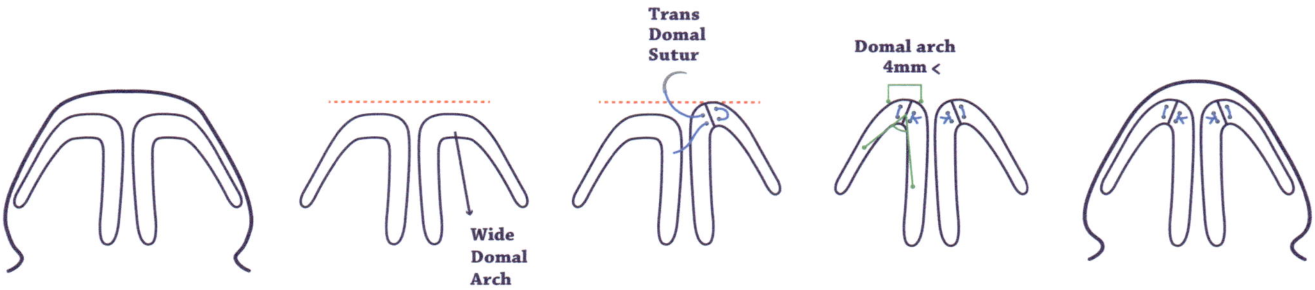

Fig. 13.13 Transdomal sutures reposition the domal cartilage subunits into proper shape and position

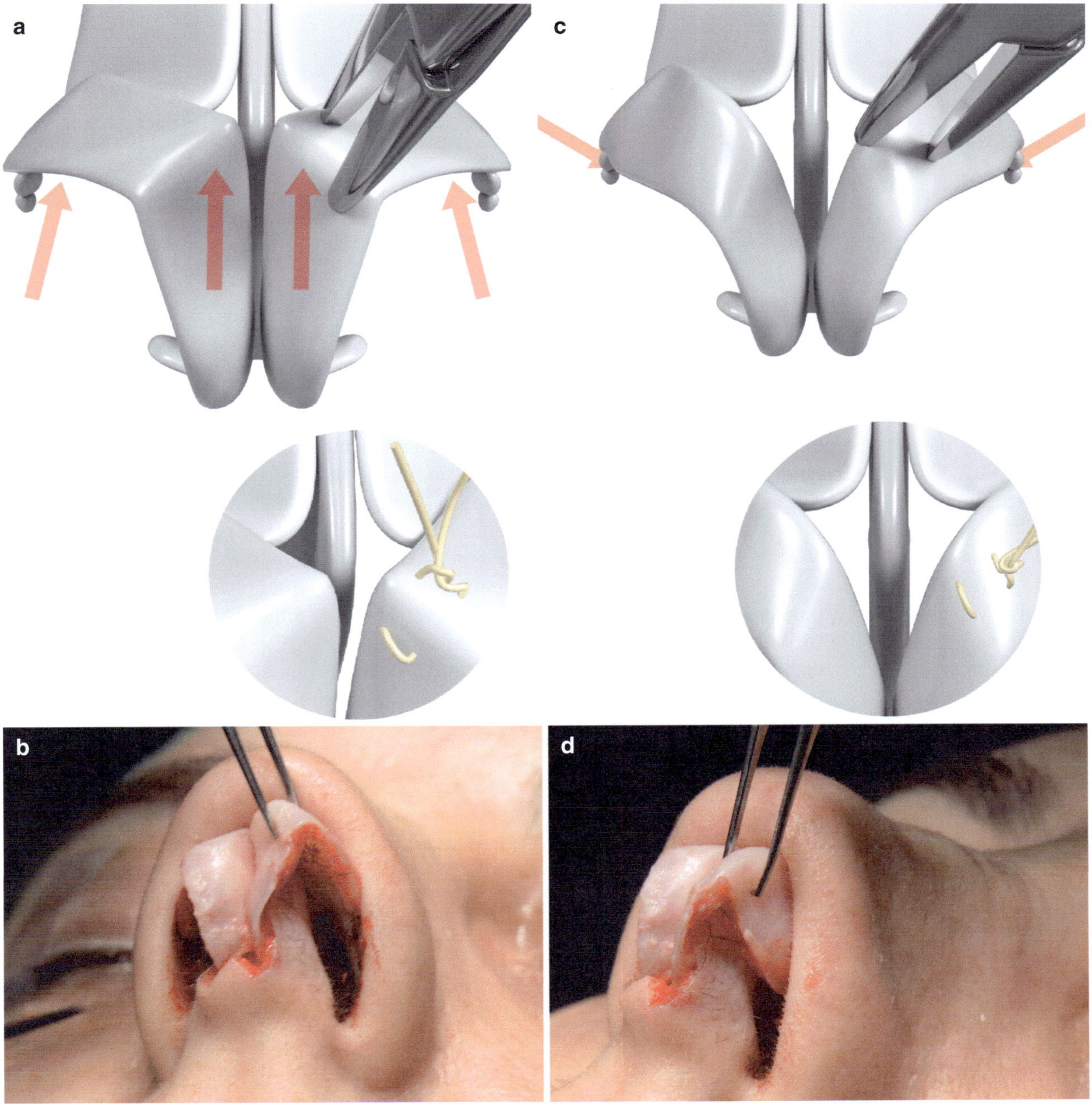

Fig. 13.14 (**a**, **b**) The favorable caudal–cranial relationship created when the forceps are held correctly. (**c**, **d**) The unfavorable caudal–cranial relationship created when the forceps are held incorrectly

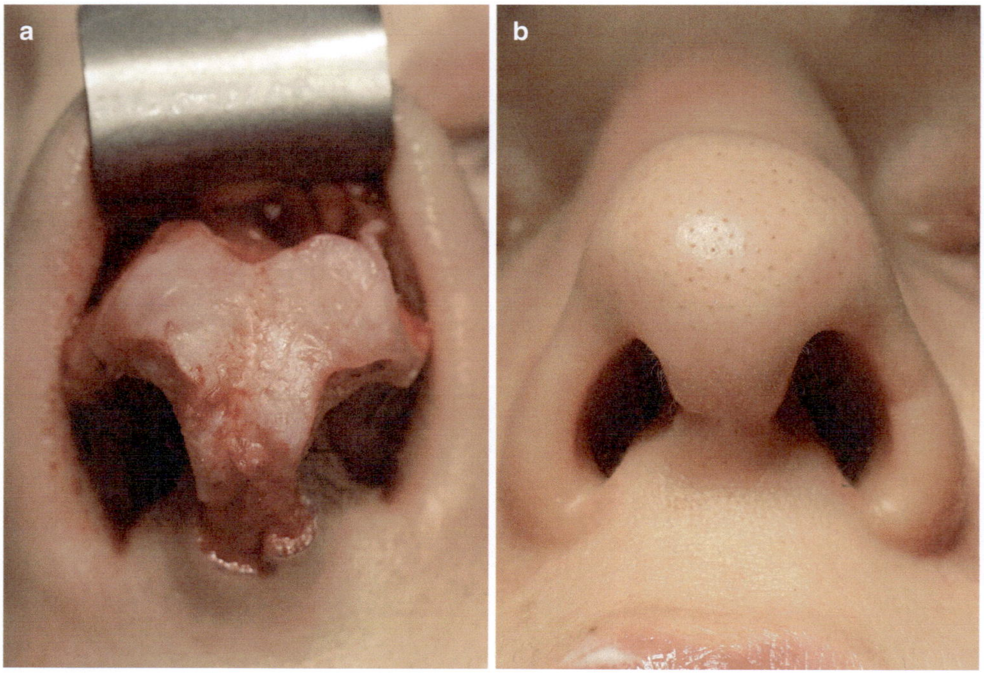

Fig. 13.15 (**a**) An intraoperative view of the cartilages reveals that the caudal margin of the lateral crus lies well below the cephalic margin. (**b**) A view from below the nasal tip reveals an isolated, wide tip lobule and a pinched tip

were used. The outcome 2 years after surgery is seen in Fig. 13.22.

13.2.2.2 Case 2

In this case with a wide nasal tip and bifid lobule, the domes are rounded. The patient desired a smaller or more elegant nose (Fig. 13.23). Basic tip techniques were implemented. Preoperative and 2-year postoperative photographs are seen in Fig. 13.24.

13.2.2.3 Case 3

This is a case with a wide and asymmetrical nasal tip, and no history of nasal trauma (Fig. 13.25). The steps of nasal tip surgery are seen in Fig. 13.26 and 2-year postoperative photographs are shown in Fig. 13.27.

13.2.2.4 Case 4

Use of these five tools (cephalic trimming, transdomal suture, dome-equalizing sutures, columellar strut, and cap grafting) afforded satisfactory long-term results. Ten-year postoperative photographs are shown in Fig. 13.28.

13.2.2.5 Case 5

Another example that used basic techniques. Long-term results are shown in Fig. 13.29.

13.2.3 Modified Transdomal Suturing

In this section, some situations requiring modification of transdomal suturing will be discussed. The modified transdomal suturing techniques shown below are valuable options for the surgeon to consider.

13.2.3.1 Transdomal Suturing with Dome Trimming

After transdomal suturing, the tip is visually inspected and palpated to ensure that the new dome is symmetrical and anatomically correct and to observe whether the tip looks natural. If unilateral asymmetry is evident, the suture should be removed and replaced until the positioning is correct. If asymmetry persists even after replacing the suture, the transdomal suture should be removed and unilateral dome trimming performed (Fig. 13.30).

Technical Pearl: If dome symmetry cannot be achieved by placing a transdomal suture, dome trimming is required.

Case 6

An example of transdomal suturing with dome trimming is shown in Fig. 13.31.

Two-year postoperative photographs are shown in Fig. 13.32.

13.2.3.2 Transdomal Suturing of an Overlapping Medial Crura

After transdomal suturing, the tip projection and rotation, and the columellar configuration, are reassessed intraoperatively. As discussed above, the transdomal suture contributes slightly to tip projection and rotation. If suturing is associated with excessive projection/rotation, or if the medial crural configuration is impaired, overlapping may be necessary, particularly in patients with long medial

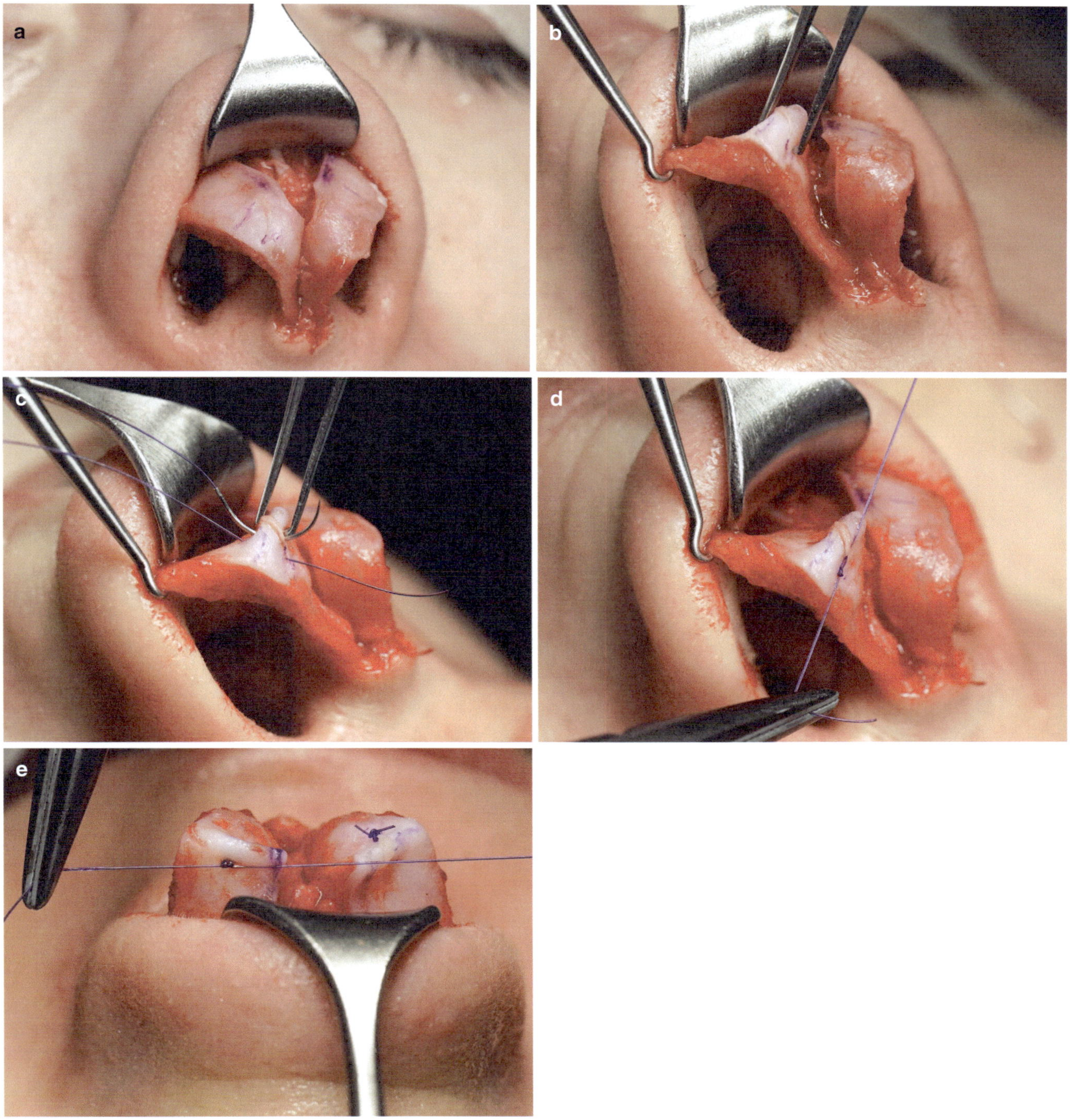

Fig. 13.16 (**a**) The position of the new (ideal) dome is marked with a pen. (**b**) The marked points are squeezed between the two ends of the forceps. An assistant elevates the caudal edge of the lateral crus using a hook or a pair of forceps. (**c**) The caudocranial axis is brought to the ideal position and sutured. The mattress suture extends mediolaterally and terminates in the lateral direction. The suture corrects the caudocranial axis, thus any disturbance to an axis that is already in the correct position is avoided. (**d**) Axis correction not only creates a narrow, refined tip but also strengthens the nasal wall, reducing the need for an alar rim. (**e**) Idealized dome and alar cartilage anatomy after bilateral sutures. (**f**) Illustration shows the desired suture effect: a convex dome with a concave area positioned just laterally to it, while maintaining a flat surface along the lateral crura. The surgeon should avoid applying excessive tension when knotting the suture, as this may cause cartilage deformities

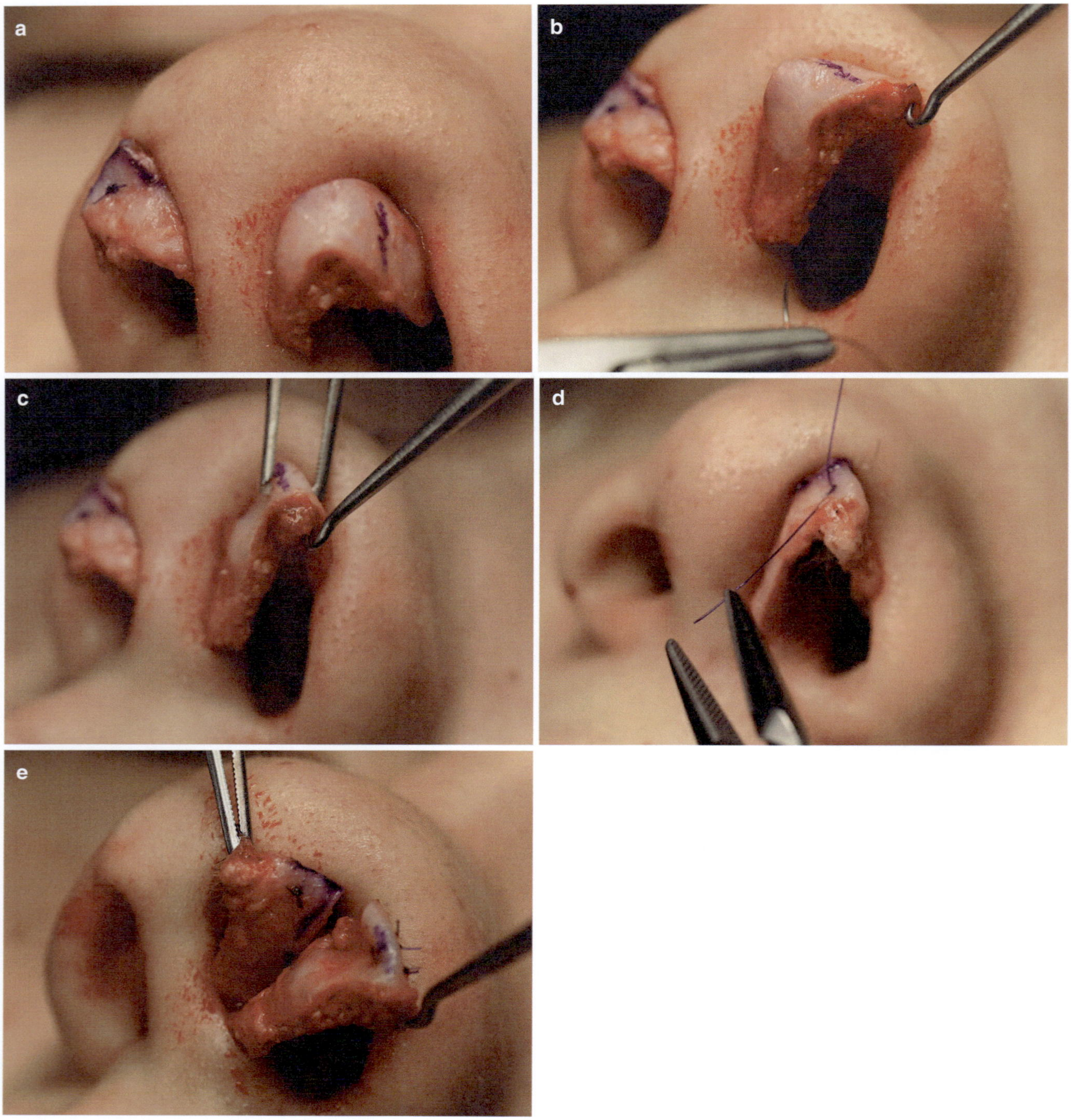

Fig. 13.17 (**a–e**) Traditional tip rhinoplasty techniques, such as cephalic trim and transdomal sutures, can easily be performed using endonasal rhinoplasty. Each new dome should be created in different nostrils

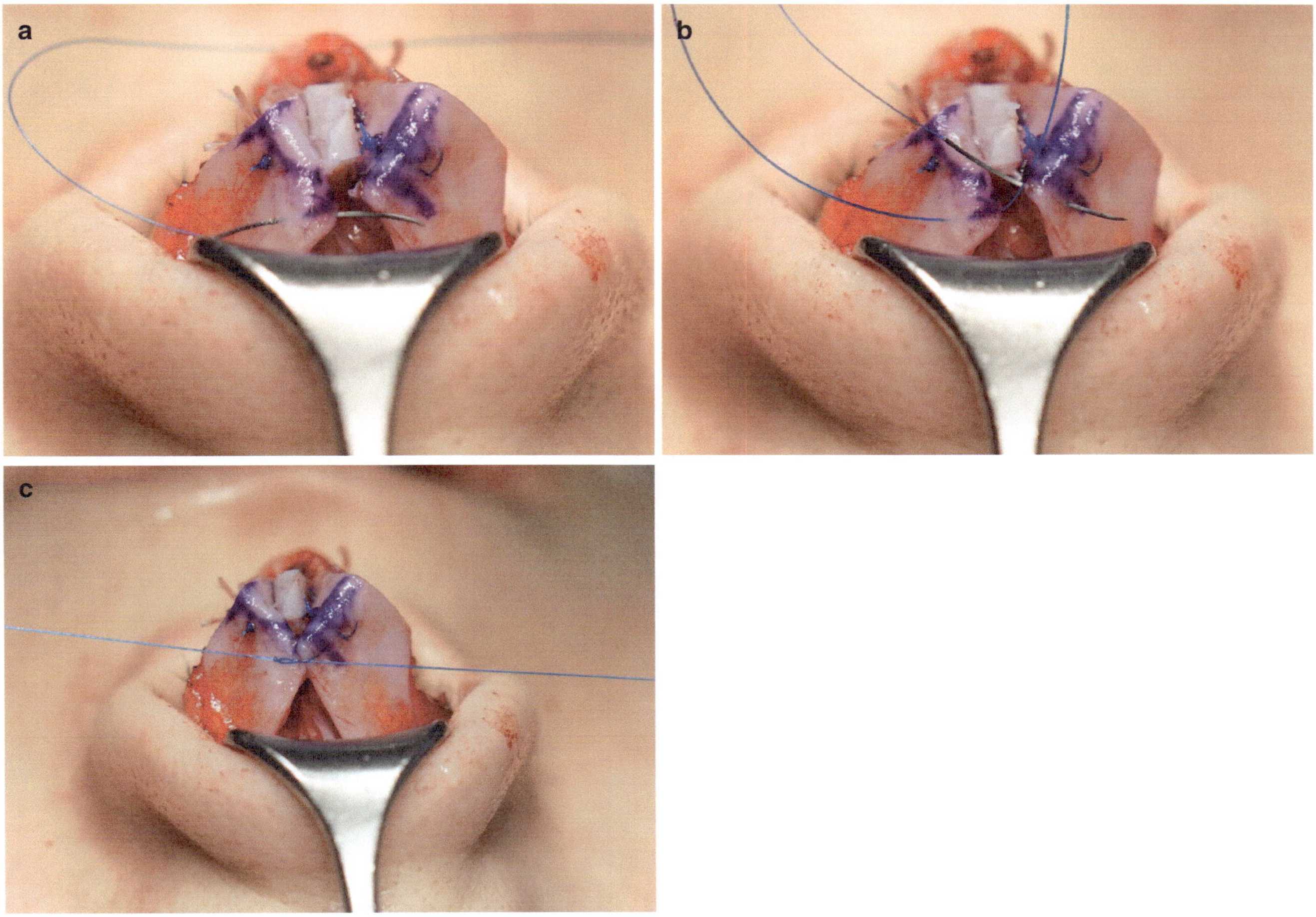

Fig. 13.18 (a–c) The dome equalizing suture provides tip strength and symmetry and contributes to establishing the favorable relationship between edges of lateral crus. The domal separation angle is controlled by the dome equalizing suture

crura. Medial crural overlapping reliably and predictably corrects horizontally positioned crura, with adjustment of projection and rotation (Fig. 13.33).

Case 7

A case of this issue: When viewed laterally, exhibit remarkable "hanging" columellae that reflect long medial crura. Medial crural overlapping may be necessary to address this problem; transdomal suturing can exacerbate the issue (Fig. 13.34; Video 13.10).

With diagnosis established, the next step is to choose an approach. A closed rhinoplasty was preferred in this case. Let's review the surgical steps.

The surgery was started with transdomal mattress sutures that are shown in Fig. 13.35.

After transdomal suturing, the alar arch deformed. Therefore, medial crural overlap is required (Fig. 13.36).

Preoperative and 1-year postoperative photographs are shown in Fig. 13.37.

13.2.3.3 Transdomal Suturing with Placement of a Subdomal Apex Graft

Case 8

The domal segment is usually quite short and is often the thinnest, most delicate, and narrowest region of the entire alar cartilage arch. In some patients, the domal segment may be too thin and weak for suture passage (Fig. 13.38; Video 13.11).

If a subdomal graft is placed prior to transdomal suturing, the graft serves as a block underneath the dome, preventing distortion. The subdomal graft behaves as two separate grafts that lie independently under each dome. The subdomal graft is carved from straight septal cartilage. Each graft is usually 4–5-mm long and should be about 1.5 mm thicker in the caudal than the superior aspect. The graft thus pushes the caudal margin of the lateral crus superiorly. Such reorientation is very important to create a favorable nasal tip contour. A wide and strong lateral crus

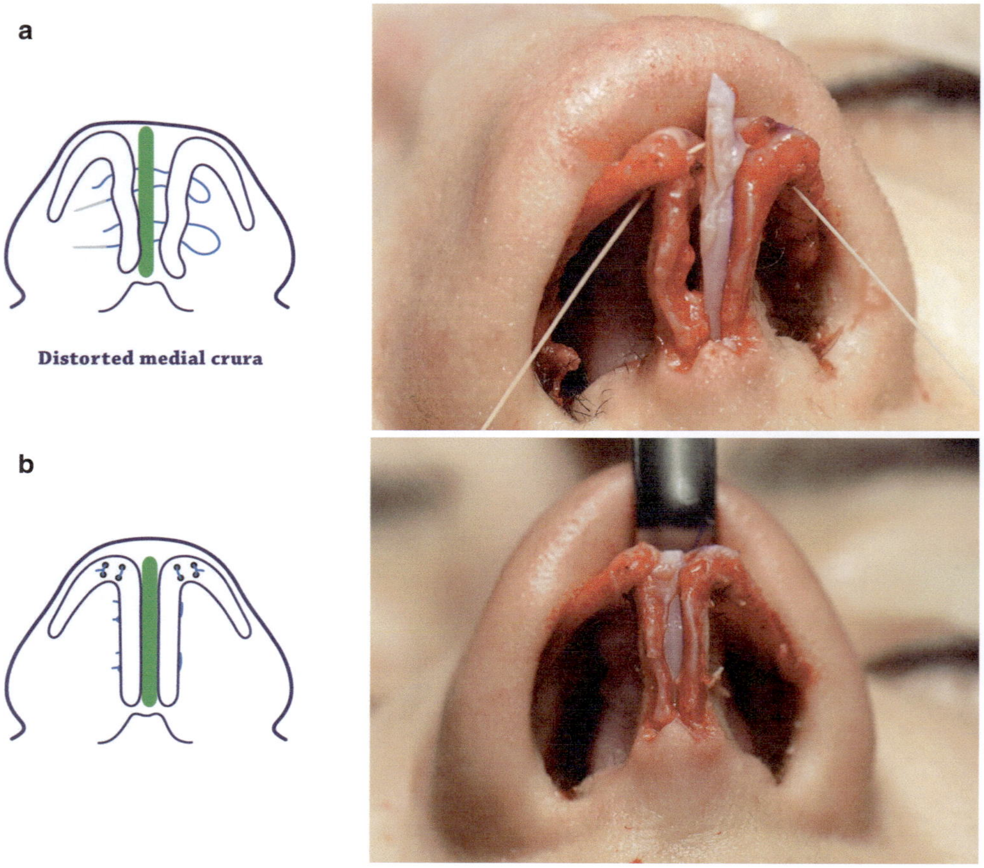

Fig. 13.19 (**a**, **b**) Placement of strut graft into a pocket created between the medial crura. The graft is secured in place with a nonpermanent mattress suture. Illustrations of how the strut acts as a scaffold onto which buckled medial crura may be sutured and thereby straightened. After strut placement, the alar cartilages close up and looks narrower

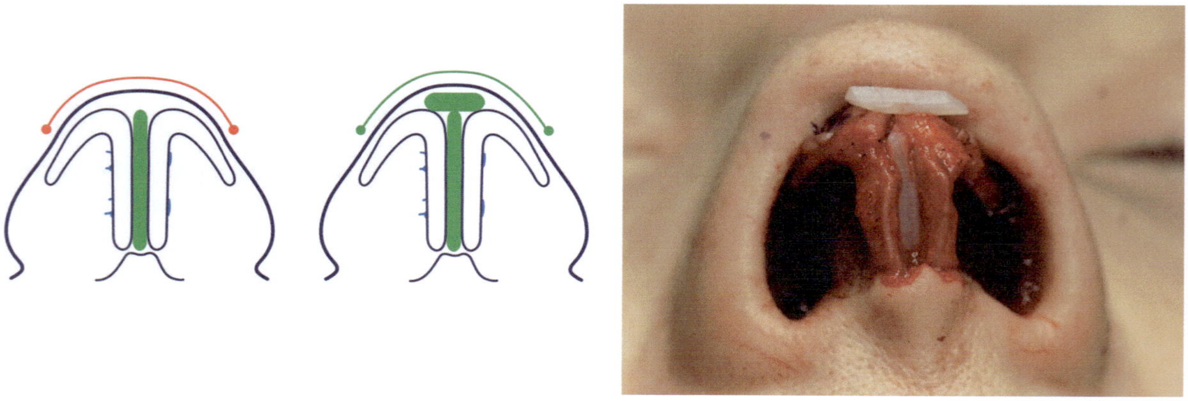

Fig. 13.20 The cap graft also changes the tip shape, providing a new dome, defining points in tips that lack definition. After placement, the tip looks narrower. The graft rests directly over the domes. It is sutured in place using absorbable sutures

is followed by a thin, weakly concave segment. A transdomal suture placed after strengthening the domal segment with a graft is effective for refining the tip. To this end, straight iris scissors are used to open a bilateral subdomal pocket between the domes and the nasal lining. The graft is inserted under one dome and a transdomal suture is placed as described above. The redundant portion of the graft (over the dome) is resected (Fig. 13.39).

Preoperative and 1-year postoperative photographs are shown in Fig. 13.40.

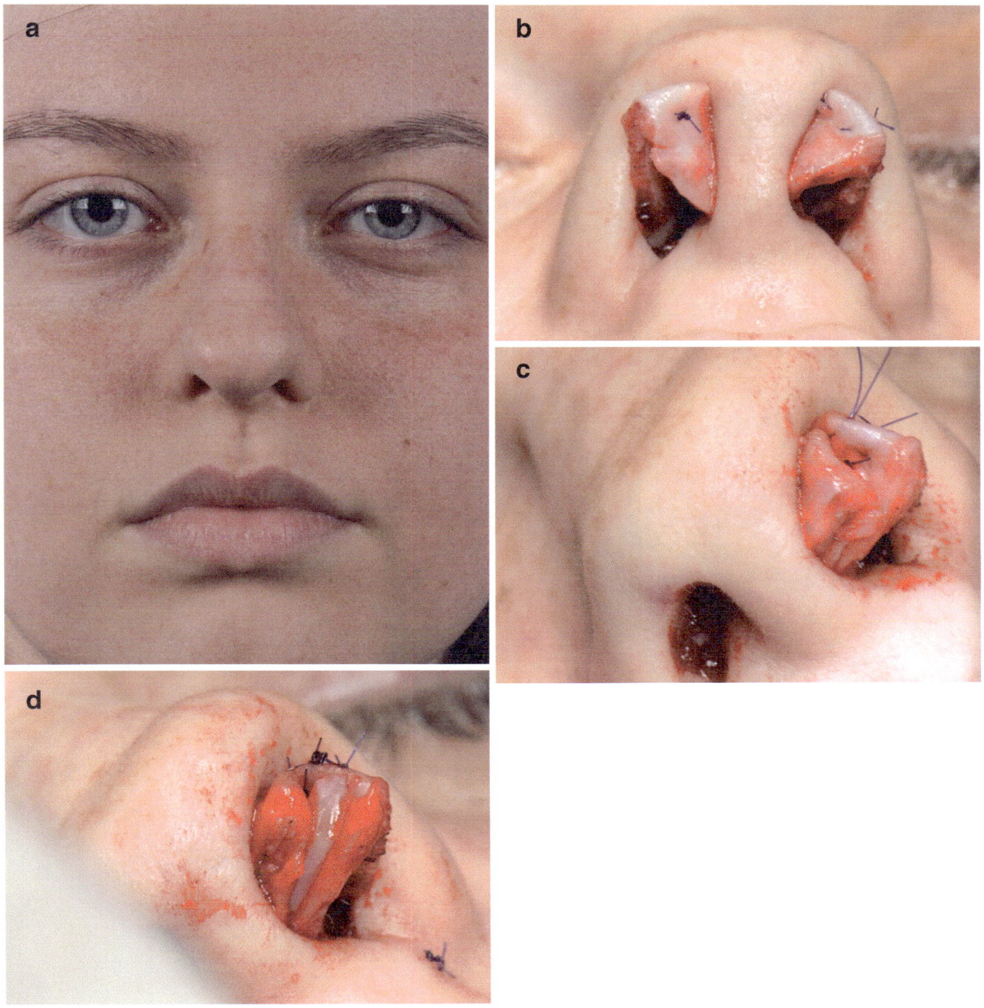

Fig. 13.21 (**a–d**) A closed approach was used. Cephalic resection, transdomal and dome equalizing suturing adequately repaired the cartilage configurational deformities that caused the wide nasal tip. A columellar strut was used to stabilize the tip

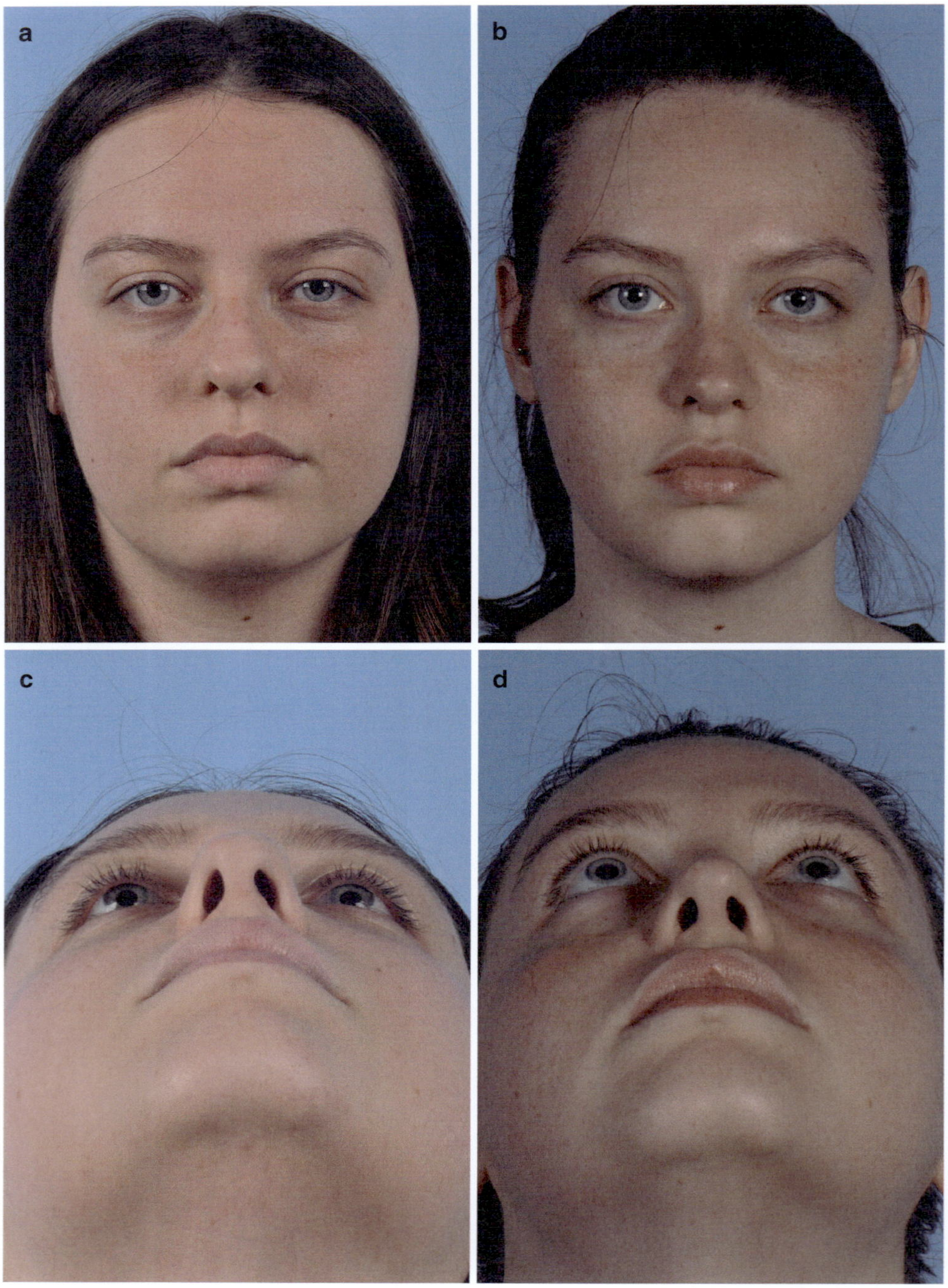

Fig. 13.22 (**a–d**) The nasal tip definition has been improved. On base view the tip is now triangular rather than trapezoidal

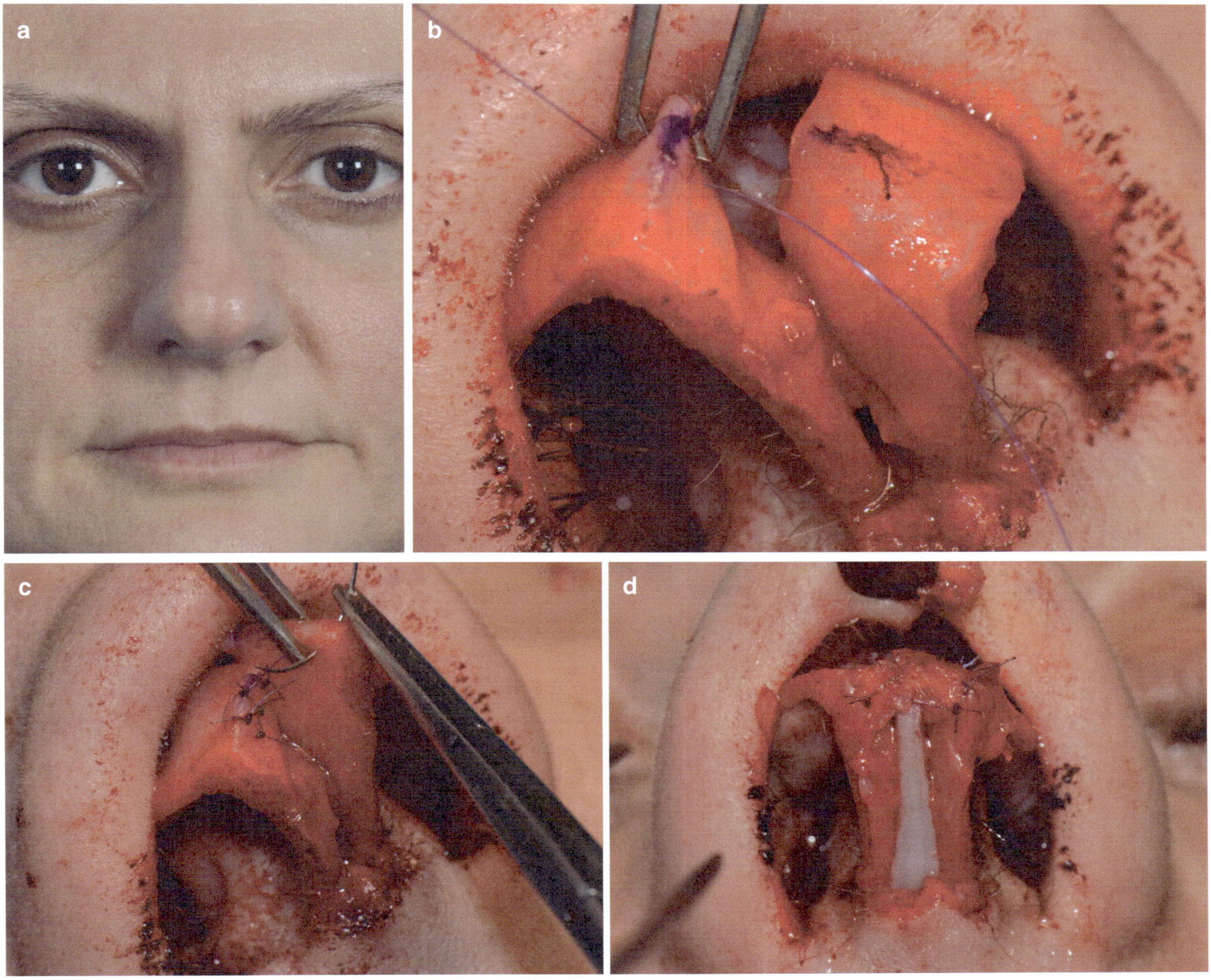

Fig. 13.23 (**a–d**) The open approach was used. Both transdomal and dome-equalizing sutures were placed. After columellar strut placement, a thin cap graft was used

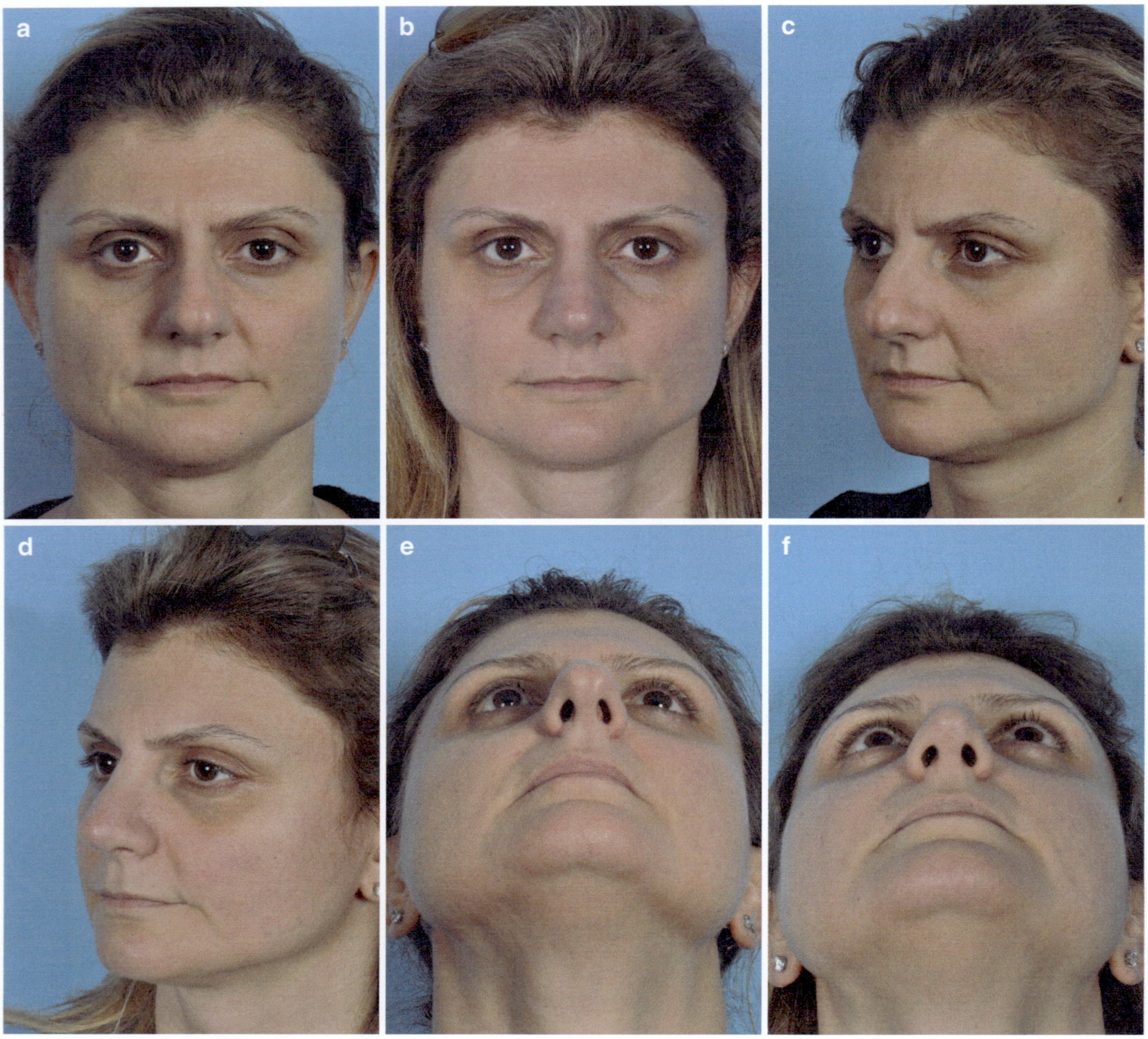

Fig. 13.24 (**a–f**) Tip definition is greatly improved. The bifidity is also corrected

Fig. 13.25 (**a**, **b**) Moderately large alar arch with bulbous, bifid, and less defined tip. Excessive width between the domes and caudal septal deviation are noted on the basal view

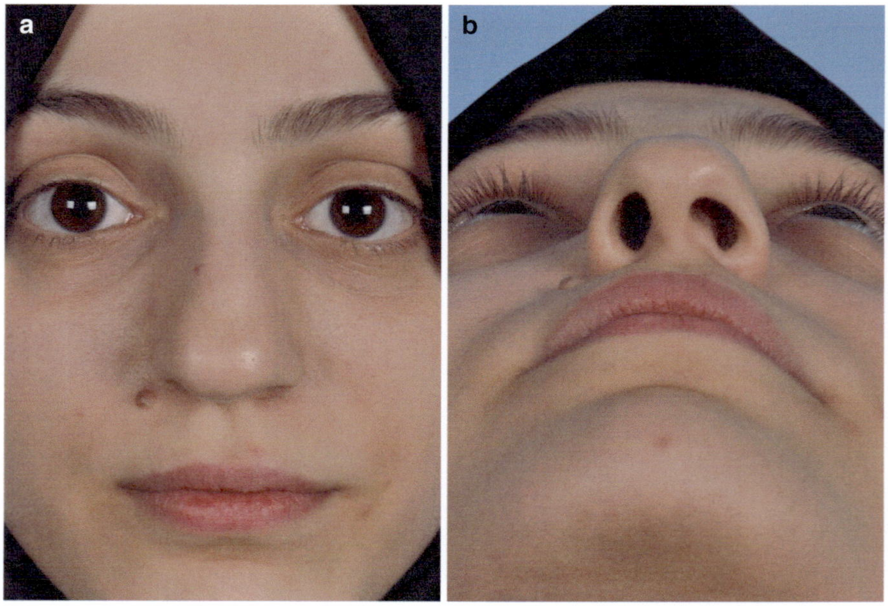

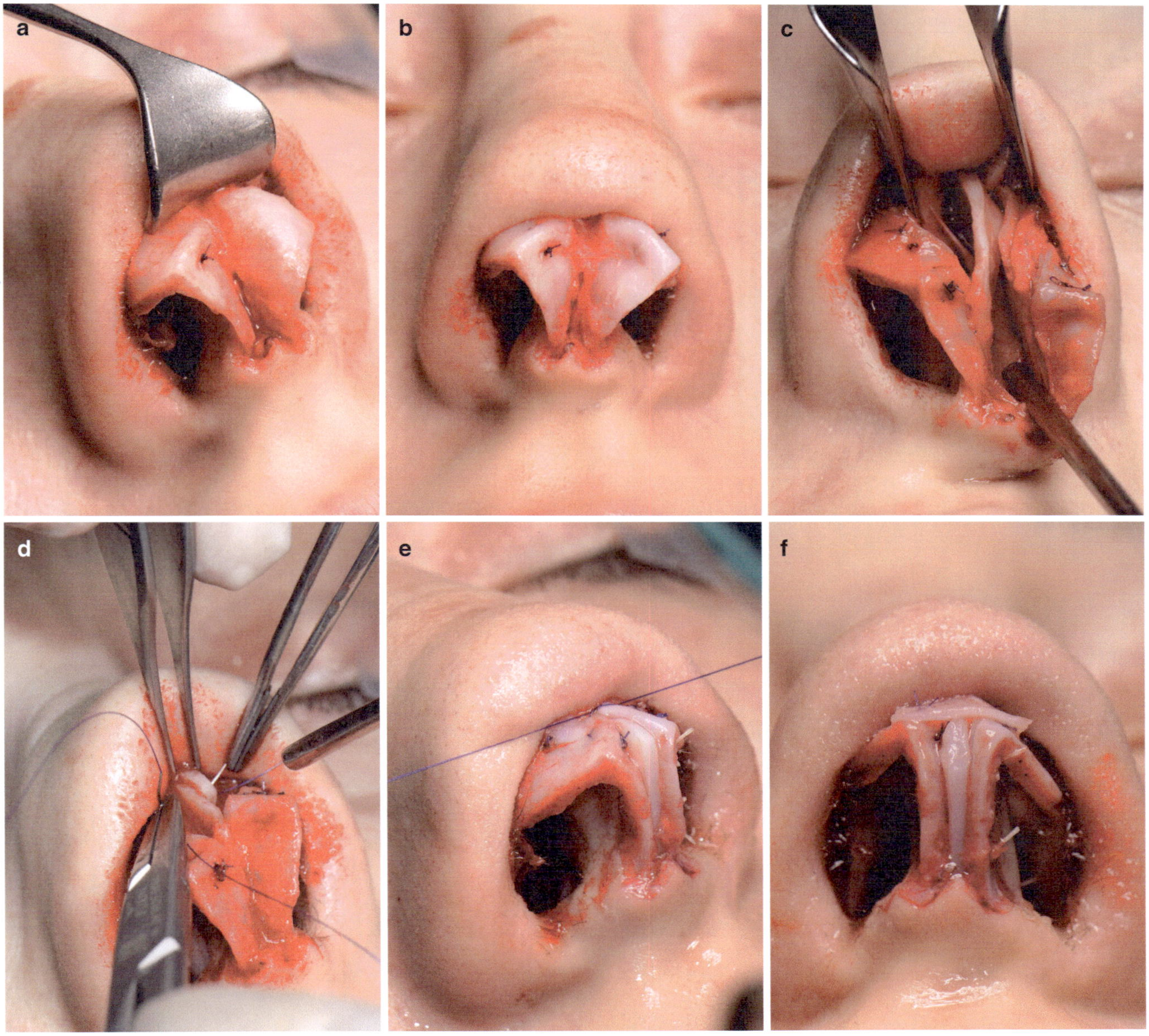

Fig. 13.26 (**a**) Compare the right side (where the transdomal suture was placed) to the left side. The lateral crural plane was corrected. (**b**) The bilateral transdomal suture. (**c**, **d**) The tip asymmetry caused by caudal septal deviation was resolved using right spreader and septal batten grafts. (**e**) The dome-equalizing suture and columellar strut. (**f**) The small cap graft placed to enhance definition

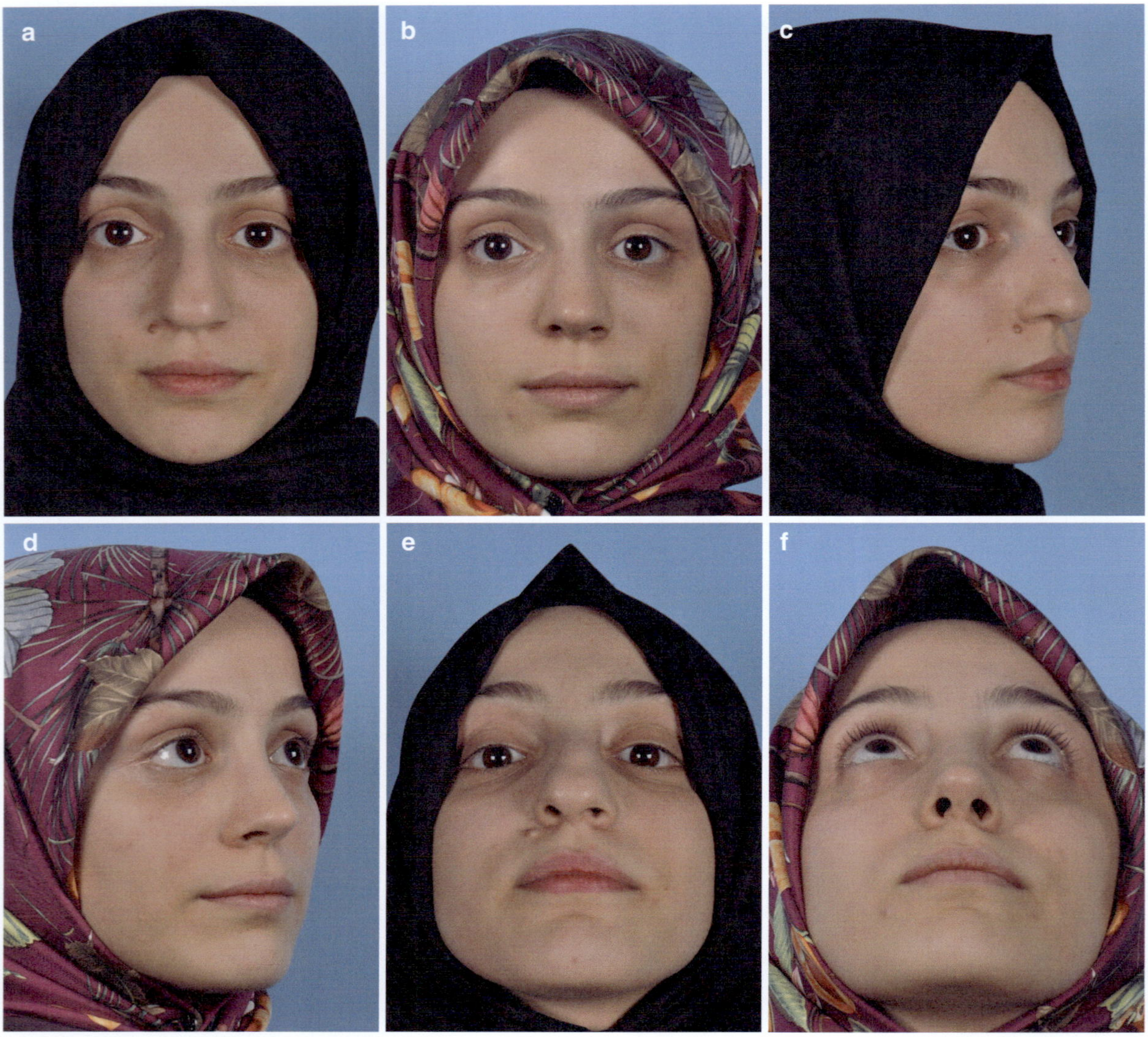

Fig. 13.27 (**a–f**) Nasal tip is more defined and more symmetric on front view. Interdomal distance has diminished

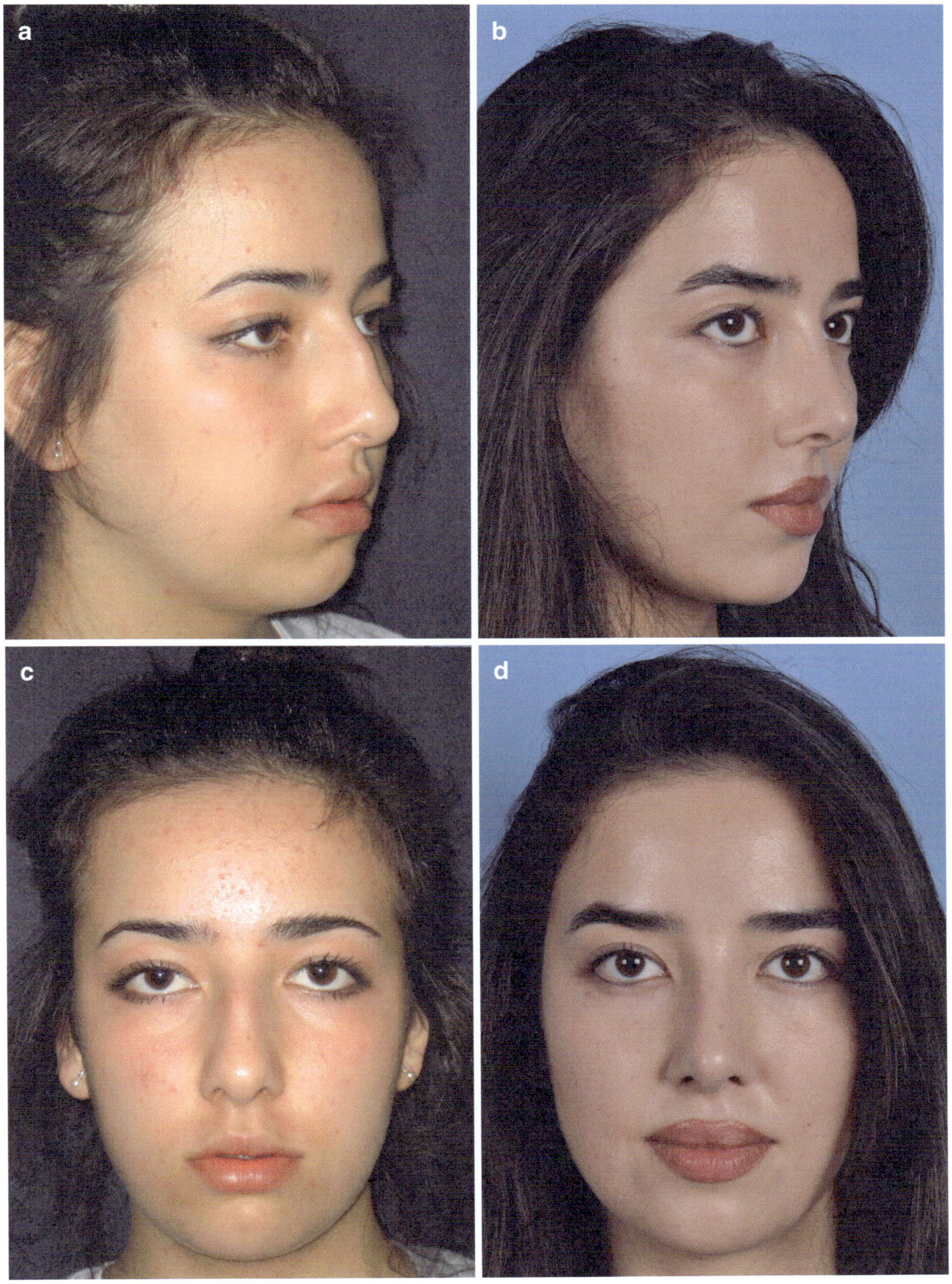

Fig. 13.28 (**a–d**) The nasal tips have not deteriorated

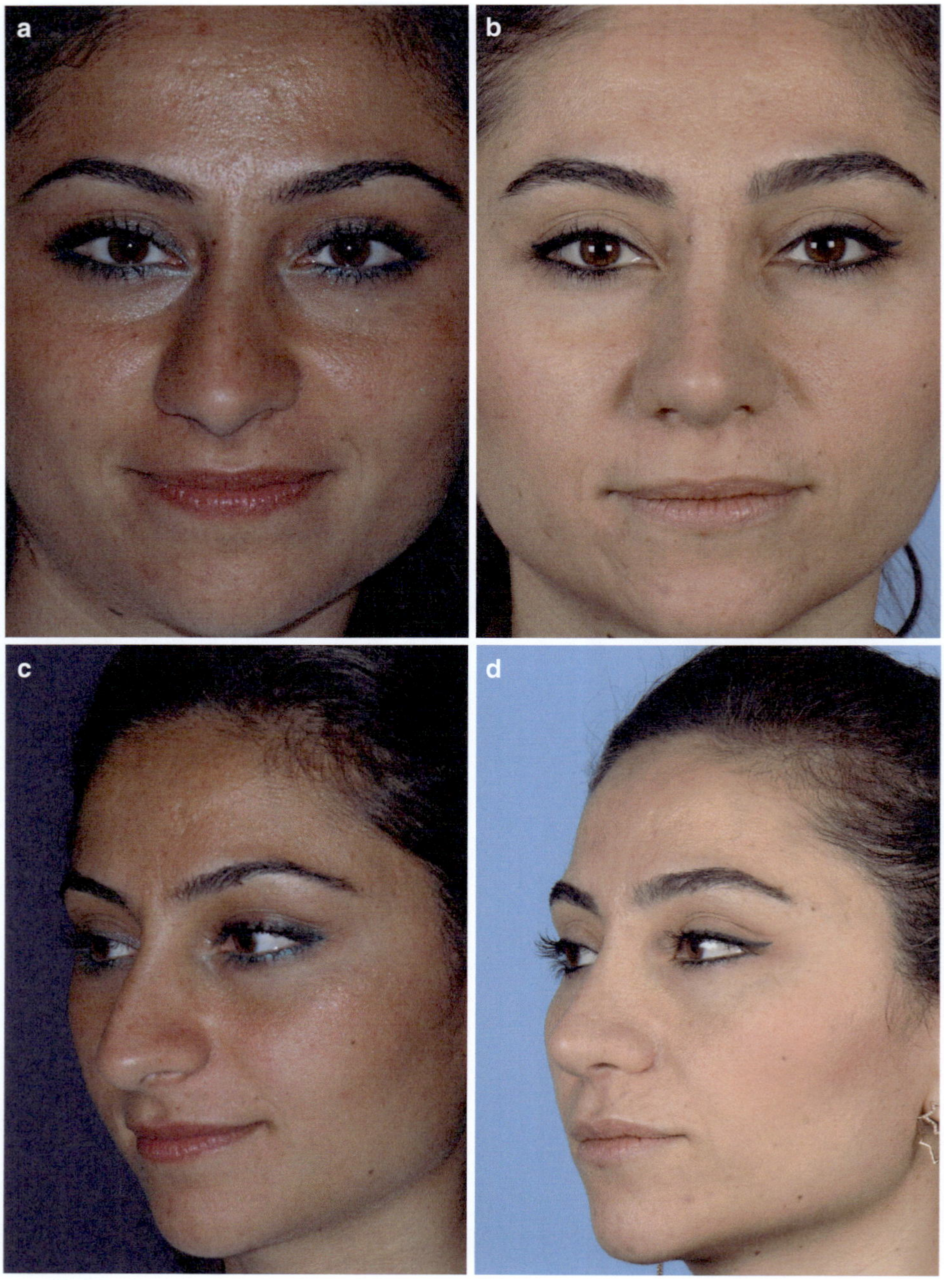

Fig. 13.29 (a–d) The 11-year postoperative photographs. The tips are satisfactory in terms of both form and shape

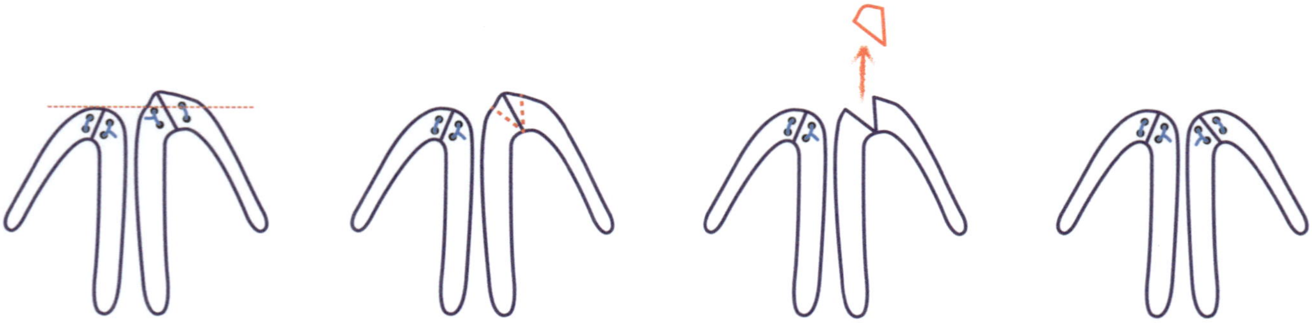

Fig. 13.30 The excised part should be triangular. Cranial-based triangular excision is done. Continuity of the dome is reestablished using absorbable sutures

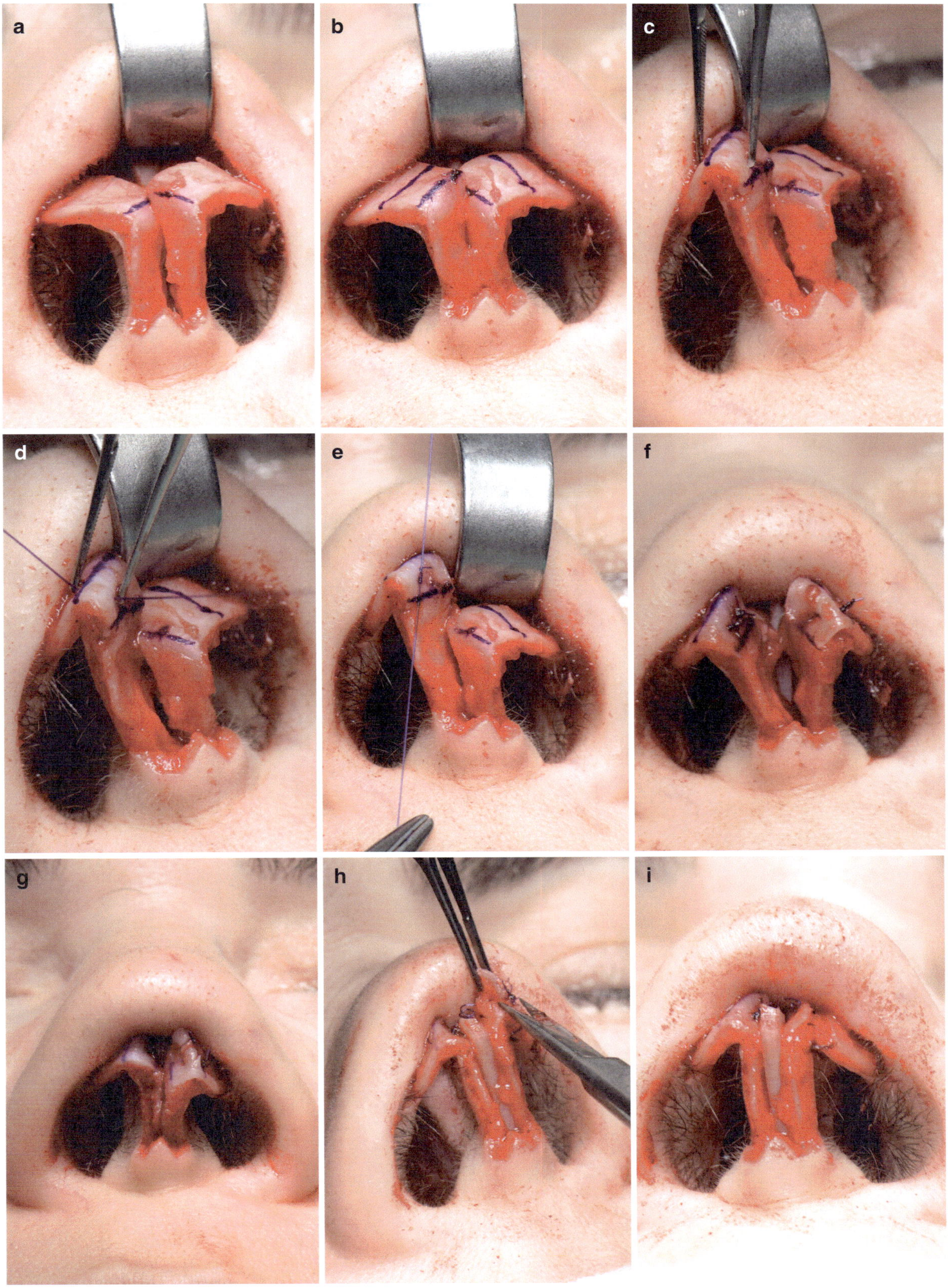

Fig. 13.31 (**a**) The anatomical dome points. (**b**) The new dome points. (**c**) The position of the forceps. (**d**) The transdomal suture. (**e**) Projection and rotation have increased on the right. (**f**) The opposite side is similarly sutured. (**g**) The left dome remains higher than the right dome. (**h**, **i**) The dome is divided via a vertical incision. Excess cartilage is removed. (**j**, **k**) Edge-to-edge suturing follows; the separated cartilages are reapproximated using 6–0 polydioxanone sutures. (**l**–**n**) Dome-equalizing suturing is then performed

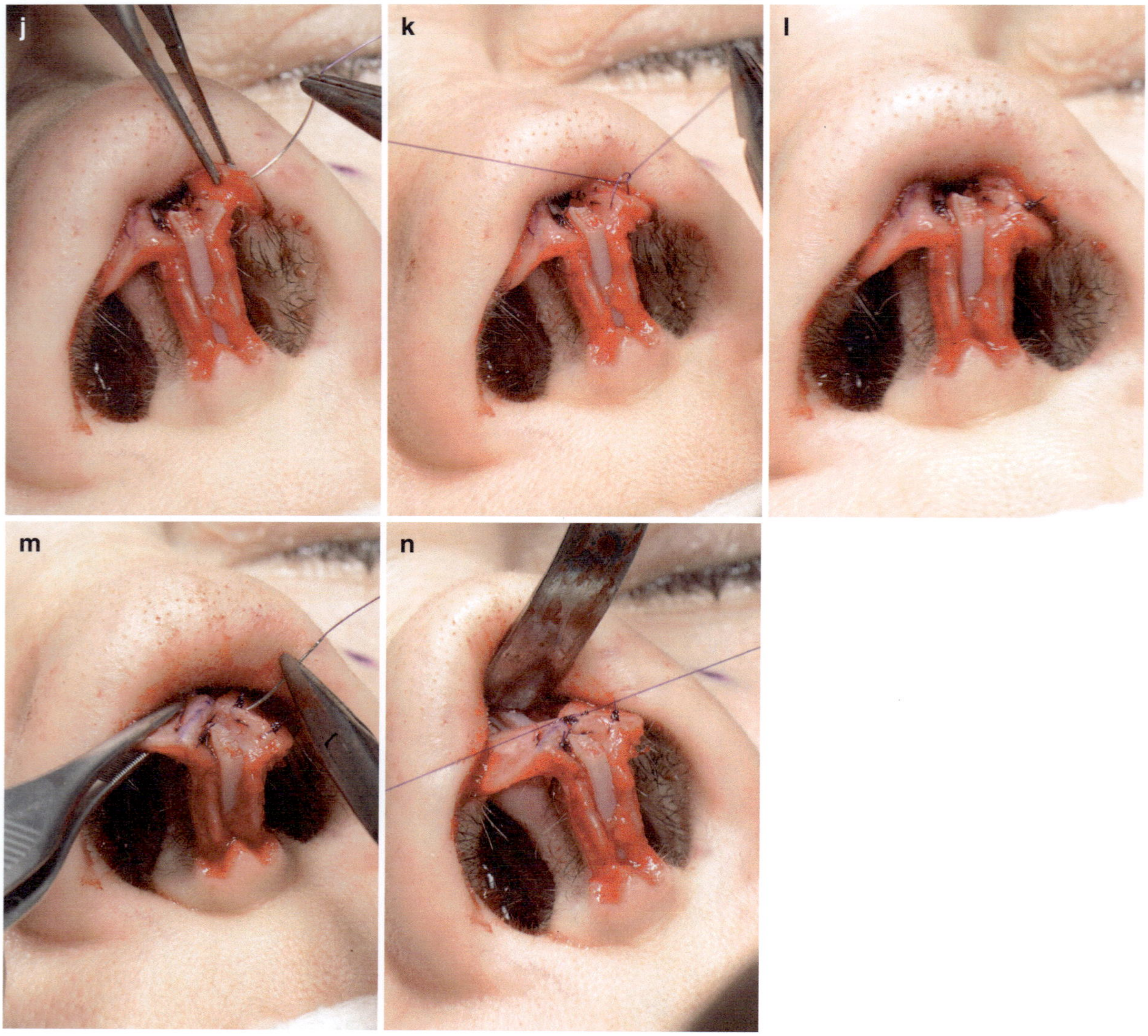

Fig. 13.31 (continued)

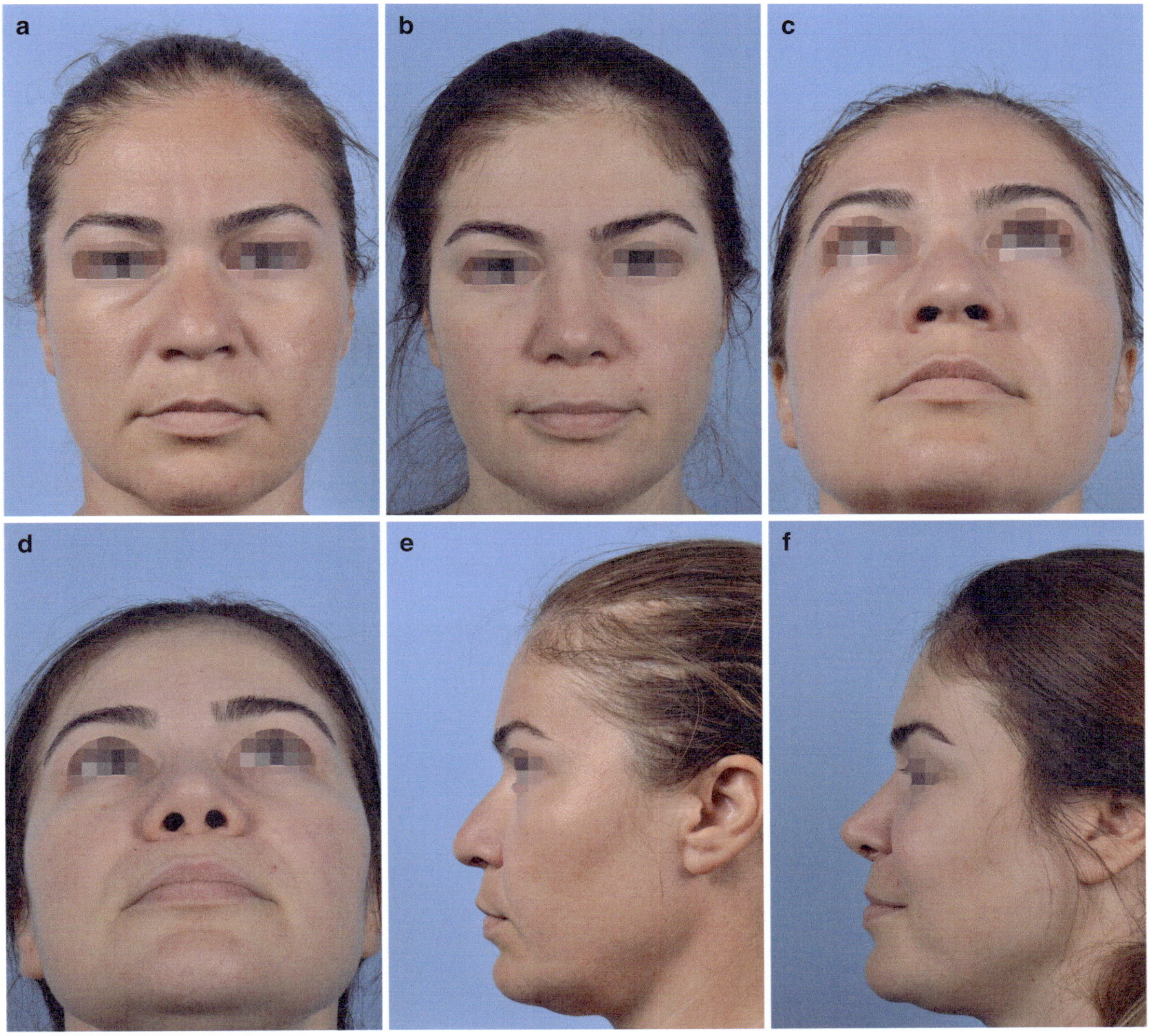

Fig. 13.32 (**a–f**) The tip is narrower and the brow-tip aesthetic line is better defined. The base view shows improved triangularity to the tip. The tip is slightly rotated superiorly

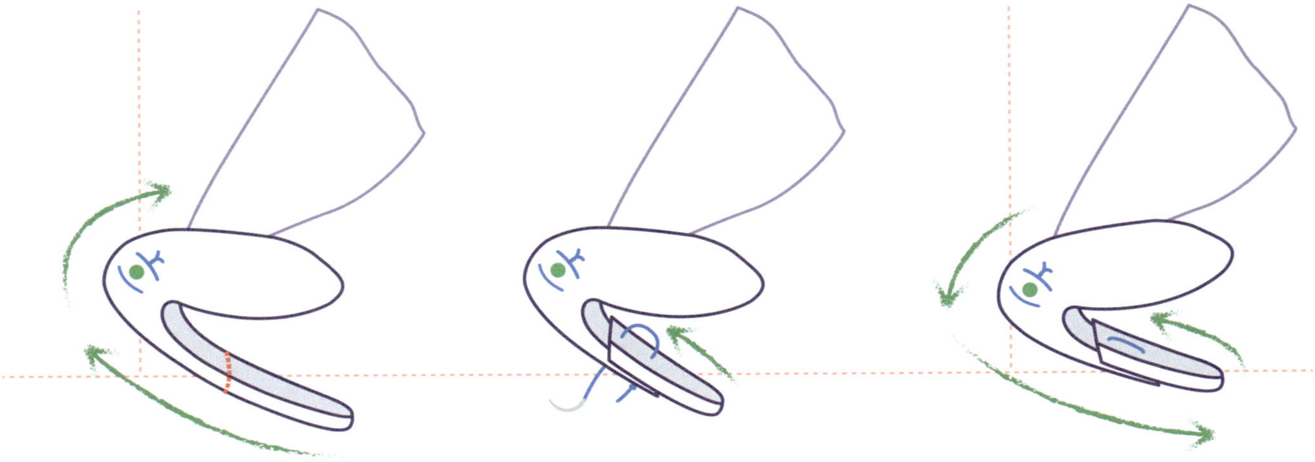

Fig. 13.33 Division and overlap of the medial crus lead to shortening its length. Medial crus being shortened can affect nasal tip rotation, projection, or symmetry

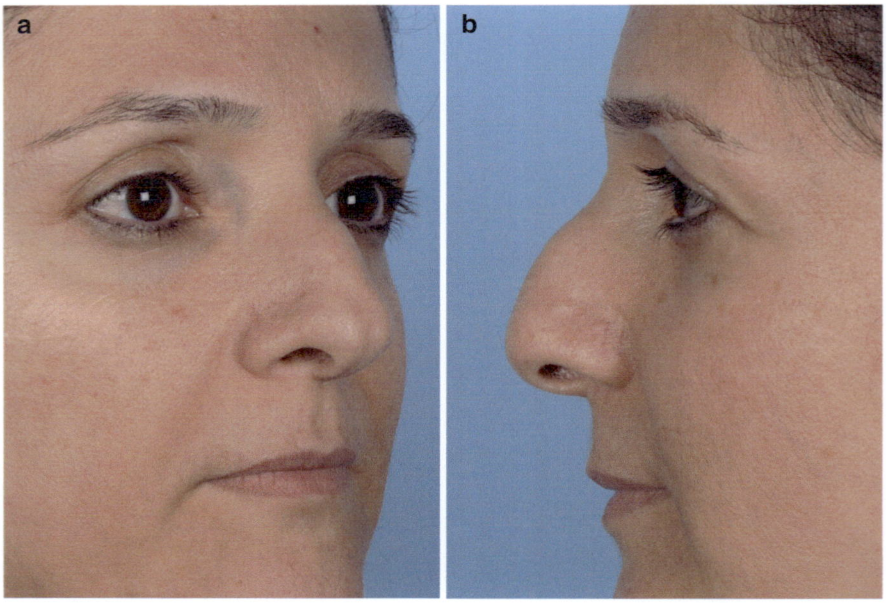

Fig. 13.34 (**a**) A wide bifid tip (oblique view). (**b**) A hanging columella

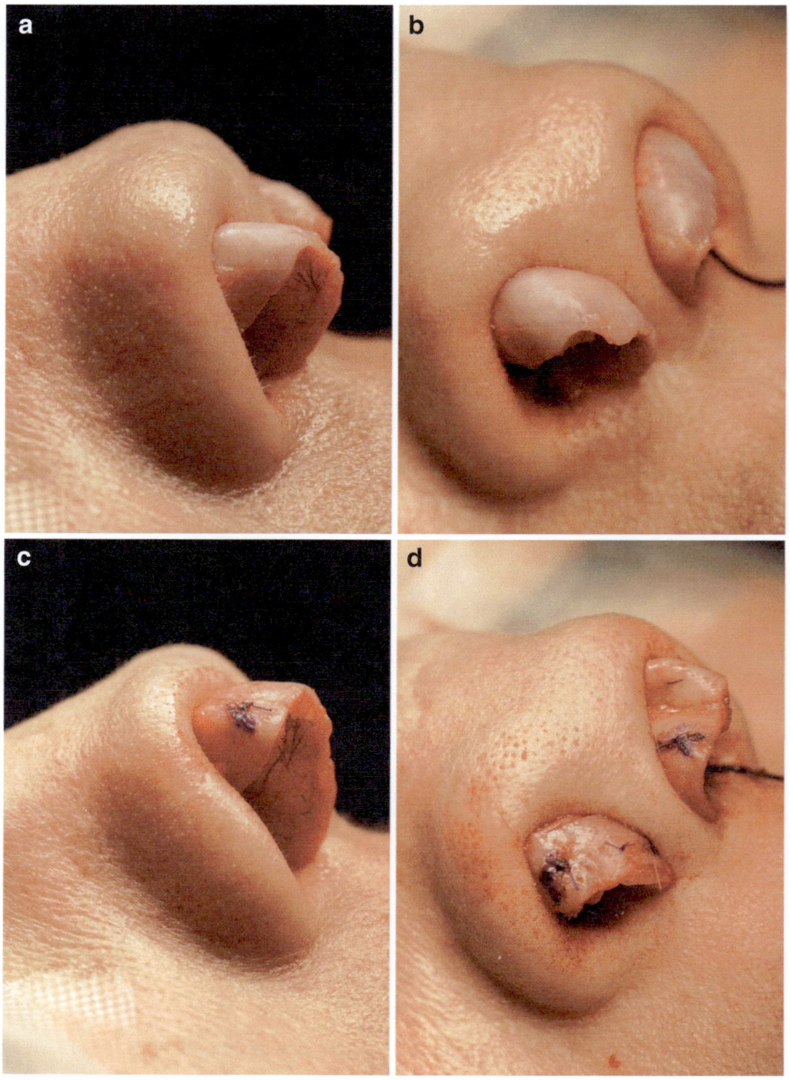

Fig. 13.35 (**a**, **b**) Before transdomal mattress suturing. (**c**, **d**) Notice after transdomal mattress suturing, medial crura became longer and misconfigured

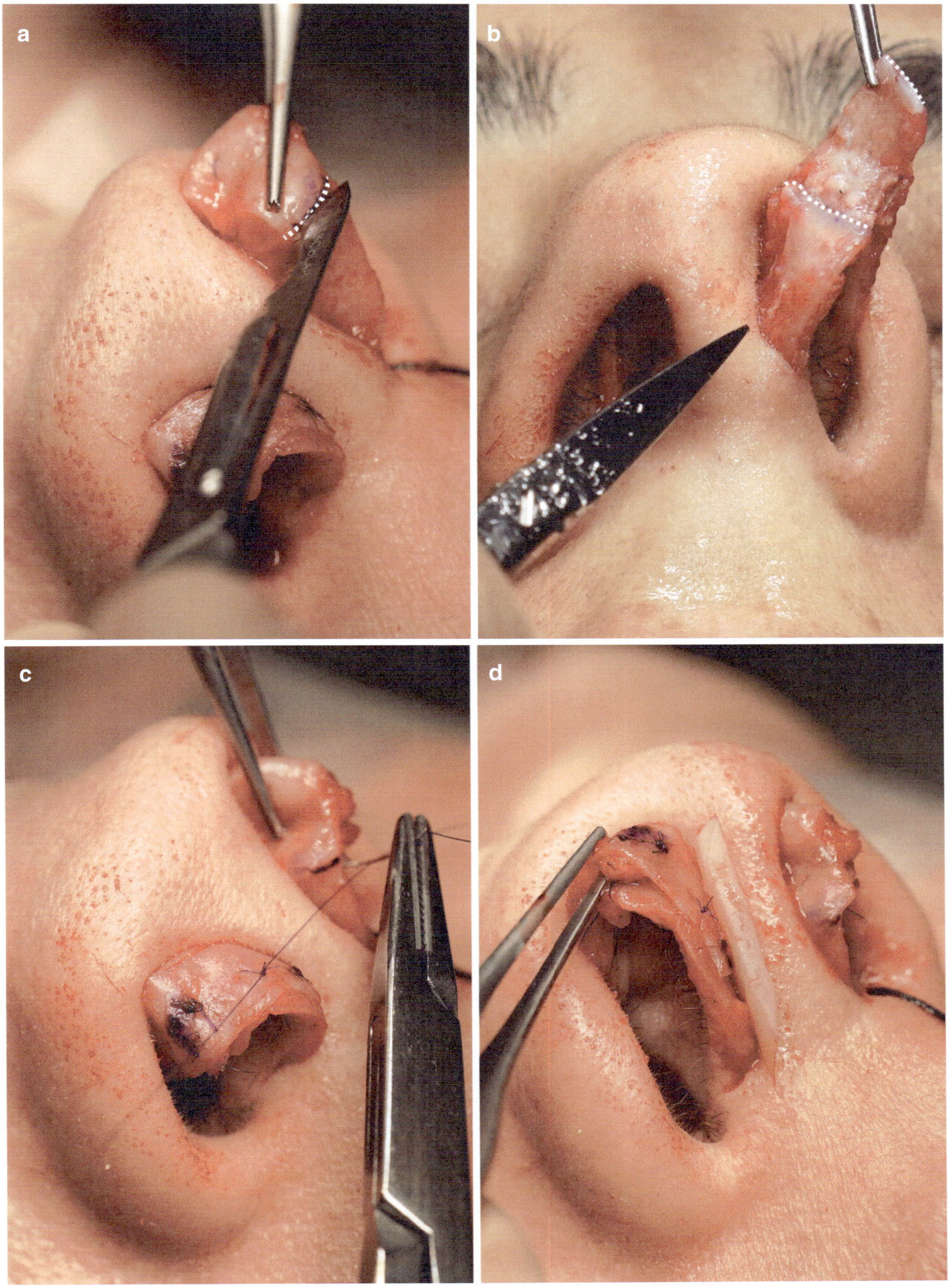

Fig. 13.36 (**a–d**) After incising the medial crus, the most projecting proximal portion was dissected from the vestibular skin and transposed over the distal segment. The overlapped ends were fixed and stabilized with mattress sutures. After overlapping the contralateral side, tip surgery was completed by placing a columellar strut and a cap graft

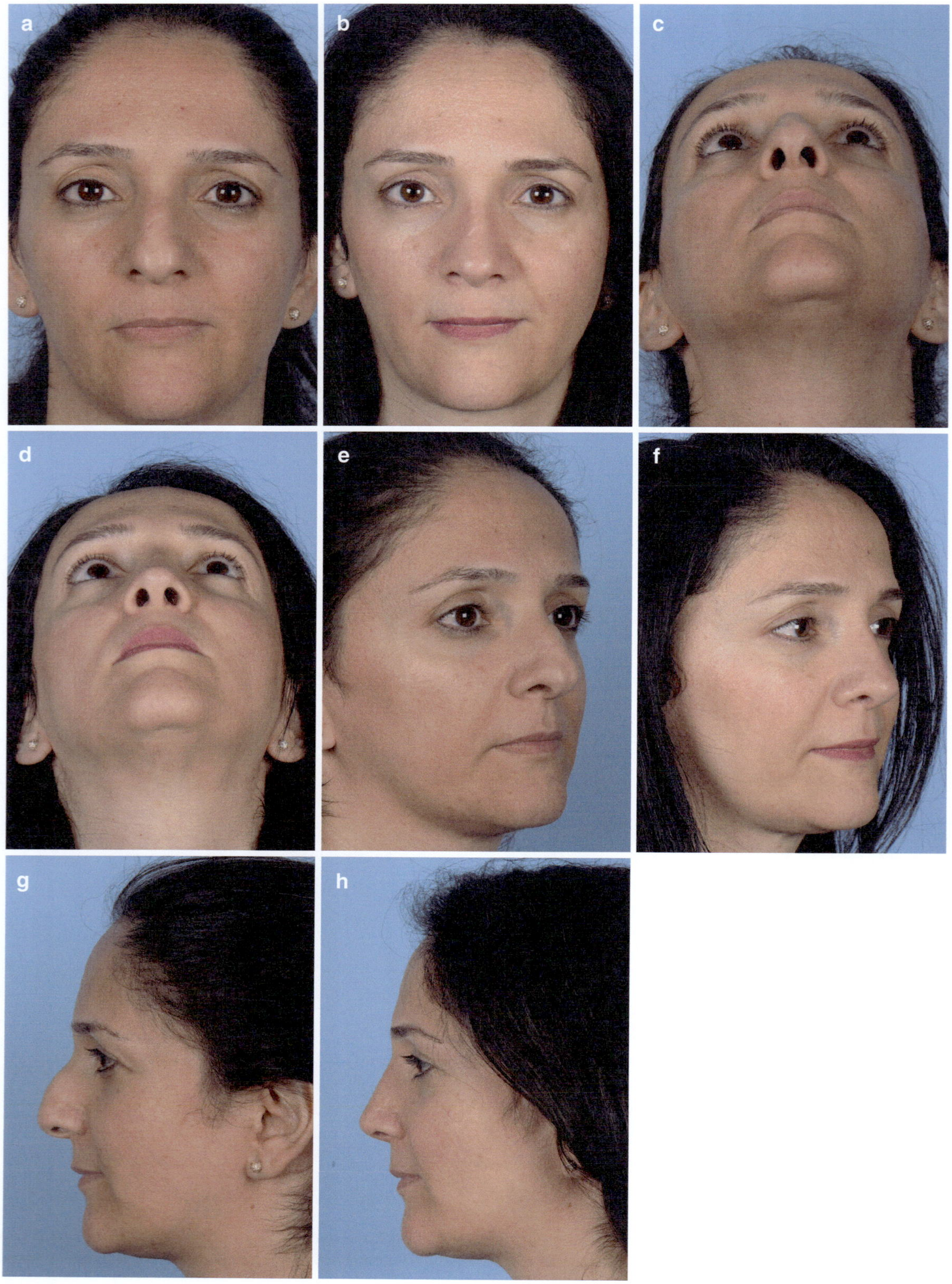

Fig. 13.37 (**a–h**) Wide tip and bifid lobule corrected. Less frontal nostril show

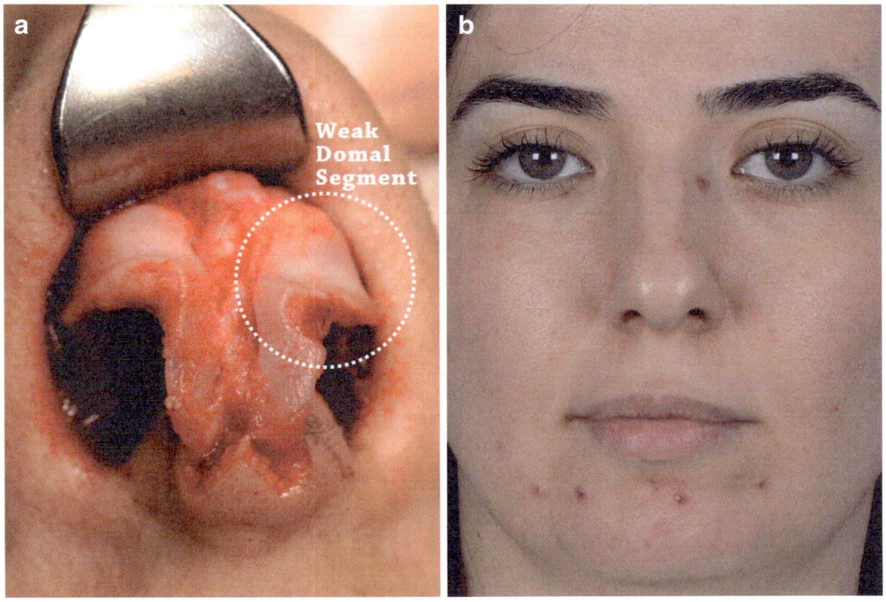

Fig. 13.38 (**a**, **b**) Dome suturing can be unpredictable in patients that have weak alar cartilages

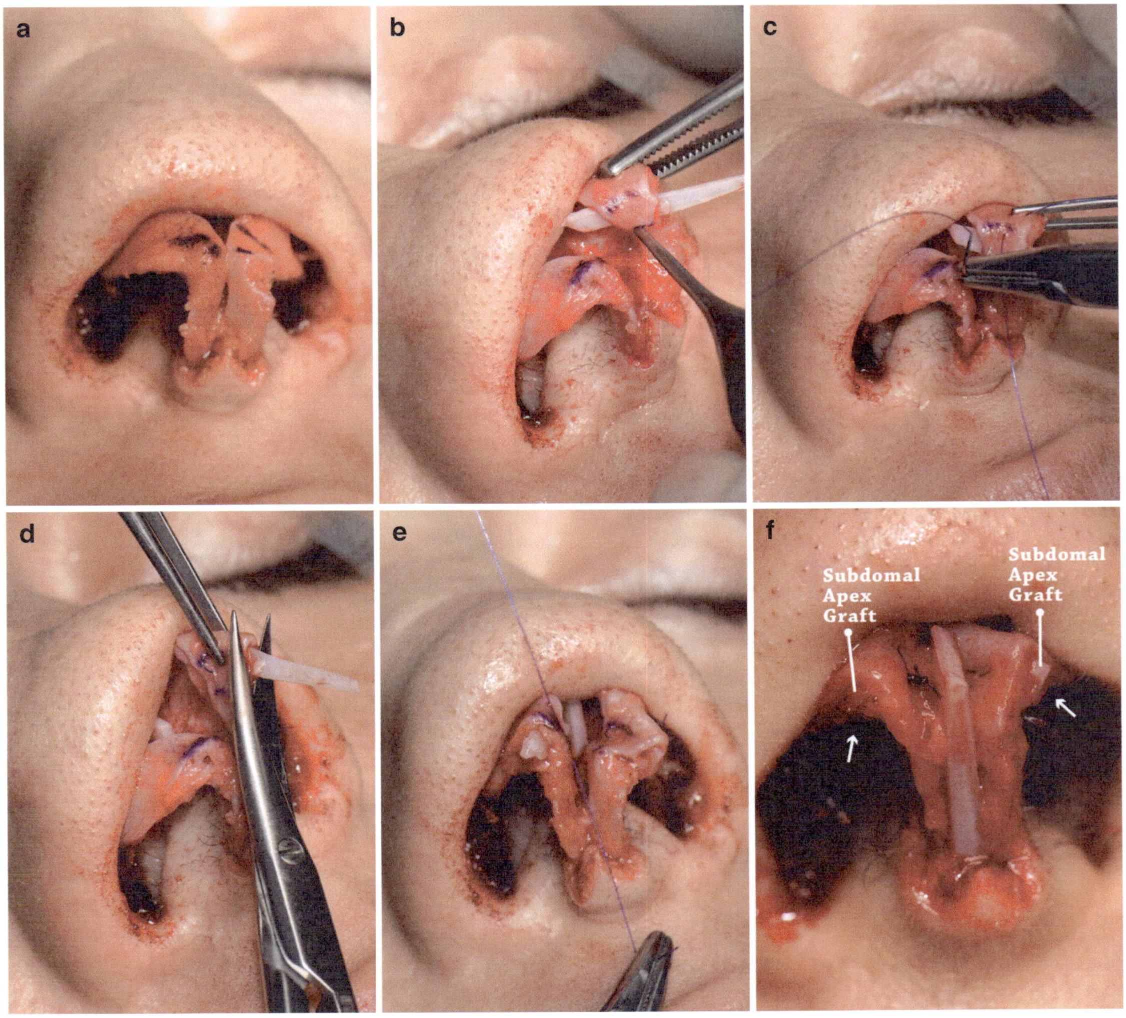

Fig. 13.39 (**a–f**) Subdomal apex graft that is placed through both domes to create symmetry and stabilize the dome structure just before transdomal matrix suture. After placement of the subdomal apex graft, the caudal edge of the lateral crus moves superiorly that is a favorable position for the caudal margin. (f) The white arrows show how the caudal margins of the lateral crura have been rotated superiorly

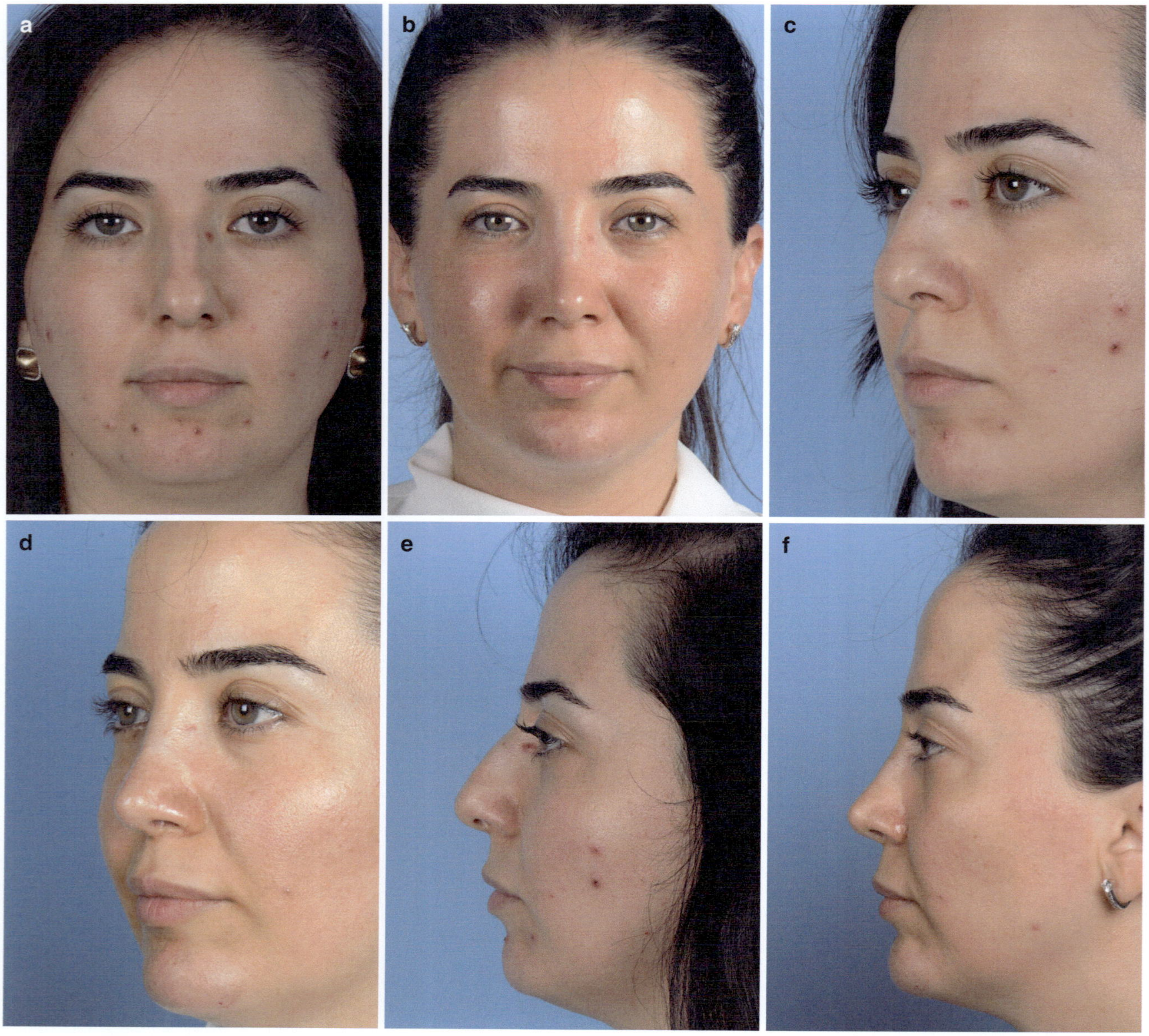

Fig. 13.40 (**a–f**) The transdomal mattress sutures with a subdomal apex graft across the tip-defining points decreased the broadness of her tip

13.3 Intermediate Techniques

Even if all the basic surgical steps have been executed appropriately, any persistent lateral crural convexity may result in a wide nasal tip. In such cases, the work of the surgeon is not complete. Two types of problems cause persistent convexity: pseudo-convexity of the lateral crus or real convexity of the lateral crus.

13.3.1 Pseudo-Convexity of the Lateral Crus (An Extrinsic Issue)

Although a lateral crural convexity is corrected via transdomal suturing, the convexity may still be evident because of alar sidewall concavity; this is termed as pseudo-convexity of the lateral crus. The solution is simple: place an alar batten graft on the concave aspect of the lateral nasal wall (Fig. 13.41; Video 13.12).

What is an alar batten graft? *Alar* refers to the nasal ala and *batten* is a nautical term that refers to a thin flexible strip of wood that provides support in bad weather. Alar button grafts are prepared using different sources of cartilage, depending on the individual's requirements. Any lateral crus excess is an ideal source of graft material. The graft is placed precisely over the area of maximal collapse and appropriately oriented. The pocket should be no wider than the graft for a good fit, and to minimize migration; fixing is unnecessary. The convex graft surface is optimally oriented in the lateral direction (Fig. 13.42).

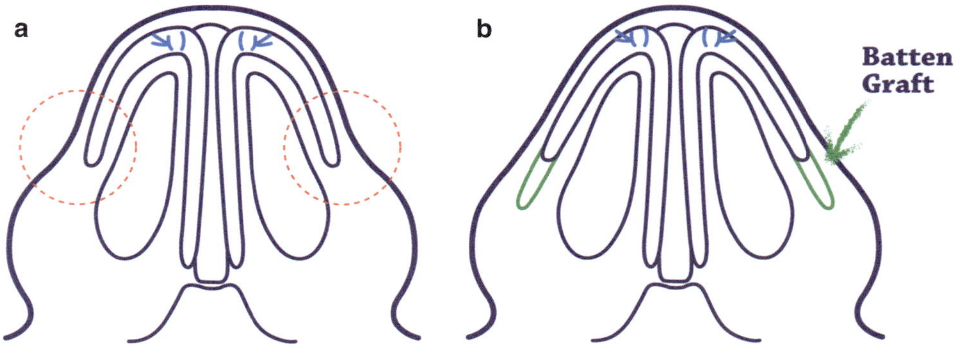

Fig. 13.41 (**a**) Although transdomal suturing has corrected the lateral crural convexity, the crus still appears to be convex. (**b**) Placement of an alar batten graft

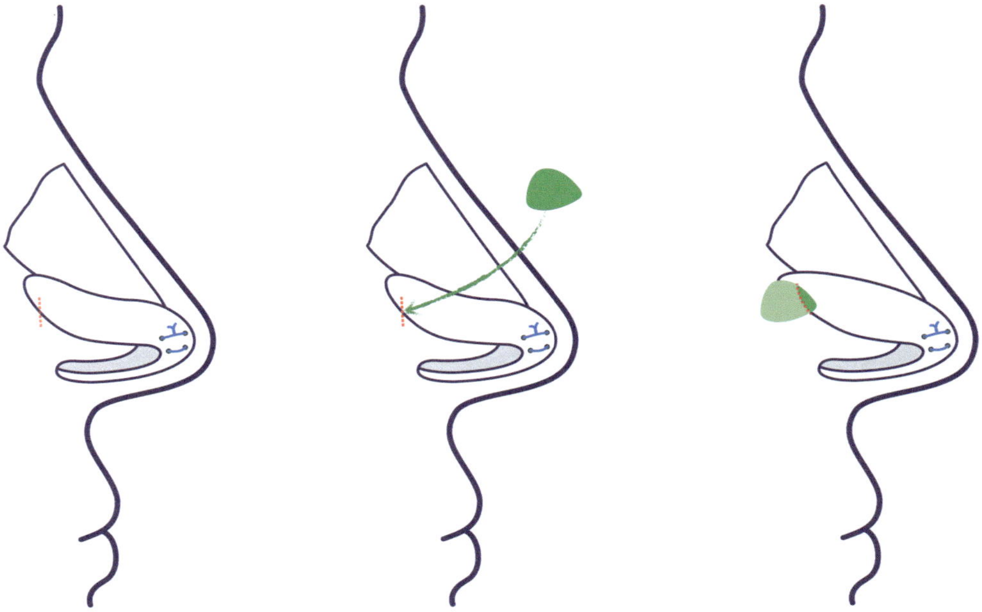

Fig. 13.42 Alar batten graft placement. This method is simple and highly effective to treat pseudoconvex lateral crus caused by a weak lateral alar wall

13.3.1.1 Case 9

In patients with pronounced lateral crural convexity, the lateral nasal wall must be meticulously examined intraoperatively. If any concavity is evident just below the convexity, that concavity is avoided when creating the ideal tip. A 1 × 1.5-cm cartilage graft prepared from the cephalic excess of the lateral crus is placed in a pocket opened in the lateral sidewall. The surgeon must place the graft as deep as possible in the nasal wall with the convex surface facing outward (Fig. 13.43).

This case's preoperative and 1-year postoperative photographs are shown in Fig. 13.44.

13.3.2 Convexity of the Lateral Crus Is (An Intrinsic Issue)

Lateral crural convexity may persist despite suturing; a transdomal suture may fail to reduce convexity. In such a case, there is residual convexity of the lateral crus. A graft sutured directly under (an underlay or ventral graft) or over (an overlay or dorsal graft) the lateral crus corrects the residual convexity and eliminates any crural irregularity. The logic is simple: a combination of two planes creates a straight plane. Thus, graft cartilage sutured directly under or over a convex lateral crus eliminates convexity; the lateral crus is anatomically near-ideal (Fig. 13.45; Video 13.13).

What is a lateral crural graft? In the literature, a graft prepared using septal and costal cartilage is termed a lateral crural strut graft if it is sutured under the lateral crus, and a lateral crural graft if it is sutured over the crus. We do not make this distinction; in practical terms, any cartilaginous graft sutured in a self-parallel manner is a lateral crural graft. Such grafts can be prepared using:

- Septal cartilage.
- Costal cartilage.
- A cephalic portion of alar cartilage.

Auricular cartilage should never be used to create a lateral crural graft for correcting convexity. However, if the lateral crus exhibits concavity or some other deficiency, auricular cartilage may serve as a strut graft.

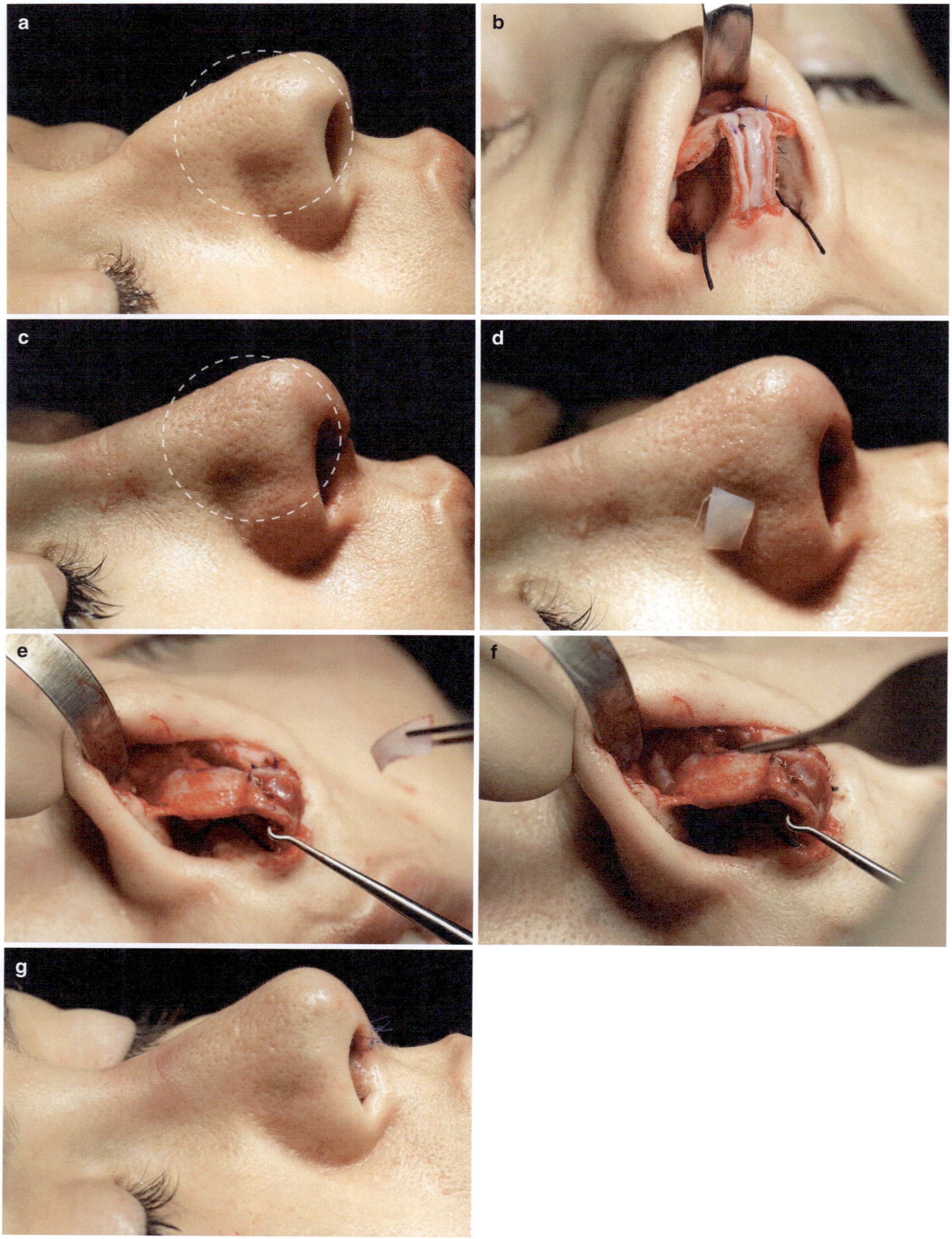

Fig. 13.43 (**a**) The circled areas indicate convex lateral crura. (**b**) Transdomal suturing repaired the lateral crural convexity. (**c**) Although the convexity was eliminated, pseudo-convexity developed because of the hollow regions described above. (**d–g**) Alar batten grafting corrected the pseudo-convexity and narrowed the tip

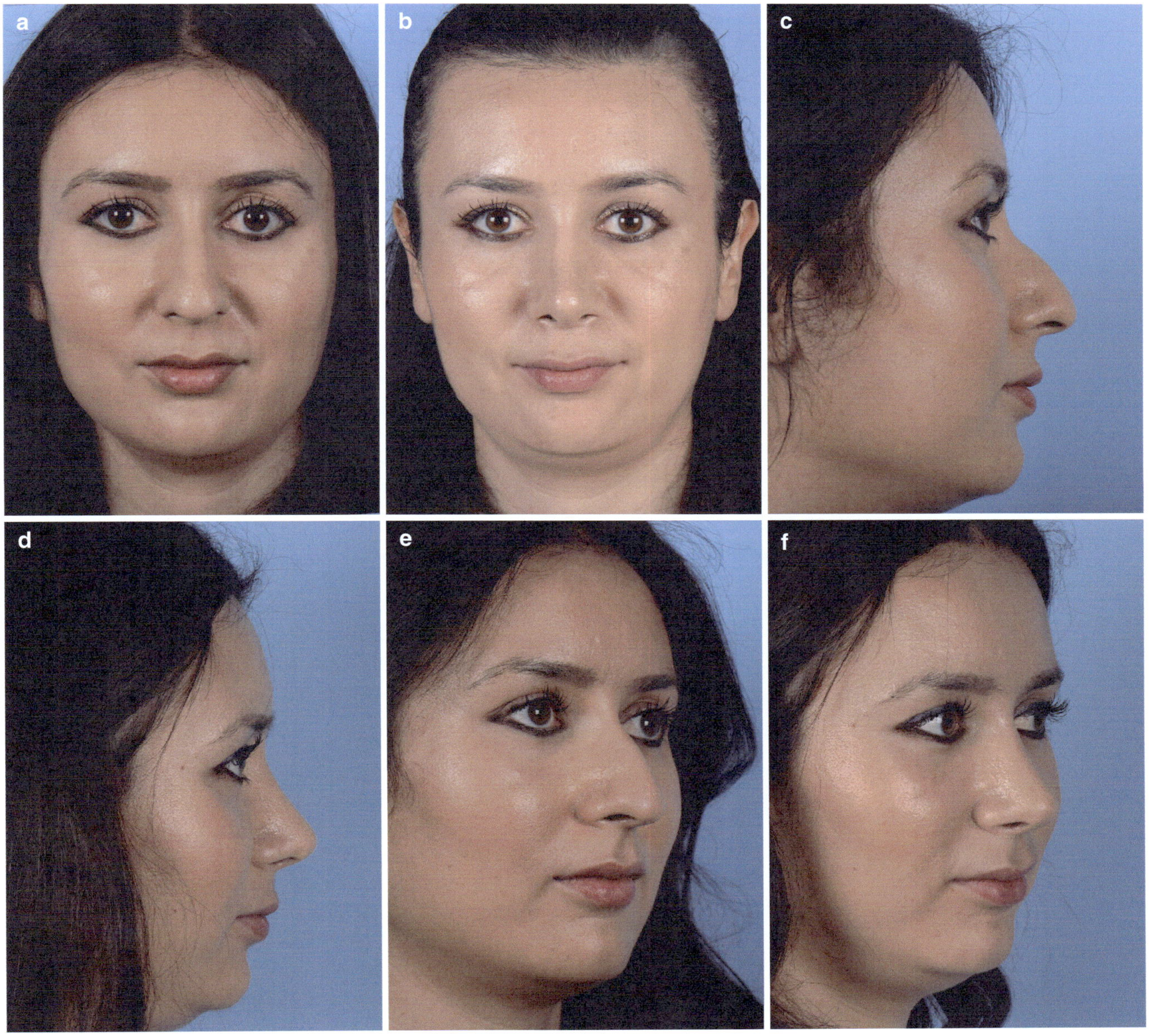

Fig. 13.44 (**a–f**) Osteocartilaginous hump has been lowered and radix has been raised to a pleasing dorsal profile. Nasal tip has more definition and interdomal distance is more symmetric and narrower with suture and bilateral alar batten grafts

It is inappropriate to standardize the length of a lateral crural strut, as this is case-dependent. However, the width must be 4–5 mm. Also, thick struts must be avoided; a thickness of 1–2 mm is ideal. Most struts are placed bilaterally, but unilateral placement is perfectly acceptable.

Examples showing how convex lateral crura are reshaped using lateral crural grafts follow, commencing with a septal lateral crural graft.

13.3.3 Septal Lateral Crural Graft

The graft is prepared from septal cartilage and fixed directly under or over the lateral crus. In terms of strut placement:

- If lateral crural convexity persists after transdomal suturing (i.e., if the lobule remains wide), the graft should be fixed under or over the lateral crus. In such a case, the graft length should extend from immediately lateral to the dome to a point slightly beyond the convex portion.
- If alar strengthening is required in terms of external valve functionality, the graft should extend to the pyriform aperture (this enhances stability). The graft is usually oriented along the long axis of the crus, with its long axis pointing the outer canthus and the lateral end is placed in a pocket created superficial to the alar sidewall.
- If an underlay is used, a cartilaginous graft placed between the vestibular skin and the lower surface of the lateral crus should be fixed to the crus at several points. Inexperienced

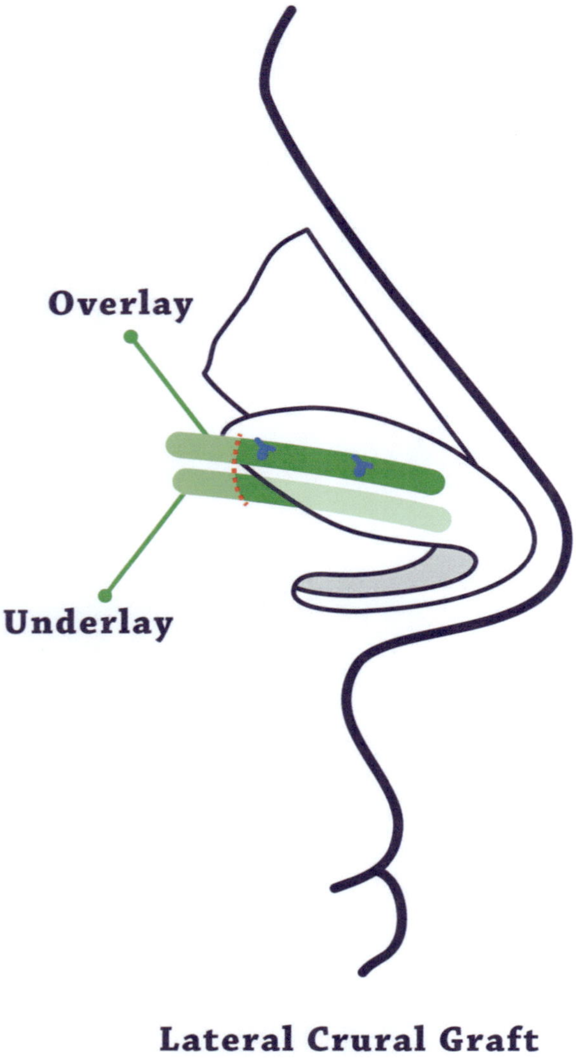

Fig. 13.45 Overlay: lateral crural graft placed over the existing lateral crus as onlay graft. Underlay: graft placed in undermined pocket between undersurface of lateral crus and skin

surgeons may find it difficult to dissect the vestibular skin from the crus; dissection beginning at the caudal edge of the lateral crus is recommended. However, the vestibular skin may tear; suture placement may increase tearing, but the tear will heal (Fig. 13.46).

- If an overlay is to be used, the lateral crural graft is placed directly onto the lateral crus and fixed using nonabsorbable sutures (Fig. 13.47).

13.3.3.1 Overlay or Underlay?

- No general rule on overlay/underlay choice during wide nasal tip surgery has emerged. However, the author generally prefers to place underlays in thin-skinned patients and overlays in thick-skinned patients.

13.3.3.2 Case 10

Clinical outcomes of underlay placement are seen in Fig. 13.48 (Video 13.14), and preoperative and 1-year postoperative photographs of this case are shown in Fig. 13.49.

13.3.3.3 Case 11

Another example of underlay placement is seen in Fig. 13.50. Preoperative and 1-year postoperative photographs are shown in Fig. 13.51.

13.3.3.4 Case 12

Long-term results of underlay placement are seen in the 13-year postoperative photographs in Fig. 13.52.

Overlay placement is generally preferred for thick-skinned patients, as mentioned above.

13.3.4 Clinical Outcomes of Overlay Placement

13.3.4.1 Case 13

The major issue in this case is thick skin with wide nasal tip due to excessive convexity of lateral crura (Fig. 13.53). Lateral crural grafting can also be performed using a closed approach (Fig. 13.54). Preoperative and 1-year postoperative photographs are shown in Fig. 13.55.

13.3.4.2 Case 14

Lateral crural grafting of a thick-skinned patient is shown below.

A 20-year-old woman dislikes the appearance of her nose. She thinks the tip is too wide and she doesn't like the wide dorsum with a hump (Fig. 13.56).

In patients with wide nasal tips, if alar sidewall weakness is accompanied by prominent lateral convexity, the ala may become medialized after transdomal suturing. An overlaid lateral crural graft can prevent or correct such problems. This issue usually arises in thick-skinned patients. The alar wall must be meticulously examined preoperatively. Case 15 is a typical example of this type of wide nasal tip.

13.3.4.3 Case 15

In this patient, alar sidewall weakness was accompanied by prominent lateral convexity. Therefore, an overlaid lateral crural graft was placed.

A wide lobule may be associated with lack of lateral support for the alar sidewalls (Fig. 13.57).

Preoperative and 1-year postoperative photographs are shown in Fig. 13.58.

What might happen if a graft is not placed in patients with wide nasal tips and weak alar side walls? *A pinched tip deformity may occur.* Case 16 is a typical example.

13.3.4.4 Case 16

Preoperative photographs show a moderately wide tip and weak alar side walls. It is clearly seen postoperatively that

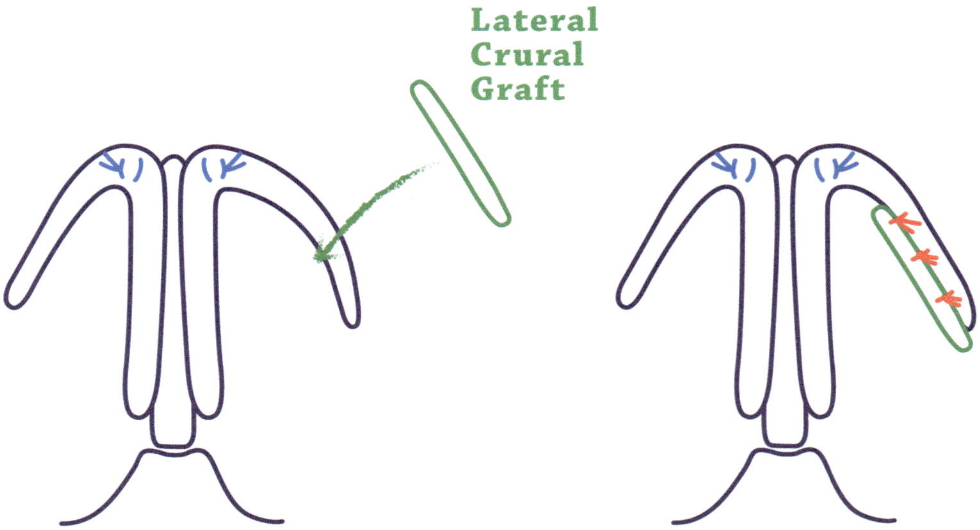

Fig. 13.46 Underlay placement of a lateral crural graft. The graft is sutured to the deep surface of the lateral crura with absorbable sutures. The graft might be extended to the accessory cartilage junction or over the piriform aperture

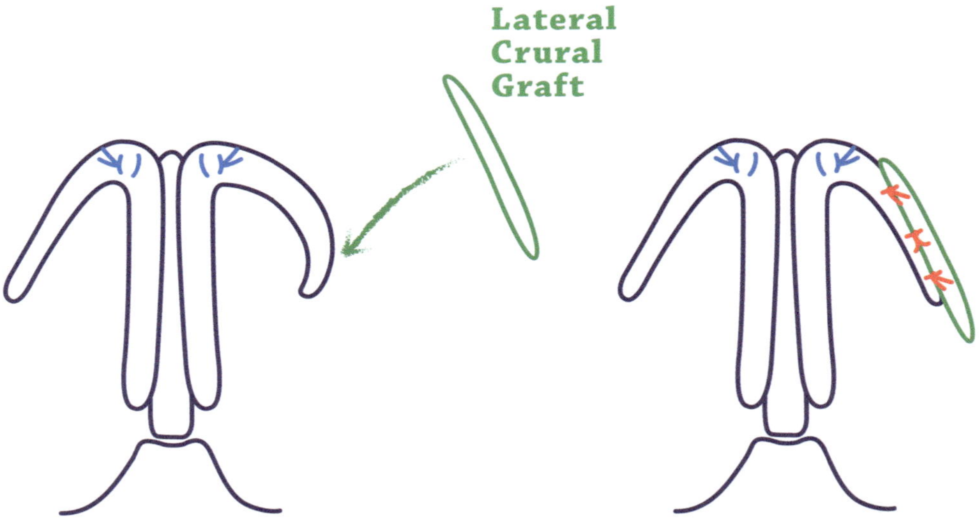

Fig. 13.47 Overlay placement of a lateral crural graft. It should start right next to the dome or cup graft. The lateral end of the strut is placed in a newly formed pocket at the outer canthus direction inside the lateral alar wall. The graft is fixated directly to over the surface of lower lateral cartilage with absorbable sutures

using basic wide tip techniques without lateral crural grafts caused a pinched tip appearance (Fig. 13.59).

Technical Pearl: The surgeon must understand that lateral strut thickness is extremely important. Excessive graft thickness will become apparent postoperatively. Graft thickness is of concern when grafts are placed as either underlays or overlays.

Case 17 is a typical example for this situation.

13.3.4.5 Case 17

She had a broad nasal tip with thick skin. In this case, a thick lateral crural graft was placed. Almost 4 years after her primary surgery, she suffered from fullness on the right alar wall.

What happened? Thick graft showed itself under the skin (Fig. 13.60).

To fix that problem, the thick part of the lateral crural graft was removed under local anesthesia (Fig. 13.61).

13.3.5 Alar Lateral Crural Grafting

To eliminate lateral crural convexity, the cephalic excess of alar cartilage may be used as a lateral crural graft. The cartilage is placed either over or under the remaining cartilage.

Lateral crural alar grafts are placed via either open rhinoplasty or tip delivery. After exposure of the lateral crura, cephalic trimming is performed to ensure that an intact piece of cartilage at least 6 mm long is preserved. Cartilage trimmed from the cephalic region is separated from the vestibular skin and removed as a free cartilage graft. This graft is then either slid below or turned under the remaining lateral cartilage. The graft is then placed on top of the remaining lateral crus, and the cartilages are sutured back-to-back using absorbable material.

The graft should be placed as an underlay if the lateral crus is excessively convex, and as an overlay in all other

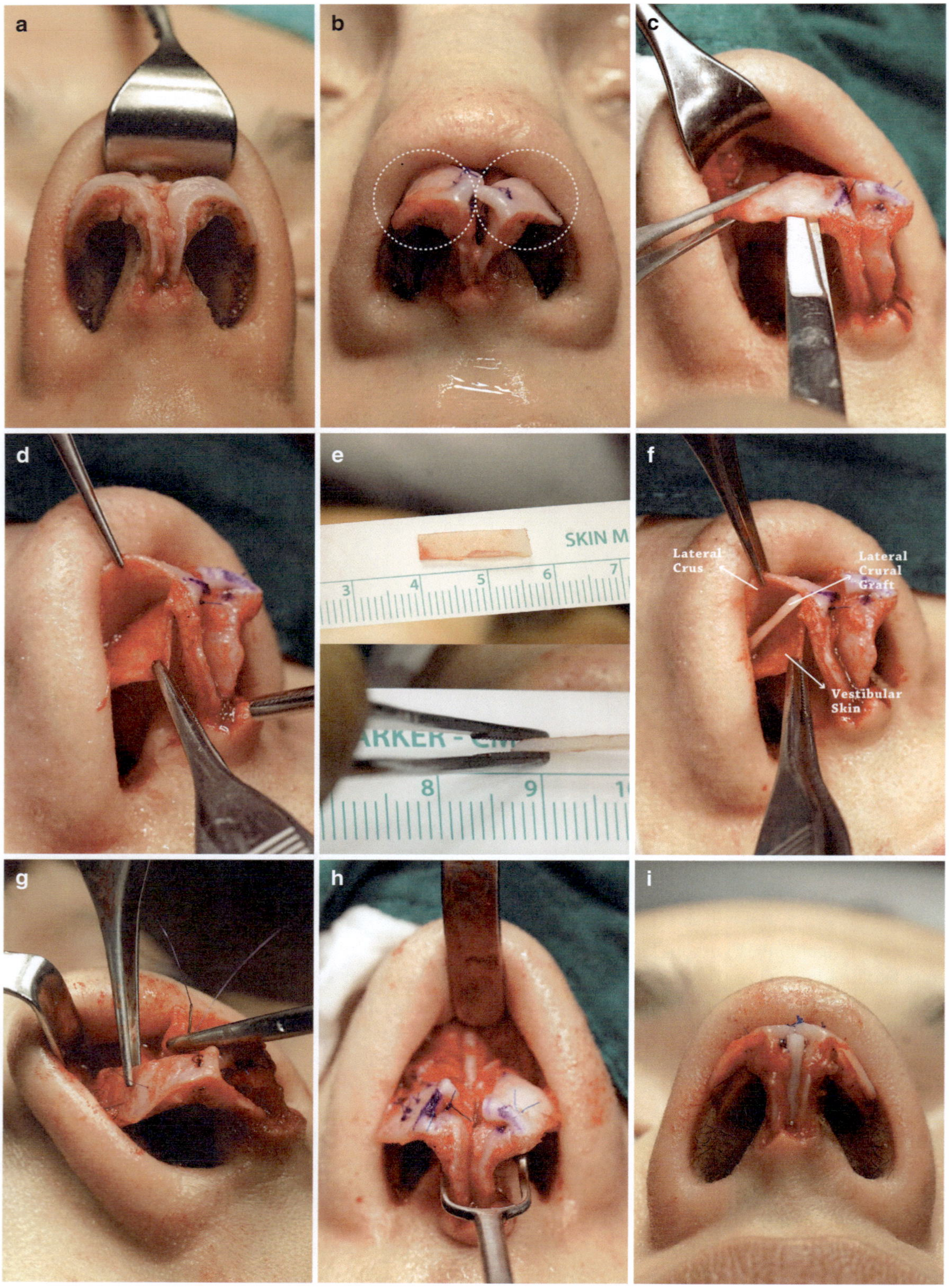

Fig. 13.48 (**a**) The open approach. (**b**) After transdomal suturing, lateral crural convexity was still evident. (**c, d**) The vestibular skin of the lateral crus was undermined and dissected from the cephalic border of the crus toward the caudal border. (**e**) The lateral crural graft was prepared from the septum. (**f**) The lateral crural graft was placed on the deep surface of the lateral crus in a pocket previously created by undermining. (**g**) The graft was secured to the crus by two or three sutures of 5/0 nonabsorbable material. (**h**) Compare the sides; the lateral crural graft was placed on the right. (**i**) The enhanced alar cartilage anatomy

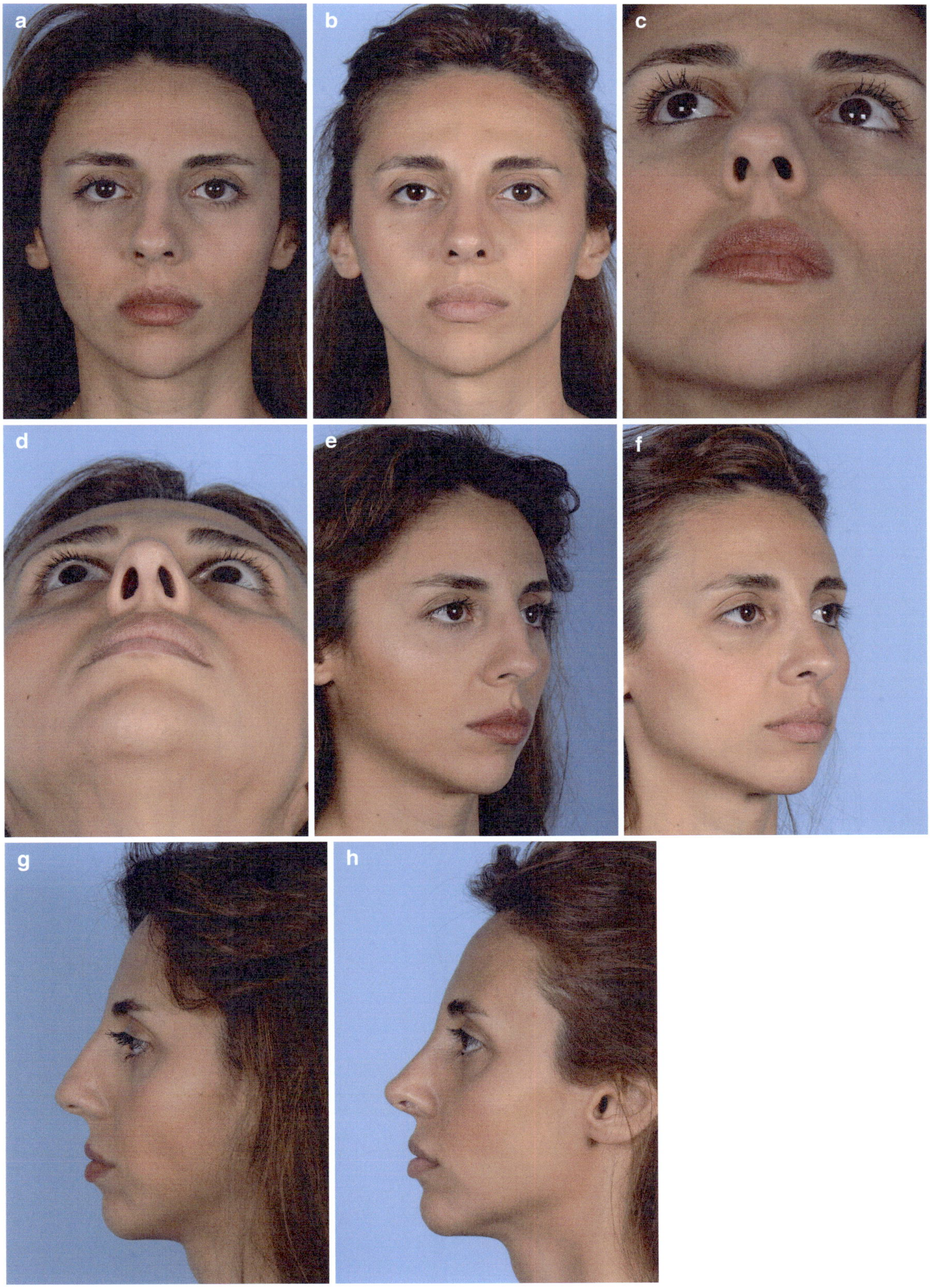

Fig. 13.49 (**a–h**) The wide tip has been corrected with the creation of aesthetically pleasing, tip-defining points and contour, using tip suturing and grafting techniques

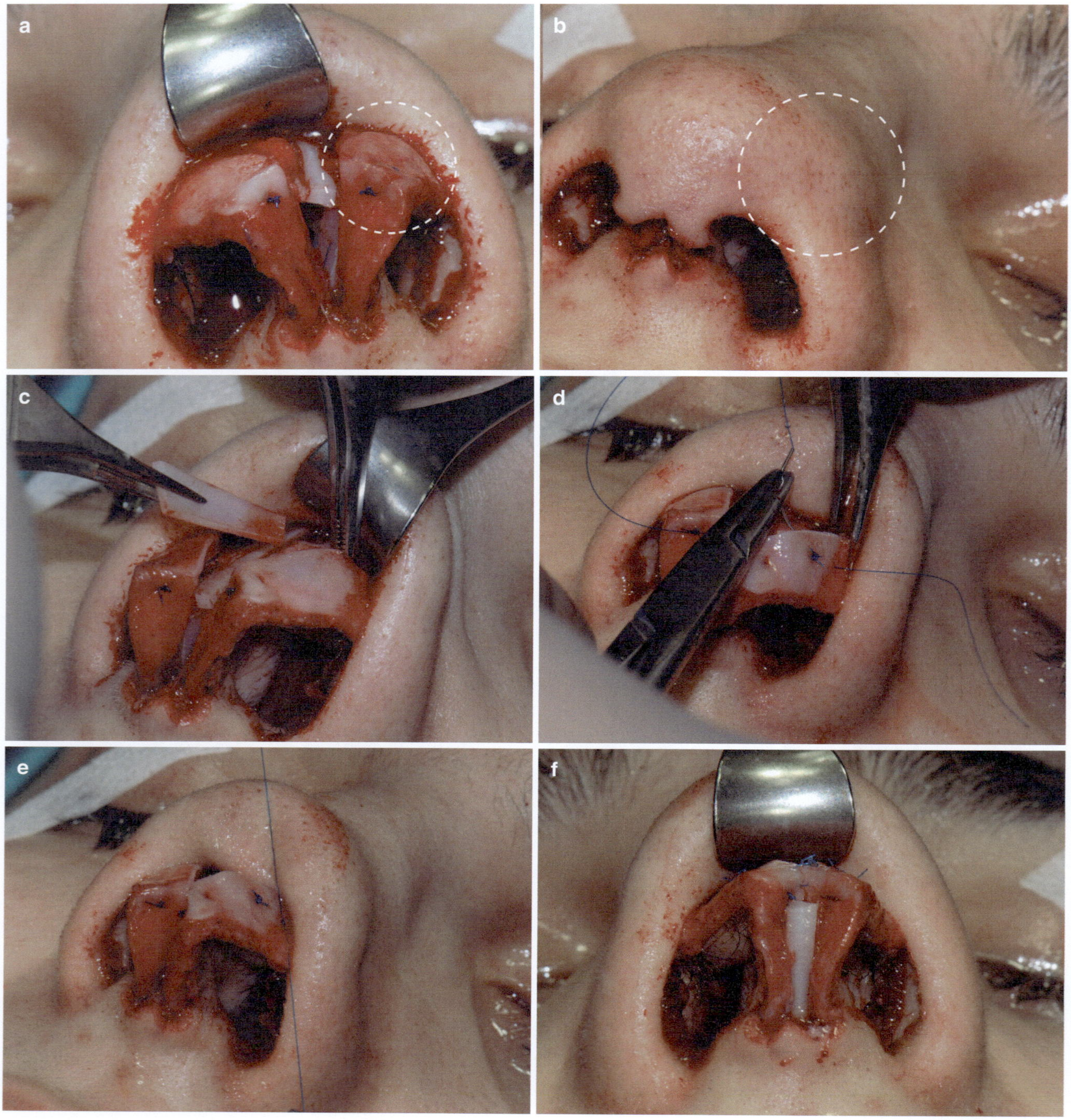

Fig. 13.50 (**a**, **b**) After transdomal suturing, the lateral crural convexity persists. (**c–f**) An underlay lateral crural graft is placed to remedy the convexity

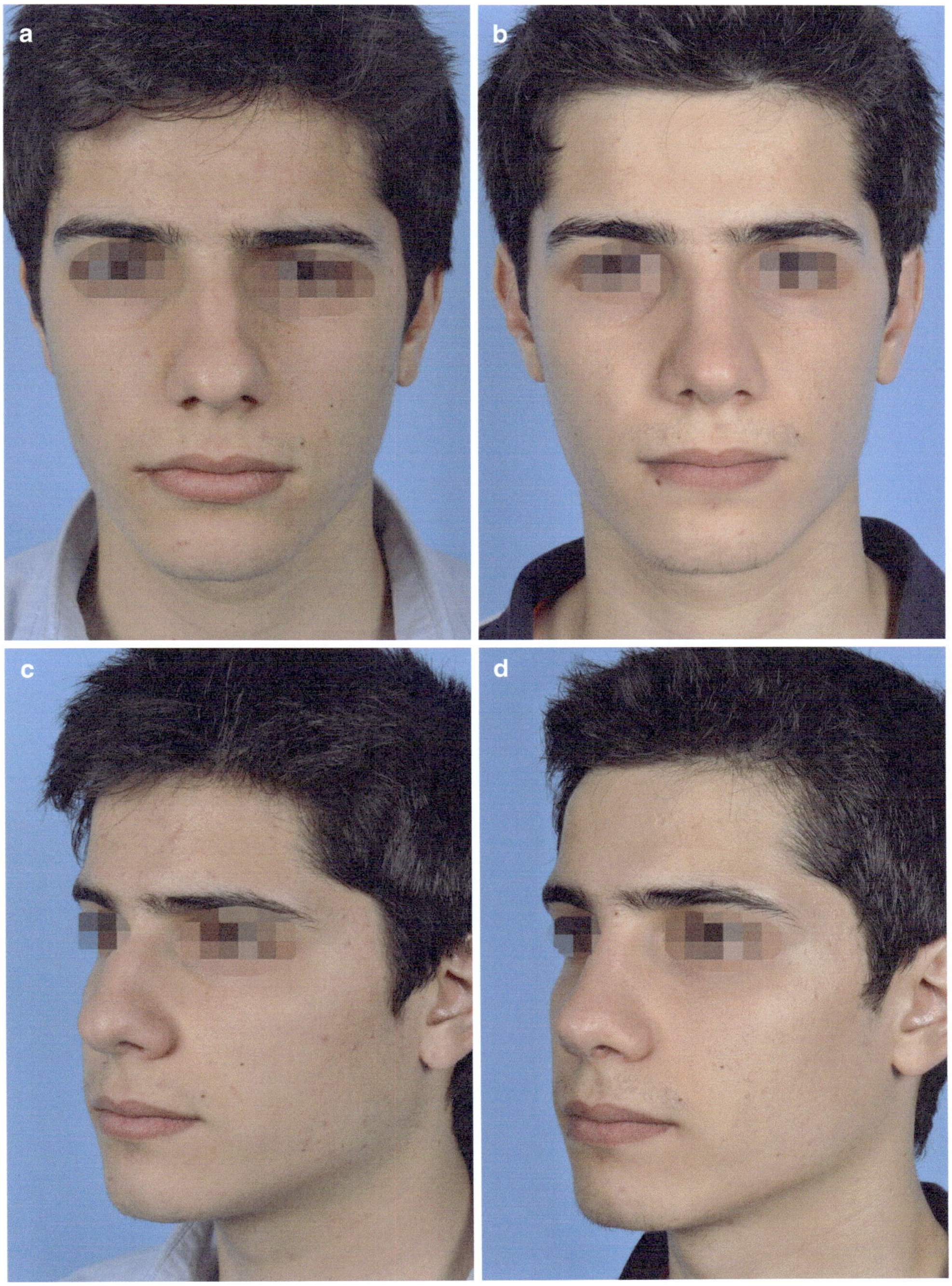

Fig. 13.51 (**a–d**) This patient with wide tip had an increased domal arch with an excessive convex lateral crus. Twelve months after the patient shows the improved aesthetic appearance of the tip. Correction of the boxy tip and the lateral alar convexity has been achieved with the placement transdomal suture and lateral crural grafts

cases. When placed as an underlay, the alar cartilage is turned and sutured to existing cartilage with the concave aspects of both cartilages apposed. Lateral crural grafting is nondestructive, reversible, and incremental; excessively convex cartilage is corrected using horizontal mattress sutures (Figs. 13.62 and 13.63; Video 13.15).

13.3.5.1 Clinical Outcomes

Representative cases featuring overlay placement of alar lateral crural grafts (via sliding) are presented here.

Case 18

A 44-year-old woman complained of a wide nasal tip. Preoperative and intraoperative photographs are shown in Fig. 13.64. Preoperative and 3-year postoperative photographs are shown in Fig. 13.65.

Case 19

A 28-year-old woman requested reduction of the size of her nose. She has thin skin; a wide tip, and bifid lobule. Preoperative and intraoperative photographs are shown in

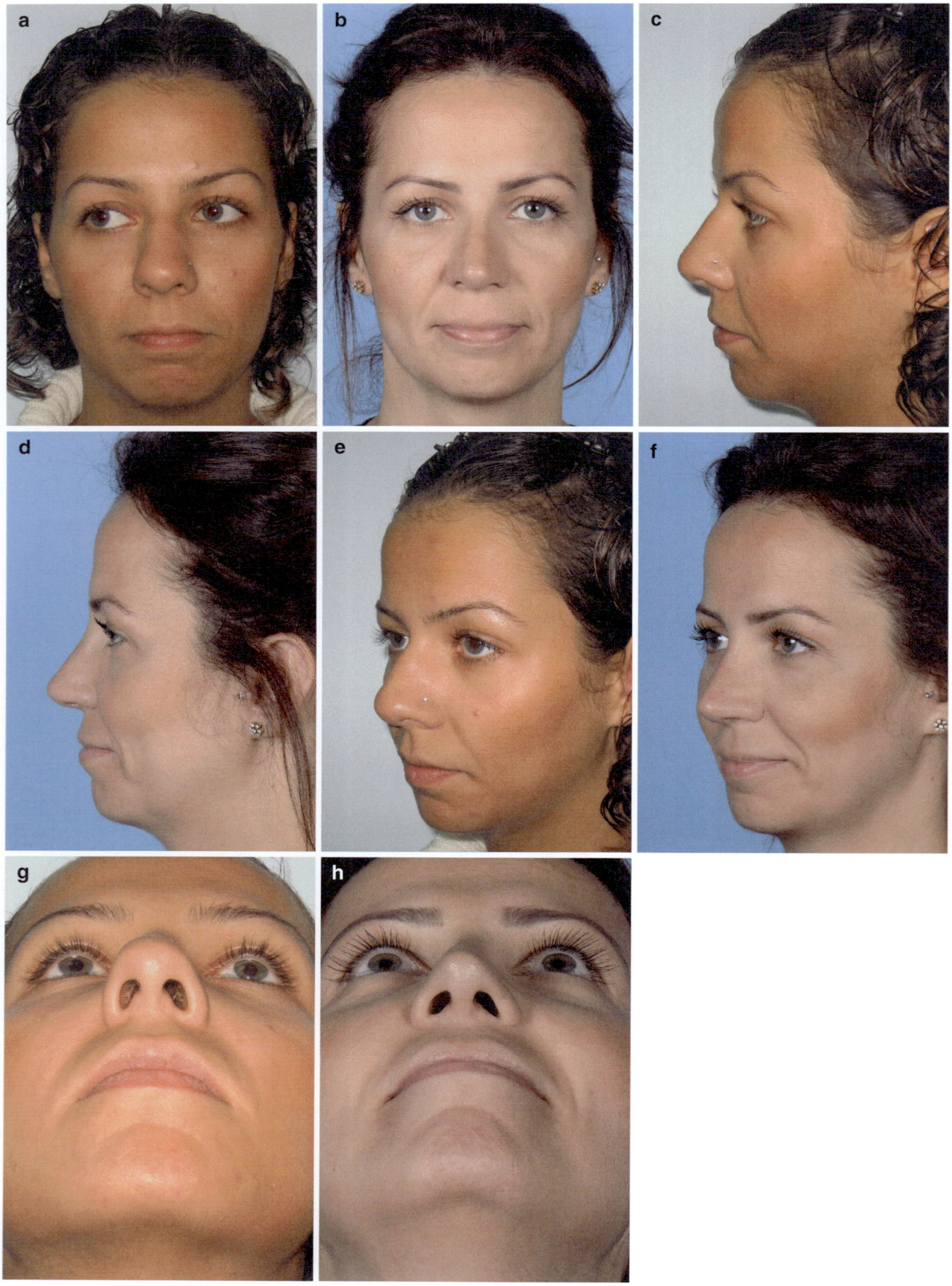

Fig. 13.52 (**a–h**) Dome suturing, cephalic trim, columellar strut, lateral crural graft, and cup graft combination has satisfactorily corrected the moderate wide nasal tip even in the long term

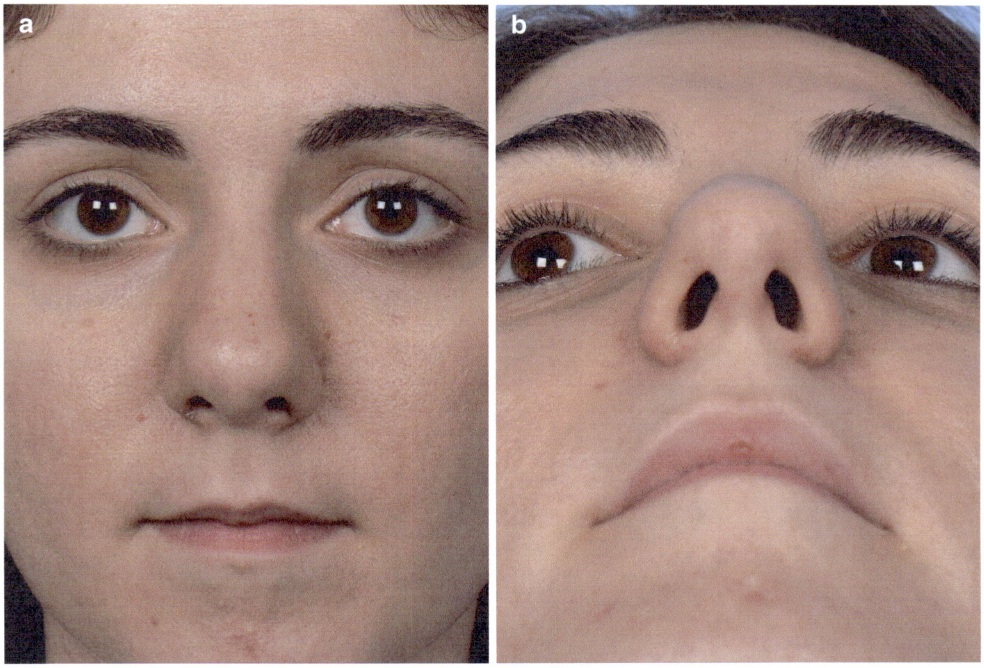

Fig. 13.53 (**a**, **b**) Moderately wide nasal tip with thick skin

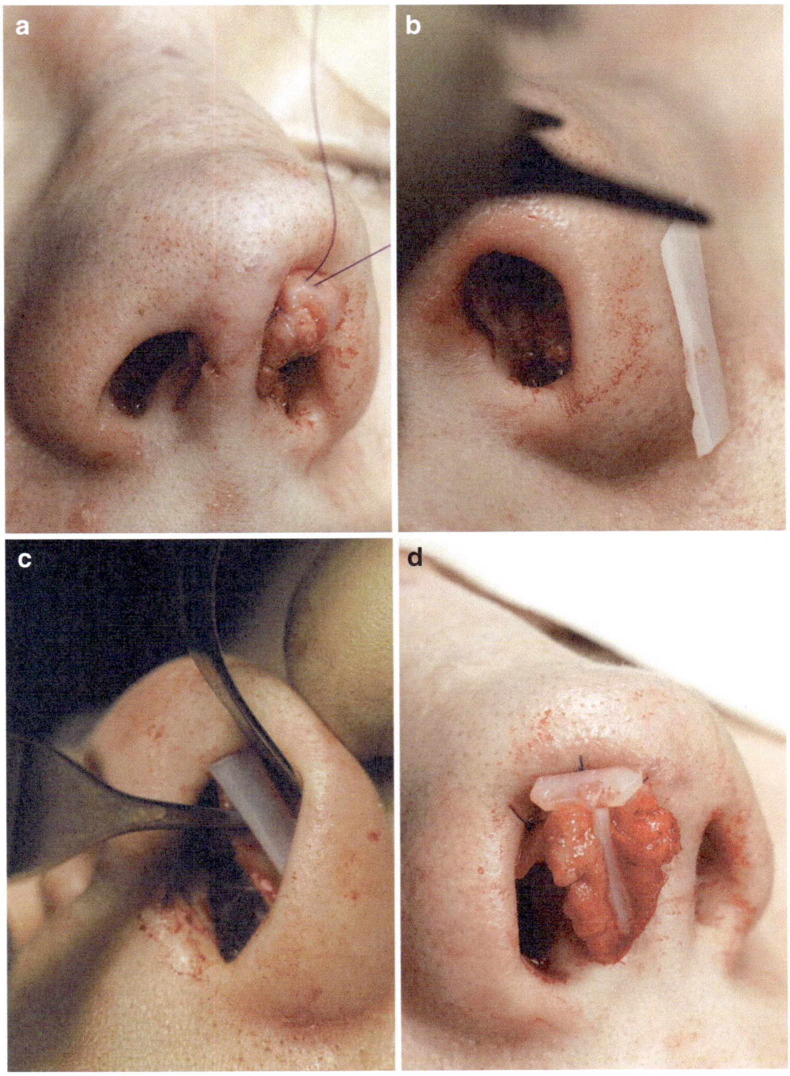

Fig. 13.54 (**a–d**) The alar cartilages are strengthened and projected via placement of columellar strut, onlay lateral crural grafts, and tip graft to "tent out" the thick overlying envelope

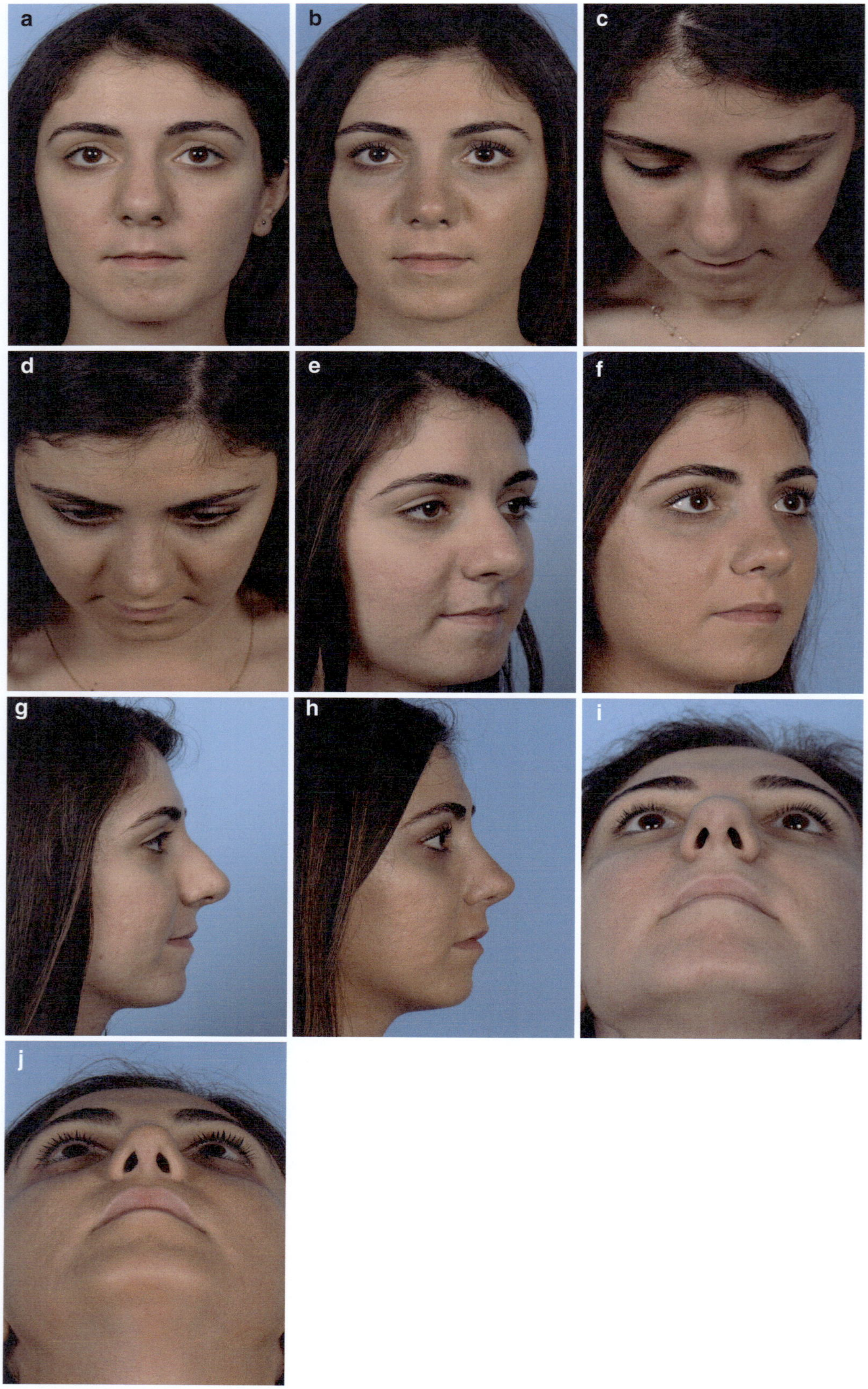

Fig. 13.55 (a–j) Transdomal suture and lateral crural grafts together solved the excess concavity of lateral crura

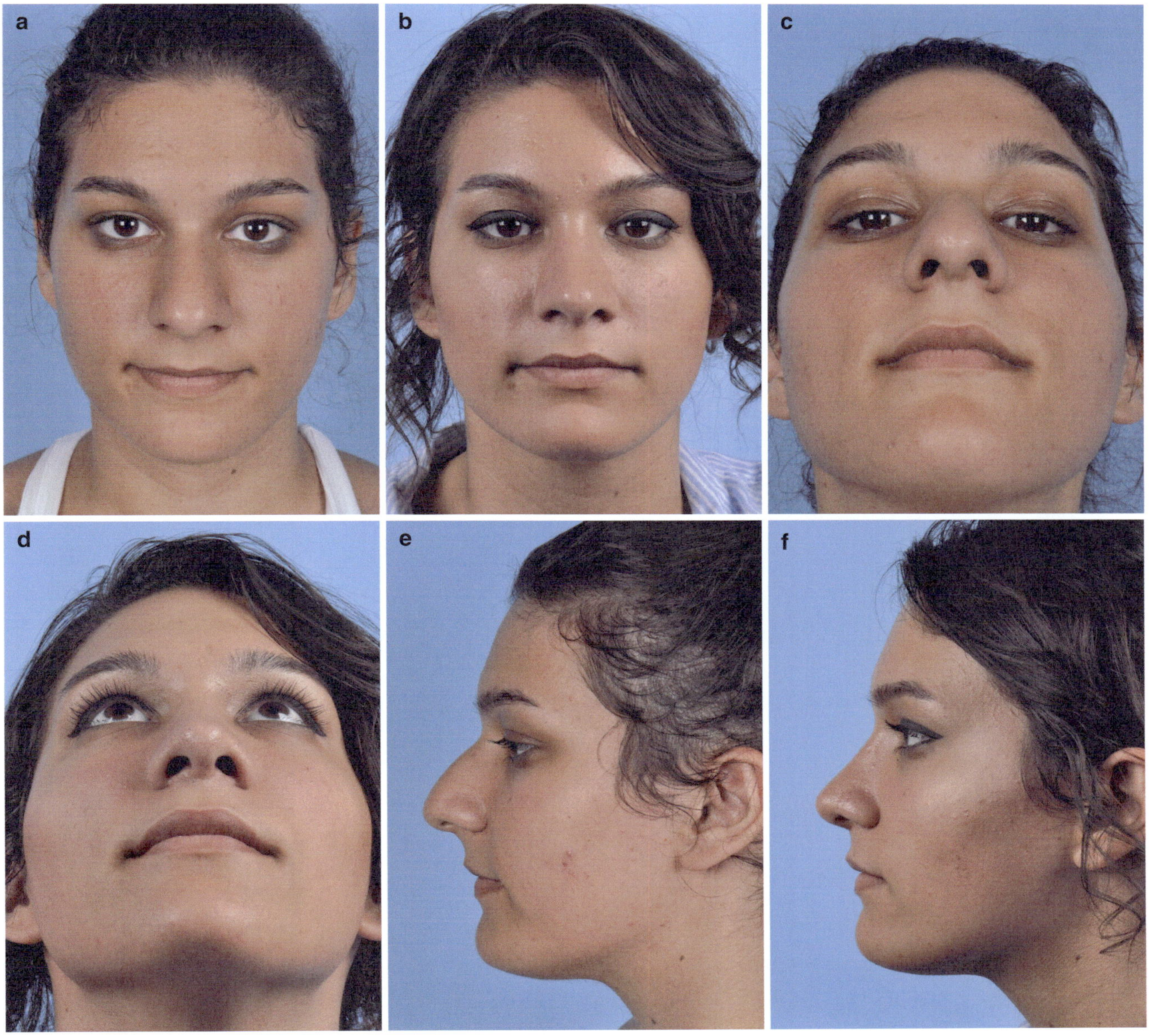

Fig. 13.56 (**a–f**) Lateral crural grafts corrected the excessive convexity of the lateral crura and transdomal sutures across the domes and narrowed the tip-defining points

Fig. 13.66. Preoperative and 1-year postoperative photographs are shown in Fig. 13.67.

The graft should be placed as an underlay if the lateral crus is excessively convex.

Representative examples of underlay placement of alar lateral crural grafts ("turning under").

Case 20

A wide nasal tip with excessive lateral crus convexity. Cephalic excess was placed under the lateral crura.

Preoperative and intraoperative photographs are shown in Fig. 13.68, and preoperative and 1-year postoperative photographs are shown in Fig. 13.69.

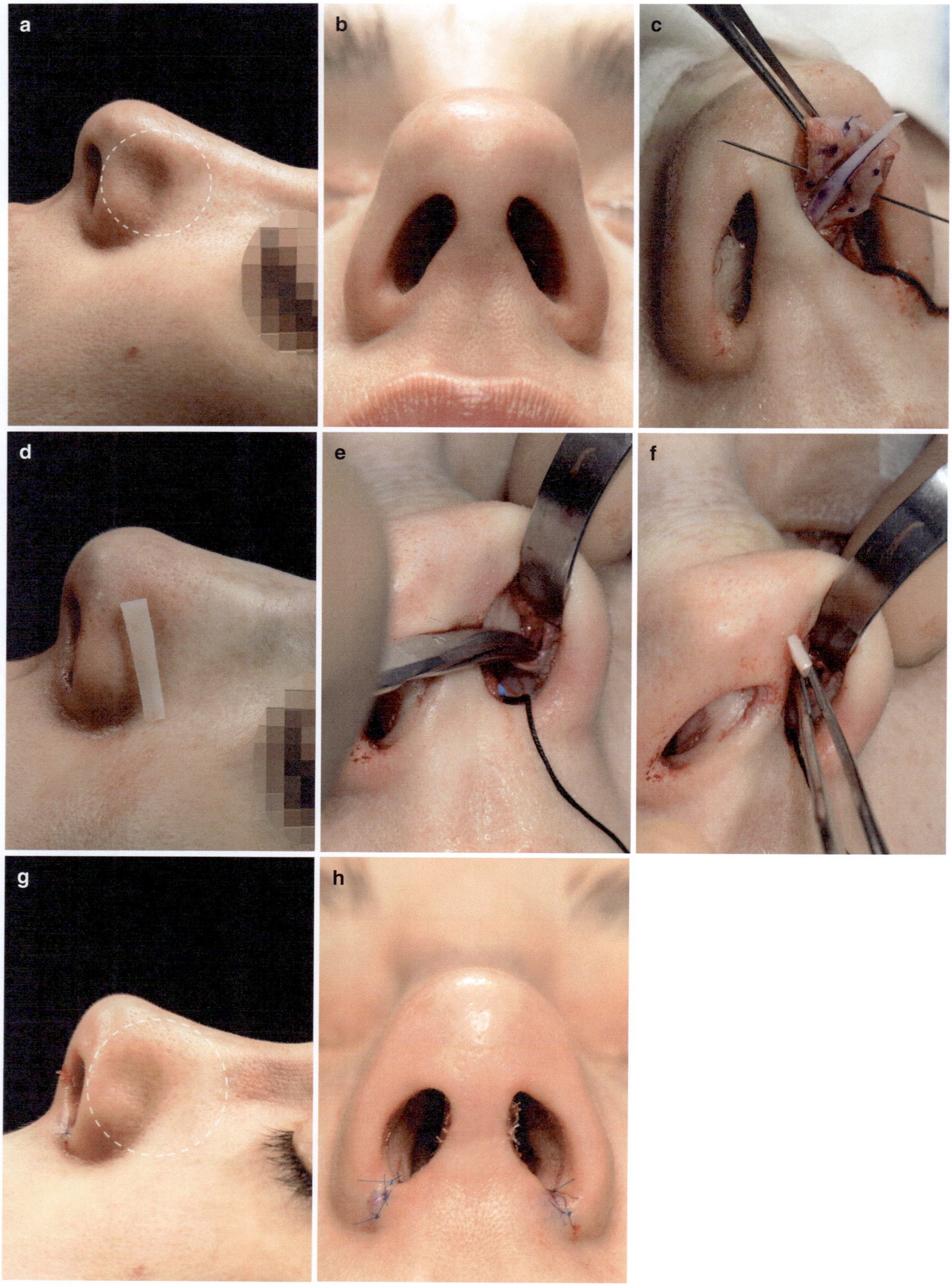

Fig. 13.57 (**a–f**) The graft should extend to the pyriform aperture to enhance stability. This strengthens the ala in terms of external valve functionality. (**g–h**) Compare with pre/op pictures. Lateral crural graft has solved the concavity of sidewall

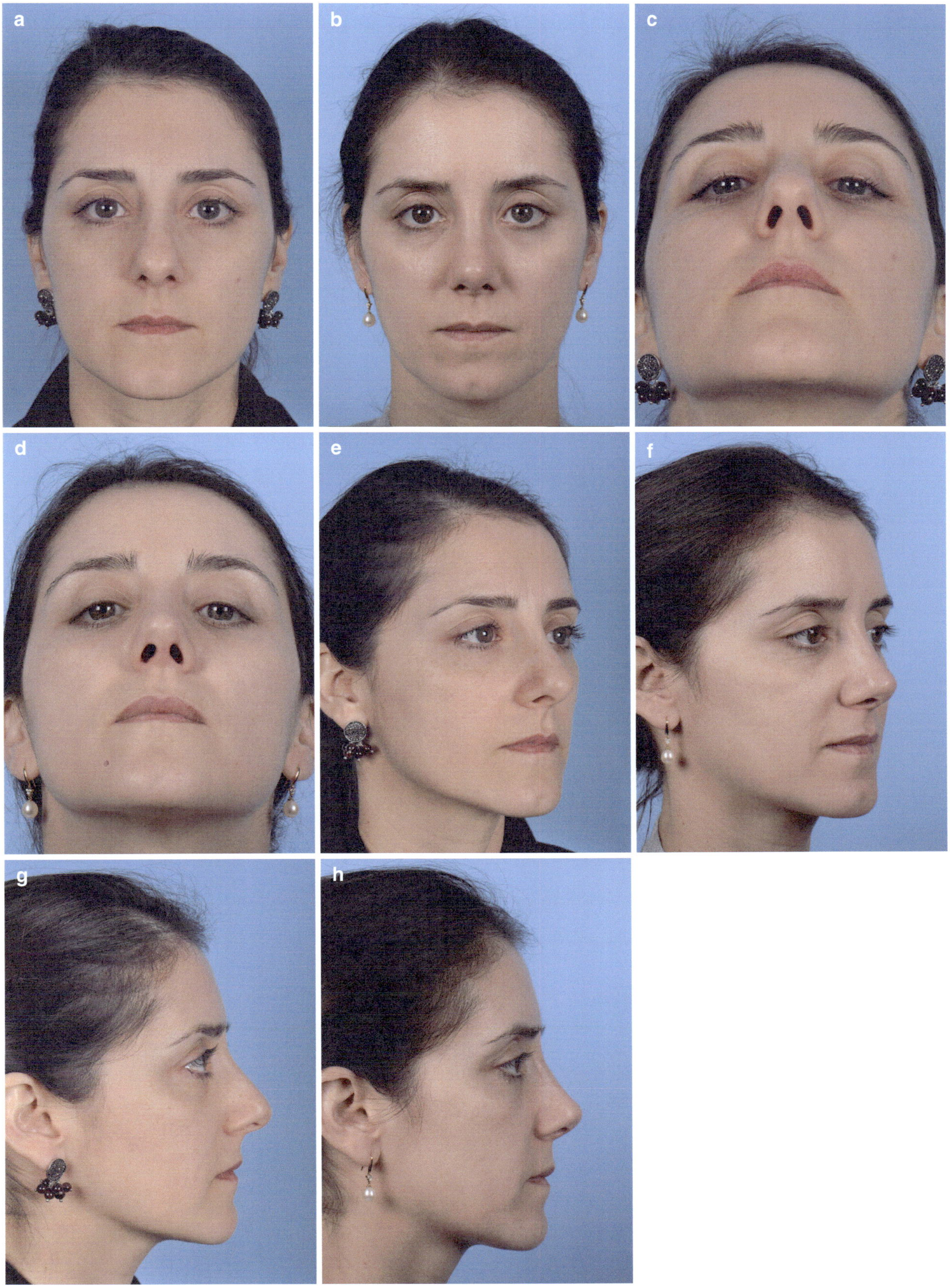

Fig. 13.58 (**a–h**) Not only is the tip narrowed but the alar side walls are also strengthened

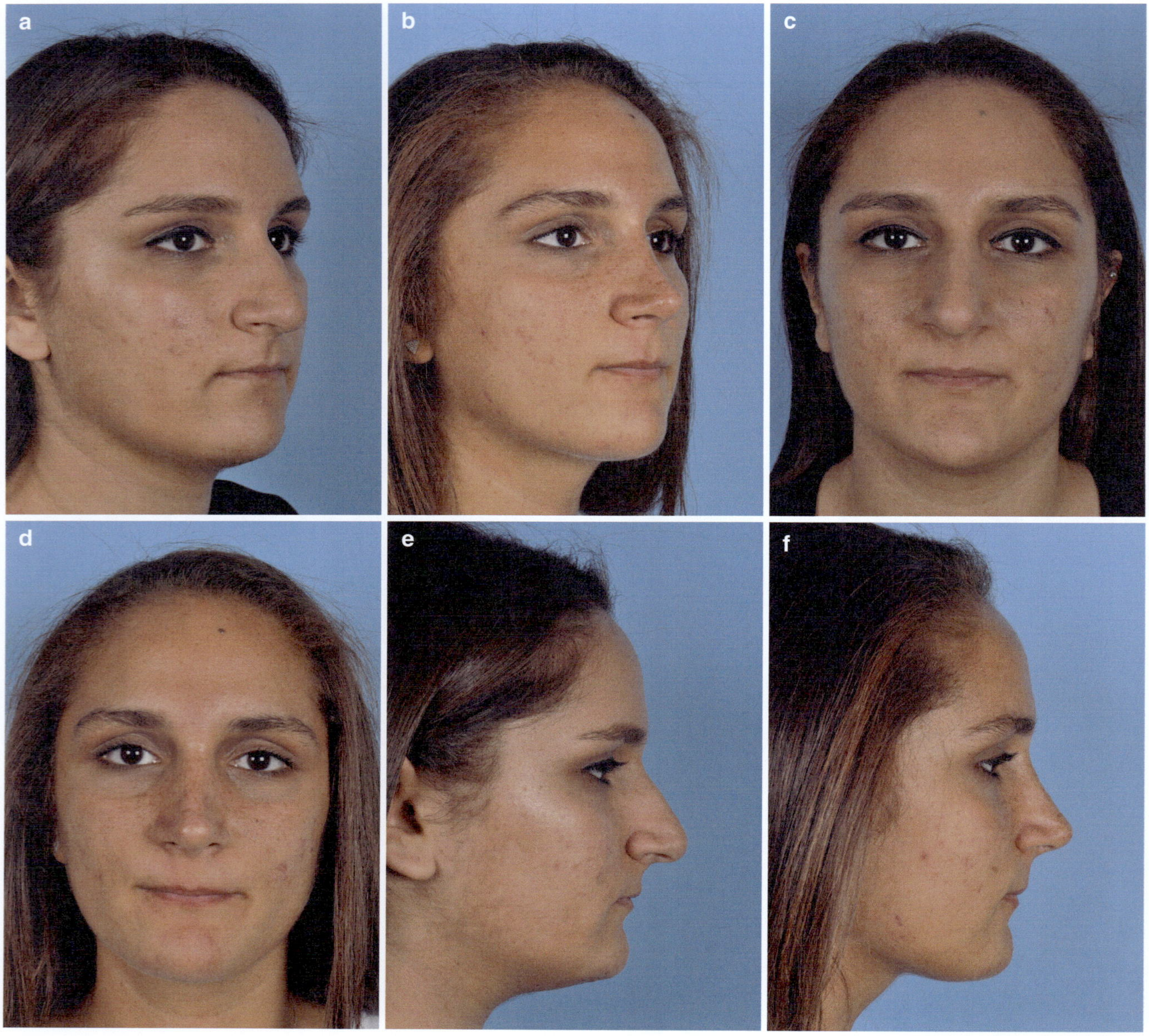

Fig. 13.59 (**a–f**) Before and after photographs. In this patient, a pinched tip appearance occurred using basic tip techniques without strengthening the alar sidewall

Case 21

The chief complaint of this 46-year-old patient with thick skin was her wide tip. Preoperative and intraoperative photographs are shown in Fig. 13.70 (Video 13.16).

In preoperative and 1-year postoperative photographs (Fig. 13.71), the patient shows improved brow-aesthetic lines as well as correction of wide tip and the lateral alar convexity with the placement of alar lateral crural grafts.

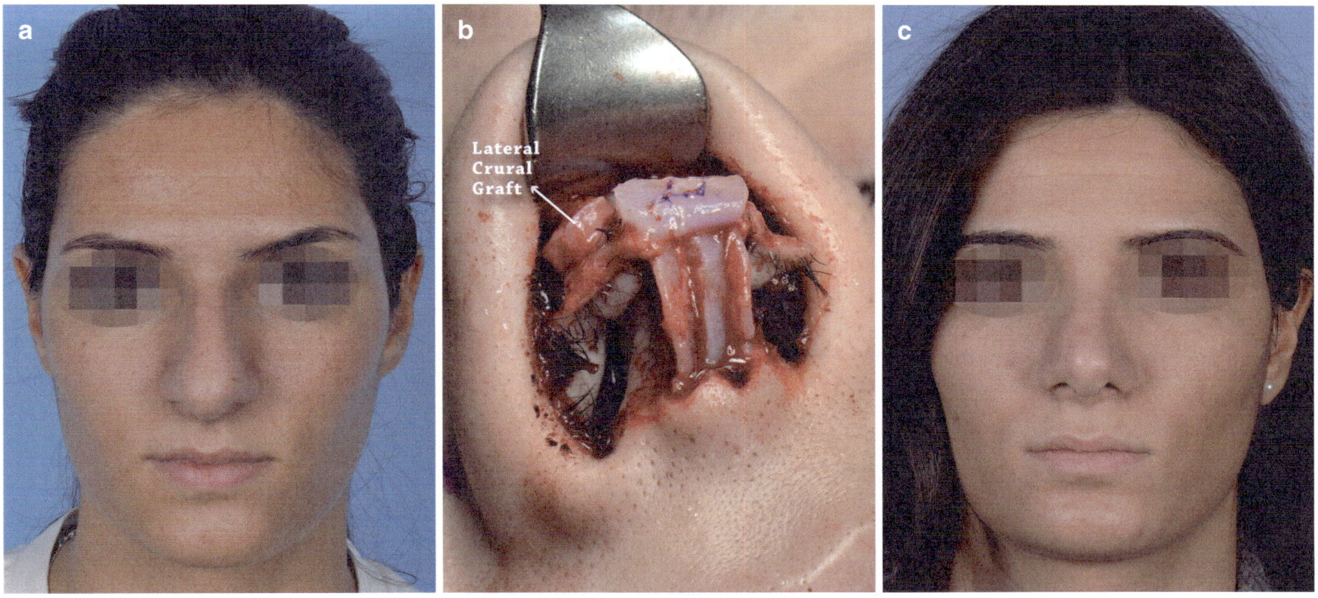

Fig. 13.60 (**a**) A preoperative frontal view. (**b**) A thick, lateral crural graft was placed as an overlay (intraoperative view). (**c**) Four years later, the tip was narrow but the thick lateral crural graft was evident as alar skin fullness on the left

Fig. 13.61 (**a**, **b**) Excision was performed endonasal under local anesthesia

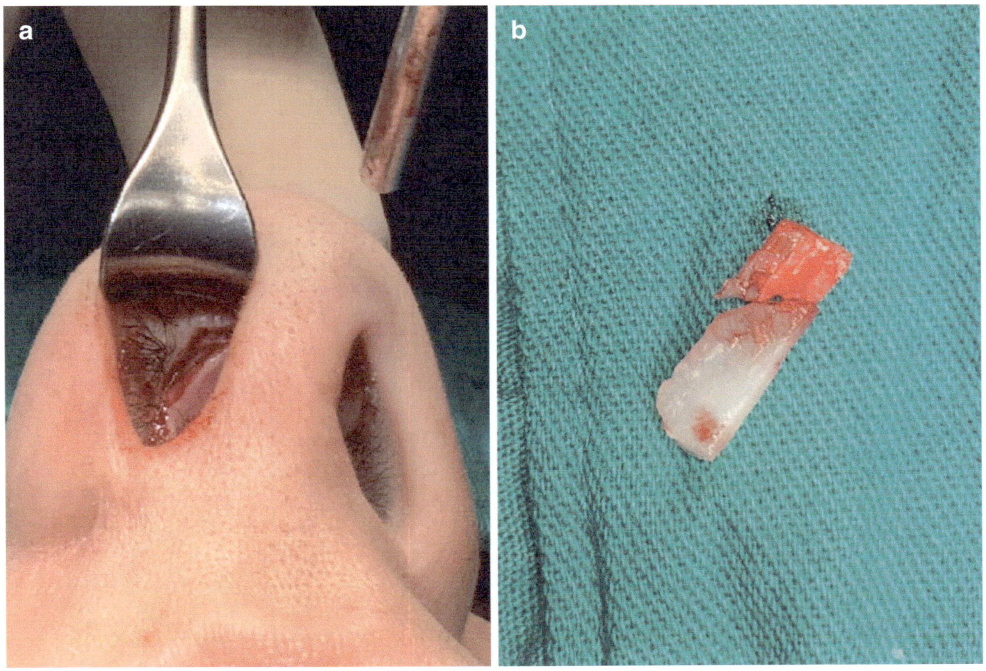

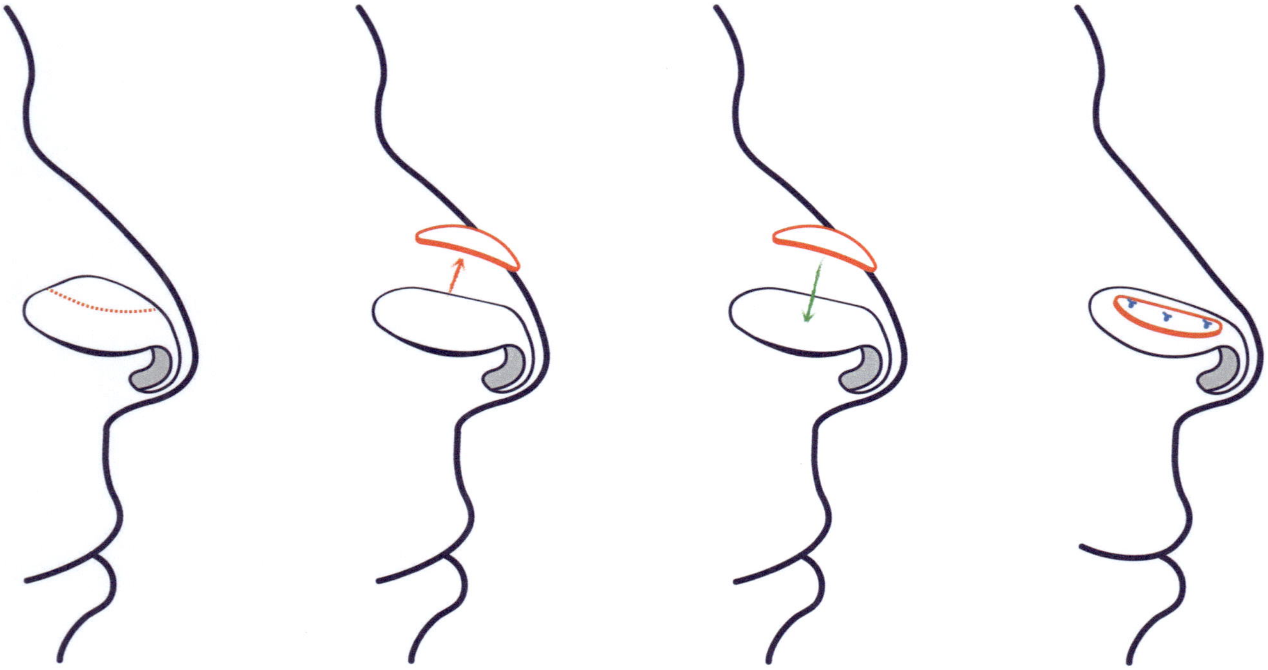

Fig. 13.62 Alar lateral crural grafting three-quarter overlay

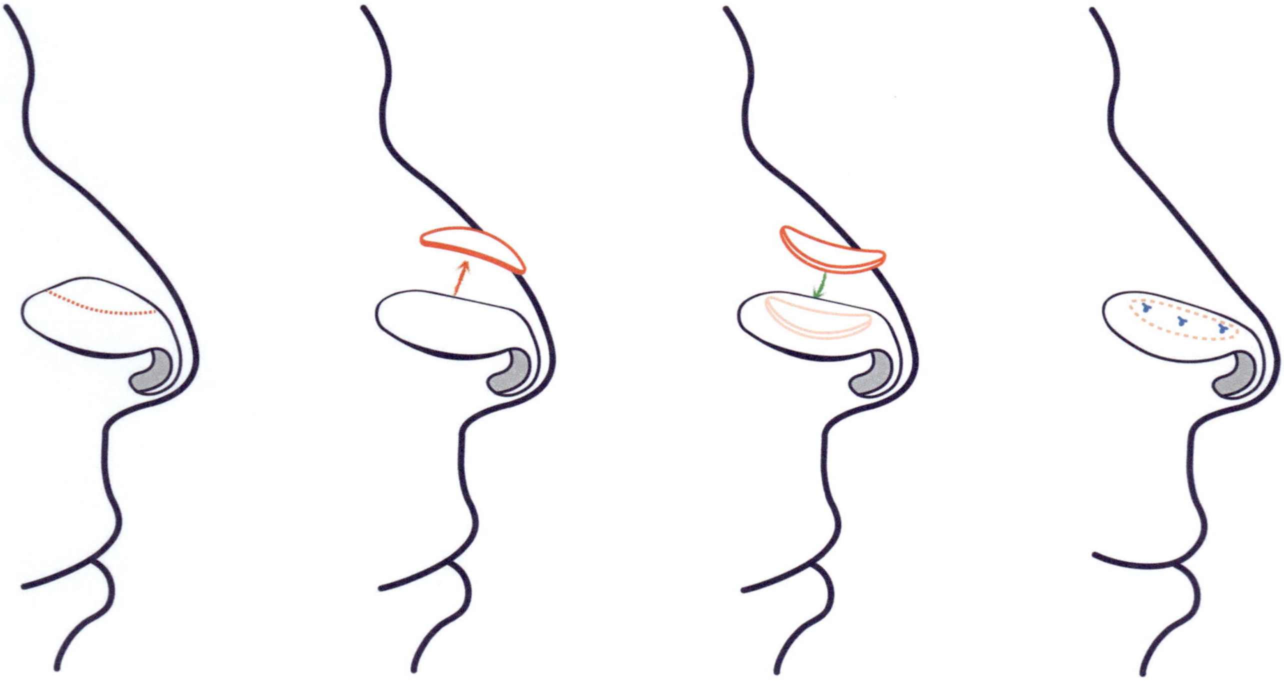

Fig. 13.63 Alar lateral crural grafting three-quarter underlay

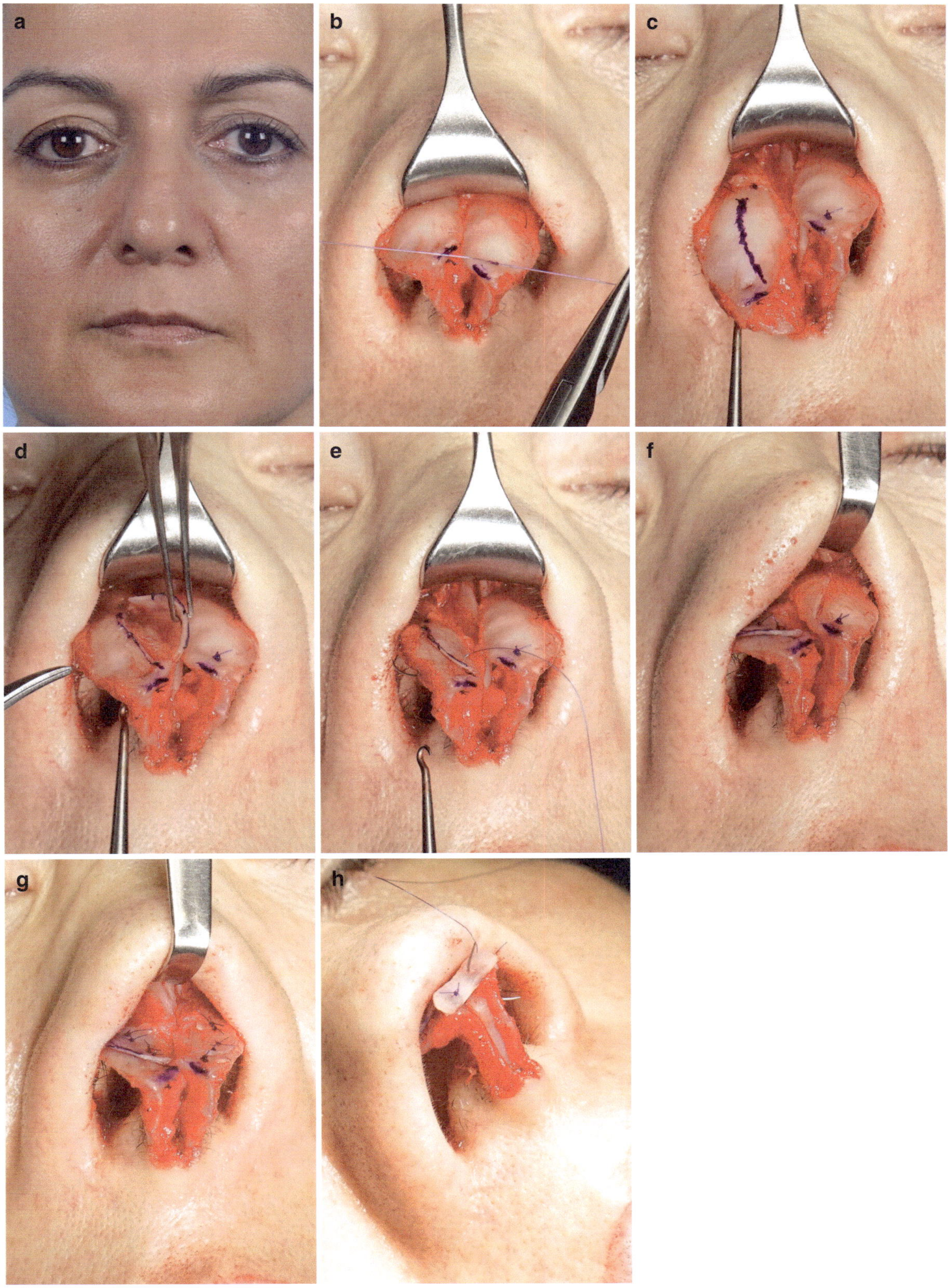

Fig. 13.64 (**a**) A preoperative frontal view. The tip is wide and bifid. (**b**) Excessive convexity is the main/key feature of lateral crura. The convexity remained after bilateral transdomal suturing. (**c**) The alar lateral crural graft is a versatile tool to fix remaining convexity. Marking. (**d**) Incision and dissection. (**e**) The cephalic excess was removed then sutured on the lateral crus. (**f**) Compare the sides. The lateral crural graft is on the right that fixed convexity. (**g**) The lateral crural graft sutured contralateral side. (**h**) Placement of a small onlay tip graft sutured over the domes

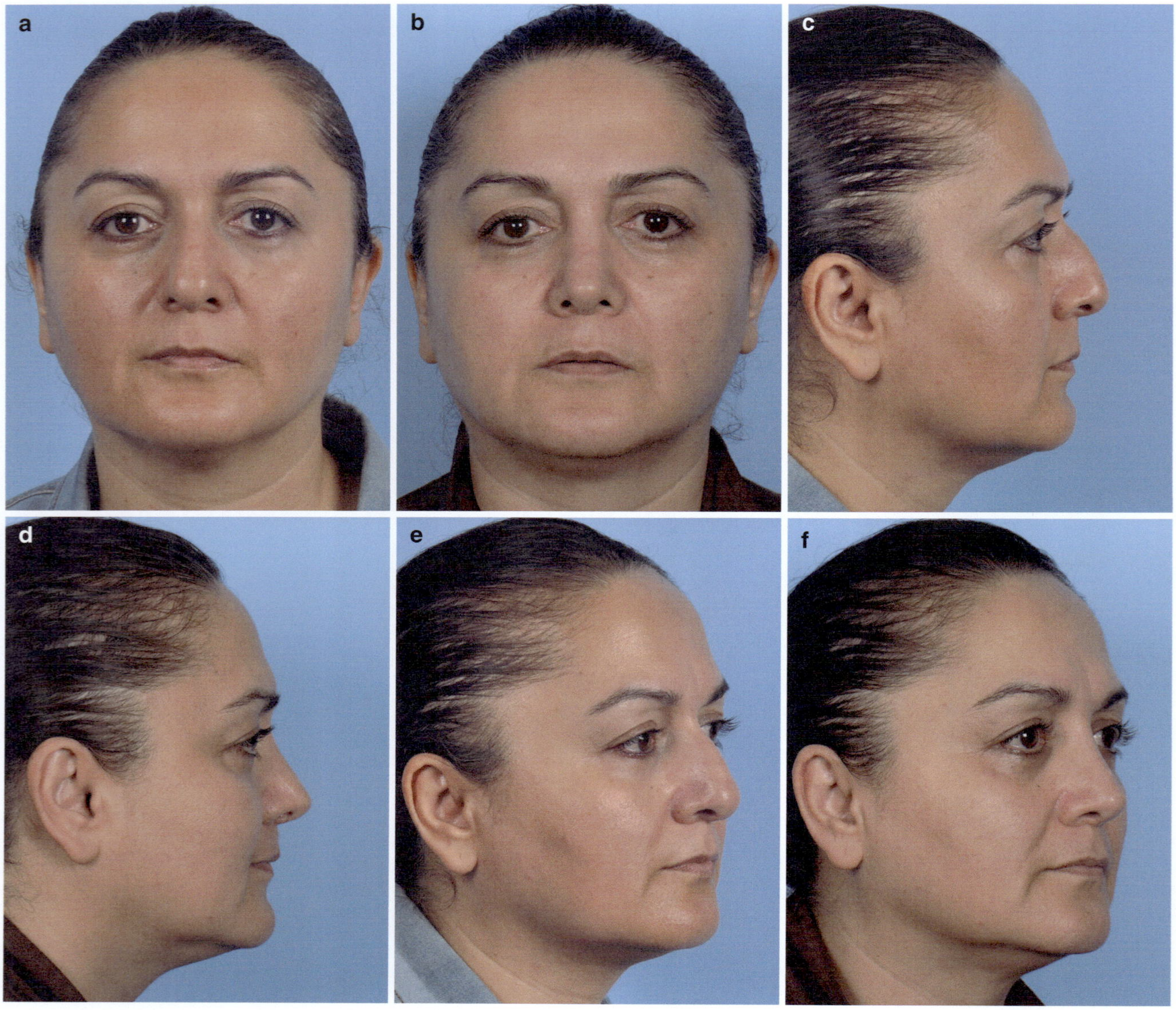

Fig. 13.65 (**a–f**) The tip shape is improved without changing rotation

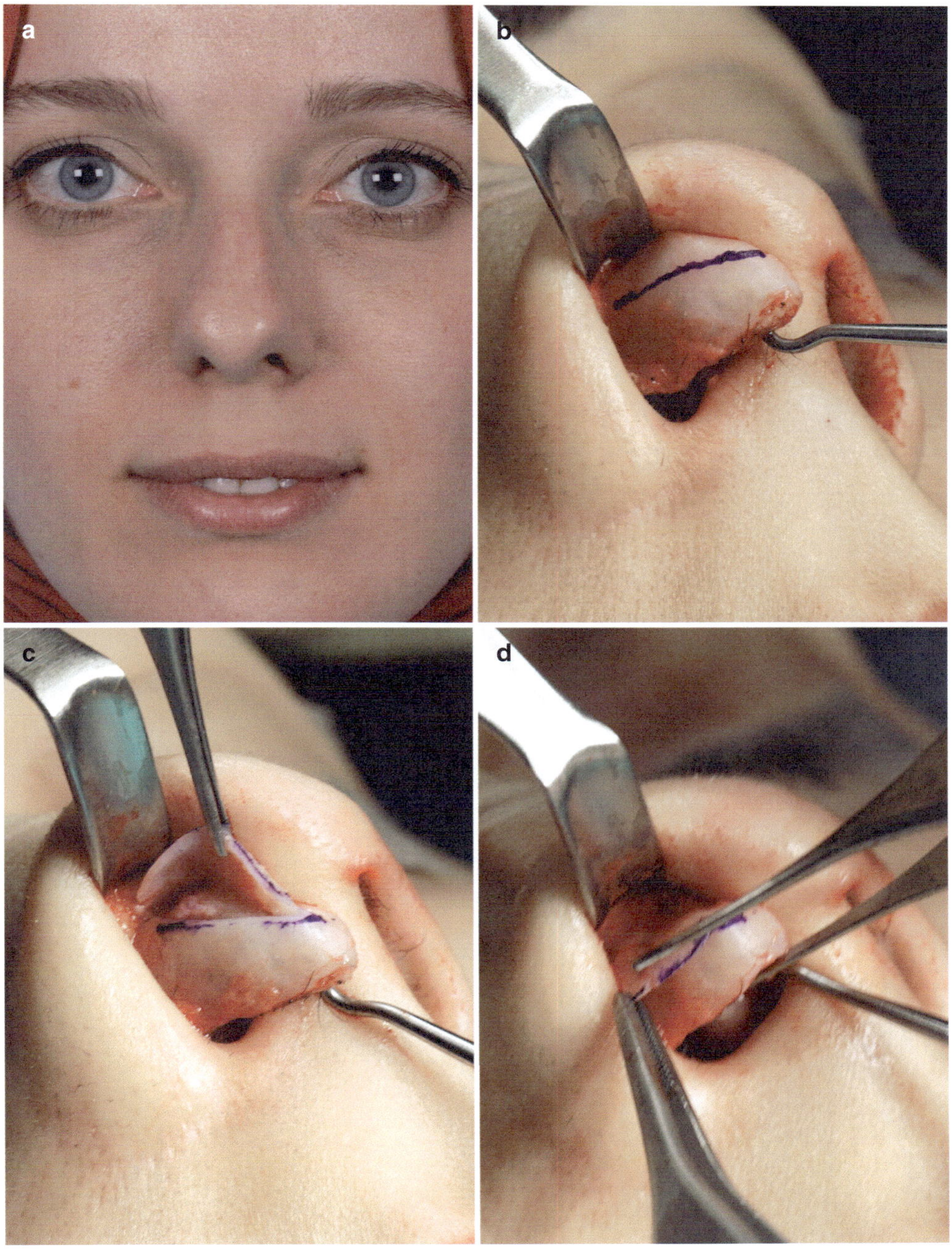

Fig. 13.66 (**a–h**) The procedure used the closed approach (overlay placement of alar lateral crural grafts)

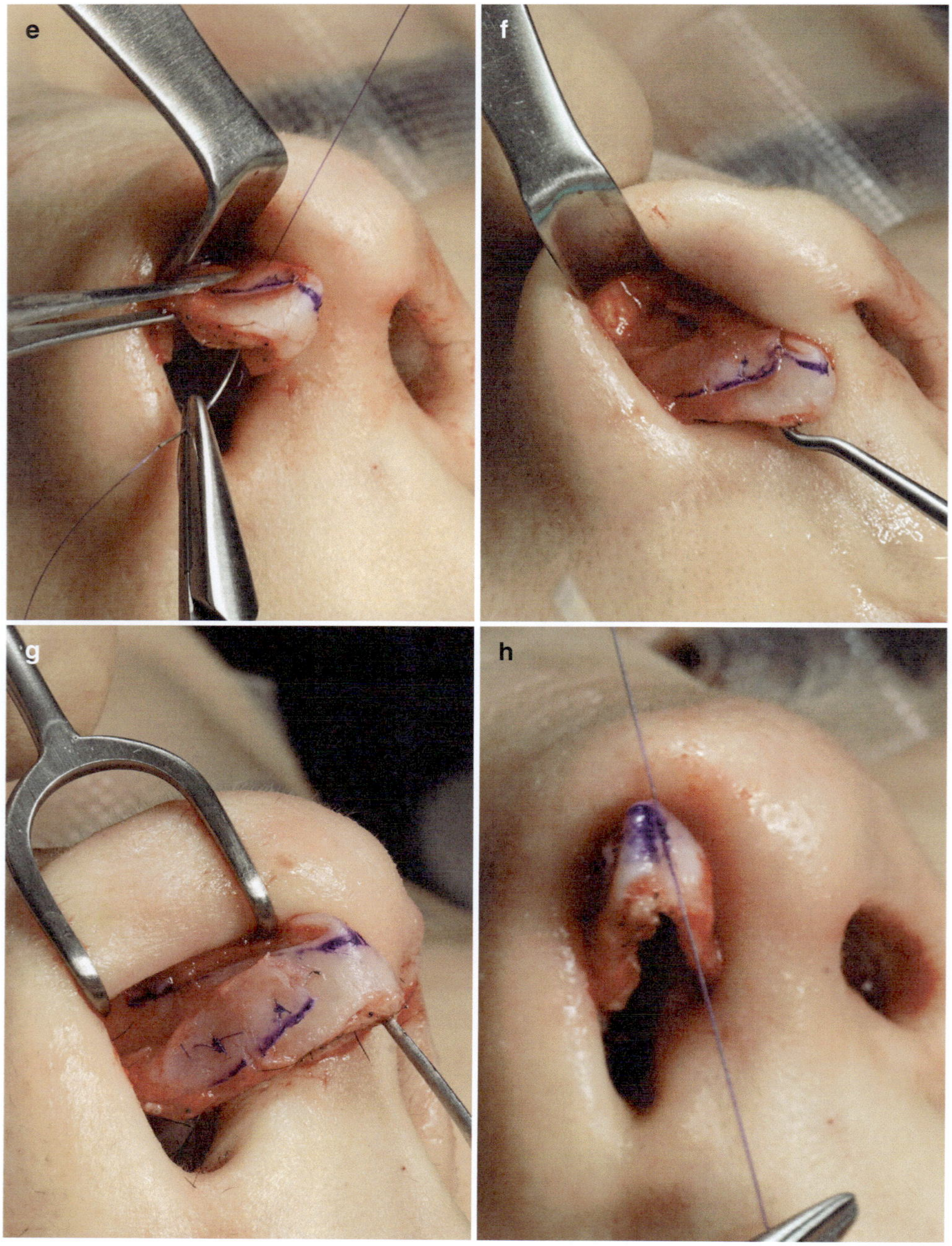

Fig. 13.66 (continued)

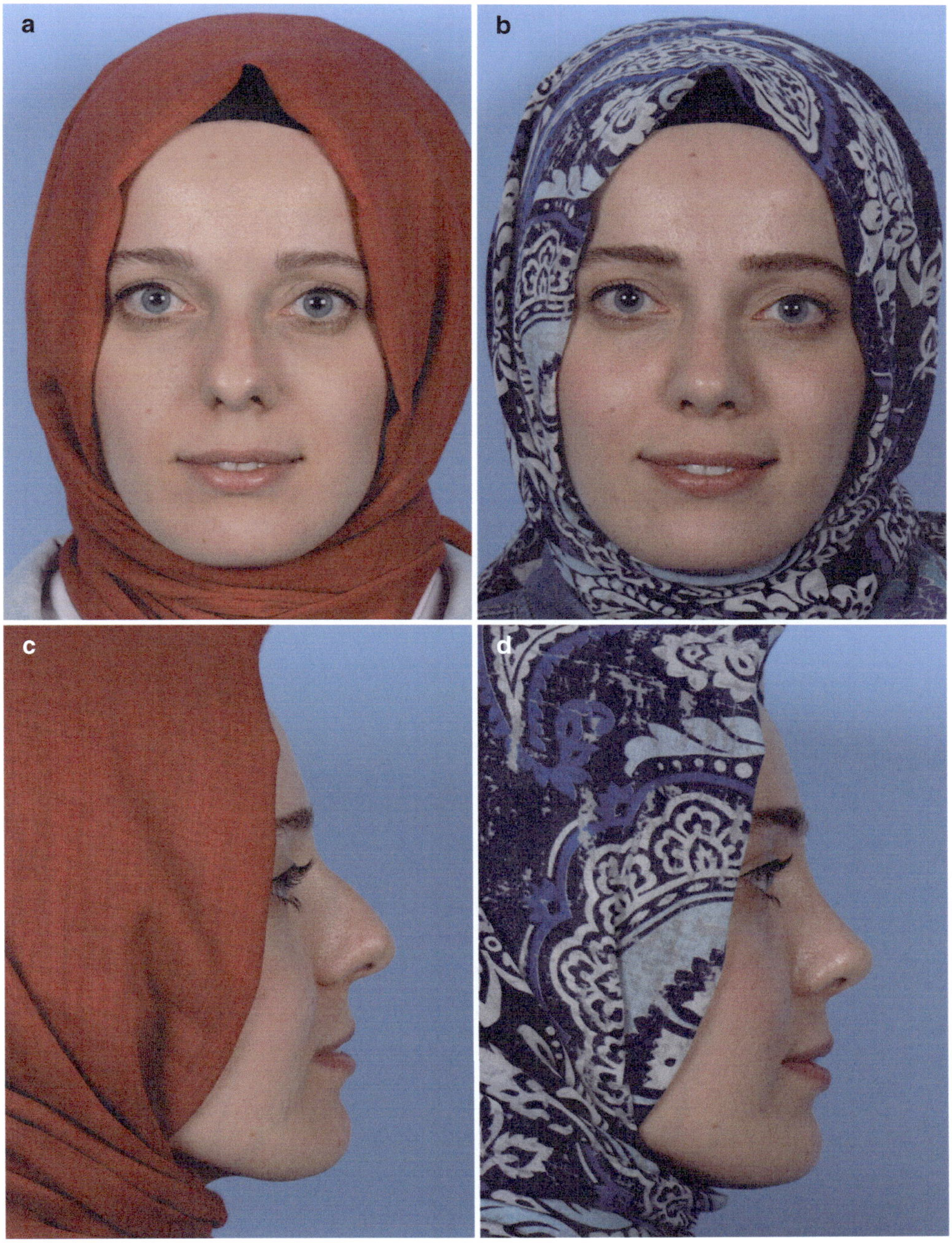

Fig. 13.67 (**a–f**) Overall the tip is narrower and the proportion between the tip and dorsum on lateral view has been established. The bifidity is also corrected

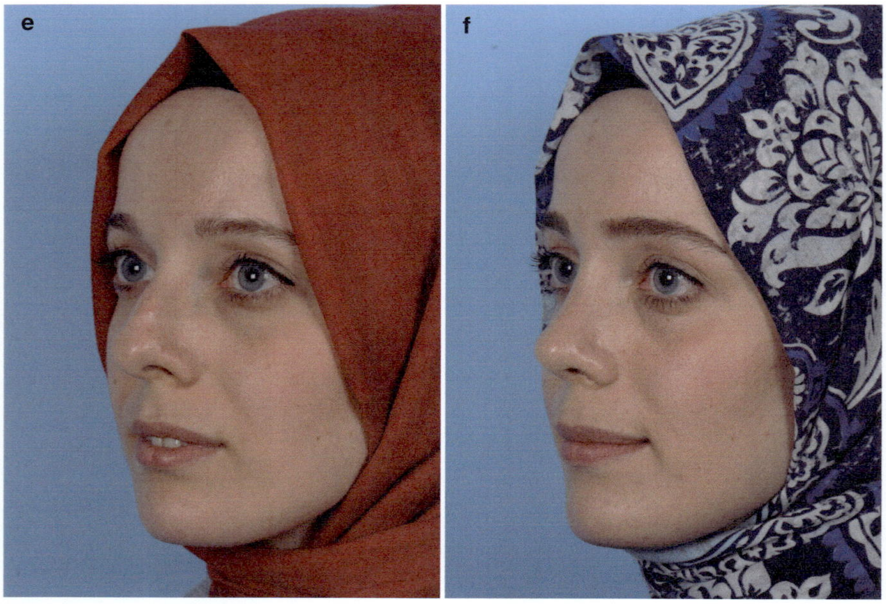

Fig. 13.67 (continued)

Fig. 13.68 (**a**) A preoperative frontal view. (**b**) The transdomal suture. (**c–f**) The lateral crus excess was placed in a pre-prepared pocket under the lateral crus. The concave sides are sutured to face each other

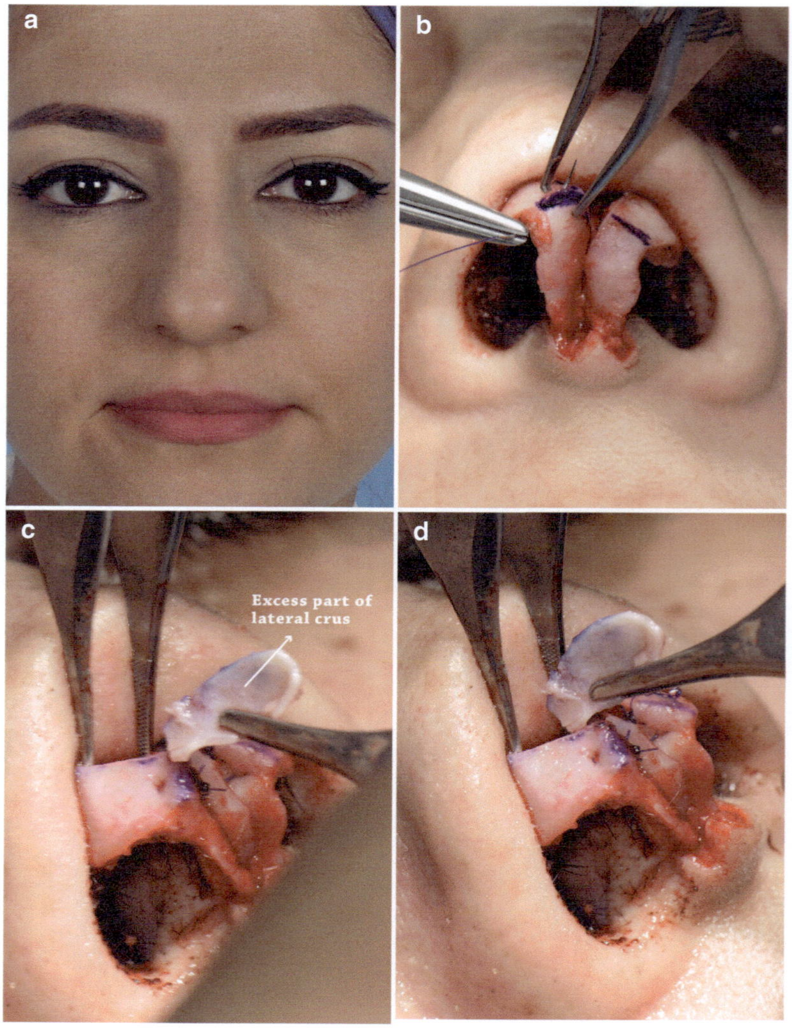

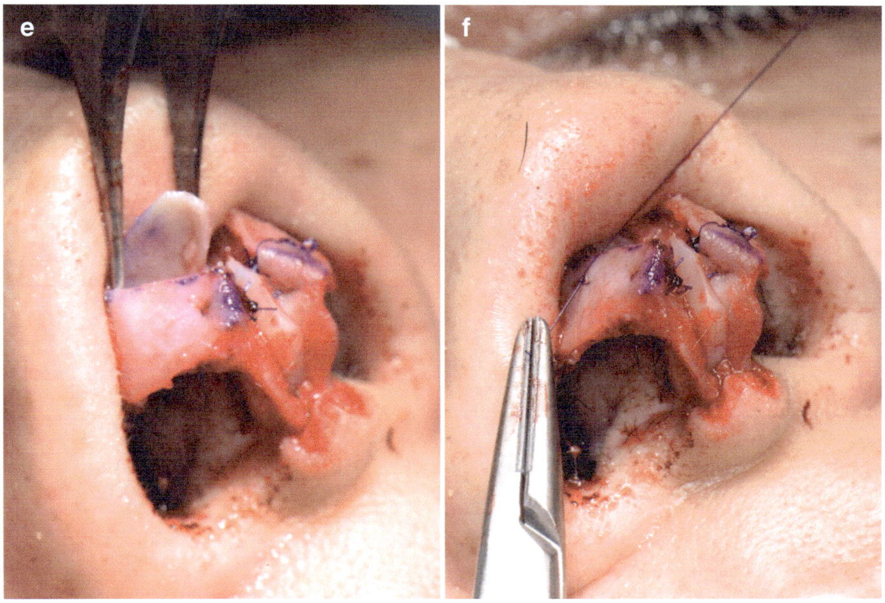

Fig. 13.68 (continued)

Fig. 13.69 (**a–d**) Note the refinement of the nasal tip. The basal view demonstrates the correction of the wide tip

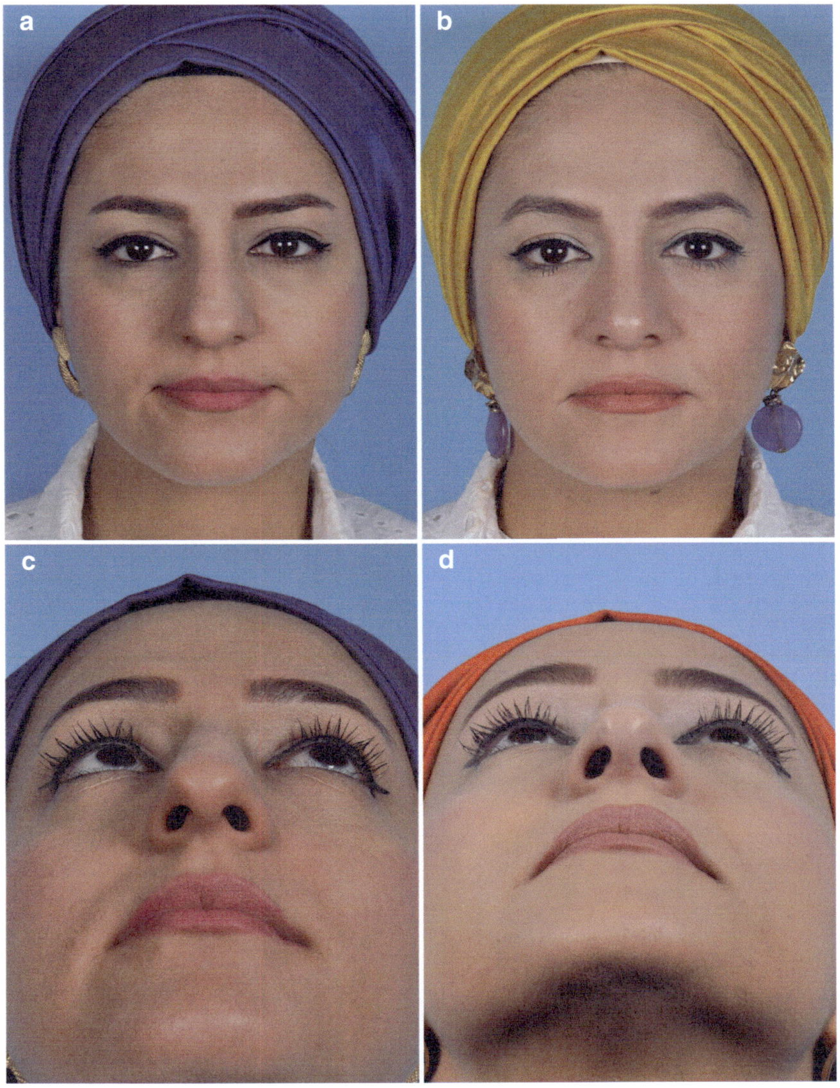

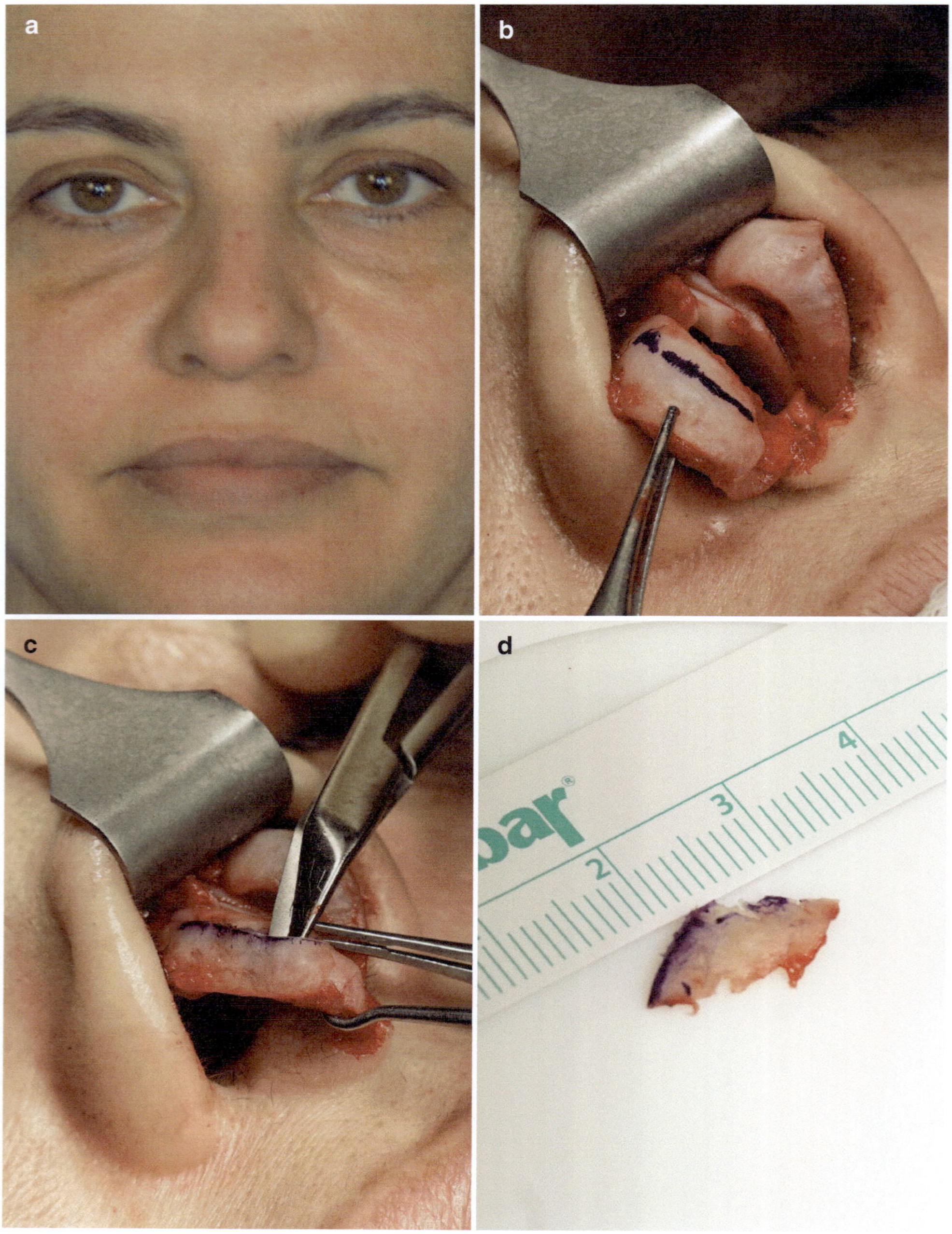

Fig. 13.70 (**a**) Wide and amorphous tip. (**b**) The cephalic resection line was marked. (**c**) After cephalic resection, a pocket was prepared. (**d**) The lateral crural excess was apparent. This served as a graft. (**e**) The graft was placed under the lateral crus. (**f**) After bilateral graft placement, the procedure is completed

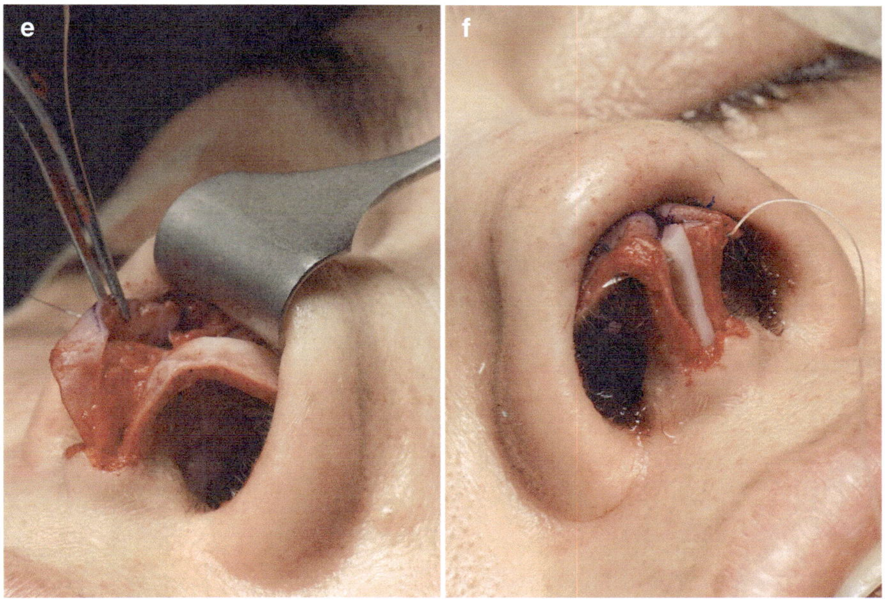

Fig. 13.70 (continued)

Fig. 13.71 (**a–f**) The results of rhinoplasty surgery are shown here. On frontal view, the nose has now been narrowed nicely to erase signs of her prior, moderately wide nasal tip. Oblique view shows how the lateral crural convexity has been corrected. This angle also appreciates that her nose has been reshaped to give a more feminine contour overall

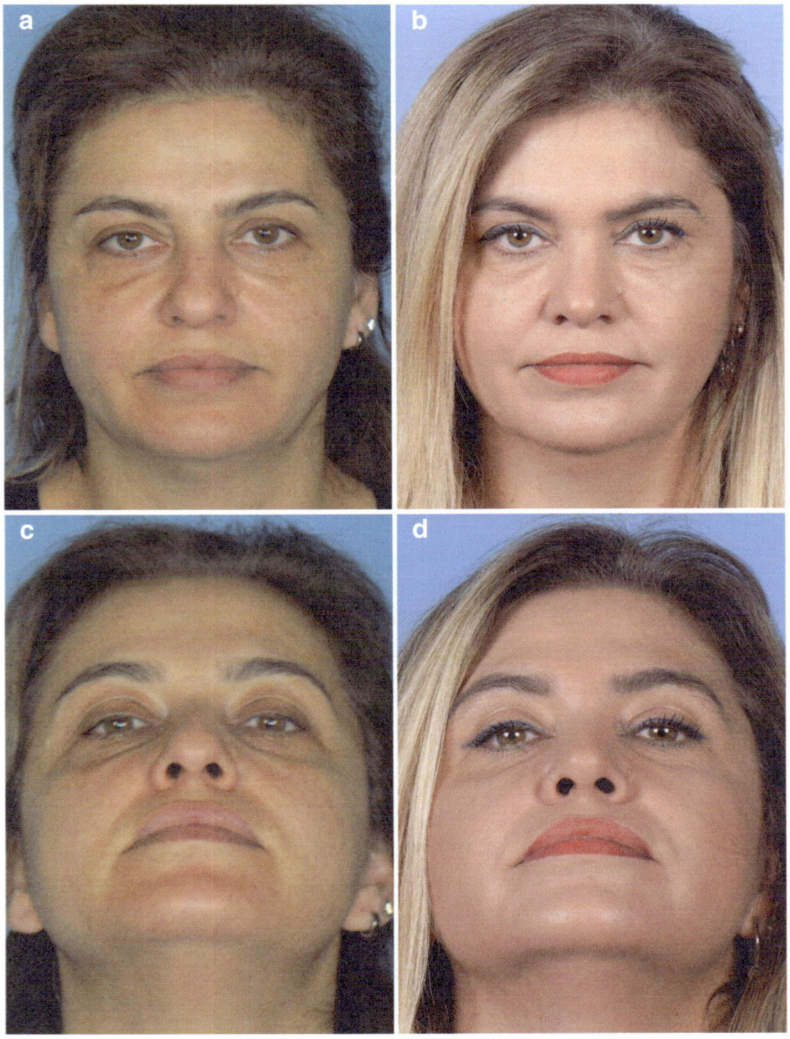

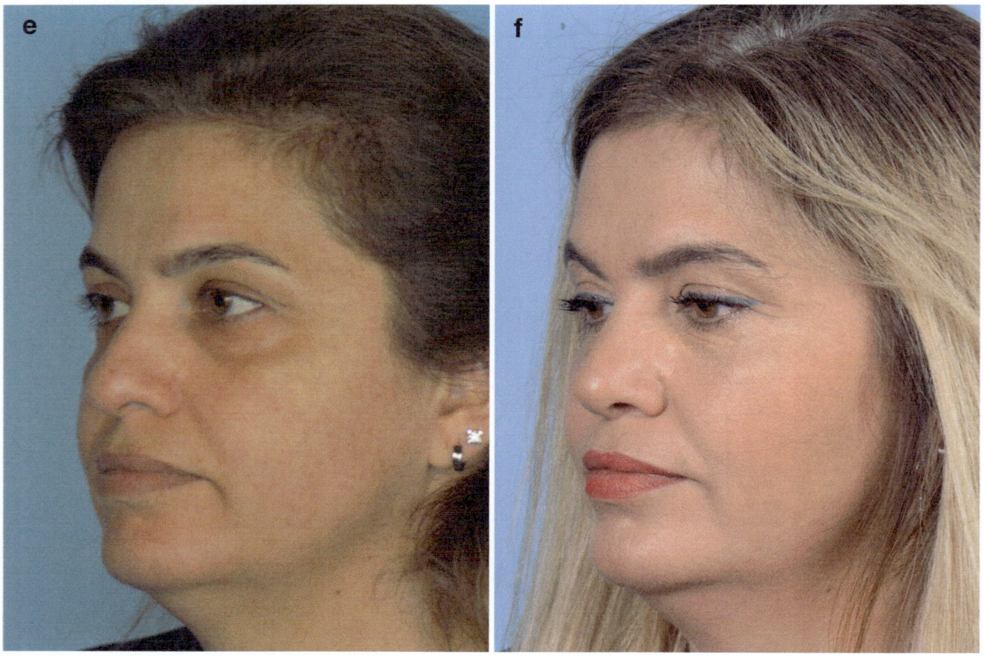

Fig. 13.71 (continued)

13.4 Advanced Techniques

Suture tip plasty and lateral crural grafting are commonly used to fix a wide tip. However, if the lateral crus is horizontally overdeveloped, suture tip plasty and lateral crural grafting may distort or deform the alar cartilages, or may simply be ineffective. In such cases, the length of the lateral crus must be reduced (Fig. 13.72).

Wide tip with long lateral crura cases. There are two ways to shorten a long lateral crus.

- Concomitant Overlap Steal Tip-plasty (COST). Lateral crural steal suturing is followed by medial crural overlap Lateral crural steal suture is a very versatile technique for shortening and shaping the lateral crus; however, rotation and projection are increased. Tip projection, rotation, and configuration of medial crura are reevaluated after suture, and the desired projection and rotation are achieved by medial crural overlap. Medial crural overlapping also fixes a malformed or deformed medial crus at the same time if it exists.
- Vertical Alar Resection (VAR). The overdeveloped portion of the lateral crus is vertically resected immediately lateral to the dome. The tip is narrowed in proportion to the extent of the resection. If additional rotation is required, additional resection is possible. VAR not only shortens the lateral crus but also corrects any malformation or asymmetry.

COST or VAR? If a long lateral crus is accompanied by a medial crural abnormality, lateral crural steal suturing with overlapping is appropriate to shorten the lateral crus and narrow the tip; overlapping corrects any malformation of the medial complex. If the lateral crus is both long and abnormal (i.e., exhibiting excessive concavity or an irregularity), VAR should be preferred. Vertical resection beginning at the lateral crus eliminates malformations.

Technical Pearl: If incision and/or excision of the alar cartilage is required, this must be performed on the segment showing configuration deformity (Fig. 13.73).

First we will discuss COST, then VAR. Examples are presented in the discussions that follow.

13.4.1 COST (Lateral Crural Steal + Medial Crural Overlap)

13.4.1.1 Case 22

Consider a patient with a large, wide nasal tip. The two principal aesthetic issues are the wide tip per se and a hanging columella visible on the lateral view (Fig. 13.74).

On intraoperative examination of the alar cartilages, the lateral crura are both strong and long, but the medial crura is malformed. The aesthetic problems are attributable to the configurational deformities. The long lateral crus explains the wide nasal tip, and the deformed medial crus accounts for the hanging columella. Therefore, the surgeon must correct these two deformities, for which COST is the technique of choice. Suturing shortens the lateral crus and overlapping resolves the columellar configurational problem.

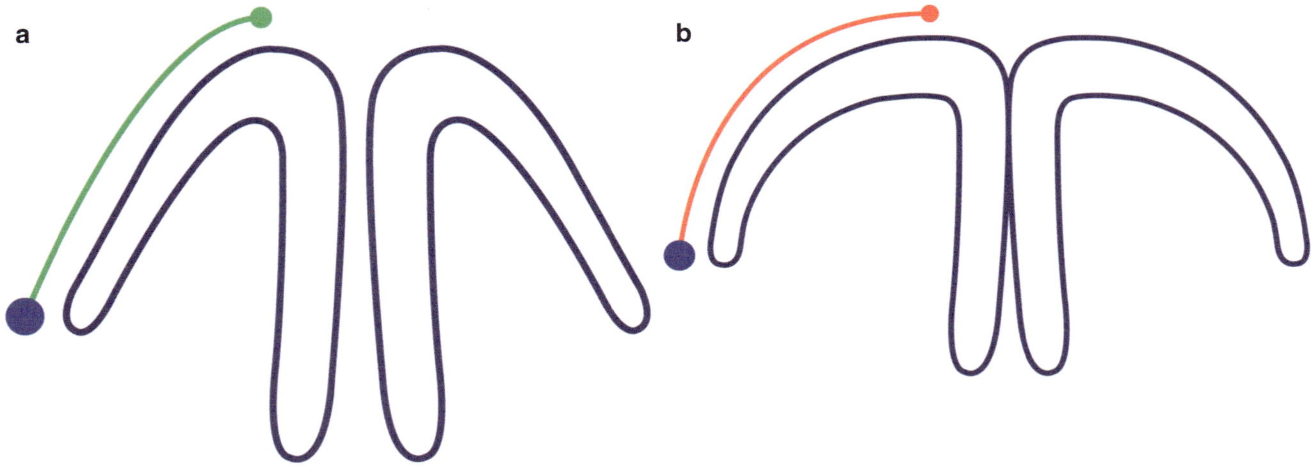

Fig. 13.72 (**a**) A normally developed lateral crus. (**b**) A horizontally overdeveloped lateral crus. This must be shortened, to achieve an outcome similar to that in (**a**)

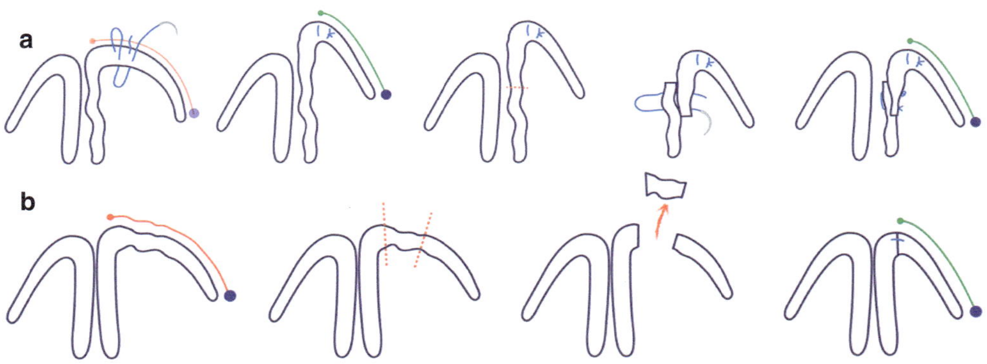

Fig. 13.73 (**a**) The combination of lateral crural steal and medial crural overlap in COST is associated with more surgical advantages in wide tip patients with long lateral crura and malformed medial crura. Lateral crural steal procedure narrows the tip because of shortening the lateral crura. Overlap of the alar cartilages in the medial crura improves alar–columellar relationship. (**b**) Long and malformed lateral crura can lead to the severe wide nasal tip. This problem can be corrected by removing the deformed part of the lateral crus bilaterally or unilaterally. Vertical alar resection technique achieves both shortening and flattening of the lateral crura simultaneously

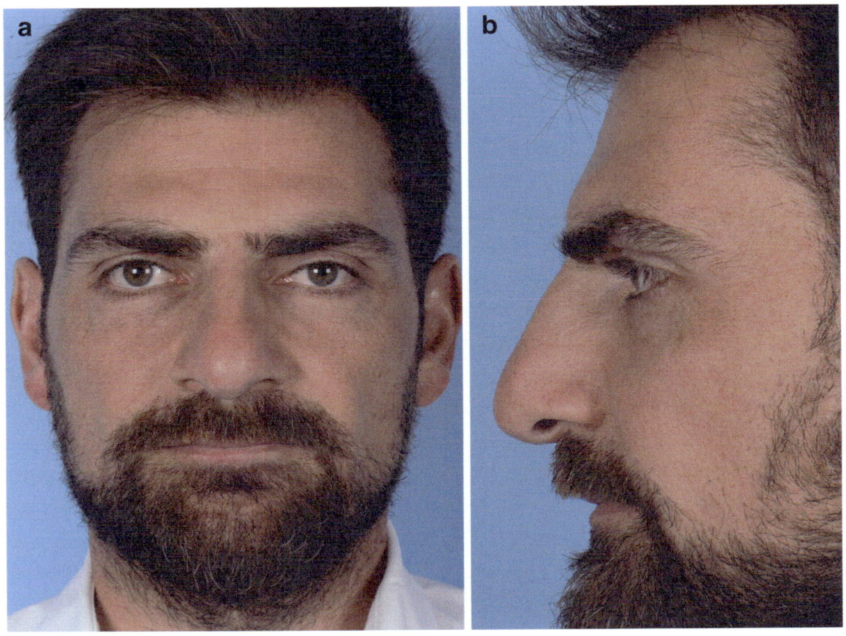

Fig. 13.74 (**a**, **b**) Preoperative photographs of a 33-year-old man who presented wide nasal tip, a hanging columella, and a drooping tip

The lateral crus exhibits only a length abnormality; therefore, it is prudent to shorten the lateral crus by steal suturing rather than excision. In fact, a steal suture is basically a transdomal mattress suture transferring lateral crus excess to the middle crus. Suturing creates a new dome lateral to the former dome. The extent of shortening required determines the extent of lateral crural stealing.

Medial crural extension reflects the amount of the lateral crus "stolen" via suturing. Medial crural elongation increases projection and rotation, further deforming an already deformed medial crus via application of tension. The surgeon must then correct the deformed medial crus via immediate medial crural overlap.

What does this mean and how is overlapping performed? Tip projection is reevaluated intraoperatively, and a transverse incision is created in the most deformed regions of the bilateral medial crura; the proximal stumps are dissected from the underlying vestibular skin. Thus, residual, curved, malformed, or unequal medial crural proximal stumps can slide freely in all directions over the distal segment (i.e., the overlap is sagittal).

The extent of overlap is automatically determined by the distance over which the proximal medial crural stumps slide. The overlapping proximal and distal stumps are stabilized by attaching them to each other, and to a columellar strut graft, via horizontal mattress sutures. In brief, steal suturing narrows the wide nasal tip associated with a long lateral crus, and medial crural overlap corrects the prior columellar deformity aggravated by steal suturing. Next, the alar cartilages, the configurations of which have been corrected, are stabilized and defined. A columellar strut is commonly employed for stabilization, but a septocolumellar suture or graft may be required for patients with thick skin. If tip definition is to be increased, an onlay tip graft can be placed (Fig. 13.75).

Preoperative and 1-year postoperative photographs are shown in Fig. 13.76.

13.4.1.2 Case 23

In this case, either an open or delivery approach may be used (Fig. 13.77; Video 13.17).

Intraoperative photographs show that the wide nasal tip is attributable principally to the strong and long lateral crus. A medial crural configurational deformity is evident (Fig. 13.78).

The lateral crura must be shortened to narrow the tip. In this case, steal suturing is preferred because the lateral crura are simply long and strong, and not deformed. However, the medial crura are deformed and an incision is required to correct the medial crural configuration. Therefore, it is wiser to employ steal suturing, using the excess cartilage to correct the medial crural deformities, rather than shortening the crura via resection (Fig. 13.79).

Lateral crural shortening increases tip projection. The prior configurational deformity in the medial crus was exacerbated (Fig. 13.80).

This was addressed by creating a vertical incision in the most prominent region of the deformity and dissecting the crus from the incision to the dome. A free cartilage flap was created and slid over the distal stump until the configurational deformity was eliminated. The flap was then fixed over the segment through which it was slid at three different points. A stable, smooth-surfaced medial crus was achieved by suturing the overlapped cartilages (Fig. 13.81).

This stabilized the tip and improved tip definition. Columellar strutting was essential and the angle between the two new domes was optimized by placing a dome-equalizing suture. Finally, onlay tip grafting enhanced tip definition and increased tip projection, depending on the length of the graft. A septocolumellar suture can be placed if tip projection/rotation losses over time is/are of concern. Results are shown 6 months postoperatively (Fig. 13.82).

13.4.1.3 Case 24

COST can also be used for the revision of certain cases.

These are photographs of a patient who underwent rhinoplasty 4 years previously but complained of a large nasal tip. There were two underlying causes. The frontal view shows the wide tip and the lateral view shows an excessive columella. The intraoperative photographs reveal that the configuration, position, and caudo-cranial relationship of the lateral crura were normal; however, the crura were too long, explaining the wide nasal tip. The columellar excess reflects deformation of the medial crura and prior use of an oversized columellar strut (Fig. 13.83).

The author employed lateral crural steal suturing to shorten the lateral crura (Fig. 13.84).

The author used the overlap technique to correct the medial crural configurational deformities, which became more pronounced after suturing (Fig. 13.85).

Finally, the author created an alar arch to fully optimize the configuration using the overlap technique (Fig. 13.86).

Tip projection, stabilization, and definition required attention after the internal problems were addressed. Alar base stability was ensured via columellar strutting; a lateral crural graft was used to guarantee lateral wall stability (the patient had thick skin), and a double-layered cap graft was placed to enhance tip definition and projection (Fig. 13.87).

Two-year postoperative photographs are shown in Fig. 13.88.

13.4.2 VAR (Vertical Alar Resection)

Vertical alar resection can also be used to correct wide nasal tips in patients with long lateral crura. When a crus is long and exhibits a configurational deformity, resection of excess crural cartilage not only shortens the crural length, but also corrects the deformity.

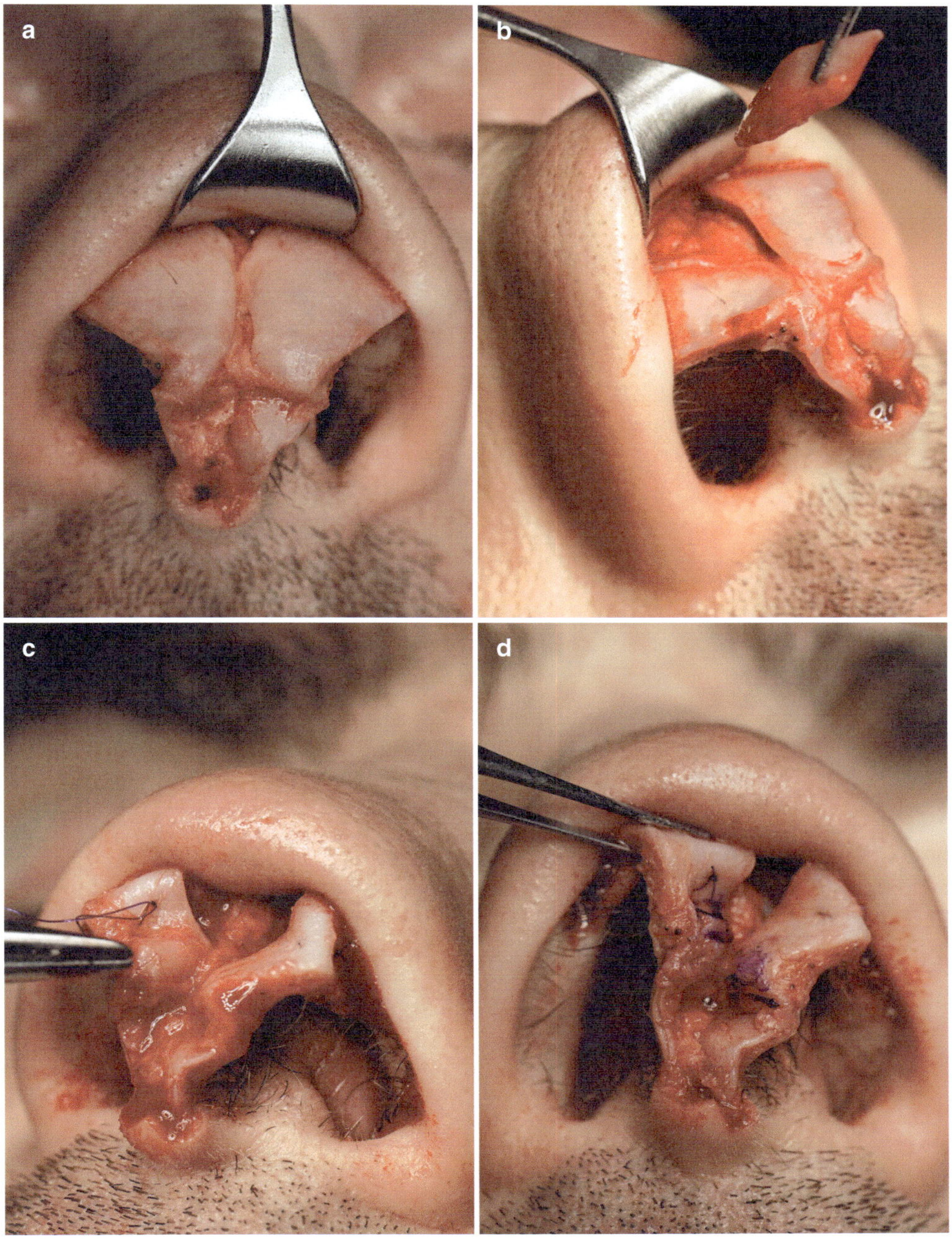

Fig. 13.75 (**a**) Frontal view of the alar cartilages. Long lateral crura and deformed middle/medial crura. (**b**) Cephalic trim. (**c**) Lateral crural steal procedure. (**d**, **e**) Medial crural division and overlap. (**f**, **g**) The new domes and medial crura were fixed to the columellar strut. Lateral crural strut, cap graft were placed

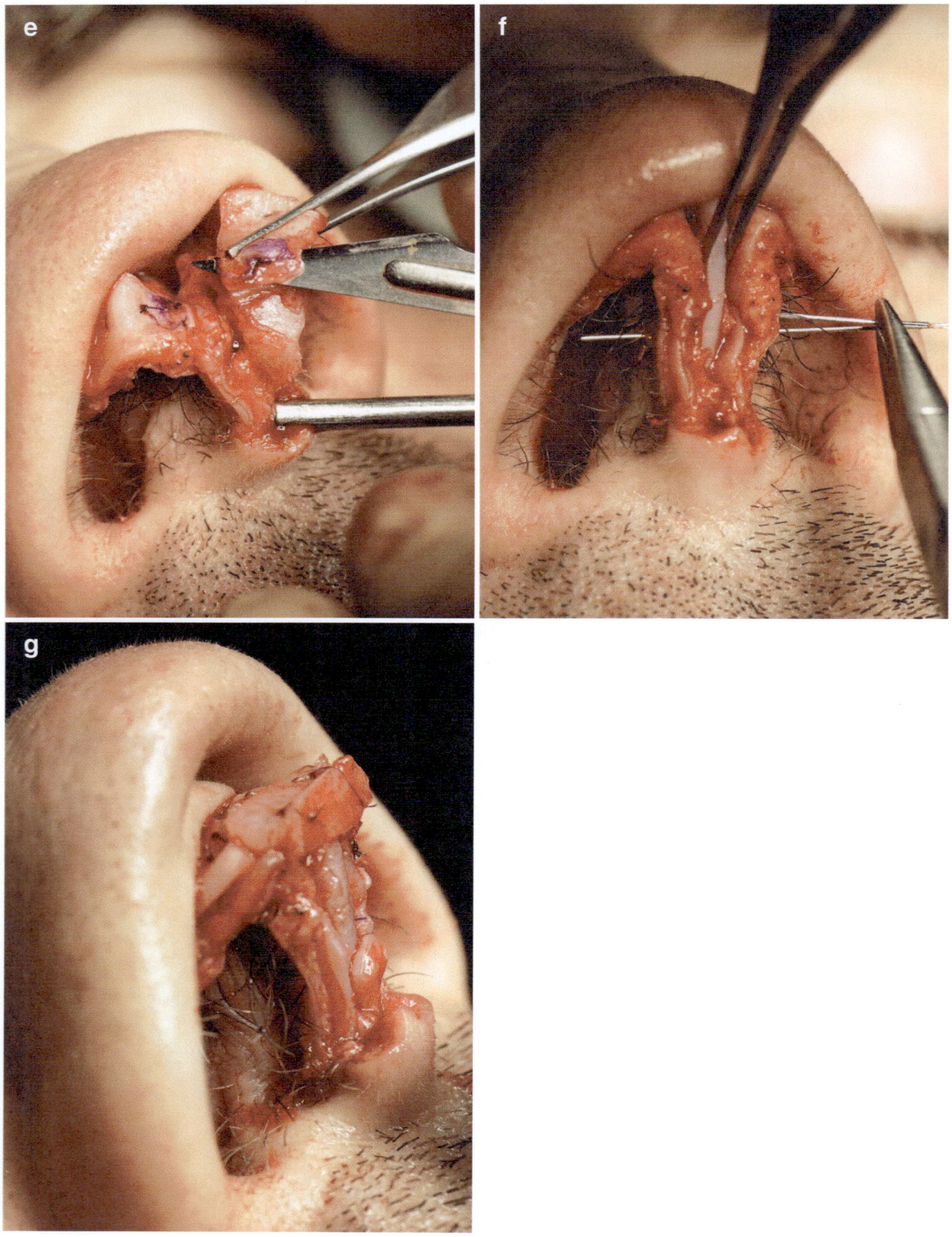

Fig. 13.75 (continued)

As shown in the illustrations below, our aim was to shorten the longer lateral crus (on the right) to render it similar to the left lateral crus (Fig. 13.89; Video 13.18).

How did we achieve this?

1. The tip-defining point was marked (Fig. 13.90).
2. The dome was cut, commencing at the dome-defining points (Fig. 13.91).
3. The lateral crus was detached from the vestibular skin and the vertical excess removed (Fig. 13.92).
4. The question is, *How much should be removed?* This varies from patient to patient. It is not a question of how much is removed, but rather, how much remains. An excessive lateral crus is always obvious. The key is to remove the excess in many small pieces (Fig. 13.93).
5. After excision, the two ends were sutured (Fig. 13.94).
6. Now that the lateral crus was shortened, the columella and lateral nasal wall must be strengthened. A columellar strut and an alar batten graft were placed. The author

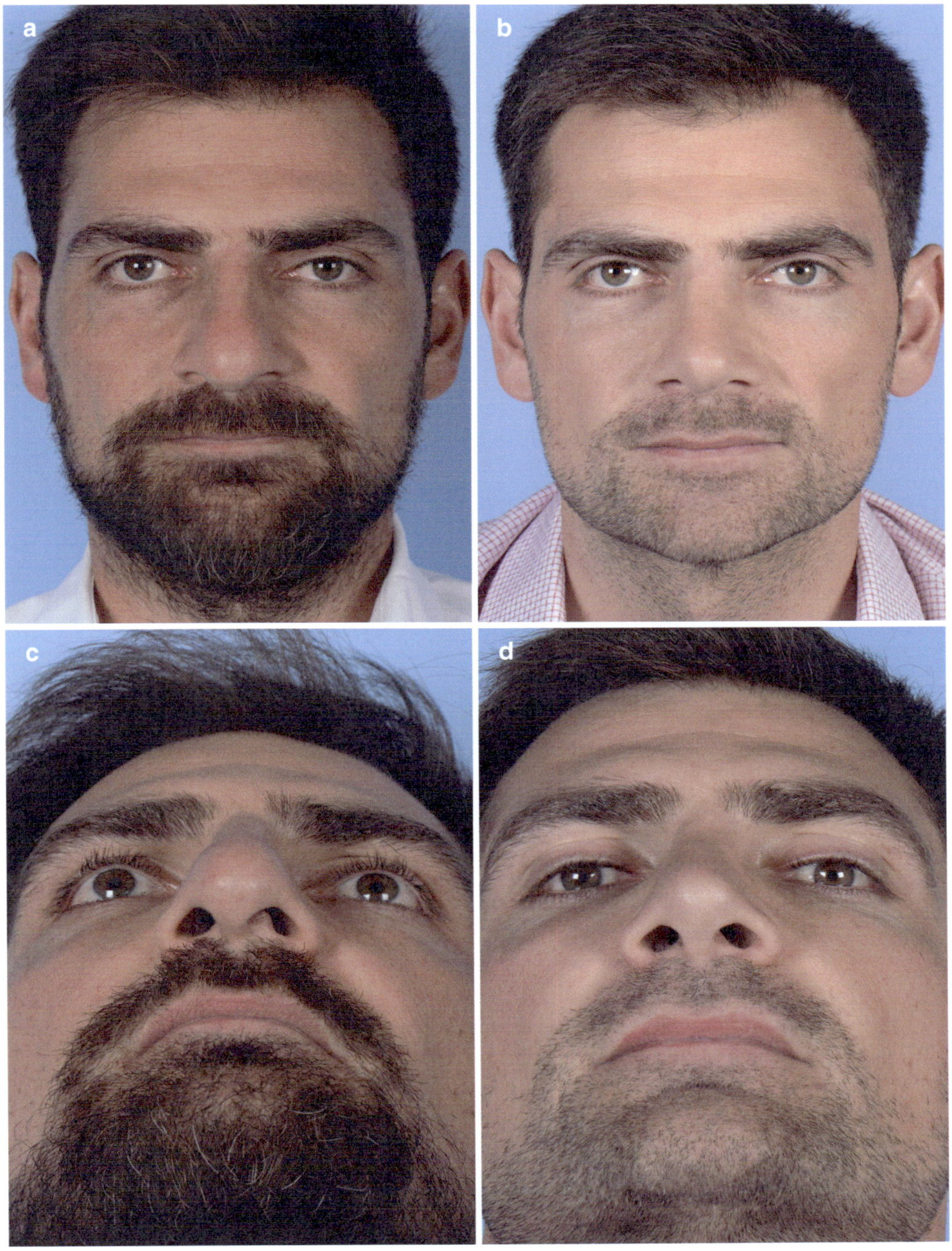

Fig. 13.76 (**a–h**) Postoperatively, the patient shows improved nasal dorsal aesthetic lines as well as correction of the wide tip and alar. Columellar discrepancy is corrected

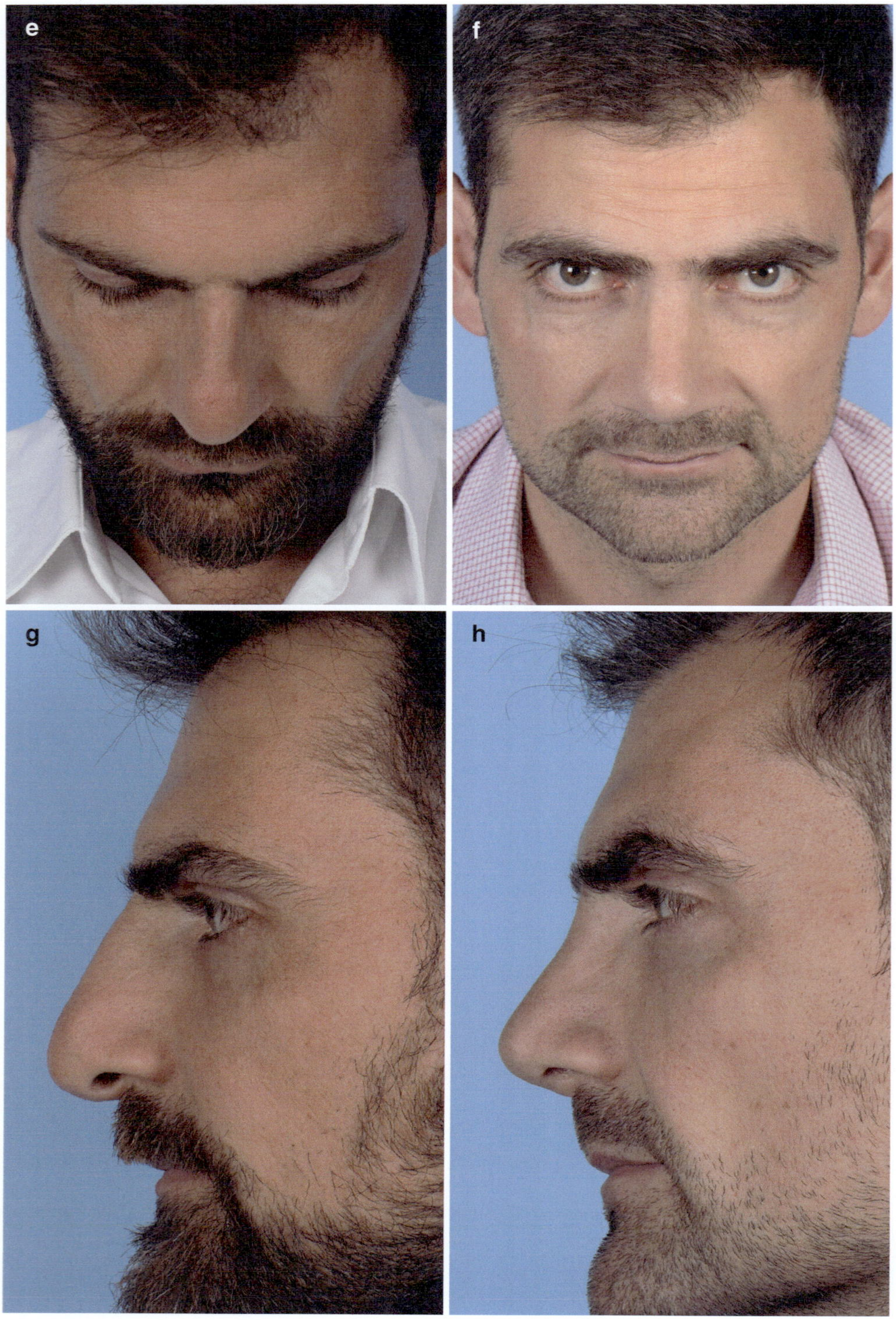

Fig. 13.76 (continued)

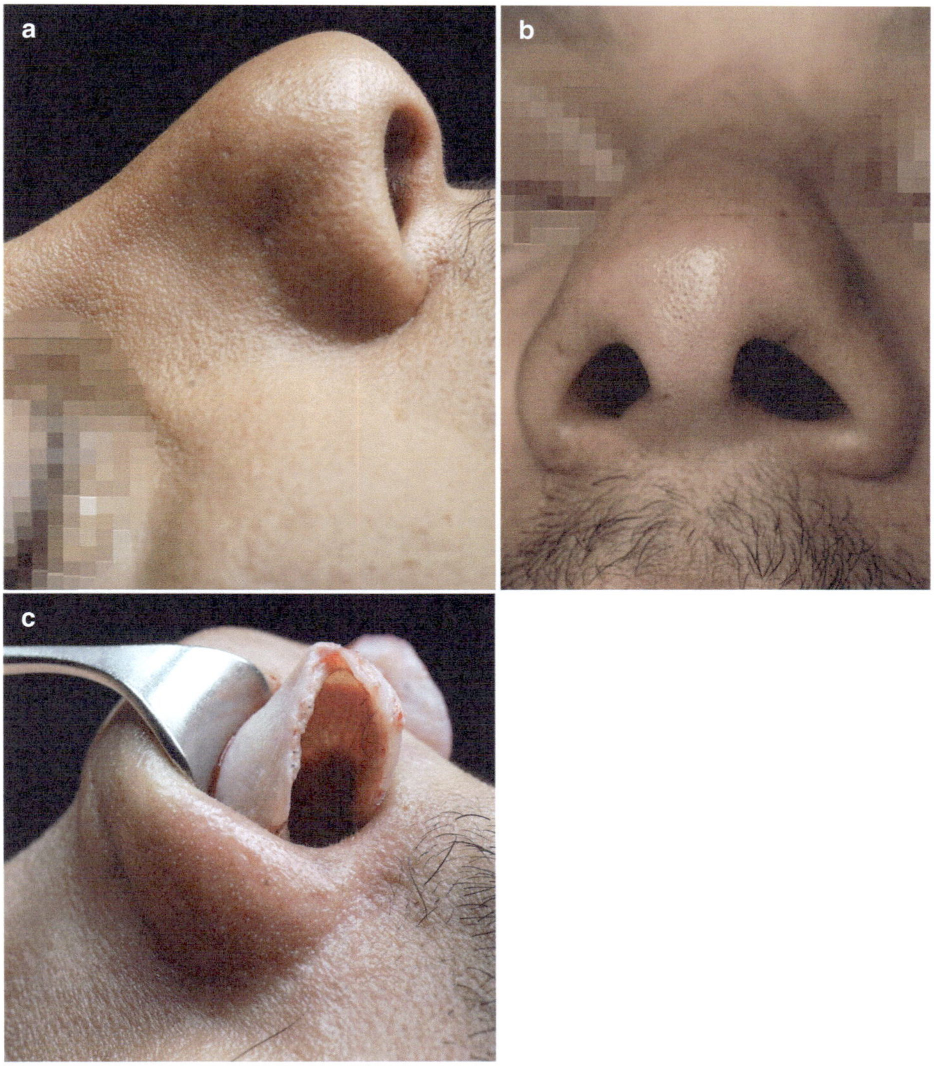

Fig. 13.77 (**a**, **b**) The long lateral crura and unfavorable configuration of middle/ medial crura. (**c**) Each alar cartilage should be shaped individually; it is best to deliver each tip through its respective nostril. To do so it is necessary to separate the middle crura from each other

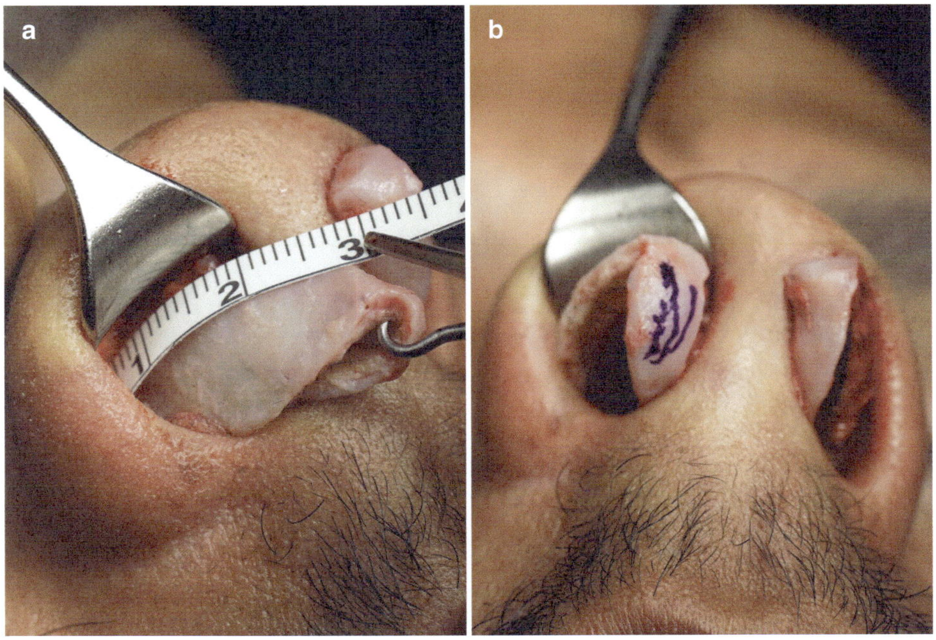

Fig. 13.78 (**a**) We do not routinely measure the lateral crus intraoperatively; the surgeon must be trained to identify a long lateral crus. However, here, we include a ruler for clarity. (**b**) Blue marked area shows malformed middle crus (excessive convex)

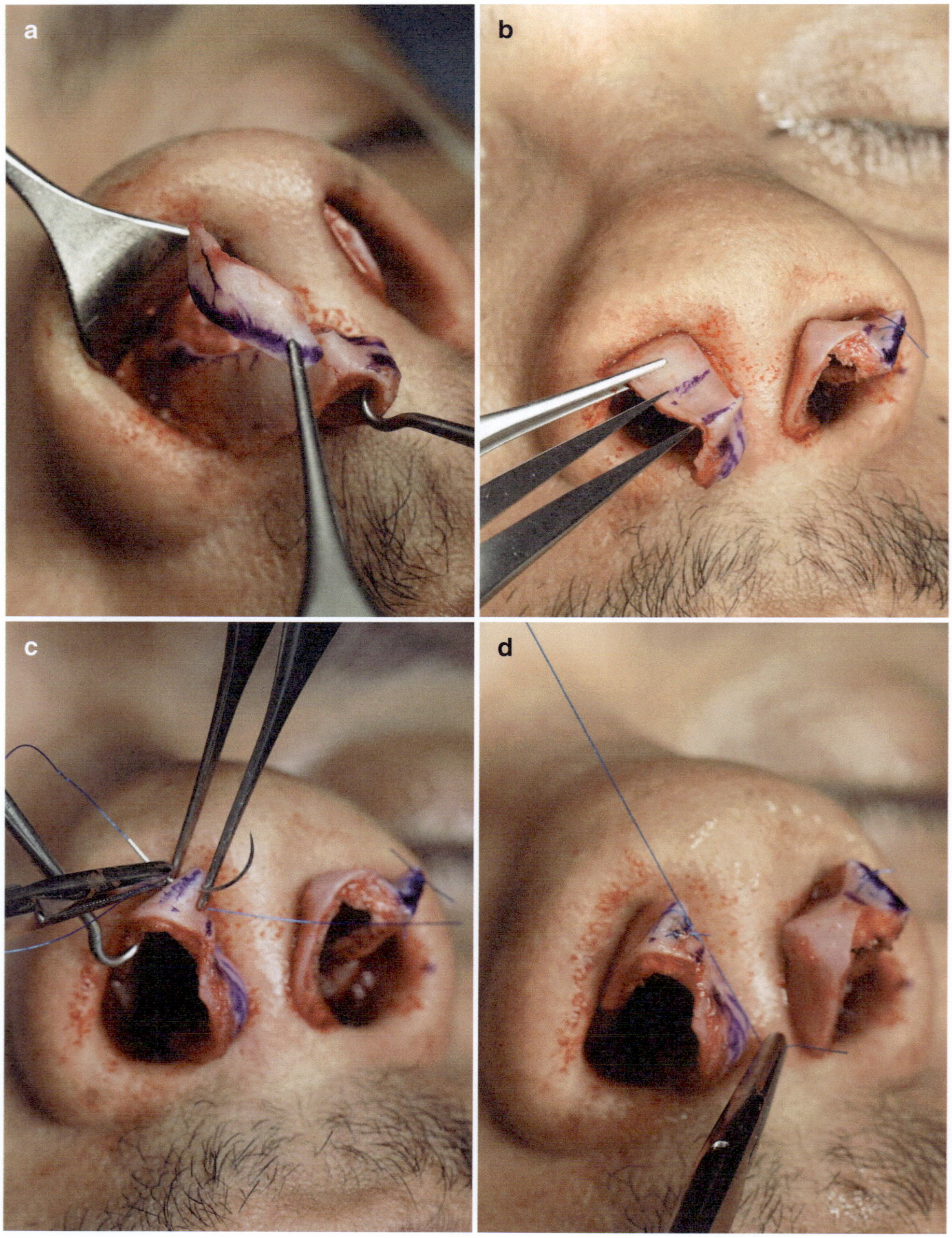

Fig. 13.79 (**a**) Cephalic trim. (**b–d**) The dome point was marked. A new dome point was created approximately 1 cm lateral to the former dome. Therefore, the lateral crus was shortened by 1 cm, and the medial crus elongated by 1 cm

always uses the patient's excess lateral crural material to create the batten graft. The grafts were placed in pockets along the alar side wall (Fig. 13.95).

7. At the end of VAR, a cap graft was added to lengthen the columella and to create new dome-defining points (Fig. 13.96).

This figure shows how the alar cartilage anatomy is enhanced after this procedure (Fig. 13.97; Video 13.19).

13.4.2.1 Clinical Outcomes

Case 25

In this case with a wide nasal tip, once the alar cartilages were exposed using an open approach, the wide tip was found to be attributable to long, hypertrophic lateral crura (Fig. 13.98).

In such cases, it is not possible to refine the nasal tip without reducing the lateral crural volume. Any attempt to shape

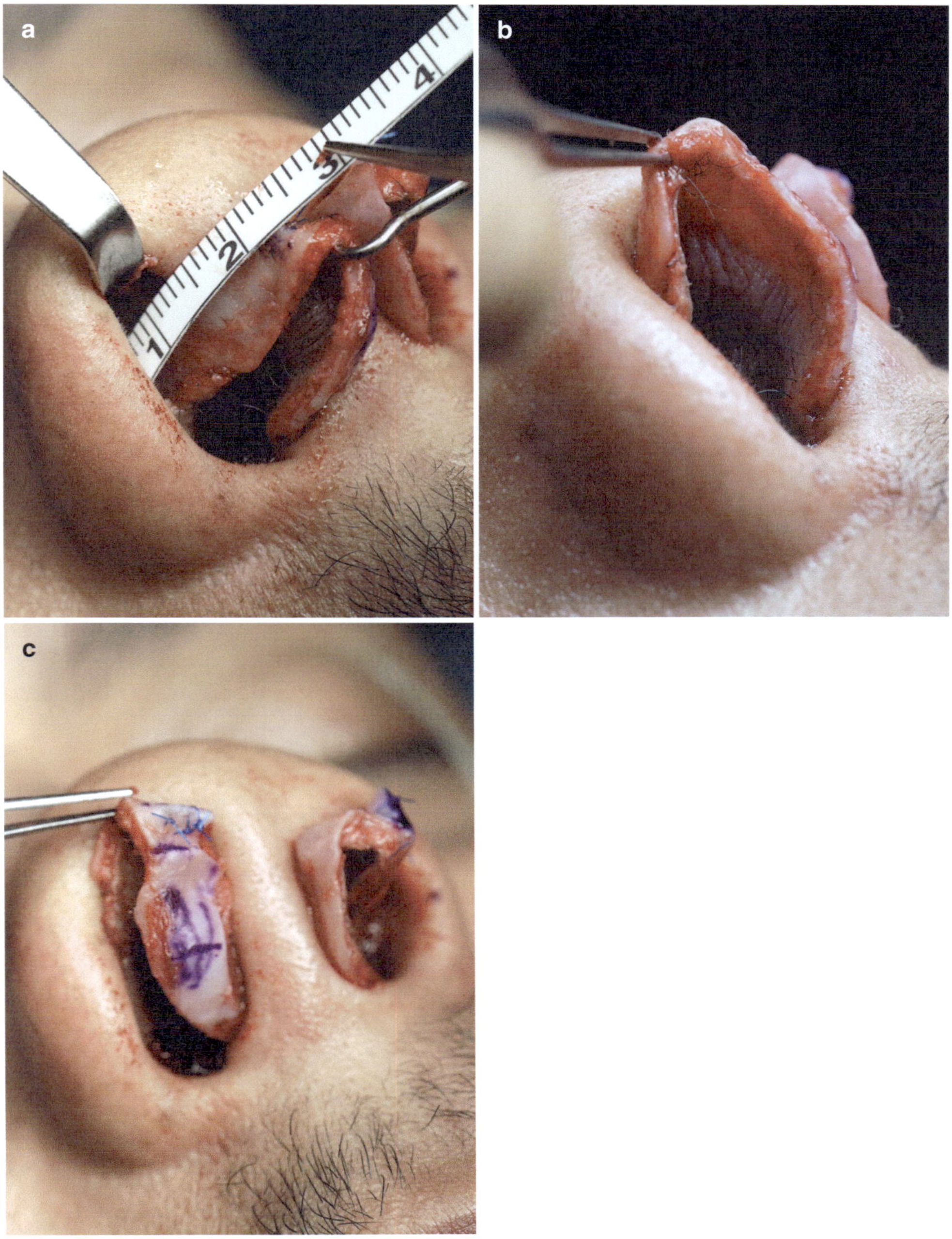

Fig. 13.80 (**a**) Compare with Fig. 13.78a how the lateral crus shortened after lateral crural steal suture. (**b**, **c**) After suture placement, the medial crura was elongated, more deformed, prolapsed caudally, and the tip became over-projected

a strong, bulky lateral crus via suturing may distort the alar cartilage.

Steal suturing combined with medial crural overlapping is not an option; it would be inappropriate to create an incision over the medial crus when the configuration thereof is near-ideal. Also, resection beginning at the lateral crus not only shortens the crus, but also resolves any configurational deformity.

The first step to reduce lateral crural volume is cephalic resection (Fig. 13.99).

The existing domal points (anatomical dome points) were marked on the rear using a pen (Fig. 13.100). Just behind the domes were incised craniocaudally with preservation of the underlying skin. Beginning at the incised dome, the lateral crura were elevated laterally by about 1.5 cm (Fig. 13.101).

Two trapezoidal pieces of cartilage were removed from regions just lateral to the two domes; the bases of the trapezoids formed the cranial edges of the lateral crus (Fig. 13.102).

After resection, excessive lateral crural regions were apparent (Fig. 13.103).

The remaining portions were sutured using 5–0 polydioxanone. The caudal edge was lifted and the identical maneuver was repeated on the other side (Fig. 13.104).

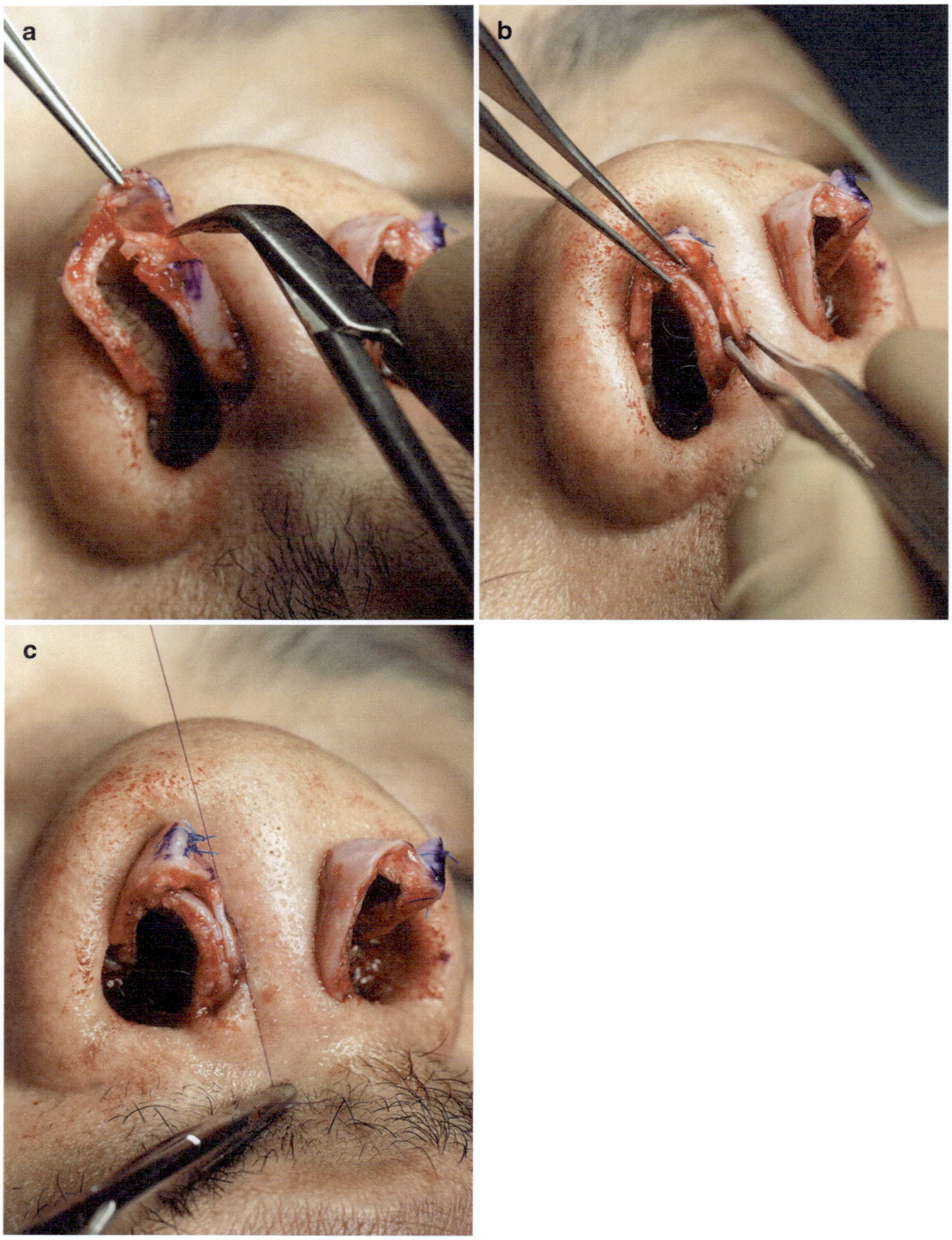

Fig. 13.81 (a–c) The over-projecting tip is corrected by transection and overlapping of the medial crus in its most prolapsed caudal aspect

The trimmed part of the lateral crus served as an alar batten graft that strengthened the lateral nasal wall (Fig. 13.105).

Interdomal sutures were inserted with preservation of dome divergence. A tip graft was placed immediately anterior to the newly created cartilage-strut complex. The leading edge of the onlay tip graft was adjusted by reference to the desired height of the new tip.

Finally, camouflage grafts (diced or crushed cartilage obtained from the excised cephalic part of the lateral crus if possible, or from a crushed/diced septum or excessive subcutaneous fibrotic tissue) were secured in place (Fig. 13.106).

By referring to the alar cartilages before and after VAR, it can be seen that (Fig. 13.107):

- The medial crural configuration is unchanged.
- The lateral crus is shortened.
- The configuration has been corrected and tip definition increased.
- The tip has been stabilized and rotation has increased somewhat.

A comparison of the preoperative and 1-year postoperative photographs reveals that the nasal tip has become more

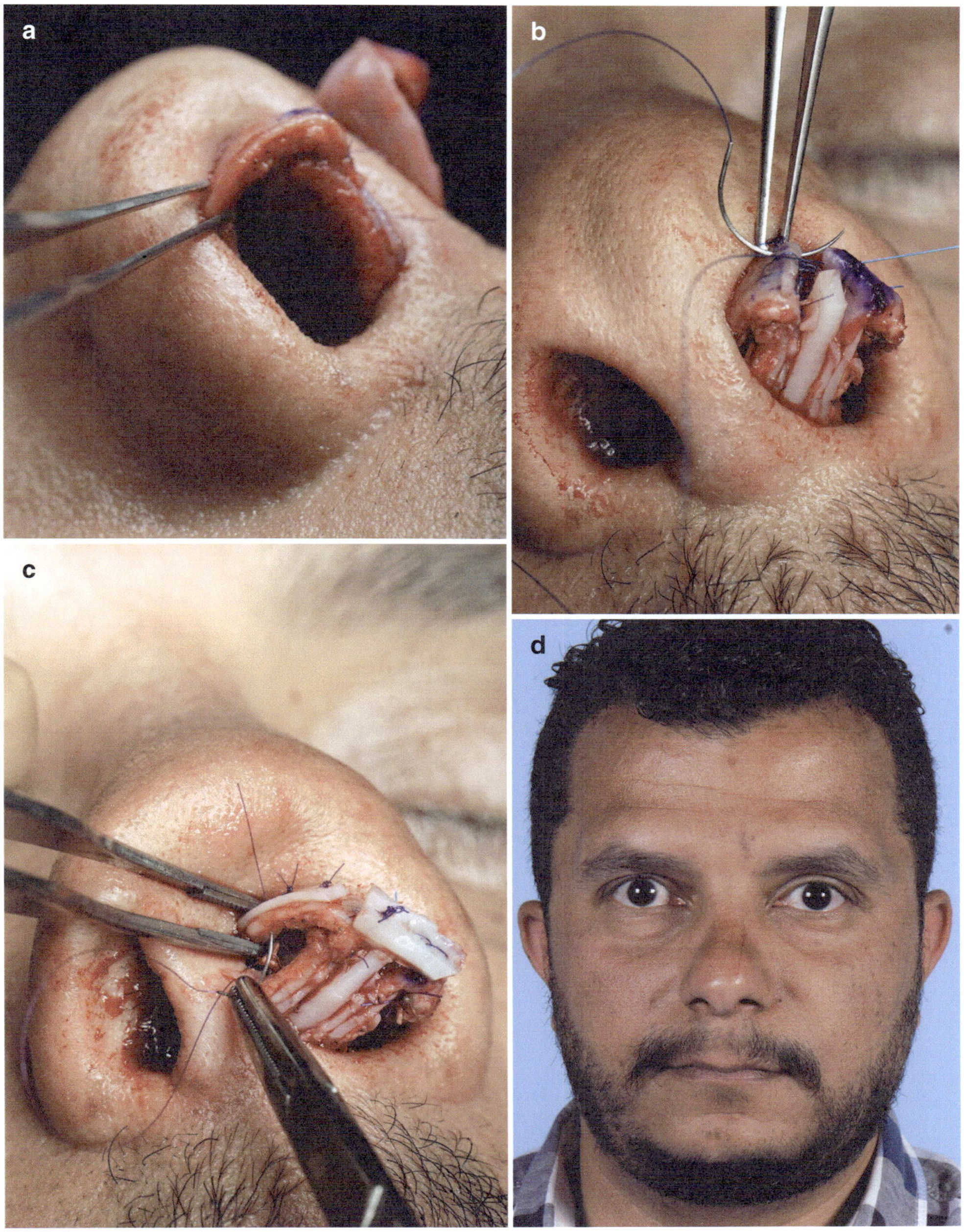

Fig. 13.82 (**a–c**) After the medial crural problem was resolved, both alar cartilages are delivered through one nostril. By visualizing two domes, it is relatively easy to decide what the shape of the tip grafts should be and where it should be located. A columellar strut and an onlay tip graft were used to restore projection. Lateral crural grafts can be employed to strengthen the lateral nasal walls of patients with thick skin, as in this case. (**d–g**) The tip was narrowed by a lateral crural steal, and springiness of the columella was fixed by overlap

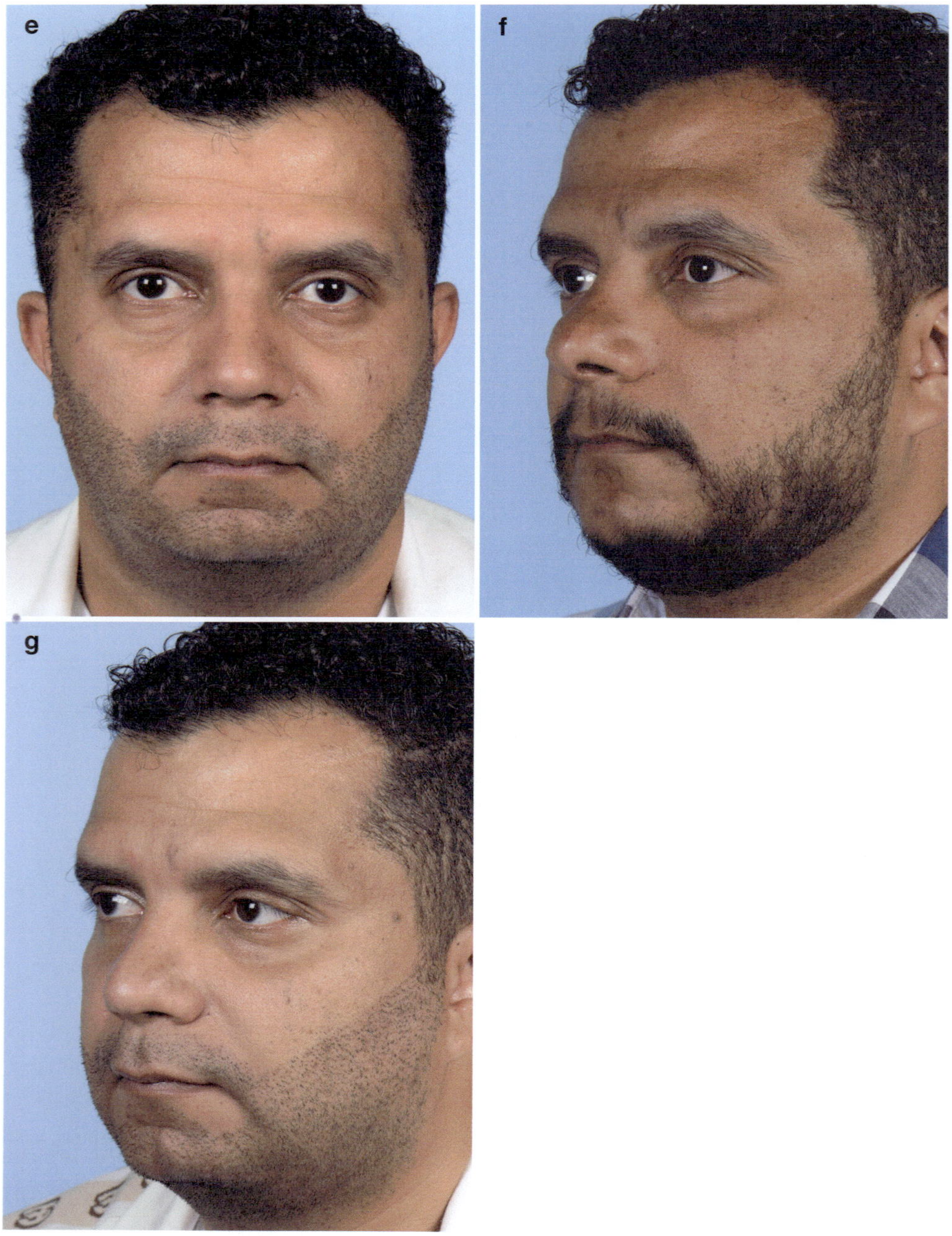

Fig. 13.82 (continued)

defined and the interdomal distance narrower and more symmetrical. The alar rims are now symmetrical and the alar base is narrower. The osseocartilaginous hump is lowered, providing a better dorsal profile. The middle third of the nose is strengthened and an aesthetically attractive curved line runs from the eyebrow to the tip-defining point (Fig. 13.108).

Case 26

For selected cases, the long-term outcomes of VAR are satisfactory. This young woman is the sister of the patient in Case 25. They exhibited similarly shaped noses. We treated this nose 10 years previously via VAR. Preoperatively, the domes were rounded and broad with full, underrotated infratip lobules and slightly over-projecting tips. Slight bony cartilaginous humps were apparent. The skin and soft tissue envelope were thick and sebaceous (Fig. 13.109).

Ten years postoperatively, tip definition has greatly improved and the infratip lobule is no longer unaesthetic. The hump is eliminated, and the tip rotated to a more satisfactory position (Fig. 13.110).

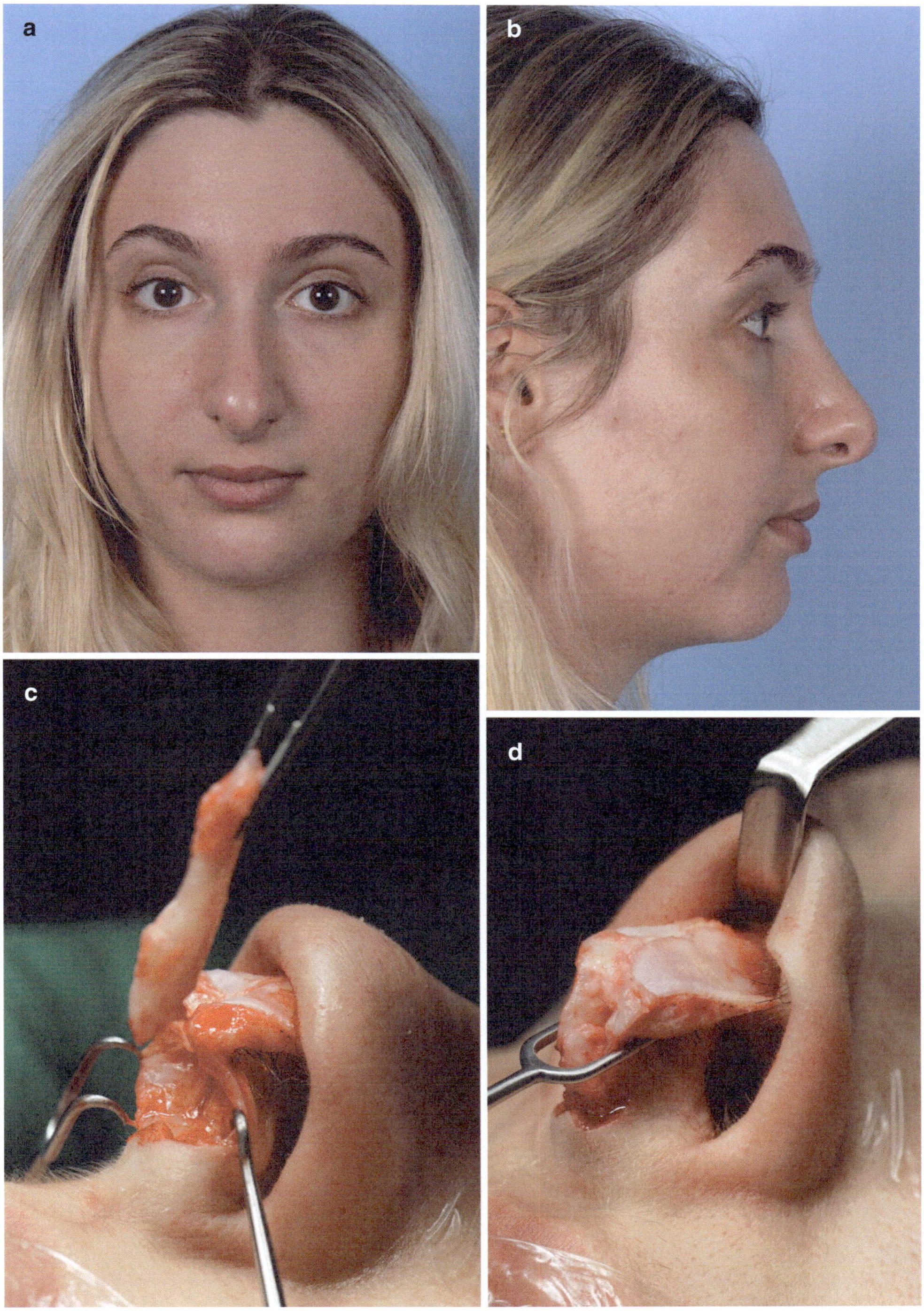

Fig. 13.83 (**a**, **b**) This patient presented requesting secondary rhinoplasty to correct a hanging infratip lobule, alar columellar discrepancy, and wide tip. (**c**) The previous columellar strut was removed. (**d**, **e**) Long lateral crura and deformed medial crura. (**f**, **g**) Actual dome and desired dome were marked

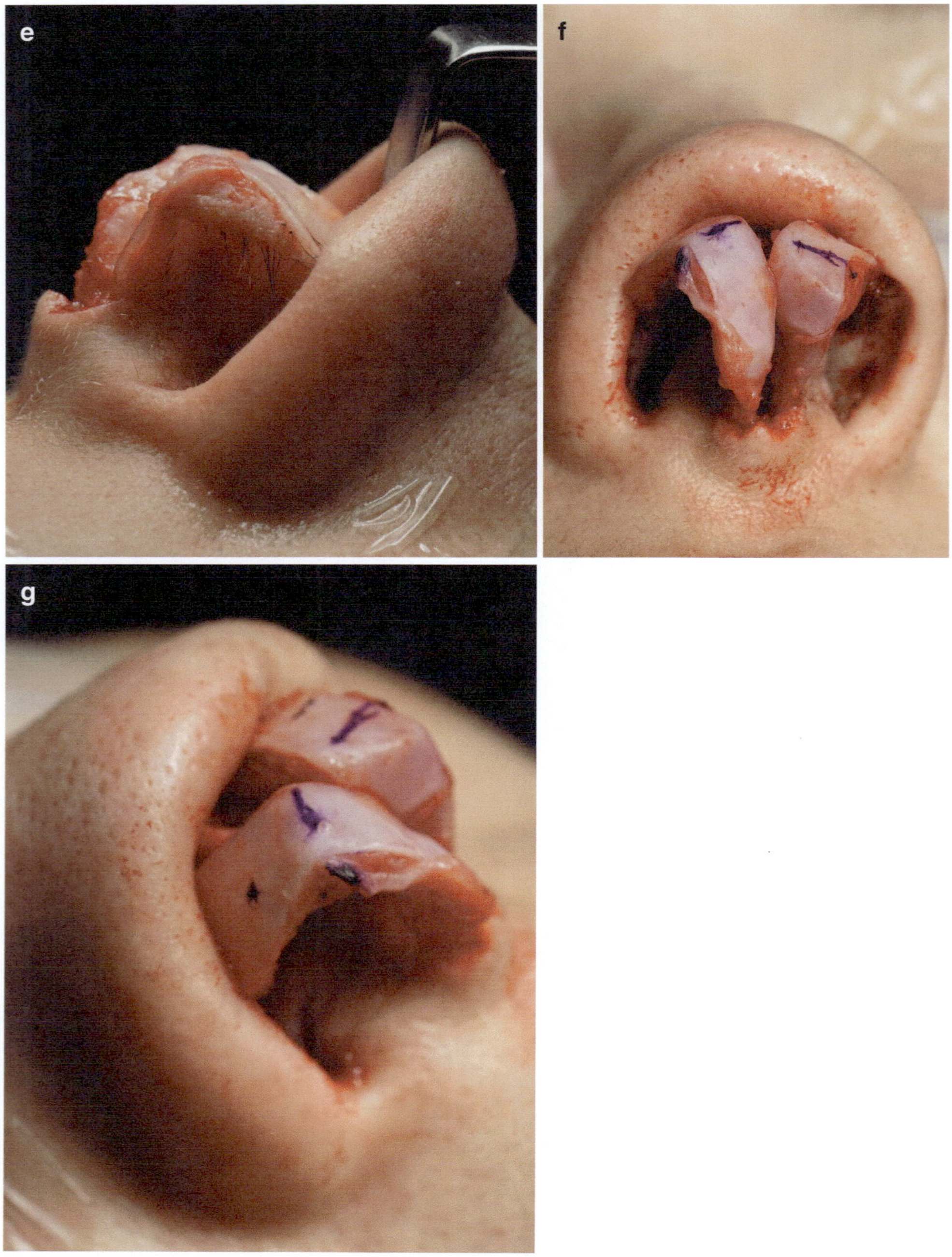

Fig. 13.83 (continued)

Case 27

The primary advantage of VAR is the versatility of the approach; it is possible to vary the location of division and the extent of cartilage resection, and to precisely contour the tip. VAR is most useful for patients with wide nasal tips that are both over-projecting and inferiorly rotated; resection of the cut segments (excessive part of lateral crura) narrows a wide domal arch and reduces projection and/or rotation. This case required moderate rotation; a wide nasal tip and a prominent over-projection are apparent (Fig. 13.111).

Intraoperative images revealed that all lateral crura were hypertrophic (Fig. 13.112; Video 13.20).

To create a narrower nasal tip, the first step is to reduce the lateral crus surface. Next, the desired dom point to initiate the var technique is identified and marked (Fig. 13.113).

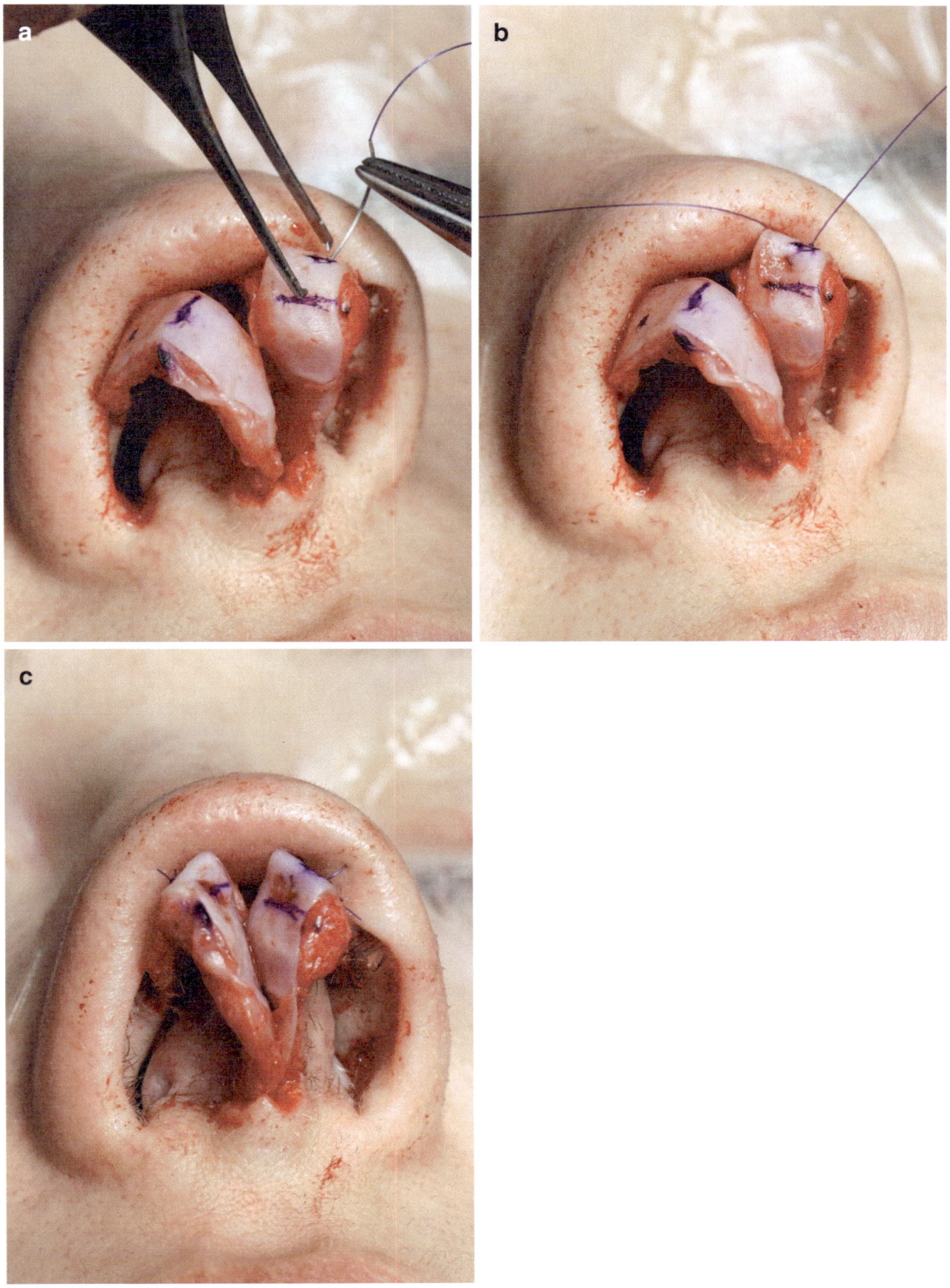

Fig. 13.84 (**a–c**) Lateral crural steal procedure

After bilateral division, the lateral crus was again dissected bilaterally from the vestibular mucosa (Fig. 13.114).

After the elevation, the excessive parts of the lateral crura were revealed. A bilateral trapezoidal excision was performed on these areas (Fig. 13.115).

Immediately after resection, the tension on the alar cartilage was reduced, and the cartilages were moved to their ideal locations. Resection should never lower the alar cartilage below the level of the dorsum. Transdomal mattress suture was placed, and suturing connected the two ends (i.e., restructured the dome) (Fig. 13.116).

The alar cartilages are now anatomically near-perfect. Resection narrows the tip, decreases projection, and increases rotation (Fig. 13.117).

Next, the tip was stabilized and defined by placing a columellar strut, a dome-equalizing suture, and alar button and cap grafts (Fig. 13.118).

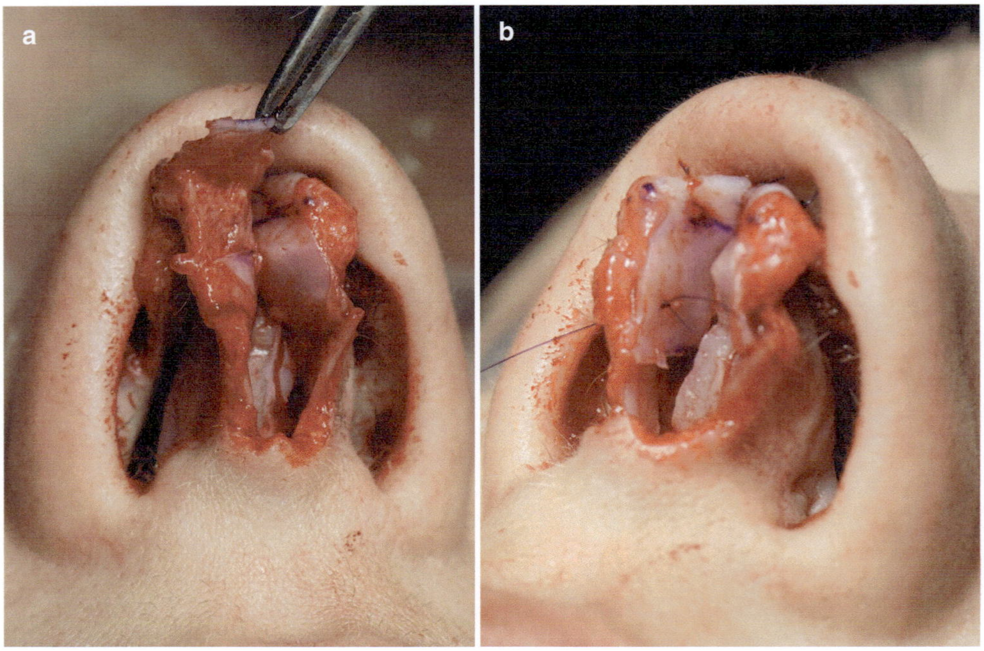

Fig. 13.85 (**a**, **b**) Division of the medial crura with overlap and suture fixation

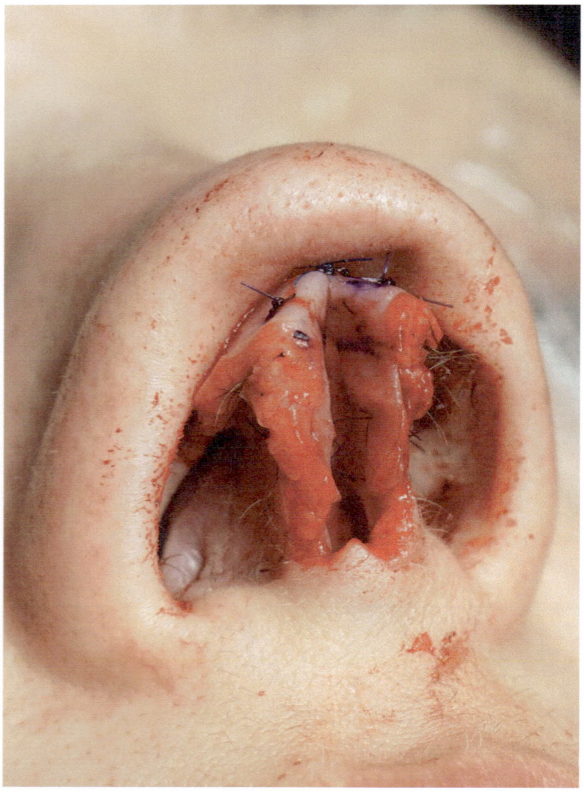

Fig. 13.86 Enhanced alar cartilages anatomy

A lateral crural graft must also be placed, regardless of the basic technique chosen, in patients with thick skin. In this case, tip surgery was completed by placing lateral crural and camouflage grafts (Fig. 13.119).

After the skin incision line was closed, diced cartilage was injected to fill the dead spaces in the tip. Bilateral sill excision was performed, and surgery was terminated (Fig. 13.120).

Preoperative and 4-year postoperative photographs are shown in Fig. 13.121. The profile is improved with straightening of the nasal dorsum. The nasal tip is deprojected and rotated upward. Also, there is an improvement in tip definition.

Case 28

This case involved tip features similar to those of Case 27 (a wide and over-projected tip). In addition, tip asymmetry was evident.

VAR technique was used for tip plasty. Postoperatively the patient shows improved nasal tip contour with less projection. There is a symmetric bidomal tip shape postoperatively. Preoperative and postoperative photographs of the patient are shown in Fig. 13.122.

Case 29

A 28-year-old woman requested reduction of the size of her tip. VAR technique was provided, resulting in a greatly improved tip definition. A preoperative frontal view and intra-

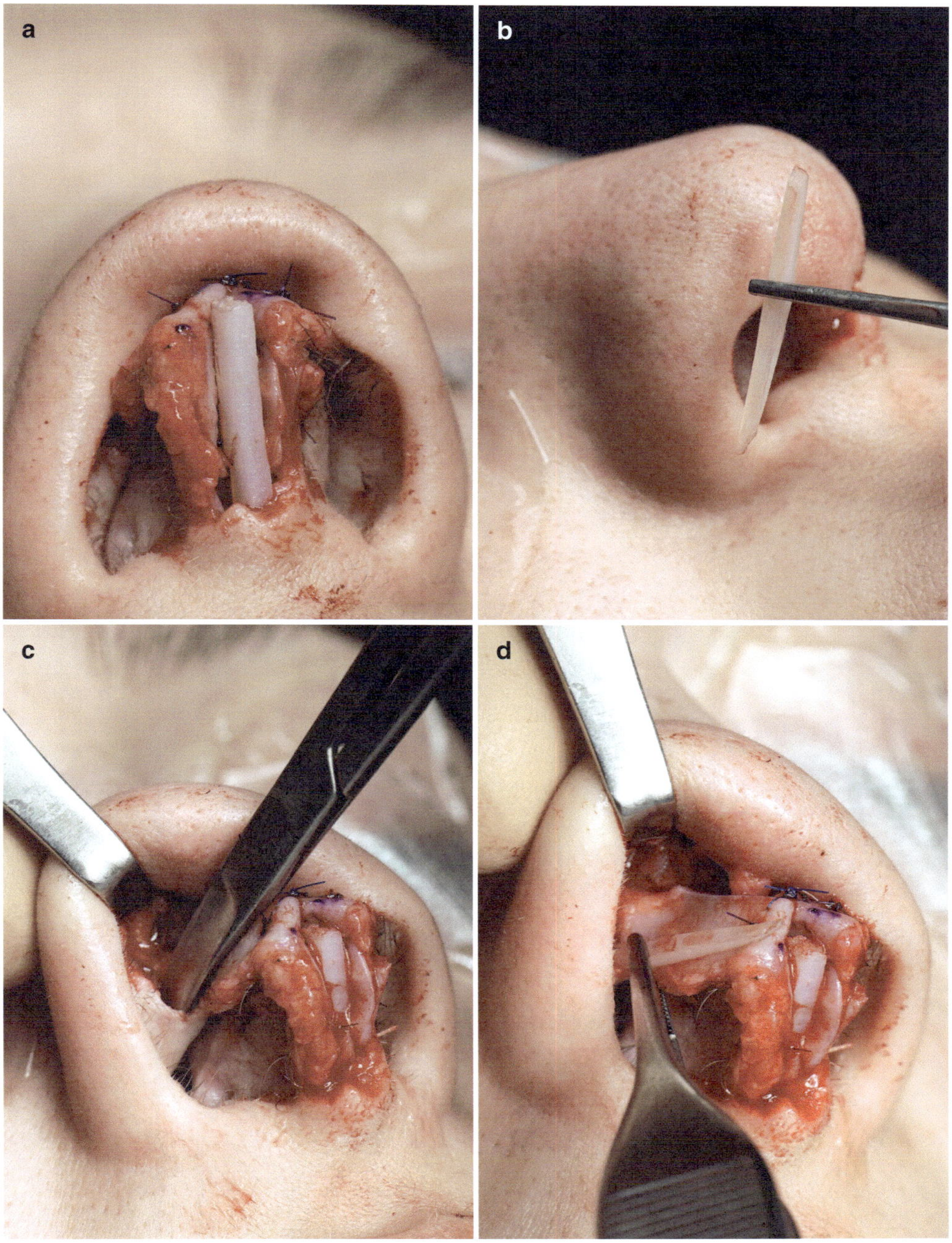

Fig. 13.87 (**a–e**) Columellar strut, onlay grafts over the lateral crura, cap, and camouflage graft

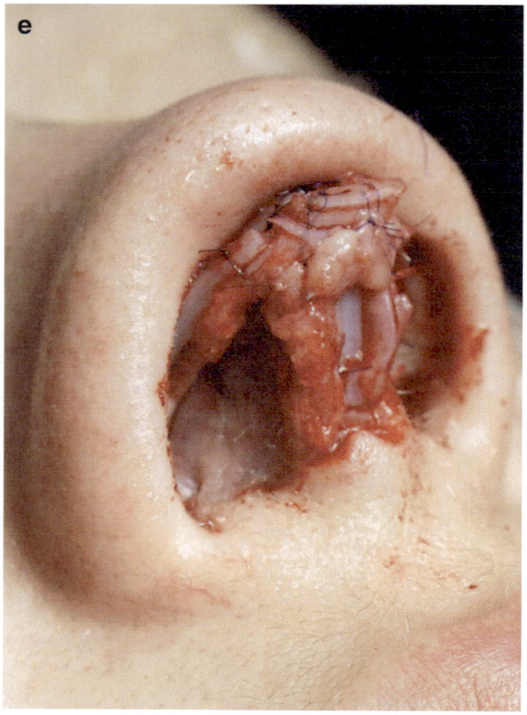

Fig. 13.87 (continued)

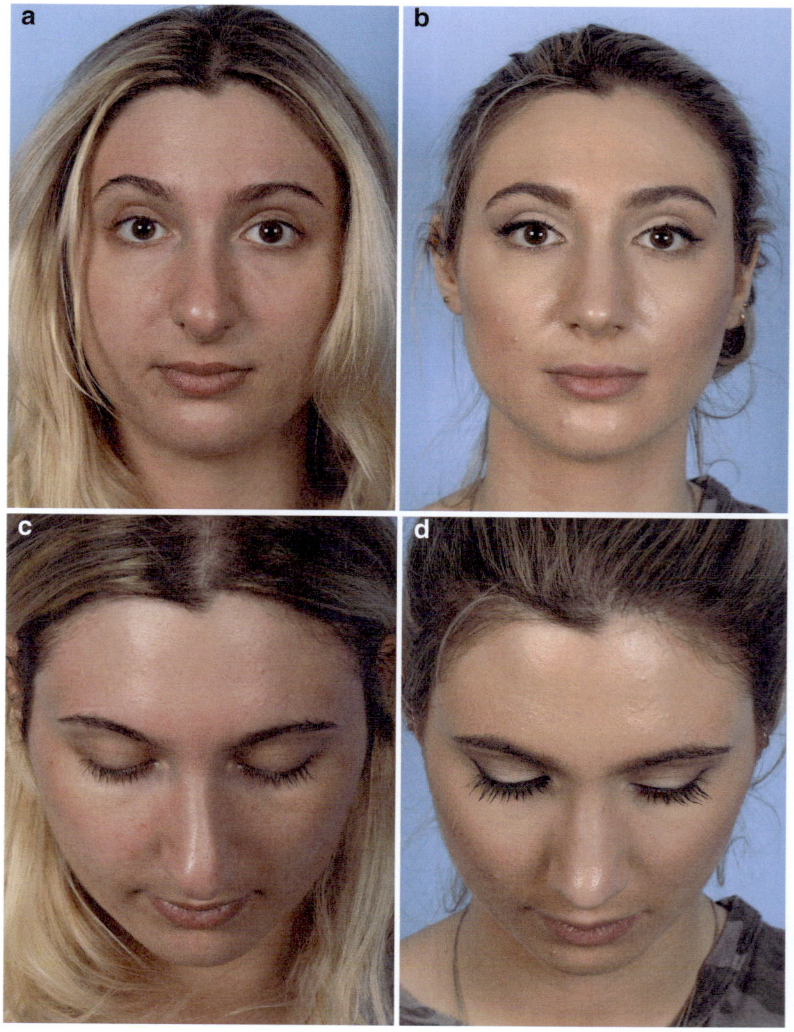

Fig. 13.88 (**a–h**) Lateral crural shortening resolved the wide nasal tip issue. The medial crural configuration deformity that was prominent in the lateral preoperative image was effectively corrected using the overlap technique. The author employed COST for this patient because the patient's excessively long lateral crus was accompanied by a medial crural malformation

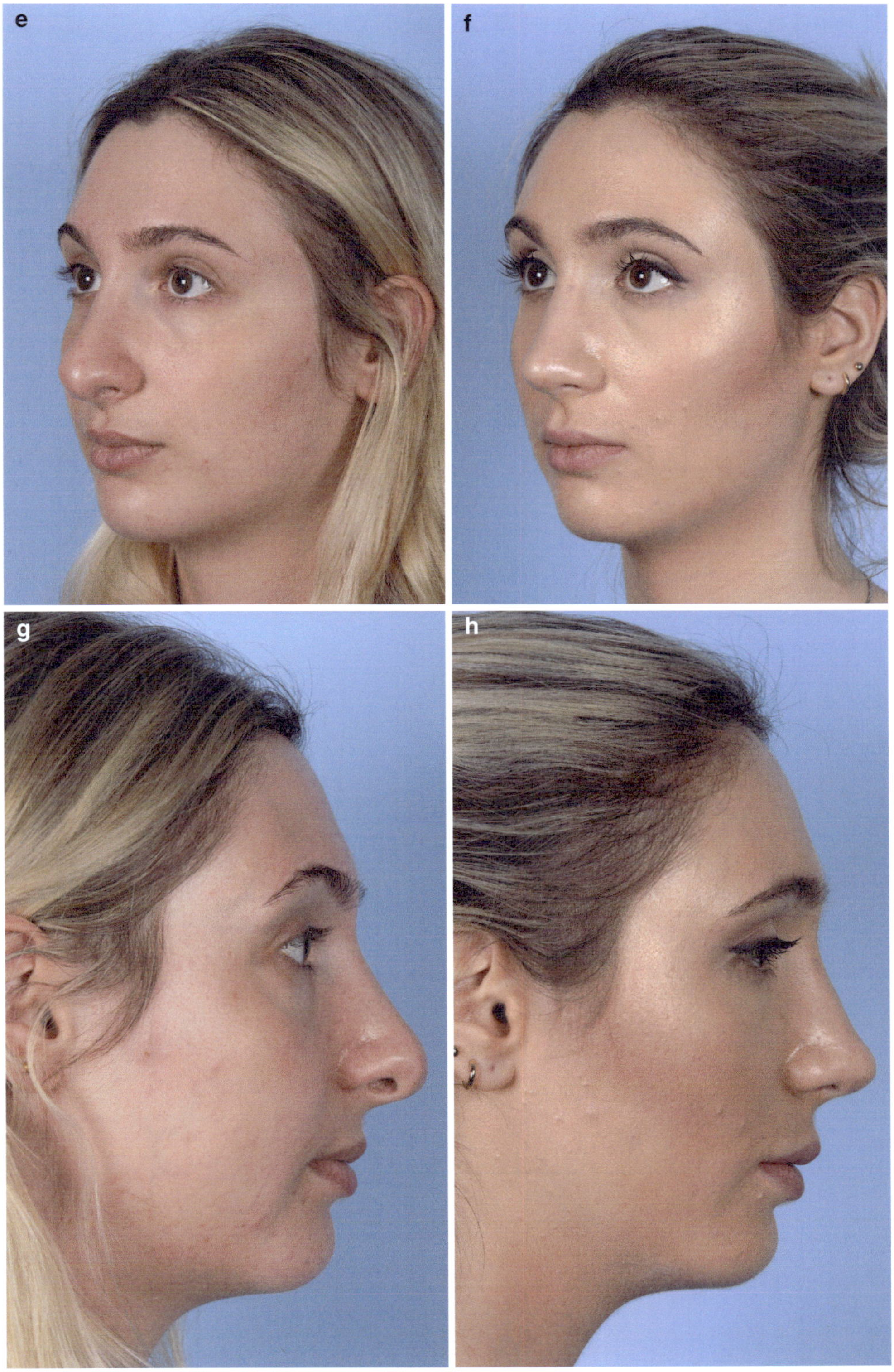

Fig. 13.88 (continued)

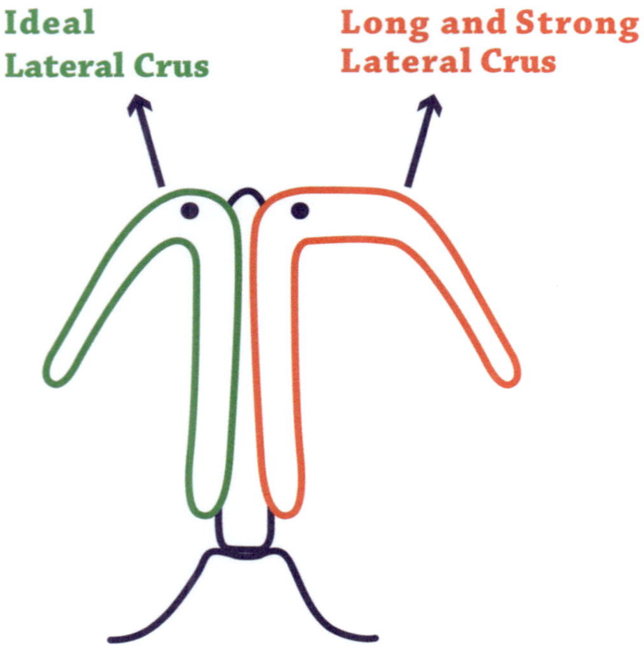

Fig. 13.89 Our aim must be to shorten the long and strong lateral crus and make it similar to the ideal one

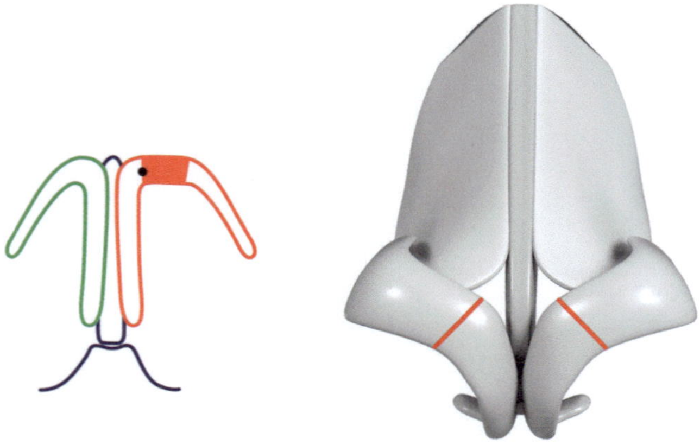

Fig. 13.90 The segment to be excised from the lateral crus

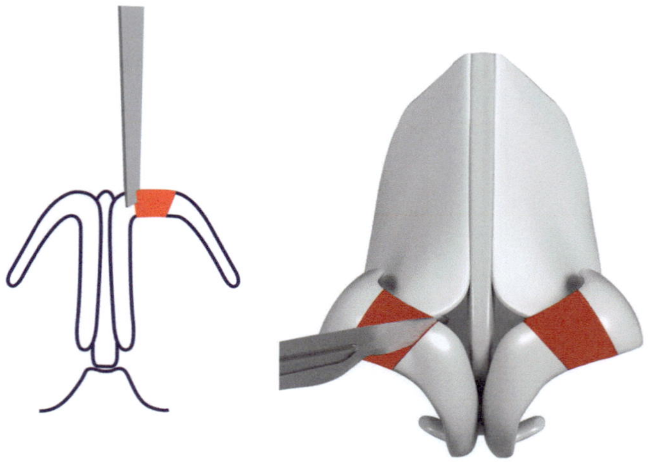

Fig. 13.91 Divide the alar cartilages just behind the dome by vertical incision

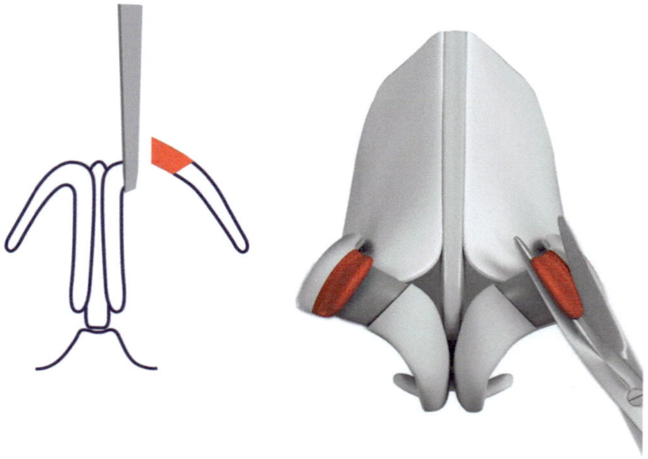

Fig. 13.92 Detach the lateral crus from vestibular skin

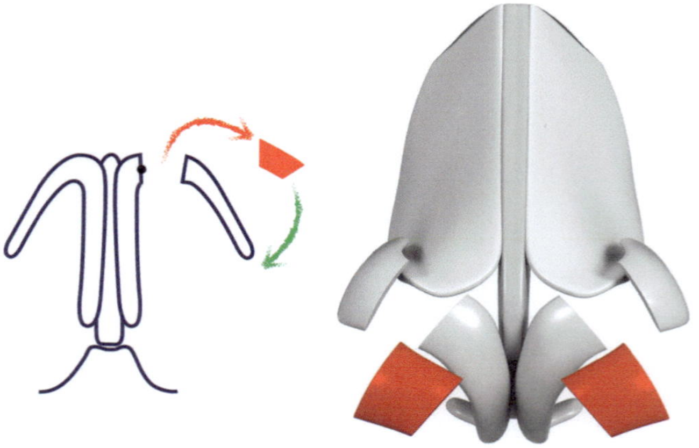

Fig. 13.93 Remove the triangle or trapezoid-shaped pieces of cartilage from both lateral crus. The base should be at the cranial edge of the crus. This way, we ensure lifting the caudal margin

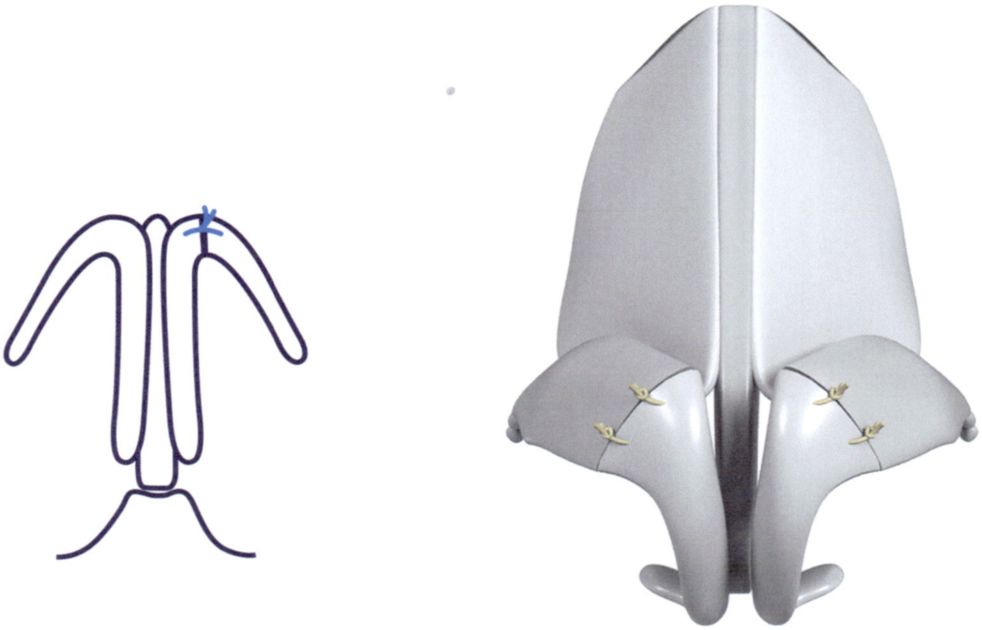

Fig. 13.94 Suture re-approximation of divided alar cartilages, undertaken with simple interrupted stitches

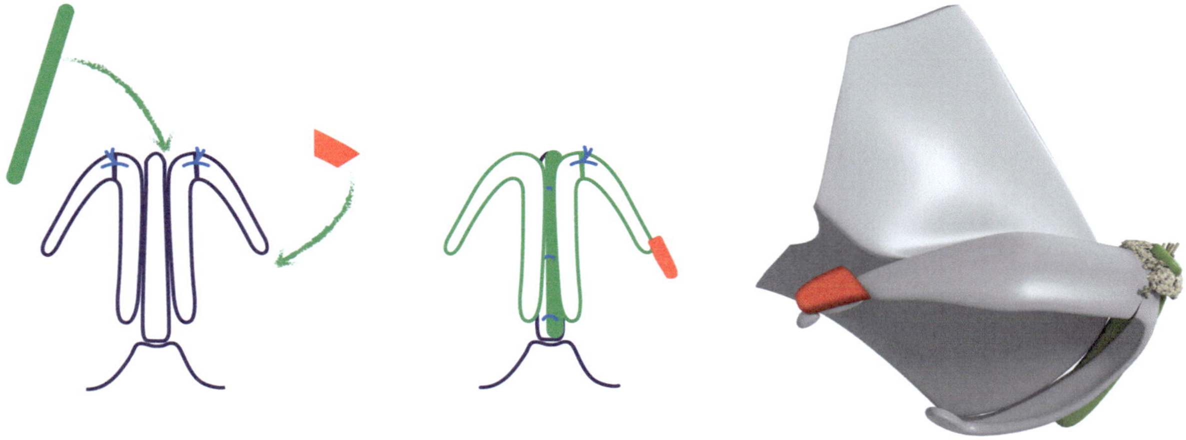

Fig. 13.95 Cap graft, columellar strut, and alar batten graft. The resected excess part of lateral crura can be preferred like alar batten graft

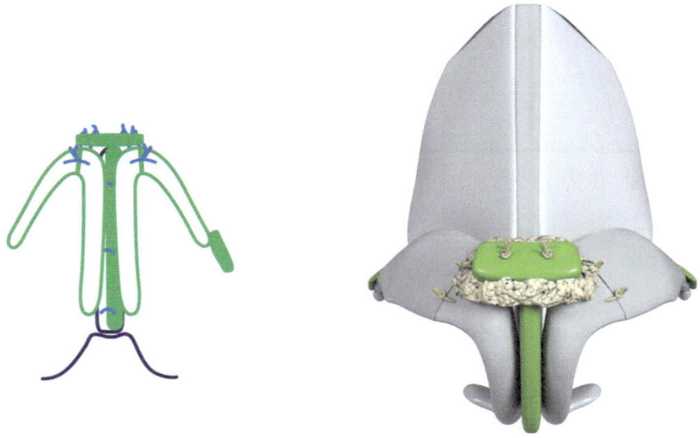

Fig. 13.96 If the patient is thin-skinned, the cap graft should be camouflaged

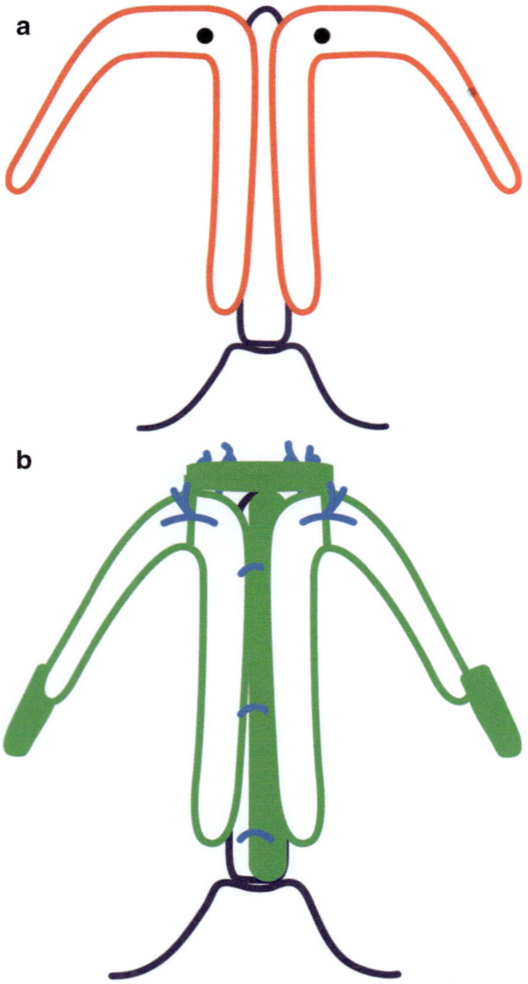

Fig. 13.97 (**a**, **b**) Alar cartilage anatomy before and after VAR technique

operative photographs are shown in Fig. 13.123 (Video 13.21). Six-year postoperative photographs are shown in Fig. 13.124.

Case 30

This technique can also be applied using the closed approach. This patient has wide nasal tip and prominent hanging infratip lobule VAR technique is a versatile tool in such cases (Fig. 13.125; Video 13.22).

Postoperatively the patient showed improved nasal tip contour with less infratip lobule prominence (Fig. 13.126).

Case 31

Technical Pearl: If the VAR technique is used to treat thick-skinned patients, overlay placement of a lateral crural graft is useful to ensure long-term tip stability and alar rim definition.

A patient with wide tip and thick skin is presented in this case.

The tip was wide and lacked definition. The goals of surgery were to narrow and sculpt the nasal tip using VAR technique (Fig. 13.127).

The preoperative and 10-year postoperative photographs demonstrate that after 10 years the tip is still stable, symmetric, and well defined. VAR technique and lateral crural grafts worked well together in this patient (Fig. 13.128).

Case 32

VAR may also be used for revision. As mentioned above, inappropriate primary transdomal suturing may deform the alar cartilages, not only narrowing the tip but also widening the lobule; the lateral nasal wall and alar rim now lack support and the nasal tip may widen postoperatively (Fig. 13.129).

During revision of such a case, it is necessary to correct the lateral crus in terms of its craniocaudal relationship, which is distorted after suturing. However, it is very challenging to reshape cartilage via suturing only. VAR can be used to correct the craniocaudal relationship. A trapezoidal resection was created immediately lateral to the dome; the wide edge lay caudally. Next, the two edges were sutured end-to-end. The caudal edge moved upward on resection and suturing (Fig. 13.130; Video 13.23).

On the 5-year postoperative photograph, nasal tip definition is improved and there is no interdomal gap (Fig. 13.131).

Case 33

If a surgeon cannot initially decide on which technique to use, basic and intermediate techniques should be attempted. However, if the results are not satisfactory, the strategy can be changed intraoperatively; advanced techniques can be employed to obtain satisfactory results.

Here is an example. The surgeon should not complete the surgery if the intraoperative result is poor (Fig. 13.132).

Two-year postoperative photos demonstrate that the patient showed improved appearance of the tip (Fig. 13.133).

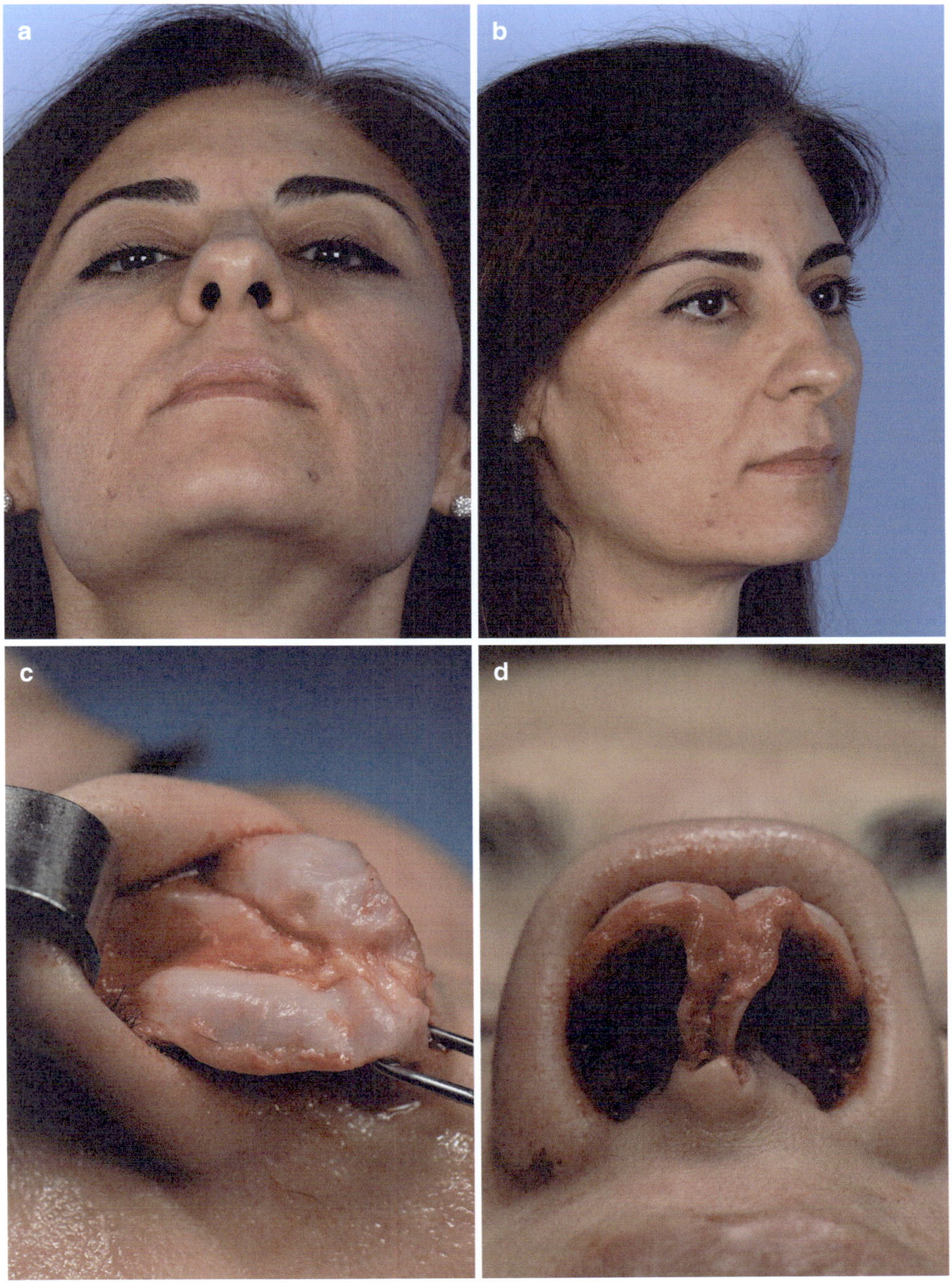

Fig. 13.98 (**a**, **b**) Wide, boxy tip with adequate rotation and projection. (**c**, **d**) The lateral crura were extremely long and convex but the medial crura were normal

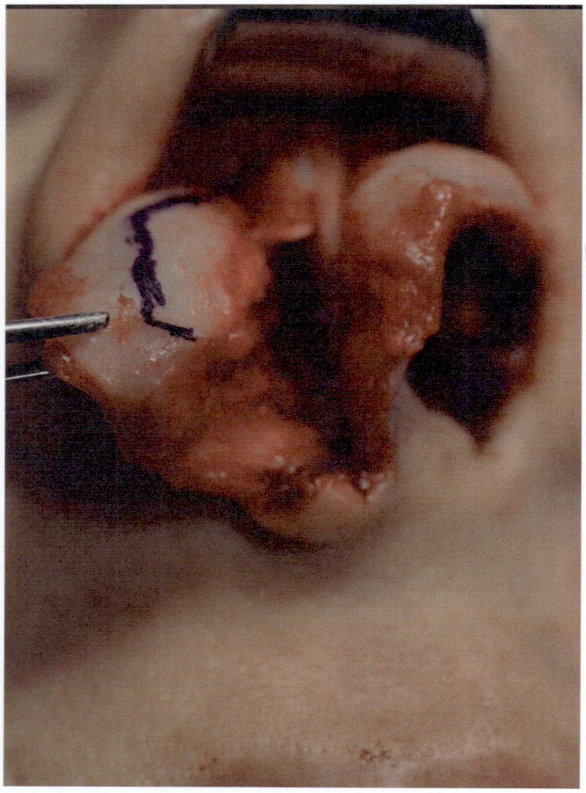

Fig. 13.99 Cephalic trim of the lower lateral cartilages, extending the domes

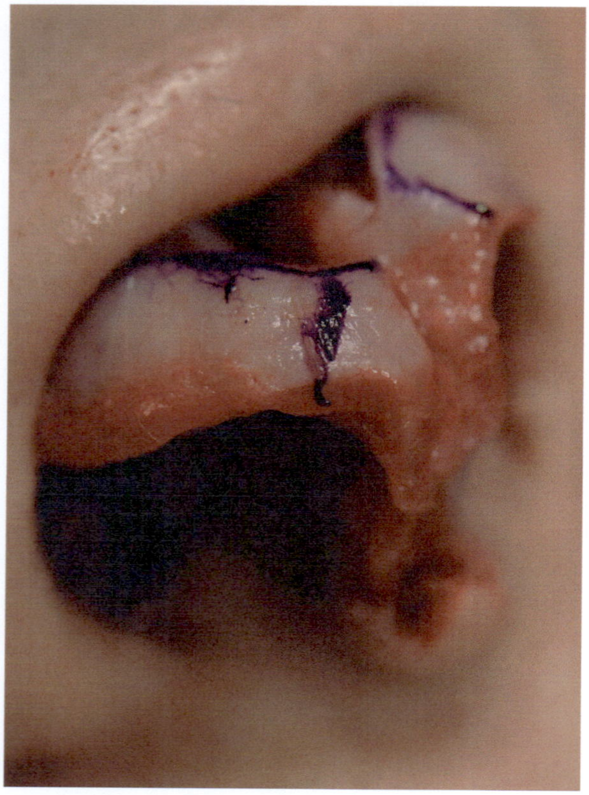

Fig. 13.100 The division line was marked

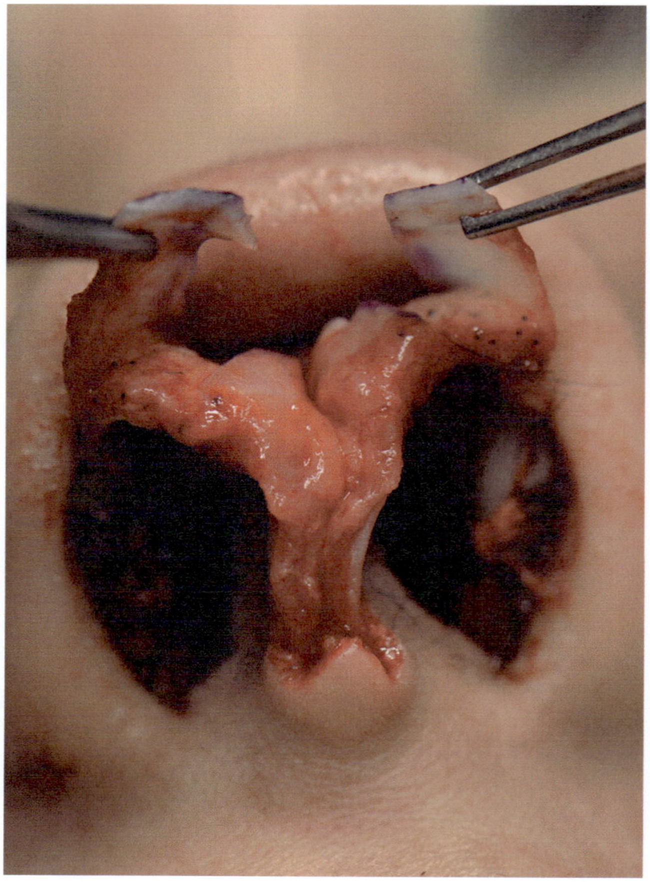

Fig. 13.101 Freeing the cartilage from the skin

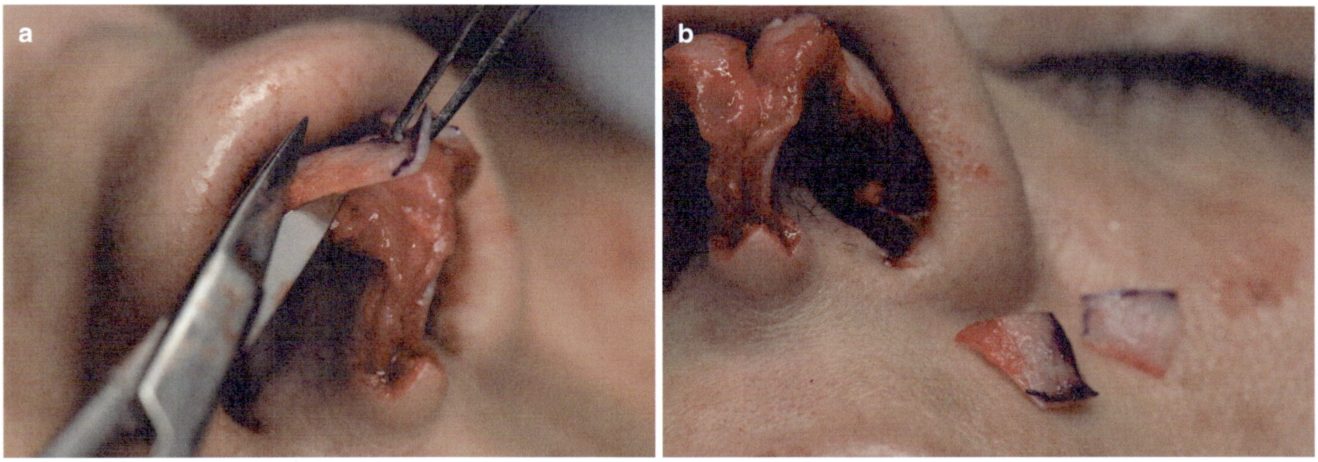

Fig. 13.102 (**a**, **b**) Vertical alar resection

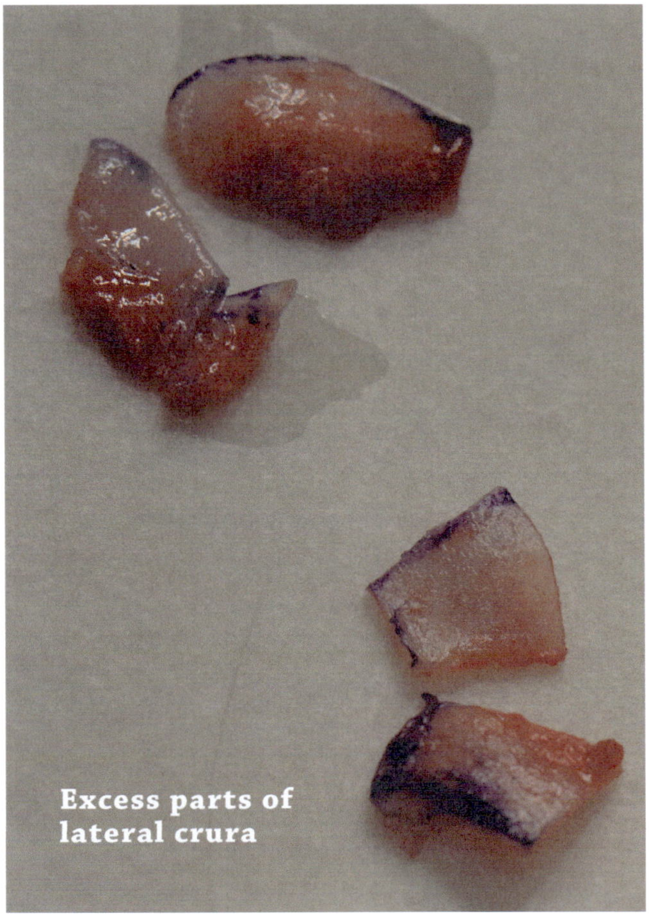

Fig. 13.103 Excess parts of lateral crura (cephalic excesses and vertical excesses)

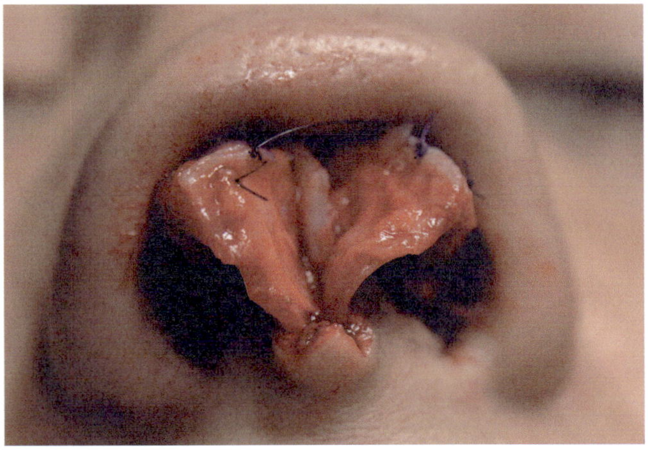

Fig. 13.104 Reapproximate the divided cartilages with suture

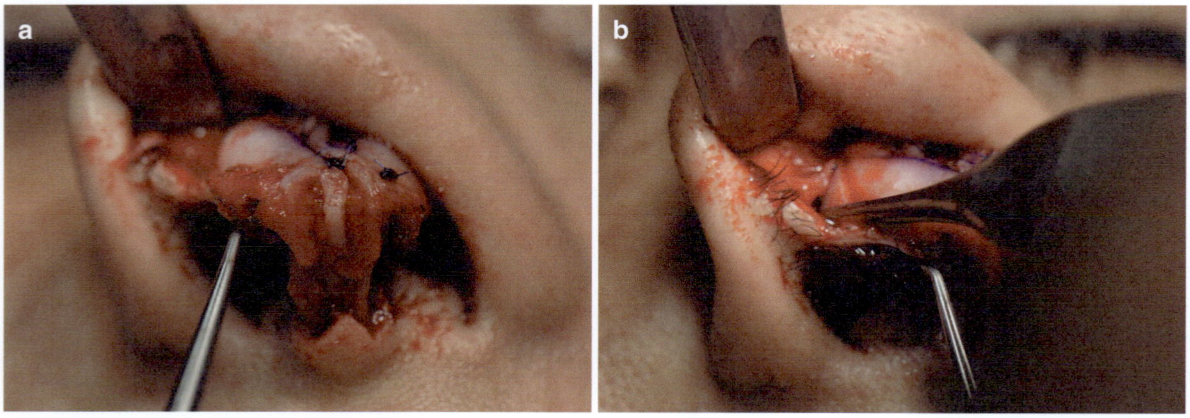

Fig. 13.105 (**a**, **b**) Scissors were used to create a small pocket in the lateral alar sidewall. The trapezoidal segment from the same side was placed inside the pocket. Fixation was unnecessary as the graft fitted well

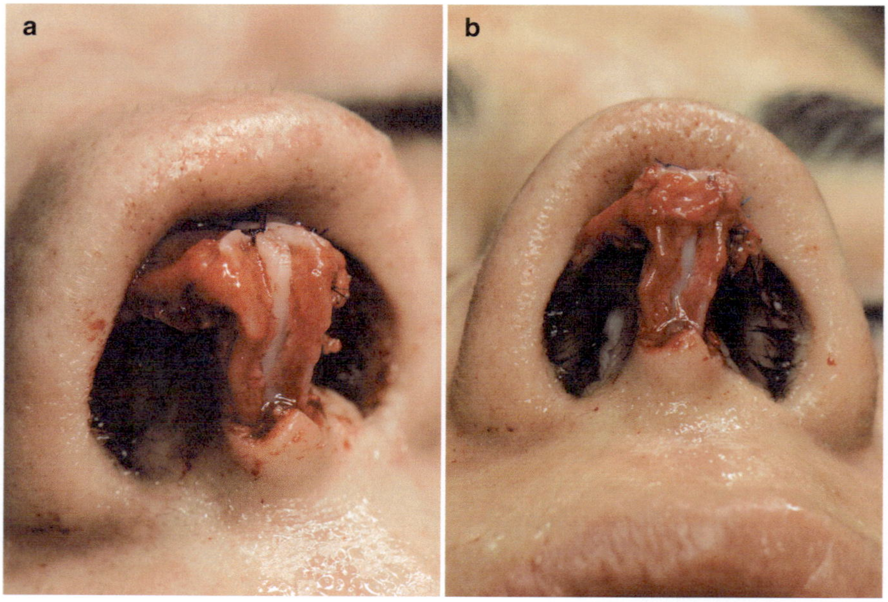

Fig. 13.106 (**a**, **b**) Columellar strut, cap graft, and camouflage grafts

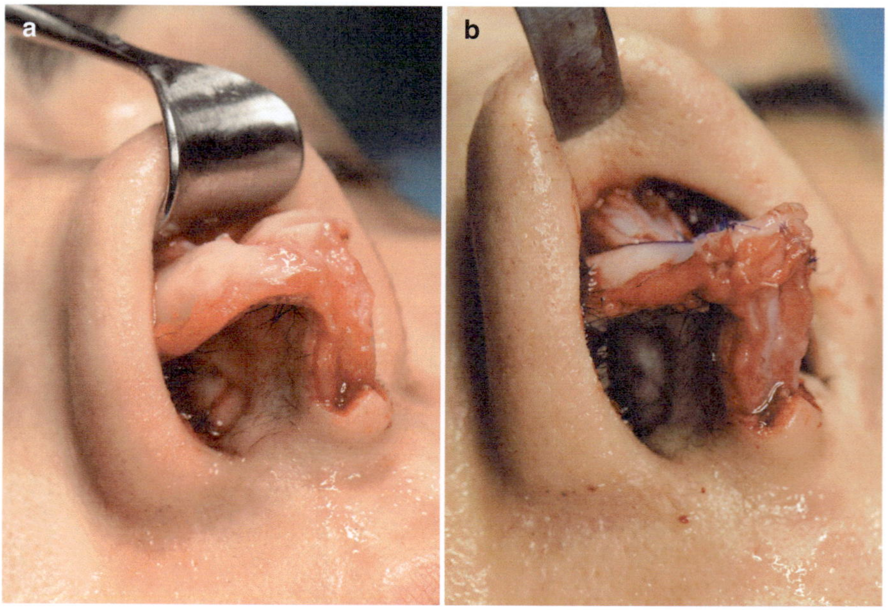

Fig. 13.107 (**a**, **b**) Compare images before and after the procedure

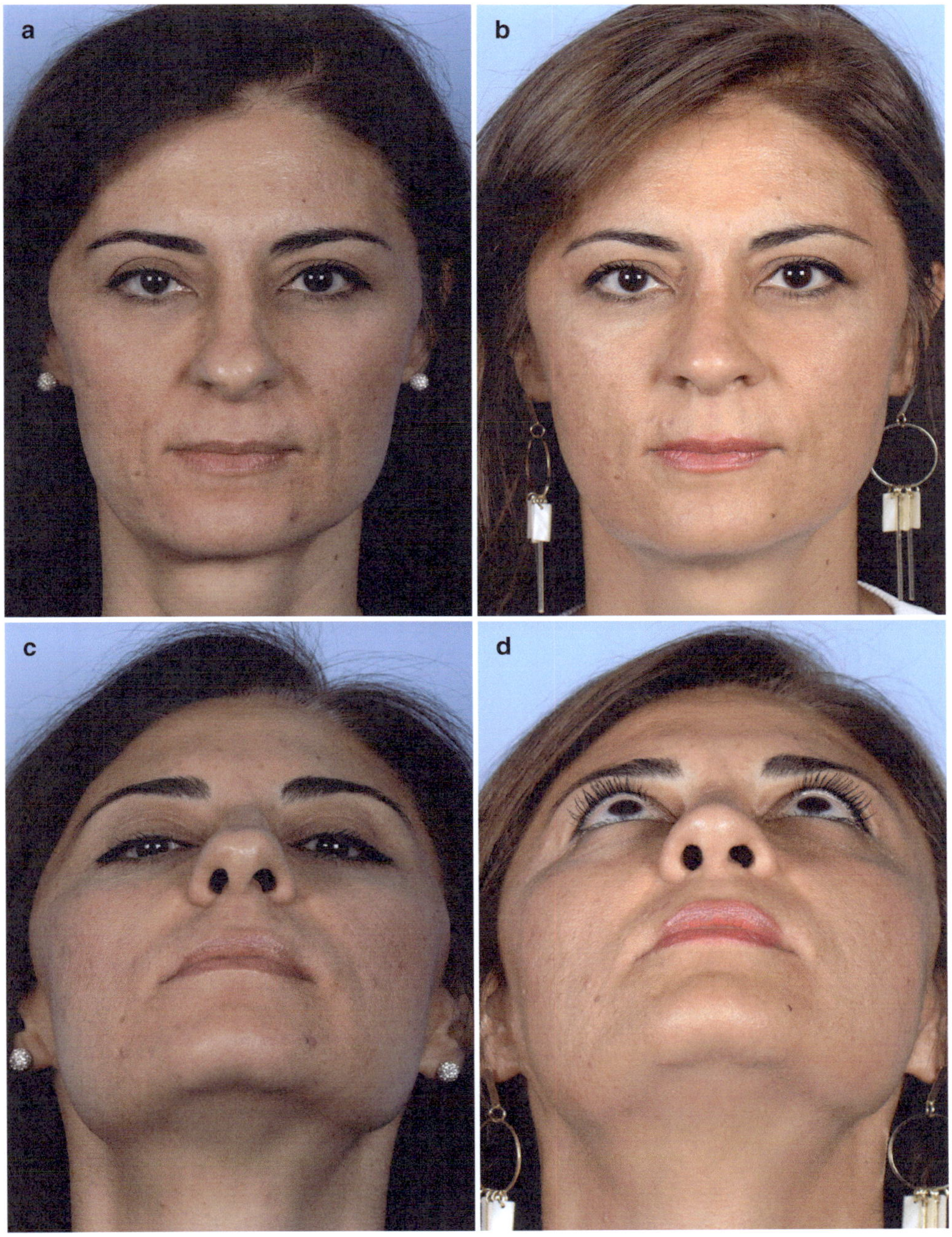

Fig. 13.108 (**a–h**) Preoperative and postoperative photographs. The tip is more defined and the domal angle has diminished. Note the improvement in lateral crural convexity, best seen on base view

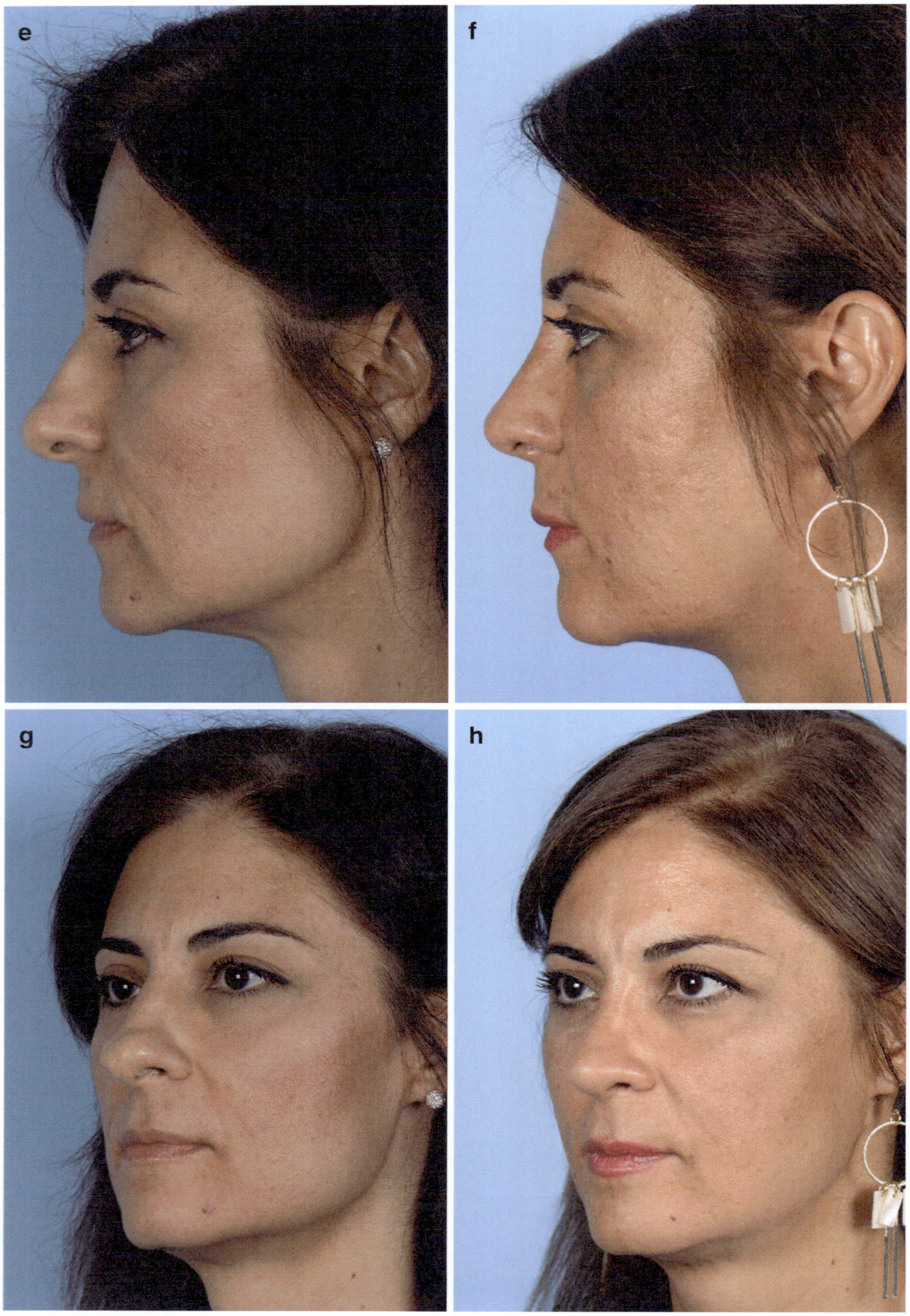

Fig. 13.108 (continued)

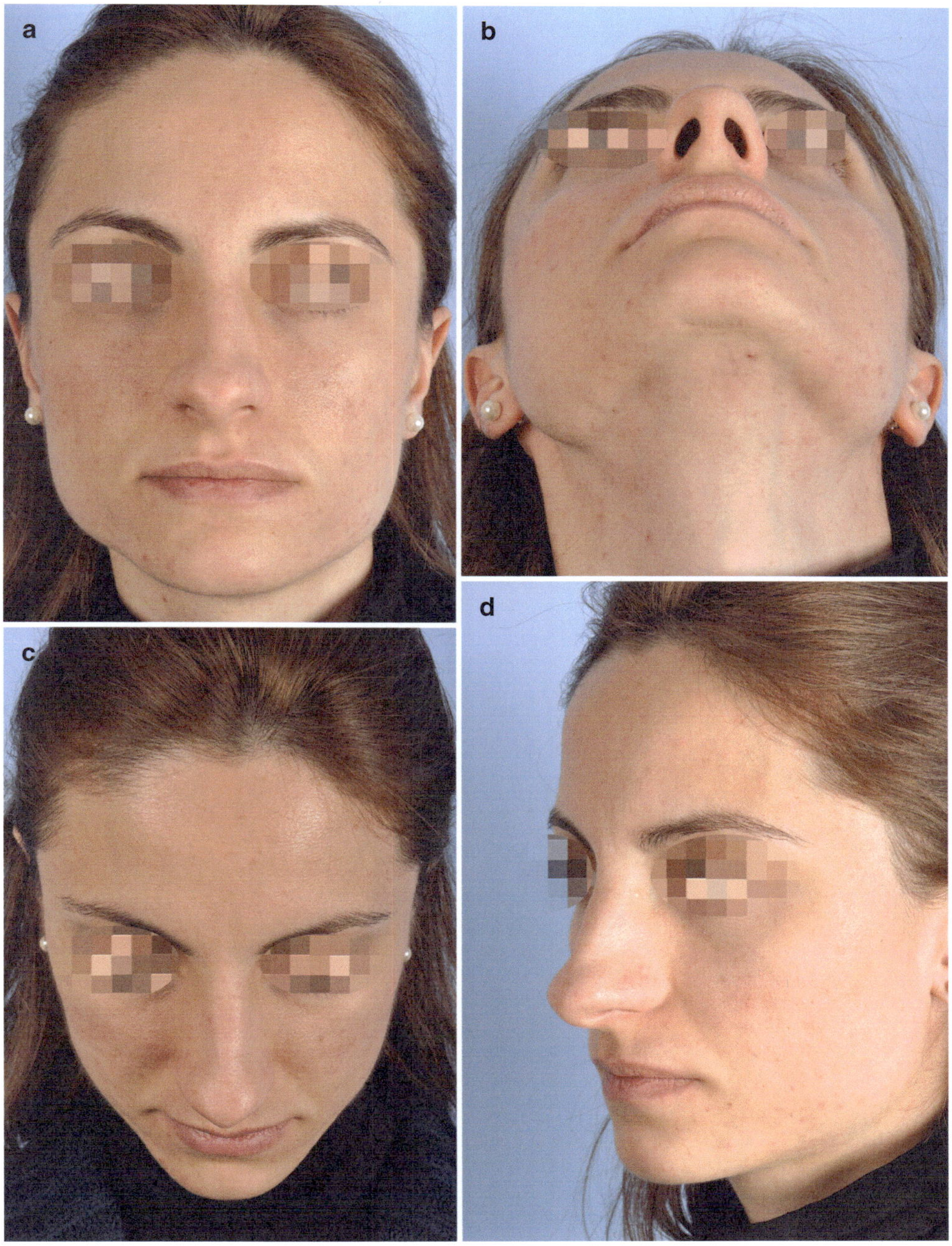

Fig. 13.109 (**a–d**) Patient with wide, nasal tip with wide domal angles

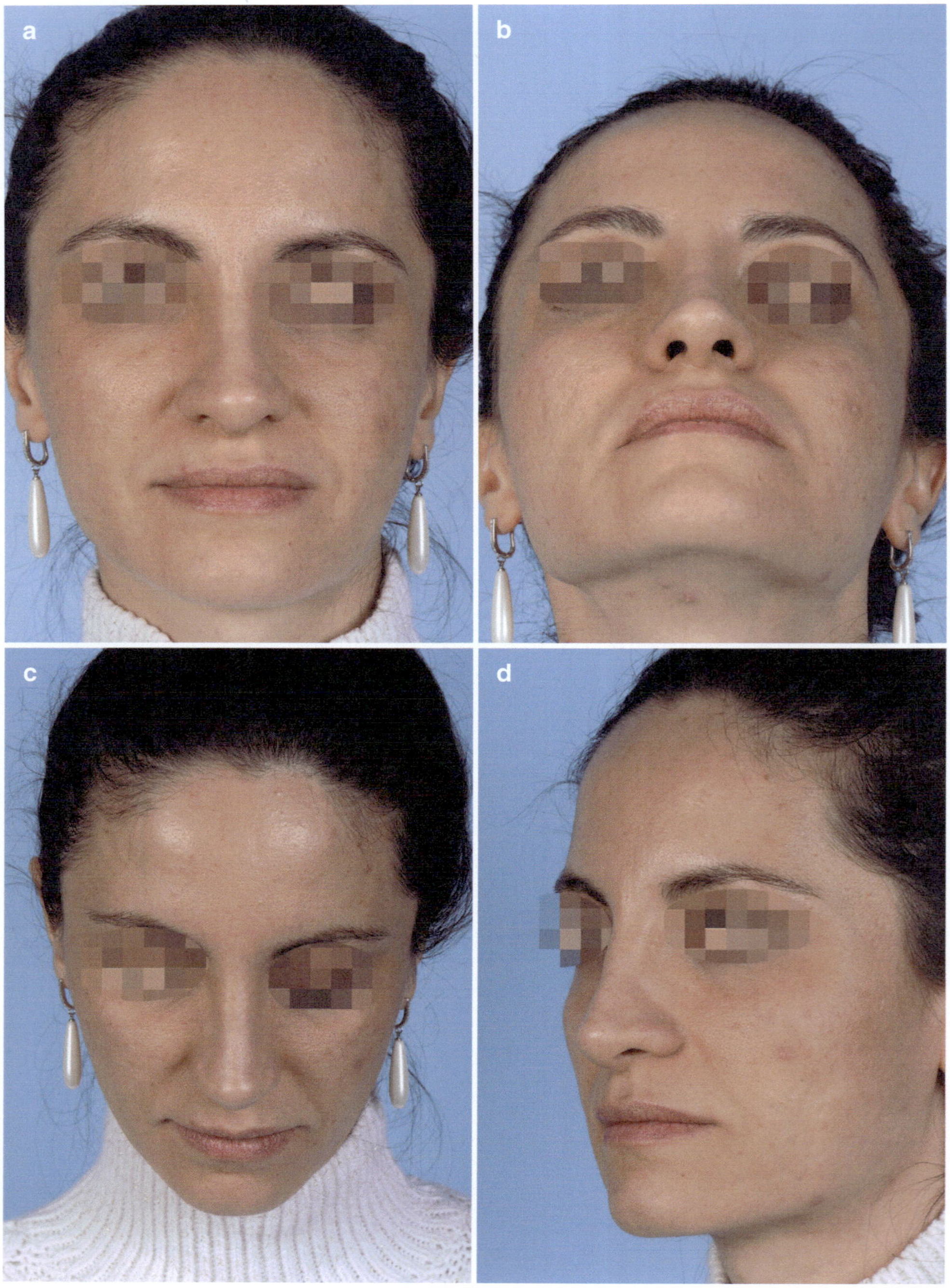

Fig. 13.110 (**a–d**) Long-term result. Width of the tip was normalized using the VAR technique. There has been no deteriorating on the tip in years

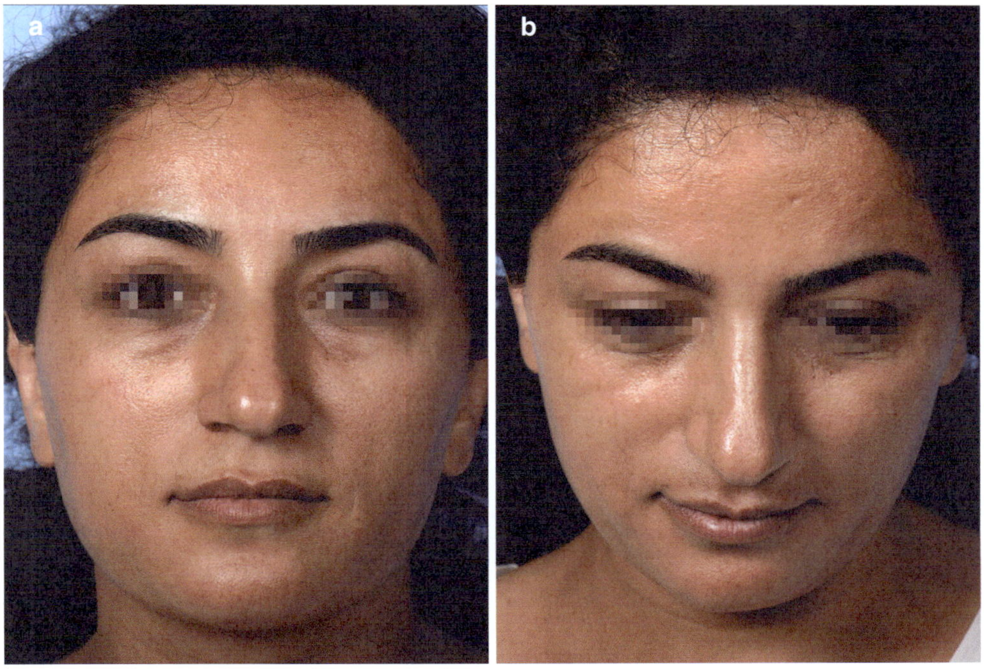

Fig. 13.111 (**a**, **b**) This 38-year-old patient complains of a large nose. The preoperative photographs show a wide nasal tip with a prominent dorsal hump

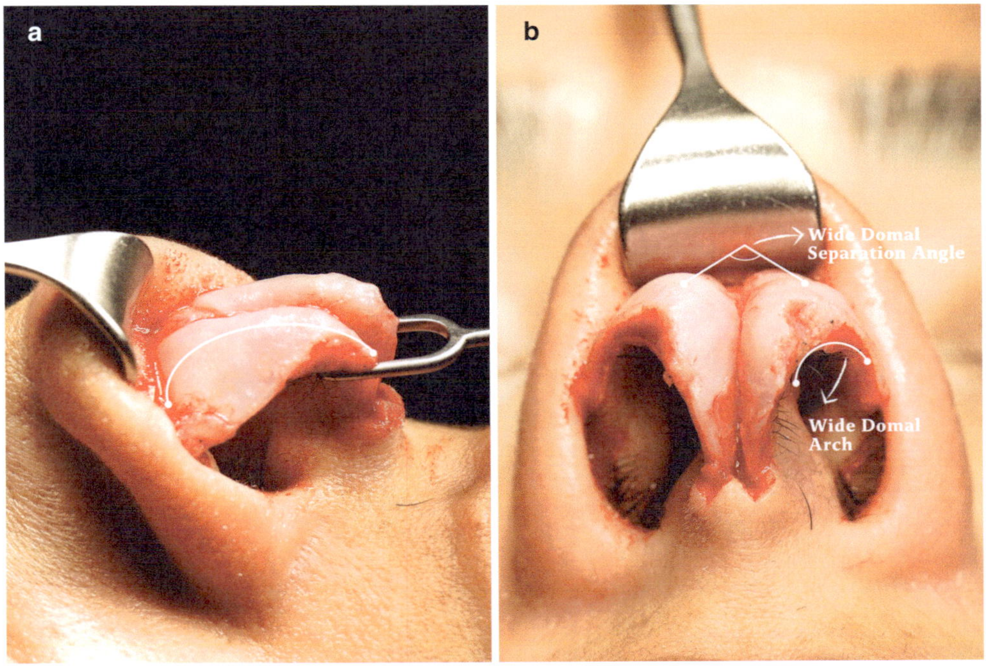

Fig. 13.112 (**a**, **b**) This photograph shows the length of the lateral crus and the hypertrophic extent thereof. Also, although the lateral crus exhibits a configurational deformity (being excessively convex), the configuration of the medial complex is good

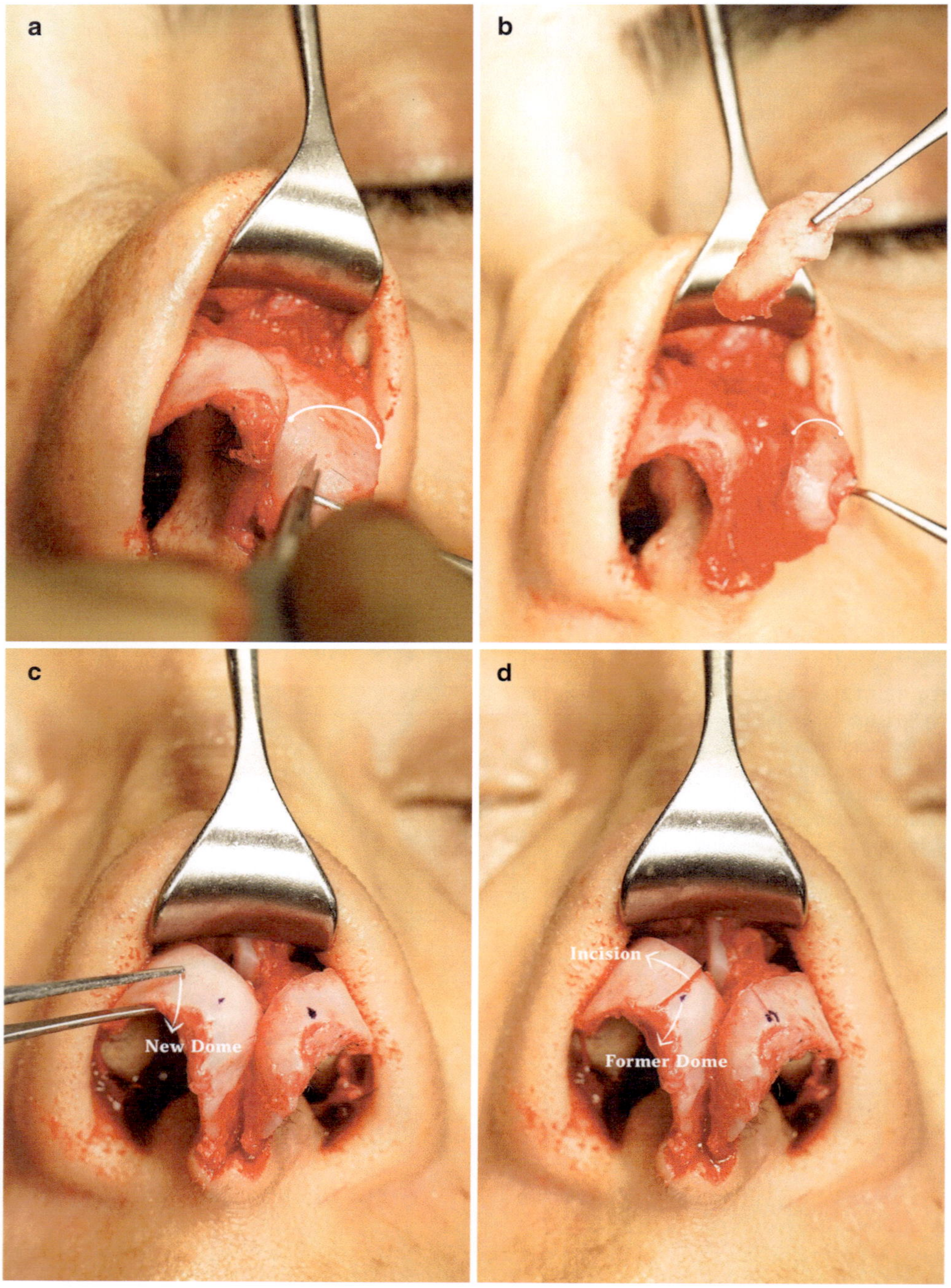

Fig. 13.113 (**a**, **b**) Compare the surface (**a**) before cephalic trimming (**b**) after cephalic trimming (**c**, **d**) The lateral crus was divided vertically just next to the marked ideal dome point

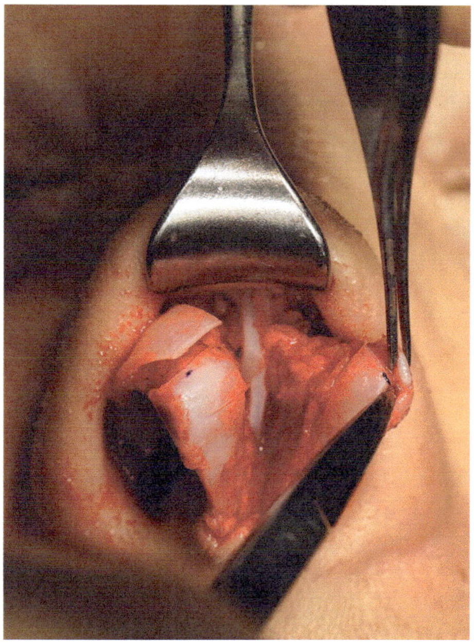

Fig. 13.114 Great care must be taken to perform this technique symmetrically

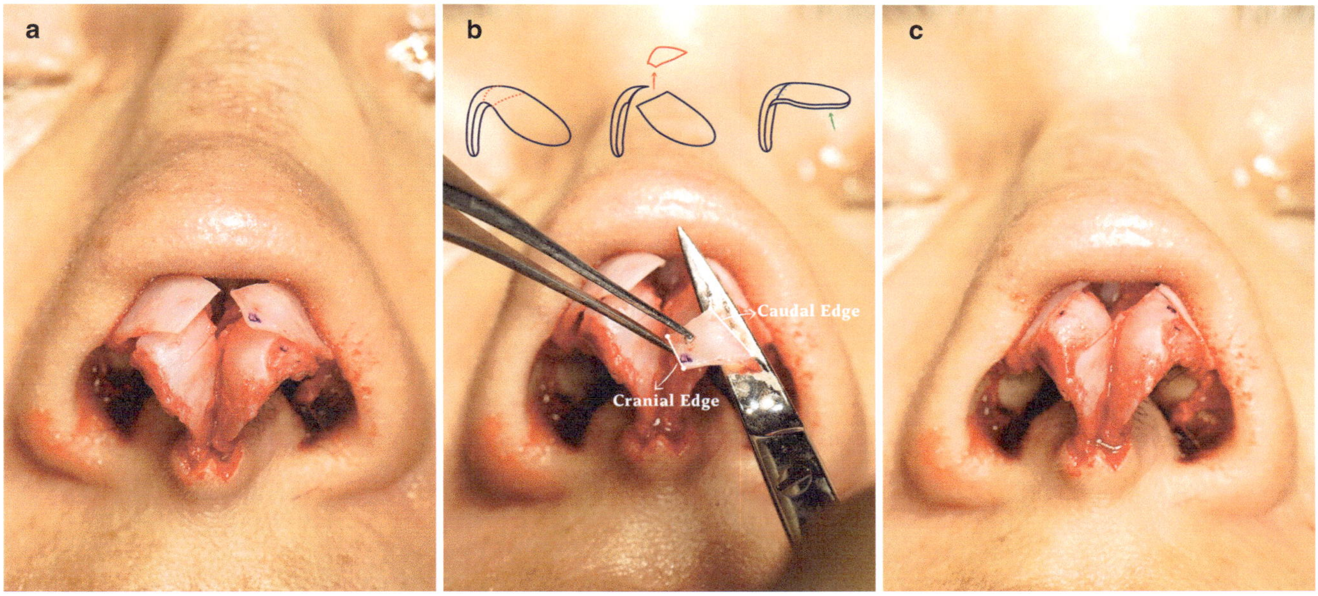

Fig. 13.115 (**a–c**) Pay attention to the shape of the removed part; to reach the ideal anatomy after suturing, the cranial edge should be longer than the caudal edge

Fig. 13.116 (**a**, **b**) Suture stabilization with mattress sutures

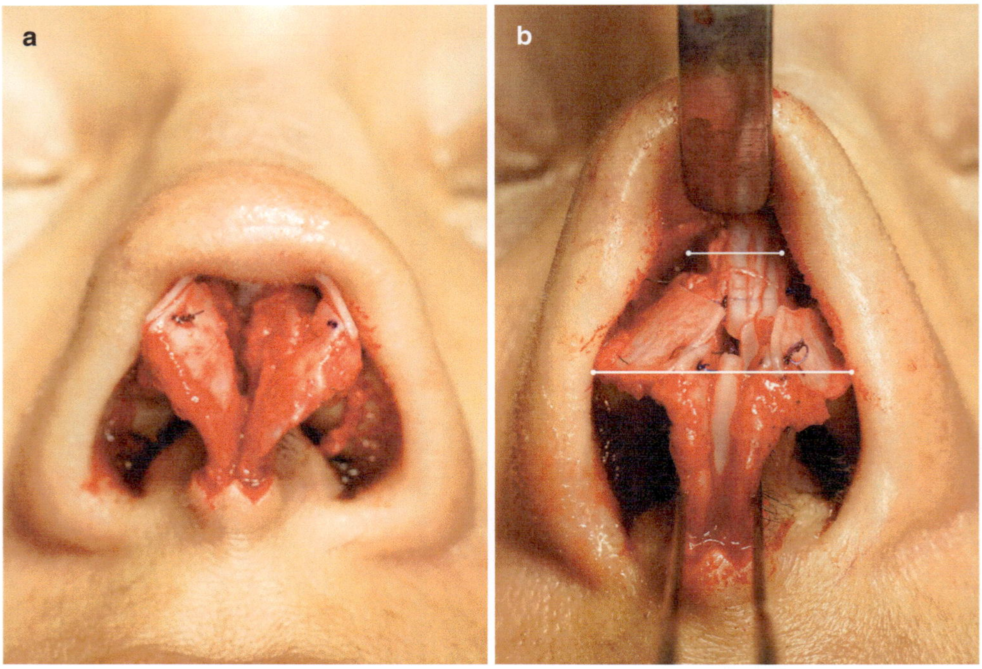

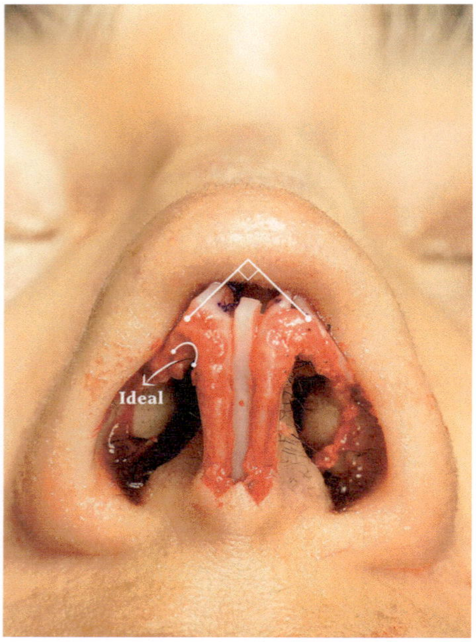

Fig. 13.117 Final view shows the degree of narrowing domal arch and deprojection achieved

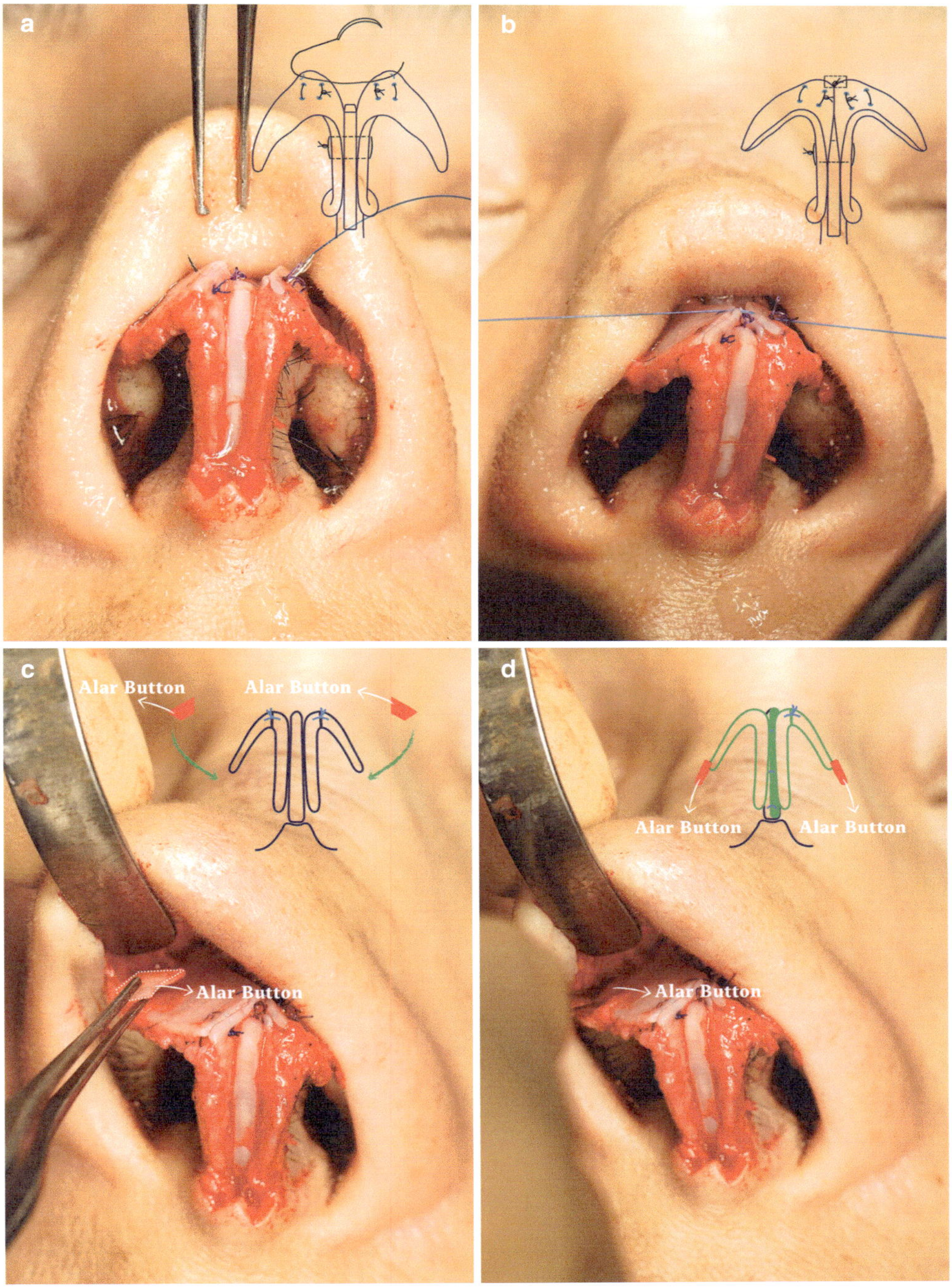

Fig. 13.118 (a–d) Approximately 1.5–2 mm thick cartilage grafts obtained from the septum cartilage were sutured to the caudal part of the lateral alar crura of the lower lateral cartilage as an onlay on the right and left with 5–0 pds sutures. Thus, using LACG, the caudal part of the lateral crura of the lower lateral cartilage was ideally positioned higher than the level of the cephalic part, and the external nasal valve was strengthened. The low the caudal part of the lateral crura of the lower lateral cartilage was elevated with LACG and the downward convex appearance of the lower lateral cartilage was corrected

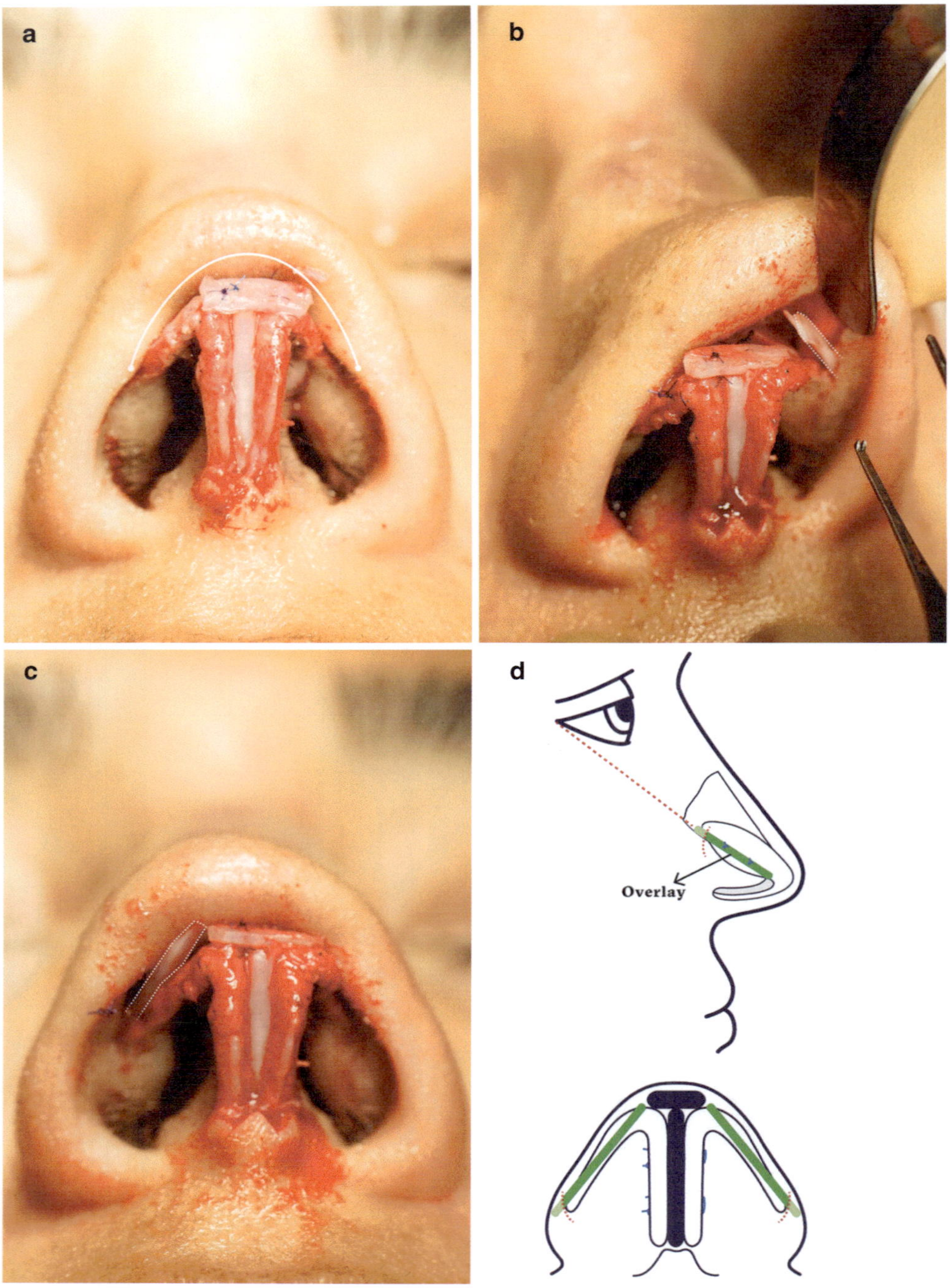

Fig. 13.119 (**a**, **b**) Septal lateral crural graft placement. (**c**) Immediately after surgery

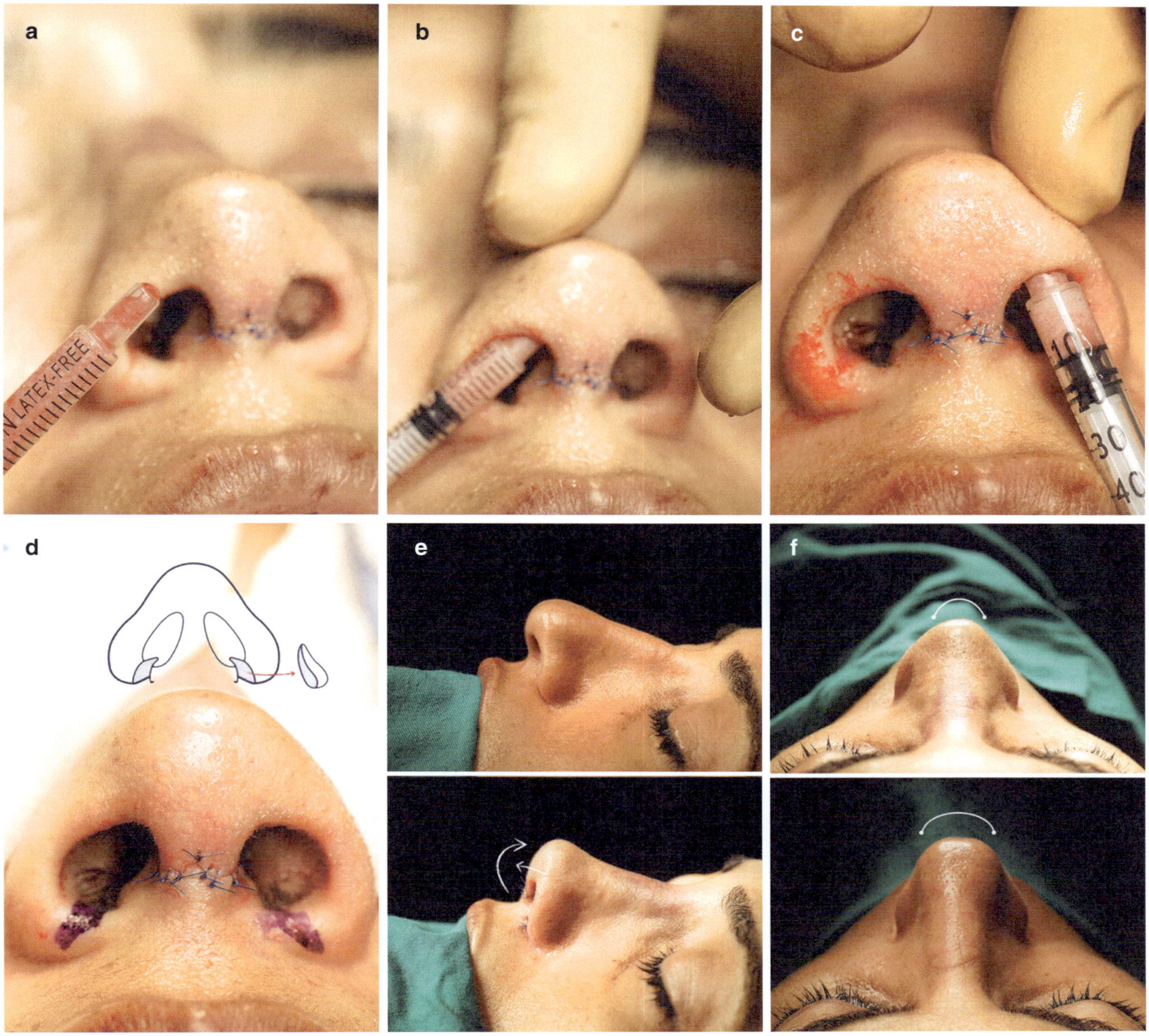

Fig. 13.120 (**a**, **b**, **c**) Injection of diced cartilage with insulin needle (**d**) Sill excision (**e**, **f**) Effects of VAR technique. Compare different views of the tip before and at the end of the procedure

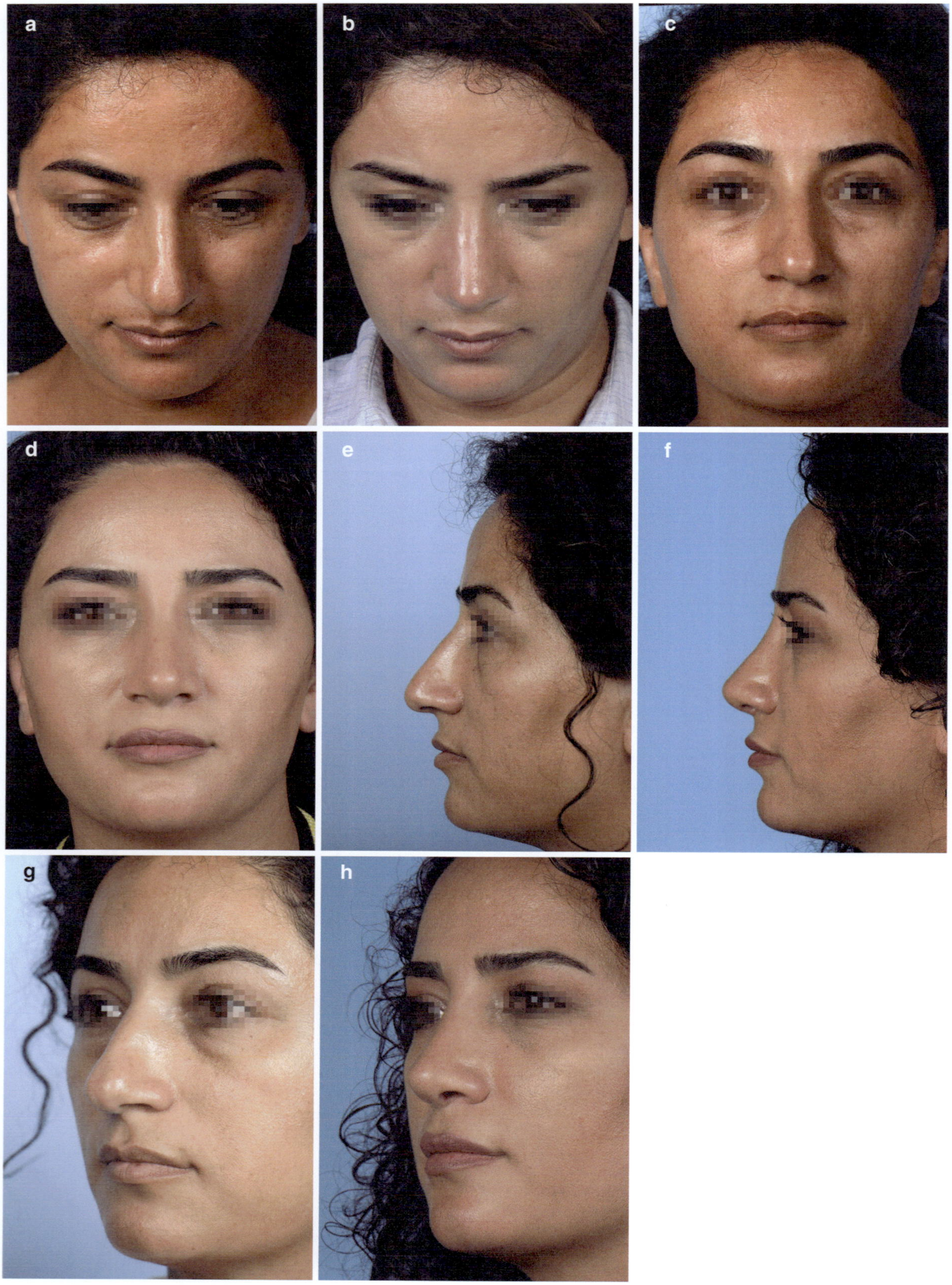

Fig. 13.121 (**a–h**) Preoperative views demonstrate thick skin envelope with a very wide bulbous and overprotected nasal tip. Postoperatively the tip has been narrowed and deprojected by shortening the lateral crura mainly with VAR technique

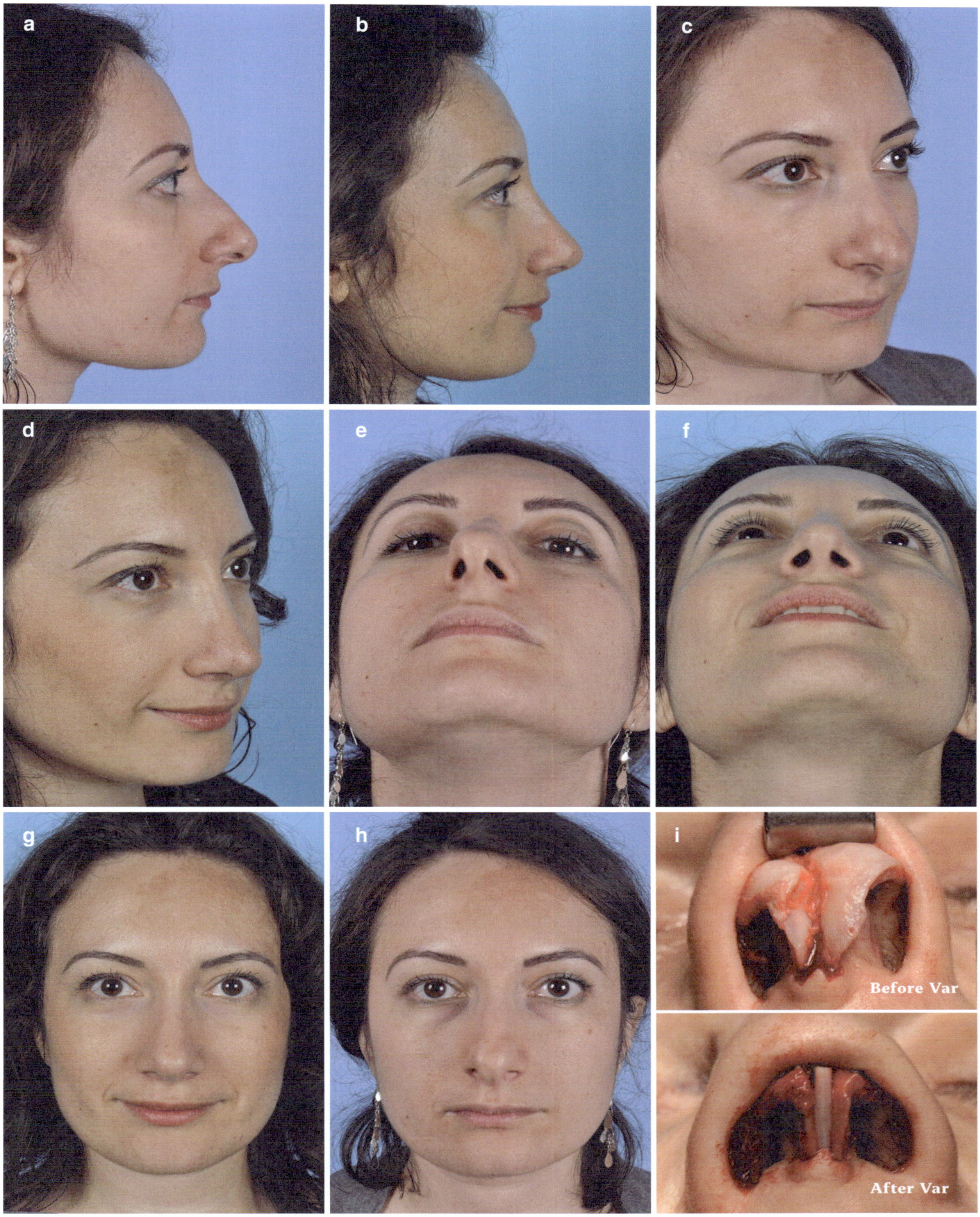

Fig. 13.122 (**a–h**) This 25-year-old woman desired a smaller, symmetrical nose. She had a broad, slightly over-projected, asymmetric nasal tip, and long infratip lobule due to prolonged and asymmetrical lateral crura. Vertical alar resection was performed to shorten and make the lateral crura symmetrical. A columellar strut was placed to maintain projection, and a dome-equalizing suture was placed for further lobule refinement and stability. Alar batten and cap graft also were placed standardly. Postoperatively, the tip is narrower, and the proportion between the tip and dorsum on the lateral view has been established. On base view, the tip is now triangular and symmetrical. The infratip lobule is no longer anesthetically dependent and the columella lobular angle has been corrected. The bifidity is also corrected

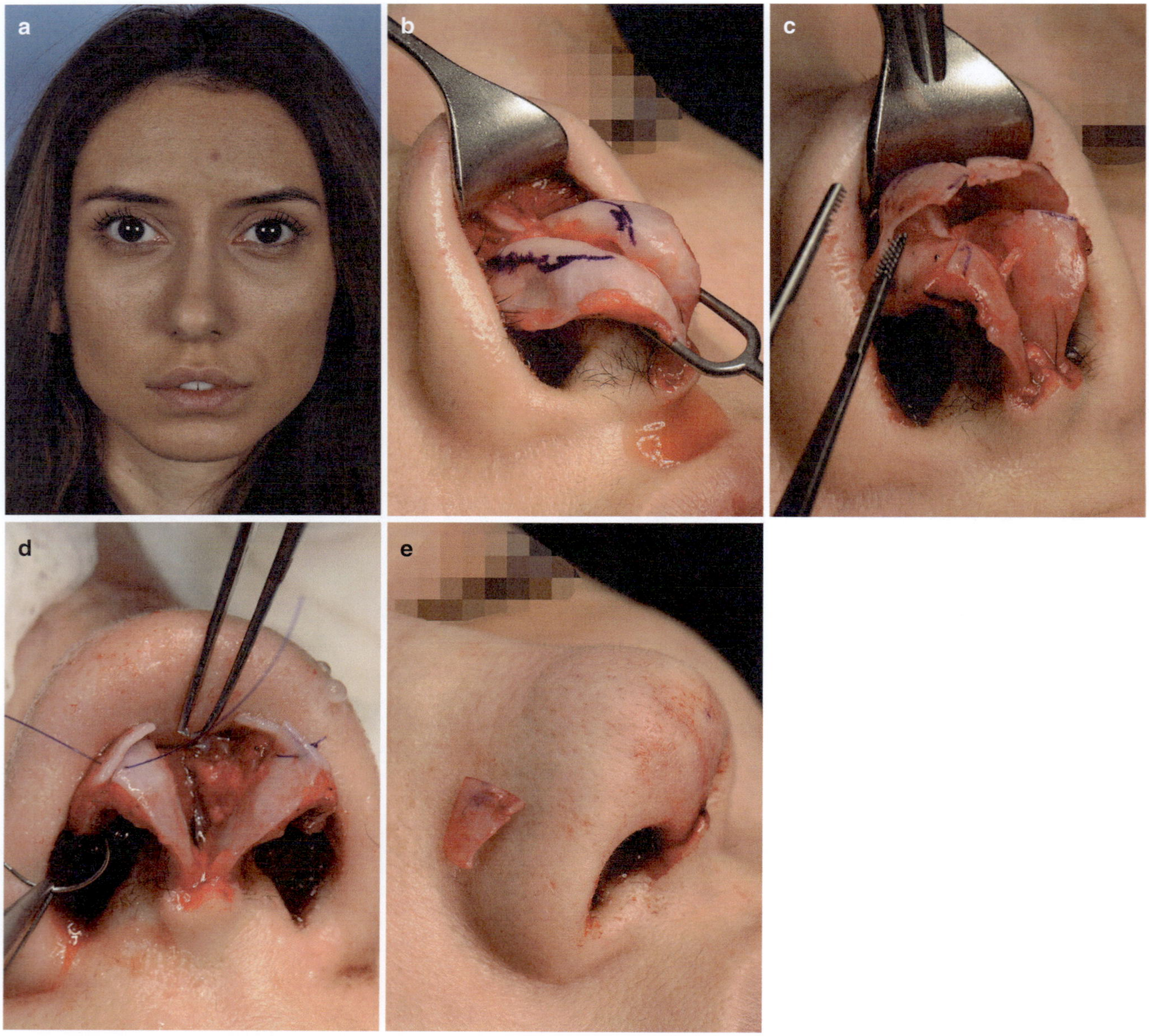

Fig. 13.123 (**a–e**) The lateral crus was horizontally overdeveloped and configurationally deformed, whereas the medial crus was not deformed. Thus, the VAR technique was preferred

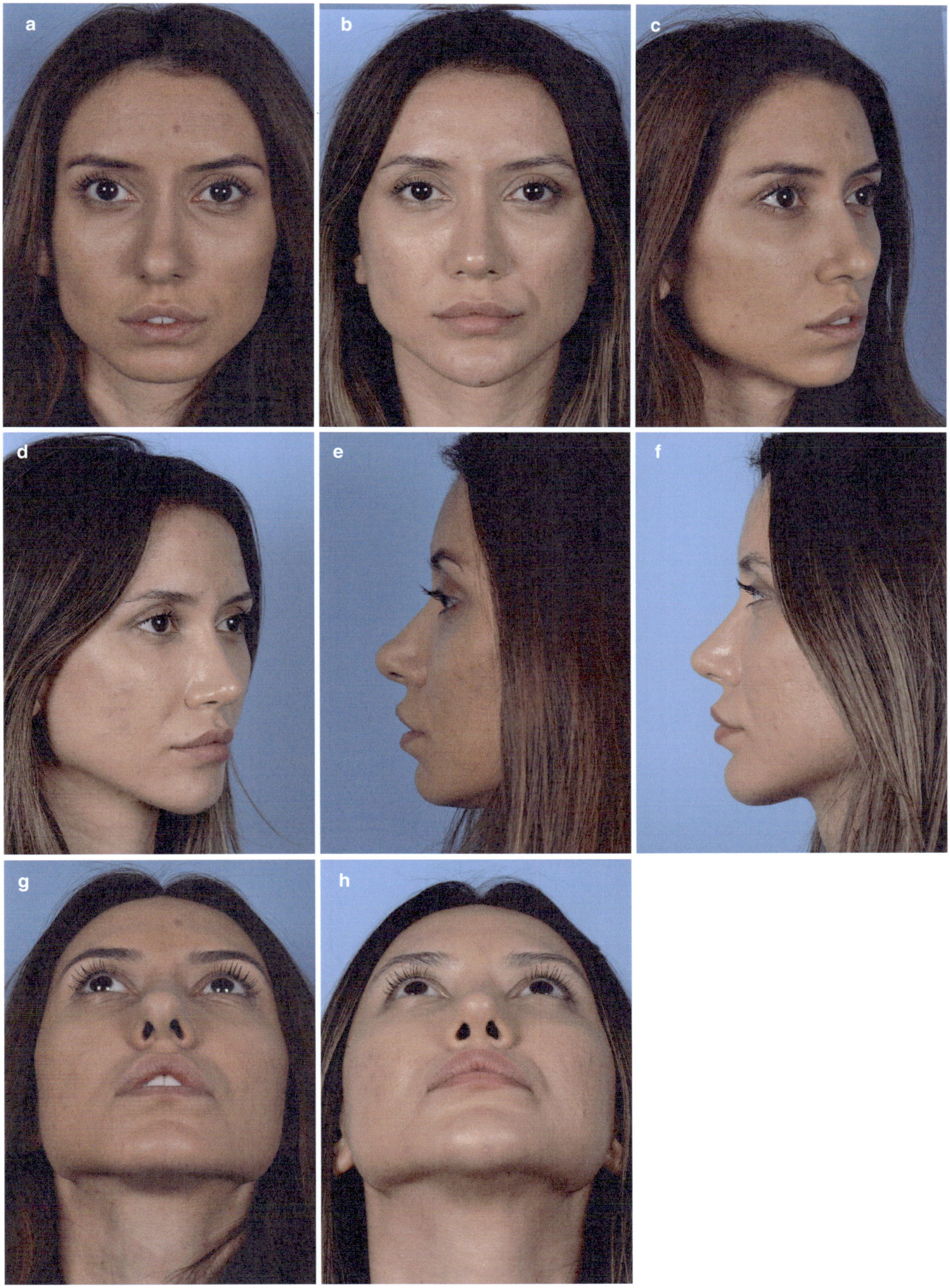

Fig. 13.124 (**a–h**) Preoperative and postoperative photographs. After the VAR technique, note differences between before and after nasal tip contour

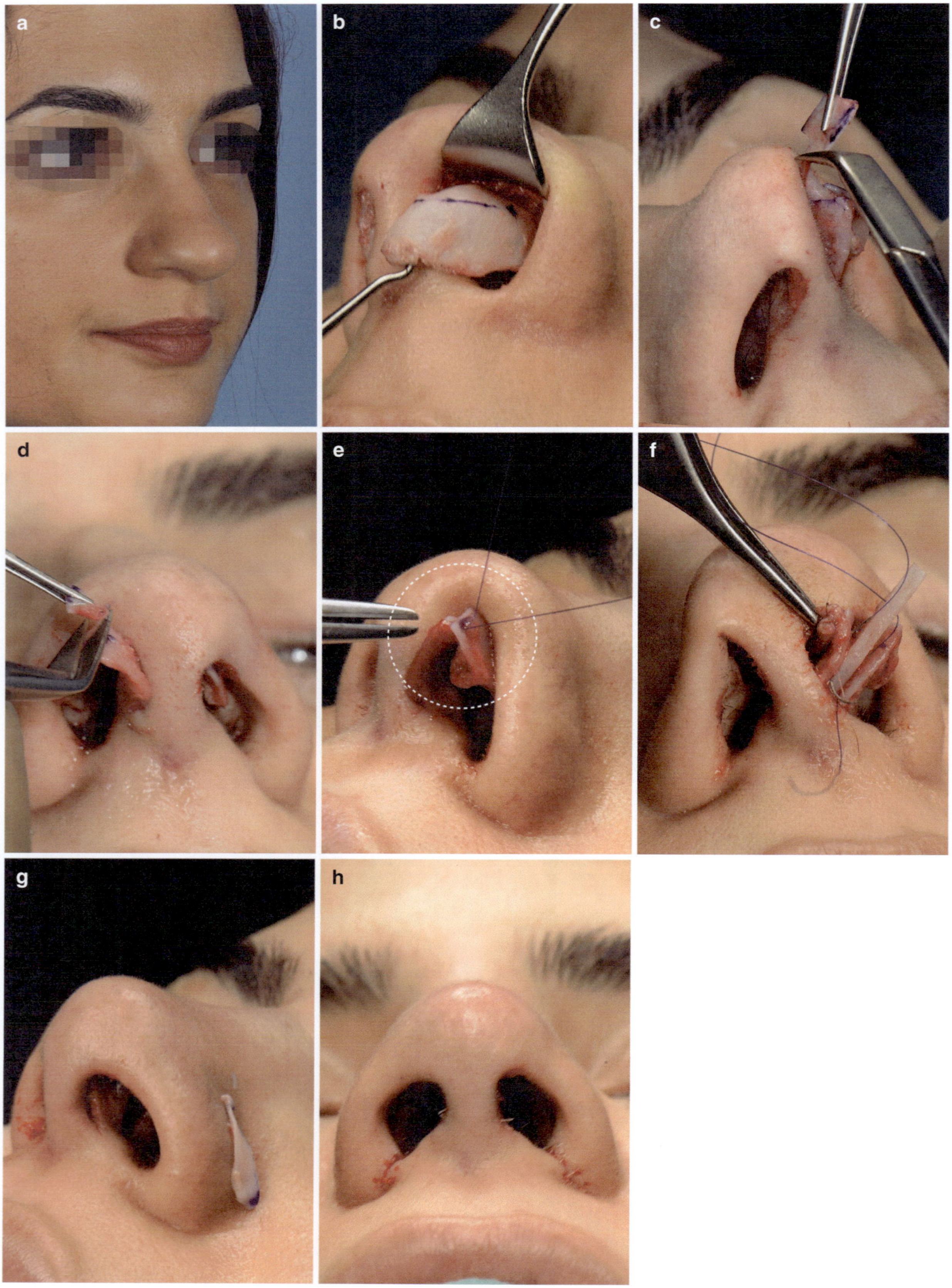

Fig. 13.125 (**a–h**) Clearly seen lateral crura are overdeveloped. The lateral crura in each nostril should be resected separately. Remaining steps are exactly the same as those of the open approach

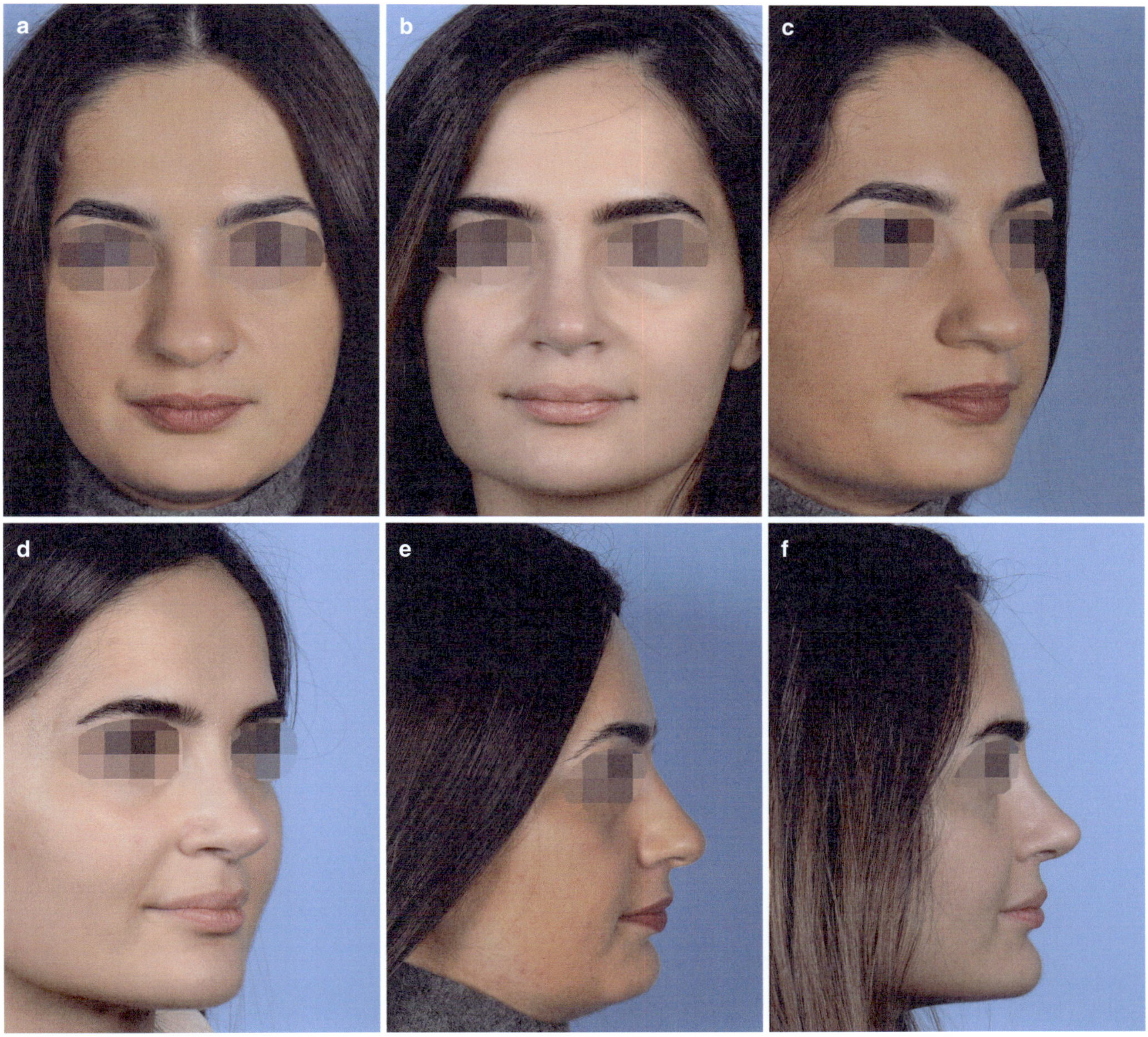

Fig. 13.126 (**a–f**) Slight lateral crural reduction and tip grafts have created an elegant and more balanced nasal tip

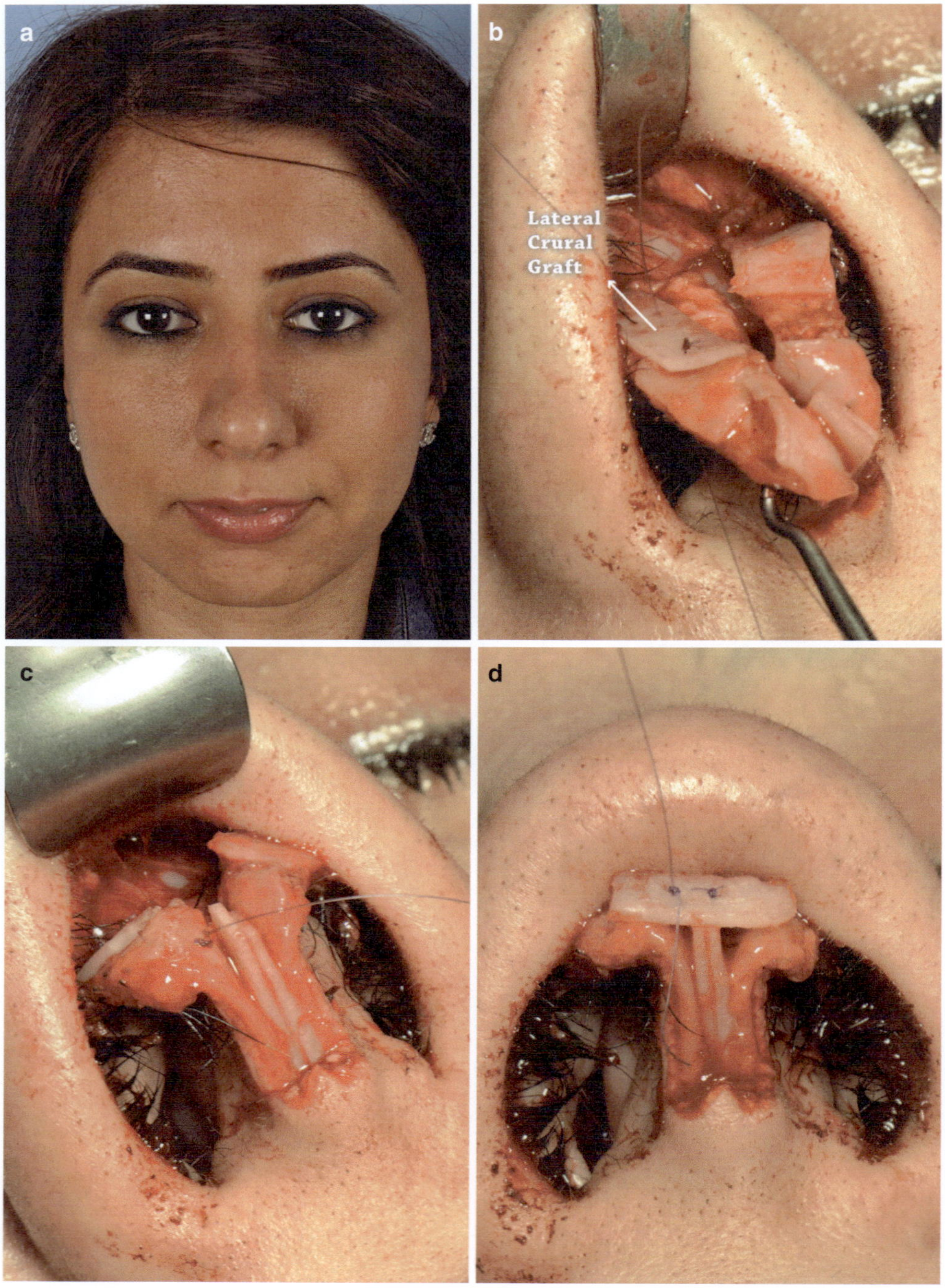

Fig. 13.127 (**a**) Frontal view of a wide tip with thick skin. (**b**, **c**) Overdevelopment Lateral crus was shortened by vertical alar resection. A lateral crural graft was fixed over the lateral crus. (**d**) A cap graft was placed. In thick-skinned patients, a cap graft does not require camouflage

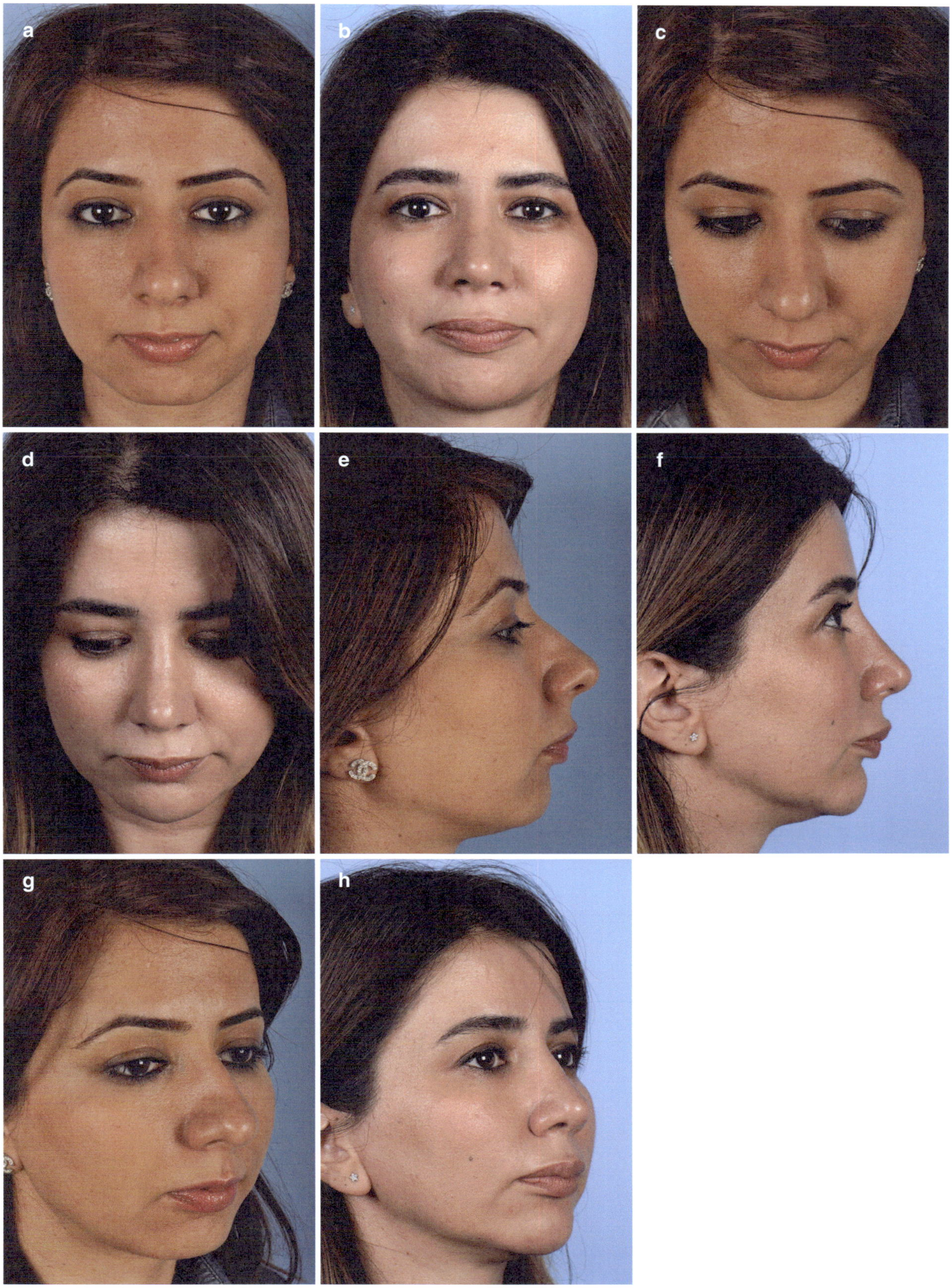

Fig. 13.128 (**a–h**) Long-term success has been achieved. To achieve the goals of a natural, refined, aesthetically flattering appearance, the tip has adhered to certain guiding principles: reconstruction of favorable structural components, reorientation, and augmentation of selected areas

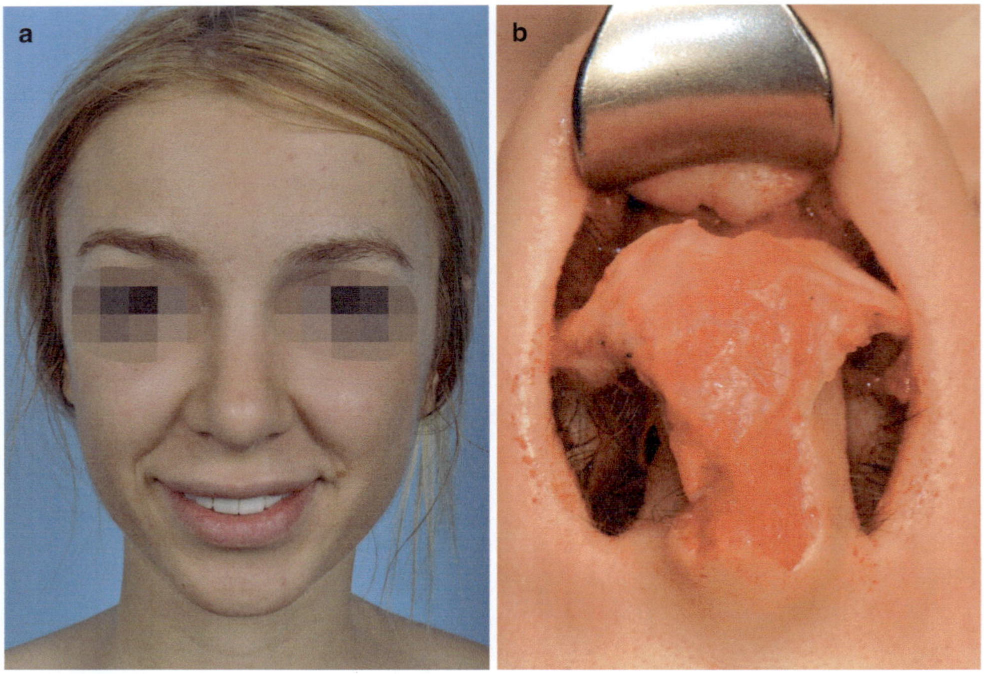

Fig. 13.129 (**a**) A preoperative frontal view; the patient had undergone rhinoplasty 3 years prior. The tip is amorphous and wide. (**b**) Intraoperative photographs show an unfavorable craniocaudal relationship of the lateral crus

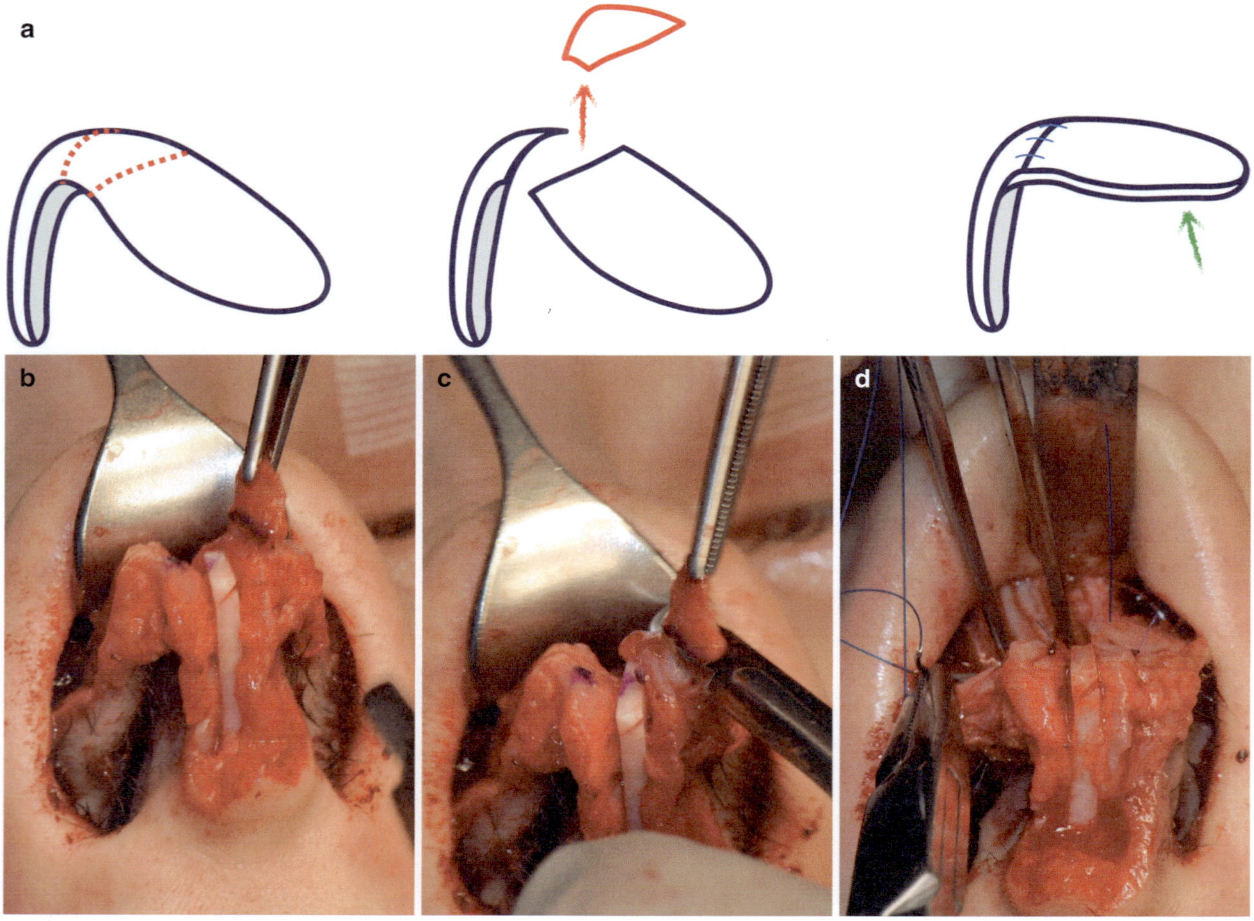

Fig. 13.130 (**a**) A trapezoidal incision was created immediately lateral to the dome, allowing the caudal edge to move upward; this was followed by end-to-end suturing. (**b–d**) A columellar strut and a cap graft were also placed. Careful examination of the lateral crura showed that the caudocranial relationship had been corrected

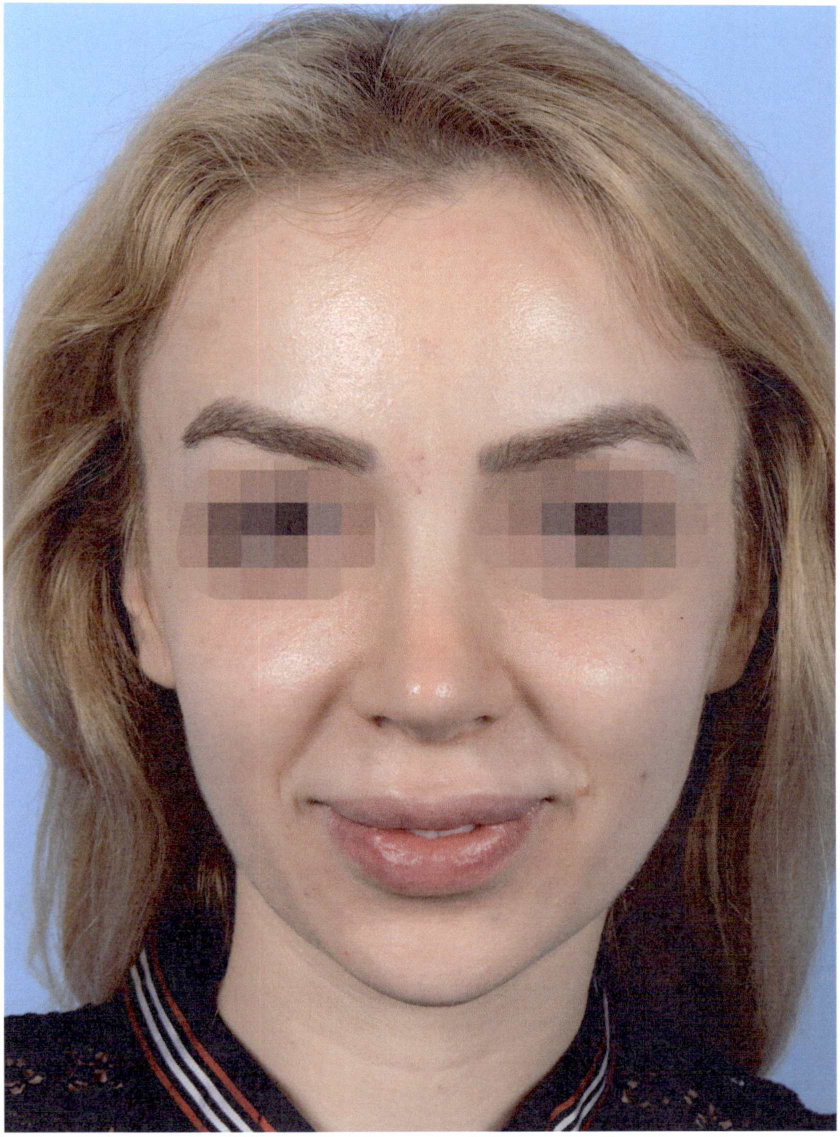

Fig. 13.131 Note that placement of the lateral crural plane in the ideal position not only enhanced tip definition but also strengthened the lateral wall

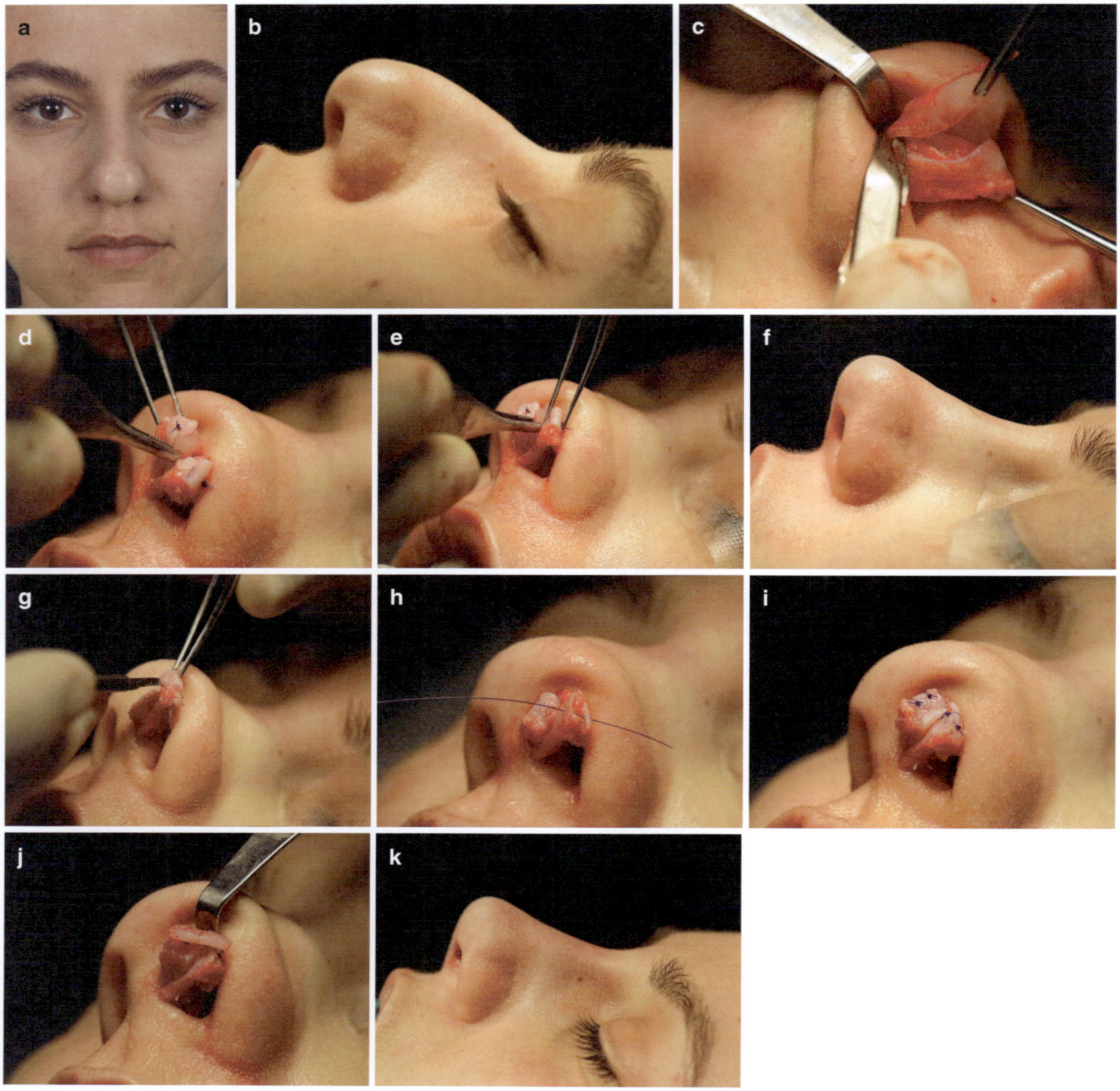

Fig. 13.132 (**a**) A preoperative frontal view. A prominent, wide nasal tip is apparent. (**b**) Intraoperative lateral view. (**c–e**) Cephalic resection, transdomal suturing, and placement of a columellar strut and a lateral crural graft. (**f**) After intermediate techniques were used, the wide nasal tip was narrowed. However, if this is not satisfactory, the strategy should be changed. (**g–j**) The suture was removed. The tip was wide because the excess lateral crus had not been resected. This was done, and a columellar strut and cup graft were placed. (**k**) More satisfying results were achieved intraoperatively

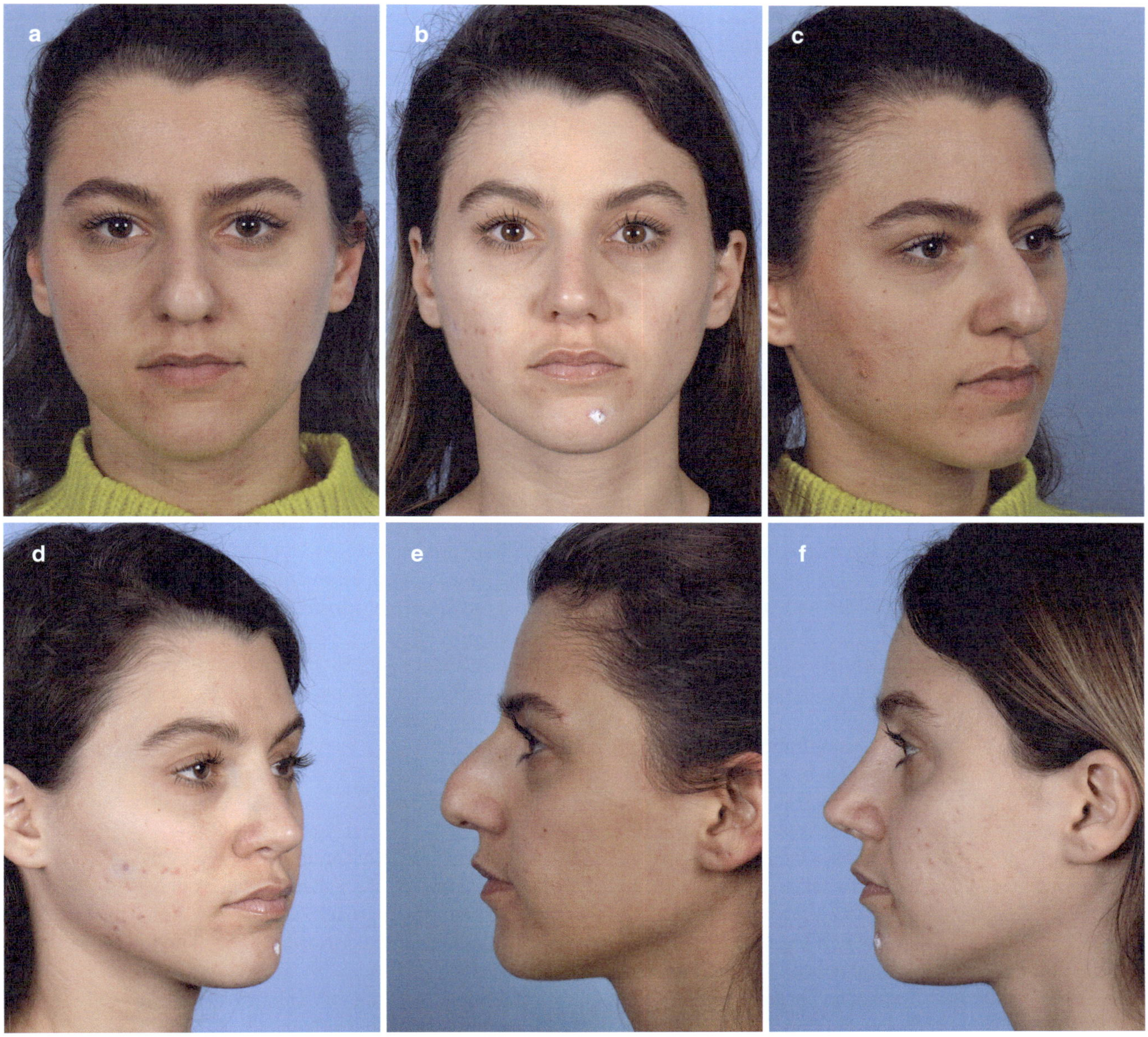

Fig. 13.133 (**a–f**) Pre- and postoperative photographs

13.5 Repositioning of the Lateral Crus

Lateral crural malpositioning can cause a wide nasal tip. The surface anatomy of a nose with cephalically malpositioned lateral crura is suggestive of a parenthesis-like deformity; shadows are apparent lateral to the nasal tip, which is wide; furthermore, the alar rims are notched, and the nose is almost square when viewed from below.

Repositioning of the lateral crus corrects these problems and can also be used to modify tip projection and rotation. In either case, the principle is the same; the lateral crura are completely released from the vestibular skin and placed into caudally oriented pockets. This can be performed with lateral crural grafting; grafts solve lateral crural deformities and reinforce the lateral nasal wall.

Surgery involves four steps:

1. The lateral crura are dissected from the vestibular mucosa. The dissected cartilage is turned, folded, and reinforced by suturing the layers, to help correct crural configurational deformities. If the patient has neither sufficiently strong nor wide lateral crura for folding, septal or costal cartilage strips can be used.
2. Pockets are opened in the alar sidewalls in the direction of the lateral canthus, and the newly formed lateral crura are inserted; the deeper the insertion, the greater the increase in tip rotation.

3. A new domal point is created via transdomal suturing. As is also true when lateral crural stealing is employed, the dome can be moved laterally to increase projection, if necessary.
4. Finally, for all patients undergoing surgery to treat malpositioning, the tip is linked to the septum via a septocolumellar strut or a suture to ensure stability.

Repositioning of cephalically oriented lateral crura can be accomplished either endonasally or via an external approach.

13.5.1 Case 34

Preoperative photographs of a patient complaining of a wide nasal tip are shown. A clear parenthesis-like deformity is evident on the frontal view, and demarcation of the tip and dorsum is apparent on an oblique view, indicating malpositioning (Fig. 13.134).

The intraoperative photographs show that although both lateral crura run in the direction of the medial canthus, they are parallel. The optimal 30° difference is absent, confirming that the wide nasal tip is associated with lateral crural malpositioning (Fig. 13.135).

Repositioning surgery then commenced. Both lateral crura were completely elevated from the vestibular skin and mobilized (Fig. 13.136).

Before repositioning, the configurational deformity was corrected, and stability thus enhanced. A midline incision was created in the crus (the residual portion was 7 mm in length), and the cephalic segment was turned, folded, and fixed at three points (Fig. 13.137). (Cephalic turn-in flap.)

The crus was inserted into a pocket created in the direction of the lateral canthus (Fig. 13.138).

A new domal point was defined via transdomal suturing and the nasal projection was checked. This was acceptable because the columellar strut that had been previously sutured between the medial crura was fixed to them, thus ensuring columellar base stability (Fig. 13.139).

After ideal projection and rotation were achieved, stabilization was addressed. Septocolumellar suturing commenced in the caudal segment of the right medial crus, crossed the septum, and terminated at the left medial crus (Fig. 13.140).

After the crus was repositioned, a gap was evident at the former crural position; this was filled with diced cartilage (Fig. 13.141).

Lateral nasal splinting is always required postoperatively; this case underwent repositioning surgery because of prior malpositioning. Patient-specific plastic splints were placed inside and outside both nostrils. Overtightening must be avoided when fixing the splints with sutures; otherwise, skin necrosis may develop. The splints and cast were removed 1 week later. If splints are not used, the recovery time is prolonged, and patients may suffer from long-term nasal congestion and vestibular swelling. The 2-year postoperative photograph shows that repositioning surgery reduced the width of the nasal tip, increased rotation, and somewhat decreased projection (Fig. 13.142).

13.5.2 Case 35

Here is a similar case; both lateral crura were completely released via open rhinoplasty. Each crus was fixed at three different points after turning and folding portions longer than 7 mm. New pockets were opened in the direction of the lateral canthus and the lateral crura were inserted. Standard suture plasty followed. A new dome was created via transdomal suturing. Columellar base stability was ensured by placing a columellar strut and a septocolumellar suture. Unlike in the previous case, gaps in the lateral nasal wall were filled by delivery of diced cartilage using an insulin syringe, followed by closure of all incisions. The gaps show where the lateral crura were removed (Fig. 13.143; Video 13.24).

The 1-year postoperative photographs show that all tip-related problems were corrected using a single basic maneuver (Fig. 13.144).

Repositioning surgery can also use a delivery approach, depending on the training, experience, and personal preference of the surgeon.

13.5.3 Case 36

Figure 13.145 displays an intraoperative view (from below) of a wide nasal tip; the patient had thick skin.

An endonasal approach was used to straighten both alar cartilages. The lateral crus runs in the direction of the lateral canthus (Fig. 13.146).

The lateral crus was completely dissected from the vestibular skin using scissors (Fig. 13.147).

Supraperichondrial dissection and release of both LLCs followed (Fig. 13.148).

The lateral crus is not wide; the excess region cannot be turned and folded. Therefore, cephalic resection was completed in a highly conservative manner, and lateral crural grafts were placed on both sides and sutured to the undersurfaces of the lateral crura (Fig. 13.149).

The new crura were placed into pockets that were more caudally positioned than normal. The operation was completed by placing a transdomal suture, a columellar strut, and a septocolumellar suture (Fig. 13.150).

Preoperative and 1-year postoperative photographs are seen in Fig. 13.151: The parentheses, which are pathognomonic of malposition of the lateral crura, have been ablated. A minimal reduction of the dorsum has preserved the well-proportioned size of the patient's nose.

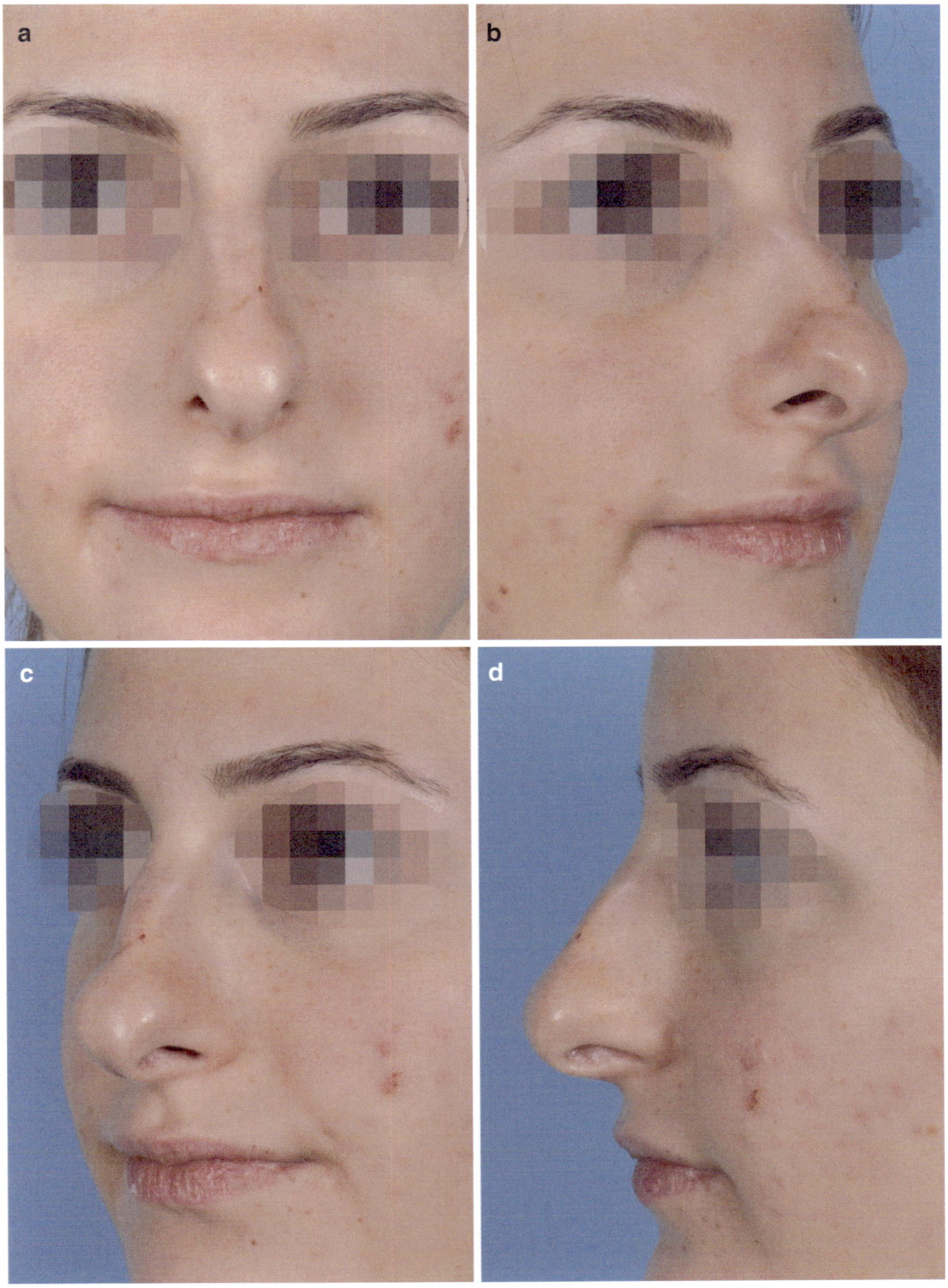

Fig. 13.134 (**a–d**) Note the demarcation between nasal subunits and parenthesis appearance

Fig. 13.135 The parenthesis deformity seen intraoperatively

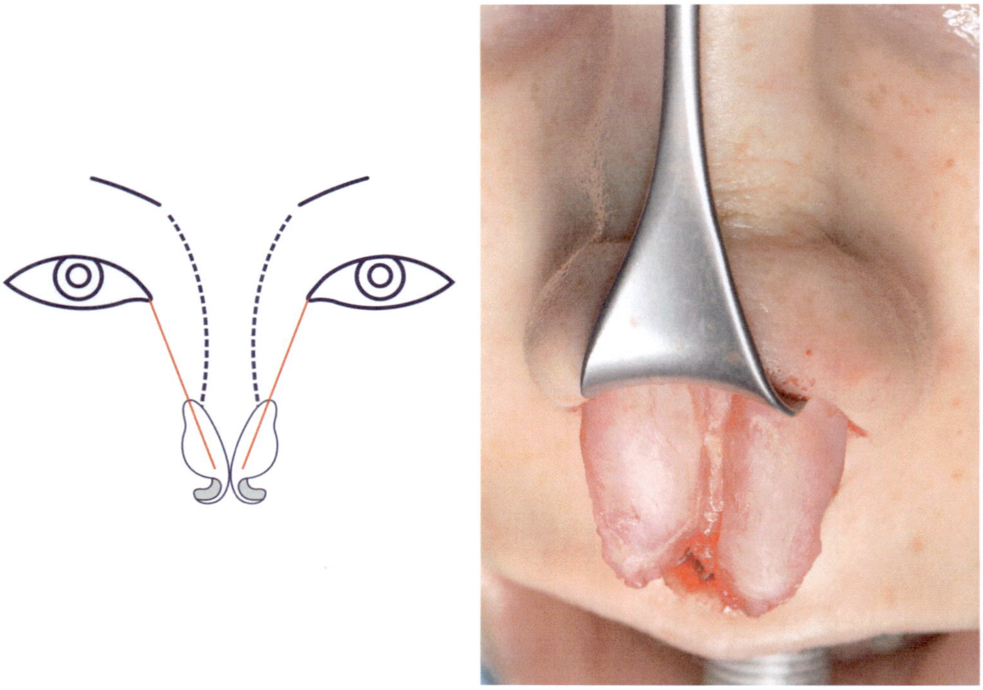

Fig. 13.136 Complete separation of the lateral crura from the skin

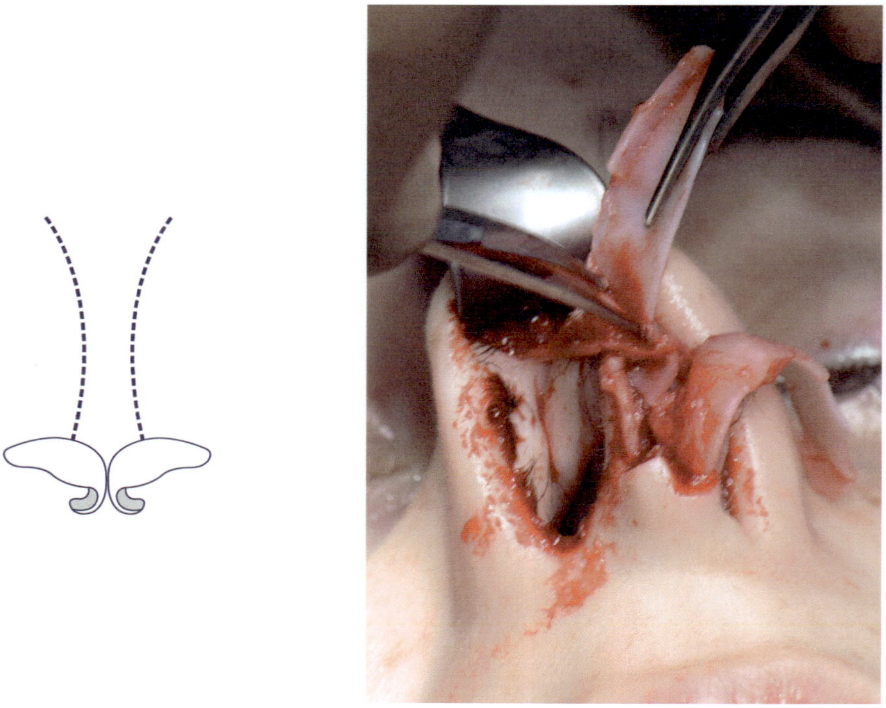

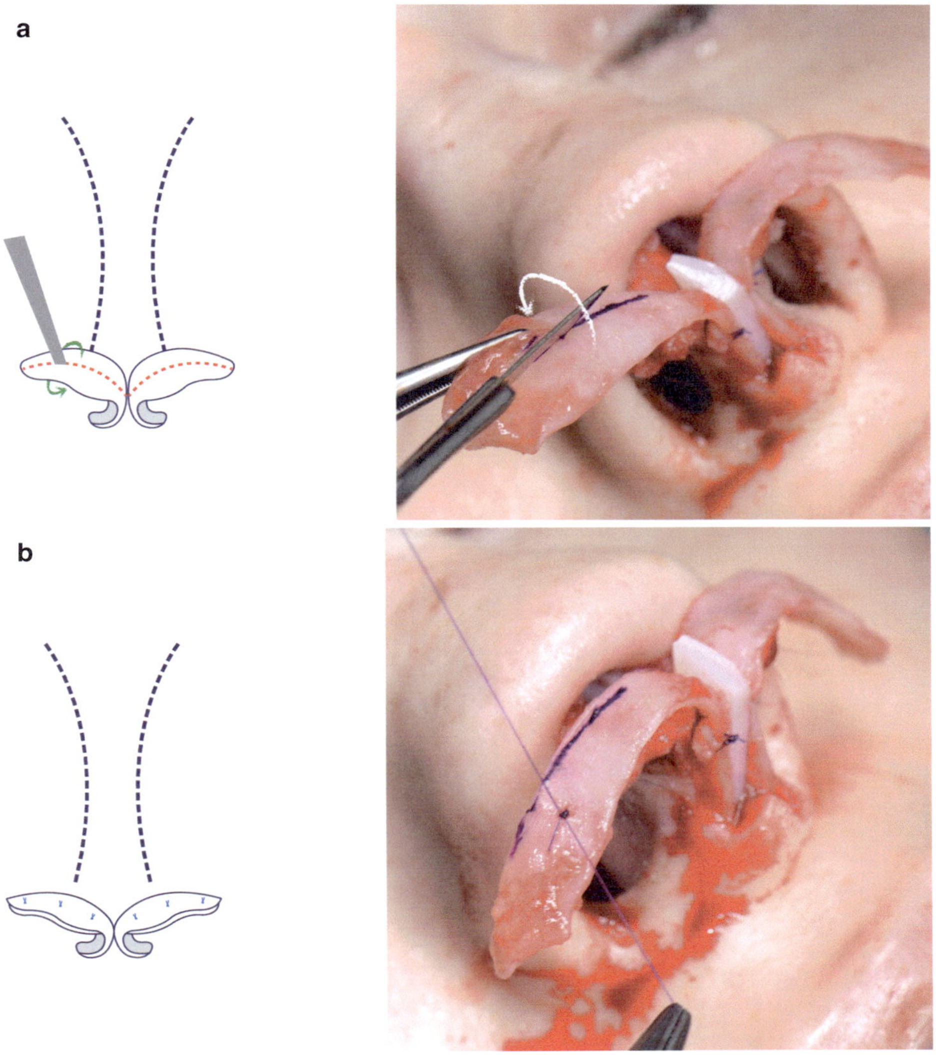

Fig. 13.137 (**a**) Lateral crura was divided horizontally. (**b**) The cranial part (flap) was turned in. The turn-in part is secured with 5–0 absorbable sutures, with the knot placed on the dorsal surface

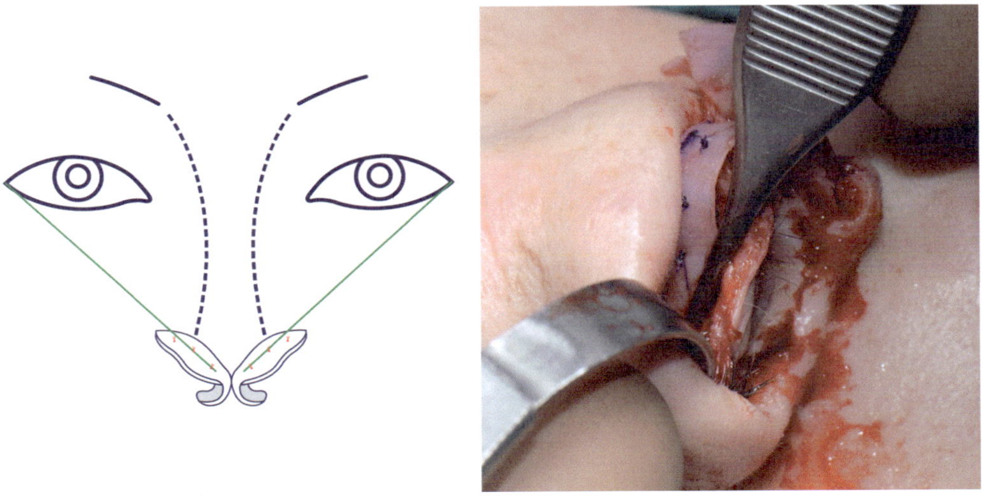

Fig. 13.138 Placement of the newly formed lateral crura into caudally dissected pockets

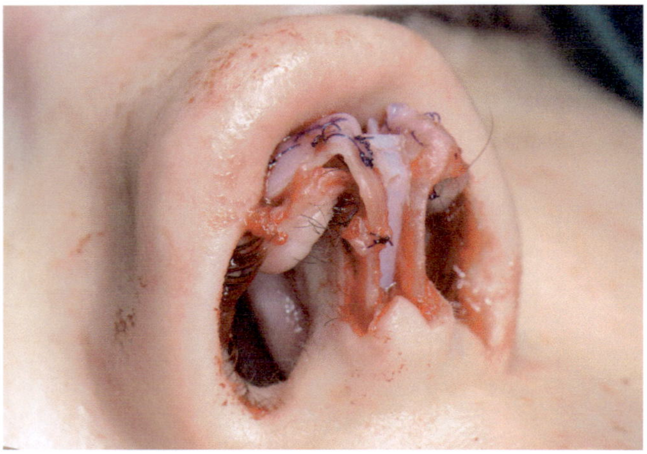

Fig. 13.139 Transdomal sutures were placed

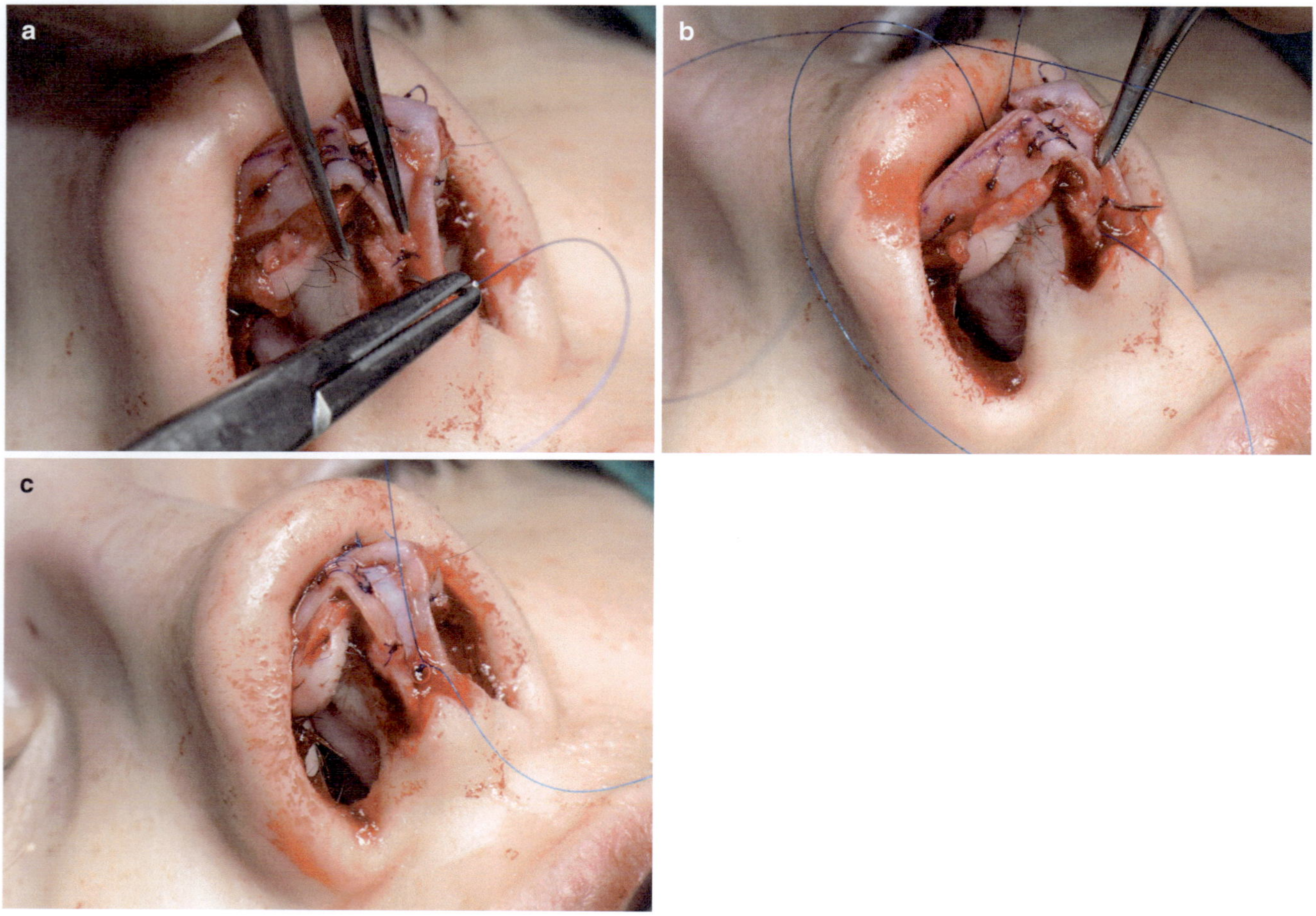

Fig. 13.140 (**a–c**) Septocolumellar suture was placed to create extra support for the newly shaped nasal tip

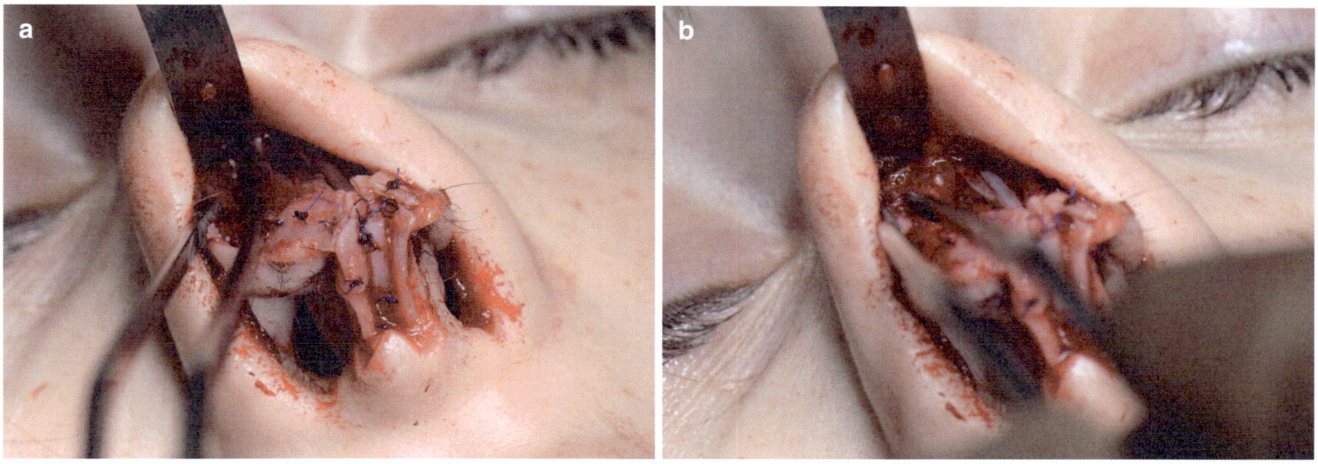

Fig. 13.141 (**a**, **b**) Diced cartilages were placed to fill gaps

Fig. 13.142 (**a–h**) In the case above, the wide nasal tip was caused by malpositioning of the lateral crura. Correction of the crural direction resolved not only the tip issue but also tip asymmetry and alar notch retraction

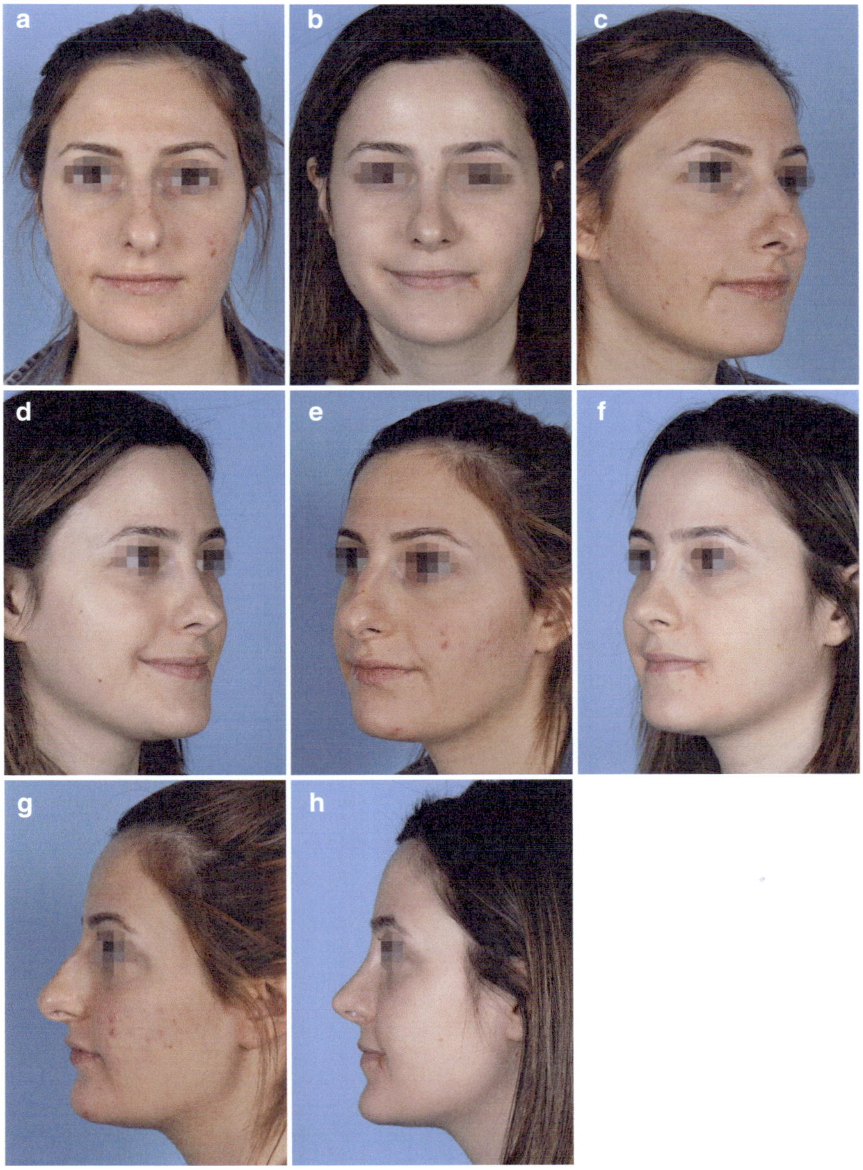

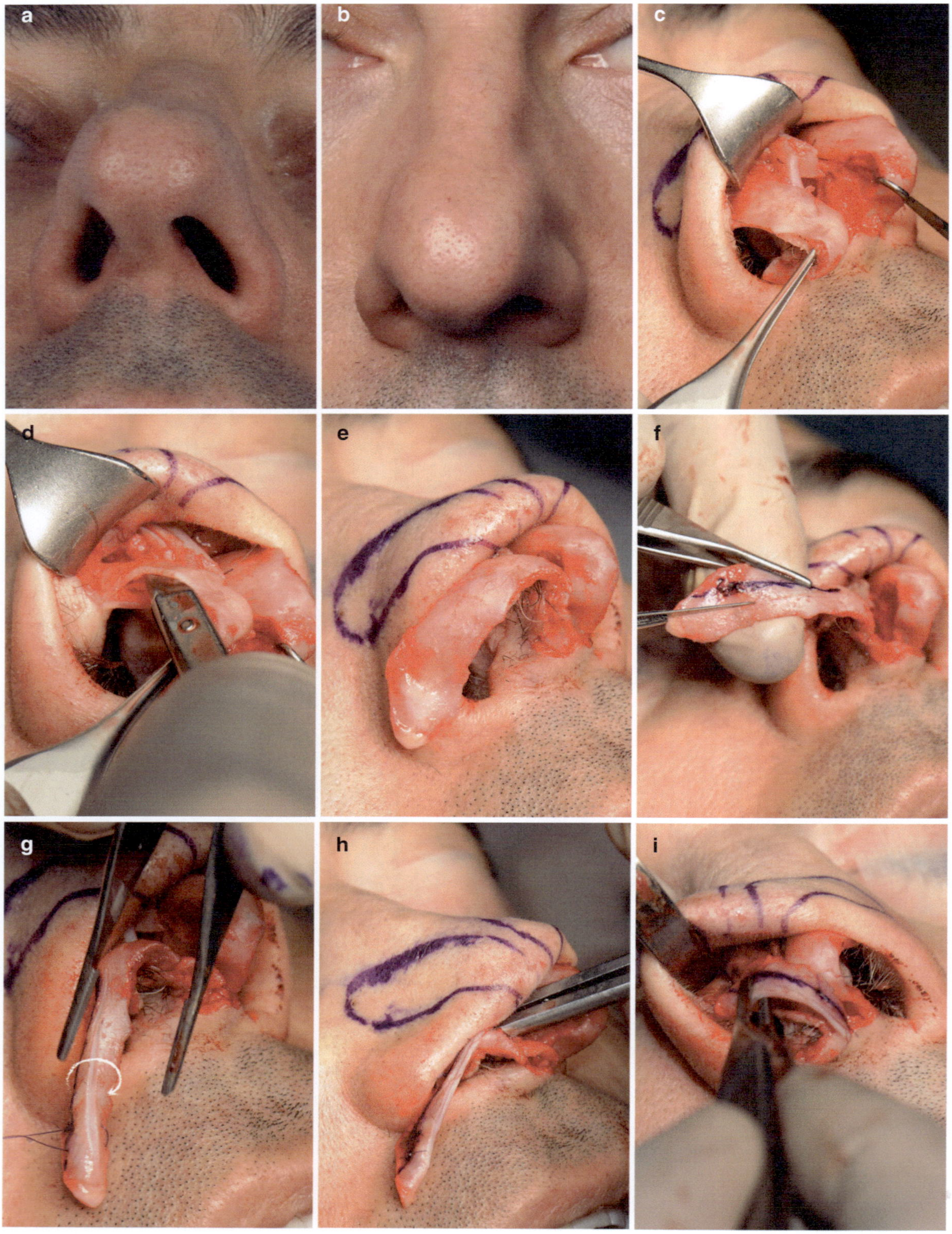

Fig. 13.143 (**a–c**) The parenthesis deformity seen here is characterized by malpositioned lateral crura and weak lateral alar wall support. Any resection or suturing of this little support will promptly cause to collapse and obstruction. Repositioning of the lateral crura must be a primary surgical maneuver. (**d–o**) The first lateral crura were detached from vestibular skin. Each one was then subdivided into two segments: caudal and cranial. In this case, the caudal flap was turned in. The caudal turn-in flap was secured at three points with two to three 5–0 PDS sutures. This folding is flattened preexisting concavities of the LLC and served as structural support for it. Once the changes to the lower lateral crura are complete, a soft tissue pocket was created bilaterally to the outer canthus within the alar lobule. Finally, the lateral crura were inserted into the newly formed soft tissue pockets. After bilateral relocation, new dome points were created. Columellar strut and septocolumellar sutures were placed for strong medial tip support

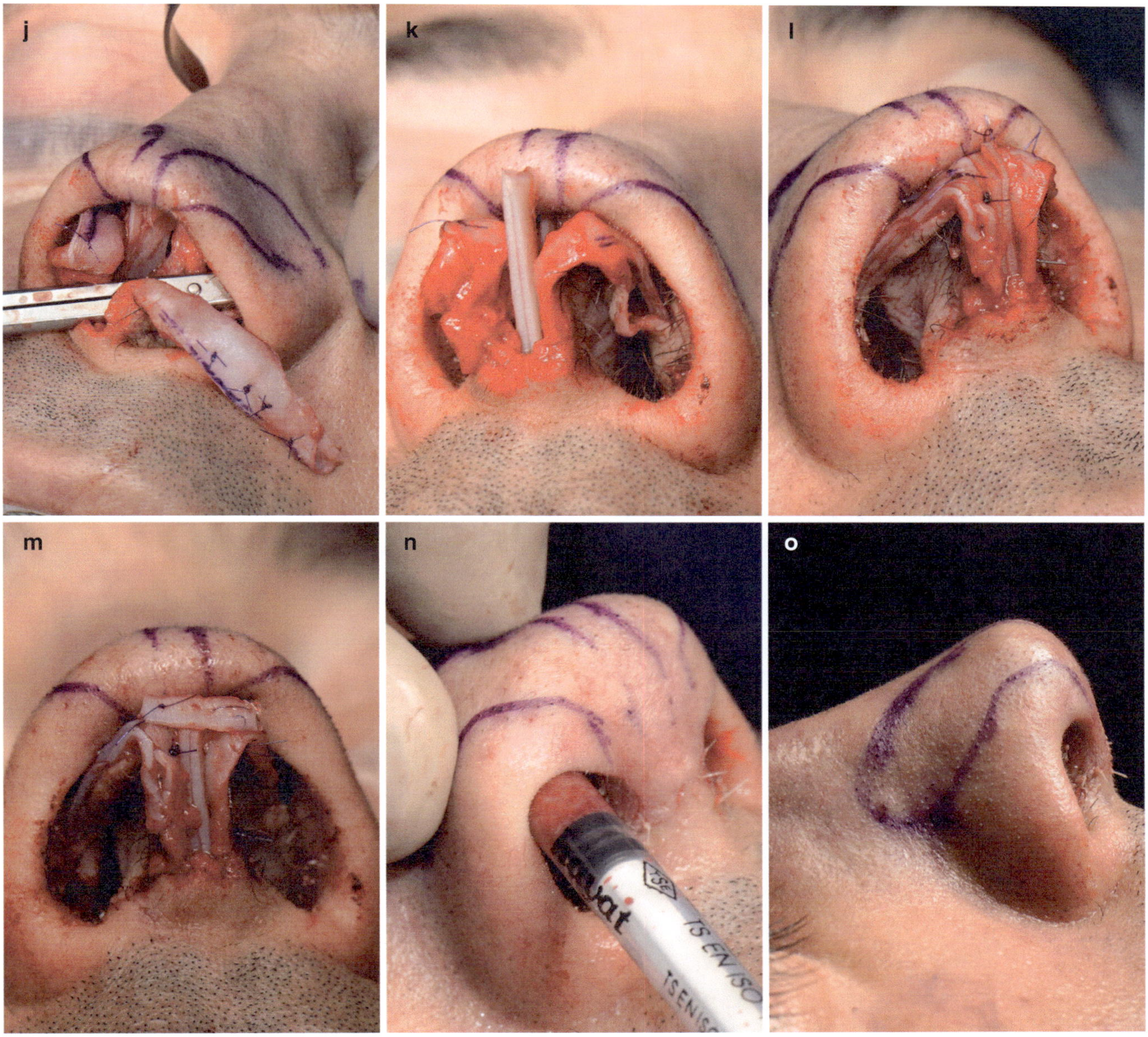

Fig. 13.143 (continued)

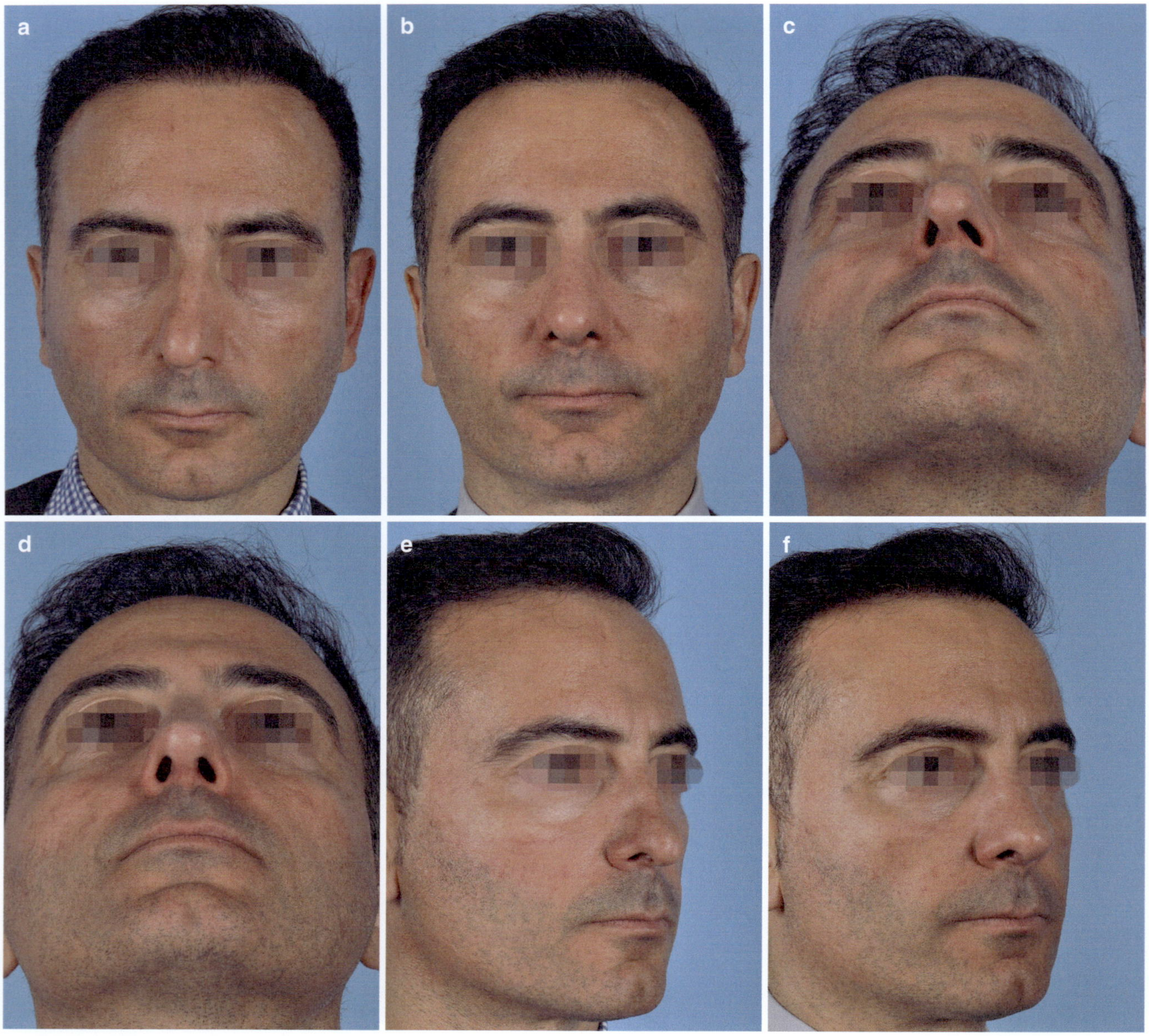

Fig. 13.144 (**a–f**) This patient above had a wide and deviated nasal type due to bilateral, convex, asymmetrical malpositioned lateral crura. He is shown 12 months after relocation of the lateral crura

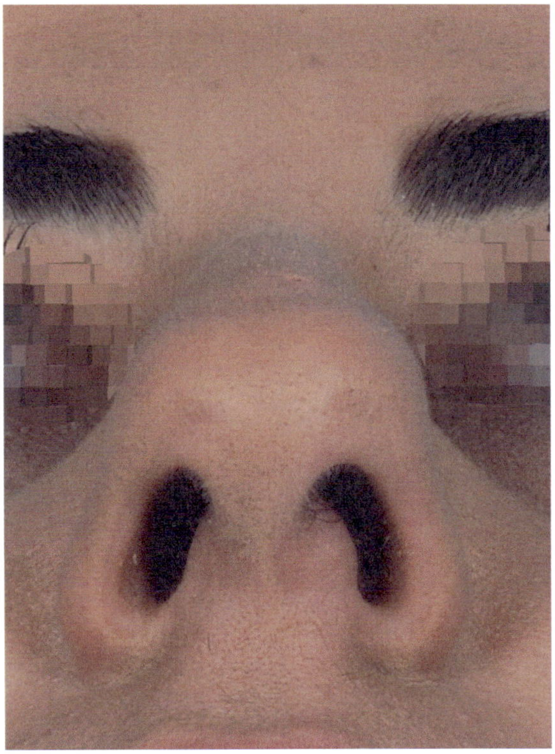

Fig. 13.145 Intraoperative views: wide nasal tip with malpositioned lateral crura

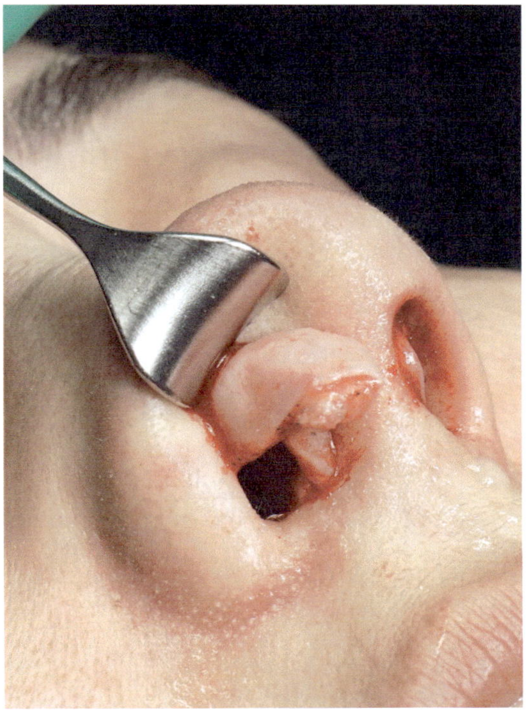

Fig. 13.146 Cartilage delivery approach. An infra cartilaginous was made at the inferior border of the lateral crus. Lateral crus was separated from the skin

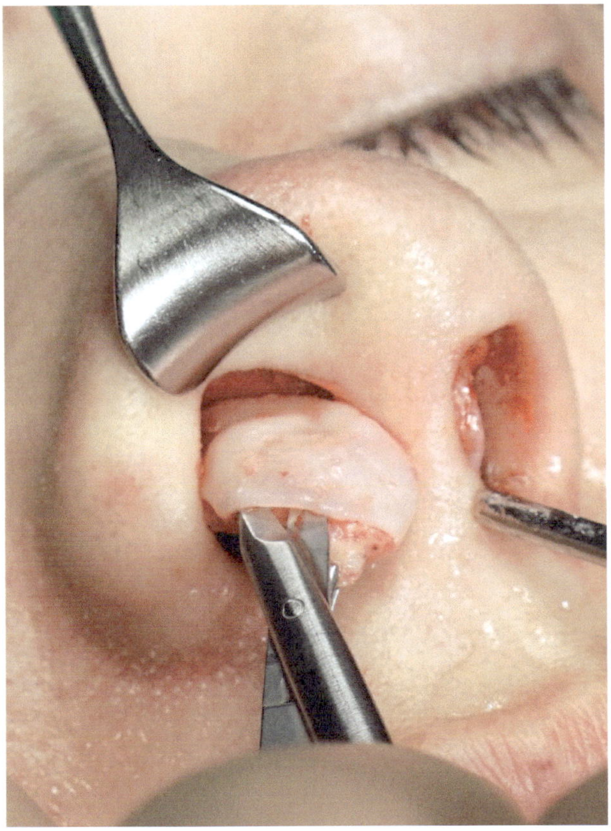

Fig. 13.147 The detachment of the lateral crus from vestibular skin with a scissor

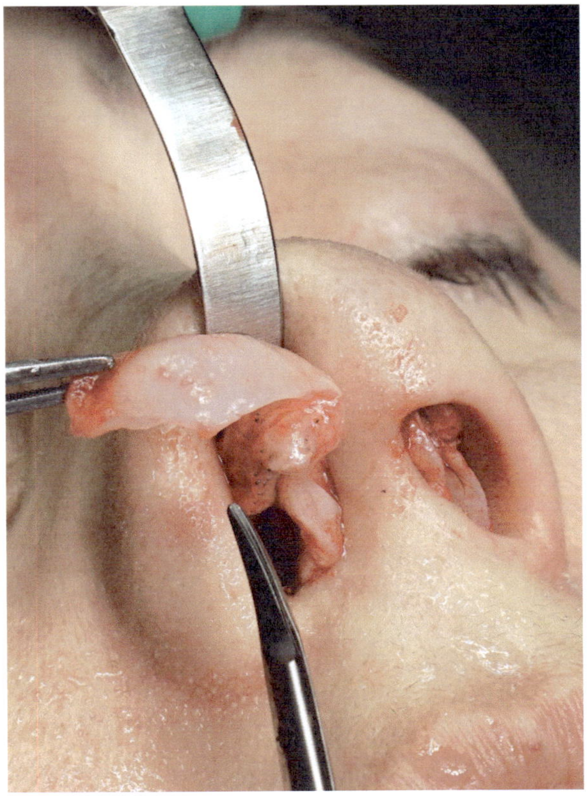

Fig. 13.148 The lateral crus is freed from its most lateral attachments. Convex but weak lateral crura were seen. The decision must be made whether a caudal or cranial flap should be done, or septal lateral crural grafting. In this case, the septal graft was chosen for the reconstruction of lateral crura

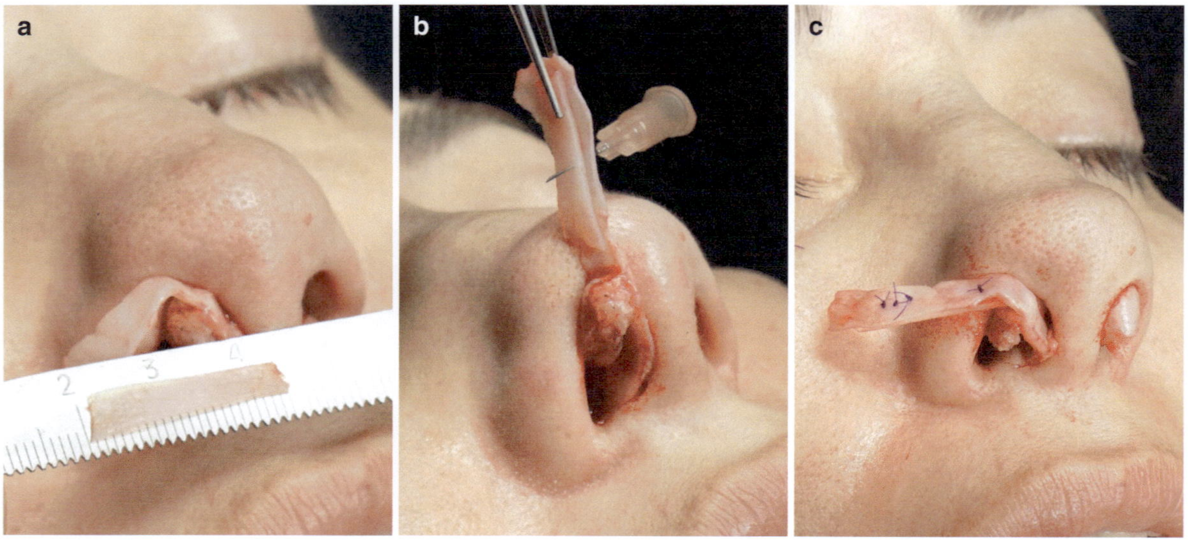

Fig. 13.149 (**a**) The lateral crural graft should be derived from the septum. (**b**) Any needle could be used for stabilization before suturing. (**c**) The graft was sutured to the undersurface of the lateral crus

Fig. 13.150 (**a**) Newly formed lateral crura. (**b**) A nonabsorbable suture was placed through the alar domes to create a dome-defining point. (**c**, **d**) A pocket was made in the skin with scissors between the intracartilaginous incision and the alar rim. Then the crus was inserted into this pocket. Columellar strut and septocolumellar suture were used for tip stabilizing

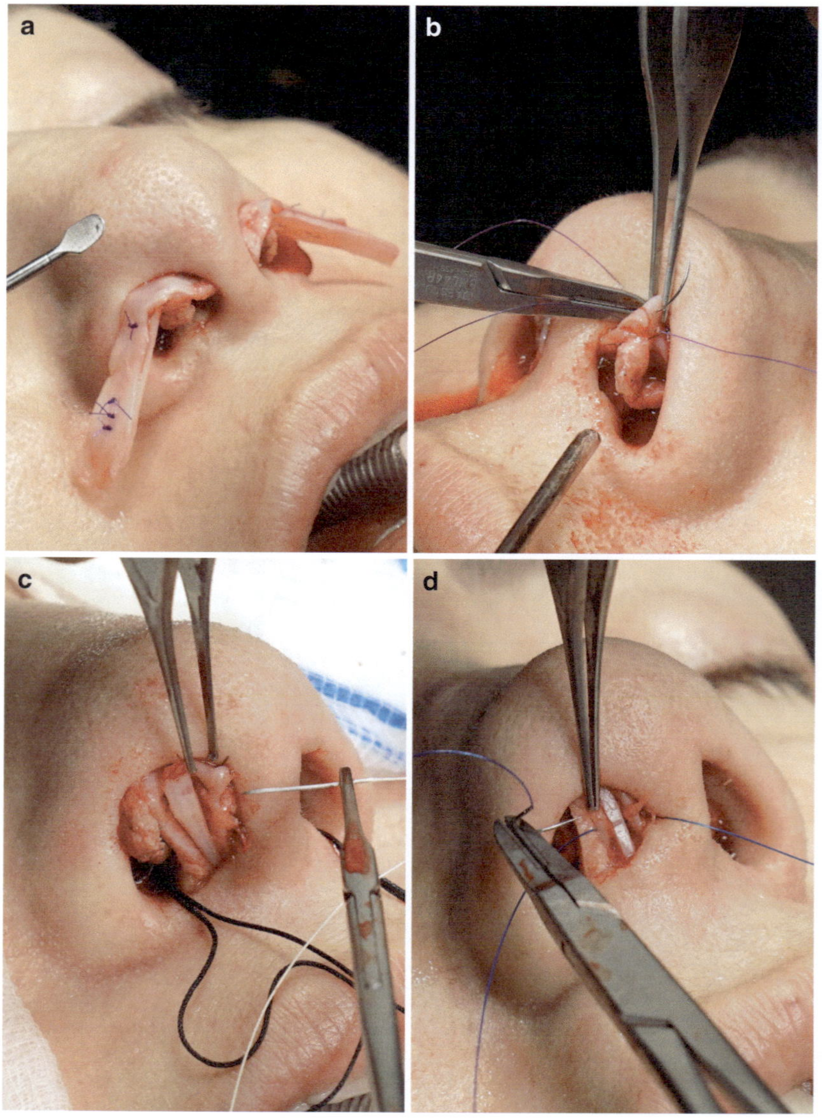

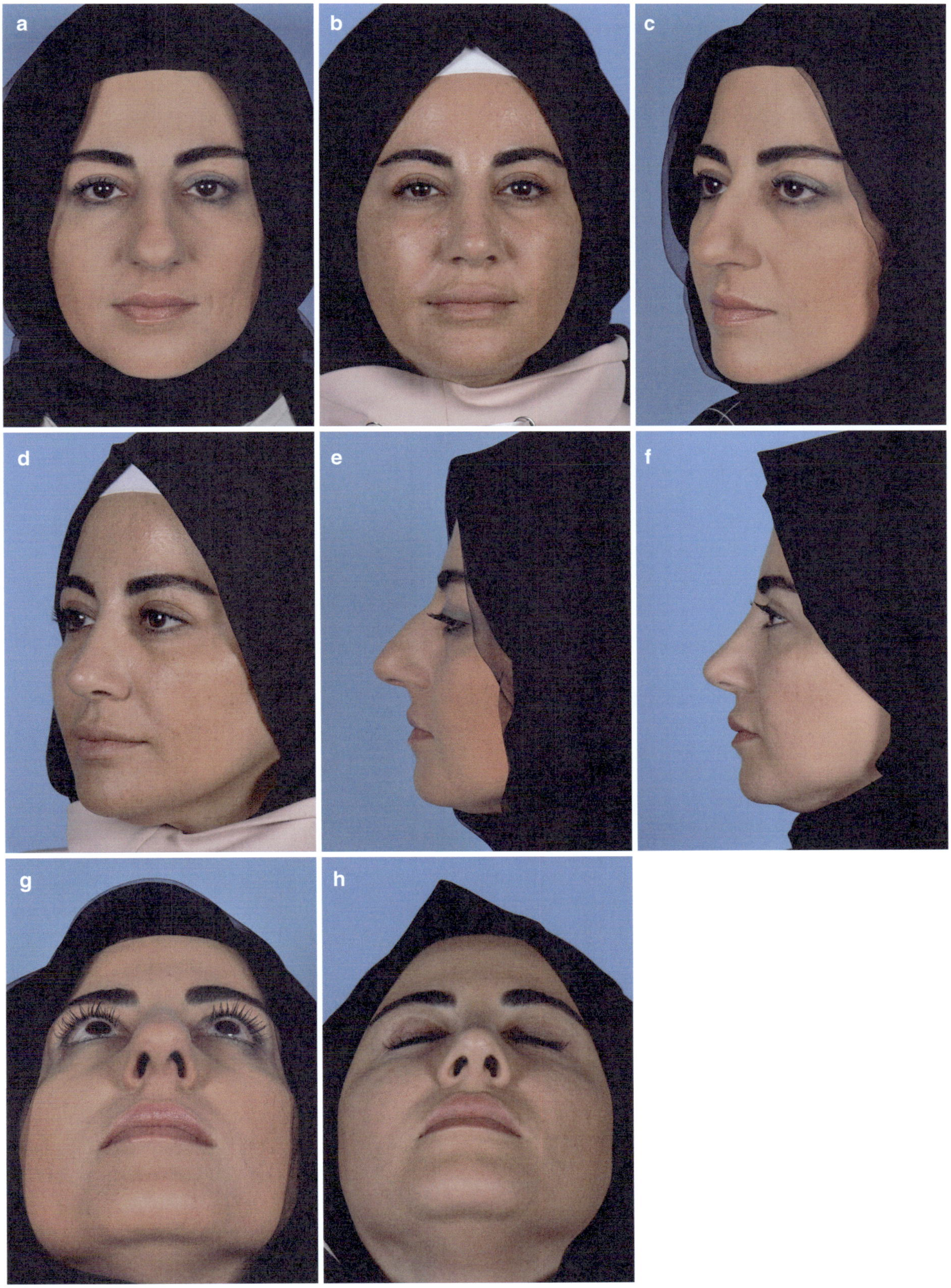

Fig. 13.151 (**a–h**) Postoperative photographs are showing closed repositioning of the lateral crura, which improved large nasal tip and removed the parenthesis tip deformity

13.6 The Alar Base

Alar base surgery is the final step when narrowing the tip; this affords a natural (balanced) outcome. An ideally aesthetic nose exhibits a harmonious relationship between the alar base and other facial features.

The alar base is the distance between the alar creases and is ideally equal to the intercanthal distance. Alar flare is the maximal alar convexity above the alar crease, which ideally should not extend to over 2 mm outside the crease (Fig. 13.152).

It is generally agreed that nasal base reduction should be considered when the interalar distance is greater than the intercanthal distance (Fig. 13.153).

During alar base reduction, the surgeon must be careful to avoid asymmetry, scarring, and over-resection. Alar base over-resection causes functional and aesthetic problems. Over-resection narrows the external nasal valve, triggering breathing problems and/or development of the hockey stick deformity (Fig. 13.154).

The alar base reduction design should be wedge-shaped, crescent, or ellipsoidal. We will look at each of these in one or more cases.

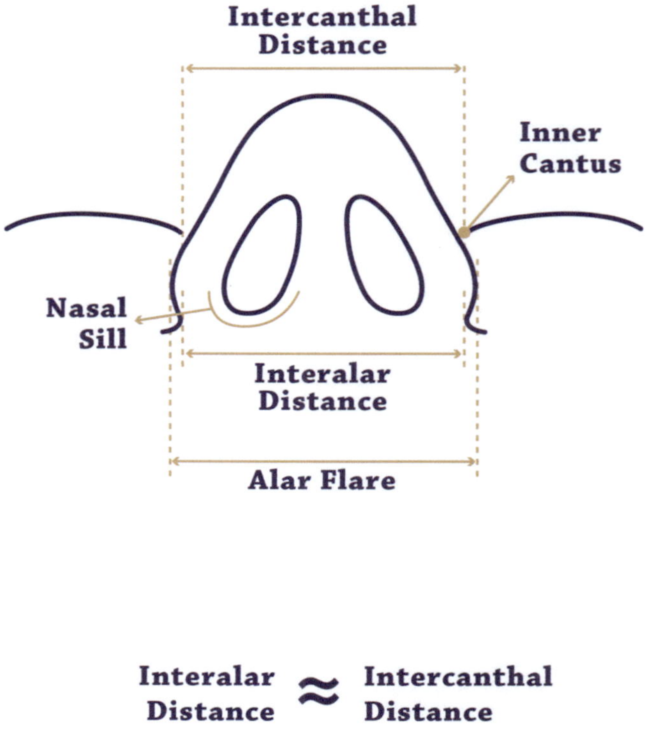

Fig. 13.152 Classic Caucasian alar base anatomy

13.6.1 Wedge-Shaped Skin Resection: Case 37

When the alar base has a wide appearance because of a wide nostril sill, and flaring is absent, the sill (only) is narrowed. Wedge-shaped skin resection commencing at the nostril sill narrows the alar base (Fig. 13.155; Video 13.25).

The preoperative photograph in Fig. 13.156 shows a patient with a wide alar base attributable to an excessive nostril sill (Video 13.26).

The narrowing of nasal tip and change in tip projection will have a direct effect on the alar base configuration. For this reason, the alar base reduction must be made at the end of tip surgery after the closure of all incisions (Fig. 13.157). The amount of sill resection is carefully measured by the caliper and then marked. It is significantly important not to disrupt the natural curve of the alar base (Fig. 13.158).

Medial and then lateral sill incisions are made with a #11 blade and then a wedge Bilateral resection of the nostril sill is done (Fig. 13.159).

After resection, first, the subcutaneous layers were approximated with 5.0 absorbable sutures. These in-depth sutures take tension off the skin edges, thus decreasing the risk of postoperative notching (Fig. 13.160).

Then the skin was sutured with 6.0 sutures. Many primary sutures were placed after initial skin mattress suturing.

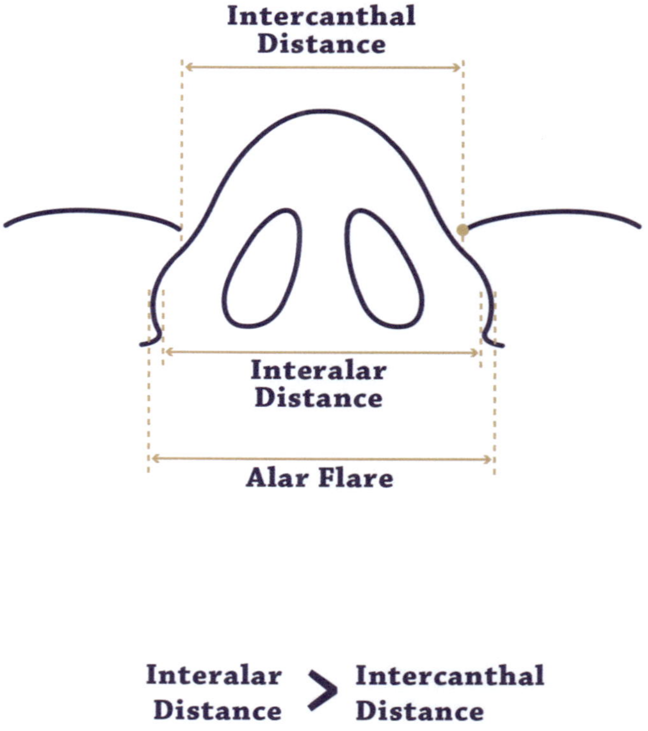

Fig. 13.153 When the inter-alar distance is greater than the intercanthal distance, an alar base reduction is needed

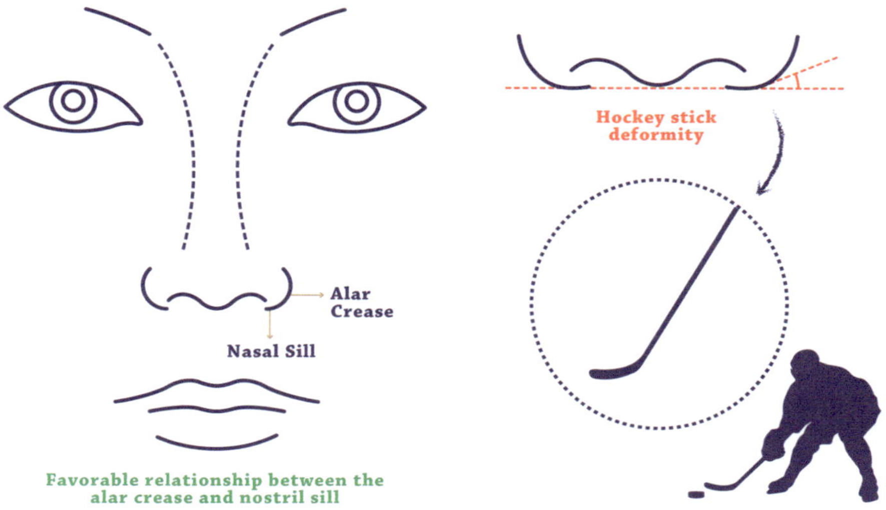

Fig. 13.154 If the curvature of the alar crease is disturbed, the angle with the nostril sill becomes excessively acute and it gives a hockey-stick appearance to the nasal base

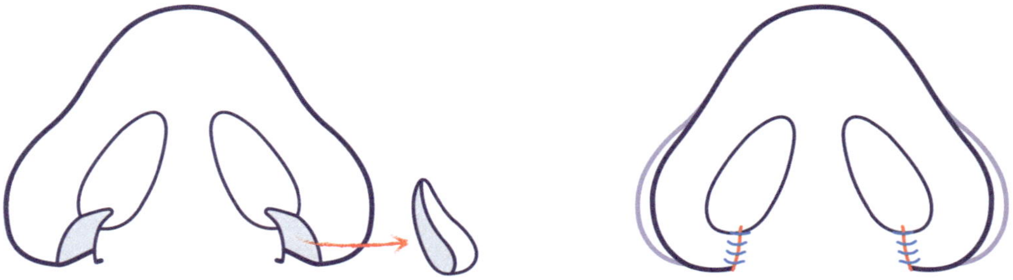

Fig. 13.155 A wide base with wide nostrils and without excessive alar flare, wedge excisions from the nostril floor will result in a narrowing of the nostrils and decrease in the nasal base width. Excision designed in a wedge shape ensures preservation of the natural curvature of the sill and ala

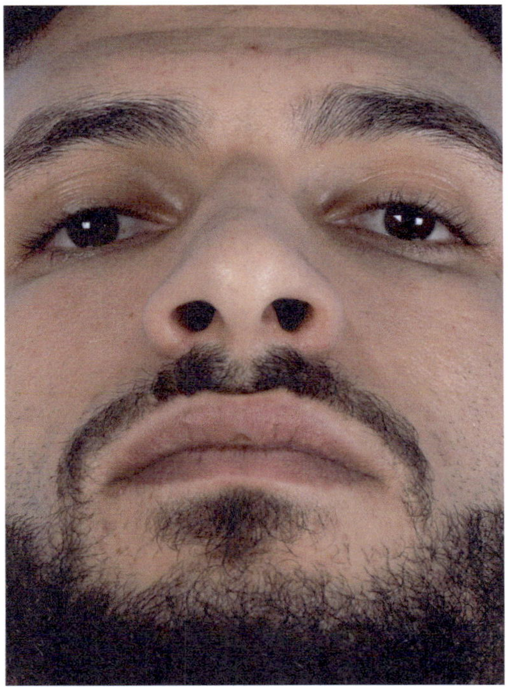

Fig. 13.156 In this case the preoperative photograph reveals a wide alar base caused by an excessive nostril sill

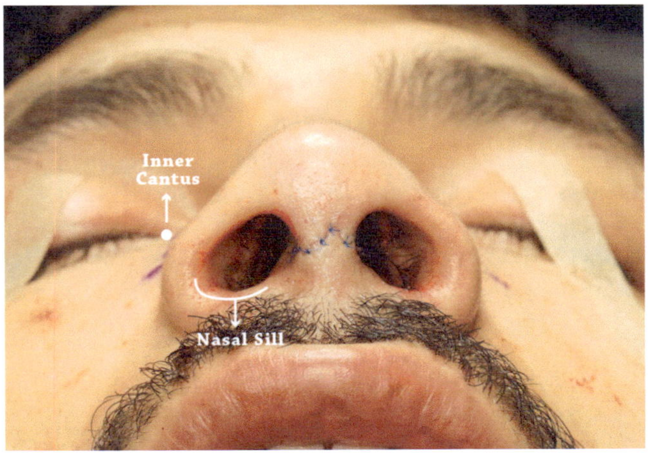

Fig. 13.157 A photograph taken at the end of surgery to correct the wide tip. Notice the long sill

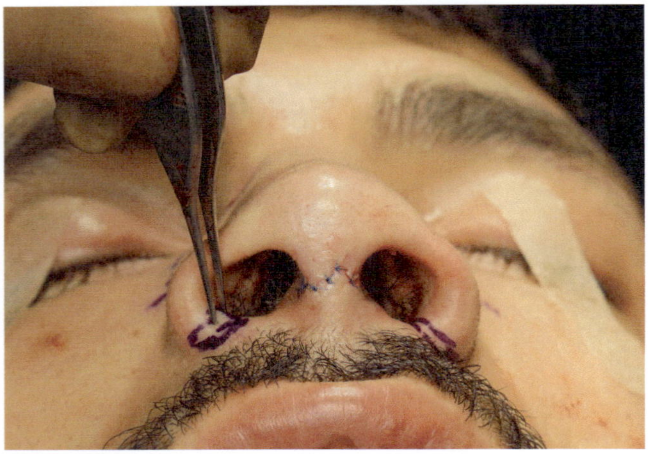

Fig. 13.158 The wedge-shaped resection line was marked

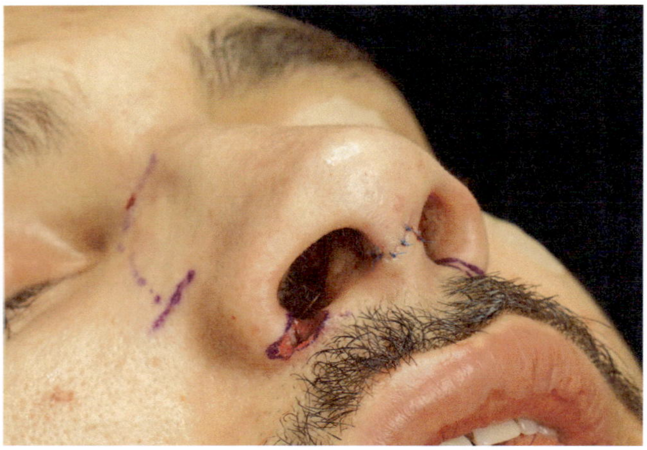

Fig. 13.159 Bilateral resection of the nostril sill

Mattress sutures can be used vertically or horizontally. These mattress sutures promote wound edge eversion and less prominent scarring (Fig. 13.161).

One year after surgery, the alar base was narrowed, and symmetry was evident. In the oblique view, nostril show was reduced (Fig. 13.162).

13.6.2 Crescential Alar Base Reduction: Case 38

When the alar base is shown wide because of excess alar flare and a long nostril sill, crescentic alar base reduction is required. The crescent-like shape is designed to narrow the alar flare maximally while reducing sill width at the same time (Fig. 13.163; Video 13.27).

Figure 13.164 shows a typical example of a patient who needs a crescentic alar base reduction (Video 13.28). A closed approach was preferred to fix wide nasal tip.

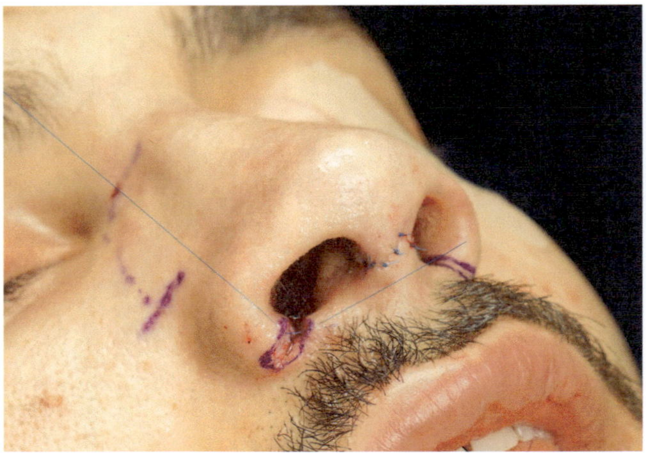

Fig. 13.160 The deep subcutaneous suture

The planned crescentic alar base reduction was marked (Figs. 13.165 and 13.166). Crescential resection was performed (Fig. 13.167).

After suturing the subcutaneous tissue, the surgical area was primarily sutured after the first mattress suture was placed in the skin (Fig. 13.168).

Postoperative views of the same patient after a crescentic alar base excision, which resulted in a decrease in the alar base width and narrower, more vertically oriented nostrils with no obliteration of the natural alar-facial crease or violation of the natural curve of the alar rim (Fig. 13.169).

13.6.3 Case 39

This is another case with a wide nasal base and a wide nasal tip. In addition, the tip was counter-rotated and overprojected, which caused the nose to appear excessively long. Crescentic alar base resection narrowed the nasal base. VAR was used for the tip. Resecting the excess part of the lateral crus corrected the tip problems. The surgical outcome is evident when compared to photographs taken before and 3 years after the surgery (Fig. 13.170).

13.6.4 Ellipsoidal Excision: Case 40

When the alar base is shown wide in appearance because of excessive alar flaring and the sill is ideal, an ellipsoidal excision is required. This ellipse width should be 2–8 mm according to the requirement (Fig. 13.171).

A patient with a wide alar base caused by excessive alar flare is shown in Fig. 13.172 (Video 13.29). The photograph in Fig. 13.173 was taken at the end of surgery to correct the wide tip.

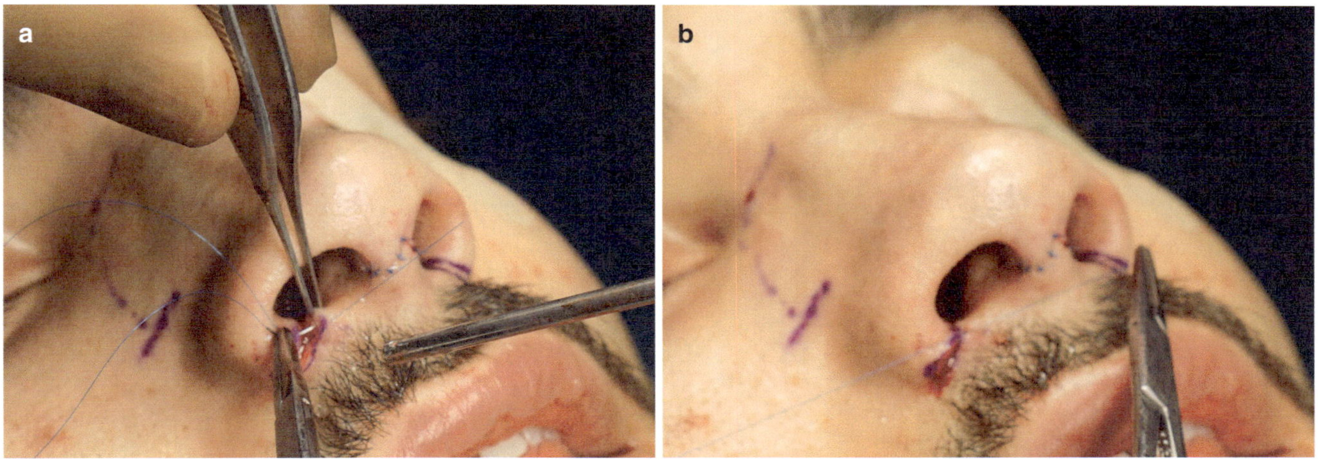

Fig. 13.161 (**a**, **b**) Vertical mattress suture; the mattress suture should be preferred for closing the skin because it provides strength and wound eversion

Fig. 13.162 (**a–d**) Pre- and postoperative photographs. Wedge excision shows a sufficient narrowing of the nasal base with elimination of the extreme nostril sill. Another positive effect of the nostril sill excision is reducing "excessive nostril show," especially on oblique view

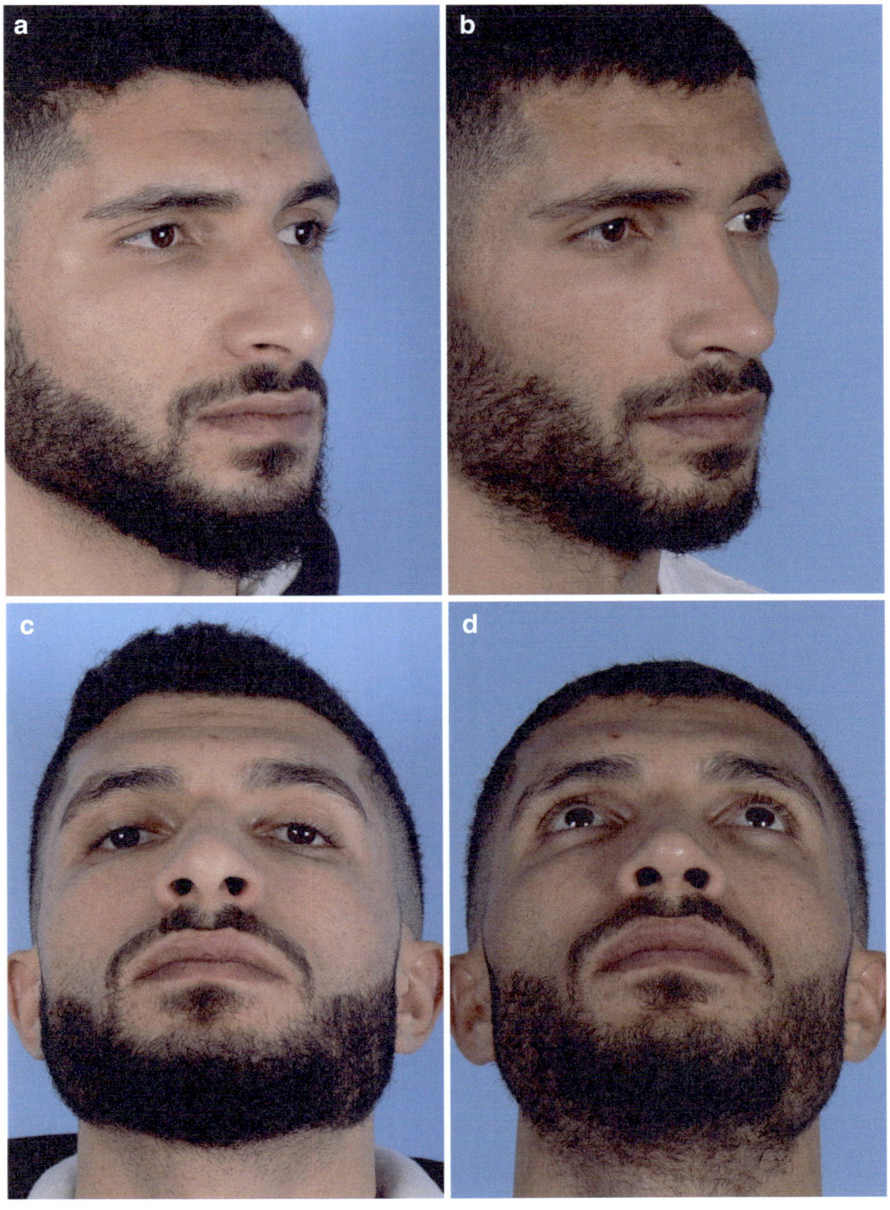

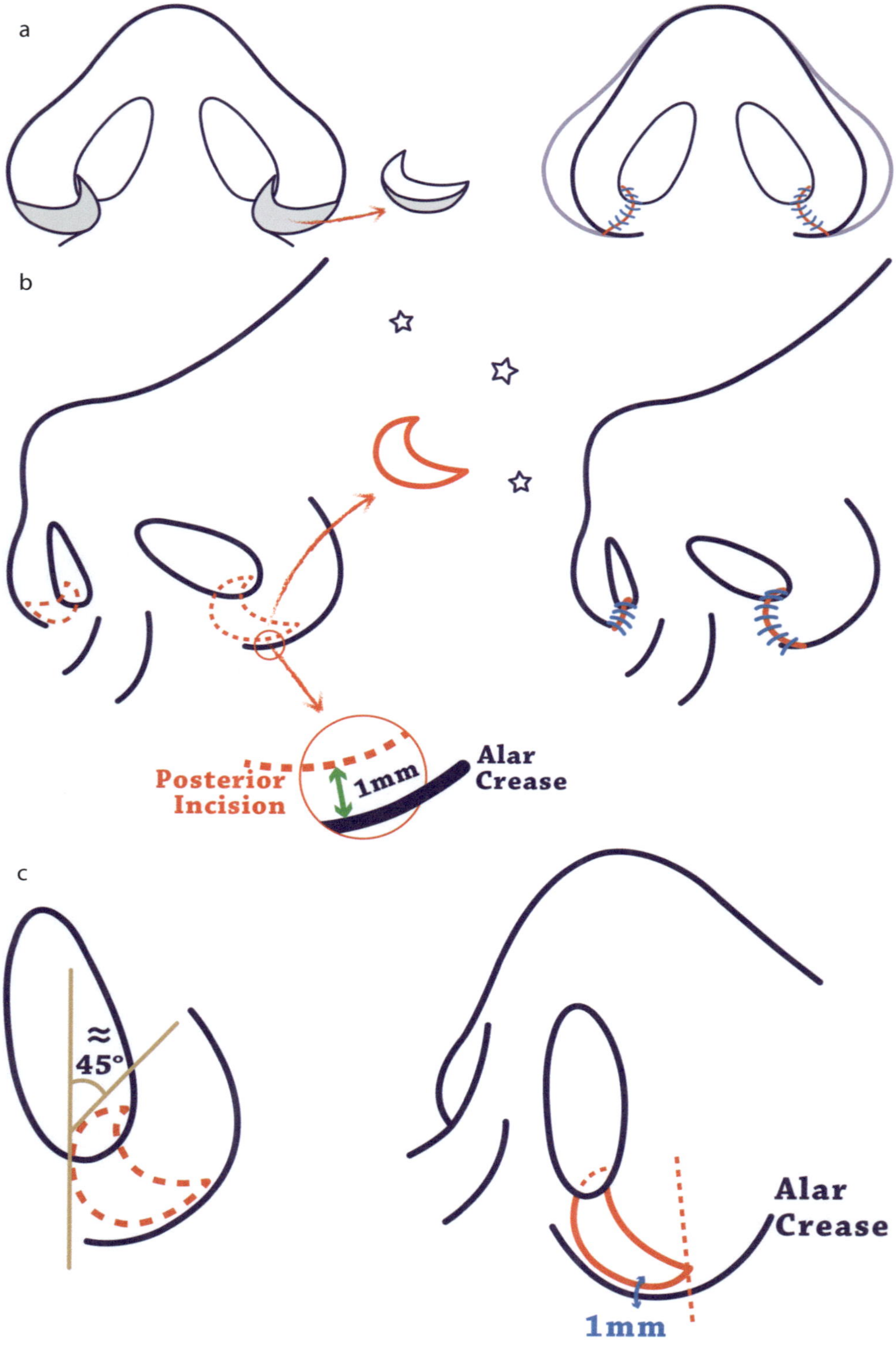

Fig. 13.163 (**a**) If the wide alar base is associated with excessive flaring and nasal sill length, sufficient nasal base narrowing can be achieved by combining the internal vestibular floor excision with an external alar wedge excision. (**b**, **c**) Schematic illustration of the crescentic alar base excision technique. The excised area includes a combination of nostril sill and alar base in varying proportion, depending on the degree of excess

The planned alar base resection was marked (Fig. 13.174).

Skin and soft tissue were removed; the mucosa was preserved (Fig. 13.175).

The first suture approximated the subcutaneous layers. Cleaning of the surgical area should be performed gently (using a syringe rather than suction) (Fig. 13.176).

Primary sutures were placed to close the surgical area (Fig. 13.177).

Bilateral alar base reduction: A symmetrical (ideal) nasal width was created intraoperatively (Fig. 13.178).

Excessive alar flaring was corrected after surgery. There is no visible scar in the resection area (Fig. 13.179).

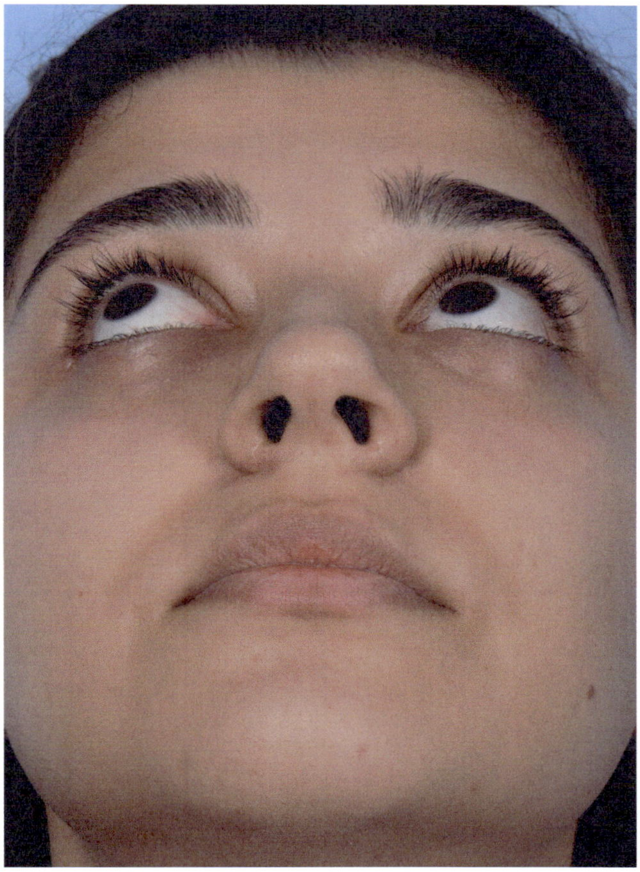

Fig. 13.164 A preoperative photograph reveals a wide alar base caused by both excessive alar flare and a wide nostril sill

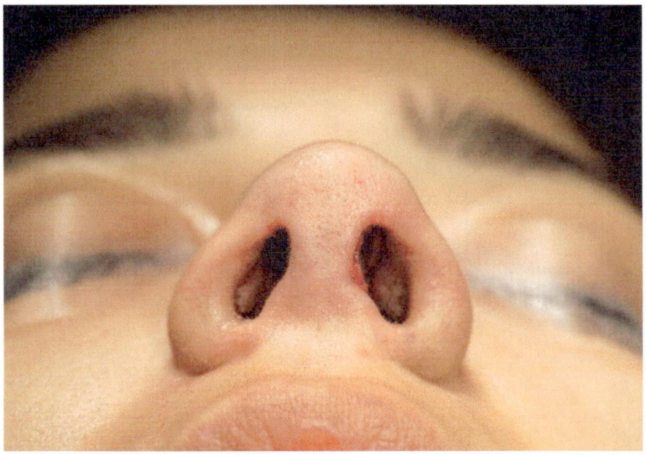

Fig. 13.165 A photograph taken at the end of closed rhinoplasty to correct the wide tip

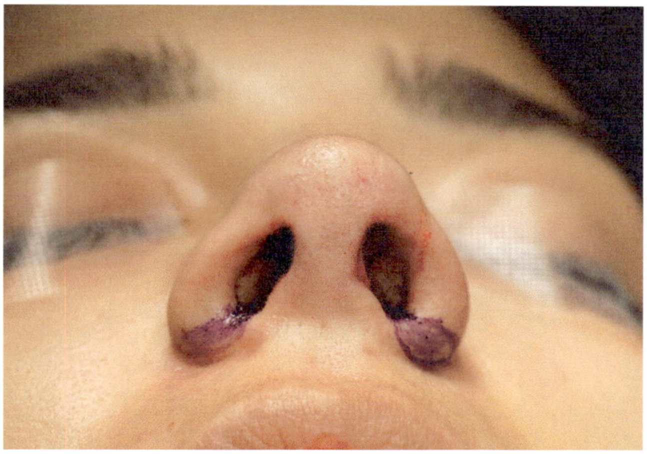

Fig. 13.166 The markings show the planned excision on the patient's alar base

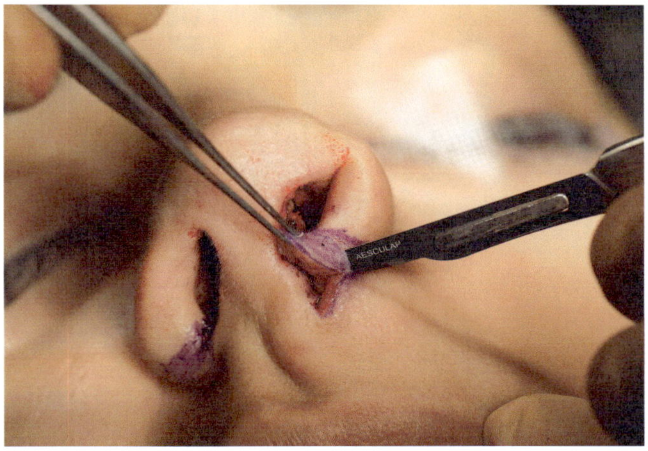

Fig. 13.167 Mainly, one draws the lower portion of the alar wedge excision around to the medial vertical wall of the nostril sill excision

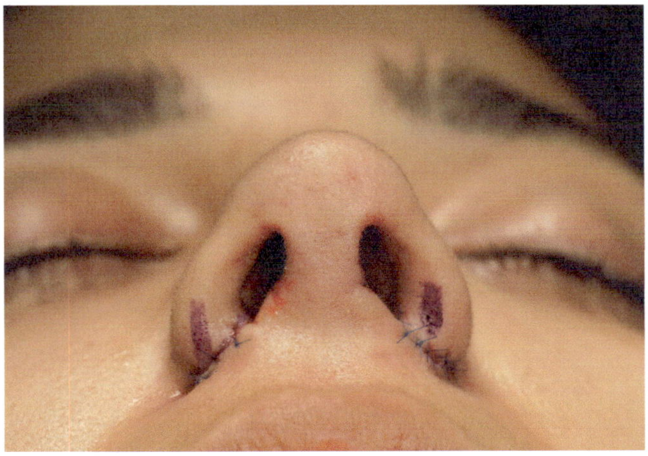

Fig. 13.168 Flare and sill reduction are completed bilaterally

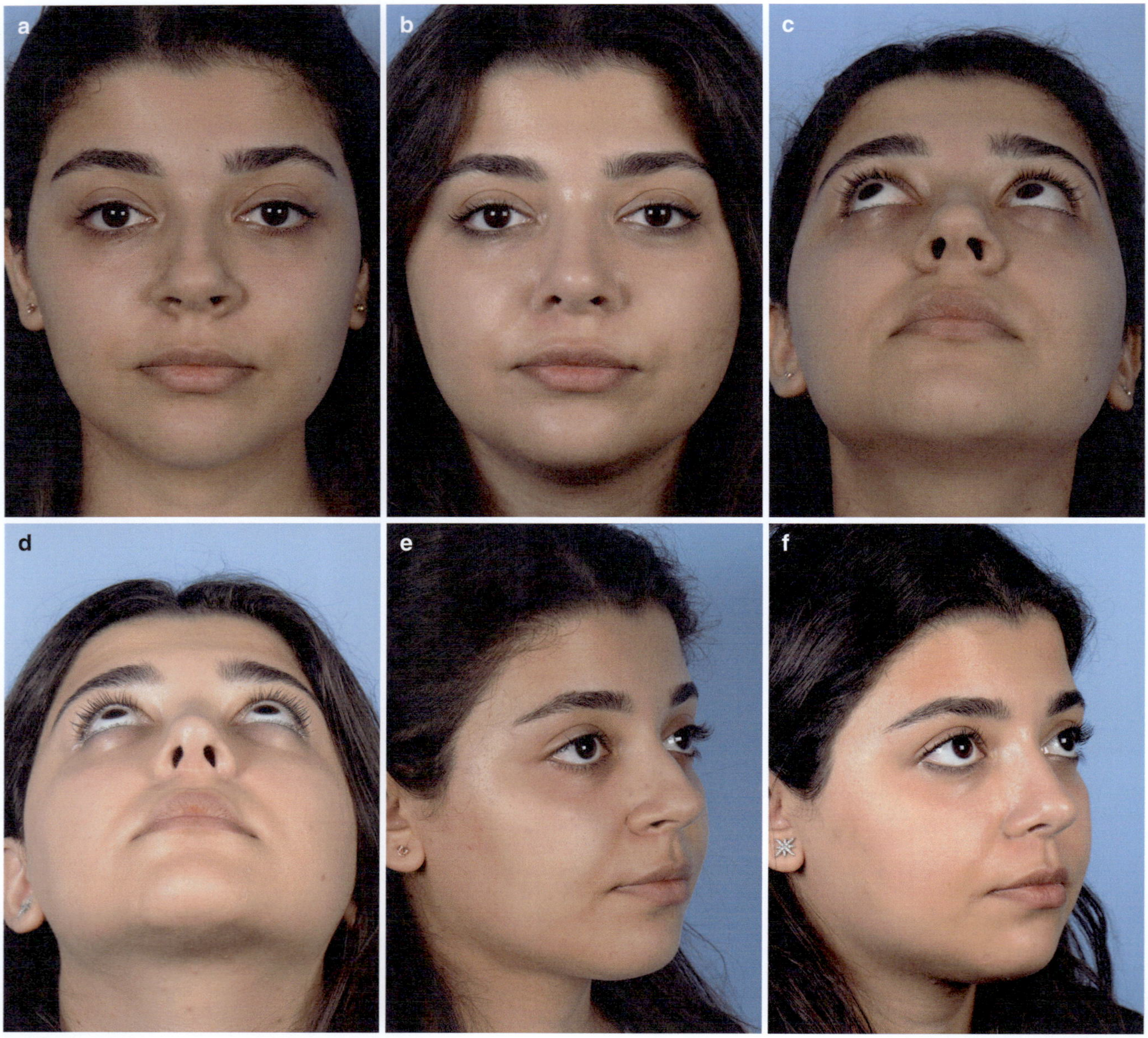

Fig. 13.169 (**a–f**) Pre- and postoperative views of the patient after a crescent alar base reduction, which effectively narrowed the nasal base, eliminated excessive flaring, and narrowed the wide nostrils. The technique preserved the natural alar-facial crease and the natural sill appearance. The broad tip with thick skin was shaped with cephalic trim, bilateral lateral crural strut, transdomal suture, dome equalizing suture, and cap graft

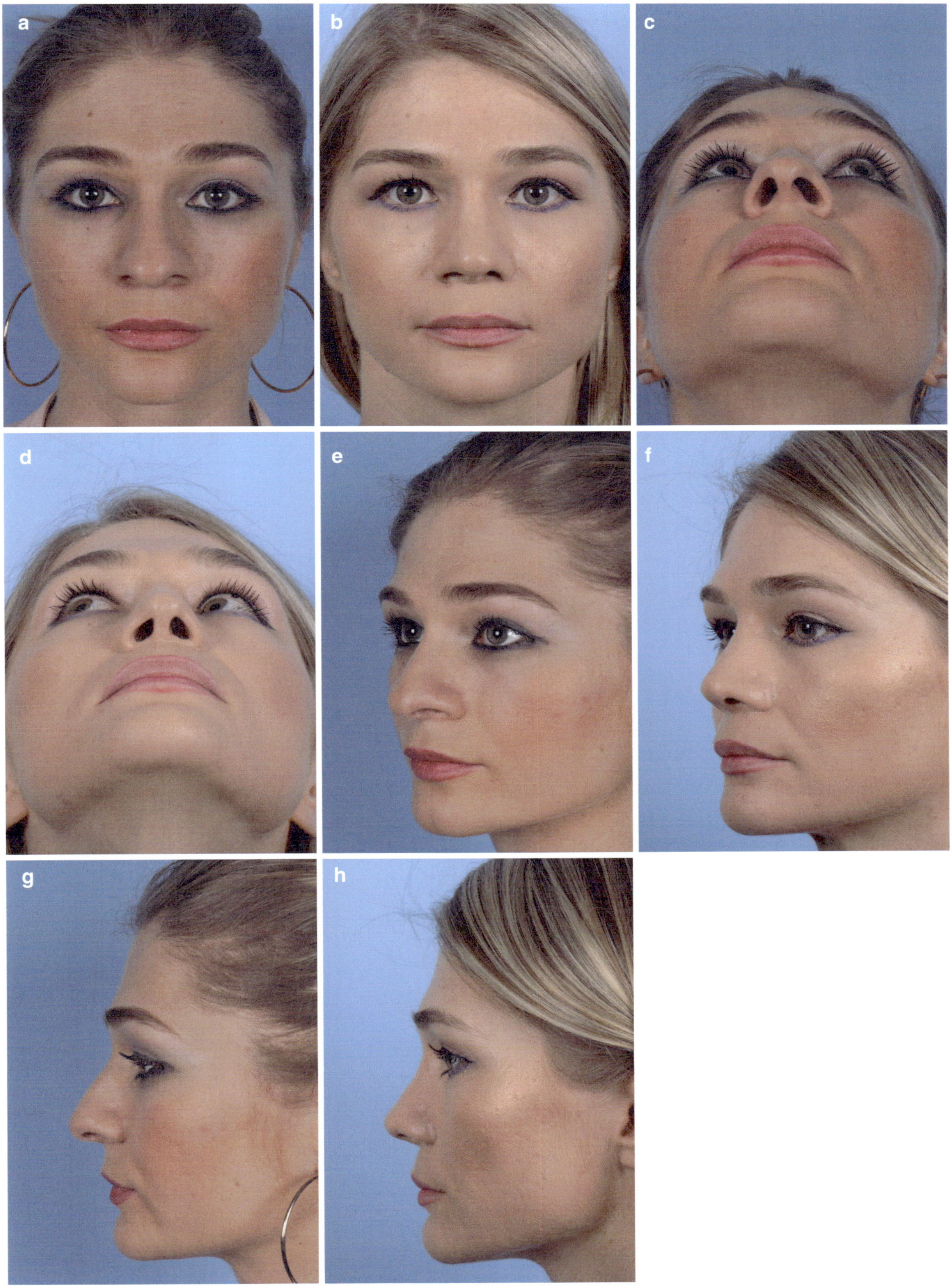

Fig. 13.170 (**a–h**) Preoperative pictures of a large nasal tip with wide alar base and excessive flare. Postoperative photographs of the same patient after a crescent alar base excision resulted in a decrease in the alar base width and a more elegant appearance. The tip was modified with VAR technique

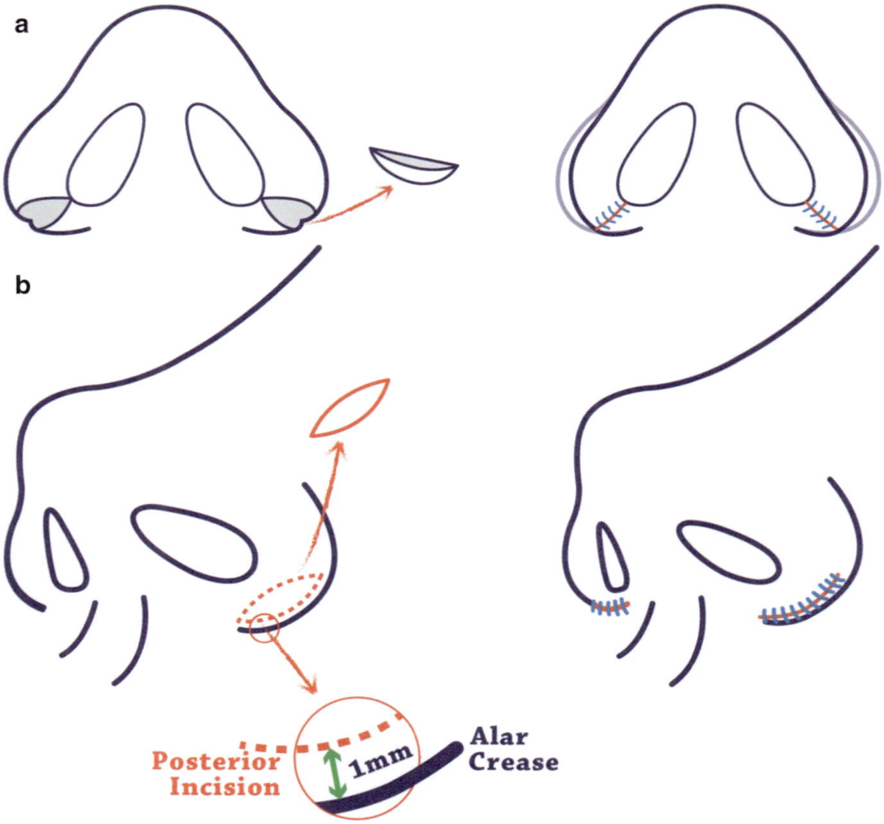

Fig. 13.171 (**a**) A wide alar base with excessive alar flare, ellipsoidal external alar excision will result in a narrower base as a result of the decrease in the widest diameter of the nasal base. (**b**) If no sill excision is indicated, stop the cutaneous excision below the nostril sill. It is important to place the posterior incision just above the crease (within 1 mm), because if it is placed too high, the scar may be quite obvious

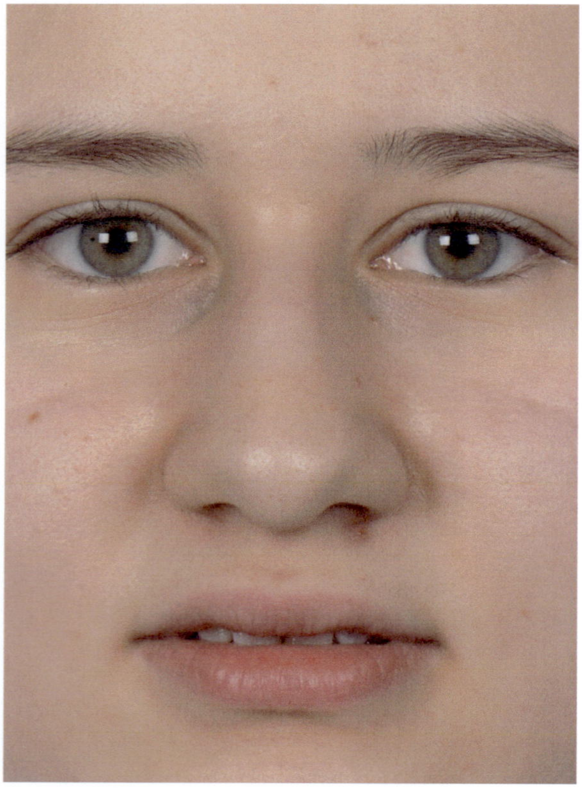

Fig. 13.172 A wide alar base caused by excessive alar flare

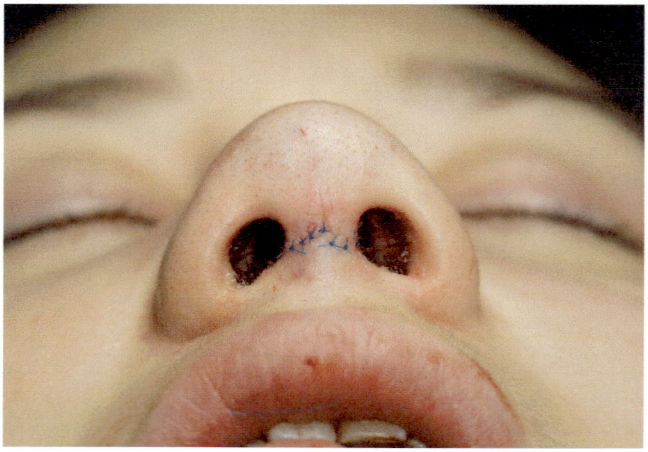

Fig. 13.173 Tip surgery completed

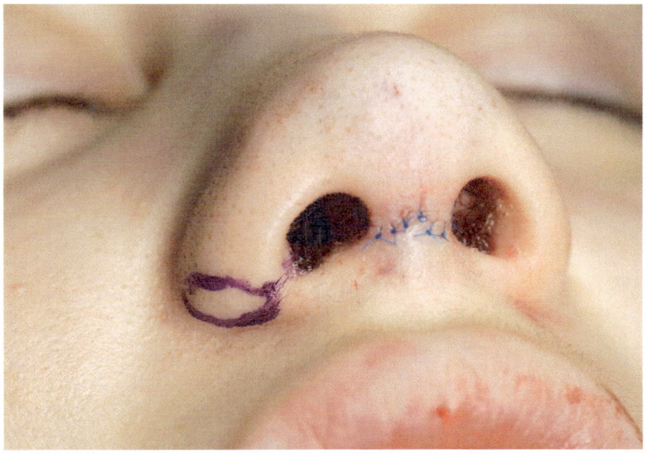

Fig. 13.174 The incision in the alar-facial groove, and the preservation of the nostril sill

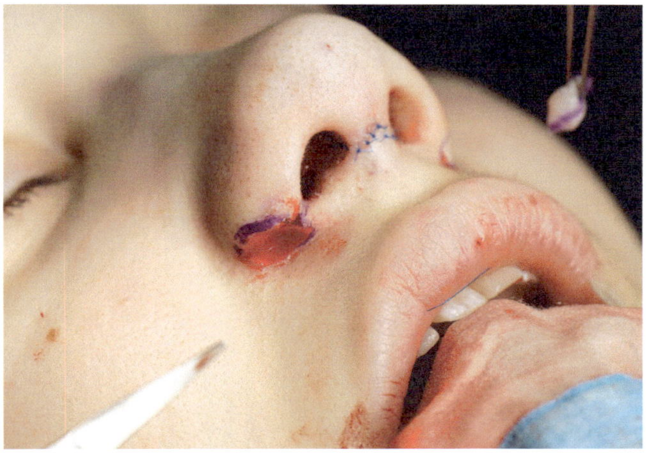

Fig. 13.175 An elliptical excision was made down to the mid-muscle level but without passing the underlying vestibular skin

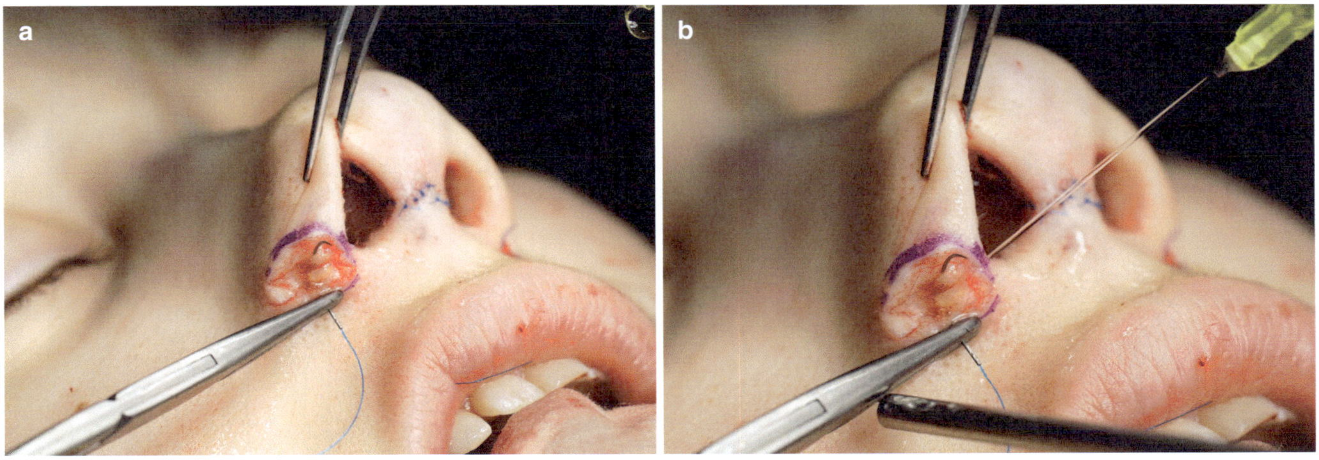

Fig. 13.176 (**a**, **b**) Placement of deep stitch

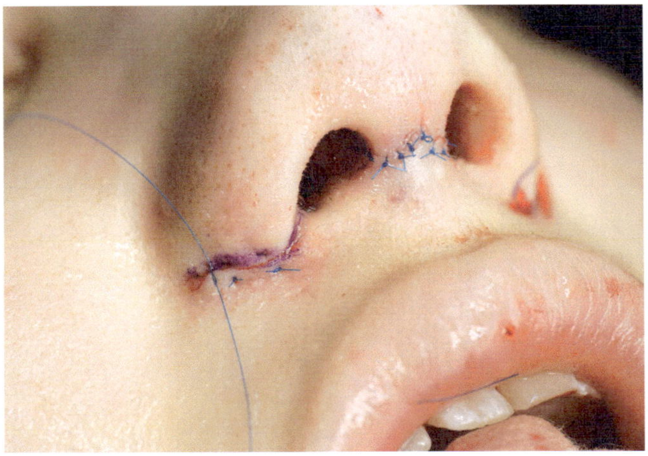

Fig. 13.177 Interrupted closure with vertical mattress sutures

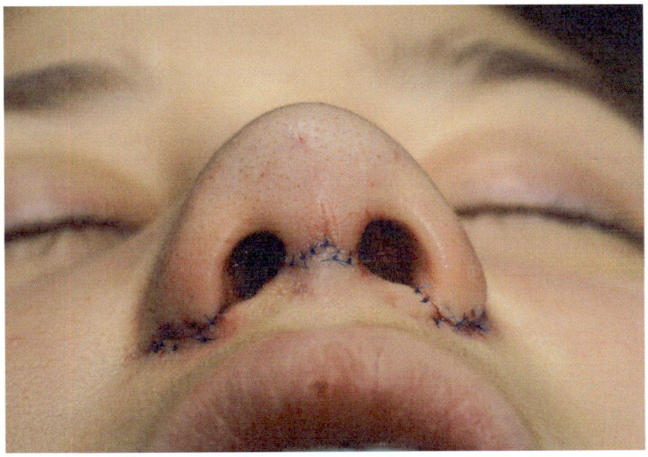

Fig. 13.178 At the end of the procedure, bilateral resection was finished

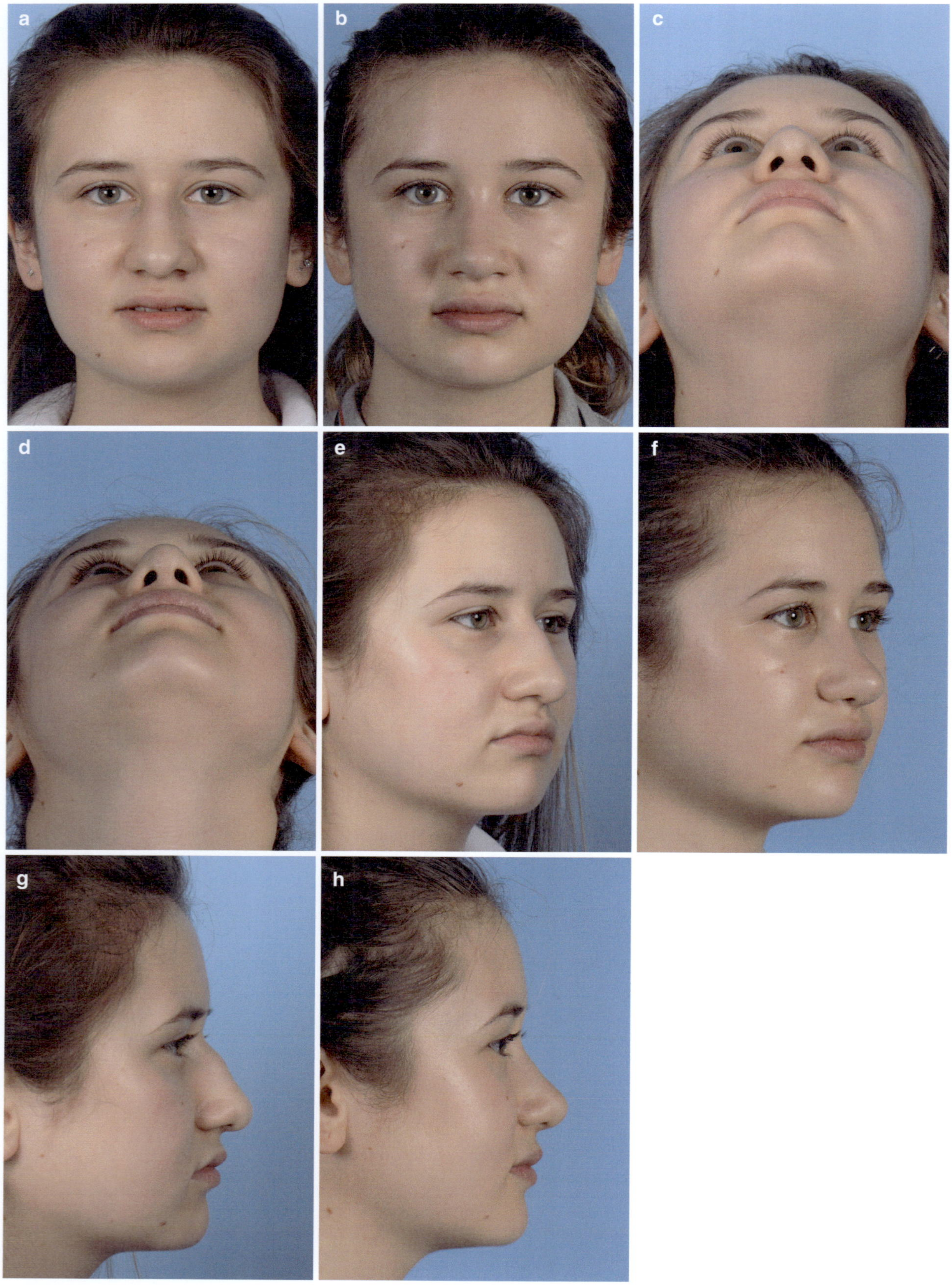

Fig. 13.179 (**a–h**) Preoperative and postoperative photographs. There is no excess nasal flare. The tip was narrowed with the COST technique. Septocolumellar strut graft was placed for long-term tip stabilization due to thick skin

13.7 Conclusions

Refining a wide nasal tip is one of the challenges of cosmetic nasal surgery. The reestablishment of a natural tip configuration is fundamental. The Introduction lists seven anatomical features required for a natural tip configuration. The focus of all surgical maneuvers is to idealize these features.

Based on difficulty, we classify wide tip surgery into basic, intermediate, and advanced procedures. Most wide nasal tips can be treated using the basic and intermediate techniques. Both feature transdomal suturing, which refines mildly and moderately wide tips. However, an important, but unrecognized, drawback of aggressive transdomal suturing is secondary deterioration of the nasal tip dynamics. Consequently, difficult cases may require advanced techniques (Fig. 13.180).

We present five cases requiring basic, intermediate, and advanced procedures using pre-, intra-, and postoperative photographs.

The basic procedures were used in the first case. The tip was slightly wide and bulbous. The width of the nose was normalized and the tip was defined using the basic procedures mentioned in Fig. 13.181.

In the second case, there was an obvious lateral crural convexity in the oblique view. In addition to the basic procedures, a lateral crural graft (intermediate technique) was used to improve the tip contours (Fig. 13.182).

In a case with an overly wide tip, vertical alar resection (advanced technique) was performed. Postoperatively, the nasal tip was more defined and the interdomal distance was decreased (Fig. 13.183).

In another case with wide tip, COST technique was performed. An advanced technique is preferred because of the long lateral crus accompanied by medial crural deformity (Fig. 13.184).

An important aspect of wide tip surgery is that the advanced technique is used not only because of the severity of the case but also because of the malposed tip. The last case is an example of this (Fig. 13.185).

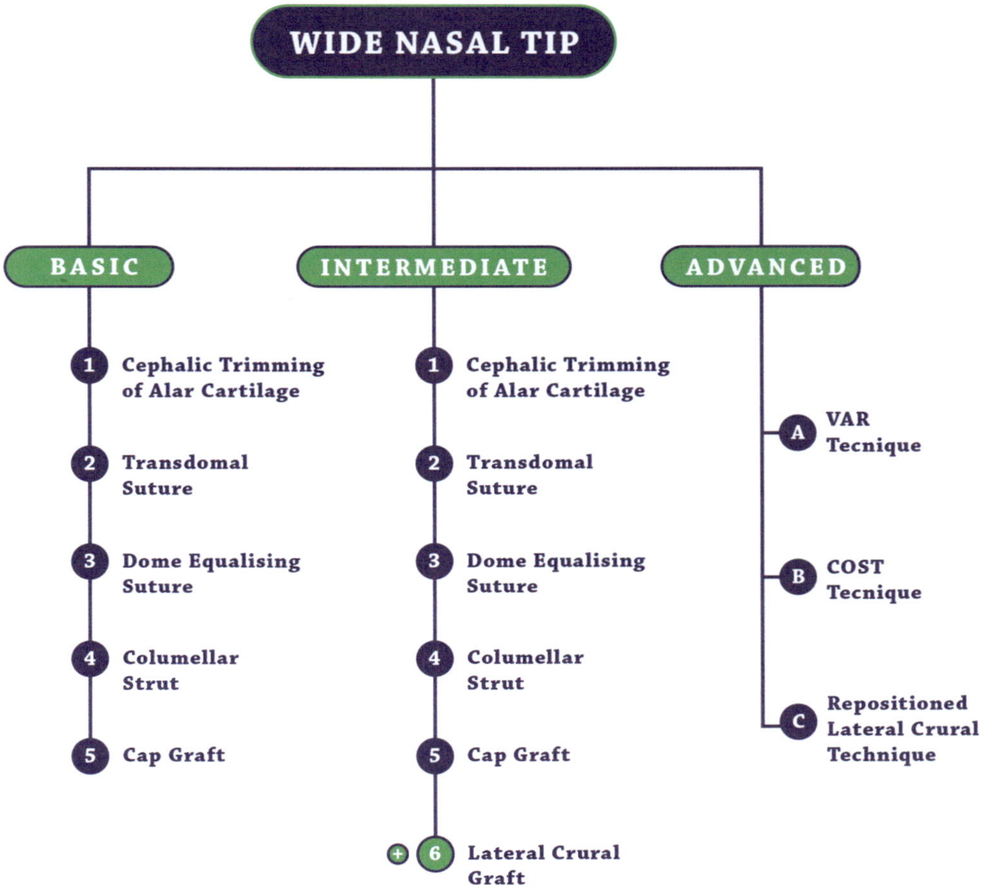

Fig. 13.180 Our algorithm for the correction of the wide nasal tip

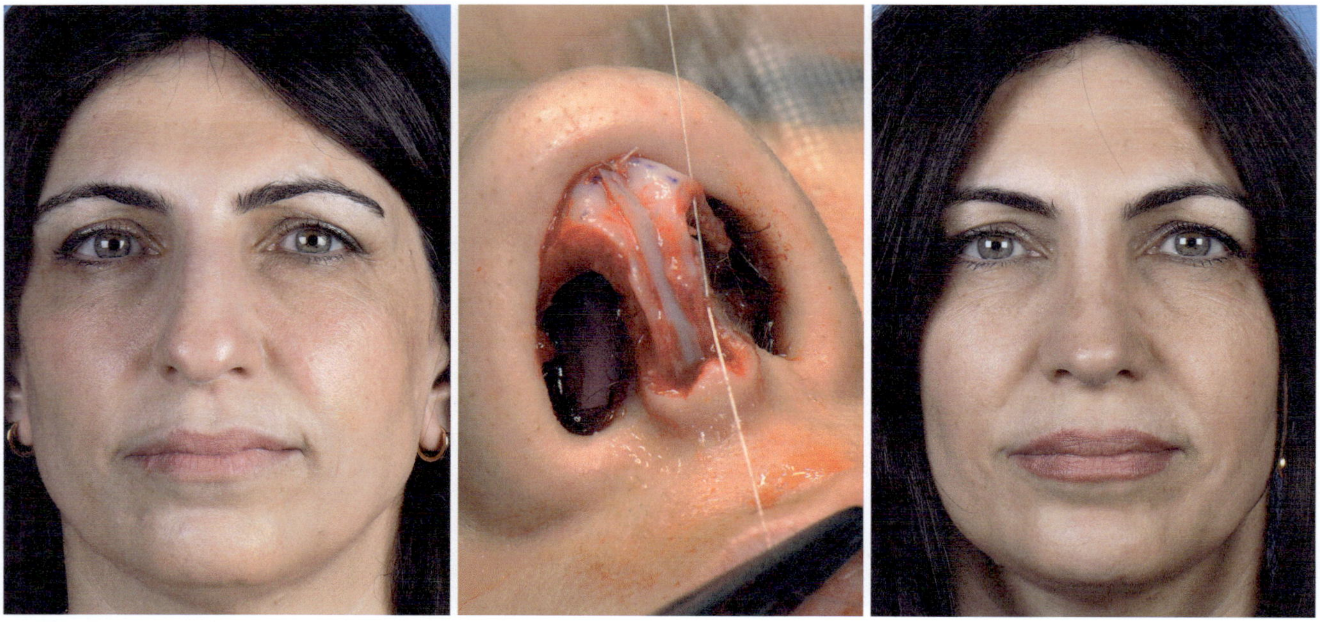

Fig. 13.181 Basic technique. Pre-, intra-, and postoperative photographs

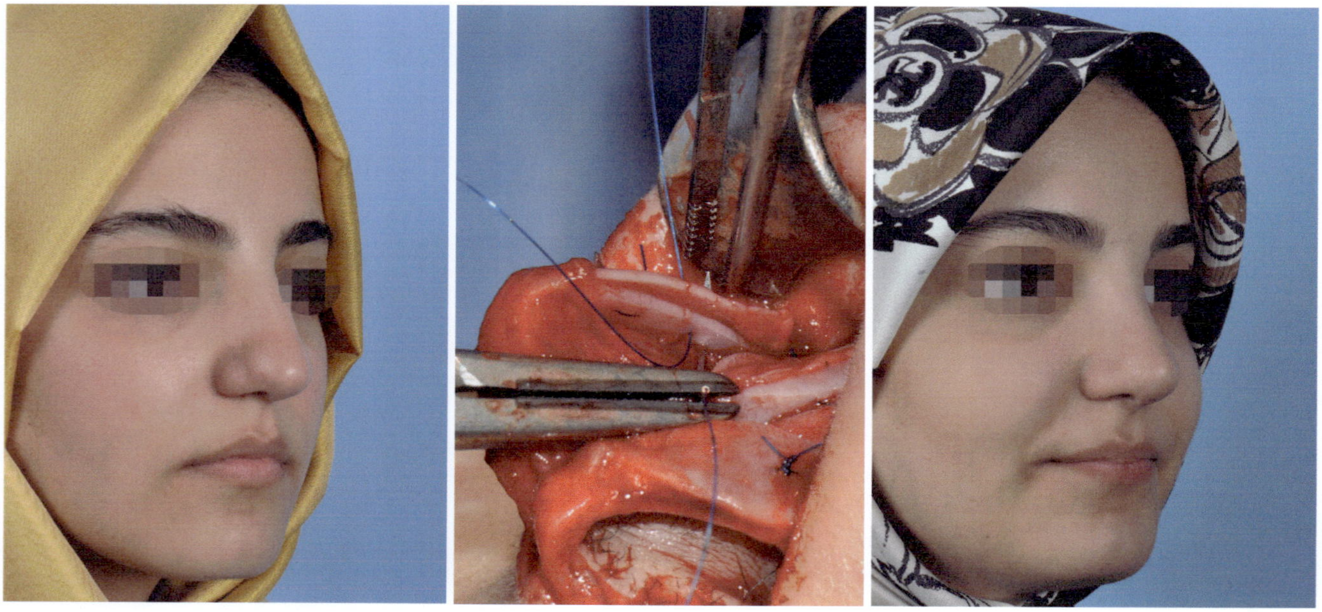

Fig. 13.182 Intermediate technique. Pre-, intra-, and postoperative photographs

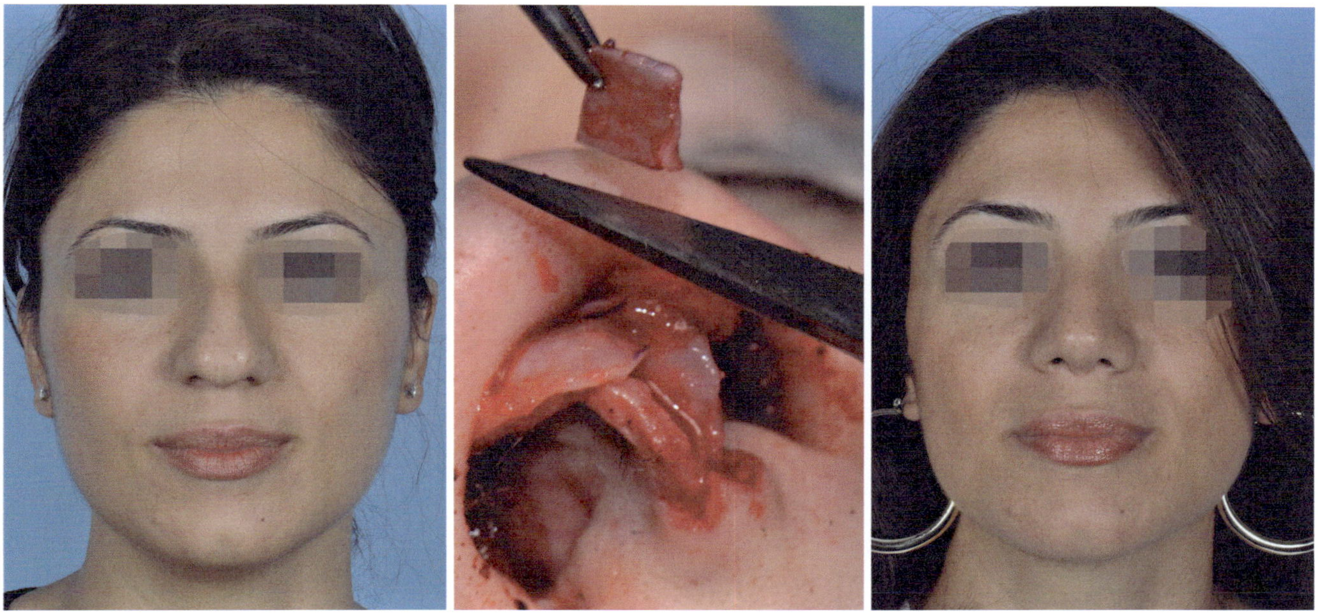

Fig. 13.183 Advanced technique. Pre-, intra-, and postoperative photographs

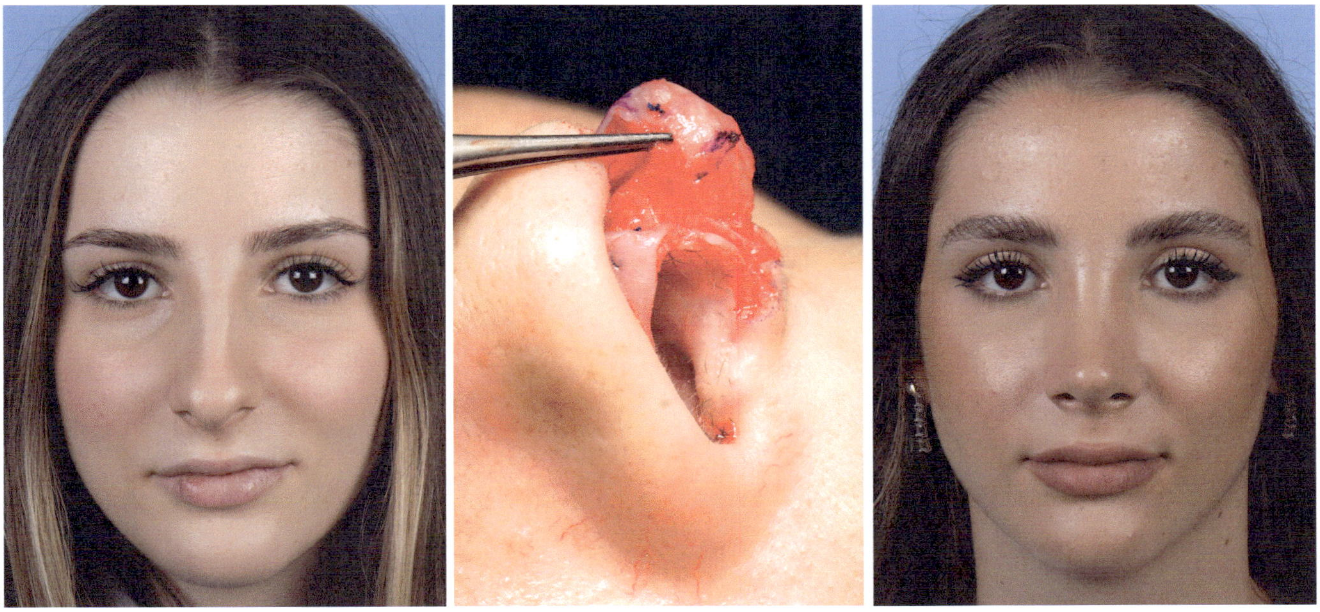

Fig. 13.184 While steal suture provided definition of the tip, overlap solved hanging infratip lobule in the frontal view. Pre-, intra-, and postoperative photographs

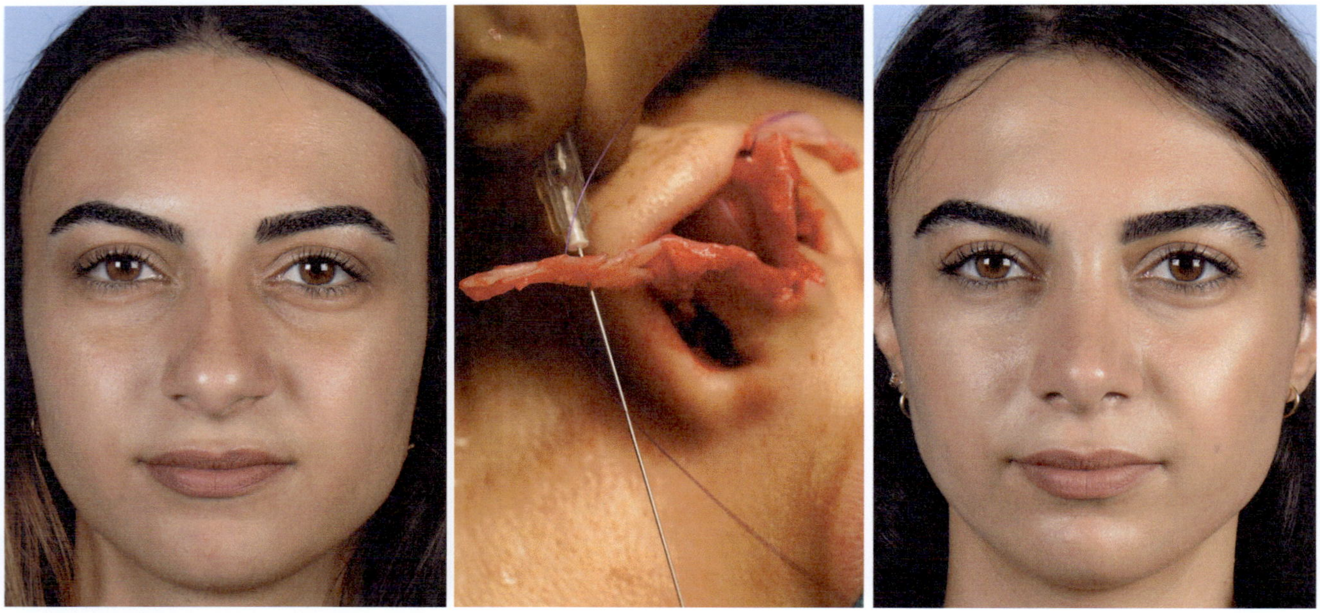

Fig. 13.185 Advanced technique. Pre-, intra-, and postoperative photographs

Disclosures The author reports no conflicts of interest or funding requiring disclosure.

Further Reading

Apaydin F. Nasal valve surgery. Facial Plast Surg. 2011;27(2):179–91.

Constantian MB. The boxy nasal tip, the ball tip, and alar cartilage malposition: variations on a theme—a study in 200 consecutive primary and secondary rhinoplasty patients. Plast Reconstr Surg. 2005;116(1):268–81.

Copcu E, Metin K, Culhaci N, Ozkök S. The new anatomical viewpoint of the nose: the interdomal fat pad. Aesth Plast Surg. 2003;27(2):116–9.

Dhir K, Ghavami A. Reshaping of the broad and bulbous nasal tip. Clin Plast Surg. 2016;43(1):115–26.

Garramone RR, Sullivan PK, Devaney K. Bulbous nasal tip: an anatomical and histological evaluation. Ann Plast Surg. 1995;34(3):288–90; discussion 290–1

Gruber RP, Friedman GD. Suture algorithm for the broad or bulbous nasal tip. Plast Reconstr Surg. 2002;110(7):1752–64; discussion 1765–8

Hamilton GS. Form and function of the nasal tip: reorienting and reshaping the lateral crus. Facial Plast Surg. 2016;32(1):49–58.

Hamra ST. Repositioning the lateral alar crus. Plast Reconstr Surg. 1993;92(7):1244–53.

Ilhan AE, Saribas B, Caypinar B. Aesthetic and functional results of lateral crural repositioning. JAMA Facial Plast Surg. 2015;17(4):286–92.

McKinney P. Management of the bulbous nose. Plast Reconstr Surg. 2000;106(4):906–17; discussion 918–21

McKinney P, Stalnecker M. Surgery for the bulbous nasal tip. Ann Plast Surg. 1983;11(2):106–13.

O'Connor GB, McGregor MW, Shapiro RL, Tolleth H. The bulbous nose. Plast Reconstr Surg. 1967;39(3):278–81.

Perkins S, Patel A. Endonasal suture techniques in tip rhinoplasty. Facial Plast Surg Clin North Am. 2009;17(1):41–54. vi

Pitanguy I, Salgado F, Radwanski HN, Bushkin SC. The surgical importance of the dermocartilaginous ligament of the nose. Plast Reconstr Surg. 1995;95(5):790–4.

Reitzen SD, Morris LG, Davis RE. Prevalence of occult nostril asymmetry in the oversized nasal tip: a quantitative photographic analysis. Arch Facial Plast Surg. 2011;13(5):311–5.

Rohrich RJ, Liu JH. Defining the infratip lobule in rhinoplasty: anatomy, pathogenesis of abnormalities, and correction using an algorithmic approach. Plast Reconstr Surg. 2012;130(5):1148–58.

Sazgar AA. Horizontal reduction using a cephalic hinged flap of the lateral crura: a method to treat the bulbous nasal tip. Aesth Plast Surg. 2010;34(5):642–5.

Şeneldir S, Altundağ A, Dizdar D. Cutting the holy dome: the evolution of vertical alar resection. Aesth Plast Surg. 2018;42(1):275–87.

Seneldir S, Durna YM. An innovative and easy dome holding technique for transdomal suture in rhinoplasty. J Craniofac Surg. 2018;29(6):e585–8.

Slupchynskyj O, Cranford J. Quantitative measurements of the bulbous tip in ethnic rhinoplasty. Ann Plast Surg. 2017;78(5):569–75.

Slupchynskyj O, Rahimi M. Revision rhinoplasty in ethnic patients: pollybeak deformity and persistent bulbous tip. Facial Plast Surg. 2014;30(4):477–84.

Tasman AJ, Helbig M. Sonography of nasal tip anatomy and surgical tip refinement. Plast Reconstr Surg. 2000;105(7):2573–9; discussion 2580–2

Toriumi DM, Asher SA. Lateral crural repositioning for treatment of cephalic malposition. Facial Plast Surg Clin North Am. 2015;23(1):55–71.

Toriumi DM, Checcone MA. New concepts in nasal tip contouring. Facial Plast Surg Clin North Am. 2009;17(1):55–90. vi

14 Narrow Nasal Tip

14.1 Introduction: Brief Clinical History

Rhinoplasty surgery is used to correct problematic alar cartilage anatomy. Aesthetic and functional problems can be addressed with anatomical solutions; these are best designed using appropriate techniques based on characterization of the patient's anatomy. Structural support of the lateral alar wall is provided by the lateral crus. Thus, the lateral crus can be a cause of a narrow nasal tip if it is too weak to hold the lateral nasal wall. The anatomical problems discussed below can result in a narrow tip due to lateral crura.

14.1.1 Lateral Crus Malposition

If the end point of lateral crus is directed to the inner canthus, the lateral nasal wall is no longer supported because the lateral crus, which is required to support the nasal wall, has moved to a different location. This malpositioning explains the weak alar sidewall and should be considered in cases of a primary narrow nasal tip. Alar cartilage malpositioning is also a common anatomical characteristic of secondary rhinoplasty patients. When the primary surgeon fails to recognize malpositioning, residual tip deformities persist. If the primary surgeon narrows the nose using standard surgical techniques without placing malpositioned cartilage into the ideal position, additional deformities develop even though the goal of narrowing the nose is achieved; a pinched appearance can occur (Fig. 14.1).

14.1.2 Problematic Inner Configurations

The primary configurational abnormality is a concave lateral crus. Patients with this condition present with an omega-shaped cartilaginous dome with a visible external depression near the tip, or a weak lateral crus with an undulating shape. There is no discontinuity in the alar cartilage integrity. Thus, in cases of mild and middle concavity, especially in the oblique view, this defect presents as a cavity in the lateral nasal wall, which is a cosmetic problem. In cases with severe concavities, which are quite rare, the lateral crus may prolapse into the nose cavity. This can result in functional problems in addition to cosmetic concerns (Figs. 14.2 and 14.3).

14.1.3 Weak and Deformed Lateral Crus

A weak and deformed lateral crus is generally caused by prior rhinoplasty surgery. Usually, uncontrolled cephalic resection of the lateral crus to narrow the nose can result in a weak or deformed lateral crus (Fig. 14.4).

14.1.4 Unfavorable Relationship Between the Caudal and Cranial Edges of the Lateral Crus

The relationship between caudal and cranial edges of the lateral crus may be distorted due to previous surgeries. If the caudal edge of the lateral crus is under the cranial edge, support of the lateral nasal wall weakens, a wide lobule and a depression in the alar sidewall may form, and the nose appears narrow, especially in the oblique view. This relationship is also the cause of a narrow nasal tip in primary cases (Fig. 14.5).

14.1.5 Why Does Nasal Obstruction Occur with a Pinched Tip?

The lower lateral cartilages play an important role in nasal breathing because these cartilages are the primary structural elements of the external nasal valve. The external nasal valve regulates air flow through the nose and is limited by the following three walls:

Supplementary Information The online version contains supplementary material available at https://doi.org/10.1007/978-3-031-65619-4_14.

S. Şeneldir, *Photographic Atlas of Rhinoplasty*, https://doi.org/10.1007/978-3-031-65619-4_14

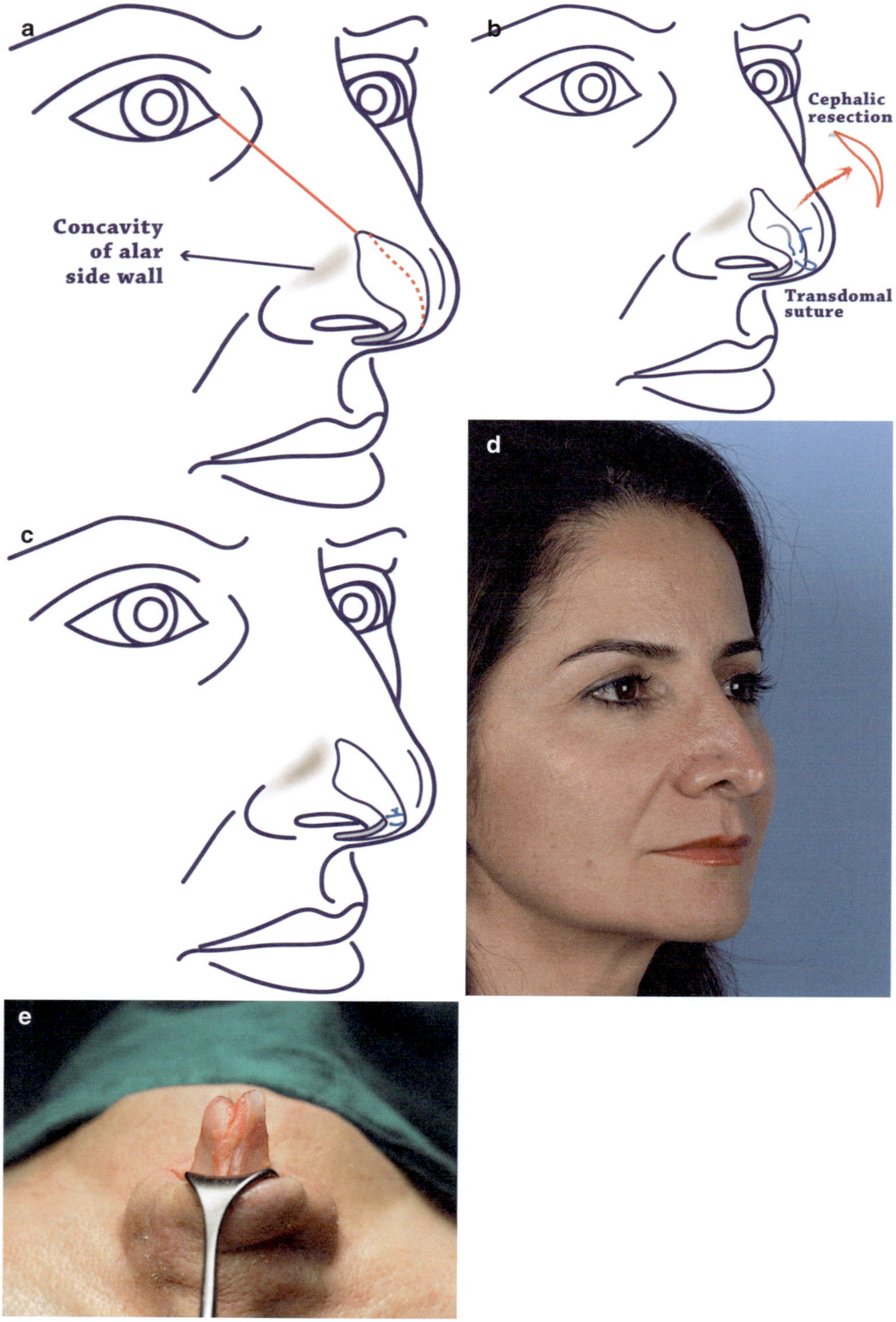

Fig. 14.1 (**a**) Primary malposed lateral crus. The shadow shows the depressed nasal tip in the oblique view. (**b**, **c**) A weak and malposed lateral crus as a result of incorrect techniques resulted in a pinched tip. (**d**) A patient who had undergone previous surgery. (**e**) Parallel lateral crura, a sign of malposition

- **Lateral wall**: Lateral crura of the lower lateral cartilage and fatty-fibrous tissue of the nasal alae.
- **Medial wall**: Membranous septum and medial crura of the lower lateral cartilage.
- **Inferior wall**: The floor of the nose. Inadequacy of the nasal valve due to insufficiency of the lateral crura may cause airway obstruction, especially in the inspirium. Sometimes in the deep inspirium, unsupported lateral nasal walls may even touch the septum (Fig. 14.6).

The exact location of the pathology must be described and noted preoperatively, because it is difficult to identify

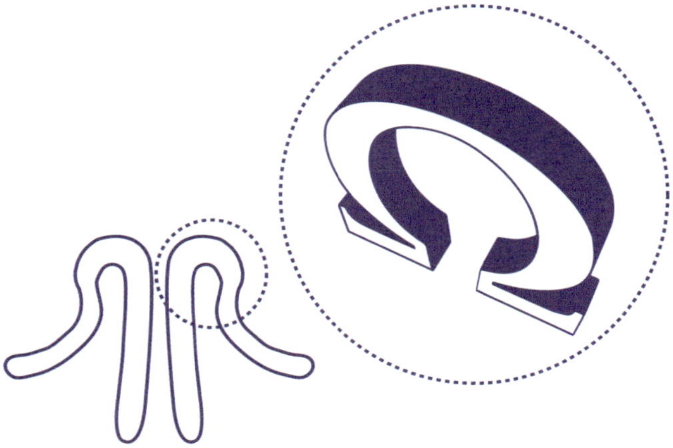

Fig. 14.2 The illustration shows omega-shaped alar cartilage

this area intraoperatively. By supporting the described points of the lateral nasal wall with a small object (such as a cerumen curette), this delicate area can be localized. However, while these areas are being supported, using a nose speculum or endoscope can result in inaccurate evaluations.

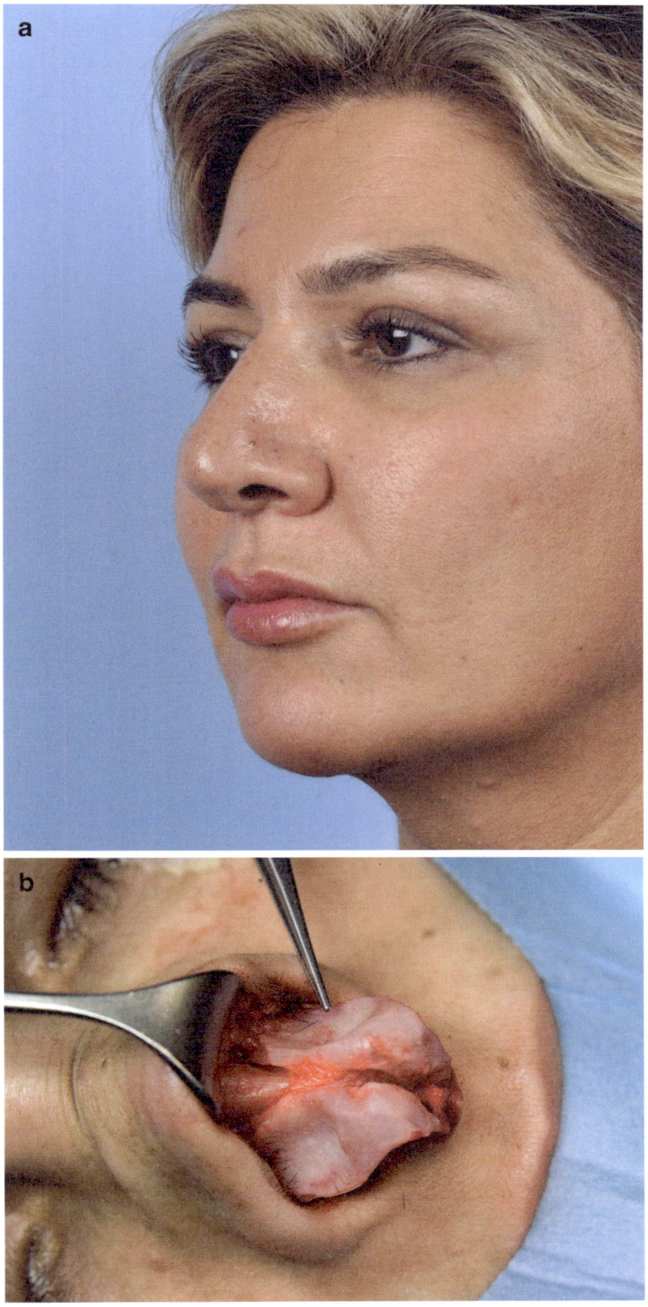

Fig. 14.3 (**a**, **b**) Clinical images of omega-shaped alar cartilages corresponding to Fig. 14.2

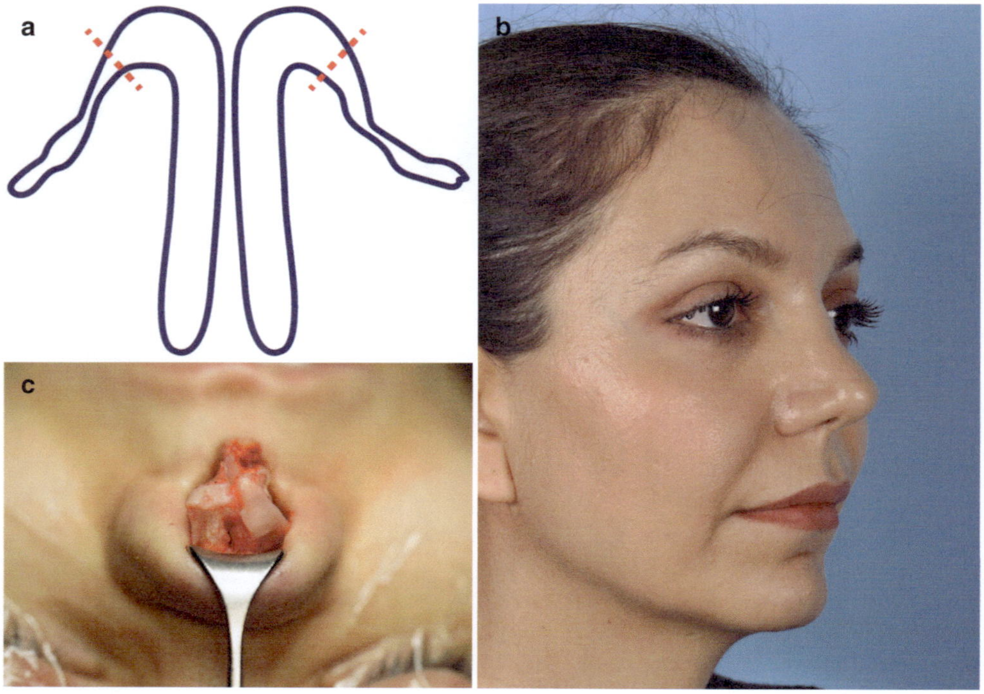

Fig. 14.4 (**a**–**c**) Pinched appearance may stem from deformed lateral crura that include buckling, disruption, asymmetric alignment

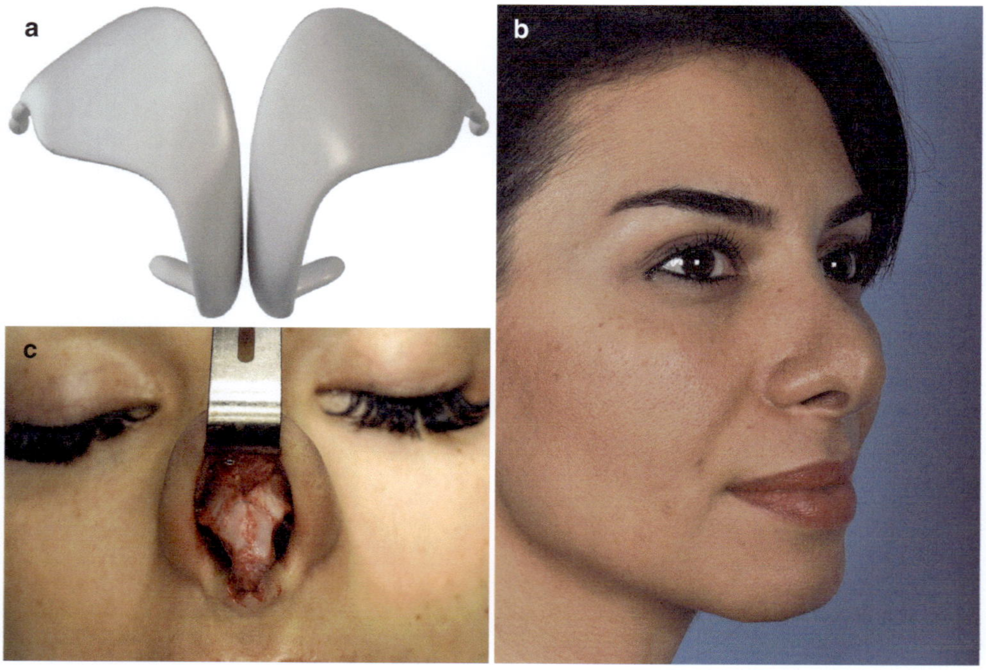

Fig. 14.5 (**a**–**c**) If the cartilage is in such an unfavorable configuration that the caudal edge of the lateral crus is significantly below that of the cranial side, this may predispose to loss of support in the lateral alar region and consequent pinched tip deformity

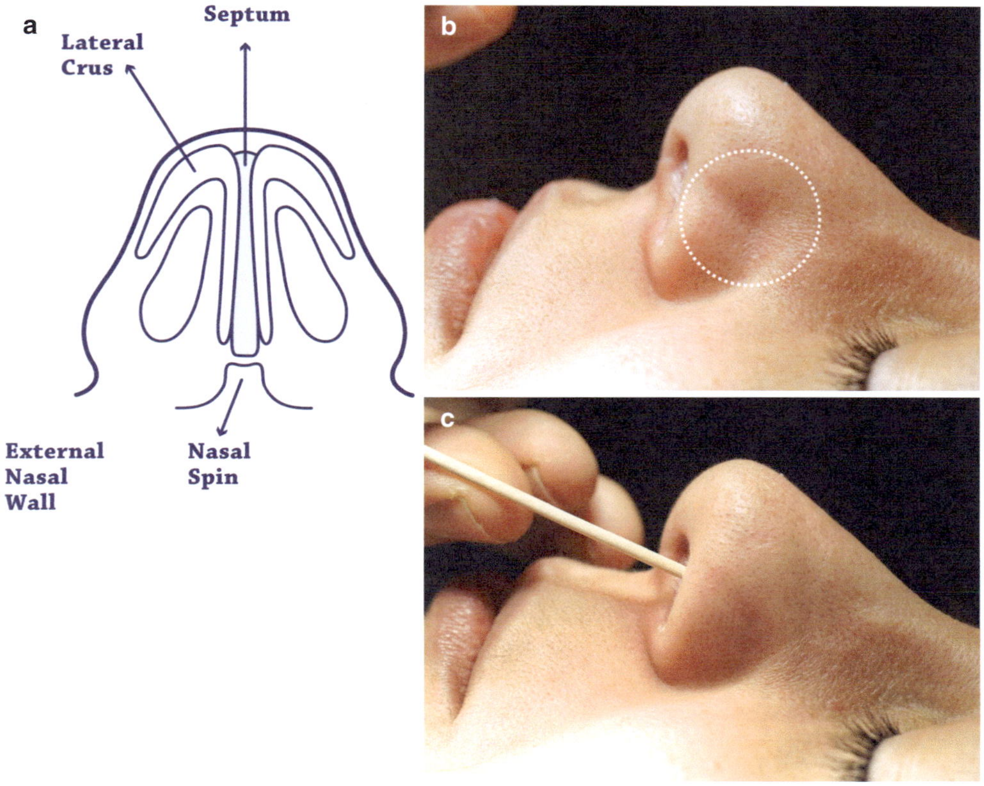

Fig. 14.6 (**a**) External nasal valve anatomy. (**b**) The dotted area shows depression of the lateral nasal wall that is affecting the external nasal wall. (**c**) By supporting the depressed part of the lateral nasal wall with a small curette, this delicate area was localized

14.2 Treatment Strategy

Addressing anatomical problems is an important step in the treatment strategy. First, any of the above anatomical problems should be identified, after which they can be addressed using appropriate techniques. Whether the issue is congenital or the result of prior rhinoplasty, the proper process from diagnosis to treatment must be followed. It is important to examine the position of the lateral crus to establish the correct diagnosis.

If a malpositioned lateral crus is present, a repositioning operation is performed (Fig. 14.7).

If the narrow tip is the result of excessive concavity of the lateral crus, a lateral crural graft can be used for treatment. This is an appropriate choice for mild and moderate concavities (Fig. 14.8).

If the malformed segment of cartilage is not suitable for reconstruction, the cartilage may be excised and a septal or costal cartilage graft can be used to reconstruct the entire lateral crus by placing a large cartilage graft in the alar lobule at the external valve (Fig. 14.9).

For a severe concavity of the lateral crura, cartilage can be excised, preserving the vestibular mucosa and flipping it over such that the concavity faces inward. It must be firmly secured to the dome (Fig. 14.10).

The lateral nasal wall can be controlled after strengthening the lateral crus. However, it may require additional support. In this situation, an alar batten graft (lateral wall batten graft) can be used. The lateral wall batten graft is placed in the area under the supra-alar crease. This small graft may provide additional structural support and recurvature to maintain alar integrity during inspiration.

In some pinched noses alar retraction may accompany. Despite strengthening the lateral nasal wall, an alar retraction may persist. In this case, auricular composite grafting can be performed.

Technical Pearl: Constructing a strong nasal tip requires constructing a strong septal vault. The caudal septum should be evaluated, especially in revision cases. Weakness in the dorsal septum may accompany the pinched tip. Reconstructions made on the tip that are not supported by a strong septum will not be durable. If there is weak septal support, the strength and resistance of the caudal septum should be enhanced using a spreader, a septal batten, or a caudal replacement graft.

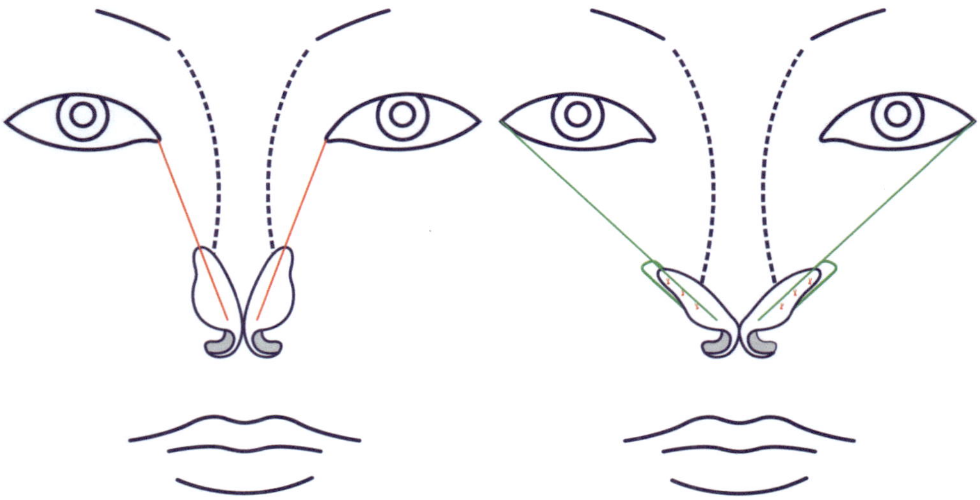

Fig. 14.7 Vector of lateral crura. Green: appropriate; red: not appropriate

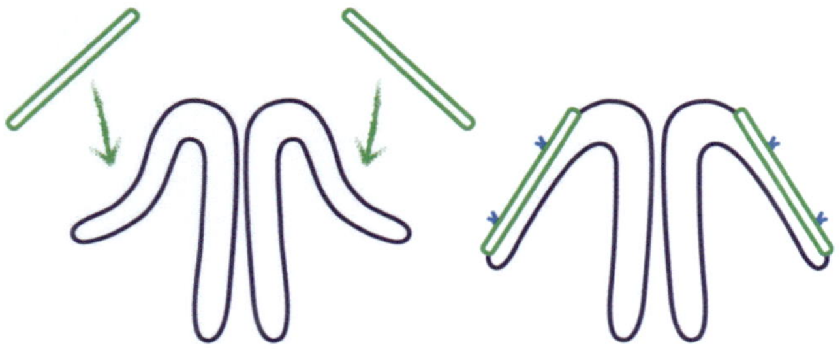

Fig. 14.8 Overlay lateral crural graft

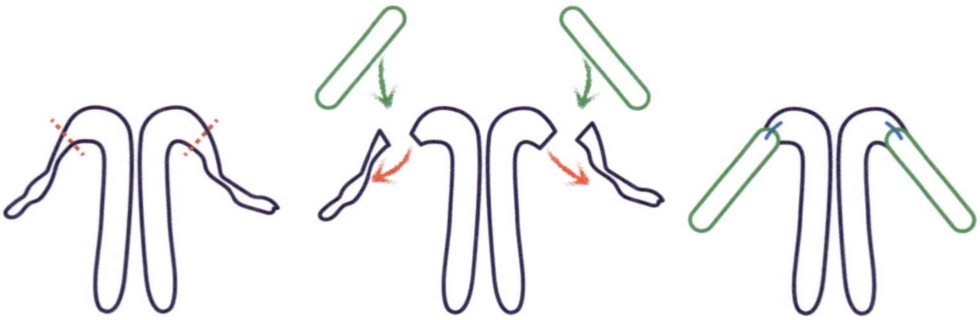

Fig. 14.9 The disrupted, buckled, and asymmetric alignment lateral crura. Resection and recreation with septal cartilage

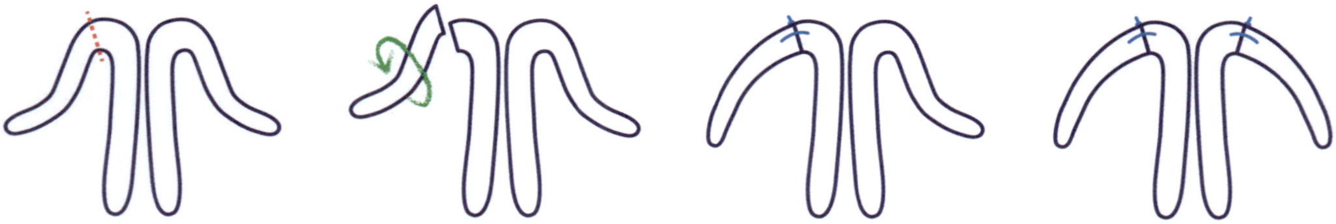

Fig. 14.10 Flip-flop technique. A pinched deformity caused by excessive natural concavity of the lateral crus may be fixed by the complete mobilization of the crus from the skin. An incision is then made just lateral to the domal area, and the lateral crus flipped over such that the concavity becomes a convexity. The rotated, reconstructed crus is then sutured to the medial segment with nonabsorbable sutures

14.3 Clinical Outcomes: Secondary Narrow Nasal Tip

In the cases presented here, the pinched or narrow nasal tip will be presented in two parts according to their cause. There are three explanations for a secondary narrow nasal tip: (1) Cephalic malposition of the lateral crus; (2) Weak and deformed lateral crus; and (3) Incorrect suturing during a previous surgery.

14.3.1 Cephalic Malposition of the Lateral Crus

Malposition is a common reason for revision tip surgery. Cephalic malposition of the lower lateral cartilages is an important cause of external nasal valve insufficiency and a pinched tip appearance. When this insufficiency is identified, treatment should be performed to reposition the lateral crura.

14.3.1.1 Case 1

In this case of previous rhinoplasty, severe nasal pinch is apparent in the profile view. Intraoperatively, we found that the underlying cause of the severe pinched nasal tip was malposed lateral crura (Fig. 14.11).

Elimination of the lobular convexity and sidewall concavity created a delicate tip and corrected the malpositioning. Because deformities caused by previous surgeries may be evident in the lateral crura, the crura must be removed and reinforced and the configurational deformities corrected. The crura must then be repositioned directly over the sutured costal cartilage grafts and finally moved to the appropriate position. Repositioning also allows us to reduce over-projection. After the tip point was fixed using a transdomal suture, the alar base was stabilized using a columellar strut and a septocolumellar suture (Fig. 14.12).

One-year postoperative photographs show that repositioning surgery not only refined the tip, but also corrected several tip-related problems. Reconstruction of septum also can lend support to the tip cartilages. Middle vault support is improved with a resulting correction of the dorsal saddling. The width of the middle third is increased with the spreader grafts (Fig. 14.13).

14.3.1.2 Case 2

In this case, the narrow tip was caused by the position of the lateral crus, which was not corrected during the primary surgery. With a suitable treatment, the results of repositioning surgery are satisfying (Fig. 14.14).

Four-year postoperative photographs are shown in Fig. 14.15. The repositioning surgery addressed the nasal pinch and other tip problems.

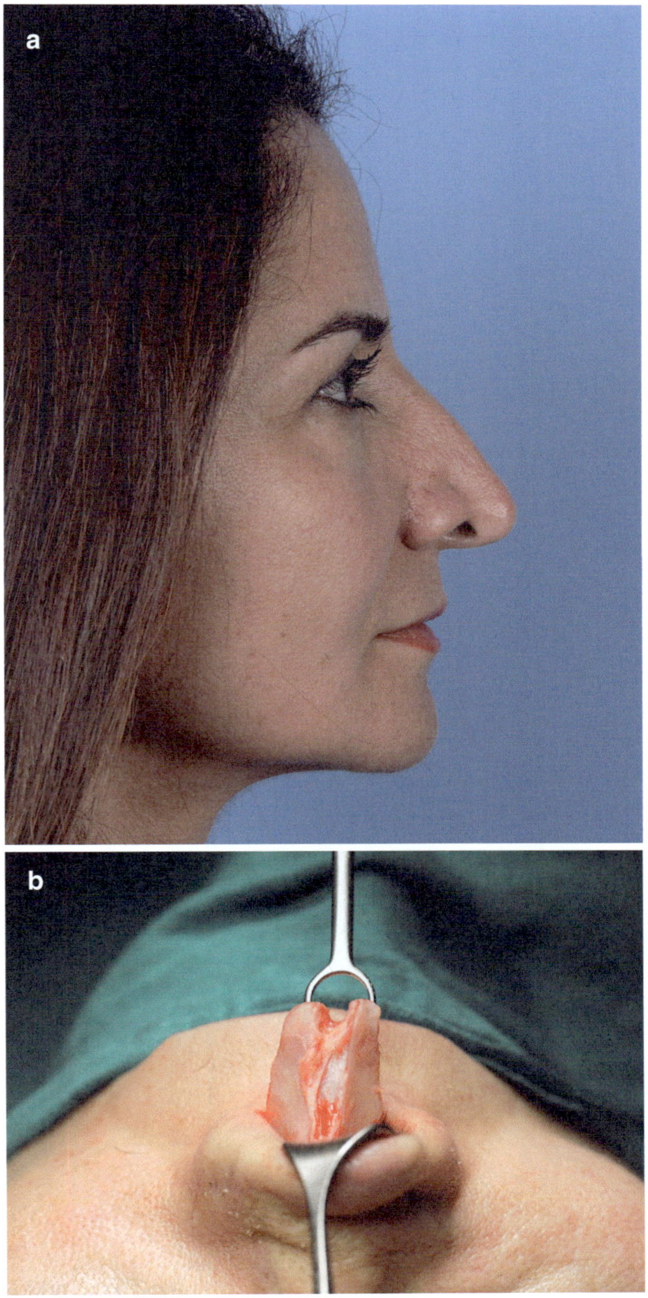

Fig. 14.11 (**a**, **b**) Pinched and over-projected nasal tip. (Supplementary Video 14.1)

14.3.2 Weak and Deformed Lateral Crus

14.3.2.1 Case 3

Case 3 is a typical example of a pinched nasal tip caused by deformed and weak lateral crura. In the basal photograph of the patient, who had undergone rhinoplasty 10 years prior, the pinched tip is evident, the external nasal valve is extremely narrowed, and the nasal passage is nearly closed (Fig. 14.16).

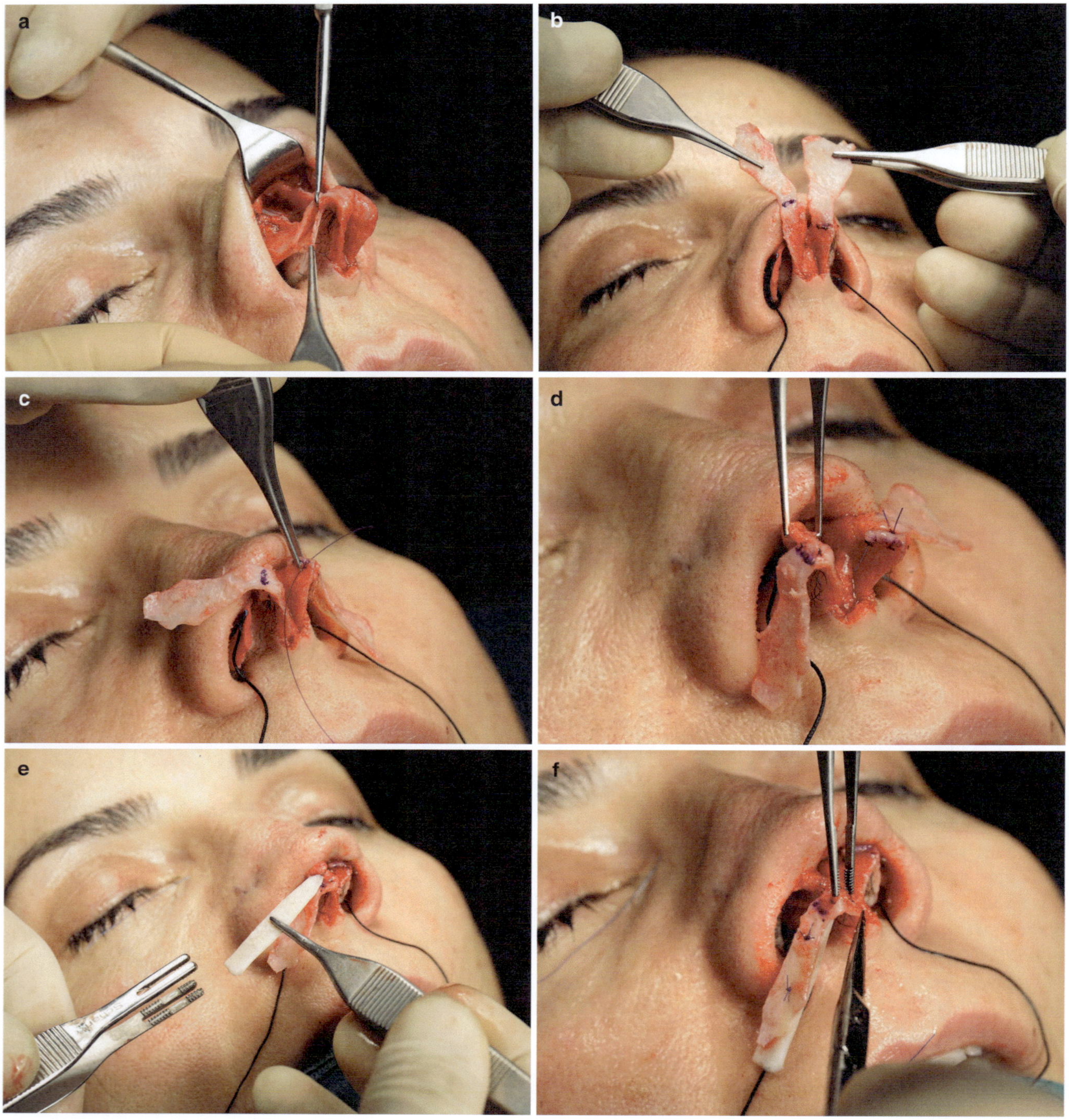

Fig. 14.12 (**a**) Caudal access is the most efficient method to detach the lateral crus from vestibular skin. (**b**) The bilateral lateral crus was freed from the vestibular skin. The right marker indicates the actual dome point, and the left shows the desired dome point. (**c**, **d**) New dome-defining points were created by suturing bilaterally. (**e**–**h**) To strengthen and correct the configuration of the lateral crura, lateral crural grafts harvested from costal cartilage were sutured under the lateral crus and placed in the opened pocket facing the outer canthus. (**i**, **j**) As mentioned previously, a strong caudal septum is important for tip stability. Bilateral extended spreader and caudal septal replacement grafts were used to reconstruct the caudal septum. (**k**, **l**) Final alar cartilage configuration. The positions of the lateral crura were ideal, resulting in a deprojected tip

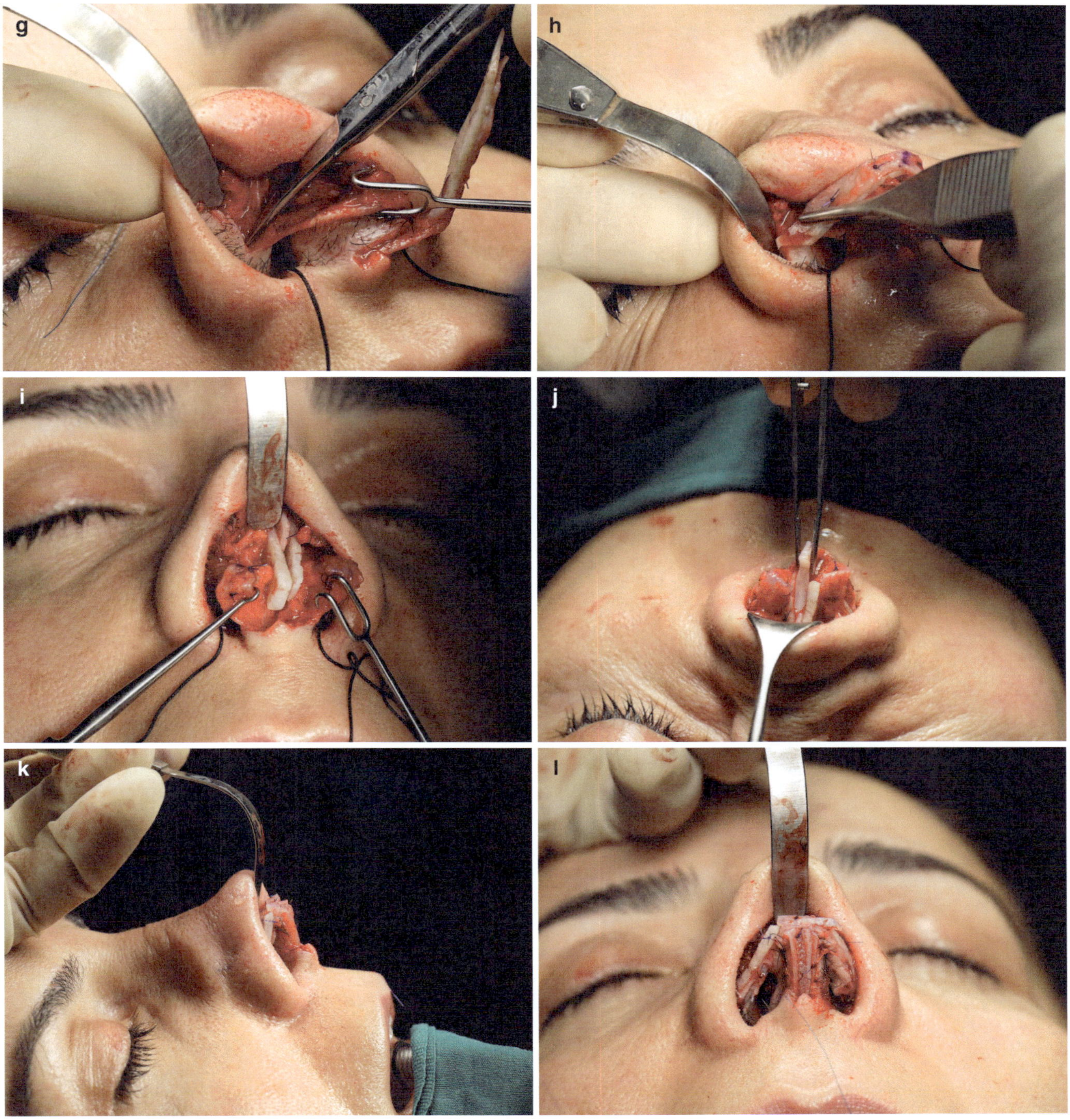

Fig. 14.12 (continued)

It may be difficult to strengthen the deformed lateral crus. To evaluate and strengthen the lateral crus extracorporeally, the lateral crus was elevated from the vestibular skin (Fig. 14.17).

Caudal septal control is important, especially in revision cases. The caudal septum in this case was not strong enough. Thus, the caudal septum was strengthened with a septal batten graft harvested from the costal cartilage (Fig. 14.18).

Because the remainder of the alar arch was strong, transdomal suturing was performed, new dome points were created, and a new and strong lateral crus from the lateral region of the new dome point was constructed (Fig. 14.19).

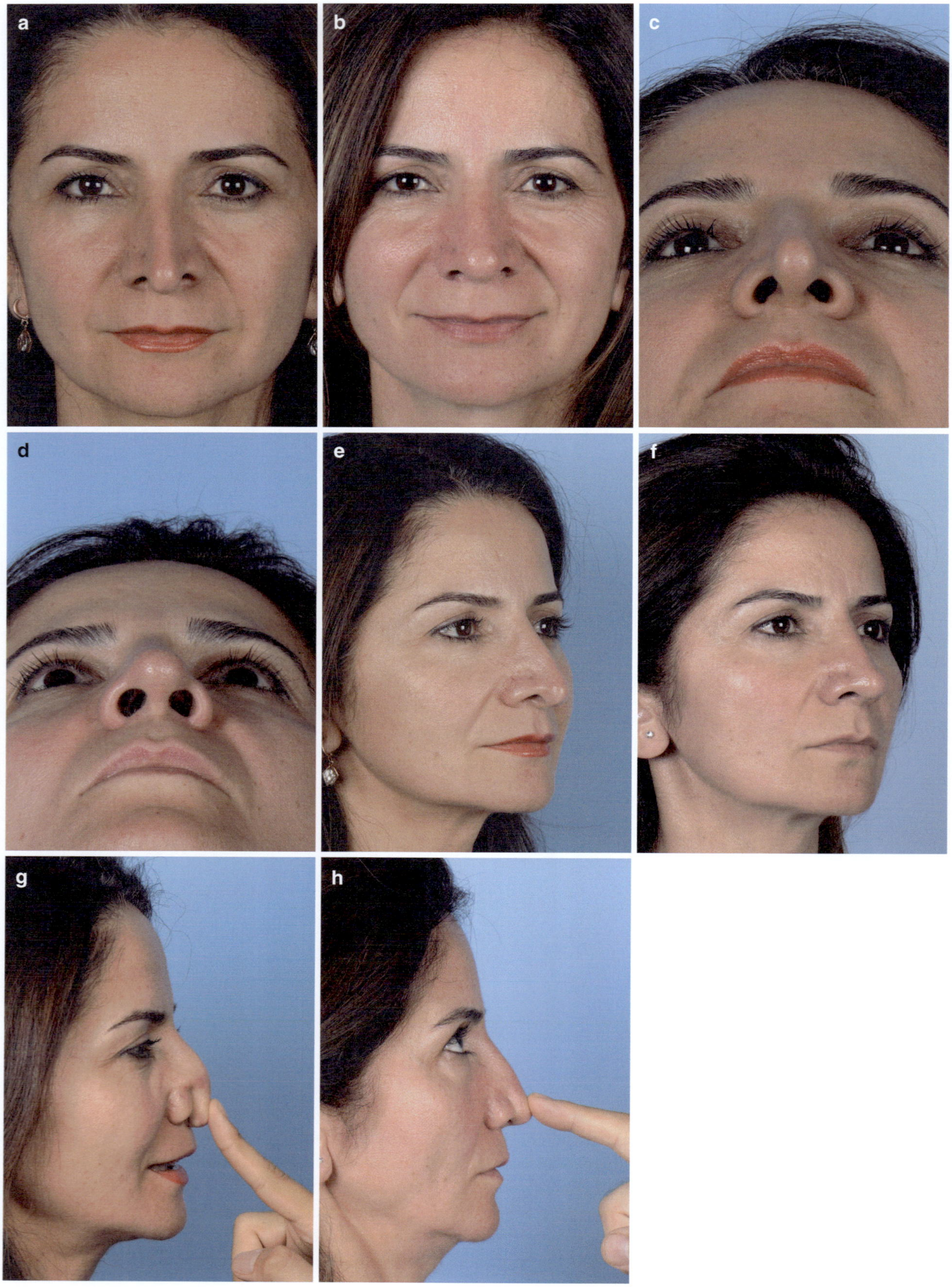

Fig. 14.13 (**a–d**) In this case, there is a total absence of septal support for the cartilaginous vault, nasal tip, and internal nasal valve. The nasal tip appeared to have a pinched configuration with a significantly over-projected tip. (**e–g**) Postoperatively, the patient was pleased with her rhinoplasty results, mainly the correction of her tip deformity. Her nasal breathing was improved, and there was no evidence of septal collapse (**h**)

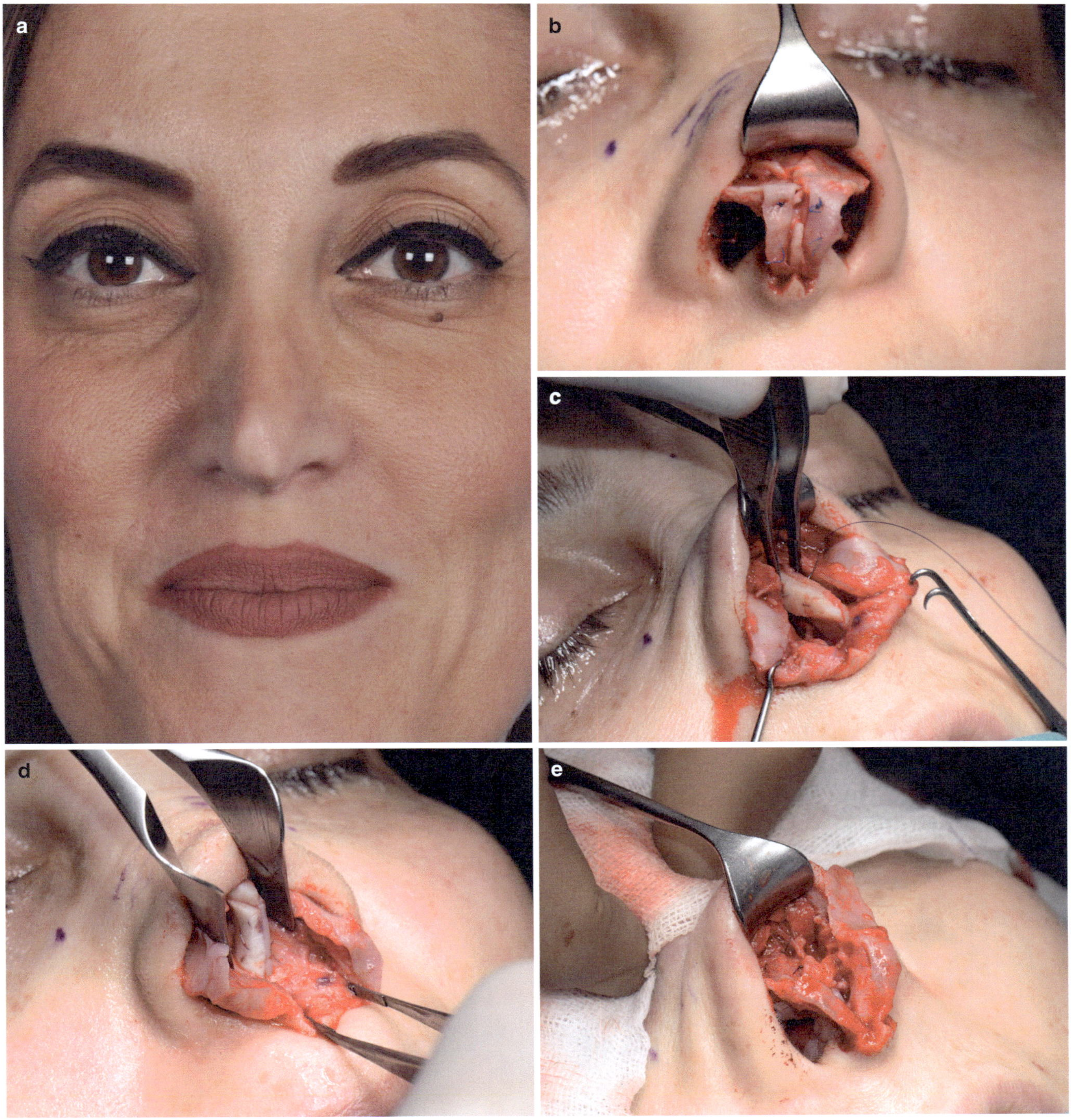

Fig. 14.14 (**a**) Preoperative frontal view. (**b**) The malposition itself caused the pinched nose. Instead of correcting the malposition of the lateral crus during primary surgery, cephalic excision and transdomal suturing were performed on the malpositioned lateral crus, which weakened it. Ultimately, a weak and malpositioned lateral crus caused the pinched tip. (**c**, **d**) Before repositioning surgery, a stable septum should be created. For this purpose, bilateral extended spreader grafts and a septal batten graft were used. (**e**, **f**) The lateral crura were repositioned. (**g–j**) During repositioning surgery, the tip should be fixed to the septum. In this case, a septocolumellar suture was used

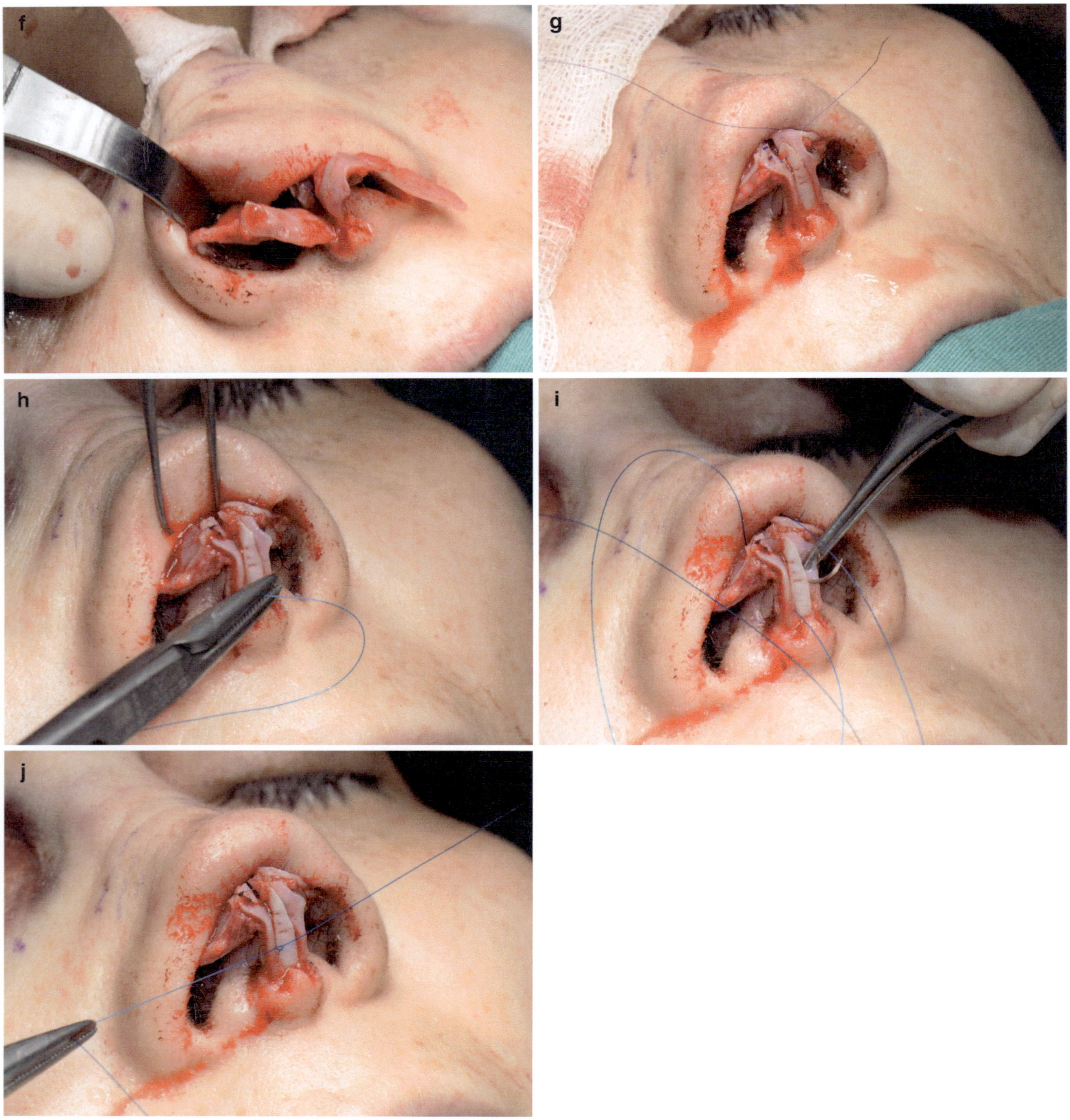

Fig. 14.14 (continued)

The graft harvested from the septum was placed in a pocket opened in a position where the lateral crus should be present. One end of the graft was sutured to the lateral region of the dome, and the other end was inserted into the pocket and opened toward the outer canthus (Fig. 14.20).

A deformed lateral crus was excised bilaterally (Fig. 14.21).

The final projection and definition were achieved by ensuring the integrity of the columellar strut and columella (Fig. 14.22).

In 1-year postoperative photographs, the pinched nasal tip was addressed, and dilation of the external nasal valve was observed (Fig. 14.23).

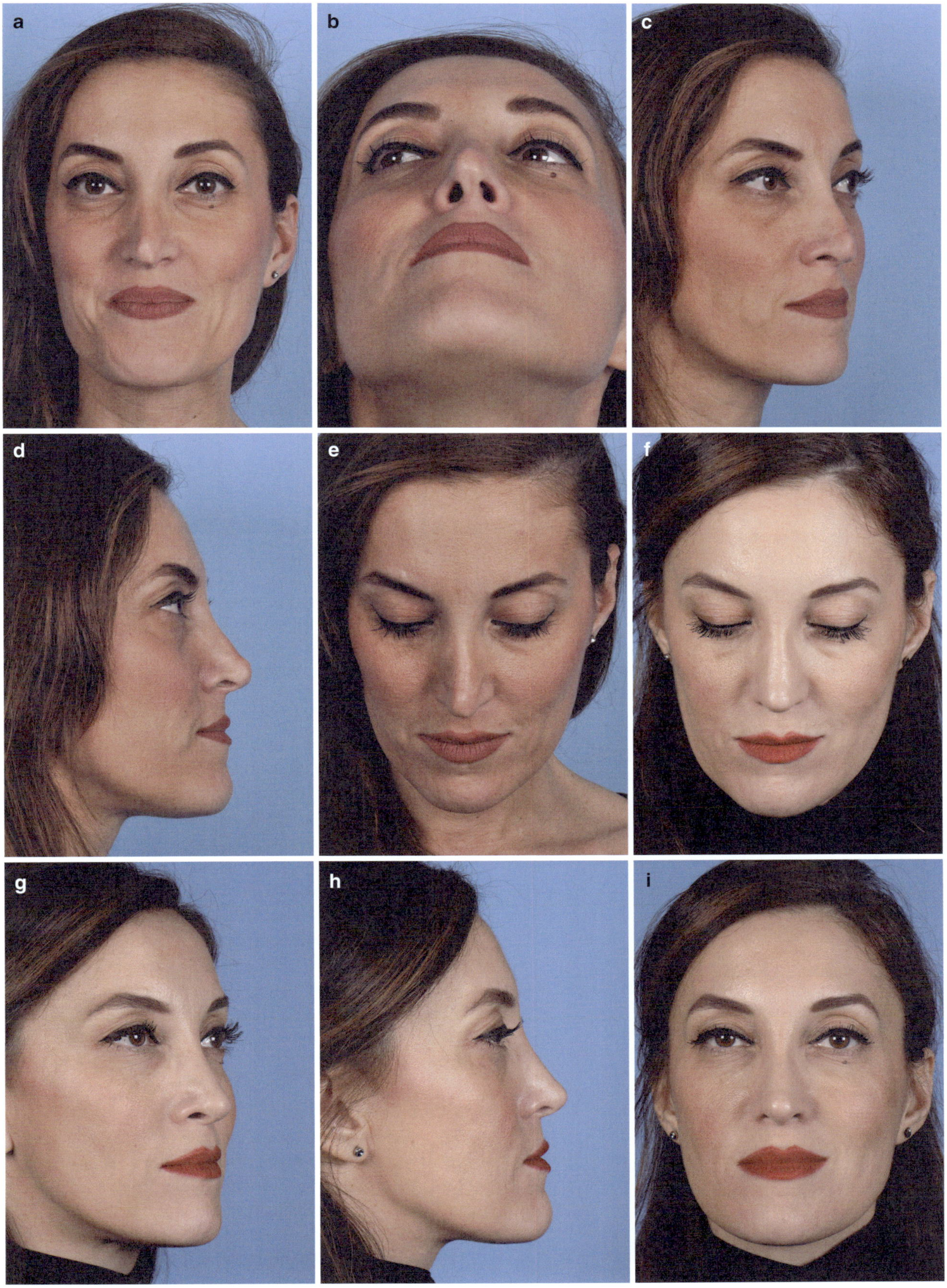

Fig. 14.15 (**a–j**) The patient is shown 4 years postoperatively. There is now ideal tip width improved symmetry with repositioning of lateral crura. The alar contour and strength is also enhanced

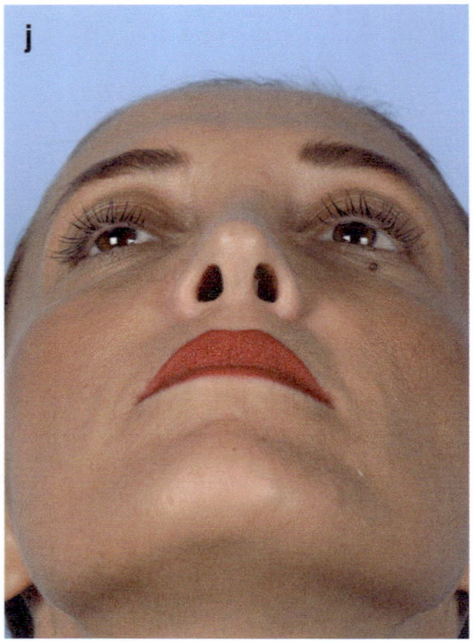

Fig. 14.15 (continued)

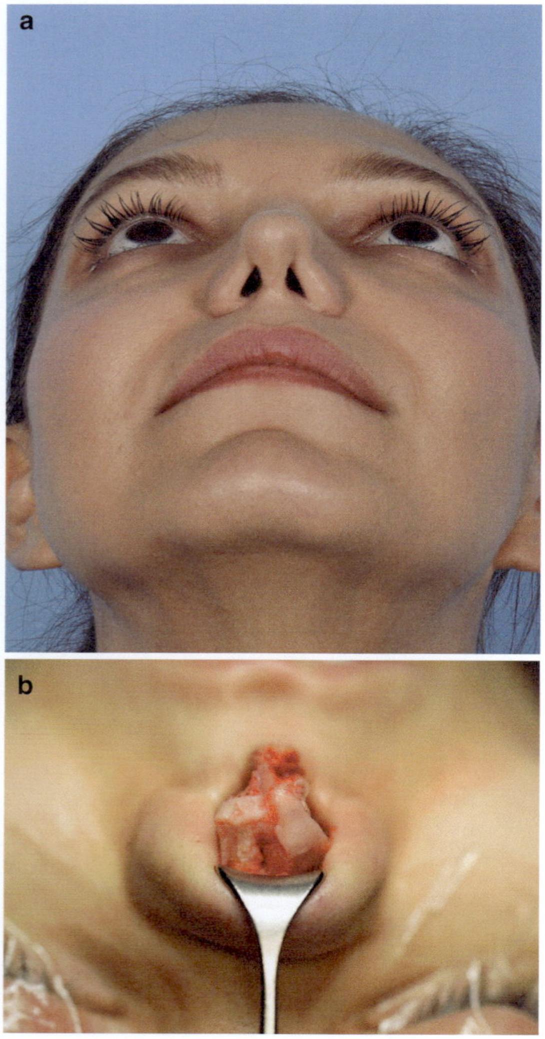

Fig. 14.16 (**a**) A patient with pinched tip. (**b**) Lateral crus weakness and deformity is evident intraoperatively

14.3.3 Incorrect Suturing During a Previous Surgery

Following tip surgery that was completed without correcting the unfavorable relationship between the caudal and cranial regions of the lateral crus, the alar lateral wall weakens. Eventually, a wide lobule and narrow alar sidewall appearance can occur.

14.3.3.1 Case 4

The preoperative and intraoperative photographs show typical examples of an unfavorable relationship between the cranial and caudal regions of the lateral crus (Fig. 14.24).

Reforming the disrupted relationship strengthens the lateral nasal wall. In revision cases, this can be corrected using the VAR technique. Trapezoidal resection from the deformed dome point provides an opportunity to reform this relationship (Fig. 14.25).

After correction of the alar arch configuration, the tip needs to be stabilized. For this purpose, the tip was fixed to the septum with a septocolumellar strut graft. The cap graft provided extra projection and definition, and bilateral lateral crural grafts provided the lateral nasal walls with extra strength (Fig. 14.26).

Two-year postoperative photographs of the case are shown in Fig. 14.27.

14.3.3.2 Case 5

Another example of an unfavorable relationship between the caudal and cranial edges of the lateral crus is seen in this case. The frontal view of this patient shows isolation of the tip lobule and a pinched appearance of the nasal tip. There is an obvious demarcation of the nasal tip, and there are visible shadows between the tip and alar lobule in the oblique view. The VAR technique was used to correct this deformity.

Fifteen-year postoperative results are satisfactory (Fig. 14.28).

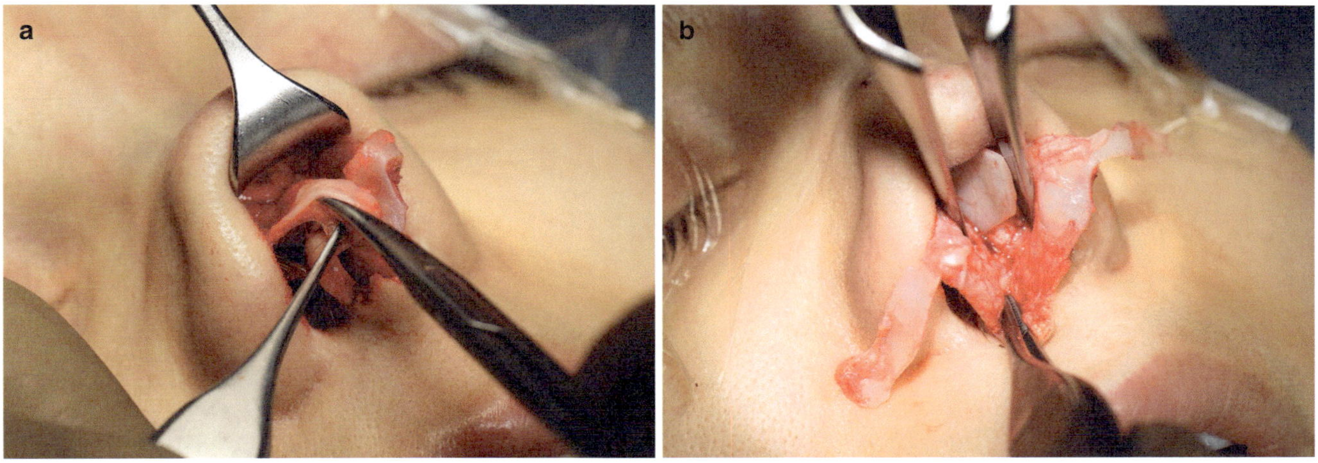

Fig. 14.17 (**a**, **b**) Both lateral crus were freed from the skin

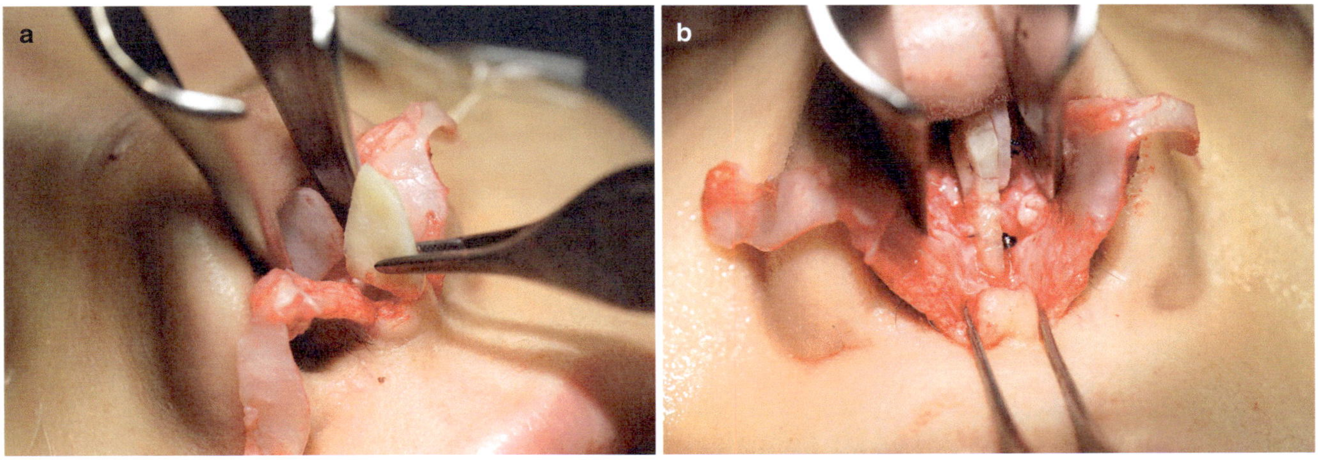

Fig. 14.18 (**a**, **b**) A strong caudal base for the newly formed alar arch was constructed using a septal batten graft

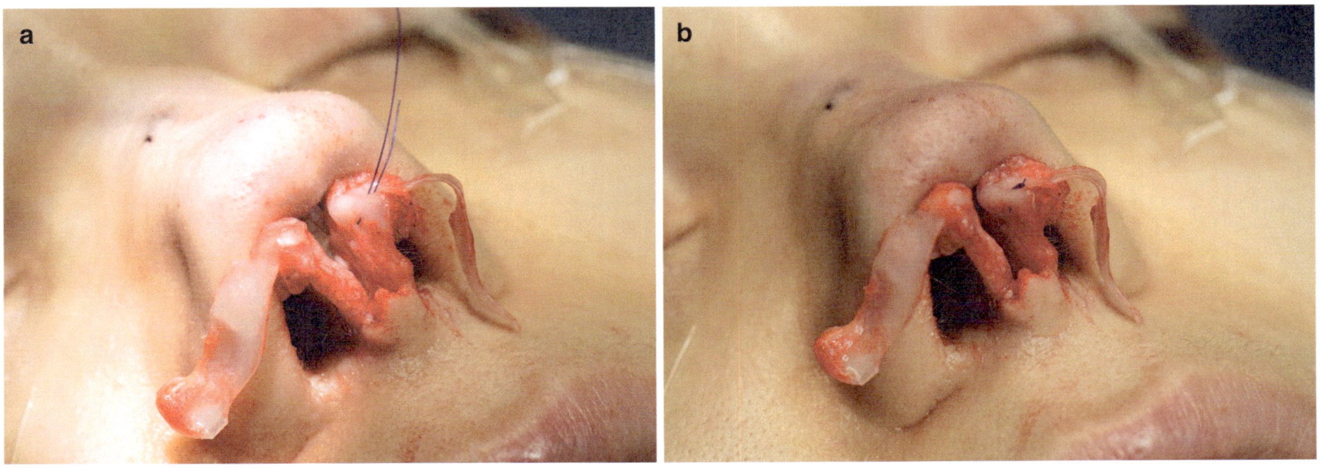

Fig. 14.19 (**a**, **b**) A bilateral transdomal suture was used. The increasing weakness in the lateral crus after new dome points were formed with transdomal sutures draws attention

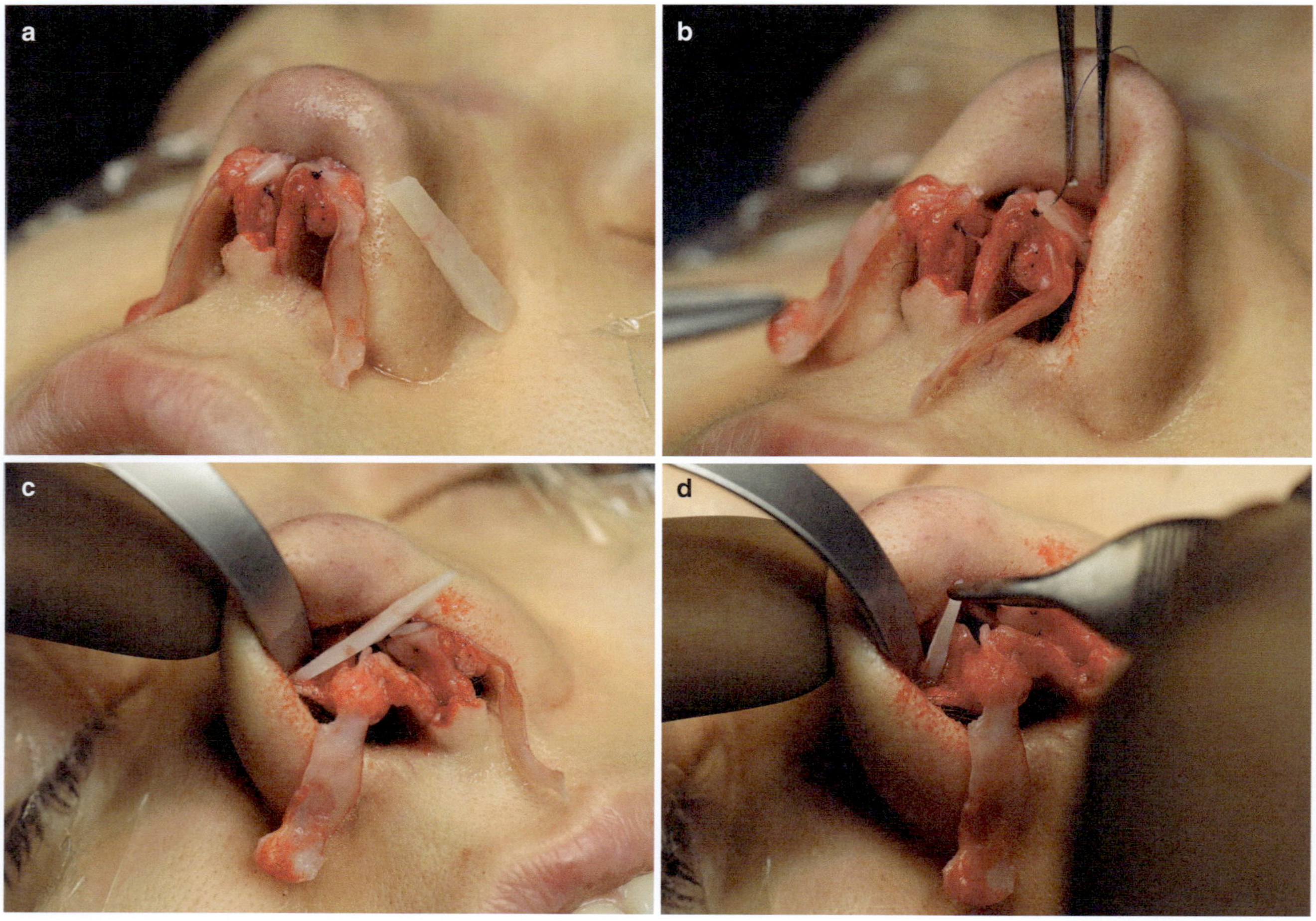

Fig. 14.20 (**a–d**) The graft was fixed to the dome with 5-0 nonabsorbable suture

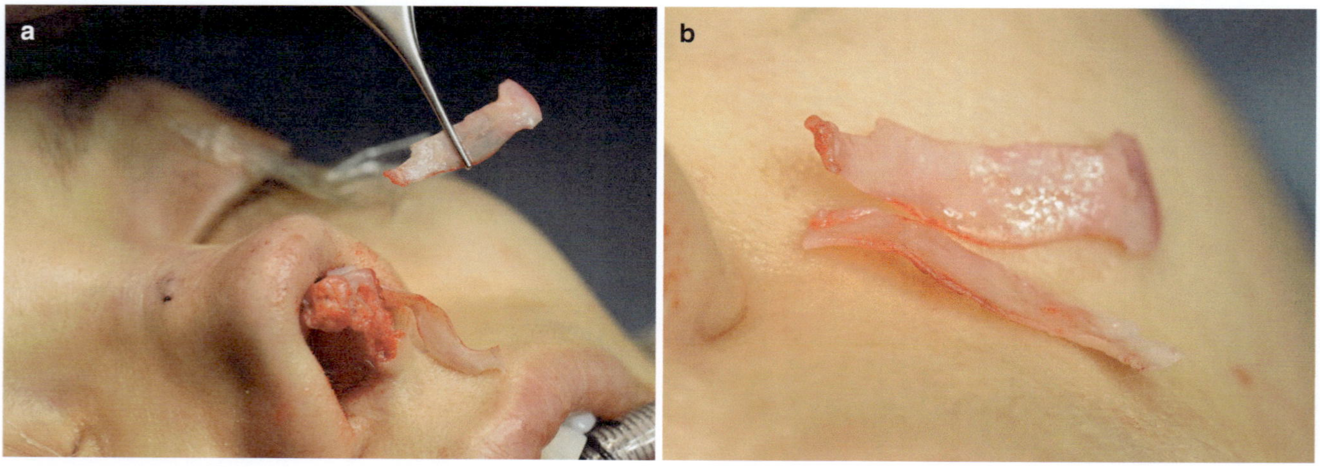

Fig. 14.21 (**a**, **b**) Deformed lateral crura were excised

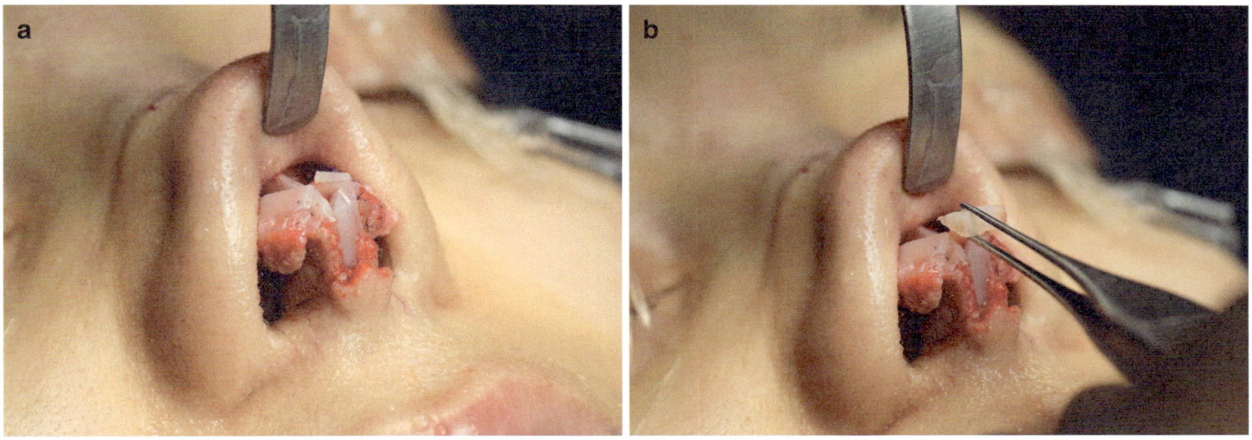

Fig. 14.22 (**a**) Lateral crura were recreated with septal cartilages. (**b**) Placement columellar strut and cap graft

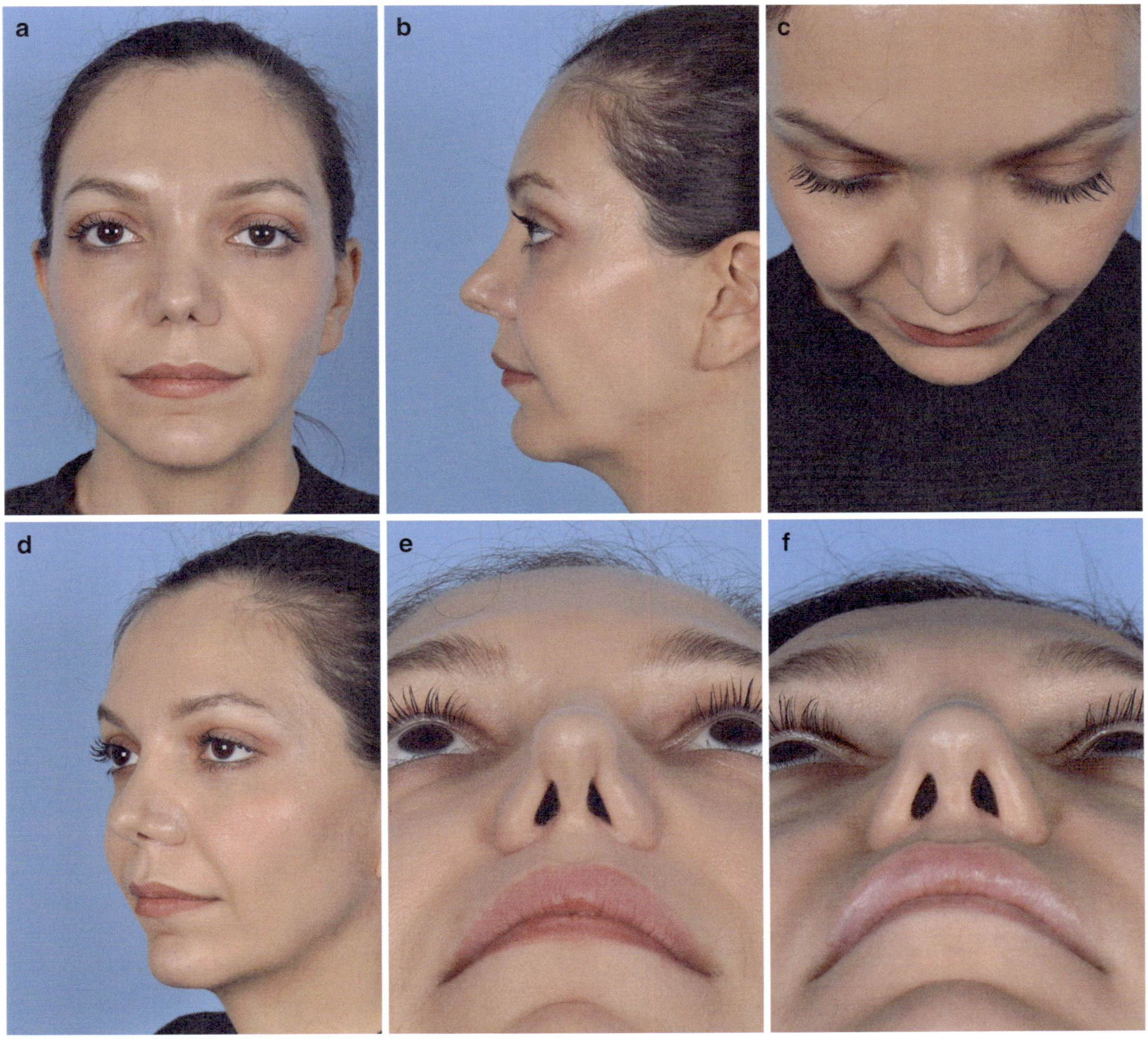

Fig. 14.23 (**a**–**j**) Postoperative photographs show symmetric nasal tip base, absence of pinching deformity, and improved nasal breathing. (**a**, **e**) preoperative pictures; (**f**, **j**) postoperative photographs show symmetric nasal tip base, absence of pinching deformity, and improved nasal breathing

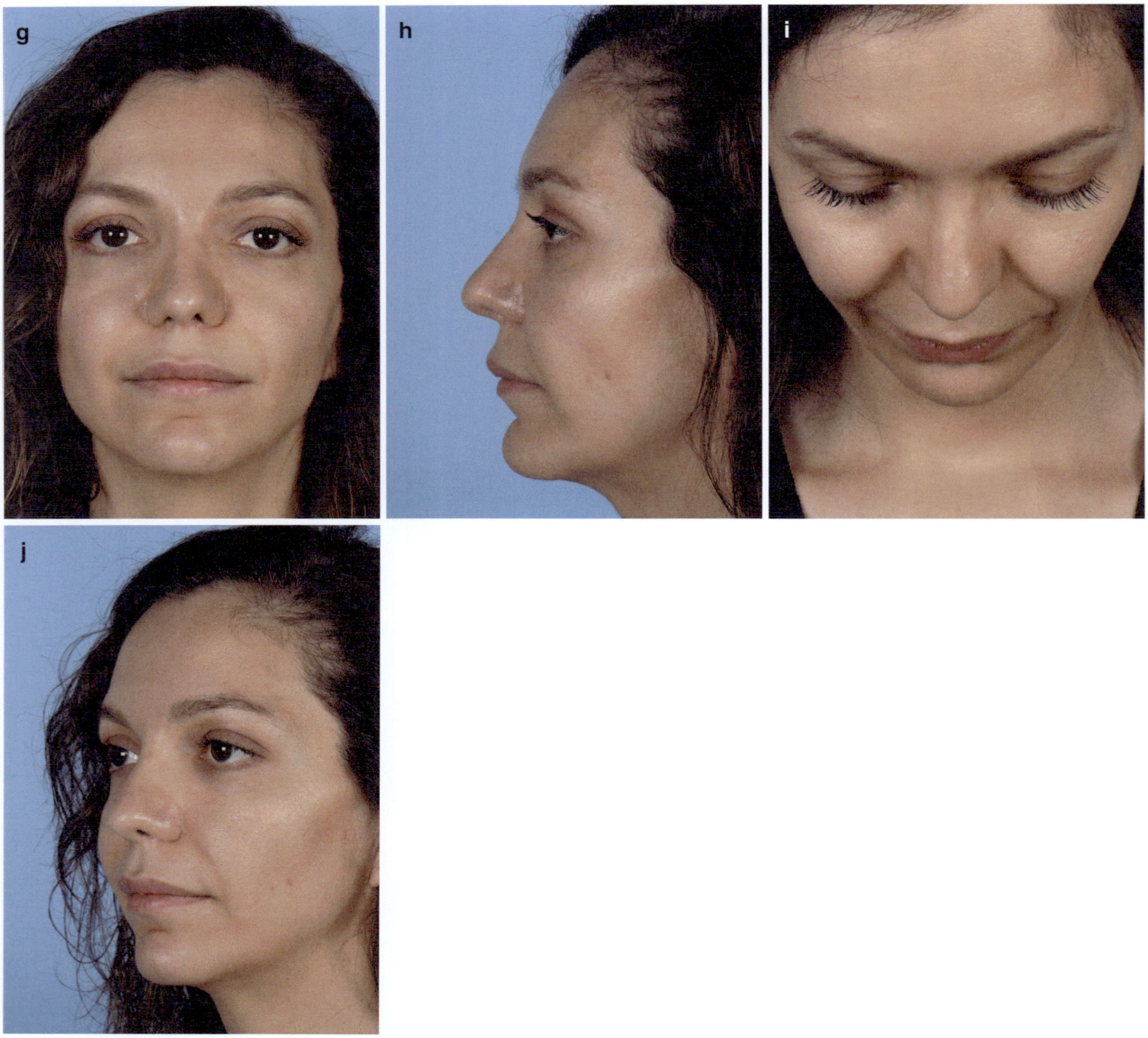

Fig. 14.23 (continued)

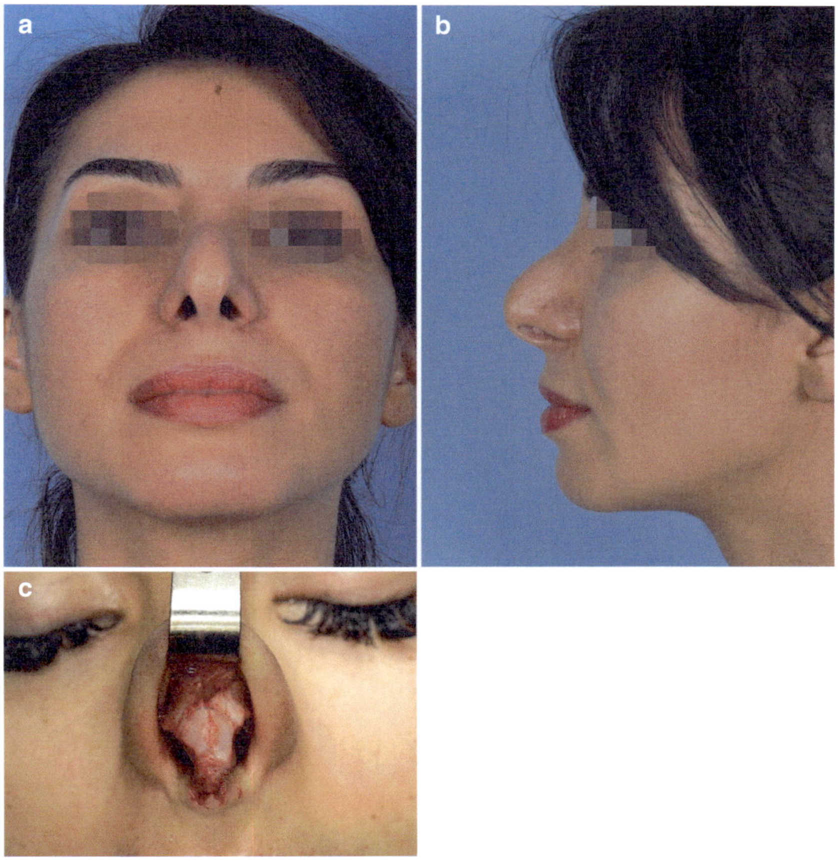

Fig. 14.24 (**a–c**) Three main tip problems were evident: a pinched appearance due to the unfavorable relationship, hanging columella due to excessive springiness, and supratip fullness mainly by the lateral crura and excess dorsal septal cartilage. (Supplementary Video 14.2)

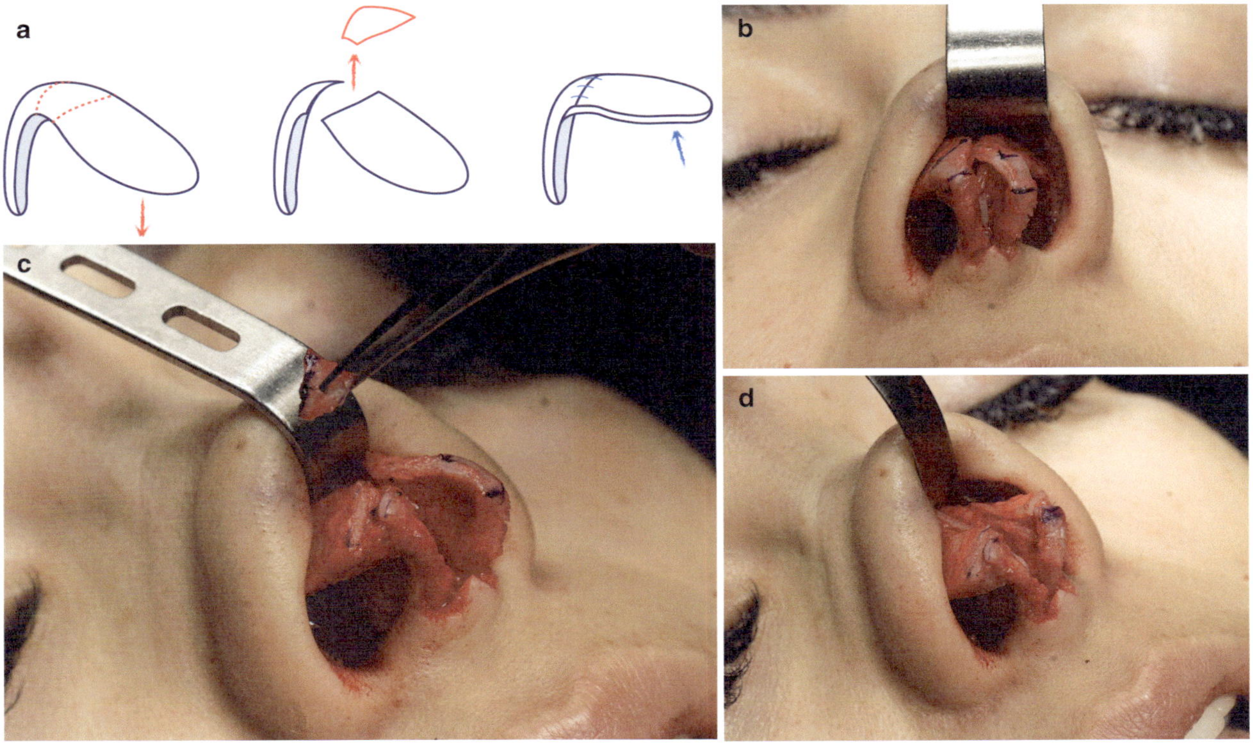

Fig. 14.25 (**a**) Schematic illustration of the effects of trapezoidal resection of crura on the degree of lateral crura configuration. (**b**, **c**) Trapezoidal resection corrected the configuration of the alar cartilage, and supratip bulging. (**d**) Reapproximate remain segments with suture

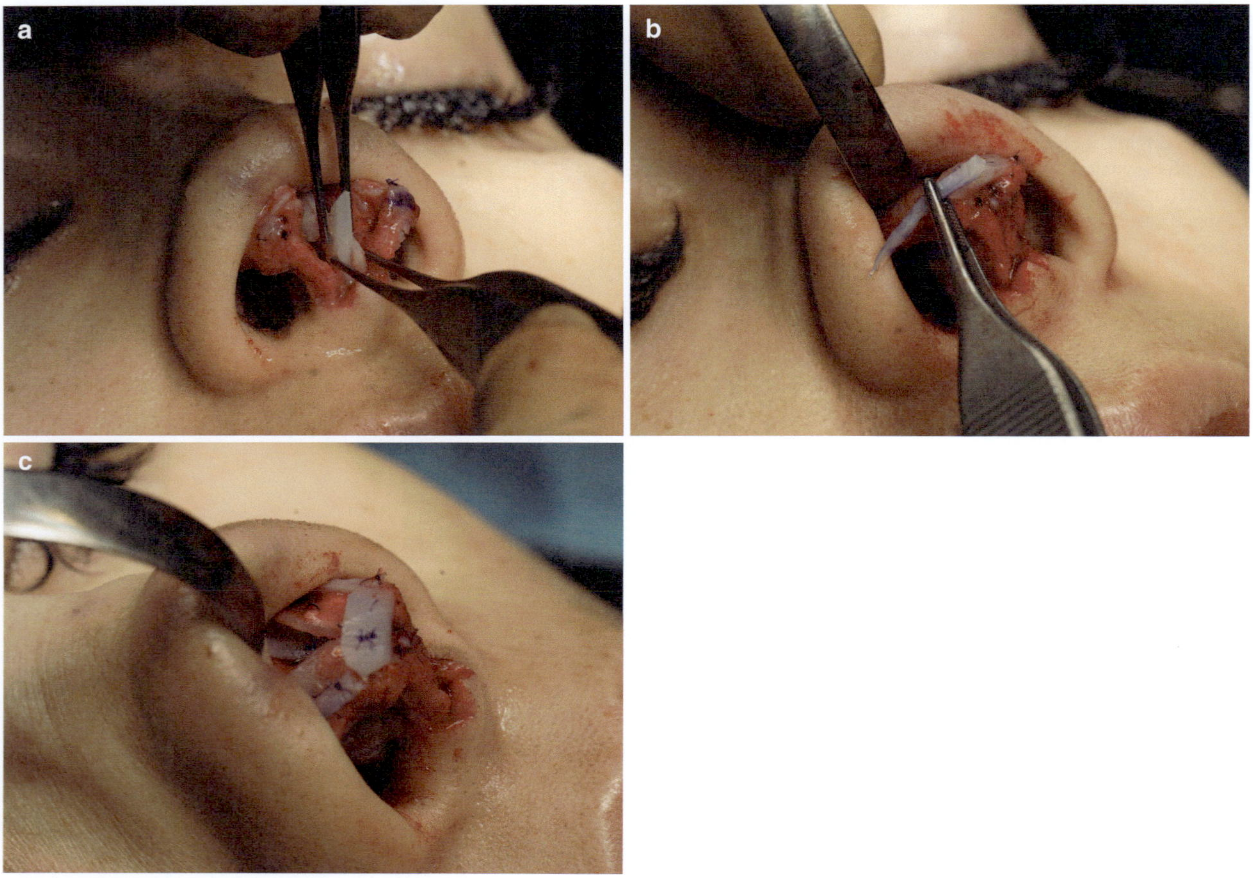

Fig. 14.26 (**a**–**c**) A thin lateral crural graft was sufficient

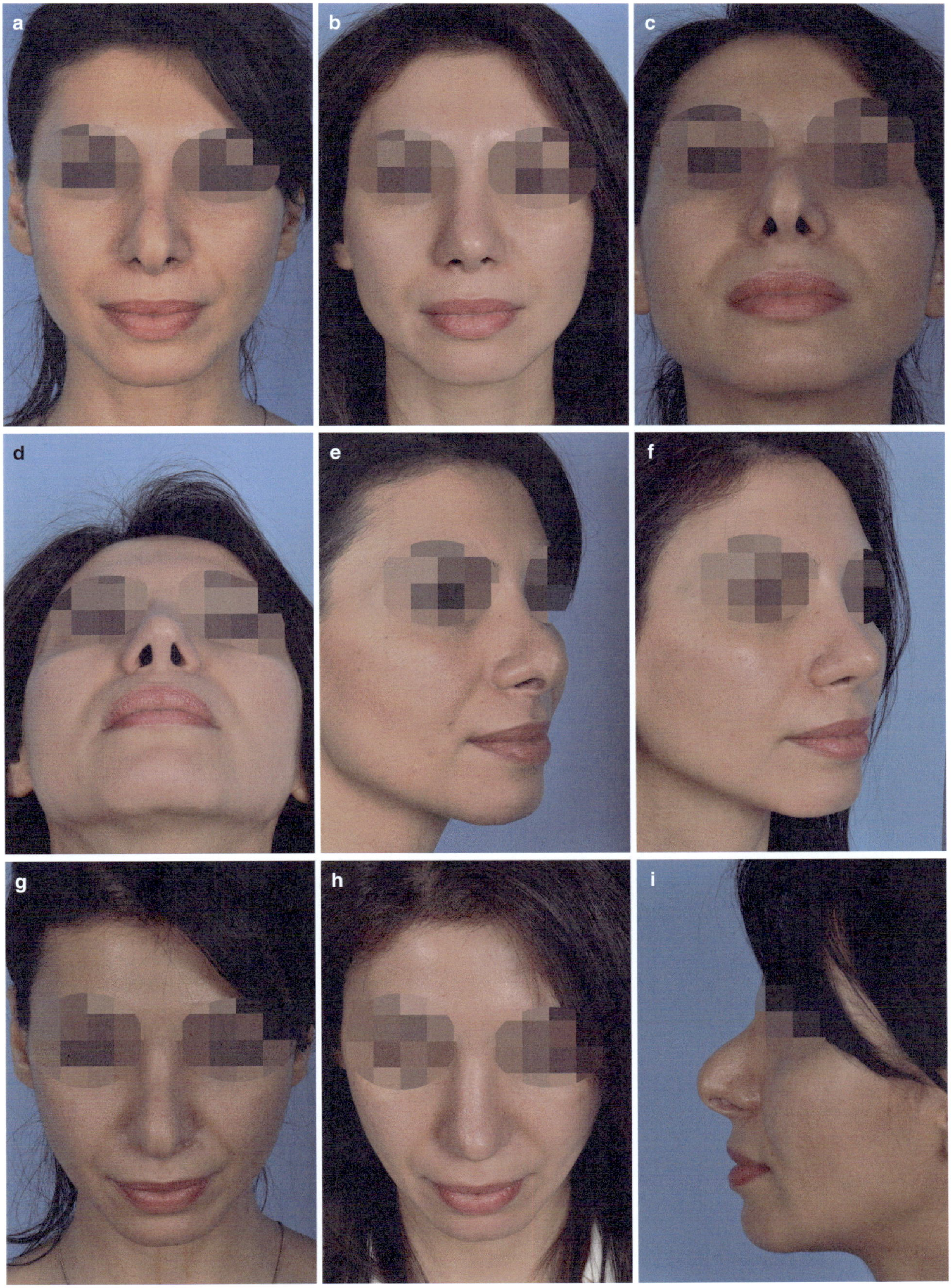

Fig. 14.27 (**a**–**j**) Pre- and postoperative photographs

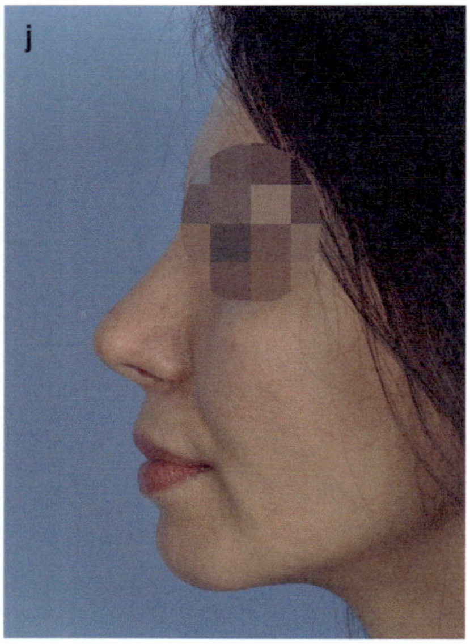

Fig. 14.27 (continued)

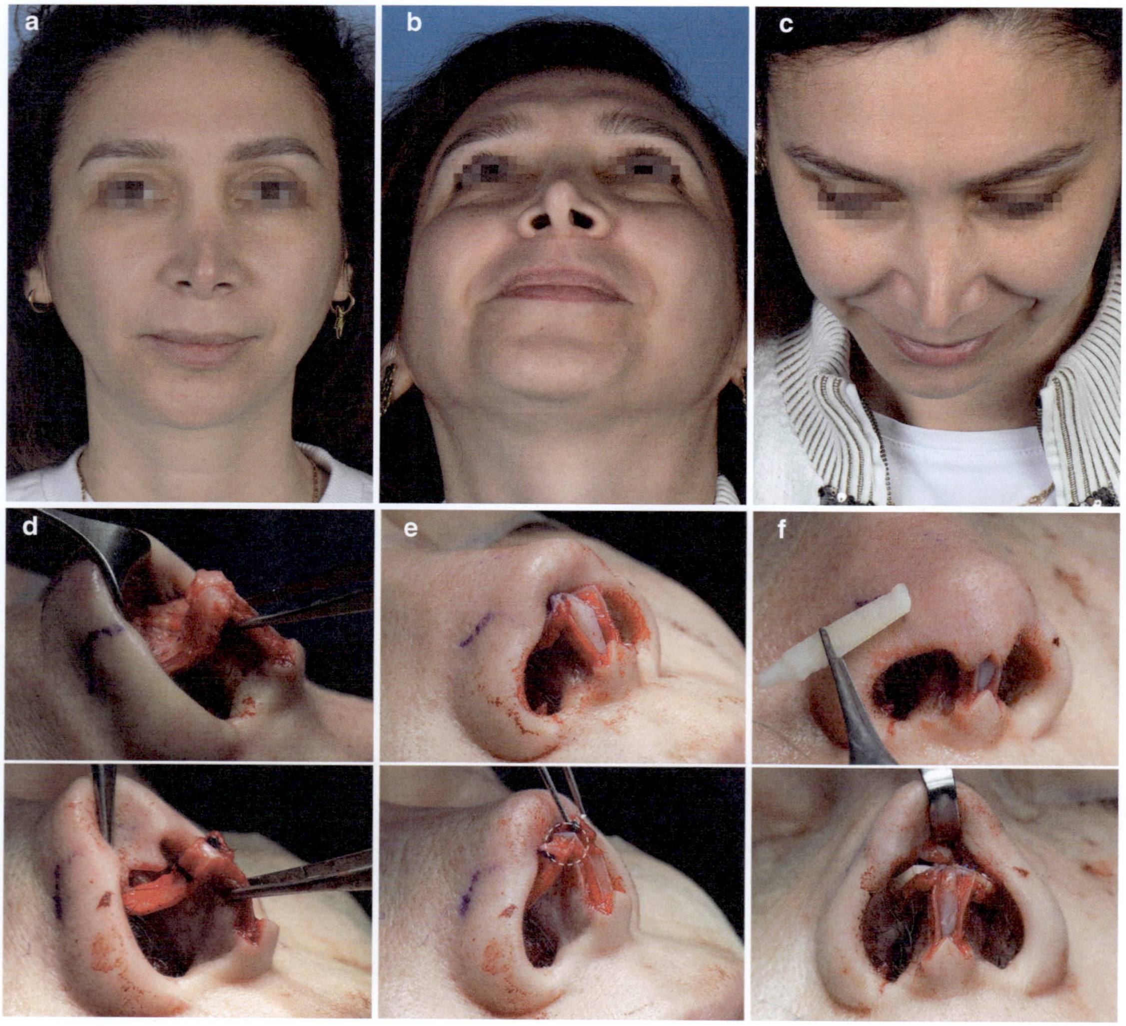

Fig. 14.28 (**a–d**) Preoperative photographs. This 26-year-old patient had rhinoplasty at age 18. In the years between that operation and the current presentation, the surgery alar sidewall became concave. The Var technique was used to restore alar cartilages on her revision surgery. (**e–h**) Long-term results: there is now an elegant tip width with improved symmetry; the alar sidewall strength is also improved

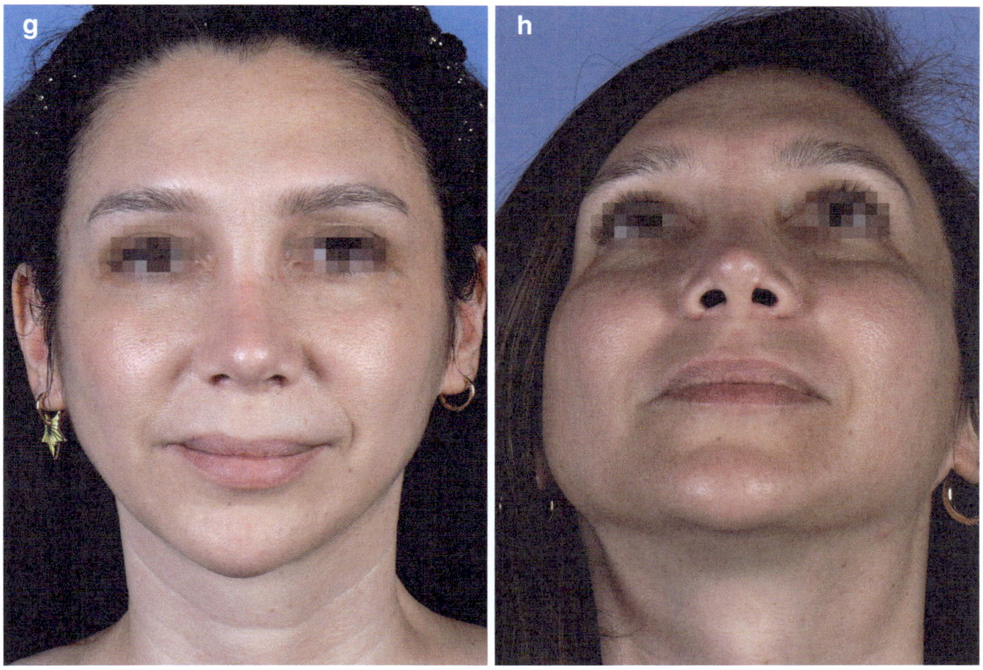

Fig. 14.28 (continued)

14.4 Clinical Outcomes: Primary Narrow Nasal Tip

In non-operated cases, narrow nasal tips are rare. This situation is mainly caused by concavity of the lateral crus. Let us examine these cases separately.

To resolve a narrow nasal tip based on a *mild concavity of the lateral crus*, it may be effective to suture a cartilaginous graft, termed a lateral crural graft, onto the lateral crus. Cephalic excess of the lateral crus should be considered as the first option. Excess cartilage is slid to and fixed on two points on the lateral crus, in a cavity elevated from the vestibular mucosa. If the surgeons observe that the concavity disappears, surgery continues (Fig. 14.29).

14.4.1 Case 6

We now examine a case with a primary narrow nasal tip. An intraoperative lateral crus image and the pinched image in the preoperative lateral view are shown in Fig. 14.30.

The surgery starts by performing a standard cephalic resection on the lateral crus. The resected part is slid to the concave area on the lateral crus and fixed with absorbable sutures (Fig. 14.31).

After the concavity had resolved, the surgery was completed using a standard suture tip plasty (Fig. 14.32).

Figure 14.33 shows preoperative and 1-year postoperative photographs. Dorsal reduction and decreased tip projection results in a nose that is more proportional to the patient's face. The concave and collapsed lateral crura have been supported with its own cephalic excess.

An illustration of a mild primary narrow nasal tip is shown in Fig. 14.34. The excess part of the alar cartilage can be used as a lateral crural graft. In contrast to the previous technique, the excess part may also be folded instead of slid; there is no difference in results when sliding or folding is used.

Let us explore an example in Case 7.

14.4.2 Case 7

A 35-year-old man is unhappy with the appearance of his nose. The nasal tip is narrow with pure definition (Fig. 14.35).

Preoperative and 1-year postoperative photographs are shown in Fig. 14.36; the lateral crural concavities have been eliminated.

The available cephalic resection material may not be sufficient to correct the concavity. In this situation, the alternative is a lateral crural graft constructed of septal cartilage. Let us look at an example in Case 8.

14.4.3 Case 8

In this case, septal lateral crural grafts were used to fix concave lateral crura. The cartilage starting next to the dome and extend-

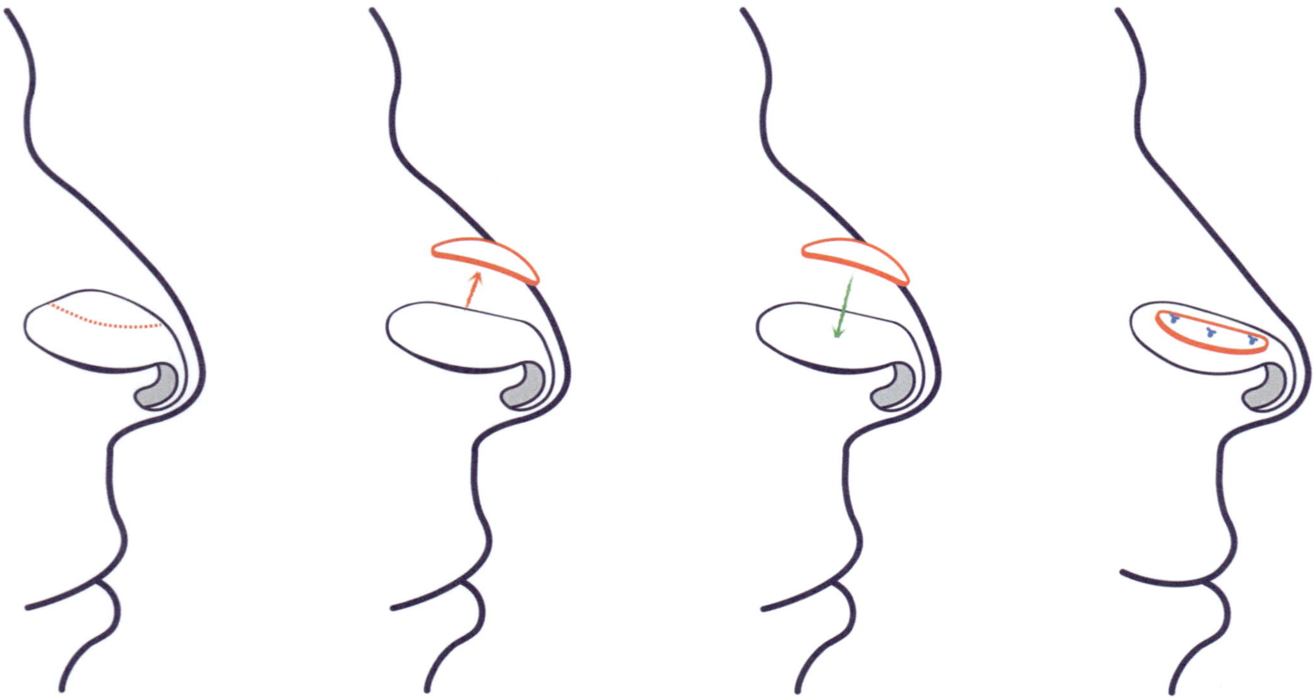

Fig. 14.29 The concave lateral crura can be strengthened with alar onlay lateral crural graft. This graft is effective in correcting the mild or moderate narrow nasal tip

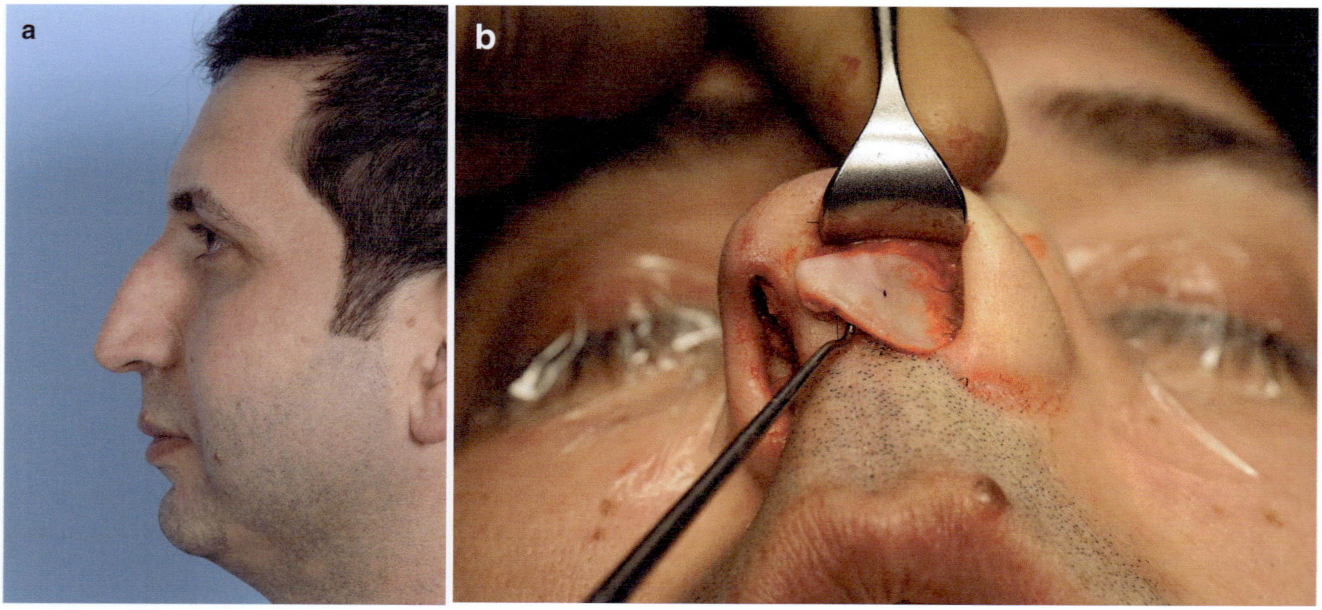

Fig. 14.30 (**a**) Mild pinched tip. (**b**) In this case, the narrow nasal tip caused mainly by the concave lateral crura

ing toward the aperture piriformis is fixed to the lateral crus at two points. Based on the need, the thickness of the cartilage must be 2 or 3 mm and the width must be 5 or 6 mm (Fig. 14.37).

One-year postoperative photographs are shown in Fig. 14.38 The lateral and frontal views show correction of the narrow tip.

14.4.4 Case 9

Another case in which the lateral crural graft was used is shown here (Fig. 14.39).

To fix the concavity, a bilateral crural graft harvested from the septal cartilage was used (Fig. 14.40).

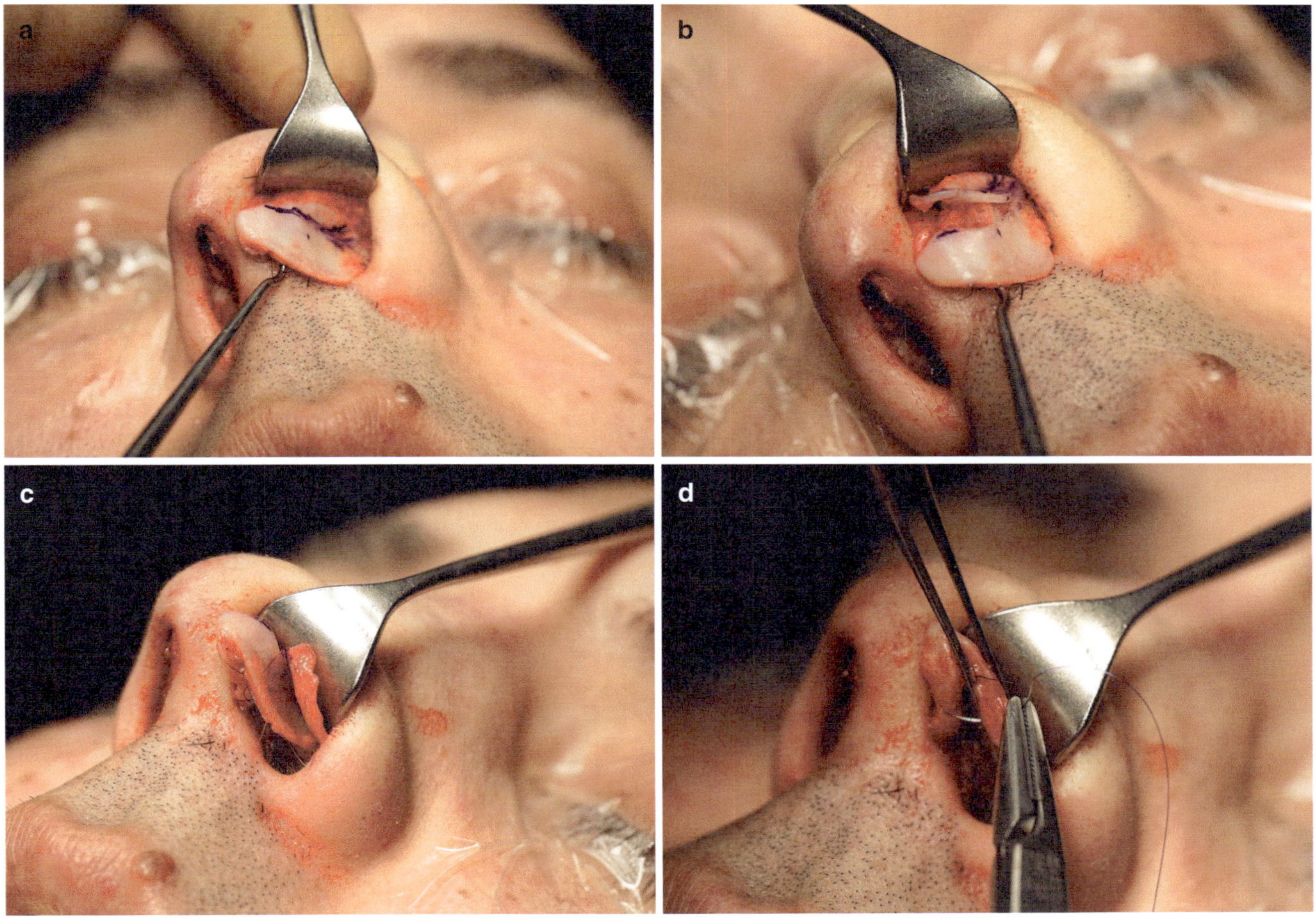

Fig. 14.31 (**a–d**) While septal cartilage can be used for correcting the pinched tip, in mild cases, cephalic excess of alar cartilages is suitable because the natural concavities recreate a more natural shape for the lateral crura

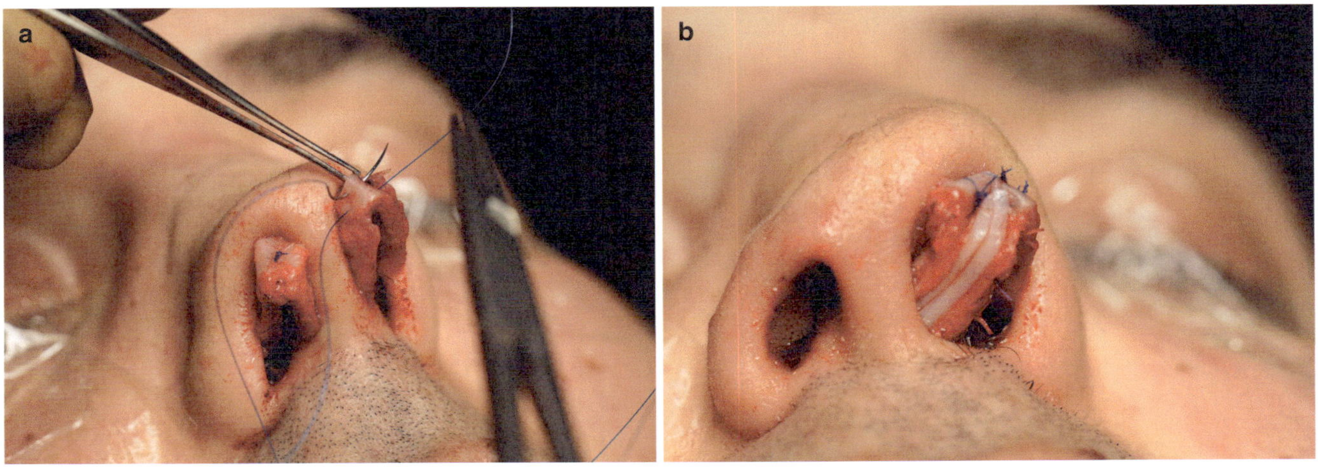

Fig. 14.32 (**a**, **b**) Transdomal suture, columellar strut

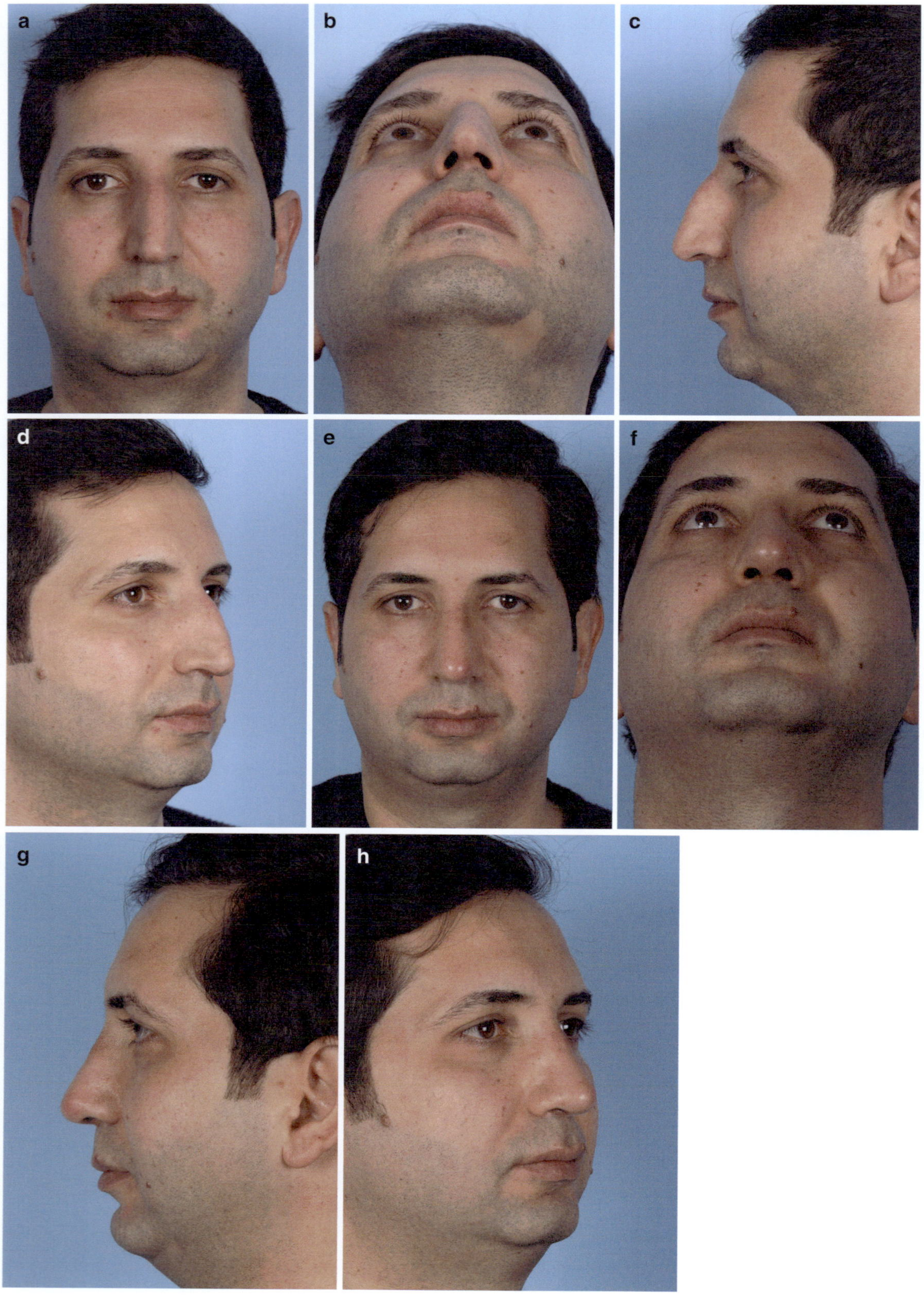

Fig. 14.33 (**a**–**h**) Pre- and postoperative views. The technique corrected the depressed alar sidewall and the pinched appearance of the nasal tip

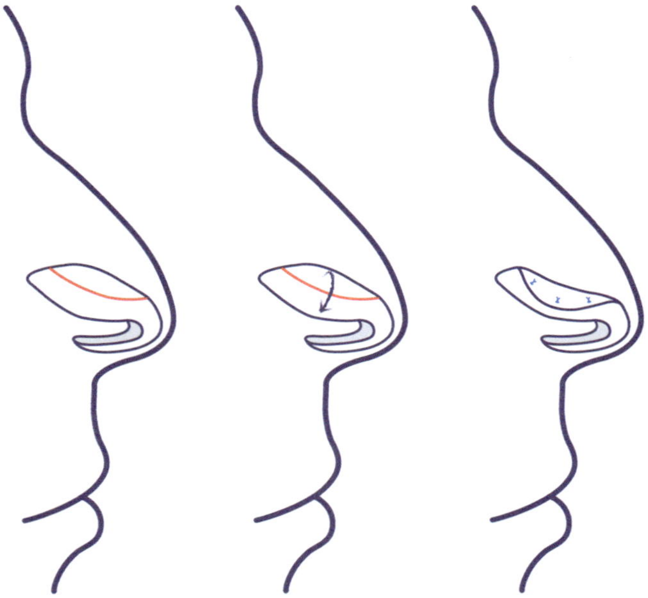

Fig. 14.34 The excess part of lateral crus may be folded to correct concavities of the remaining part of lateral crus

Preoperative and 1-year postoperative results are satisfactory (Fig. 14.41).

During tip plasty of narrow tip cases, a transdomal mattress suture is normally used. However, in some cases, transdomal mattress sutures can cause more narrowness in the nose as a side effect. Thus, this technique should be chosen on a case-by-case basis.

An example in which the transdomal mattress suture was not used is seen in Case 10.

14.4.5 Case 10

This patient was unhappy with the pinched appearance of her nasal tip. She also complained of nasal breathing. She hadn't had the previous rhinoplasty before. Preoperative and intraoperative photographs are seen in Fig. 14.42. One-year postoperative photographs are seen in Fig. 14.43.

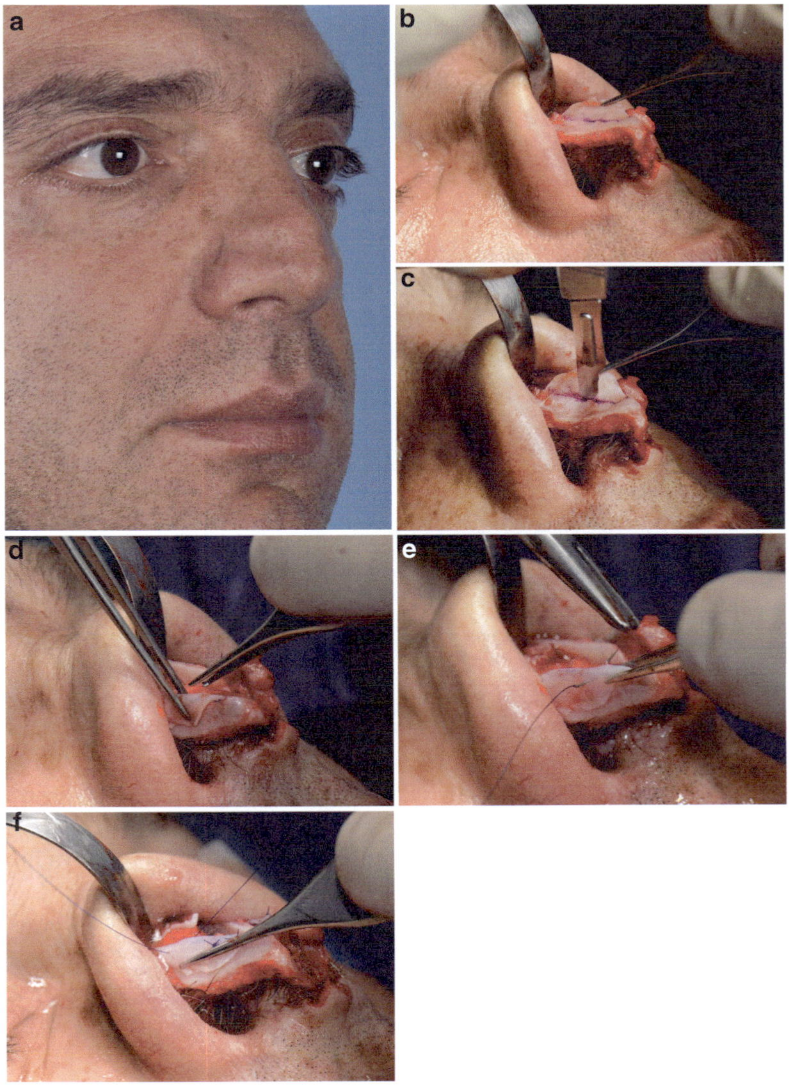

Fig. 14.35 (**a**–**f**) The excess portion of the lateral crus was dissected from the vestibular skin until 6–7 mm remained and was cut from that point and folded onto the lateral crus. (Supplementary Video 14.3)

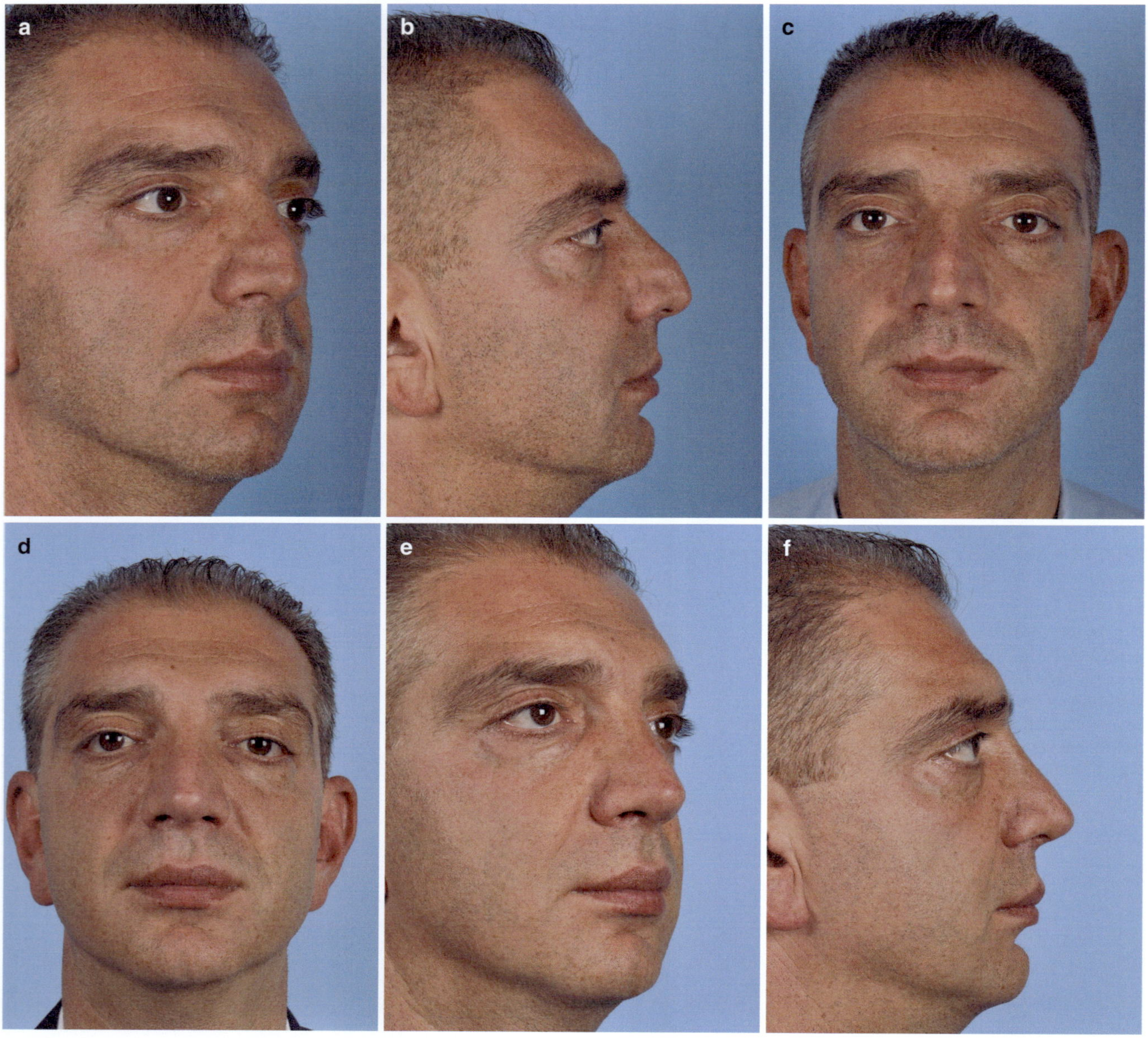

Fig. 14.36 (**a–c**) Preoperative pictures. (**d–f**) Postoperative pictures. Correction of the narrow tip problem was achieved with restoration of the alar cartilaginous strength and structure

14.4.6 Case 11

The techniques mentioned above will not be sufficient in the presence of a lateral crus that is concave enough to protrude into the nose. In this situation, different techniques must be explored. The flip/flop technique can be used to reverse the lateral crus 180° around itself, turning the concave plane into a convex plane and a convex plane into a concave plane. If the flip/flop technique is used, the desired dome point is marked and alar cartilage is cut from the marked point. The lateral crus is elevated from the vestibular mucosa, removed completely, and sutured from the same point after reversal. If the cartilage is weak or support is required and the convection of the cartilage is too significant when rotated, a straight surface is constructed using a lateral crural graft (Fig. 14.44).

Preoperative and 3-year postoperative photographs are shown in Fig. 14.45. The lateral crural concavities have been eliminated.

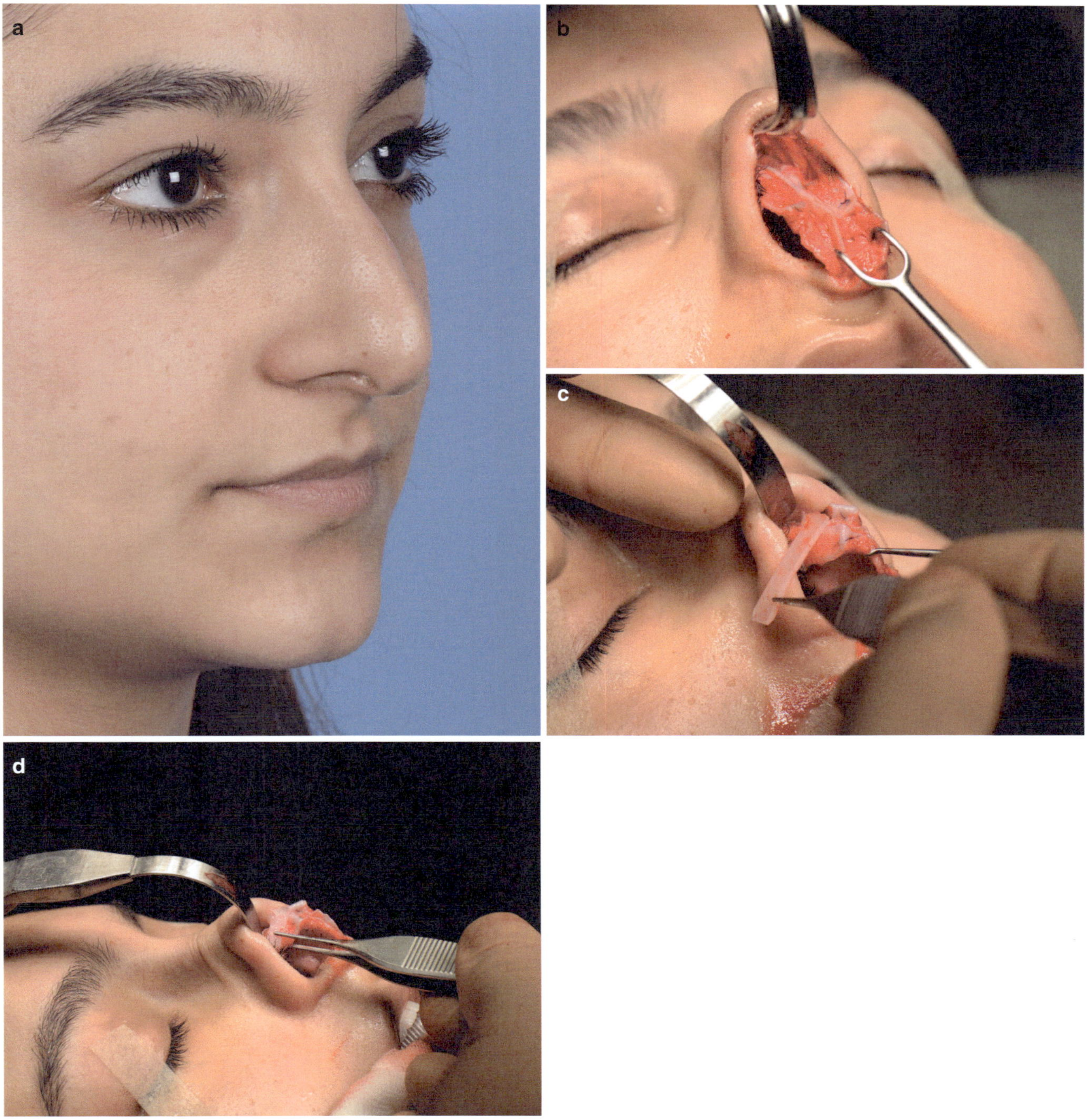

Fig. 14.37 (**a**) Narrow nasal tip and concave alar side wall. (**b**) Bilateral lateral crura are concave. (**c**, **d**) Lateral crural onlay grafts (septal cartilages) were used to strengthen the crura

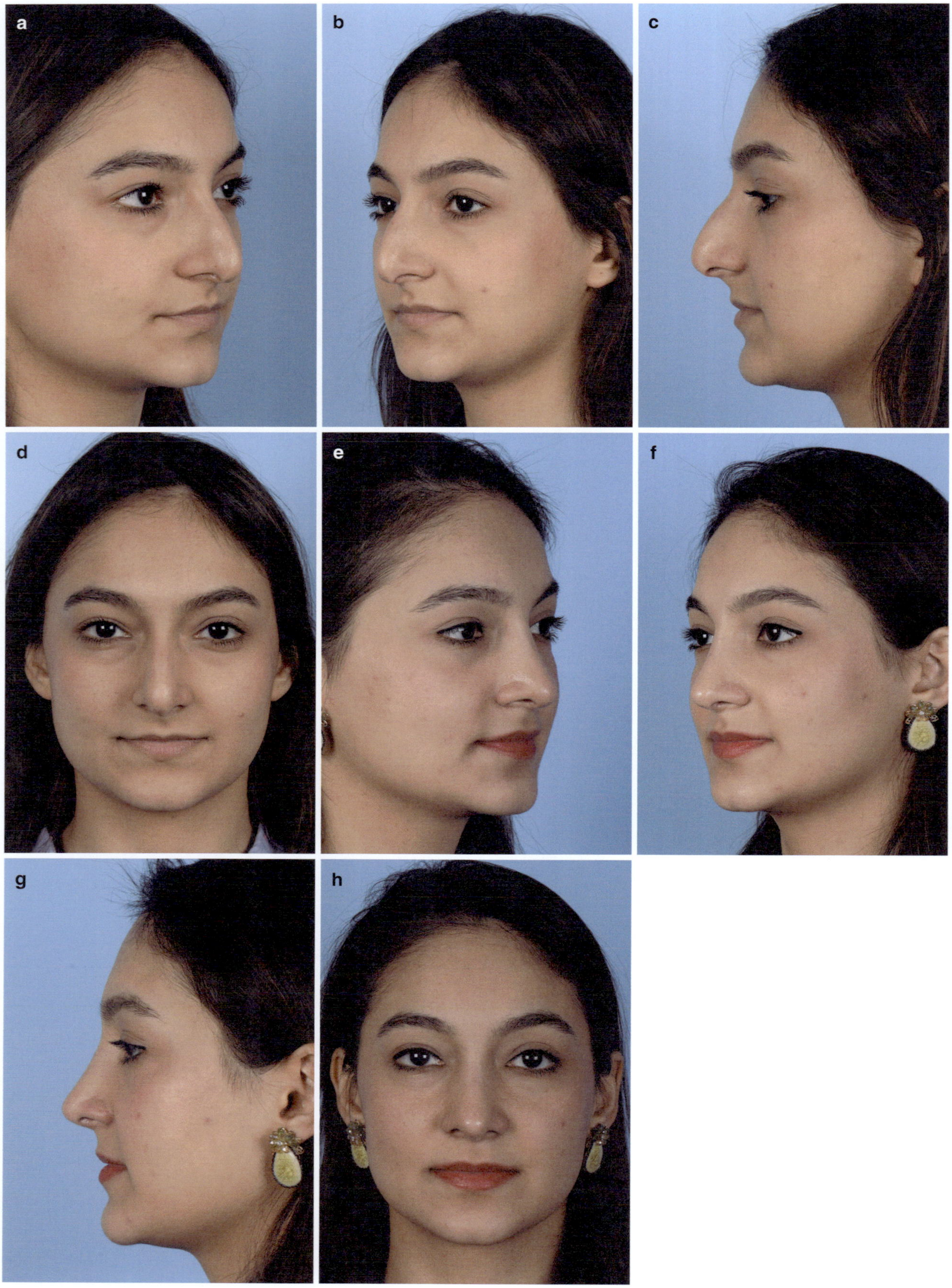

Fig. 14.38 (**a–h**) Postoperative photographs show complete correction of narrow tip and concave alar side wall

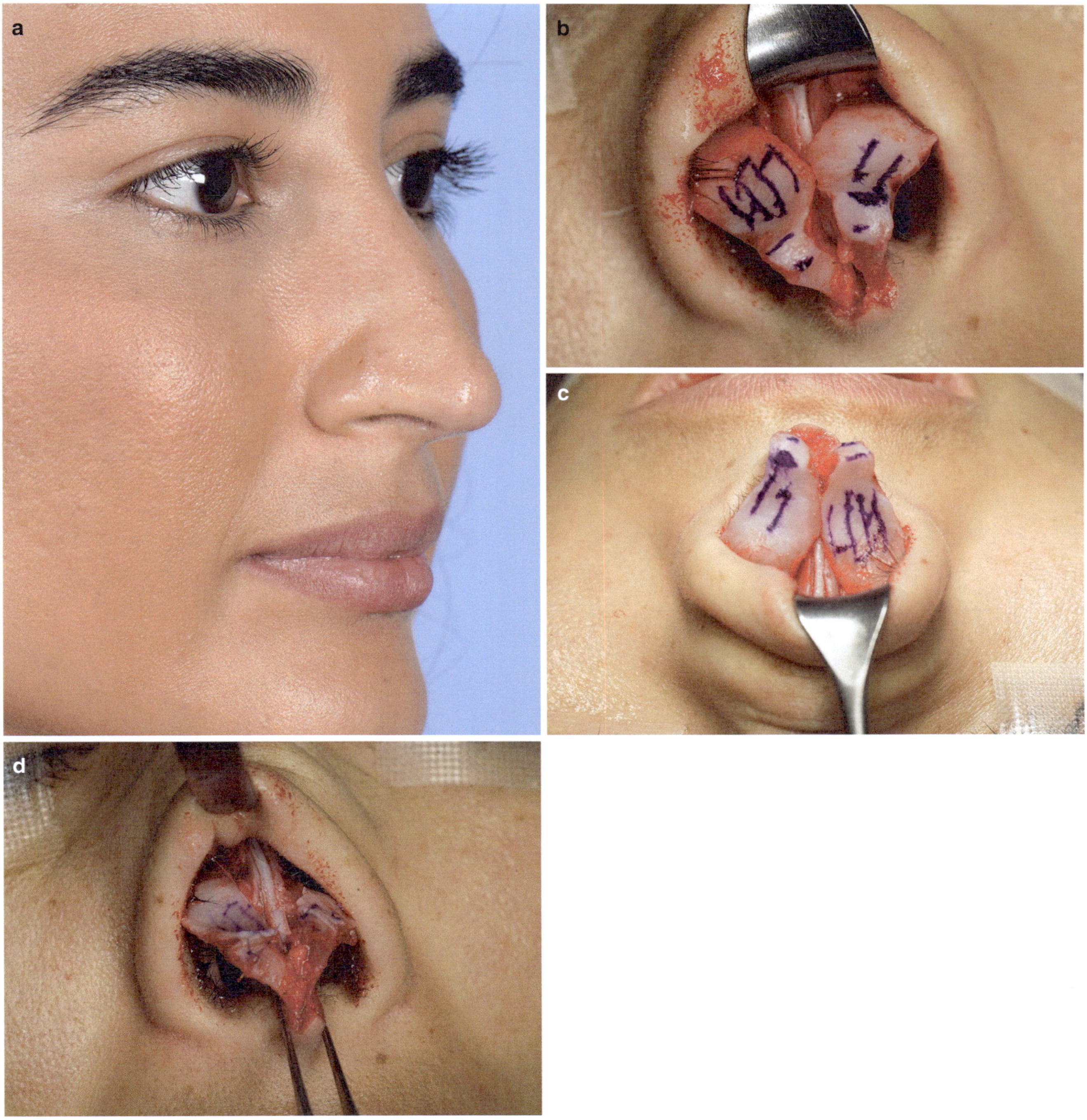

Fig. 14.39 (**a**) A concave lateral crus was evident. (**b**, **c**) A long and concave lateral crus. (**d**) The VAR technique was used to shorten the lateral crus; concavity remained. (Supplementary Video 14.4)

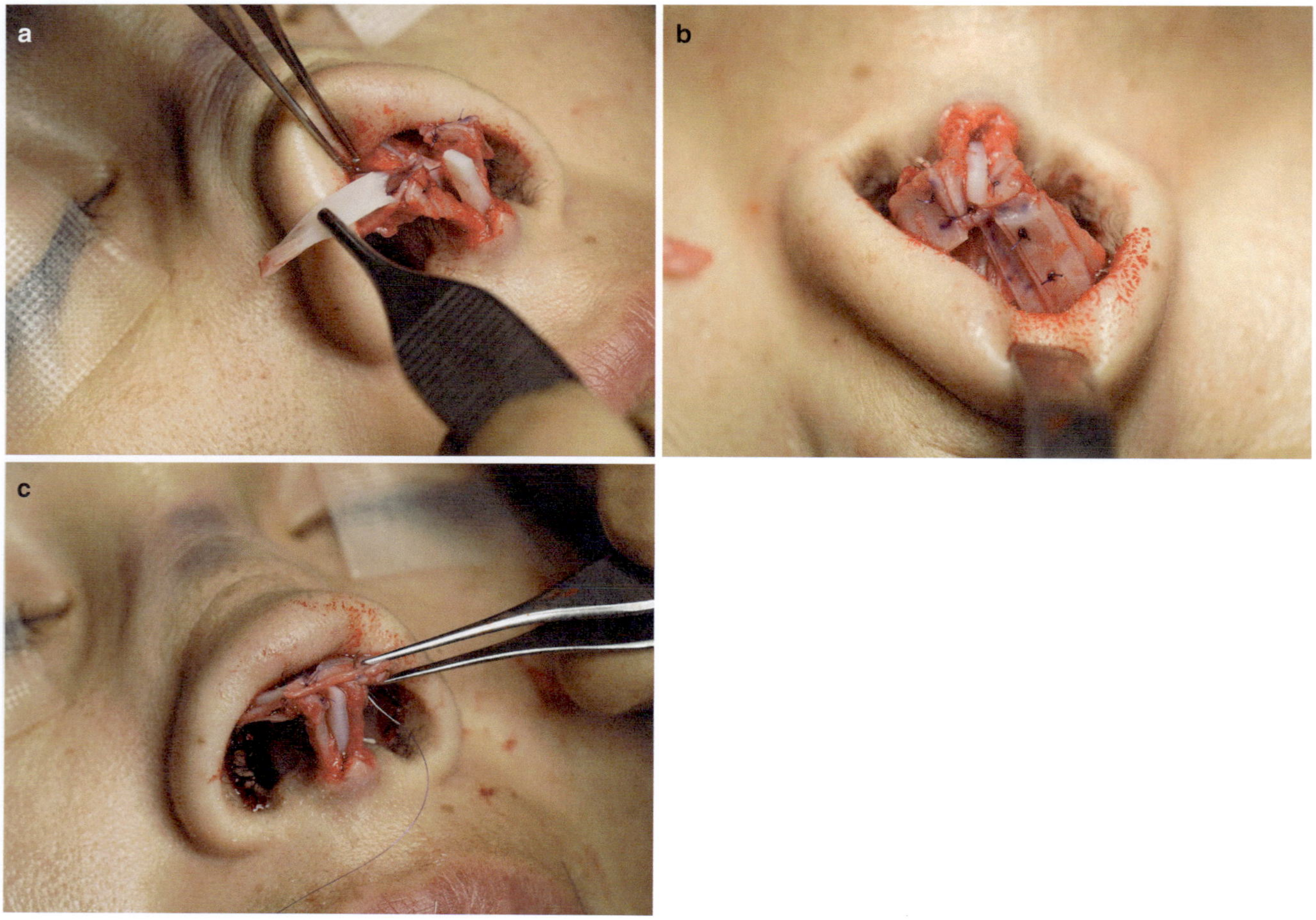

Fig. 14.40 (**a**–**c**) A bilateral septal crural graft, a columellar strut, and a cap graft were placed

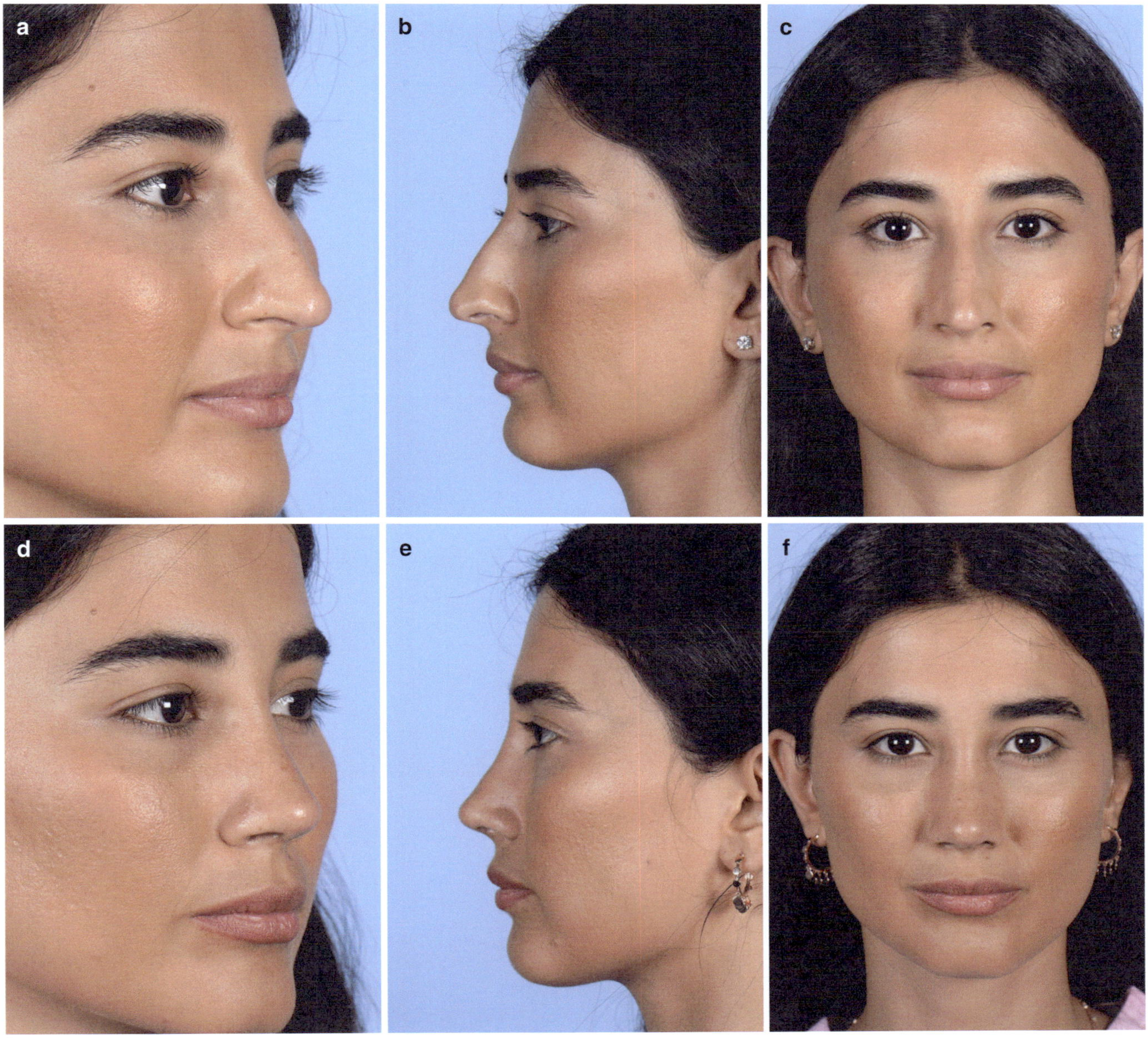

Fig. 14.41 (**a**–**c**) Preoperative photographs, pinched, slightly overprotected, and under-rotated tip. (**d**–**f**) Postoperative photographs show complete correction of the tip problems. Vertical alar resection decreased projection and resulted in superior rotation. Lateral crural grafts (septal) are flattened the crura

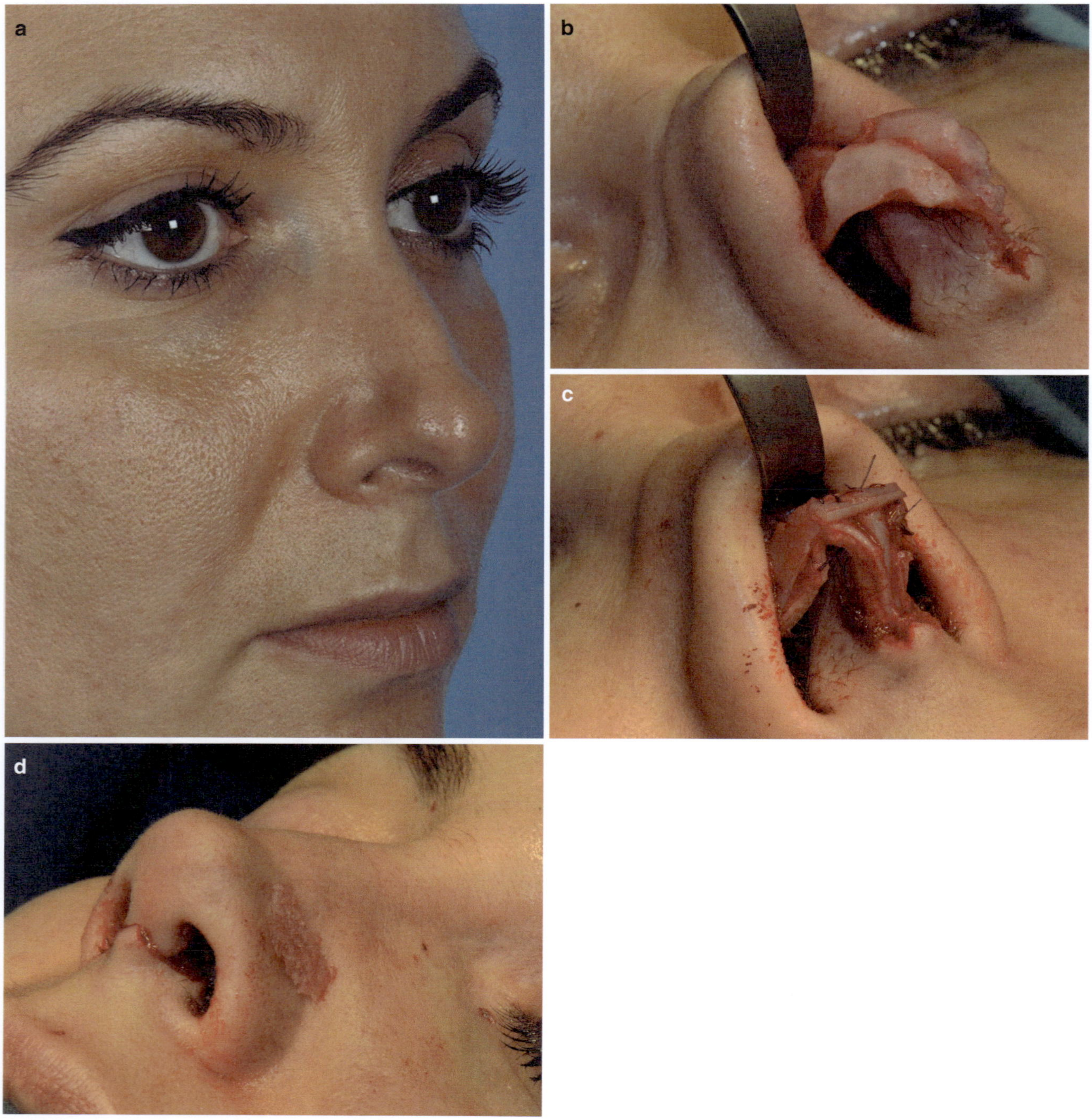

Fig. 14.42 (**a**) Preoperative photograph in the oblique view. (**b**–**d**) In this case, a cap graft was used for definition, and a bilateral crural graft was used for correcting concavities. Crushed cartilage was chosen as the bilateral crural graft

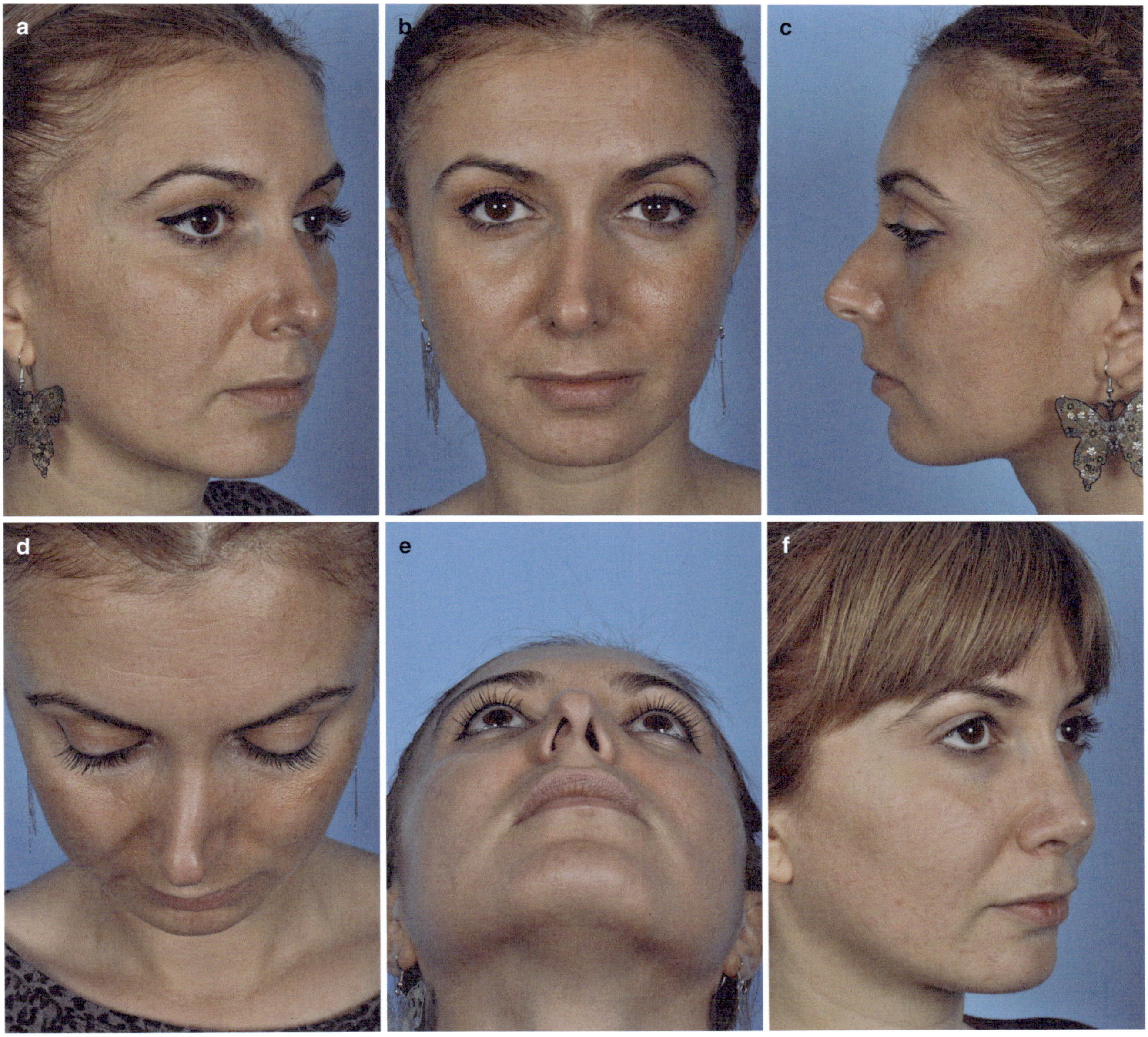

Fig. 14.43 (**a–e**) Preoperative photographs: the lateral crura are both concave; the alar arches exhibit an omega shape; a prominent tip and nostril asymmetry are seen. (**f–j**) Postoperative photographs: the tip symmetry is markedly improved; the lateral crural concavities have been eliminated; nostril symmetry is achieved by caudal septal relocation

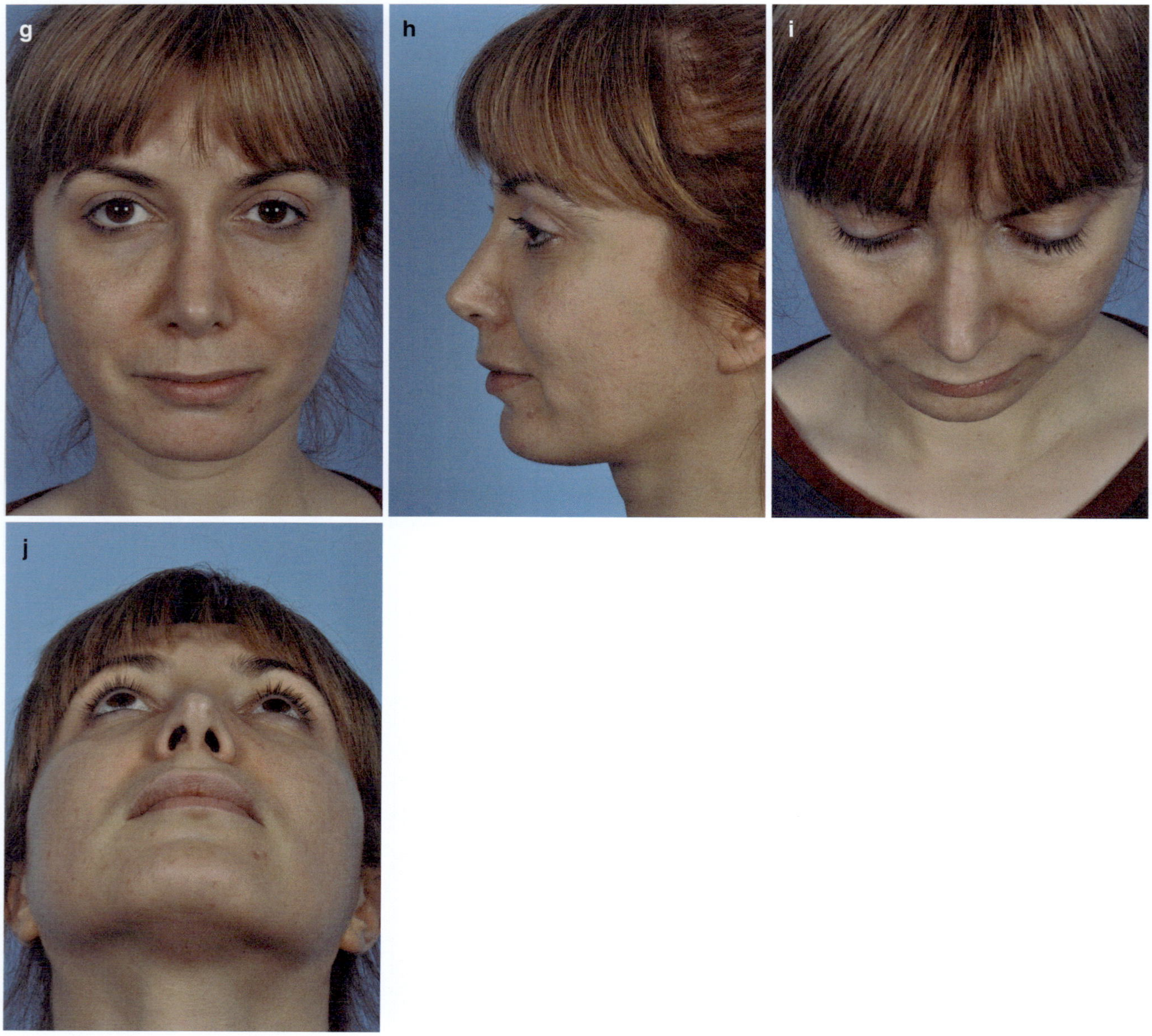

Fig. 14.43 (continued)

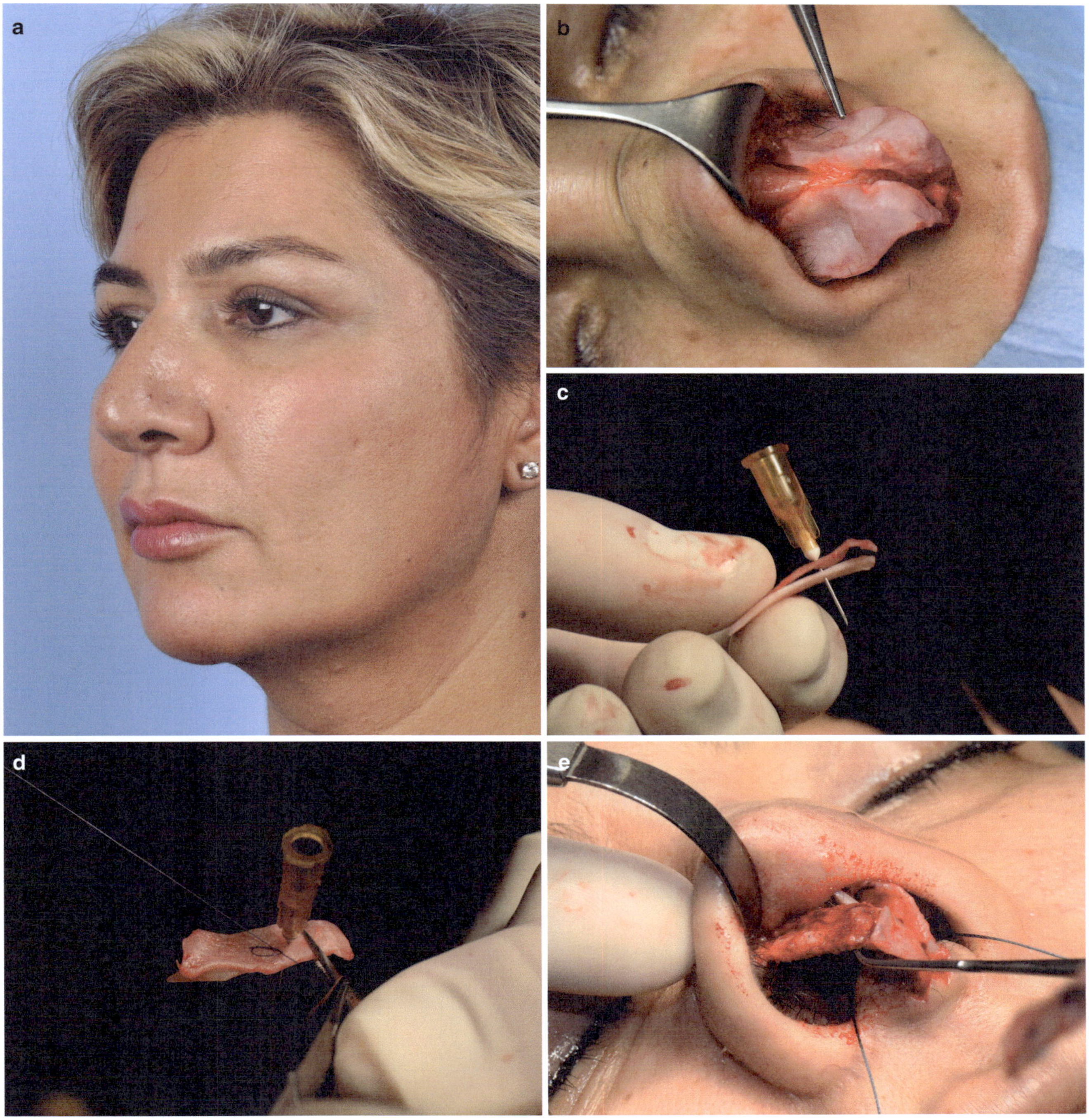

Fig. 14.44 (**a**) Preoperative oblique view. (**b**) Correspondence of the preoperative oblique view intraoperatively. The lateral crus started out convex and converted into a concave shape. (**c**, **d**) The lateral crus was completely excised from the dome point and flipped 180° around itself. The excess parts were trimmed to achieve the ideal configuration. Lastly, a septal lateral crural graft was sutured underneath extracorporally. (**e**) The bed of the lateral crus is evident. (**f**, **g**) A new lateral crus was put into its exact place bilaterally. (**h**, **i**) A new lateral crus was sutured to the dome point. (**j**) A columellar strut was sufficient to stabilize the tip. No extra stabilization material was required. (**k**) A cap graft was used for definition

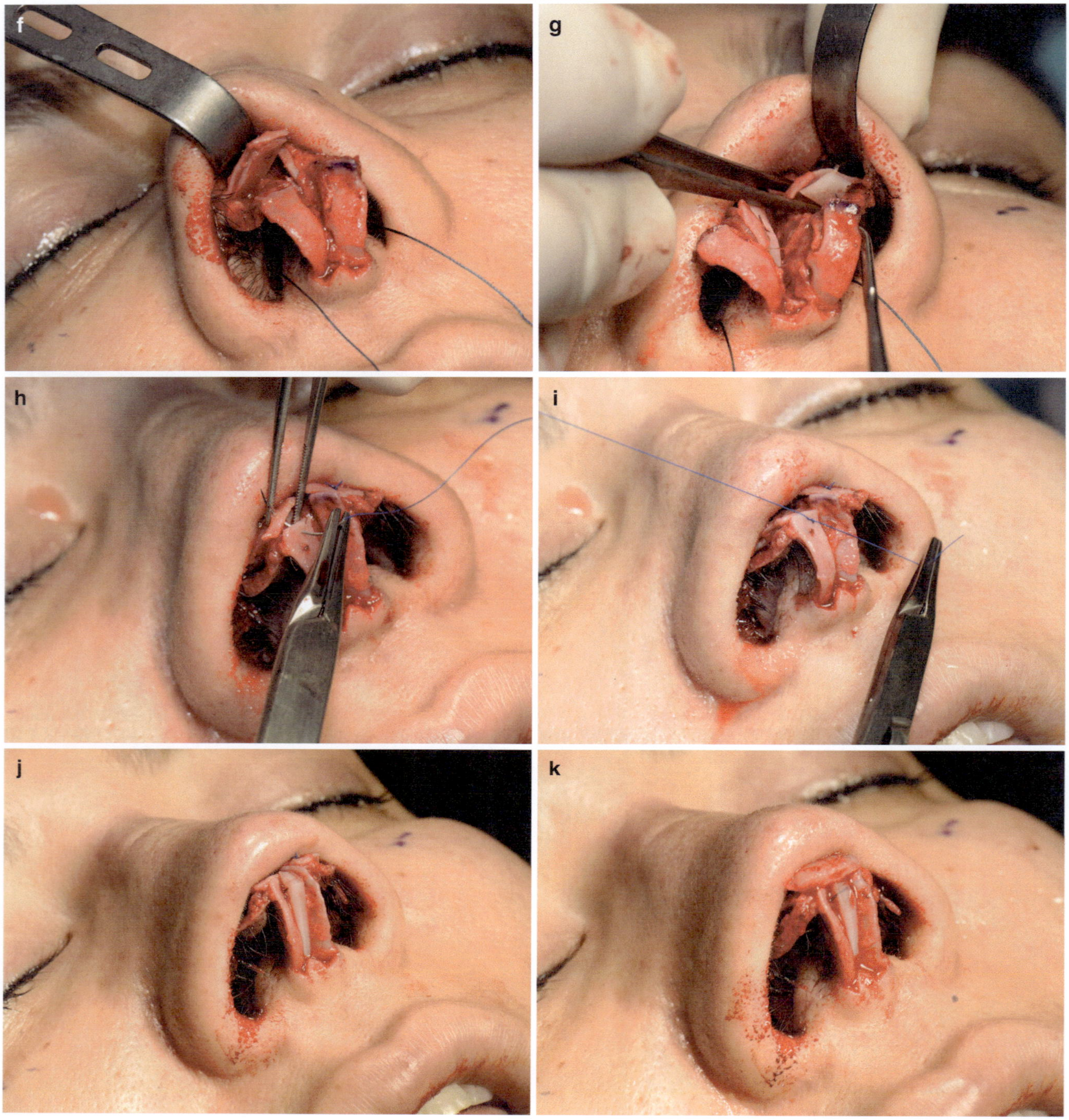

Fig. 14.44 (continued)

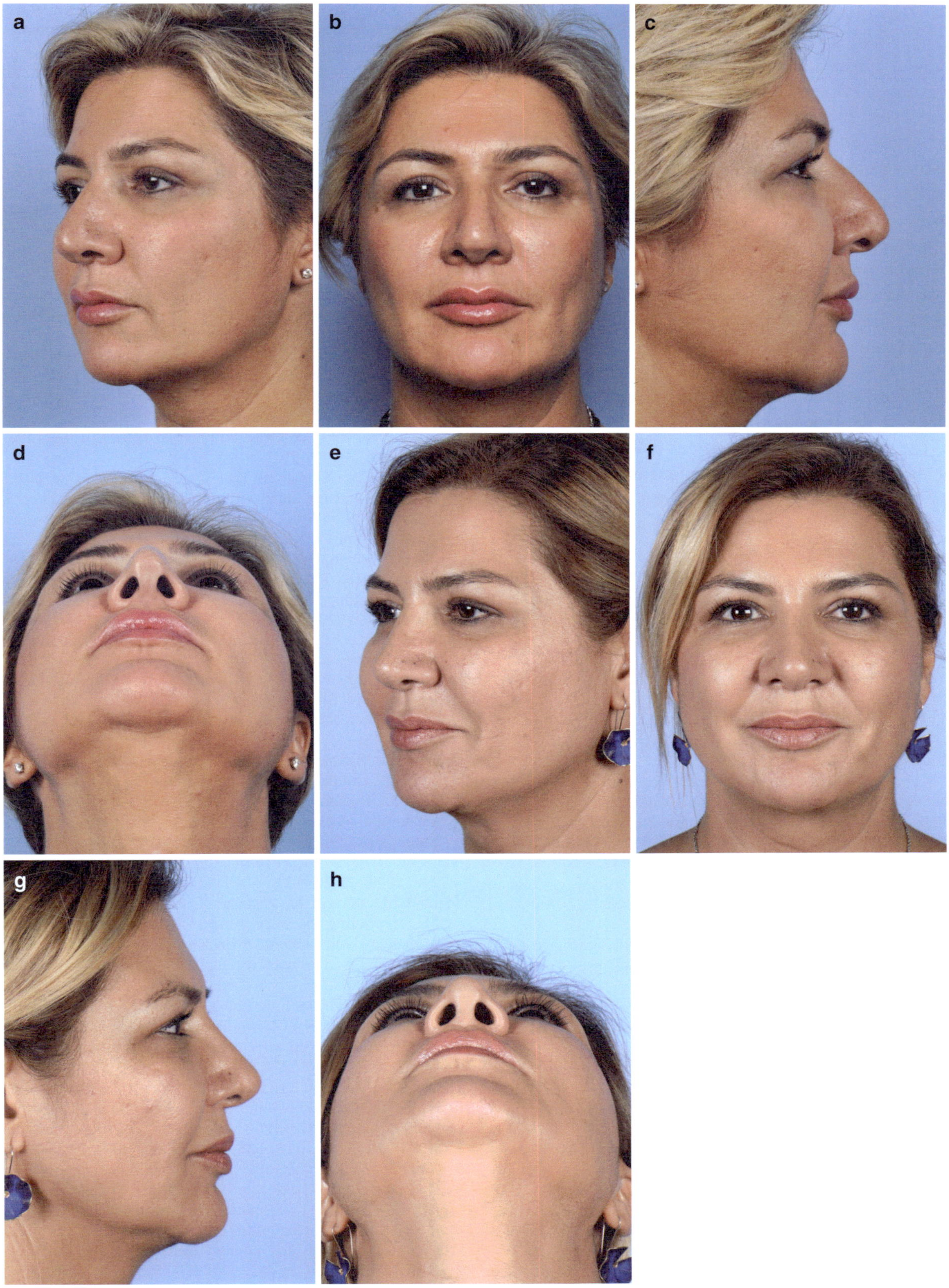

Fig. 14.45 (**a–d**) Preoperative photographs. A 41-year-old case with thick skin has a large nasal tip. The tip is broad and accentuated by concave depressions of alar sidewalls (omega shape). The patient also exhibits hanging columella on the profile view. (**e–h**) Postoperative photographs: the tip is more proportional to the rest of the nose. The concave and collapsed lateral crura have been reconstructed with the flip-flop technique. Also, reshaping of alar arches corrected the broadened tip and hanging columella

14.5 Conclusions

A narrow or pinched nasal tip can be due to primary or secondary causes. Primary cases of a pinched nasal tip are rare. In these cases, the convex dome and concave lateral crus typically have an omega shape. A lateral crural graft harvested from septal or alar cartilage is useful in mild and moderate cases. In severe cases, the flip-flop technique is a good alternative. While primary cases complain mainly of aesthetic problems, secondary cases comprise both aesthetic and cosmetic problems. In secondary cases, three main mistakes of the primary surgeon can result in a pinched tip: untreated malposed lateral crus, incorrect placement of transdomal suture, and excessive lower lateral cartilage resection. Each pathology requires a different treatment strategy. Thus, it is important to understand the underlying pathology of the pinched tip and use the appropriate technique. The result of these pathologies is external deformity and/or airway obstruction (a collapsed external valve). If weakness of the lateral nasal wall affects the alar rim, alar retraction may be present in conjunction with a narrow tip.

Disclosures The author reports no conflicts of interest or funding requiring disclosure.

Further Reading

Alexander AJ, Shah AR, Constantinides MS. Alar retraction: etiology, treatment, and prevention. JAMA Facial Plast Surg. 2013;15(4):268–74.

Ballert JA, Park SS. Functional rhinoplasty: treatment of the dysfunctional nasal sidewall. Facial Plast Surg. 2006;22(1):49–54.

Bewick JC, Buchanan MA, Frosh AC. Internal nasal valve incompetence is effectively treated using batten graft functional rhinoplasty. Int J Otolaryngol. 2013;2013:734795.

Byrd DR, Otley CC, Nguyen TH. Alar batten cartilage grafting in nasal reconstruction: functional and cosmetic results. J Am Acad Dermatol. 2000;43(5 Pt 1):833–6.

Cervelli V, Spallone D, Bottini JD, et al. Alar batten cartilage graft: treatment of internal and external nasal valve collapse. Aesth Plast Surg. 2009;33(4):625–34.

Chang CW, Simons RL. Hockey-stick vertical dome division technique for overprojected and broad nasal tips. Arch Facial Plast Surg. 2008;10(2):88–92.

Chua DY, Park SS. Alar batten grafts. JAMA Facial Plast Surg. 2014;16(5):377–8.

Cingi C, Bayar Muluk N, Winkler A, Thomas JR. Nasal tip grafts. J Craniofac Surg. 2018;29(7):1914–21.

Cochran CS, Sieber DA. Extended alar contour grafts: an evolution of the lateral crural strut graft technique in rhinoplasty. Plast Reconstr Surg. 2017;140(4):559e–67e.

Constantinides M, Liu ES, Miller PJ, Adamson PA. Vertical lobule division in rhinoplasty: maintaining an intact strip. Arch Facial Plast Surg. 2001;3(4):258–63.

Fischer H, Gubisch W. Nasal valves--importance and surgical procedures. Facial Plast Surg. 2006;22(4):266–80.

Gandomi B, Arzaghi MH, Rafatbakhsh M. The effectiveness of modified vertical dome division technique in reducing nasal tip projection in rhinoplasty. Iran J Med Sci. 2011;36(3):196–200.

Gillman GS, Simons RL, Lee DJ. Nasal tip bossae in rhinoplasty. Etiology, predisposing factors, and management techniques. Arch Facial Plast Surg. 1999;1(2):83–9.

Goodwin WJ, Schmidt JF. Iatrogenic nasal tip bossae. Etiology, prevention, and treatment. Arch Otolaryngol Head Neck Surg. 1987;113(7):737–9.

Gruber RP, Fox P, Peled A, Belek KA. Grafting the alar rim: application as anatomical graft. Plast Reconstr Surg. 2014;134(6):880e–7e.

Gunter JP, Rohrich RJ. Correction of the pinched nasal tip with alar spreader grafts. Plast Reconstr Surg. 1992;90(5):821–9.

Guyuron B. Alar rim deformities. Plast Reconstr Surg. 2001;107(3):856–63.

Guyuron B, Bigdeli Y, Sajjadian A. Dynamics of the alar rim graft. Plast Reconstr Surg. 2015;135(4):981–6.

Hirohi T, Yoshimura K. Surgical correction of retracted nostril rim with auricular composite grafts and anchoring suspension. Aesth Plast Surg. 2004;27(5):418–22.

Jang YJ, Kim SM, Lew DH, Song SY. Simple correction of alar retraction by conchal cartilage extension grafts. Arch Plast Surg. 2016;43(6):564–9.

Kalan A, Kenyon GS, Seemungal TA. Treatment of external nasal valve (alar rim) collapse with an alar strut. J Laryngol Otol. 2001;115(10):788–91.

Kemaloğlu CA, Altıparmak M. The alar rim flap: a novel technique to manage malpositioned lateral crura. Aesthet Surg J. 2015;35(8):920–6.

Kridel RW, Yoon PJ, Koch RJ. Prevention and correction of nasal tip bossae in rhinoplasty. Arch Facial Plast Surg. 2003;5(5):416–22.

Leach JL, Athré RS. Four suture tip rhinoplasty: a powerful tool for controlling tip dynamics. Otolaryngol Head Neck Surg. 2006;135(2):227–31.

Millman B. Alar batten grafting for management of the collapsed nasal valve. Laryngoscope. 2002;112(3):574–9.

Mounir A, Latimer-Sayer E. Dealing with the overprojecting pinched tip. Ann Plast Surg. 2012;68(6):549–54.

Oneal RM, Beil RJ. Surgical anatomy of the nose. Clin Plast Surg. 2010;37(2):191–211.

Orlando GJ, Marquez E. Alar rim reconstruction with autologous graft cartilage: external approach. J Craniofac Surg. 2019;30(3):868–70.

Rohrich RJ, Raniere J, Ha RY. The alar contour graft: correction and prevention of alar rim deformities in rhinoplasty. Plast Reconstr Surg. 2002;109(7):2495–505; discussion 2506–8.

Schlosser RJ, Park SS. Functional nasal surgery. Otolaryngol Clin N Am. 1999;32(1):37–51.

Soares CM, Mocelin M, Pasinato R, Berger CA, Grocoske FL, Issa MJ. Evaluating the effectiveness of the lateral intercrural suture to decrease the interdomal distance to improve the definition of the nasal tip in primary rhinoplasty. Int Arch Otorhinolaryngol. 2014;18(2):92–107.

Sufyan AS, Hrisomalos E, Kokoska MS, Shipchandler TZ. The effects of alar batten grafts on nasal airway obstruction and nasal steroid use in patients with nasal valve collapse and nasal allergic symptoms: a prospective study. JAMA Facial Plast Surg. 2013;15(3):182–6.

Toriumi DM, Josen J, Weinberger M, Tardy ME. Use of alar batten grafts for correction of nasal valve collapse. Arch Otolaryngol Head Neck Surg. 1997;123(8):802–8.

Troell RJ, Powell NB, Riley RW, Li KK. Evaluation of a new procedure for nasal alar rim and valve collapse: nasal alar rim reconstruction. Otolaryngol Head Neck Surg. 2000;122(2):204–11.

Unger JG, Roostaeian J, Small KH, Pezeshk RA, Lee MR, Harris R, et al. Alar contour grafts in rhinoplasty: a safe and reproducible way to refine alar contour aesthetics. Plast Reconstr Surg. 2016;137(1):52–61.

Wallace H, Sood S, Rafferty A. Management of the narrow nose. J Laryngol Otol. 2009;123(9):945–51.

15 Under-Projected Tip

15.1 Introduction: Brief Clinical History

Nasal tip height, also known as nasal tip projection, is the distance from the anterior most end of the tip to the level of the alar-facial groove. The author's preference, the Goode method, was used to evaluate tip projection, measured as the distance between the alar crease and the tip-defining point, and to relate it to the dorsal length. According to this method, if the length of the nose is normal (one third of the length of the face), the ideal projection would be 55–60% of the dorsal length (Fig. 15.1).

A ratio of <0.55 indicates hypo-projection or under-projection, while a ratio of more than 0.6 indicates over-projection (Fig. 15.2).

The ideal ratio differs by culture and ethnicity, and the Goode method is most applicable to Caucasian patients.

While planning for under-projected nasal tip surgery, the surgeon must be aware of all the anatomical variations, as is the case for all other surgeries. The nasal tip is formed by two main structures, i.e., two pairs of alar cartilages and the caudal septum/nasal spine on which the alar cartilages rest. The lower lateral cartilages are thrust forward toward the

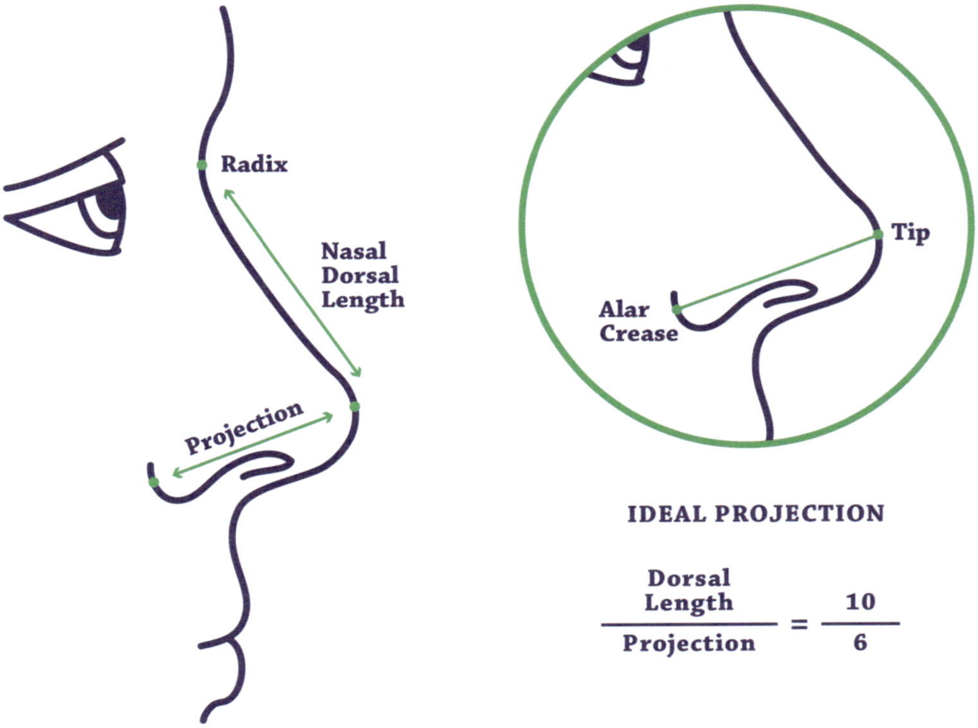

Fig. 15.1 The easy method (Goode) to calculate the ideal projection of the nose

Supplementary Information The online version contains supplementary material available at https://doi.org/10.1007/978-3-031-65619-4_15.

S. Şeneldir, *Photographic Atlas of Rhinoplasty*, https://doi.org/10.1007/978-3-031-65619-4_15

caudal septum and nasal spine. An under-projected nasal tip results from weakness, deficiency, or underdevelopment of either or both of these two anatomical structures (Fig. 15.3).

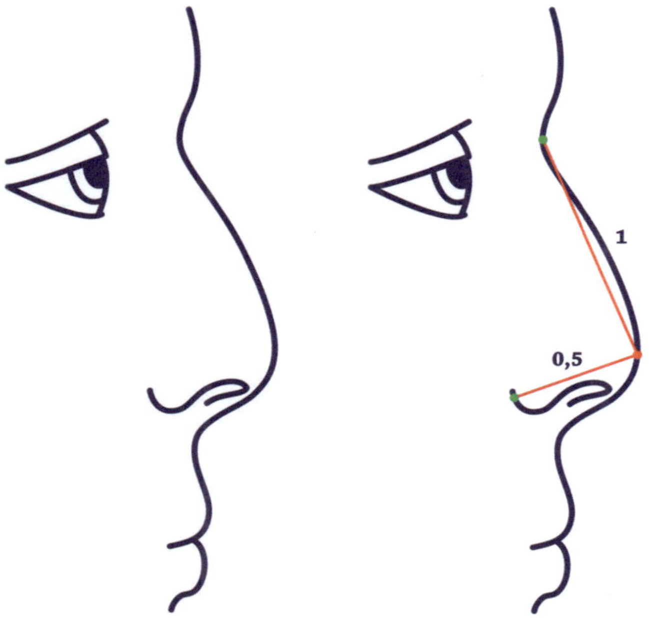

Fig. 15.2 Under-projected tip

In this context, the length and integrity of the alar cartilages are important. In particular, if the medial/middle crura are weak and short, nasal tip projection will be low; the length and strength of the medial/middle crura complex is the main factor defining tip projection. In addition, the shape and stability of the lateral crura must not be neglected while planning low nasal tip treatment. When projection is increased, the lateral crura must also be reinforced; otherwise, the newly created projection will not be stable or additional aesthetic and functional problems may arise. Moreover, the lateral nasal walls may collapse during inspiration and cause nasal airway obstruction, which is especially important in cases with thick nasal skin.

The effect of the caudal septum on tip projection also cannot be ignored. The anterior and posterior septal angles are the major points supporting the nasal tip. The caudal septum or nasal spine deficiency can cause an under-projected tip. For example, decreasing the anterior septal angle during removal of the nasal hump results in an immediately visible reduction in projection, and excessive resection of the septal angle or nasal spine results in projection loss.

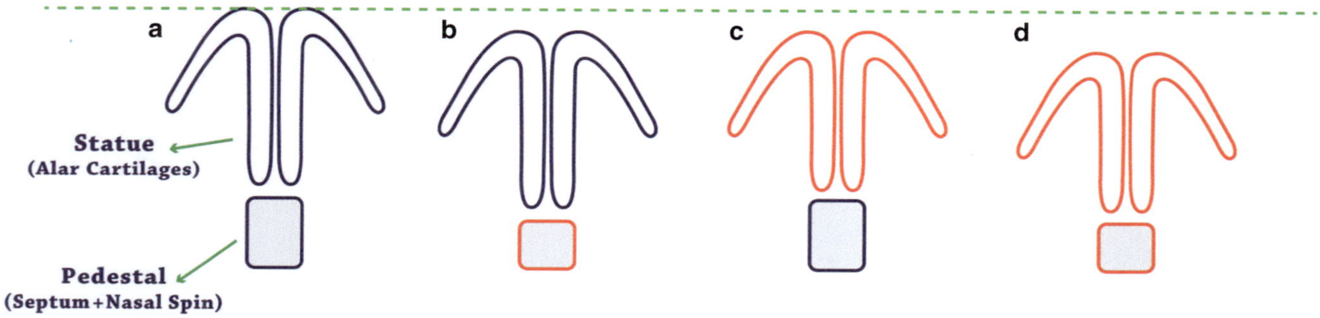

Fig. 15.3 (**a**) Normal tip projection. (**b**) Under-projection caused by deficiency of the pedestal (caudal septum and nasal spine). Lower cartilages are normal in size. (**c**) Under-projection due to weakness or underdevelopment of the lower lateral cartilages (statue). The pedestal is normal in size. (**d**) Insufficient projection due to deficient caudal septum (pedestal) and alar cartilages (statue)

15.2 Treatment Strategy

Surgical correction of an under-projected tip involves rebuilding the nasal pedestal (caudal septum and nasal spine) and strengthening and lengthening the tip cartilage using cartilaginous grafts and suturing techniques. In this context, the surgery will be discussed herein in three parts from the perspective of problem-based treatment. Under-projected nasal tip due to the alar cartilages, which is the most common cause of under-projection, will be detailed in part one; under-projection due to the septum/nasal spine, which is a less common cause, will be discussed in part two; and low nasal tip surgery due to a combination of the first two causes will be covered in part three.

15.3 Part 1: Under-Projected Tip Due to Alar Cartilage-Related Problems

15.3.1 Transdomal Suture

The first step in under-projected tip surgery is transdomal suture. This suture almost always increases projection (by an average of 2 mm) and also significantly corrects any convexity at the lower lateral cartilages. The most favorable suture material is 5-0 polypropylene suture, which has the strength necessary for permanent cartilage reformation. Thinner sutures may cut into the cartilage.

Technical Pearl: "Do not use absorbable sutures"

For each dome, the suture starts at the medial dome plane, exits and reenters it at the lateral crus, and ends at the medial side of the middle crus. The domes are mostly asymmetrical, and unwanted differences can be corrected by using the dome suture. It is not necessary to perform any mucosal dissection without tying the knot, because the suture is naturally buried under the mucosa (Fig. 15.4).

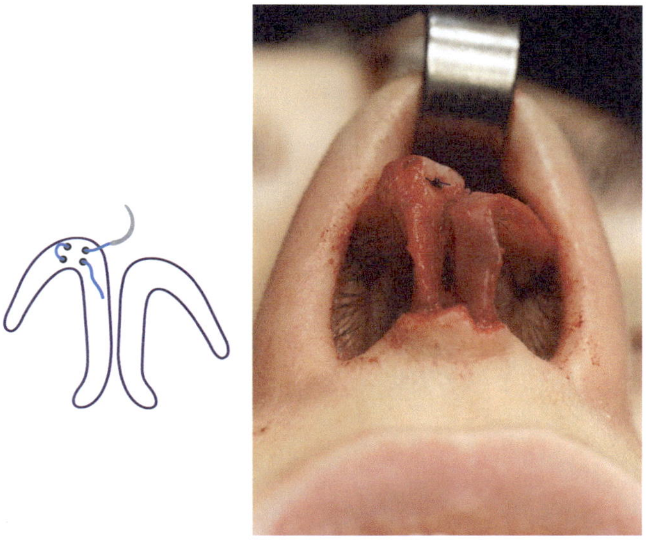

Fig. 15.4 Transdomal mattress suture is placed on the right dome. The right alar arch has gained projection; compare the left side. (Supplementary Video 15.1)

While the surgeon places the transdomal mattress suture, the assistant elevates the caudal edge of the lateral crus. This allows the caudal edge to be averted upward. Averting the caudal edge in an upward direction gives a more refined appearance to the tip (Fig. 15.5).

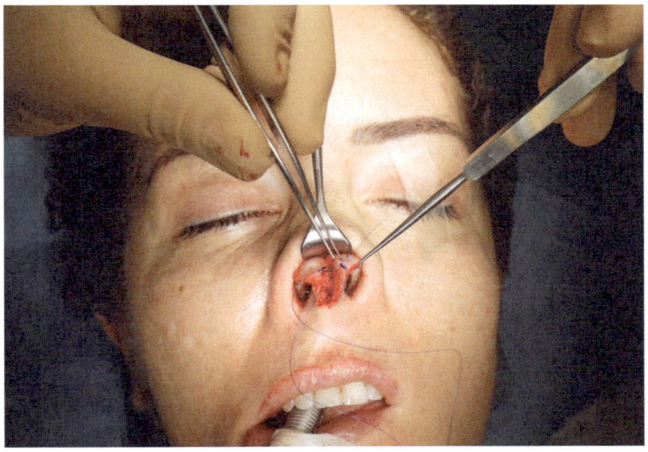

Fig. 15.5 Tip sutures may displace the caudal margin of the lateral crus well below the cephalic margin, resulting in a pinched nasal tip. To prevent this the caudal border of the lateral crus is held by an assistant with a single hook when suturing

A more lateral position of the newly created dome point with respect to the lateral crus results in greater projection (lateral crural steal suture). However, it is important to note that an increase in rotation has an impact on this suture type (Fig. 15.6).

15.3.2 Columellar Strut

The columellar strut is inserted into a pocket between the medial crura and then opened, which not only increases projection, but also corrects medial/middle crural and intercrural asymmetries (Fig. 15.7).

The ideal source for this graft is the septum. In general, an average width of 3–4 mm and a thickness of 2 mm is sufficient. If the septal cartilage is not adequate, the costal cartilage can also be used. Although the auricular cartilage can be considered as an alternative, it is less preferred because the main goal is projection, and the strength of the auricular cartilage may be insufficient to ensure columellar integrity.

The graft starts from the dome and extends to the base, but never contacts the spine. The graft is inserted between the medial and middle crura and is sutured at two different points by using a 4-0 Vicryl (polyglactin 910) straight needle suture (Fig. 15.8).

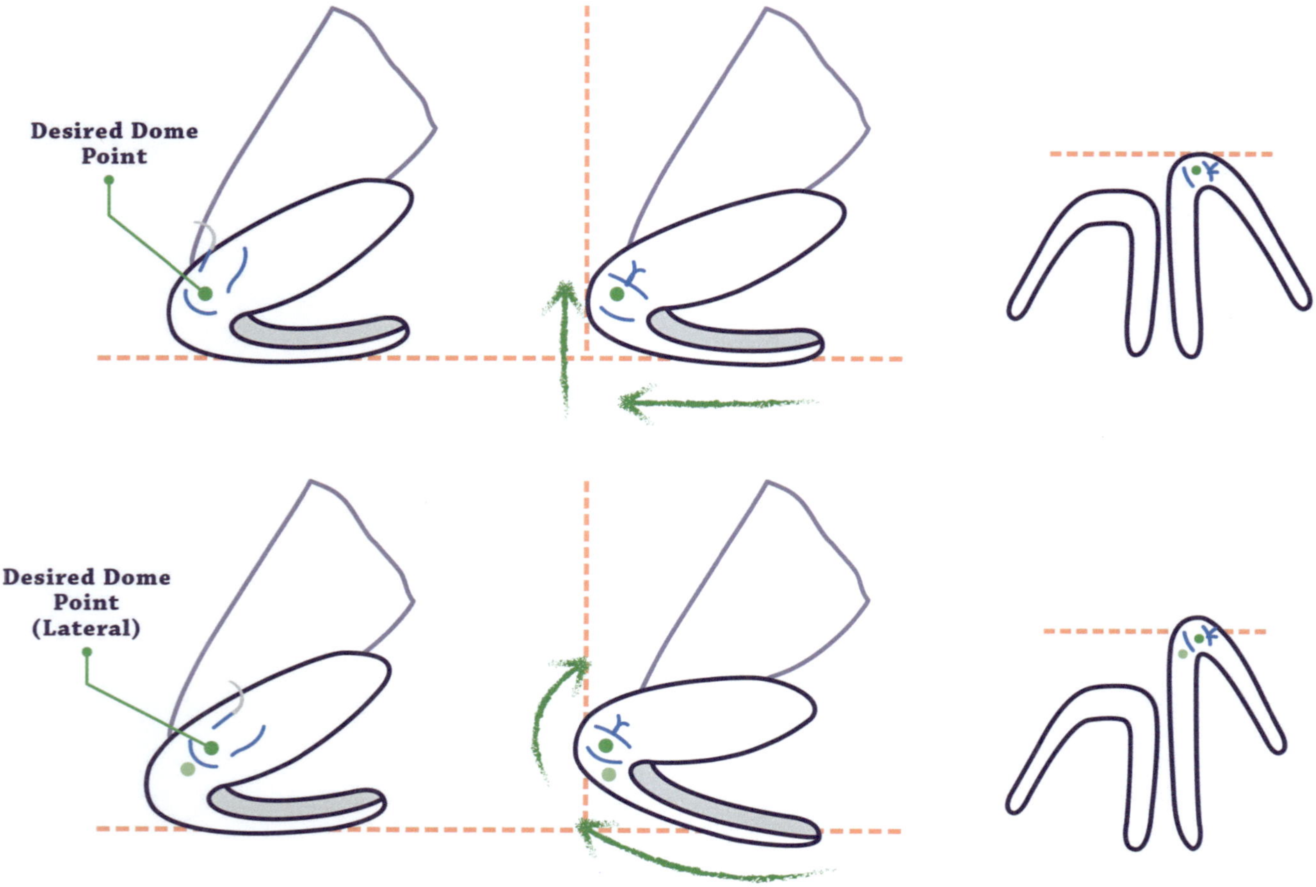

Fig. 15.6 The transdomal suture is usually placed at the dome level. If the suture is placed more lateral to the dome, it gives more projection and rotation to the tip

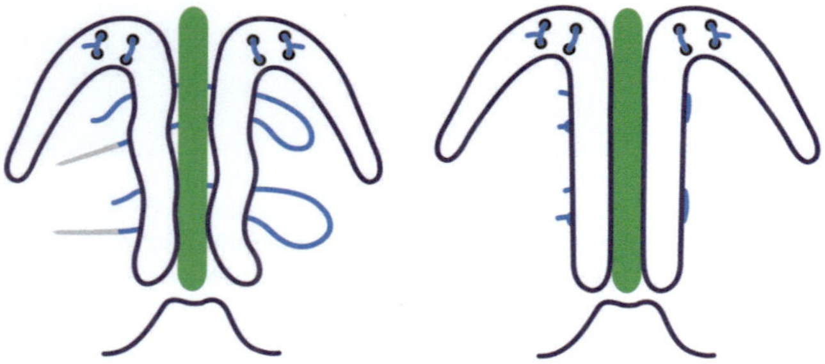

Fig. 15.7 The columellar strut is a strong and versatile graft that supports the anatomical tip to gain projection and rotation. (Supplementary Video 15.2)

Technical Pearl: If possible, the columellar strut should be designed so that it is slightly wider at the top, which facilitates the "dome-equalizing suture" and ensures an ideal dome separation angle (Fig. 15.9).

The medial/middle crural complex can be so weak and damaged that use of a columellar strut alone is not sufficient to achieve stability, particular in revision rhinoplasty or after cleft palate-lip-nose surgery. In such cases, it is necessary to repair all of the weak medial and middle crura; to do this, any thin pliable cartilage is fixed to the medial plane of the weak middle/medial crus complex, providing extra strength to the crus, followed by fixation of the columellar strut (Fig. 15.10).

15.3.3 Onlay Tip Grafts

A "cap" graft is the preferred graft for this purpose. The graft can be prepared in an oval, hourglass, or hexagonal shape and is sutured directly onto the newly built dome. The preferred width is approximately 3 mm and the length should not exceed the two dome points. The thickness of the graft is dependent on the desired projection. Septal, auricular, and costal cartilage are suitable for use as graft material. Weaker cartilage should not be used since the ultimate goal is to achieve projection. A graft prepared from weak cartilage, such as alar cartilage, provides tip definition but does not significantly contribute to projection (Fig. 15.11).

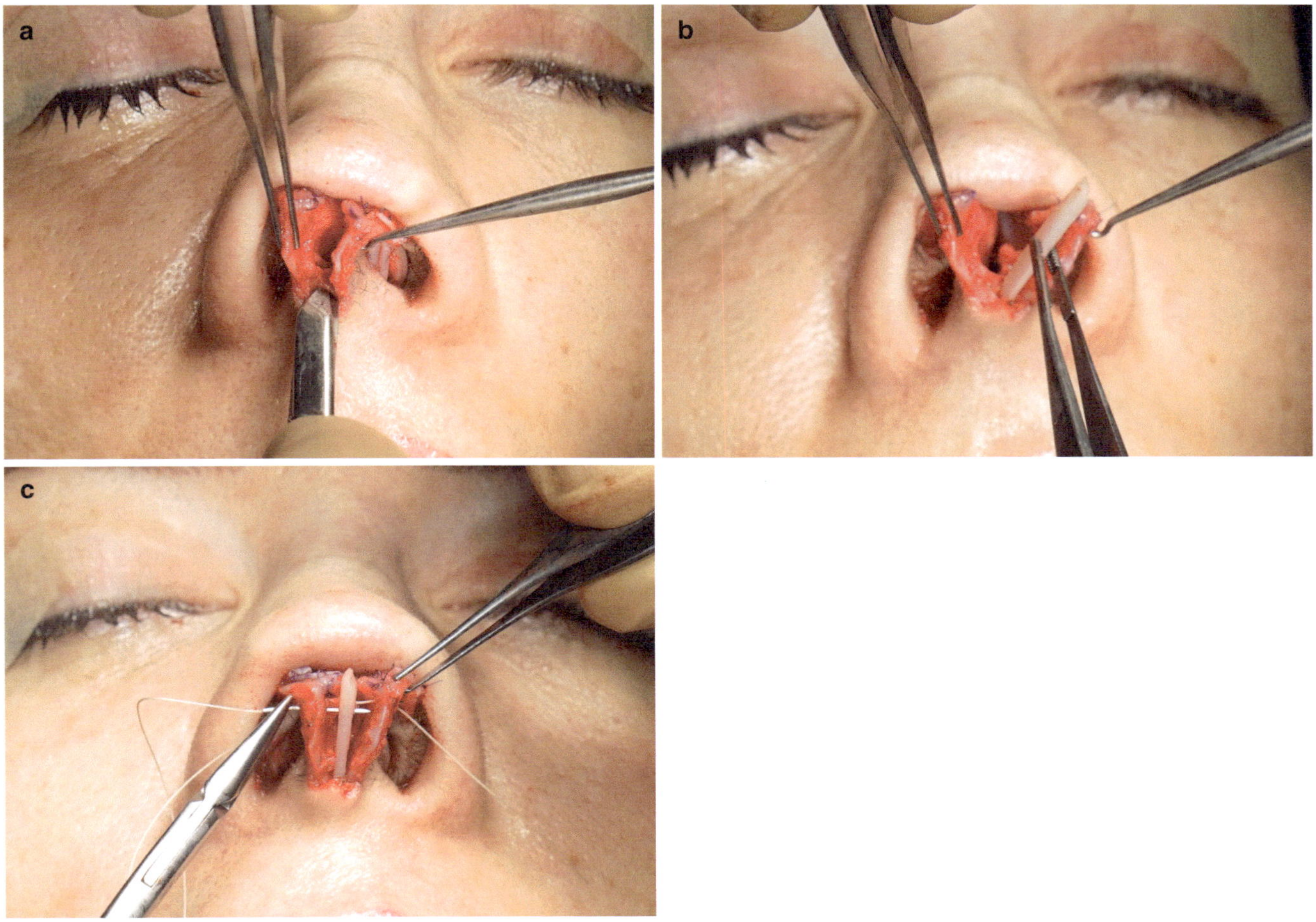

Fig. 15.8 (**a–c**) The columellar strut is placed into a pocket between the medial crura and refined with curved Stevens scissors. The graft is normally fixed in place with absorbable mattress sutures, and it must be sutured so that the anterior edge of the columellar strut is positioned posterior to the anterior edge of the medial/middle crura

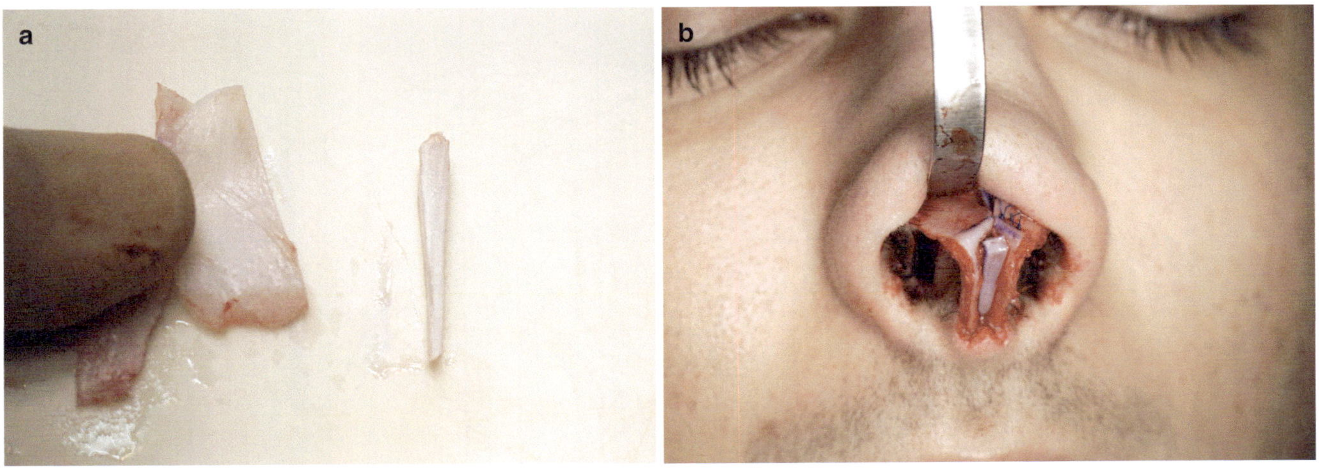

Fig. 15.9 (**a**, **b**) The columellar strut should be widened to the top

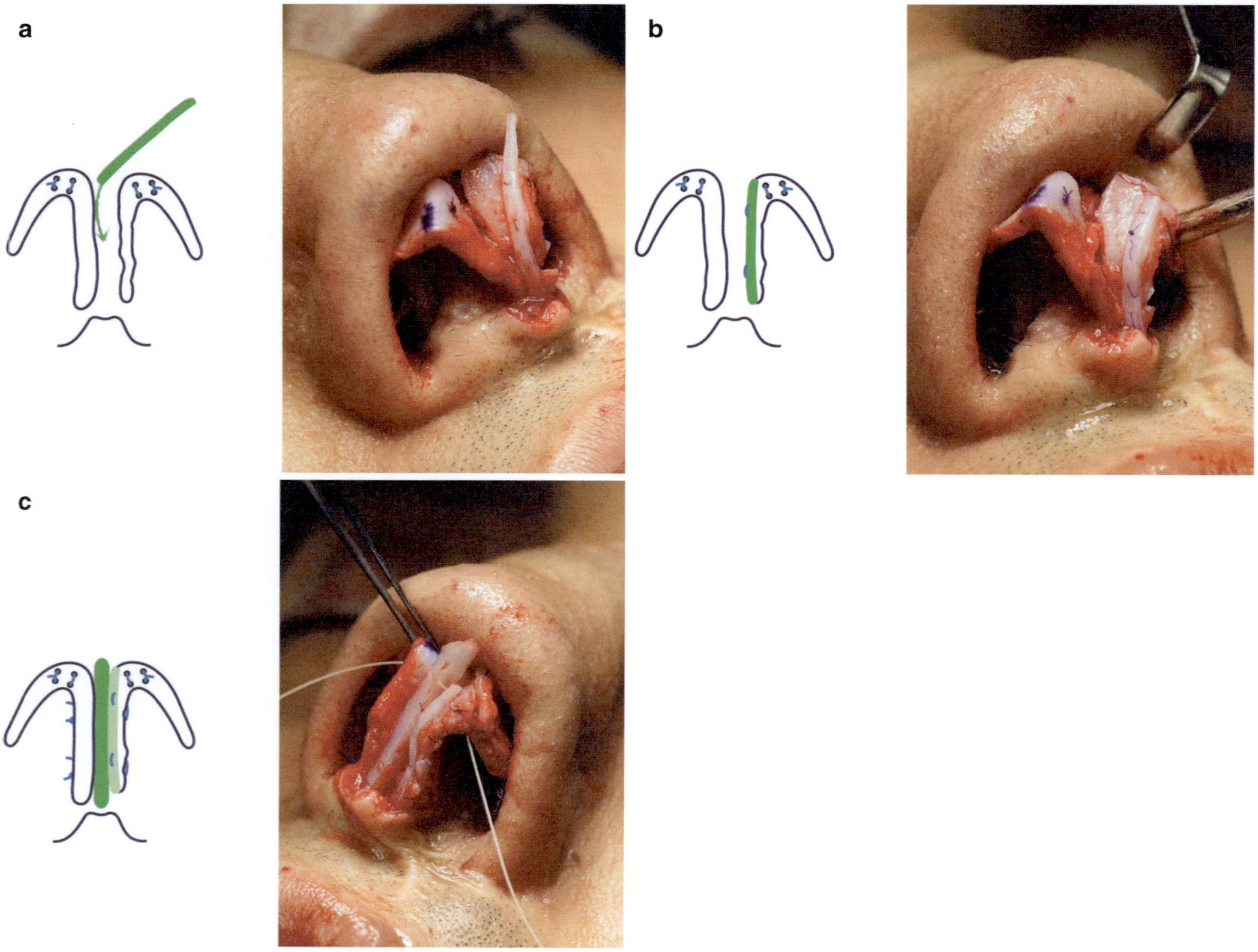

Fig. 15.10 (**a**–**c**) In the above case, the left medial crus is too weak and short, so a graft of pliable cartilage is applied to the ipsilateral side of the crus prior for fixation of the columellar strut

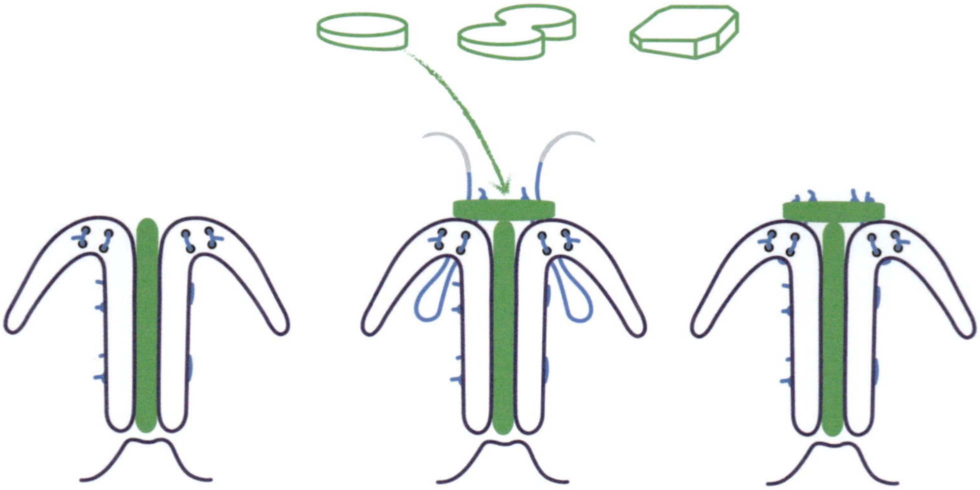

Fig. 15.11 Schematic illustrations of cup graft placement. (Supplementary Video 15.3)

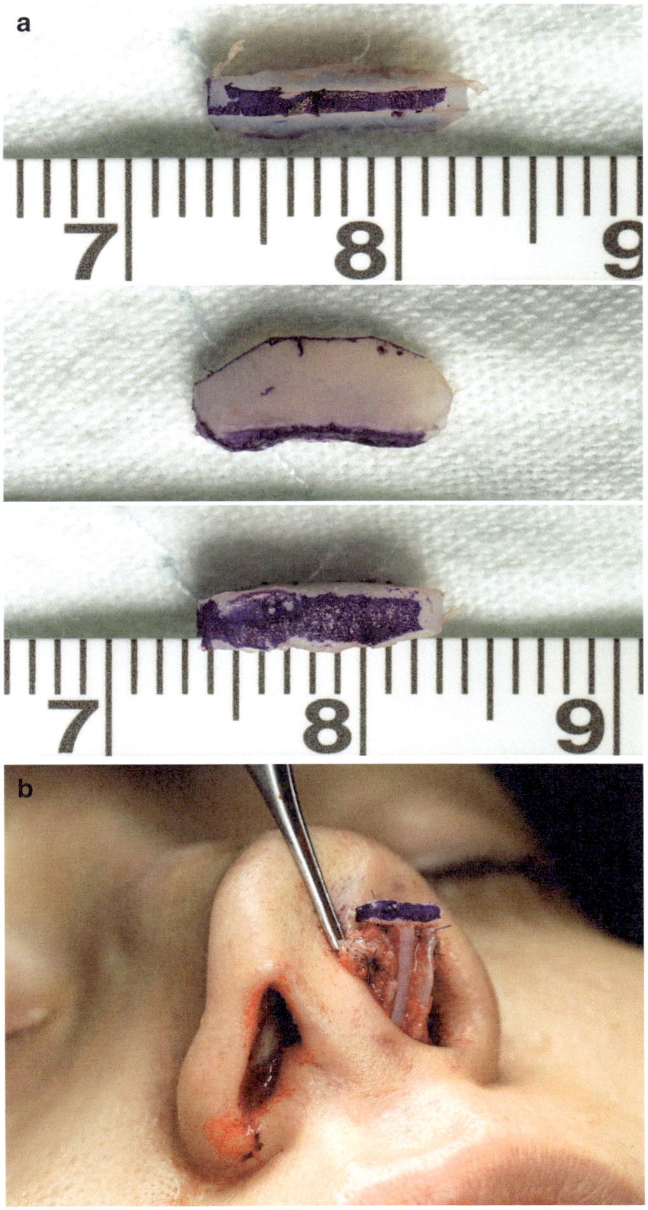

Fig. 15.12 (**a**, **b**) If possible, the cranial edge should be slightly cropped when designing the cap graft. The use of a trimmed cap graft helps to achieve a more defined dome

In addition, the caudal edge of the graft must be thicker than the cranial edge; 6-0 PDS should be used to fix the graft at two different points on each dome. The suture starts from the upper plane of the graft, passes through the dome and vestibule, returns to the dome, and finally ends at the upper plane of the graft (Fig. 15.12).

If the thickness of the cap graft is insufficient to increase projection, a layer of crushed cartilage can be placed over the cap graft. When placed over the cap graft, crushed cartilage increases projection to a certain degree and serves as a camouflage material; in contrast, when it is placed around the cap graft, it only serves as a camouflage material. Patients with thin skin who receive a cap graft are at high risk for postoperative tip irregularities and prominent leading edges caused by the underlying domal cartilage. In such cases, soft tissue, fascia, and crushed cartilage can be placed over the tip to camouflage irregularities, which may not surface for many years (Fig. 15.13).

The shield graft is another graft used, less commonly, to increase projection. This graft is placed on the middle/medial crura of the lower lateral cartilages and can increase tip projection, improve tip definition, and increase the prominence of the infratip lobule (Fig. 15.14).

Shield grafts are usually shield-shaped tip grafts carved from harvested septal cartilage, costal cartilage, or the cartilaginous segment of the dorsal hump. Cutting the graft so that it is larger at the leading edge allows for in situ carving to further refine the shape. The width generally varies from 8 mm at the leading edge. The length varies from 8 mm to 15 mm and the thickness typically varies from 1 mm to 3 mm. Standard templates of various sizes can also be used to prepare shield grafts (Fig. 15.15).

Once the graft is secured in position, it is sutured to the caudal margins of the medial/intermediate crura that have been stabilized by columellar strut and sutured in place (Fig. 15.16).

If the shield graft is used to increase projection by 3 mm or more, it must be supported by lateral crural grafts for a better transition from the tip to the alae. A buttress graft may also be required to prevent cephalic migration of the shield graft and improve its transition to the supratip (Fig. 15.17).

The author prefers the use of a shield graft rather than a cap graft to increase projection under two conditions:

- The first is for cases with an under-projected nasal tip and short or non-prominent infratip lobule, where a shield graft would be the best choice to achieve the desired projection. This is relatively common, especially in revision cases.
- The second condition refers to cases where a transdomal suture and columellar strut would not be sufficient to achieve the desired projection, such that a graft is required. A shield graft would be a good choice for these cases because it would increase the projection and length of the nose, while rendering the infratip lobule more prominent.

Technical Pearl: A shield graft can make the nose look longer. Therefore, use of the shield grafting technique is not advisable for patients with a droopy tip.

The most notable complication of this technique is an obvious tip graft contour that is visible through the skin. This complication is particularly common in thin-skinned indi-

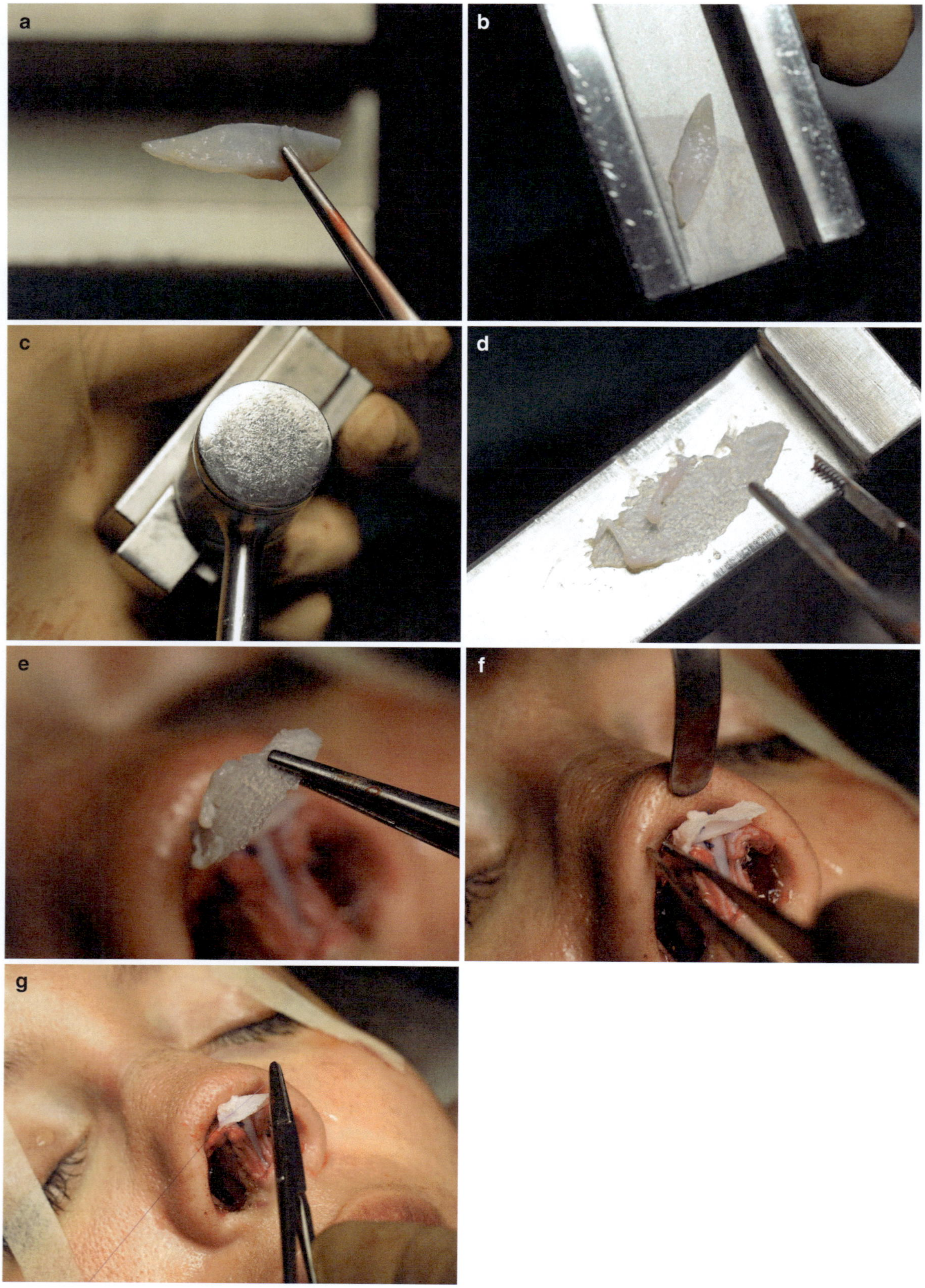

Fig. 15.13 (**a–g**) Although highly crushed cartilage has been reported to show poor long-term survival, in the author's experience highly crushed cartilage can survive, or at least meets the objective of providing long-lasting softening and camouflaging effects to the tip

viduals; to prevent it, the graft may have to be covered with soft tissues, such as fascia or the perichondrium. Another possible complication of the shield graft is migration and resultant tip deformity.

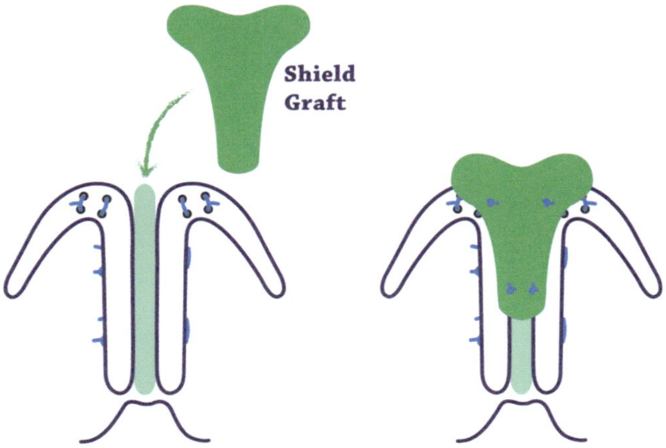

Fig. 15.14 The shield graft is a very powerful graft to increase tip projection and definition. The graft should be sutured from four points for better fixation. (Supplementary Video 15.4)

To determine if the desired level of projection has been achieved, measurement of the distance between the dorsum and the tip can serve as an intraoperative reference. The planes of the dome at the tip-defining points, and of the dorsum at the anterior septal angle, should range from 6 mm to 12 mm according to the thickness of the soft tissue. In thick-skinned noses or females, this distance should be 10–12 mm above the plane of the dorsum, while in thin-skinned noses or males it should be 6–8 mm. Once the relationship between the dorsum and the tip has been intraoperatively established, an ideal post-operative supratip break can be achieved (Fig. 15.18).

In cases where an open approach to tip surgery is used, the distance described above can be roughly measured intra-operatively (Fig. 15.19).

Less experienced surgeons are strongly advised to make this measurement during each case to gain familiarity with it. In cases where a closed approach is preferred, it is unfortunately not practicable to obtain this measurement; however, it can easily be estimated.

In patients with strong lower lateral cartilages and ideal tip-skin thickness, under-projected tip surgery can be finished without using any maneuver.

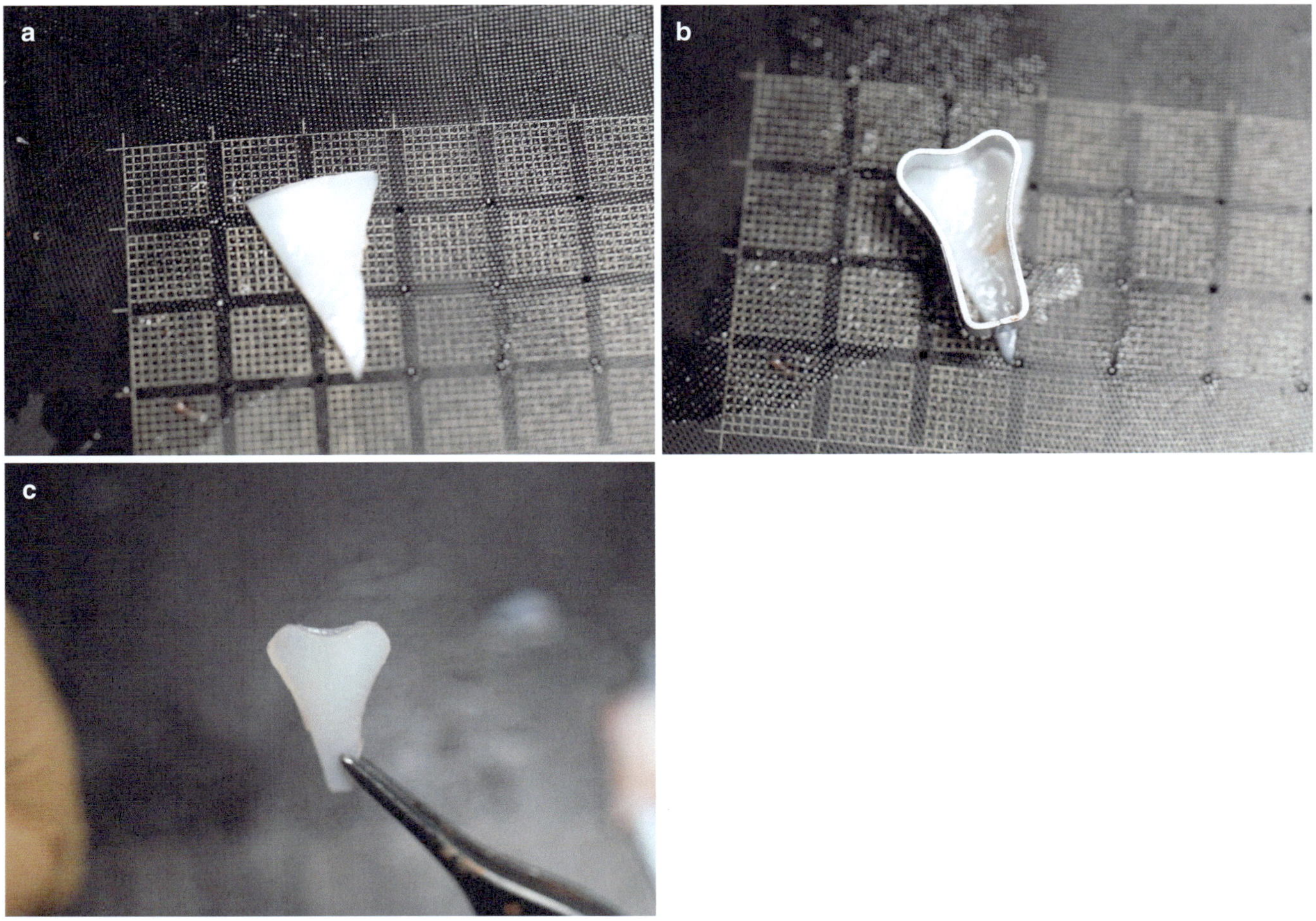

Fig. 15.15 (**a**–**c**) The shield graft is molded according to the needs of the patient

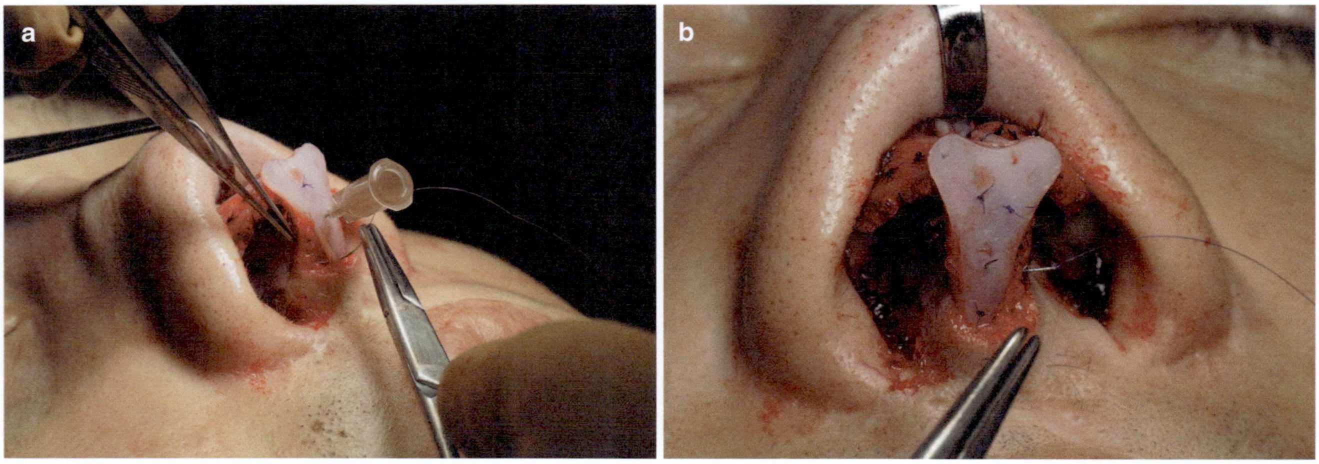

Fig. 15.16 (**a**, **b**) An insulin syringe can facilitate graft fixation. While suturing the graft, the syringe is punctured at the midline to fully secure the graft. Then the graft can be easily fixed to the medial crura at different points

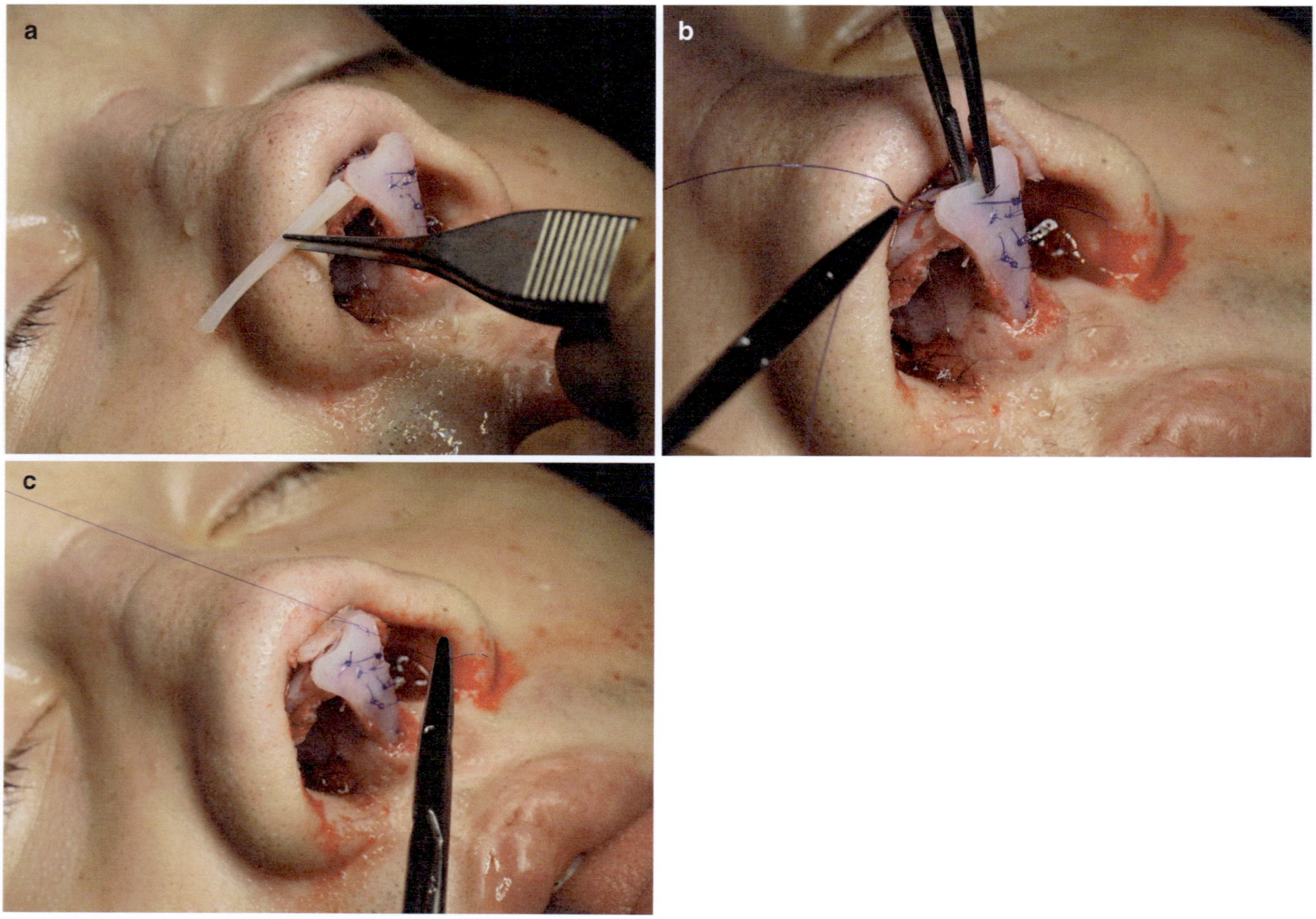

Fig. 15.17 (**a**–**c**) While a buttress graft is secured both to the dome and the shield graft with absorbable sutures, the lateral crural graft is secured over both the lateral crus and shield grafts

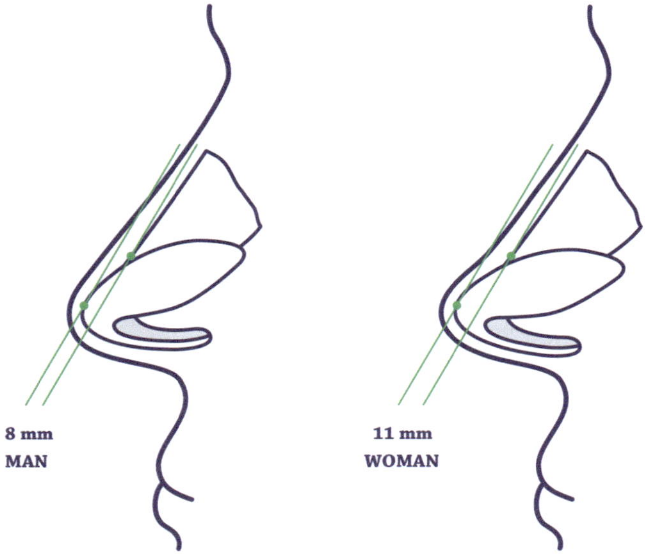

Fig. 15.18 A distance of 8–11 mm should be between the most anterior part of the cartilaginous dorsum and the newly formed dome points. (Supplementary Video 15.5)

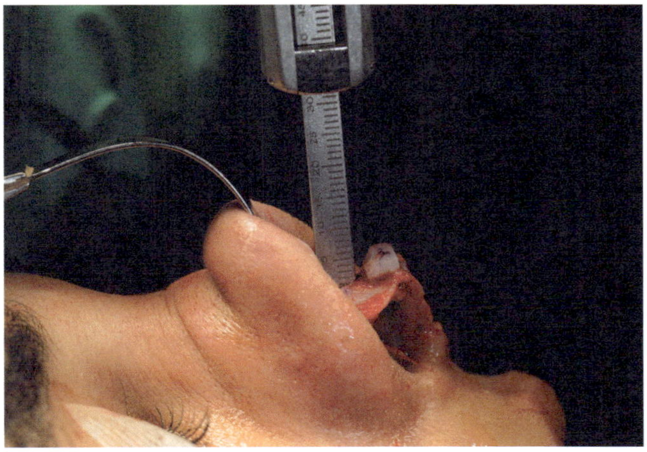

Fig. 15.19 This tool is designed by the author to measure between tip-defining point and cartilaginous dorsum

15.3.4 Clinical Outcomes

15.3.4.1 Case 1

The intraoperative lateral view shown in this case provides an example of under-projected tip surgery, the goal of which is to increase projection. In this case, a transdomal suture, columellar strut, and cap graft were used to gain projection. A gradual increase in projection was observed following use of the transdomal suture. A 1-mm-thick section of cartilage sutured over the cap graft was used to fulfill the requirement for a final, slight increase in projection. The cap graft was then camouflaged by surrounding it with crushed cartilage, because the patient was thin-skinned. After fixation of the columellar strut, the excess portion of the medial/middle crus complex was trimmed (Fig. 15.20).

One-year postoperative photographs of the patient are presented in Fig. 15.21. The photographs demonstrate that the procedures used for increasing the projection of the patient's nose were effective and sustainable in the long term. The intraoperative distance between the tip-defining point and the dorsum was 10 mm, and the significance of this distance with respect to the clinical outcome is clearly demonstrated. The lateral-view photographs of this patient demonstrate the natural-looking supratip break point.

15.3.4.2 Case 2

This 35-year-old patient desired a straighter, more defined and projected nasal tip (Fig. 15.22).

Open rhinoplasty approach is done and a columellar strut is placed. A cap graft provides volume for the tip cartilages and lengthens the tip (Fig. 15.23).

One-year postoperative photos demonstrate that the tip now projects slightly above the dorsal line and the tip definition is improved (Fig. 15.24).

15.3.4.3 Case 3

The patient complains of her nose's appearance. She feels her nasal tip is too broad, flat, and droopy, and under-projected (Fig. 15.25).

Transdomal suture, columellar strut, and cap graft were used. The nasal tip has gained rotation, projection, and strength. Seven-year postoperative photographs are shown in Fig. 15.26.

15.3.4.4 Case 4

A patient who had undergone a previous rhinoplasty complained that her nose remained under-projected and was thus too short (Fig. 15.27).

Onlay tip graft was placed more caudally to lengthen the infra-tip lobule (Fig. 15.28).

One year after, tip projection has been maintained and infratip lobule is more prominent. The dorsal cartilaginous hump has been corrected, resulting in a straight dorsum. An ideal dorsum–tip relationship has been achieved (Fig. 15.29).

Cases where the desired projection exceeds 3 mm the existing dome necessitates a shield graft. It is a good option in cases with a significant projection requirement; when the graft is transposed superiorly from the existing dome, a degree of projection will be achieved. Case 5 is a typical example of using a shield graft.

15.3.4.5 Case 5

A significant increase in projection is required for the cleft-lip-nose patient detailed in this case (Fig. 15.30).

In such cases, the thickness of the cap graft will not be sufficient to increase projection, whereas a shield graft can make the tip more projected. For these cases, a cartilaginous segment of the dorsal hump is incorporated into a shield graft and fixed to the tip (Fig. 15.31).

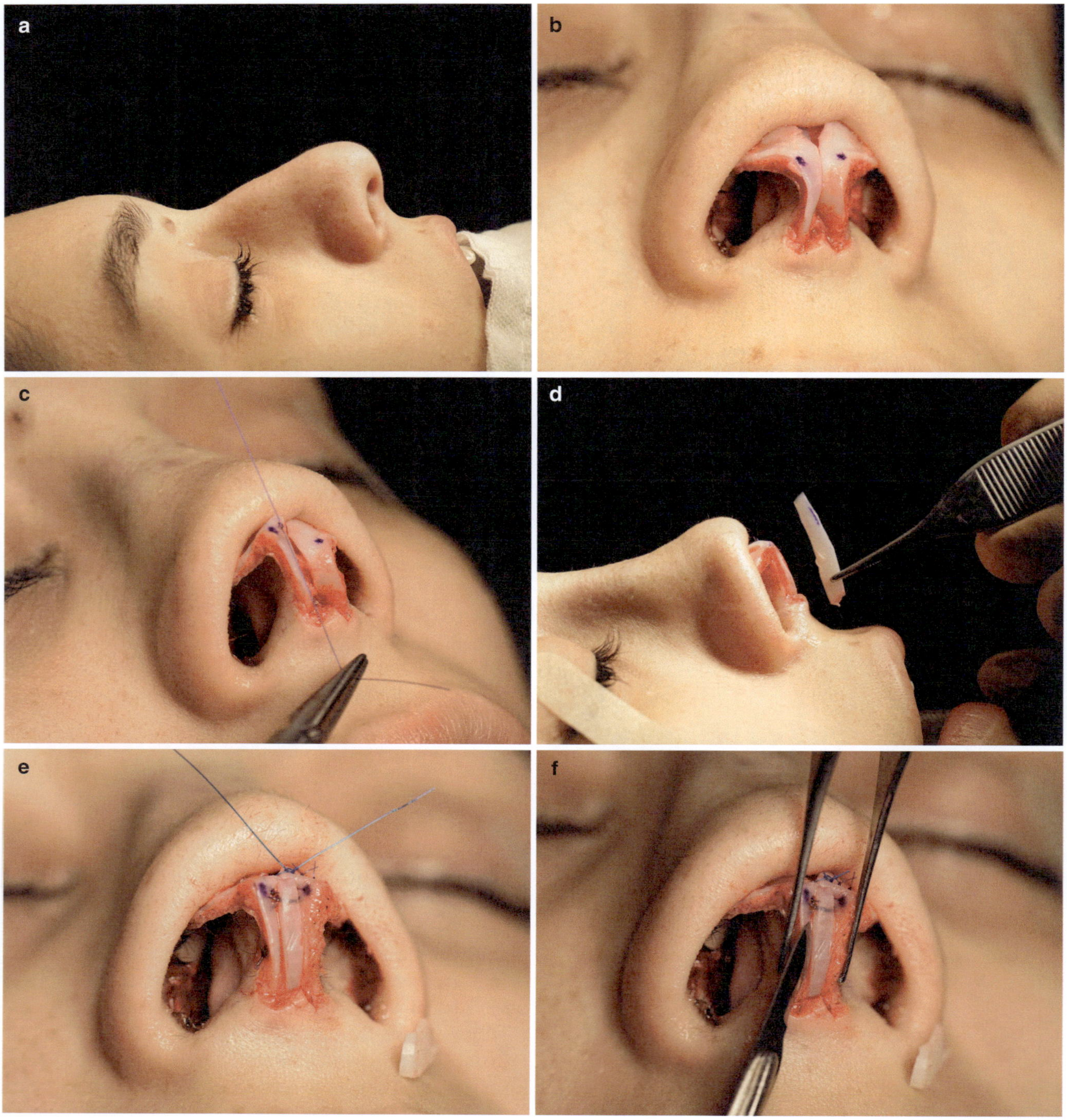

Fig. 15.20 (**a–k**) Placement columellar strut, transdomal mattress suture, cup graft. The final dome position was 10 mm above the plane of the dorsum

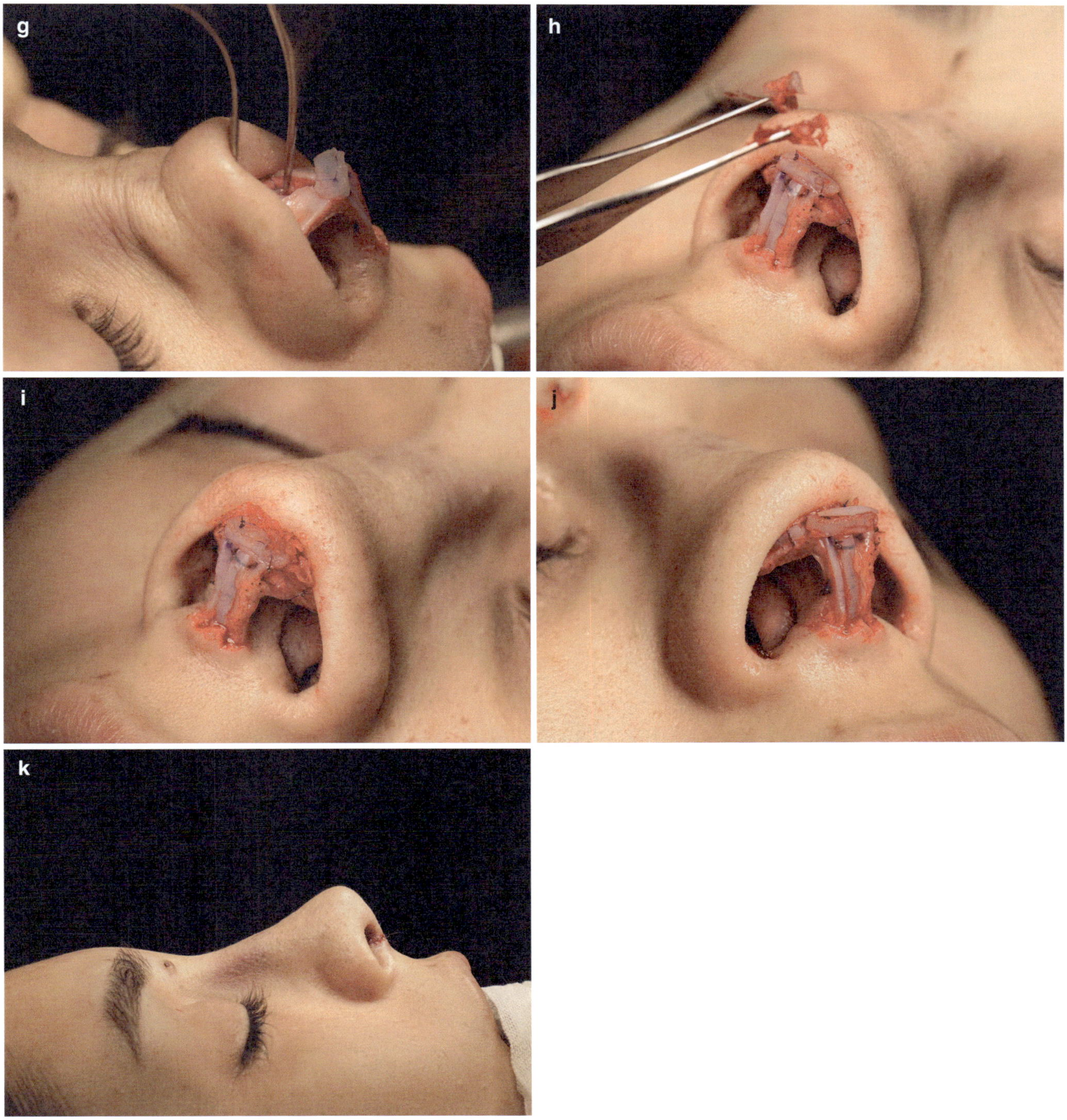

Fig. 15.20 (continued)

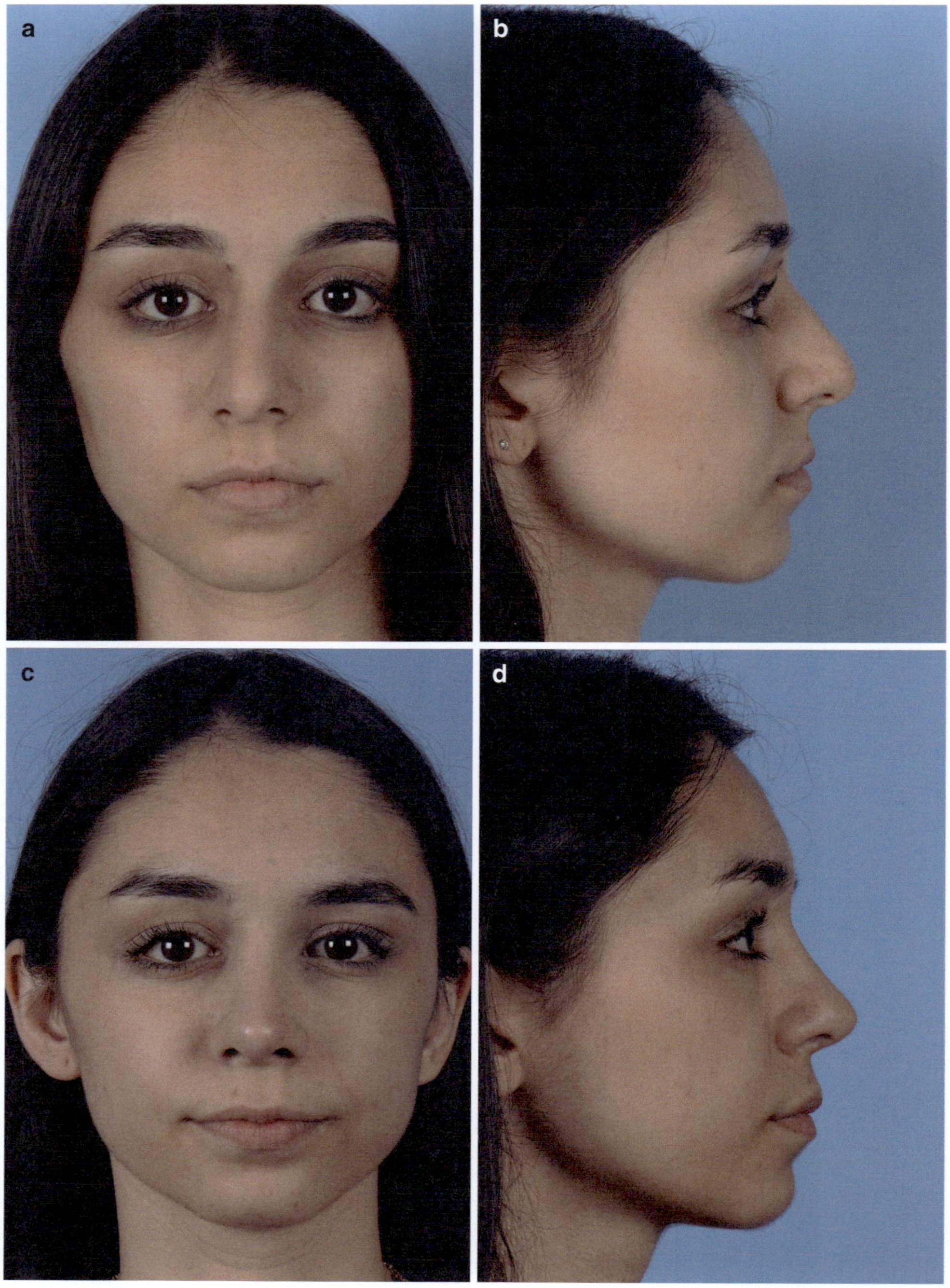

Fig. 15.21 (**a–d**) Frontal view demonstrates improved tip definition. The profile view shows that tip projection was further enhanced

One-year postoperative photographs indicate that the desired projection was achieved (Fig. 15.32).

15.3.5 Lateral Crural Graft and Septocolumellar Strut

Failure to control the projection, shape, and rotation of the nasal tip is common among patients with weak lower lateral cartilage or thick skin. For such patients, structural support is required to achieve a stable tip projection. For this purpose, two structural grafts are used in addition to the columellar strut: (1) Lateral crural graft; and (2) Septocolumellar strut.

While the columellar strut reinforces the medial/middle crura, the lateral crural graft reinforces a weak or deformed lateral crus. This helps establish a more stable alar arch; however, the weak tip must also be fixed to achieve a strong and stable septum. For this purpose, the author prefers to use a septocolumellar strut because it ensures tip stability while

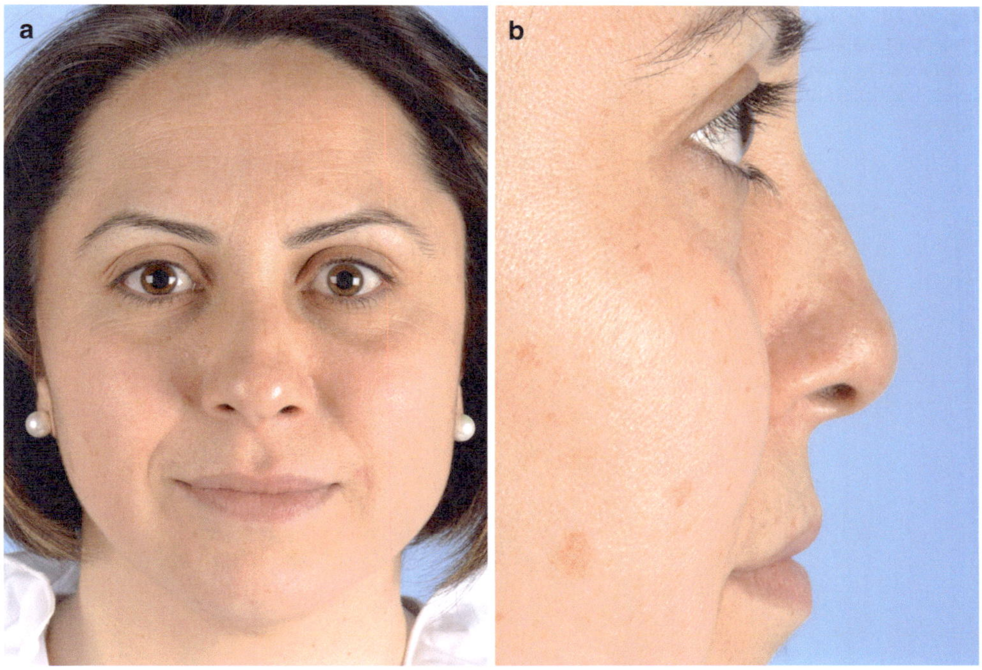

Fig. 15.22 (**a**, **b**) Preoperative photographs: the tip is under-projected and less defined with short medial crura

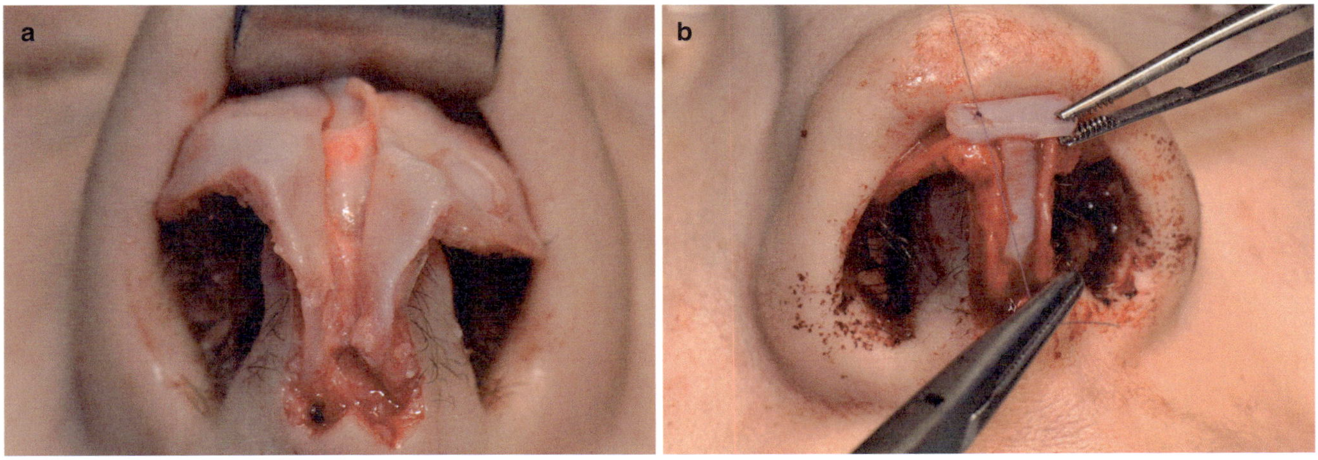

Fig. 15.23 (**a**, **b**) Columellar strut, transdomal suture, and cap graft were placed

also avoiding a rigid and immobile tip or the requirement for an excessive amount of graft material. Details of these two types of structural graft are given below.

15.3.5.1 Lateral Crural Graft

The lateral crural graft is placed over or under the existing lateral crus. These grafts are used to repair alar contour irregularities and strengthen and shape the existing lateral crura; they may also improve any external valve dysfunction. The use of overlay grafts is preferred for cases requiring a projection increase, while underlay grafts are mostly used to correct convex lateral crus or for malposition surgery (Fig. 15.33).

The graft anteriorly starts lateral to the dome. The posterior end of the graft is usually placed superficially to the pyriform aperture rim to avoid medial displacement. Graft length varies from case to case, while the width typically ranges from 1 mm to 4 mm depending on the amount of material available and the desired outcome. In addition, the graft thickness should not exceed 2 mm, or it may become visible. Another advantage of the lateral crural graft is its ability to camouflage the cap graft by softening the sharp transition from the cap graft to the lateral crus. Therefore, there is no need to camouflage the cap graft in cases where an onlay lateral crural graft is used (Fig. 15.34).

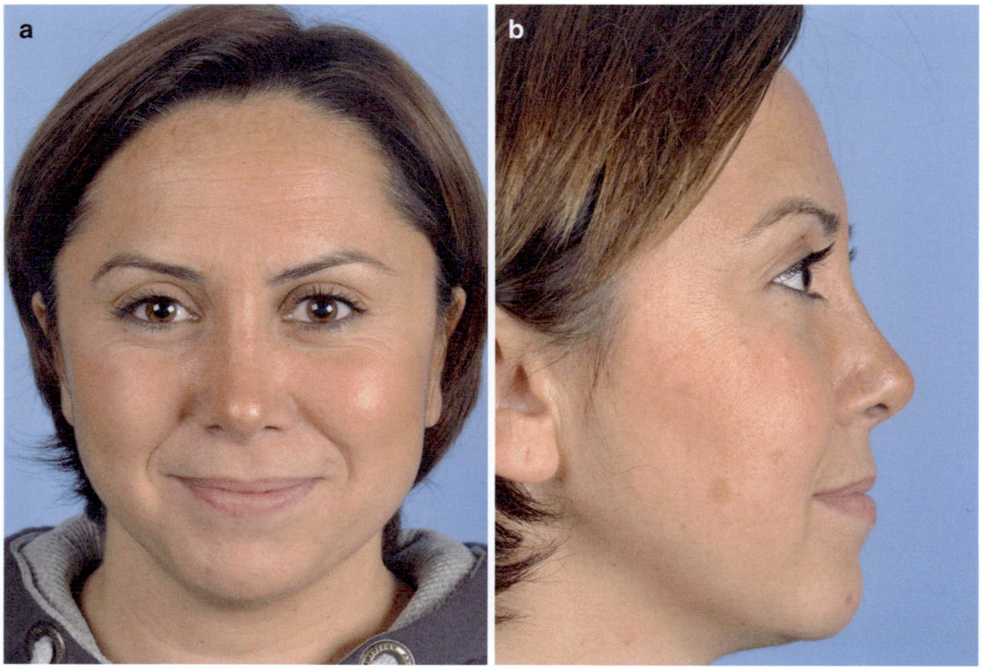

Fig. 15.24 (**a**, **b**) Tip projection has been lengthened to a more pleasant level. The tip is also better defined

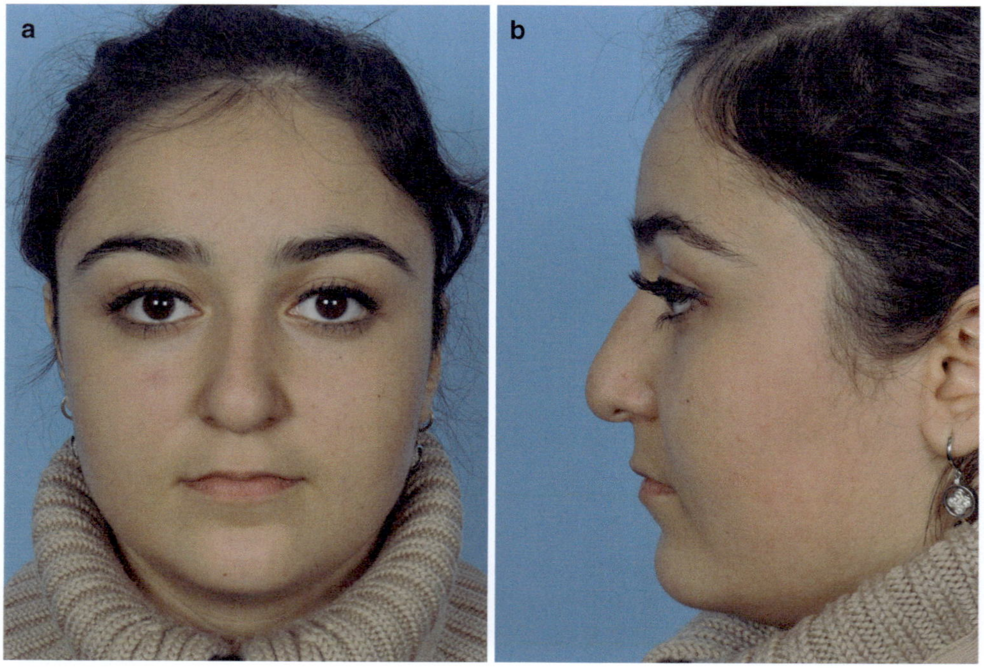

Fig. 15.25 (**a**, **b**) The tip is under-projected, slightly under-rotated, and wide

15.3.5.2 Septocolumellar Strut

It is also possible to achieve effective and permanent tip stability by inserting a cartilaginous strut between the septum and the columella (Fig. 15.35).

Typically, the septocolumellar strut is ~2 cm long and 3–4 mm wide. One end of the strut is fixed to the septum, at a minimum of two different points. The level of fixation at the septum is insignificant in practice, but it is generally appropriate to fix the strut in a relatively more concave plane. The other end of the graft extends between the two medial crura, where it is fixed to the columellar strut. Sutures thinner than 5-0 should not be used while fixing both ends, and absorbable sutures are preferred (Fig. 15.36).

15.3.5.3 Case 6

Noses with a congenitally weak alar arch are characterized by a weak midvault and drawn-up alae (Fig. 15.37).

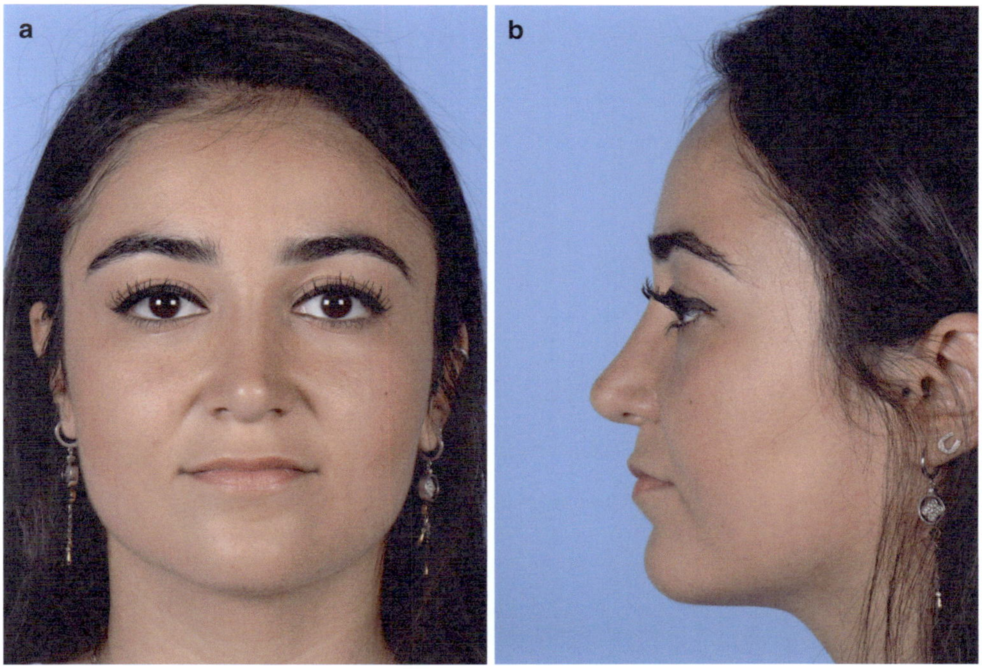

Fig. 15.26 (**a**, **b**) Projection rotation and definition of the tip have been stable, elegant, and more balanced, even long term

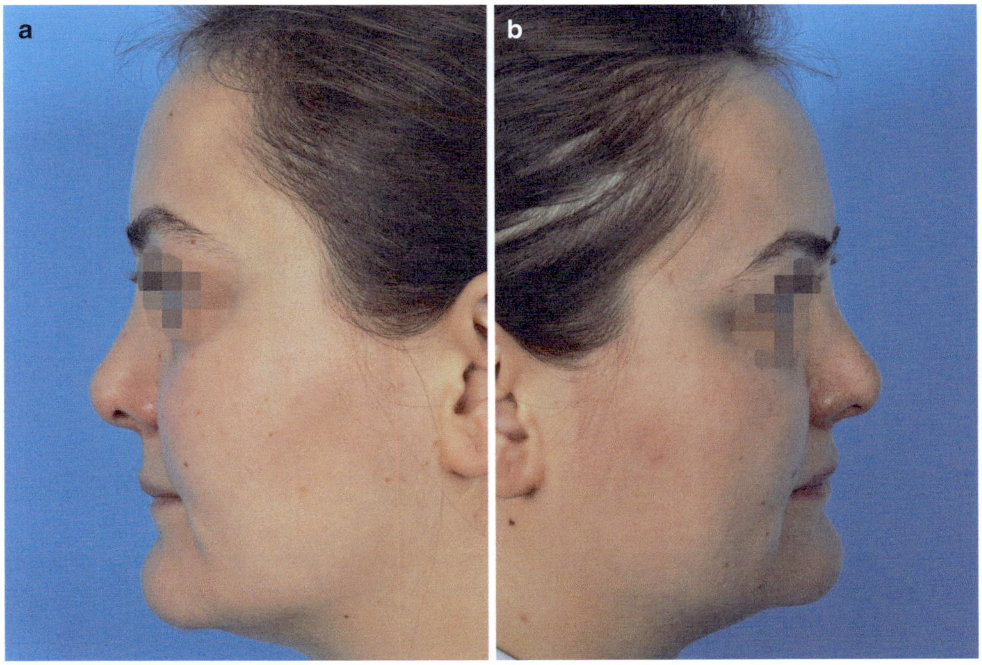

Fig. 15.27 (**a**, **b**) Short nose with under-projected tip

The intraoperative view in Fig. 15.38 illustrates weak alar cartilage and thick skin.

Surgery should begin with a transdomal suture, which is the first step to increase projection (Fig. 15.39).

The second step is to fix the tip to the septum via a septo-columellar strut and a cap graft, to achieve a slight increase in projection (Fig. 15.40).

The next step is to strengthen the weak lateral crura. For this purpose, a piece of cartilage with a width of 3 mm is harvested from the septum and sutured from the right lateral crura to the cap graft, extending through the lateral crus and ending at the pocket near the apertura piriformis in the direction of the outer canthus (Fig. 15.41).

After the desired amount of tip projection is achieved, the surgery is completed by placing crushed cartilage directly under the cap graft to make the infratip lobule more pronounced (Fig. 15.42).

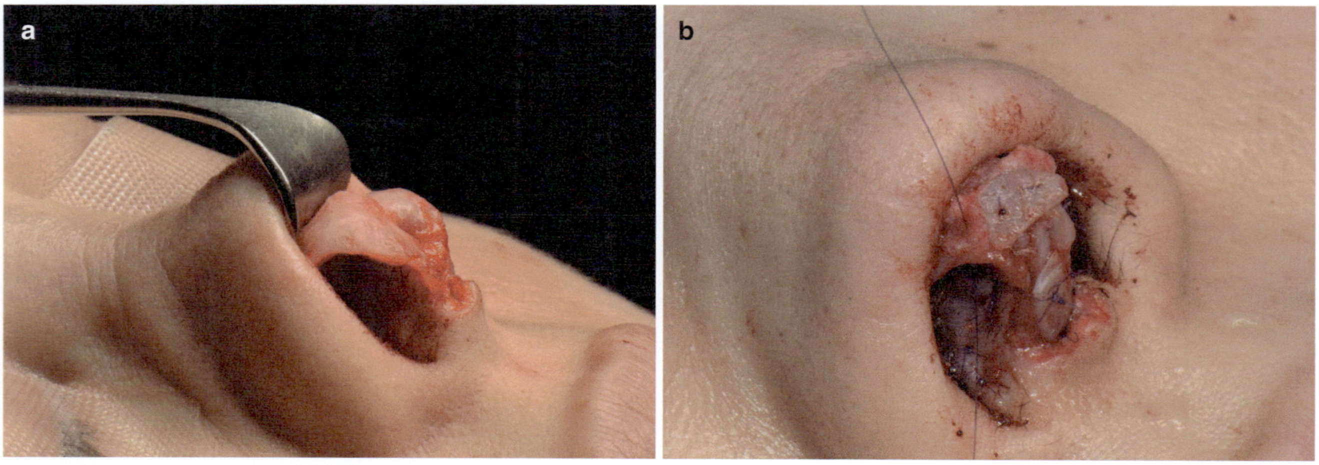

Fig. 15.28 (**a**, **b**) More caudally positioned tip graft to lengthen nose and tip together

Fig. 15.29 (**a**, **b**) Tip projection has been increased and the nose lengthened

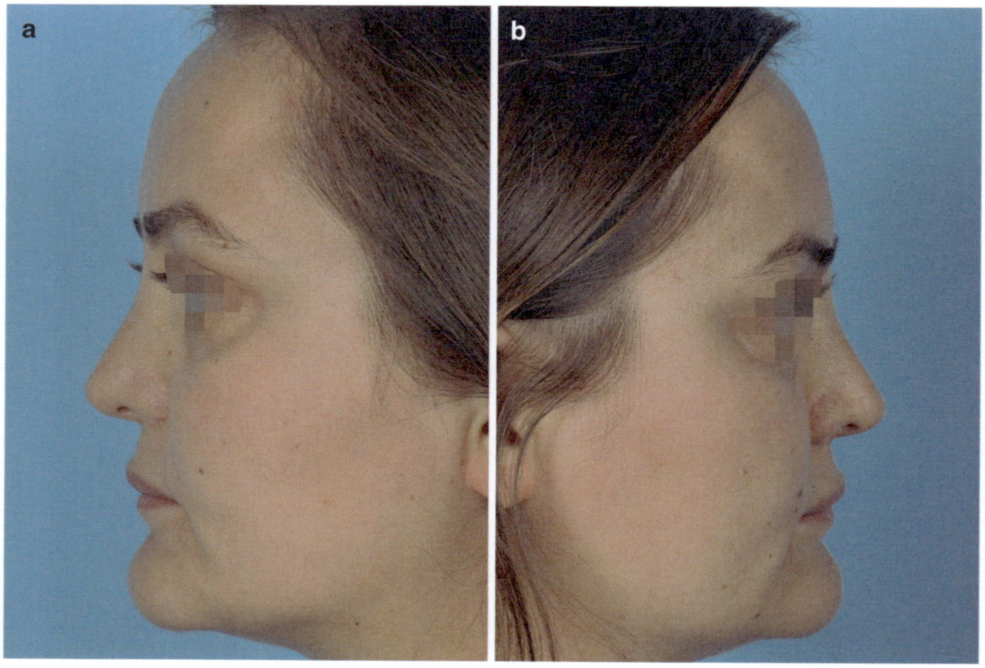

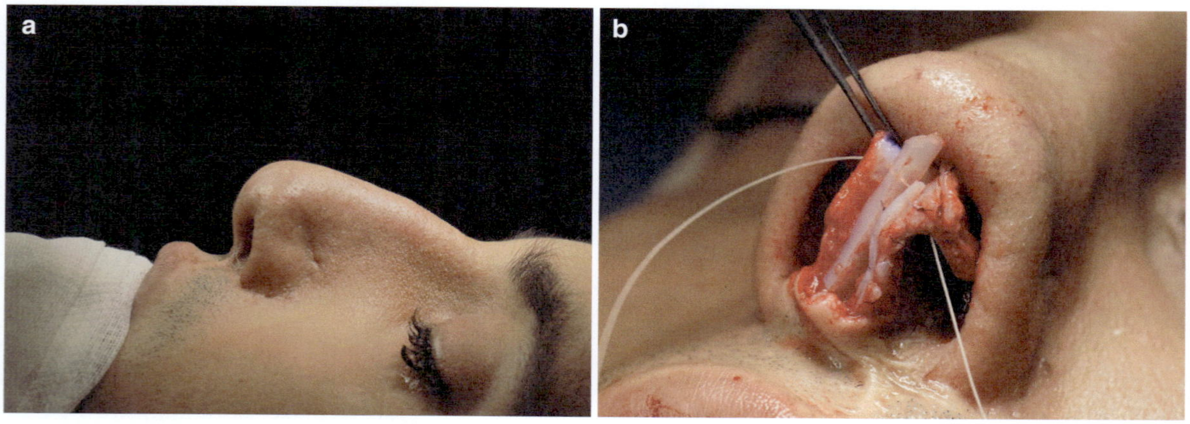

Fig. 15.30 (**a**, **b**) A substantial level of projection and nasal base stability can be achieved by repairing the left medial crus and applying a columellar strut and transdomal suture

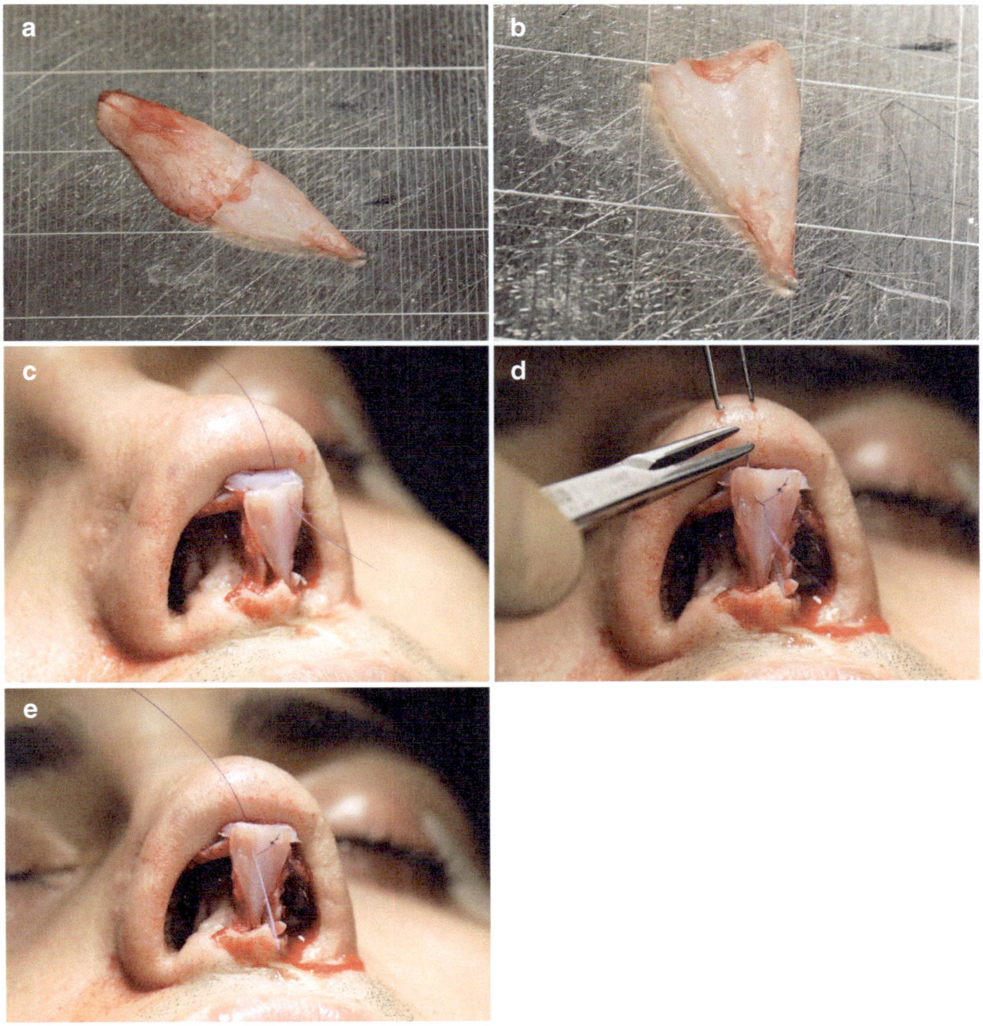

Fig. 15.31 (**a**–**e**) It is acceptable to create the shield graft from the cartilaginous dorsal hump when there is insufficient suitable material in the septum

Preoperative and postoperative photographs are shown in Fig. 15.43. The tip projection and contour are improved.

Under-projection due to weak alar cartilage is also observed in revision cases. Deformation of the alar arch by the primary surgeon is the most common reason for under-projection, and additional problems such as tip asymmetry and a pinched tip can also arise. Reconstruction of the weak and deformed alar arch not only increases projection, but also corrects other tip-related problems. In addition, fixation of the tip to the septum is essential to ensure long-term stability thereof.

15.3.5.4 Case 7

The intraoperative photo of an under-projected and pinched tip (Fig. 15.44) shows a weak and short medial/middle crus and the extent of malformation at the lateral crura.

The new dome points are defined, and the first step toward increasing projection is taken via use of the transdomal suture (Fig. 15.45).

Then, the septocolumellar strut is fixed to the concave plane of the septum, followed by the anterior septum. After that, a columellar strut is placed between the middle/medial crural complex at two different points (Fig. 15.46).

Once a stable base has been achieved, the next step is to strengthen the lateral crura. Since the position of the crura is acceptable, there is no need for any transposition. The onlay graft is harvested from the septal cartilage and sutured over the lateral crus at several points to stabilize the entire alar arch (Fig. 15.47).

Finally, a cap graft is used for final projection and definition, and fibrotic tissues removed from inside the nose are sutured under the cap graft to achieve infratip fullness (Fig. 15.48).

Photographs at 1-year postoperative photographs are shown in Fig. 15.49.

Strengthening of the alar arch and correction of its configuration increased projection and eliminated the asymmetry and pinched appearance of the nose.

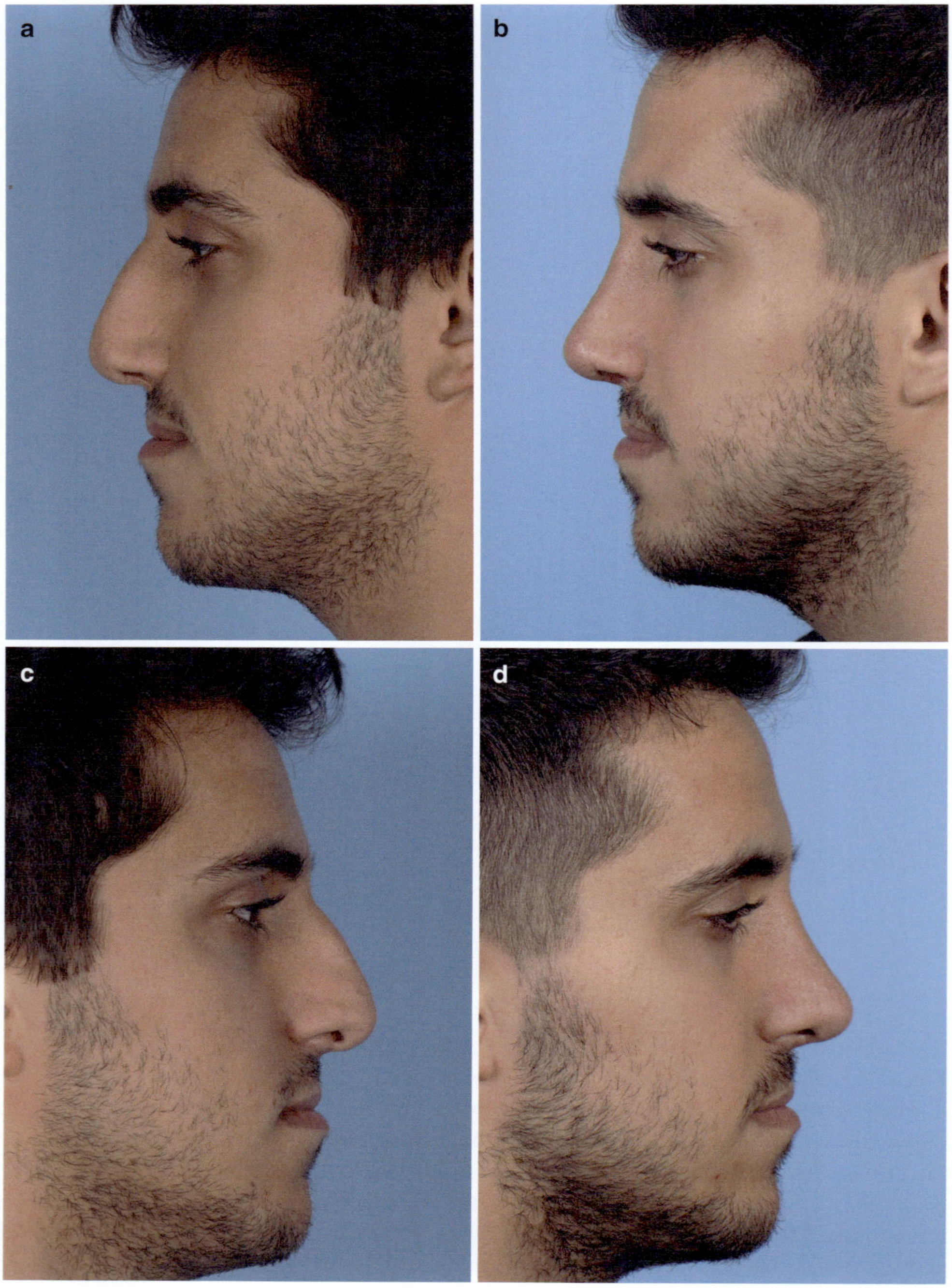

Fig. 15.32 (**a–d**) Cleft-lip patient shown preoperatively and 1 year after tip augmentation

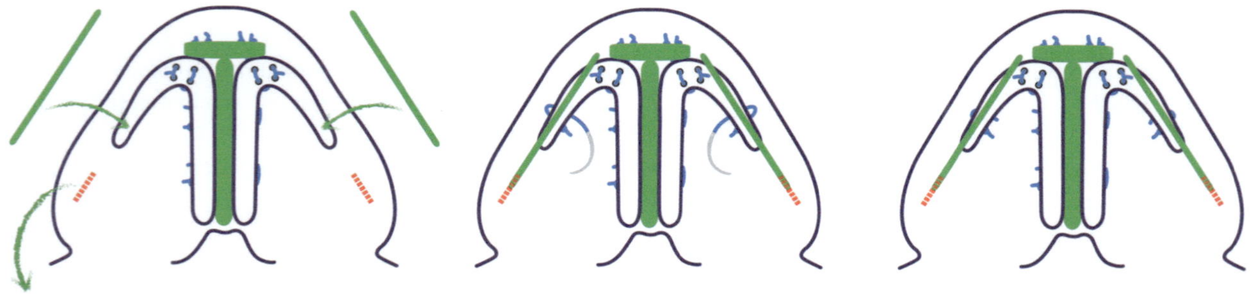

Fig. 15.33 Schematic illustrations of lateral crural graft placement

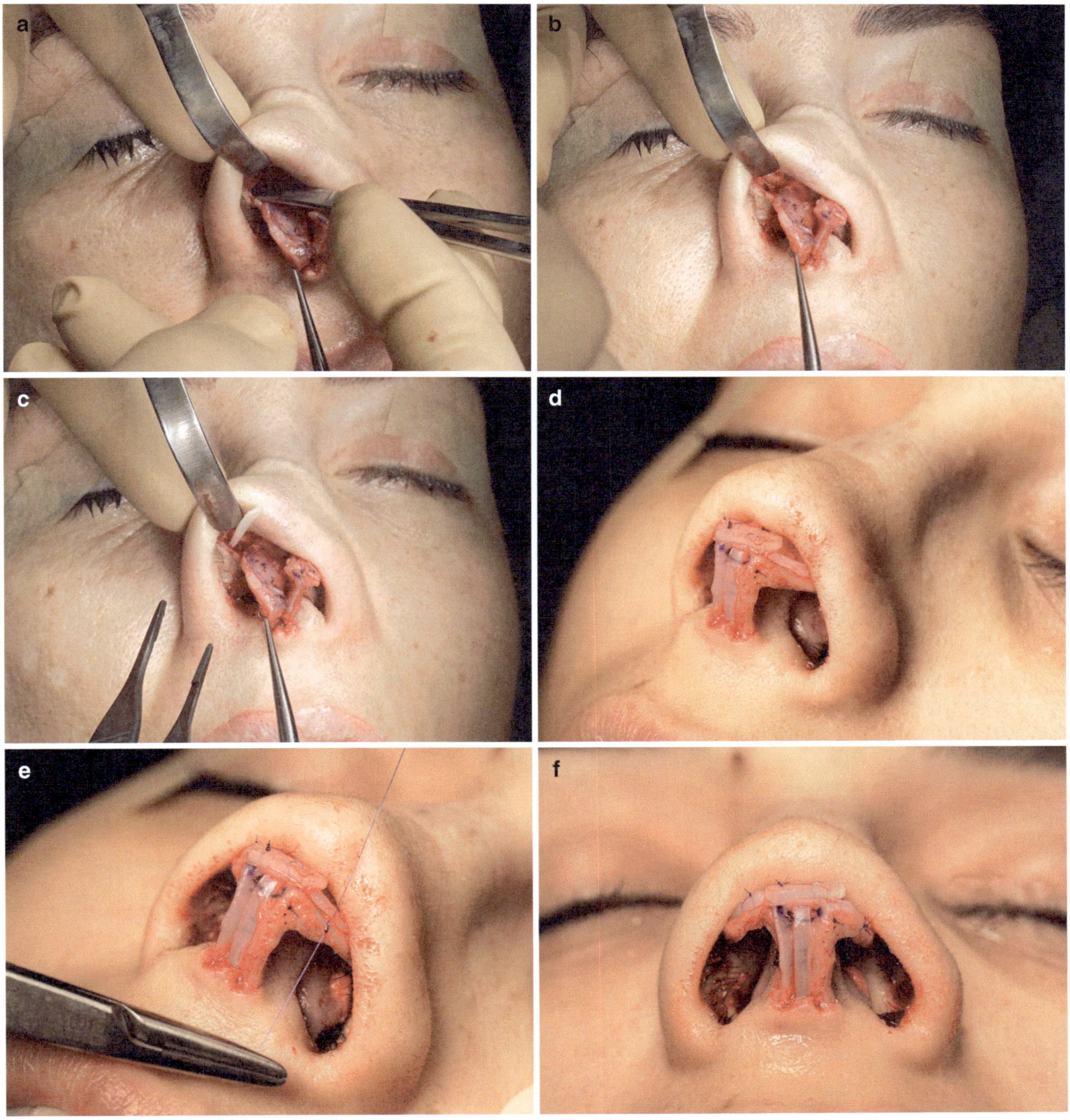

Fig. 15.34 (**a–f**) Surgical implementation of lateral crural graft placement

As mentioned previously, thick skin requires rigid and strong structural support. Even if the alar arch has normal strength and structure, it may not provide sufficient support during rhinoplasty procedures in patients with thick skin. Rather than reduction, augmentation at the midvault and dorsum should be considered in thick-skinned patients. A strong osseocartilaginous framework is essential for augmentation, to achieve safe and attractive nasal contouring and patient satisfaction.

An example of this is presented in Case 8.

15.3.5.5 Case 8

This patient has thick, lobular skin, insufficient nasal tip projection, a weak midvault, a low radix, and a slight dorsal hump. In addition to increasing tip projection, a strong dorsum and midvault are the most desirable outcomes for this patient (Fig. 15.50).

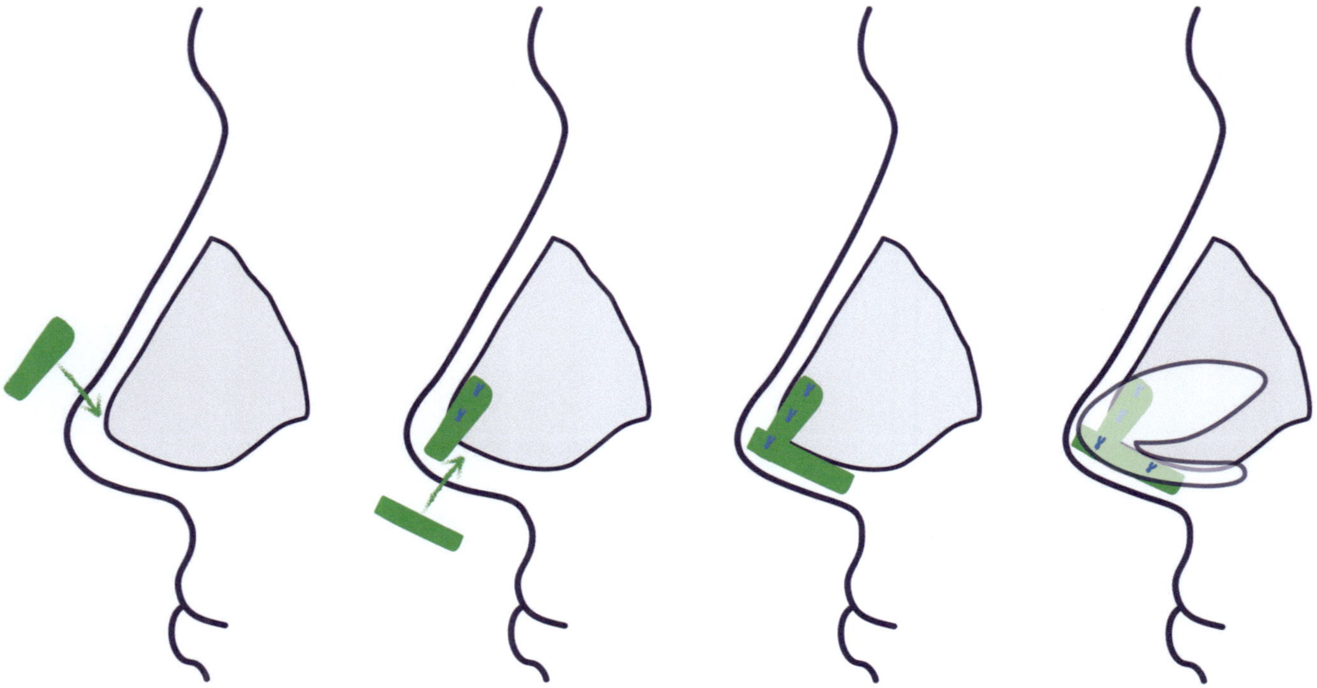

Fig. 15.35 Projection can be controlled by securing nasal tip with cartilage affixed to septum

After a moderate dorsal reduction, a strong dorsal profile was achieved via radix augmentation (Fig. 15.51).

A strong middle vault was obtained using spreader grafts (Fig. 15.52).

A transdomal suture, septocolumellar strut, columellar strut, and lateral crural onlay graft were used to achieve rigid, strong alar cartilage (Fig. 15.53).

The final projection was achieved only after the cap graft was fixed (Fig. 15.54).

Preoperative and 1-year postoperative photographs are shown in Fig. 15.55. The nasal tip now leads the dorsum with appropriate tip projection.

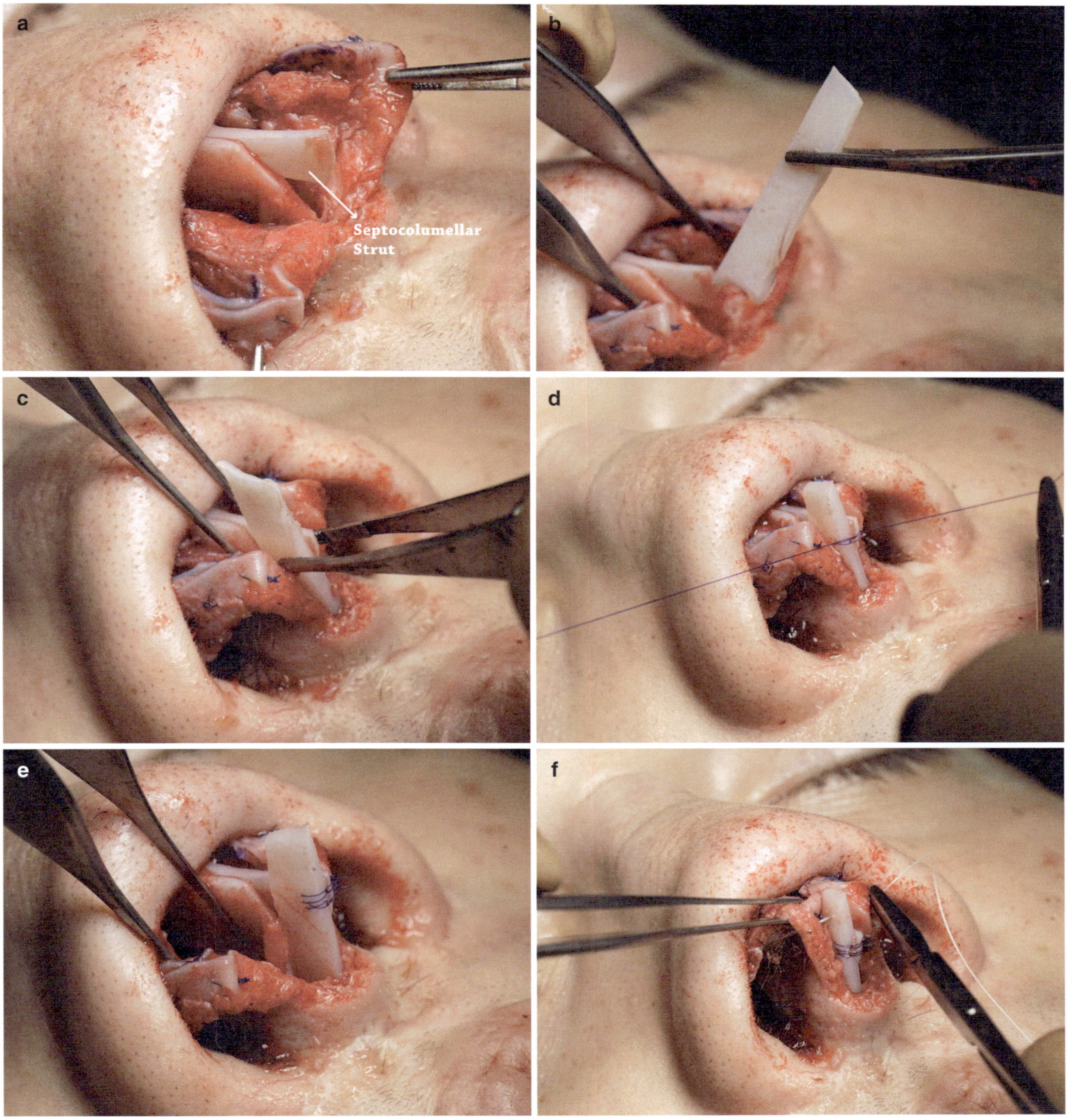

Fig. 15.36 (**a**–**f**) Septocolumellar graft placement

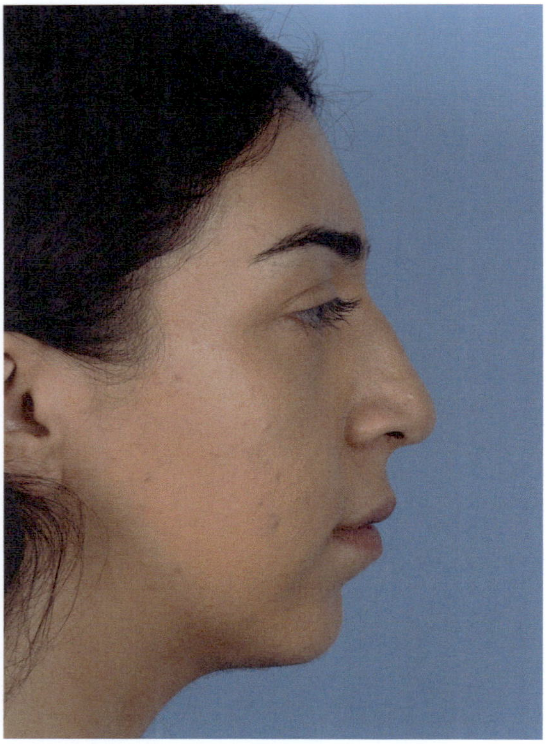

Fig. 15.37 Thick skin patient with under-projected tip. Lumping of the alae is a common sign of a weak alar arch; when observed, surgery should be planned accordingly

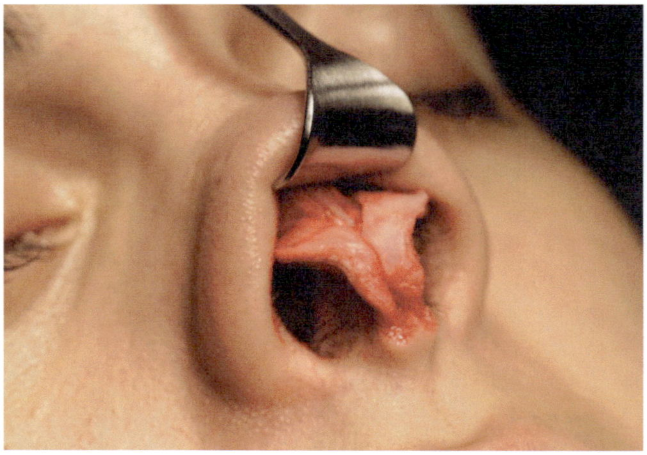

Fig. 15.38 If septocolumellar strut placement is planned, open approach is preferred

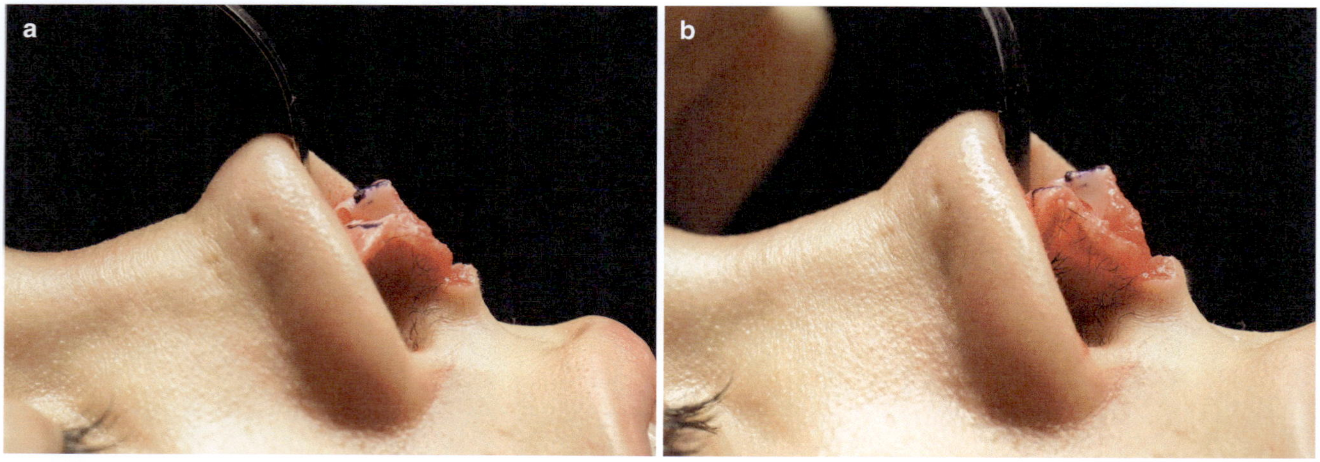

Fig. 15.39 (a, b) It is important to note any difference in projection between the sutured and unsutured domes in the first photograph. In the second photograph, an even projection is achieved via placement of a contralateral transdomal suture

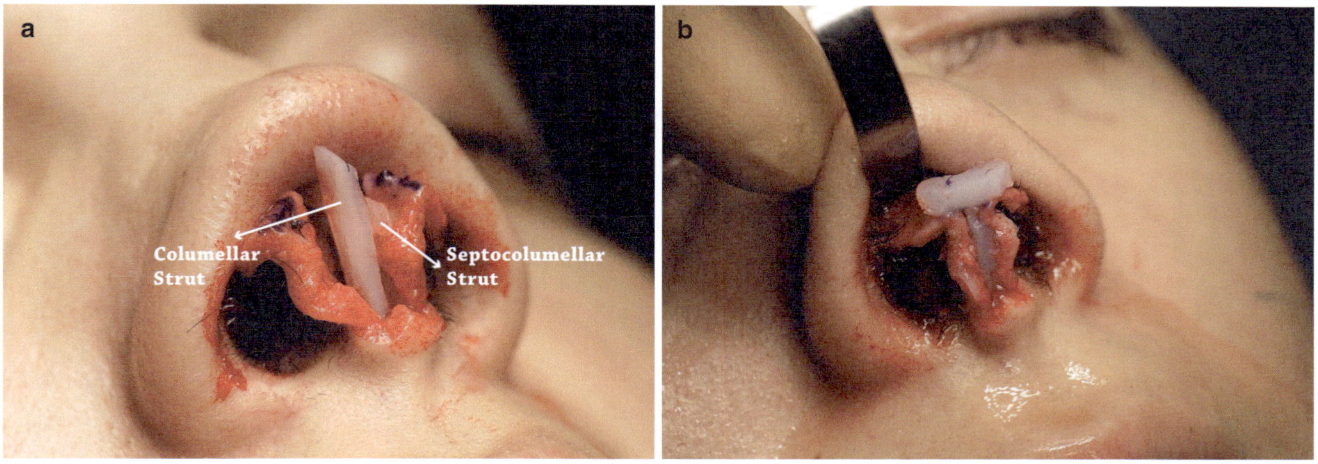

Fig. 15.40 (**a**, **b**) A strut approximately 2.5 cm in length is fixed to the septum first, followed by the columellar strut

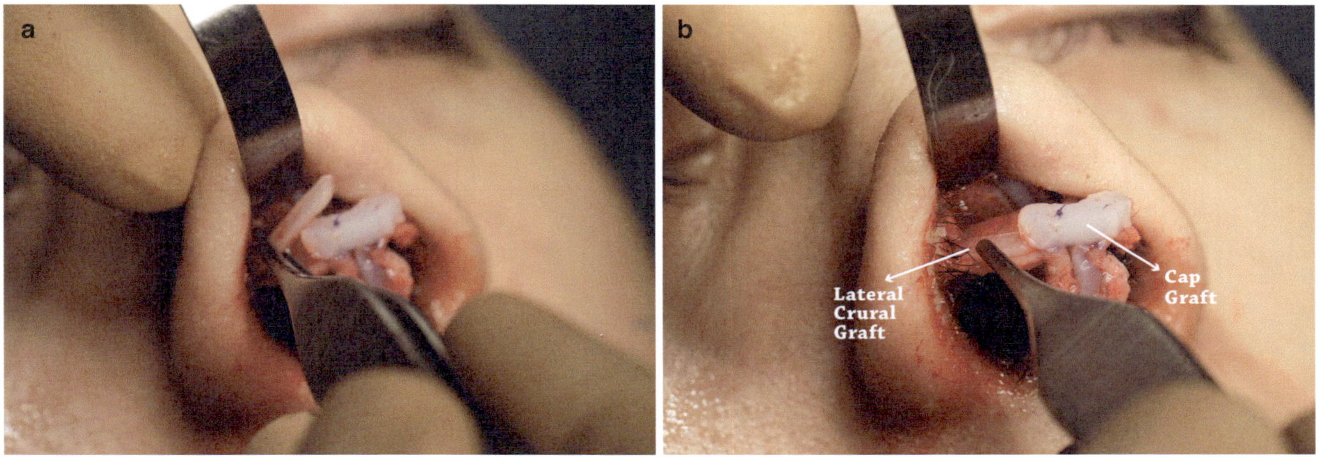

Fig. 15.41 (**a**, **b**) The lateral crural graft must continue to the caudal edge of, and be fixed to, the lateral crus at several points using a 6-0 absorbable suture

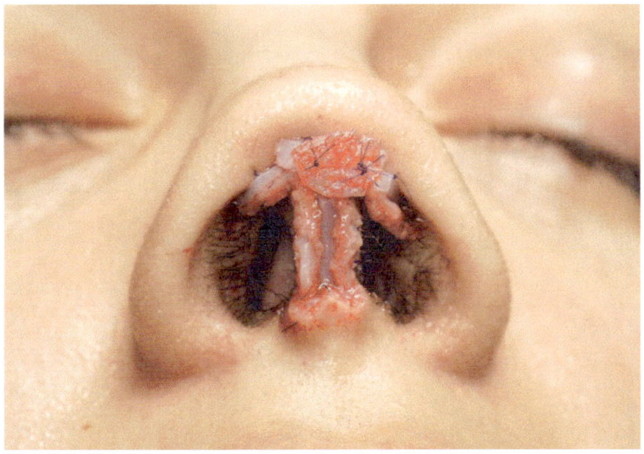

Fig. 15.42 The crushed cartilage is secured by the inferior portion of the cap graft to add volume to the infra tip lobule

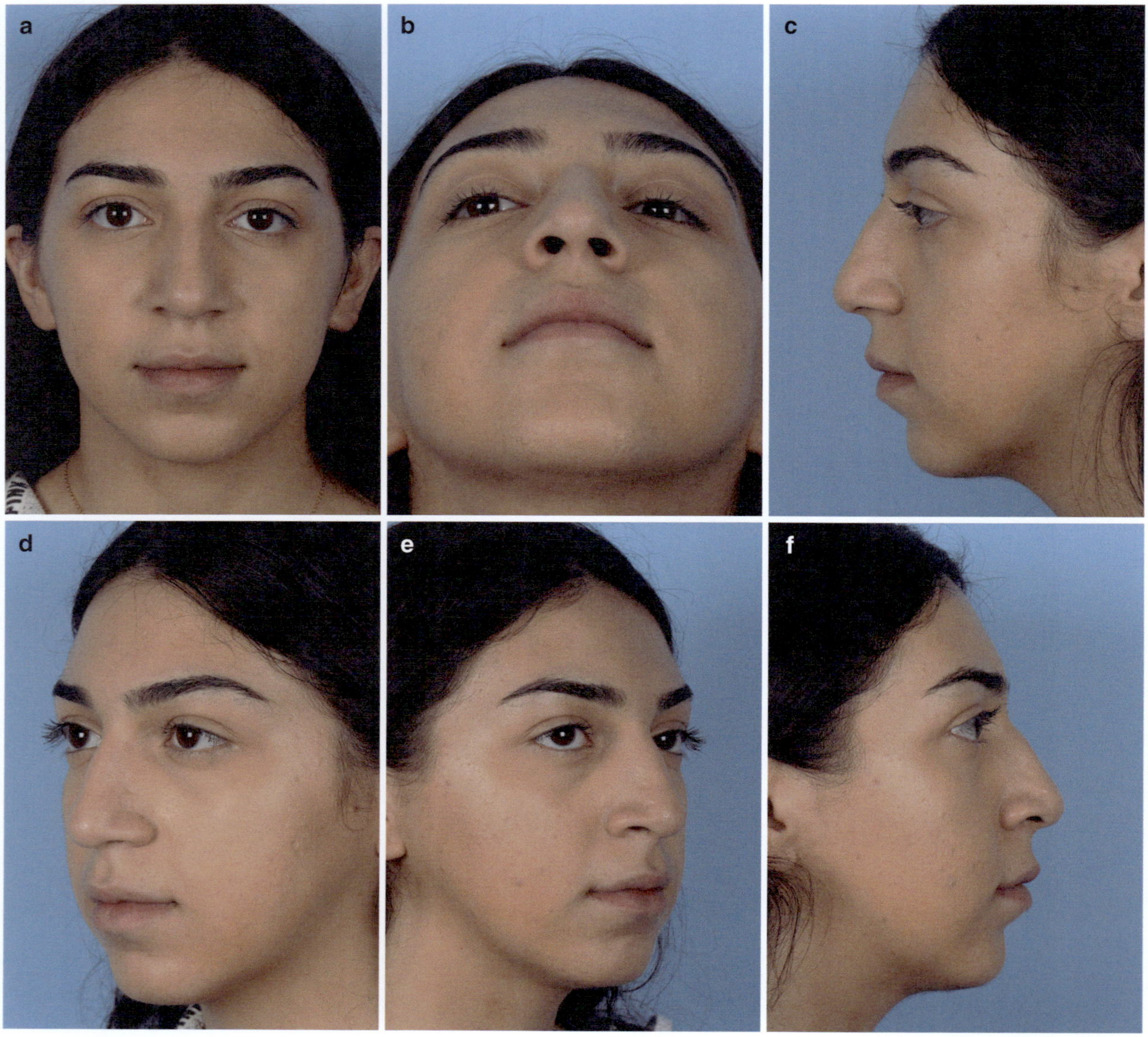

Fig. 15.43 (a–l) The patient is shown 1 year postoperatively. The tip is more adequately projected and much better supported despite thick skin

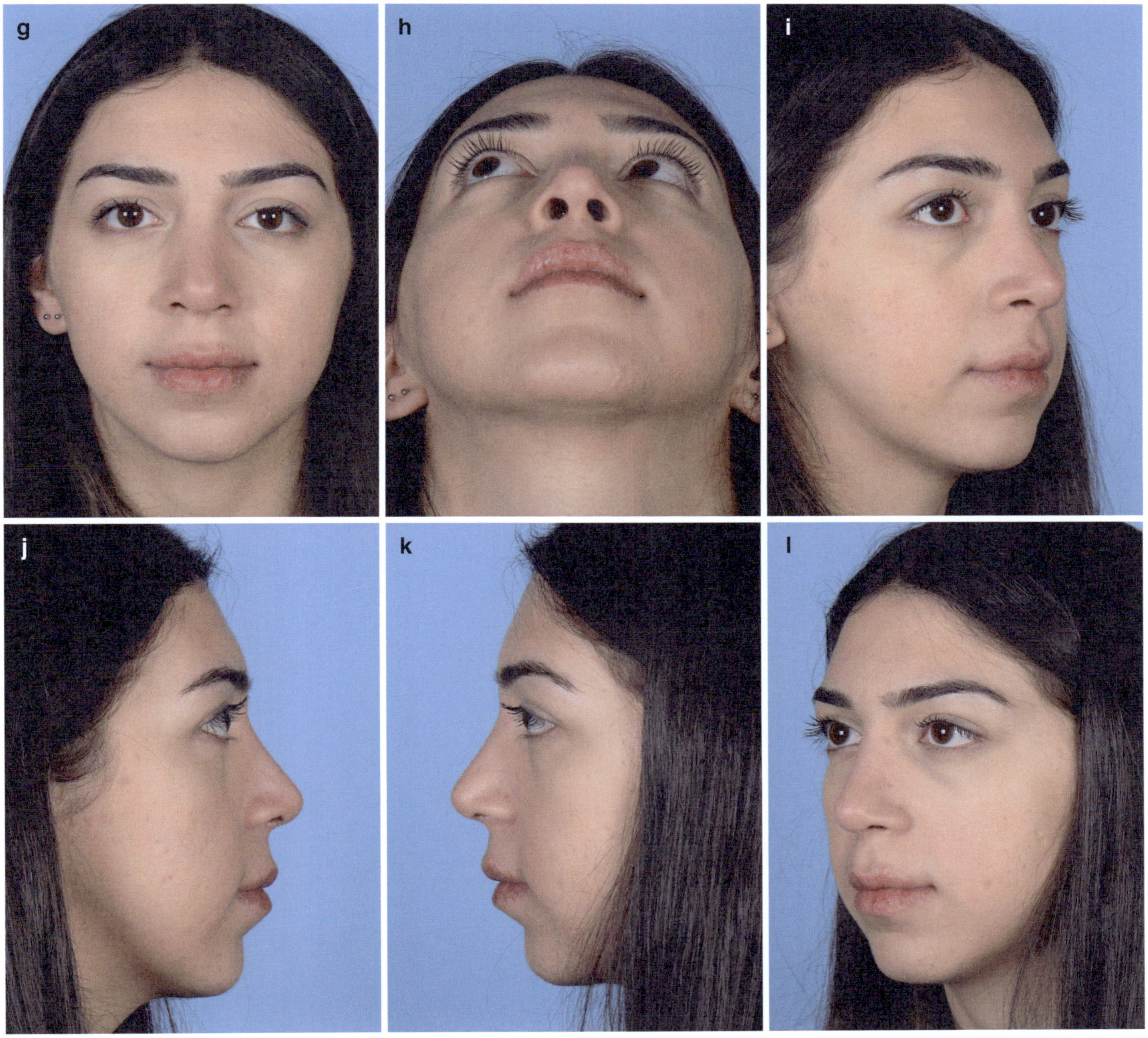

Fig. 15.43 (continued)

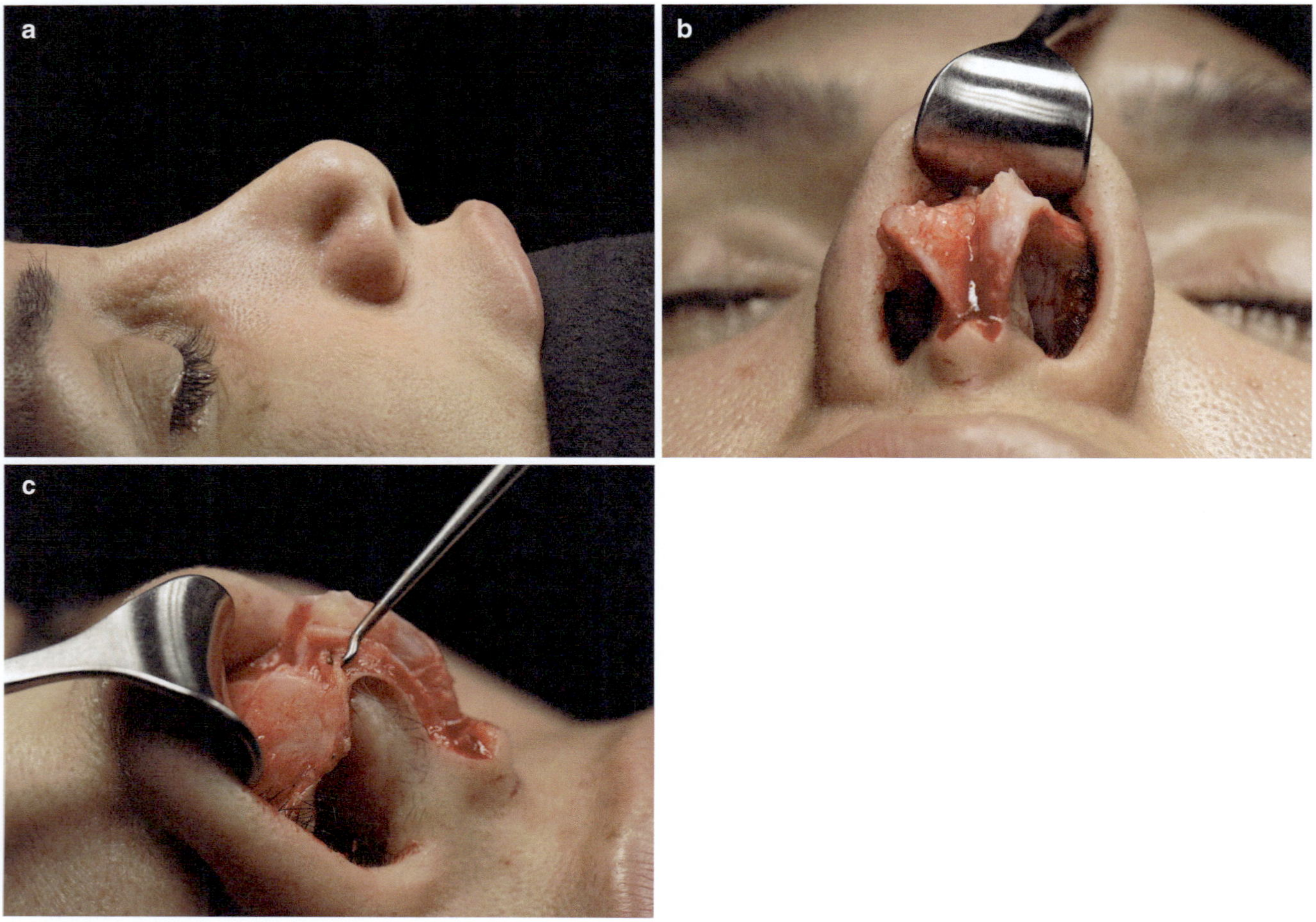

Fig. 15.44 (**a–c**) The entire alar arch is weak and malformed. Malposition of the lateral crura is very common in revision tip cases. However, after close examination, no malposition of the lateral crus was found in this case. It should be noted that if there was malposition, strengthening of the alar arch alone would not be sufficient, so additional transposition would be required

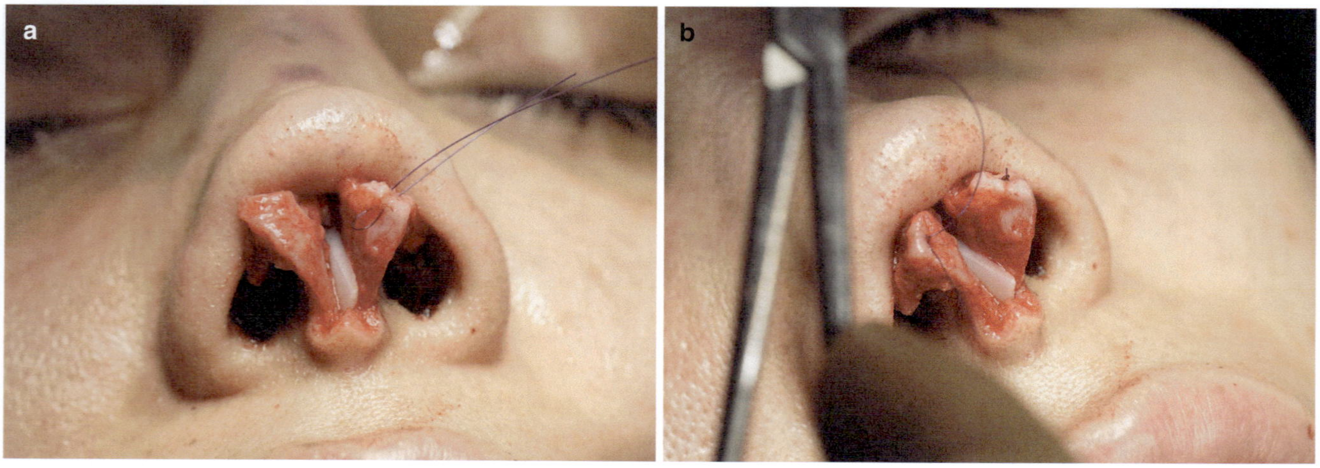

Fig. 15.45 (**a**, **b**) New dome points were created with sutures

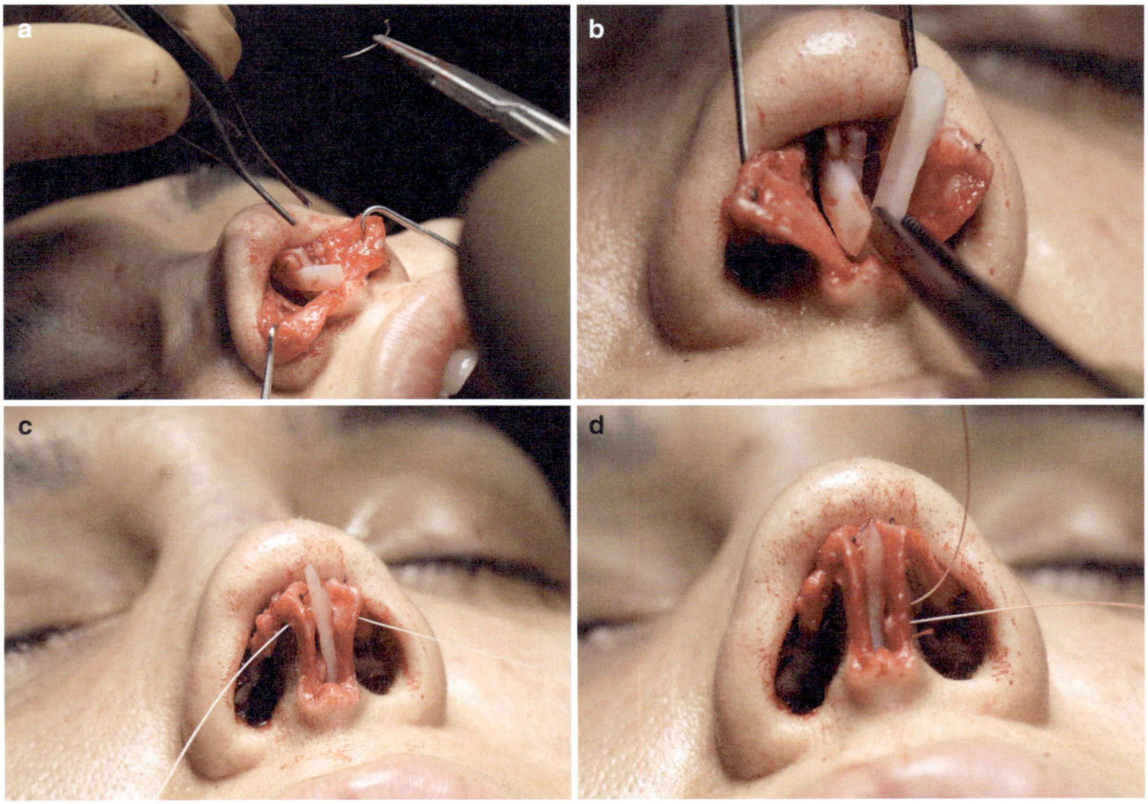

Fig. 15.46 (**a**–**d**) The septocolumellar strut is fixed directly under the spreader graft

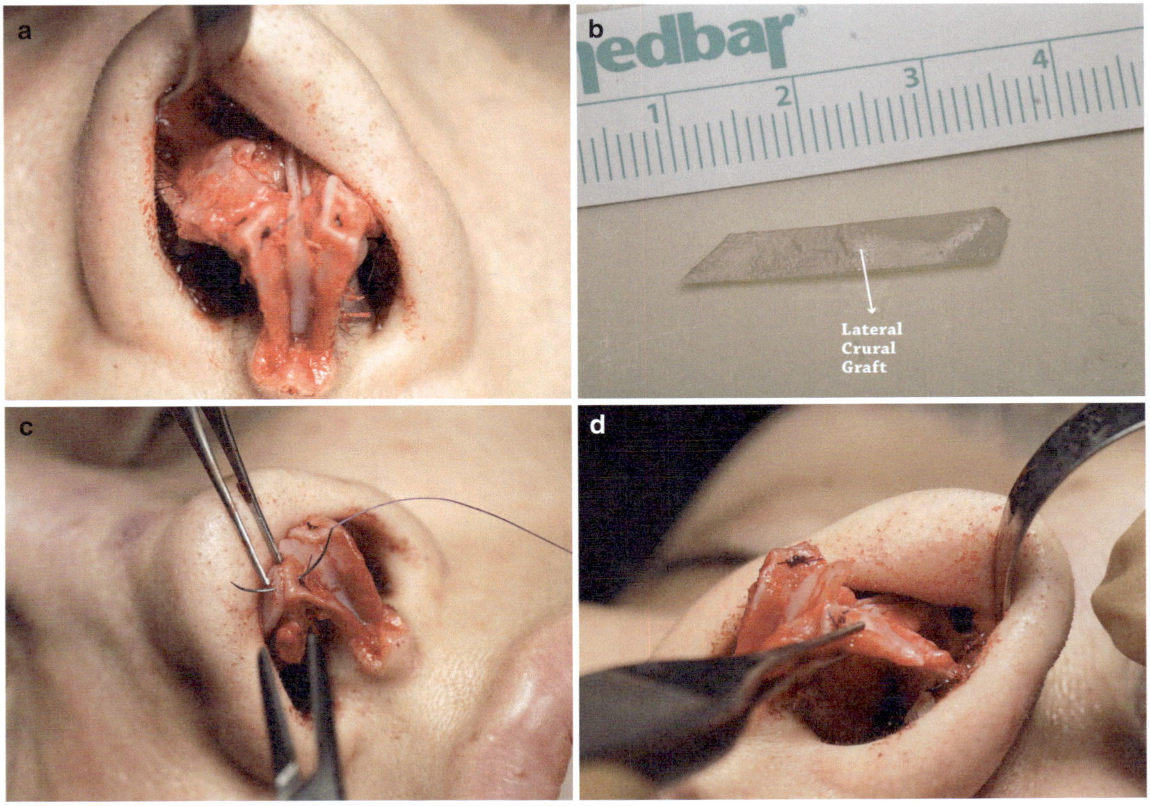

Fig. 15.47 (**a**–**d**) Lateral crural onlay graft was used to correct the disruption and buckling deformity

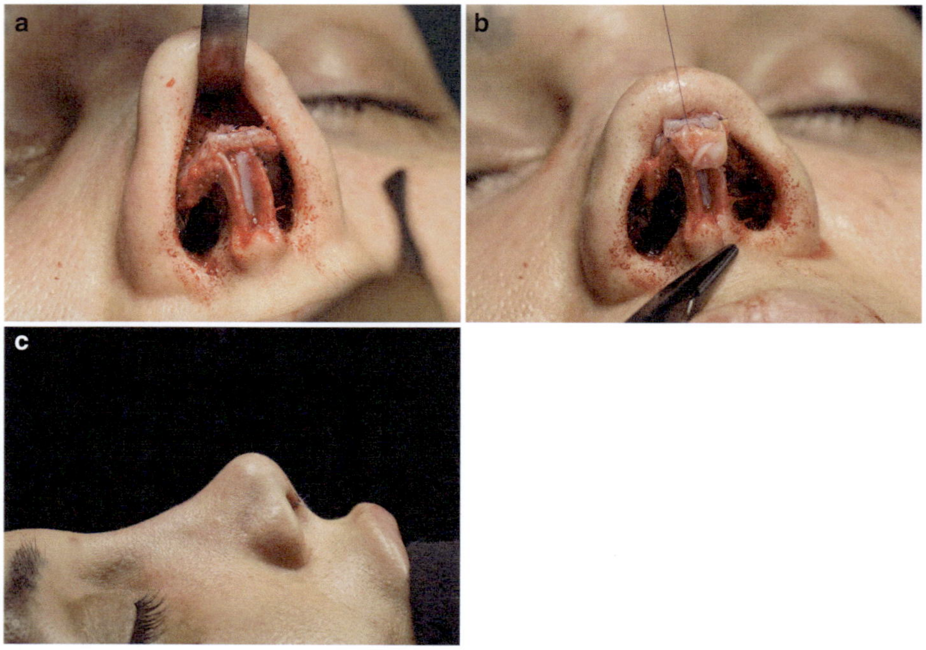

Fig. 15.48 (**a**, **b**) Cap graft and infratip lobule graft placement. (**c**) Intraoperative final view

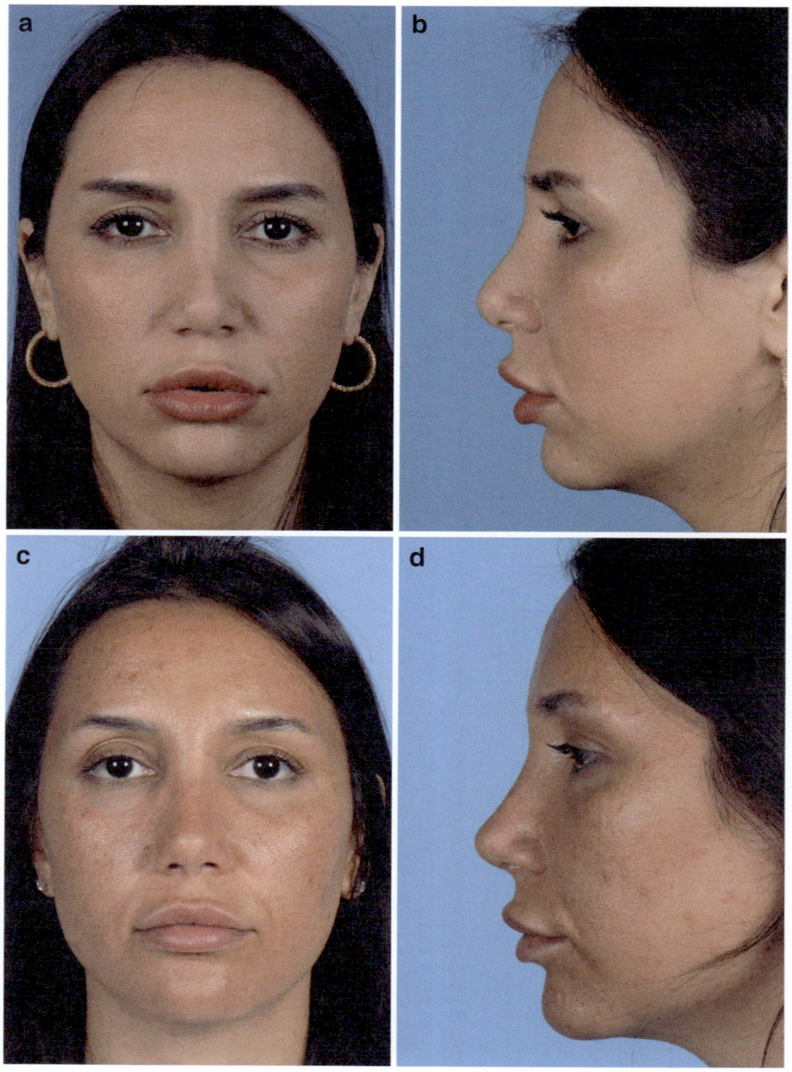

Fig. 15.49 (**a–d**) In pre- and postoperative images, the lateral view demonstrates increased nasal tip projection

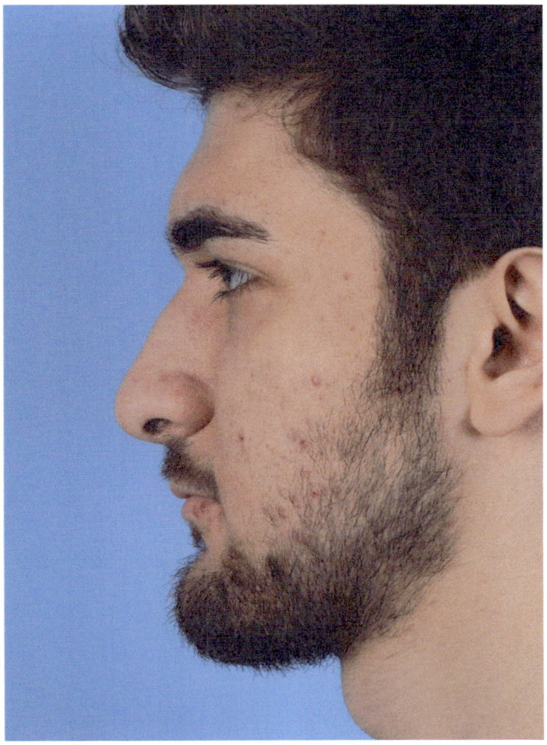

Fig. 15.50 Unbalanced profile view. Low radix, high dorsum, under-projected tip

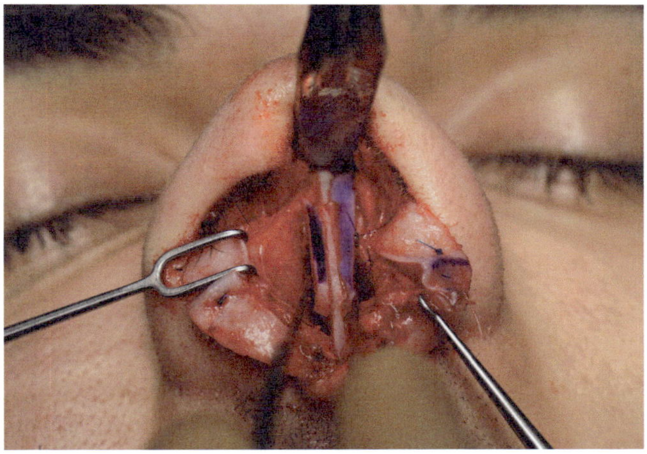

Fig. 15.52 Asymmetrical spreader grafts were used to obtain a symmetrical middle vault

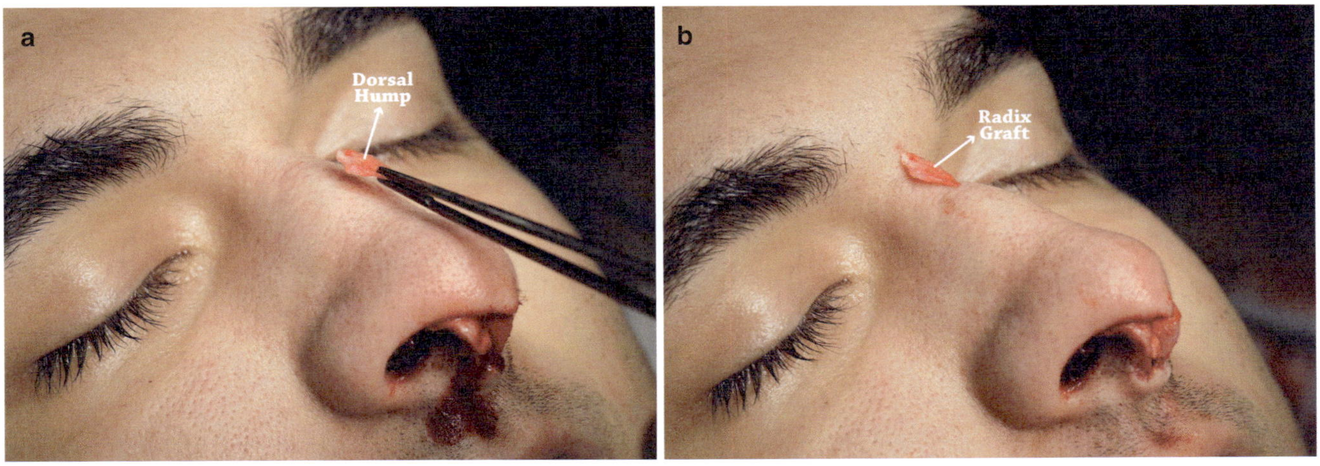

Fig. 15.51 (**a**, **b**) The primary dorsal hump material was used to augment radix

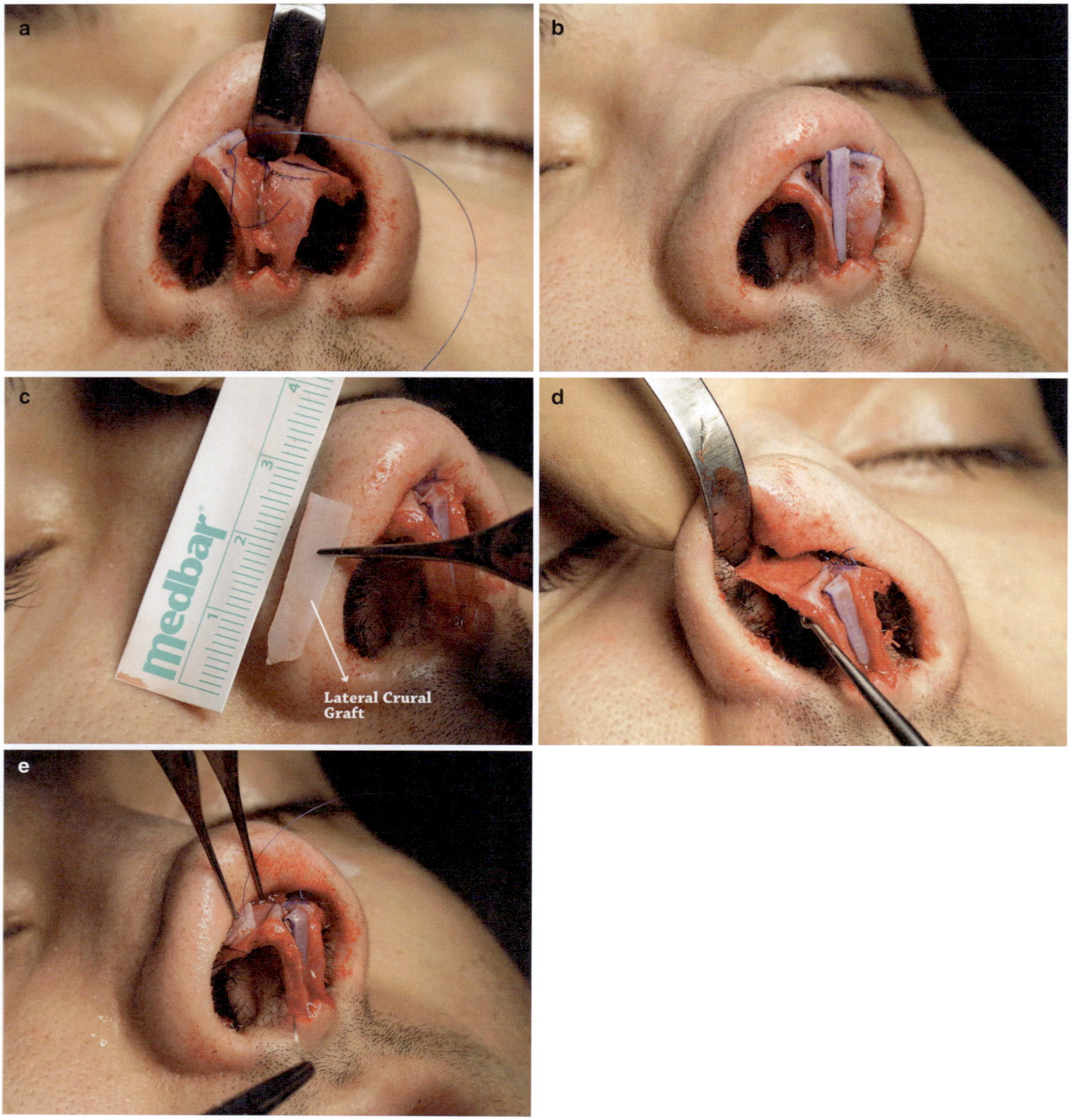

Fig. 15.53 (a–e) Lateral onlay grafts were used to give extra support

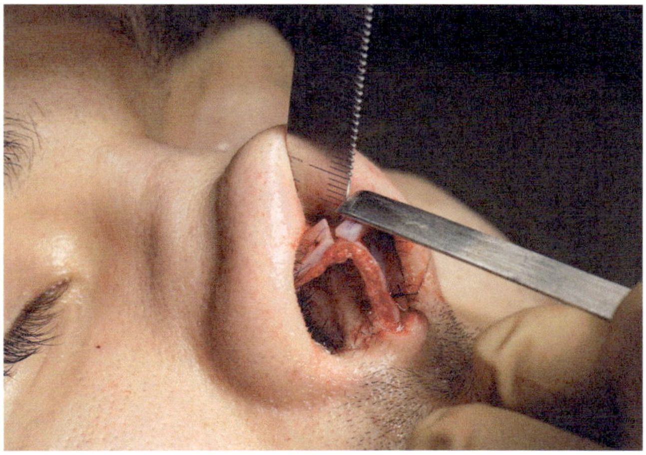

Fig. 15.54 The distance between the anterior-most end of the tip and the dorsum was 7 mm after placement of the cap graft. This distance indicates an ideal relationship between tip and dorsum

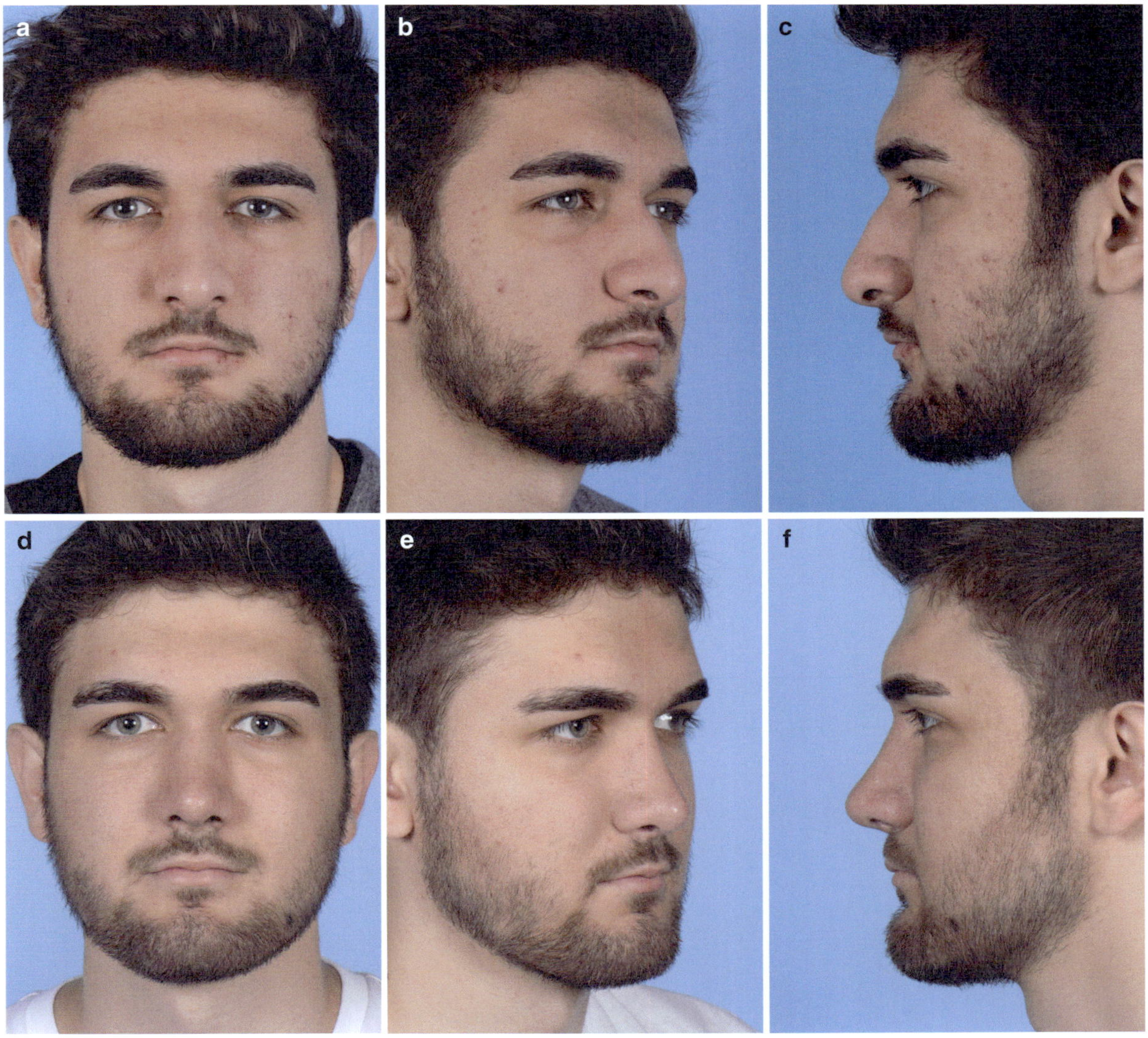

Fig. 15.55 (**a**–**f**) Postoperative photographs show a well-balanced dorsum. Note the smooth, straight dorsum and correction of the dorsal aesthetic line

15.4 Part 2: Under-Projected Tip Due to Caudal Septum and Nasal Spine

The caudal septum and nasal spine provide most of the support to the nasal tip, and weakness in these structures contributes to inadequate nasal tip projection. Re-establishing septal support is necessary to ensure proper tip projection during rhinoplasty.

There are three main causes of caudal septal deficiency: (1) iatrogenic damage resulting from a previous nasal surgery (typically septoplasty); (2) trauma; and (3) congenital defects. Regardless of the underlying cause, the first objective is to strengthen the weak, deficient, or deformed caudal septum using a caudal septum replacement (CSR) graft. Combining the graft with premaxillary augmentation increases support and provides long-term stability.

The caudal septum can be damaged during rhinoplasty, and particularly during septal surgery. The overall rate of significant change in the cosmetic appearance of the nose after septoplasty has been found to be 0.4–3.4%.

In a current study, the majority of caudal septal deficiency cases (77.5%) showed some level of premaxillary deficiency, in which the premaxilla and/or the anterior nasal spine were either underdeveloped, previously resected, or partially resorbed. In these cases, premaxillary augmentation should be performed.

Caudal septal deficiency not only results in under-projection but may also lead to the following problems: (1) retracted columella or decreased columellar show; (2) acute nasolabial angle; (3) long upper lip; and (4) supratip depression (Fig. 15.56).

Case 9 exhibited all four of these features.

A tip without any caudal septal support is depressed toward the face when the patient presses down on the tip of his or her nose. This is a very typical indicator of the need for caudal septum reconstruction (Fig. 15.57).

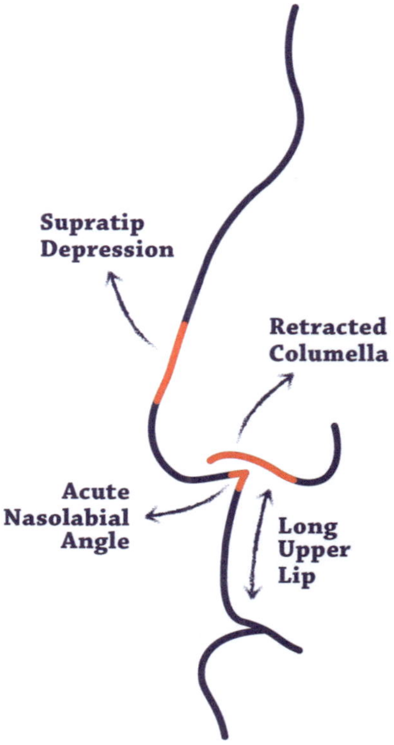

Fig. 15.56 The illustration shows signs of caudal septal deficiency

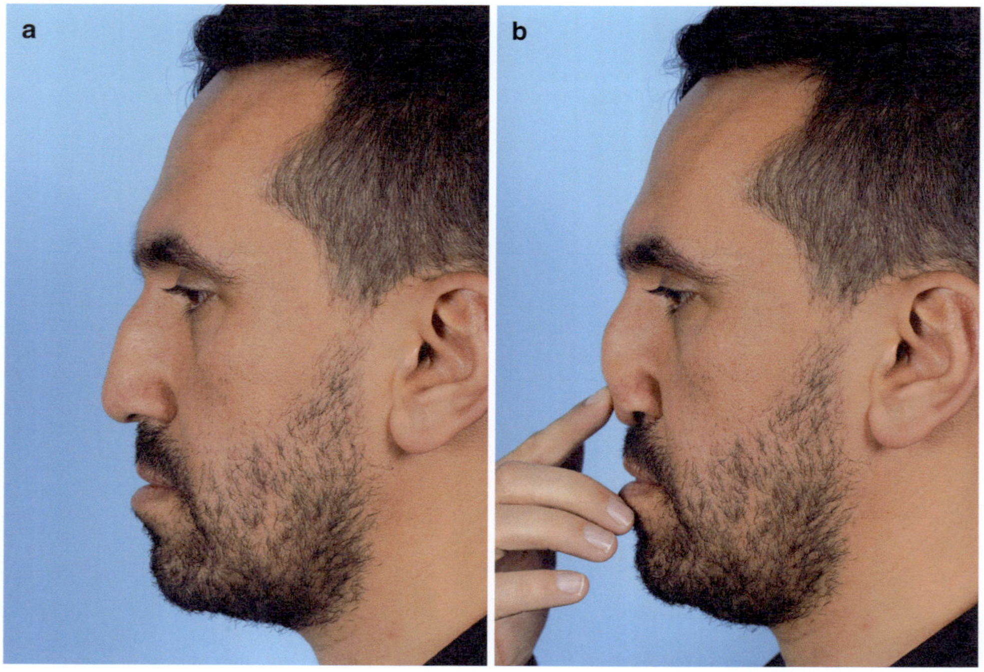

Fig. 15.57 (**a**, **b**) This test is a typical indicator of the deficiencies of caudal septum

The CSR graft should be designed to closely match the shape, consistency, and strength of the missing caudal septum; therefore, the dimensions of the graft depend largely on the size of the missing caudal segment. Donor cartilage for the CSR graft can be harvested from multiple sources, and in the absence of septal cartilage the author's personal preference is an irradiated costal cartilage homograft. The graft must be fixed at the nasal base/nasal spine and the remnant of the septum to ensure stability. The author prefers the figure-of-eight-suture using 4-0 PDS for fixation to the nasal base. The figure-of-eight-suture starts at the spine if remnant spine is available; otherwise, it starts at a nearby bony structure. If the needle cannot penetrate the bone, a small hole should be opened with a drill, piezo device, or syringe. Then, the suture is twisted back from the anterior edge of the graft and passed through the graft parallel to, and in the same direction as, the first entry site. Finally, a knot is tied at the starting point and the figure-of-eight is thus completed.

An illustration of the figure-of-eight suture is presented in Fig. 15.58.

After the CSR graft is fixed to the spine, it must be fixed to the remnant septum. The strength and size of the septum determines the method of fixation. If the remnant is sufficiently strong and large, the replacement graft and the caudal remnant should be overlapped and fixed at a number of points (Fig. 15.59).

The dorsal septum may also be weak or deformed, in which case correction frequently requires straightening or reconstituting the dorsal and caudal segments simultaneously. While the CSR graft reconstructs the caudal segment, unilateral or bilateral spreader grafts should be used to reconstruct the dorsal segment (Fig. 15.60).

Finally, if the remnant septum is not large enough to attach the CSR graph, the surgeon may use spreader grafts to attach it to the distant remnant septum. In such cases, the bilateral extended spreader grafts should first be fixed to the remnant dorsal septum, followed by fixation to the CSR graft to reconstitute the L-strut (Fig. 15.61).

The following cases are presented to illustrate the key points discussed above.

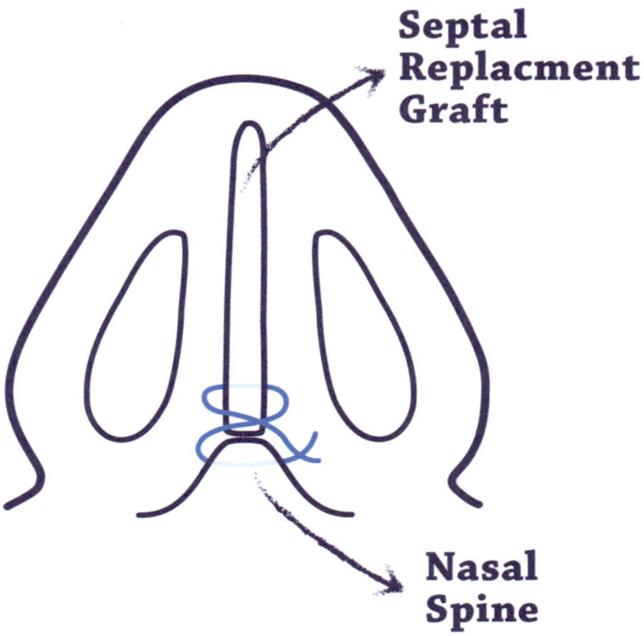

Fig. 15.58 A figure-of-eight suture is a highly secure method of affixing a septal replacement graft to the nasal spine

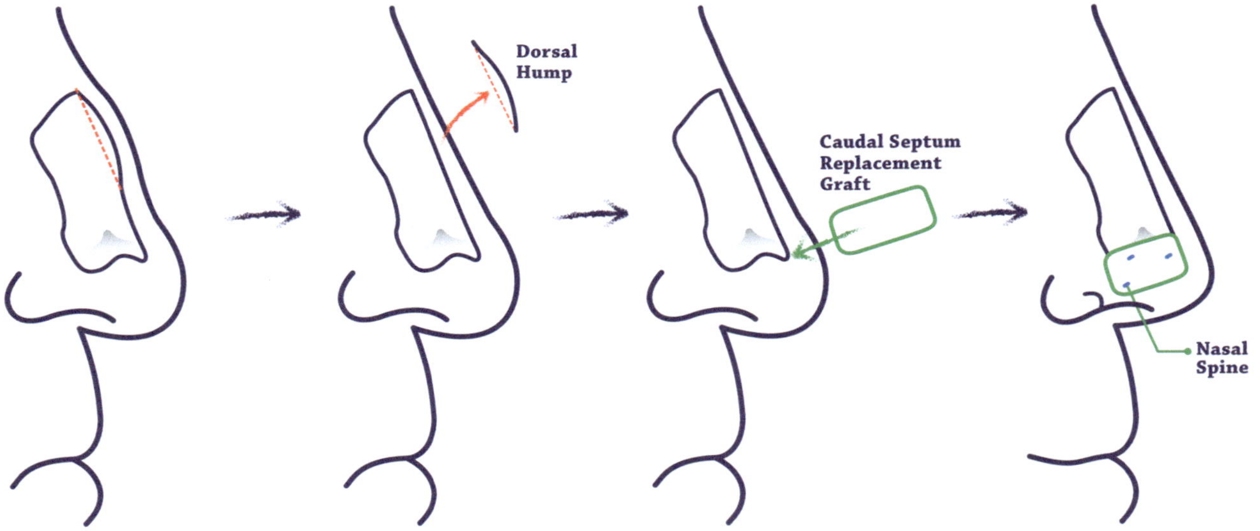

Fig. 15.59 Caudal septal reconstruction with caudal septal replacement graft

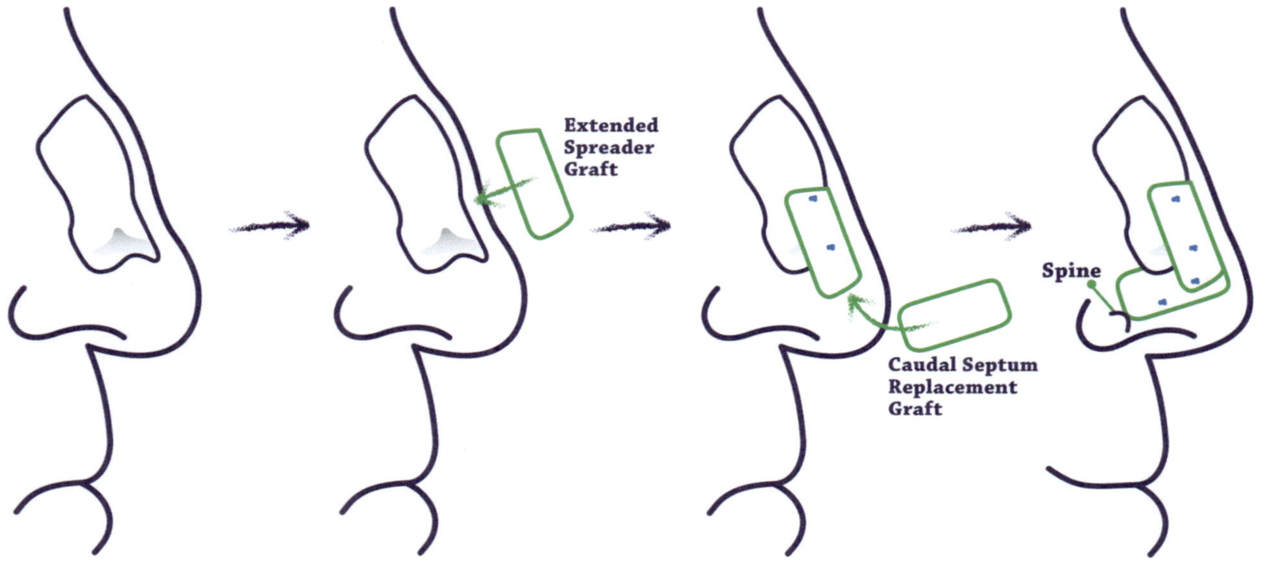

Fig. 15.60 Caudal septal reconstruction with caudal septal replacement graft and unilateral, wide, extended spreader grafts

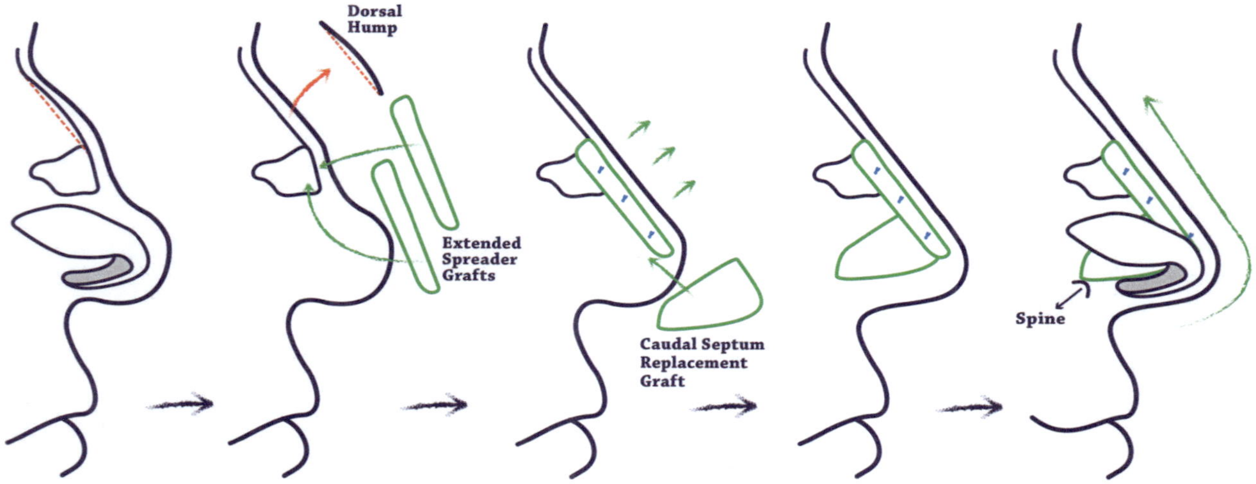

Fig. 15.61 Caudal septal reconstruction with caudal septal replacement graft and bilateral extended spreader grafts

15.4.1 Case 9

The patient in this case previously underwent a septoplasty surgery.

All the signs of caudal septal deficiency can be seen in this patient, who complained of changes in the nasal tip that surfaced a few months after the surgery (Fig. 15.62).

The external approach provides superior exposure and access to the caudal septum, and in this case, an open approach is preferred (Fig. 15.63).

Instrument palpation is used to determine how much of the caudal septum is missing (Fig. 15.64).

Irradiated costal cartilage is the preferred source for a septal replacement graft. As only the outer strips become curved, the peripheral layer must be trimmed to prevent any future distortion of the costal cartilage (Fig. 15.65).

The harvested graft is then inserted inside the nose so that the graft faces the concave plane of the remnant septum and overlaps the remnant dorsal strut. It must be fixed with three sutures to prevent pivoting or hinging. Finally, the graft is fixed to the nasal spine with a figure-of-eight suture (Fig. 15.66).

The septal replacement graft compensates for caudal septal deficiency. Once the graft is secured, under-projected tip surgery is completed via standard tip surgery procedures (Fig. 15.67).

Preoperative and 1-year postoperative photographs are presented in Fig. 15.68.

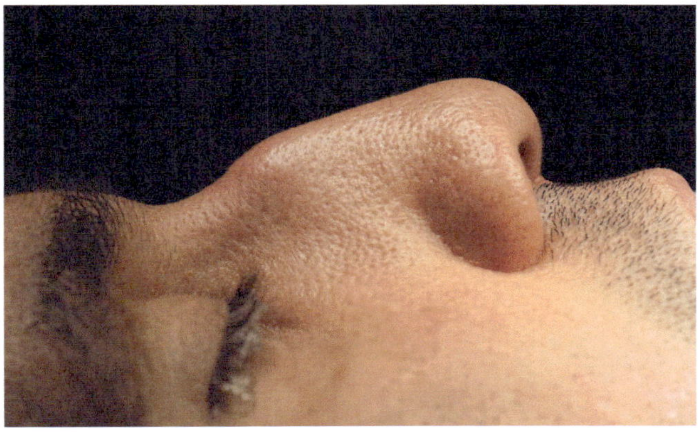

Fig. 15.62 Intraoperative lateral view of the patient in Fig. 15.17

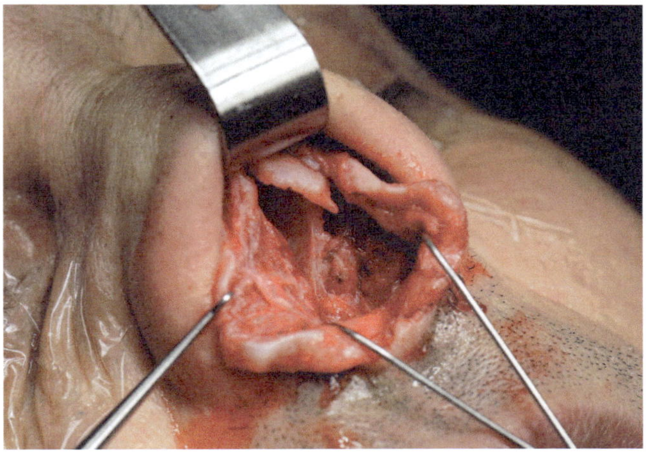

Fig. 15.63 The external approach also provides improved access to the keystone region and nasal spin

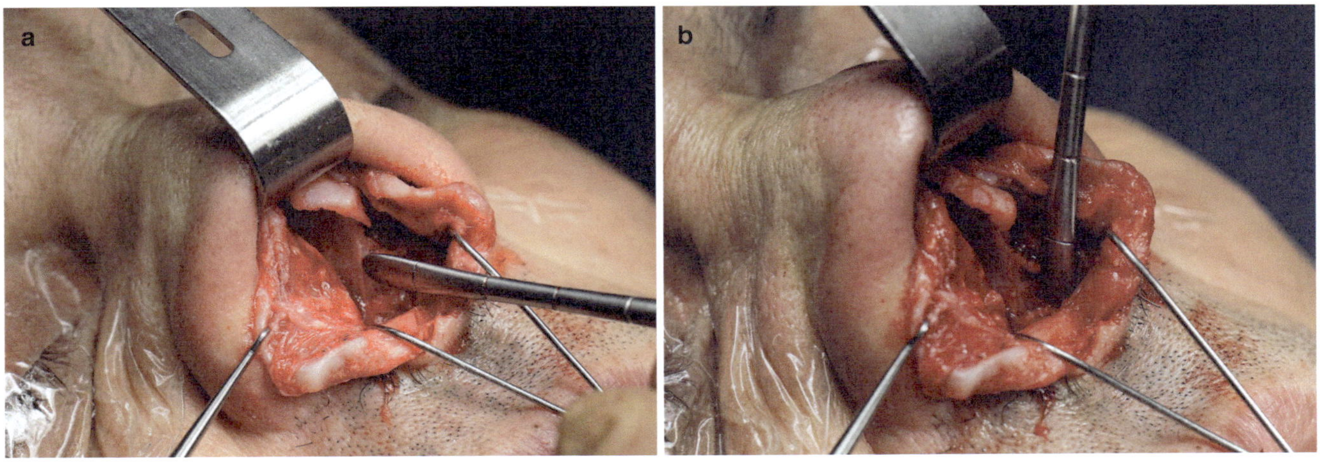

Fig. 15.64 (**a**, **b**) Measurement of deficiency area of the septum

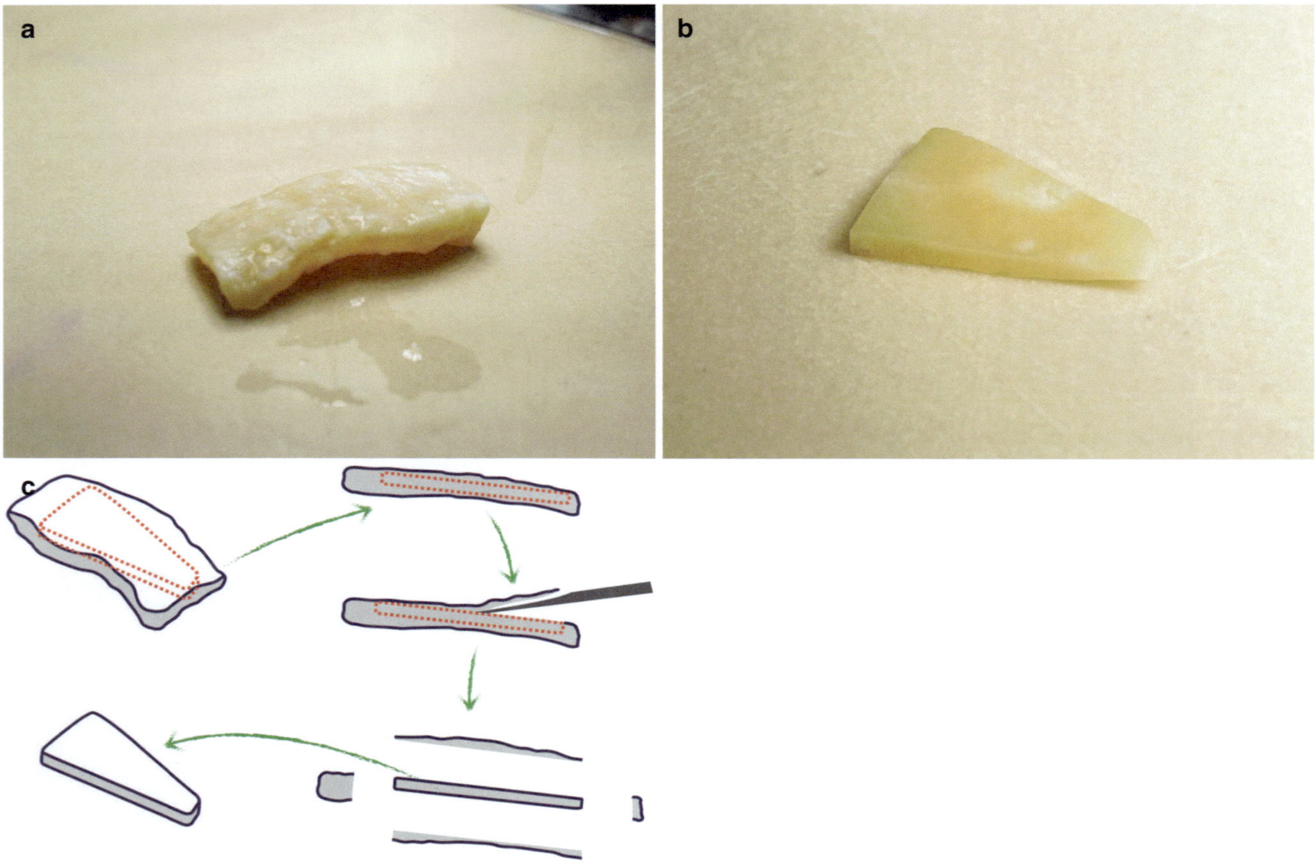

Fig. 15.65 (**a**–**c**) The cartilage should be harvested directly from the center of the costa and it must be straight to prevent distortion. The width and length of the graft vary from case to case, and the graft should be tailored to the needs of the patient. When planning to use irradiated costal cartilage, the graft must be slightly thicker than the desired septal length

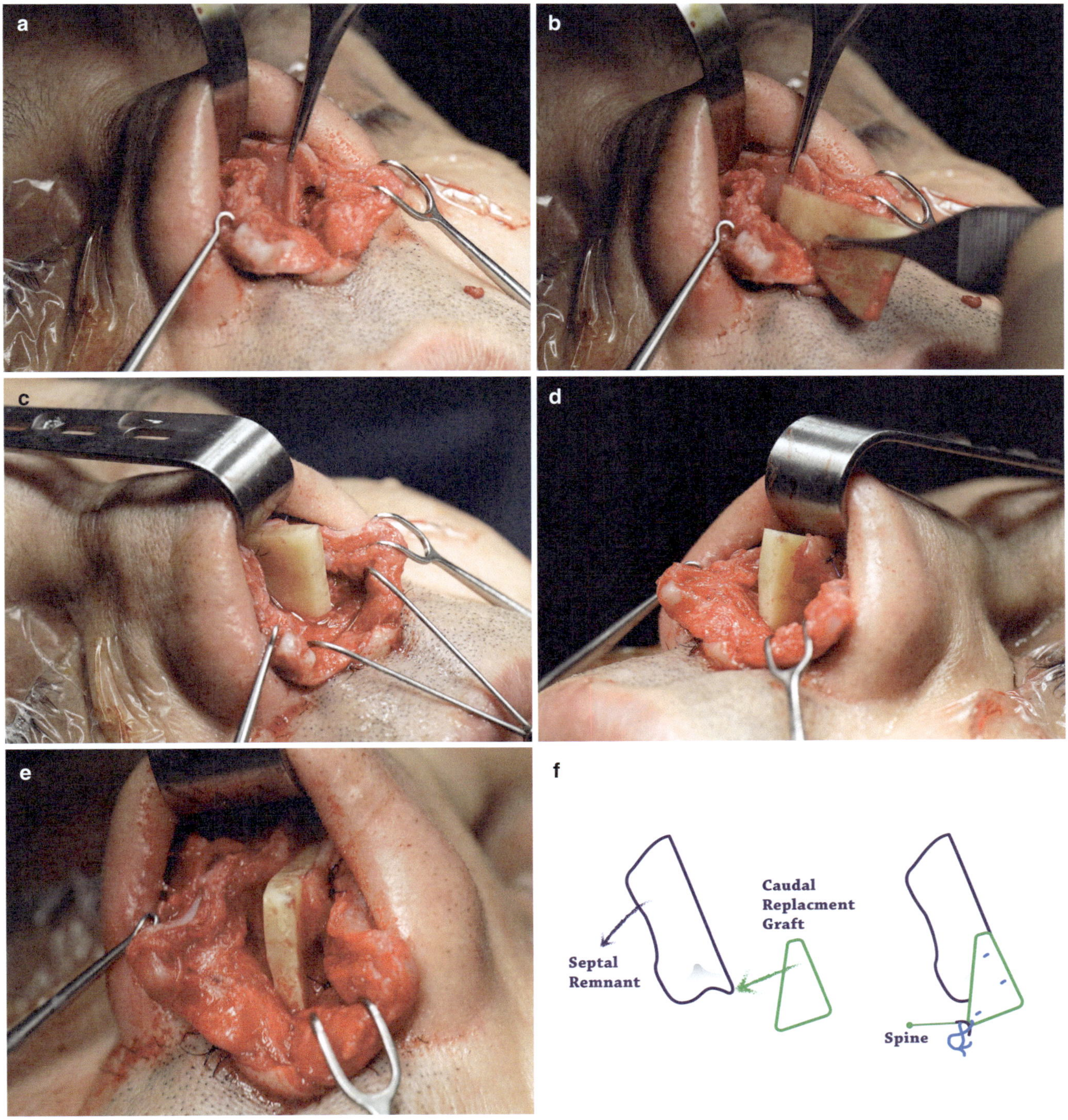

Fig. 15.66 (**a**–**f**) Placement of the caudal septal replacement graft

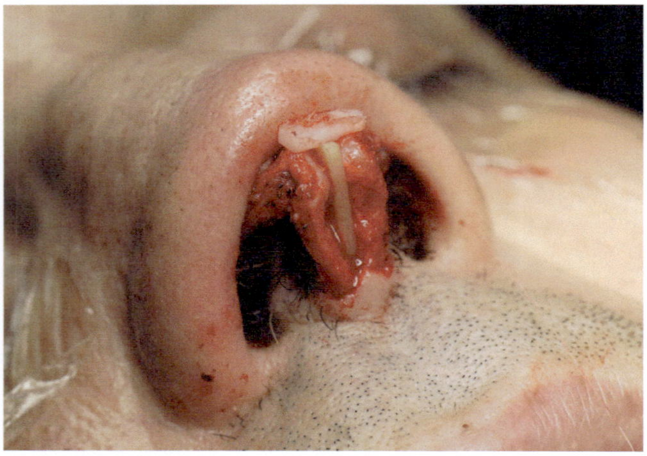

Fig. 15.67 Transdomal sutures, cap, and columellar strut grafts were used

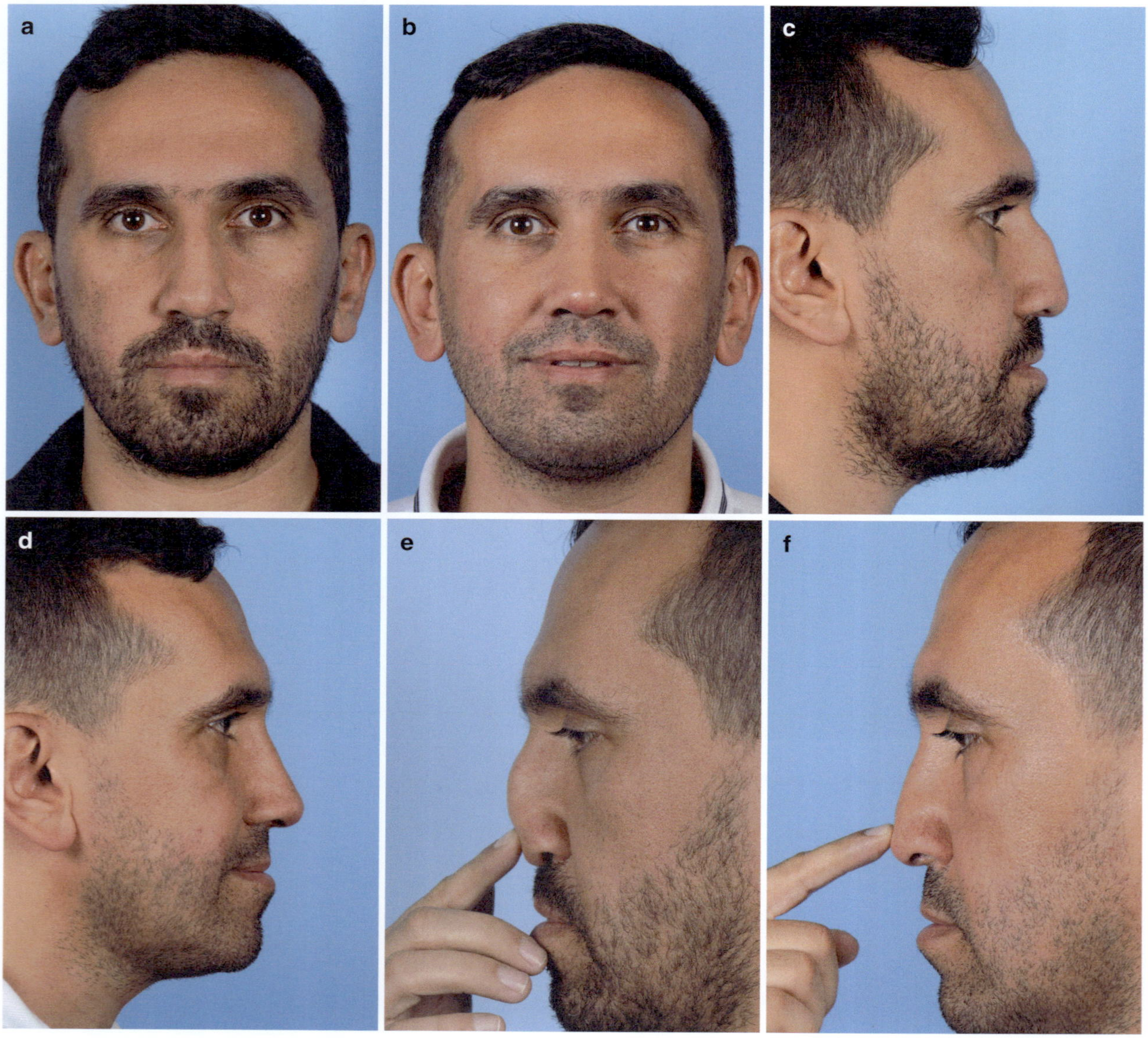

Fig. 15.68 (**a–f**) Tip projection has been maintained after reconstructing the caudal septum

15.5 Under-Projected Tip Due to Caudal Septum and Alar Cartilages

15.5.1 Case 10

This patient underwent septorhinoplasty surgery 10 years ago. In addition to under-projection, there are several additional problems, including a retracted columella, a low nasal tip, and an acute nasolabial angle (Fig. 15.69).

The intraoperative photographs demonstrate the use of an open rhinoplasty approach. The alar cartilage is very weak and deformed, and the caudal septum is deficient and frail (Fig. 15.70).

The dorsal segment of the septum also appears deformed. In this case, tip surgery should be to create a strong septal vault and alar arch. Both the dorsal and caudal segments must be reconstructed to create a strong septal vault. While a caudal septal replacement graft would compensate for the deficiency at the caudal segment, a spreader graft would strengthen the dorsal segment. The technique in Fig. 15.60 was implemented for caudal septal reconstruction (Fig. 15.71).

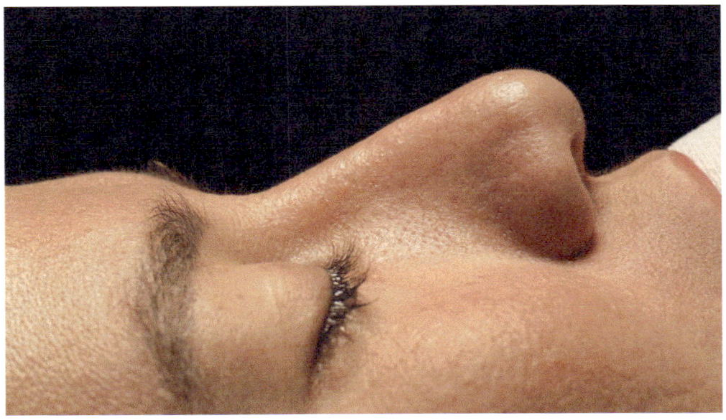

Fig. 15.69 Intraoperative lateral view of Case 10

The tip should be addressed only after all septum-related procedures are completed. First, new dome points are created using transdomal sutures, after which the alar arch is reevaluated. A columellar strut may not be sufficient to strengthen the deformed medial and middle crura, in which case cartilage grafts can be sutured on the medial plane of each crus. These grafts reinforce the limbs of the alar arch, while lateral crural grafts can be used to bilaterally strengthen the lateral crura. Using this approach, all segments of the alar arch can be reinforced (Fig. 15.72).

The final projection and tip definition are achieved with a cap graft, and the surgery is completed using camouflage grafts to ensure that the grafts are not visible through the skin (Fig. 15.73).

Some of the graft materials used in this case were redundant; in such cases, costal cartilage is preferred unless there is a large amount of septal cartilage available. The use of auricular cartilage should be avoided because it is not strong enough for satisfactory reconstruction. A large amount of graft material can be obtained using costal cartilage. An oblique incision should be used to harvest the cartilage because the resulting grafts are more likely to remain stable (Fig. 15.74).

Preoperative and 1-year postoperative photographs; the tip is more defined and projected. The columellar retraction at the nasolabial angle has been corrected (Fig. 15.75).

15.5.2 Case 11

This is a case of an under-projected tip patient who underwent a prior surgery and suffered from nasal trauma. The patient's retracted columella, acute nasolabial angle, long upper lip, and depression at the supratip are very pronounced in the lateral view. The underlying cause of these problems may be a weak caudal septal vault. Even in primary cases,

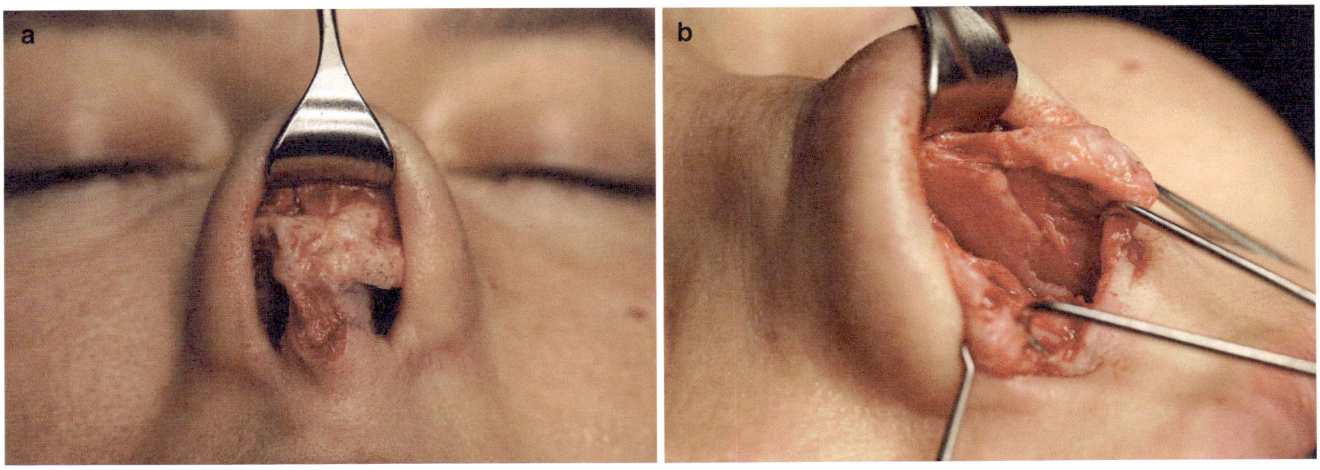

Fig. 15.70 (**a**) Deformed, weak alar arch. (**b**) Previously resected caudal septum

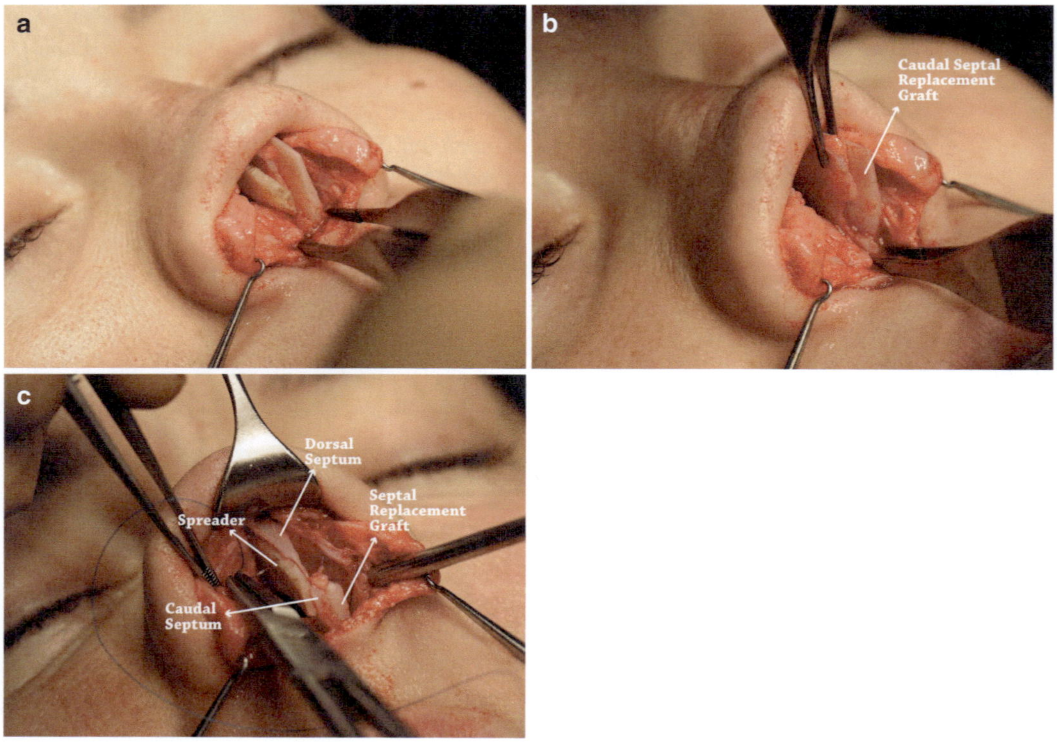

Fig. 15.71 (**a–c**) A graft to compensate for septal deficiency is sutured to the concave plane of the remnant septum and the spreader graft is sutured to the contralateral side

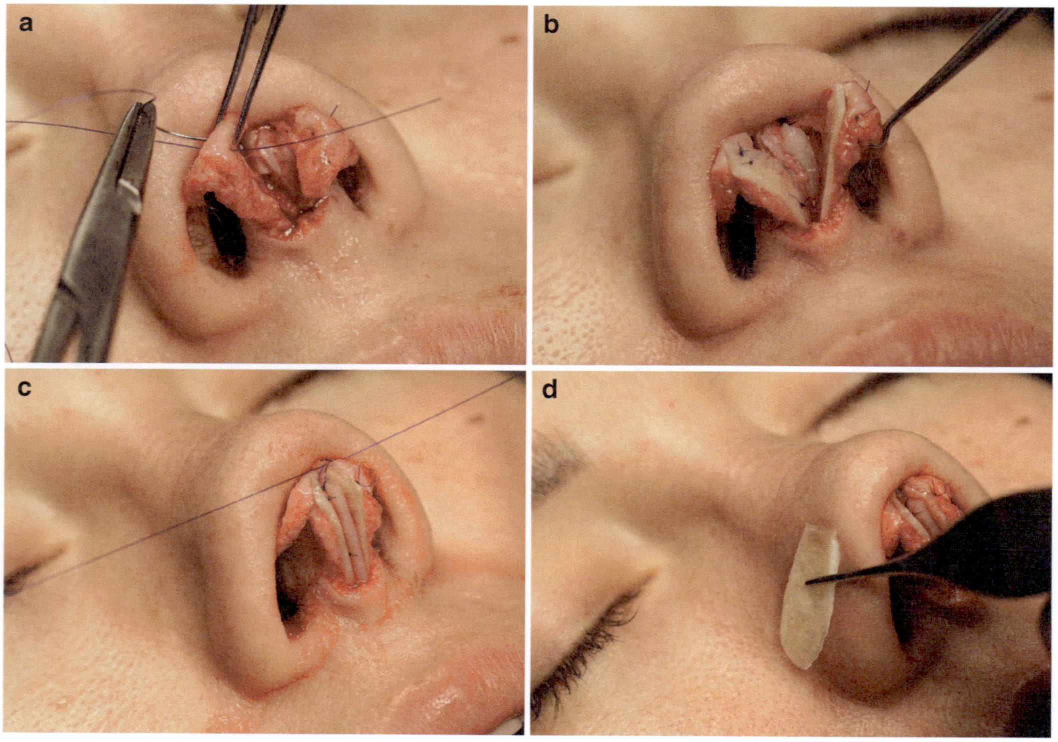

Fig. 15.72 (**a–d**) A graft thickness of 1–2 mm is sufficient to reinforce the alar base. Absorbable sutures are used for fixation to prevent them from protruding through the skin. The use of a columellar strut and dome-equalizing suture is essential. In addition, a relatively wide graft must be used to correct the configuration of the lateral crura. The graft should also be fixed to the dorsal plane of the lateral crus using absorbable suture material

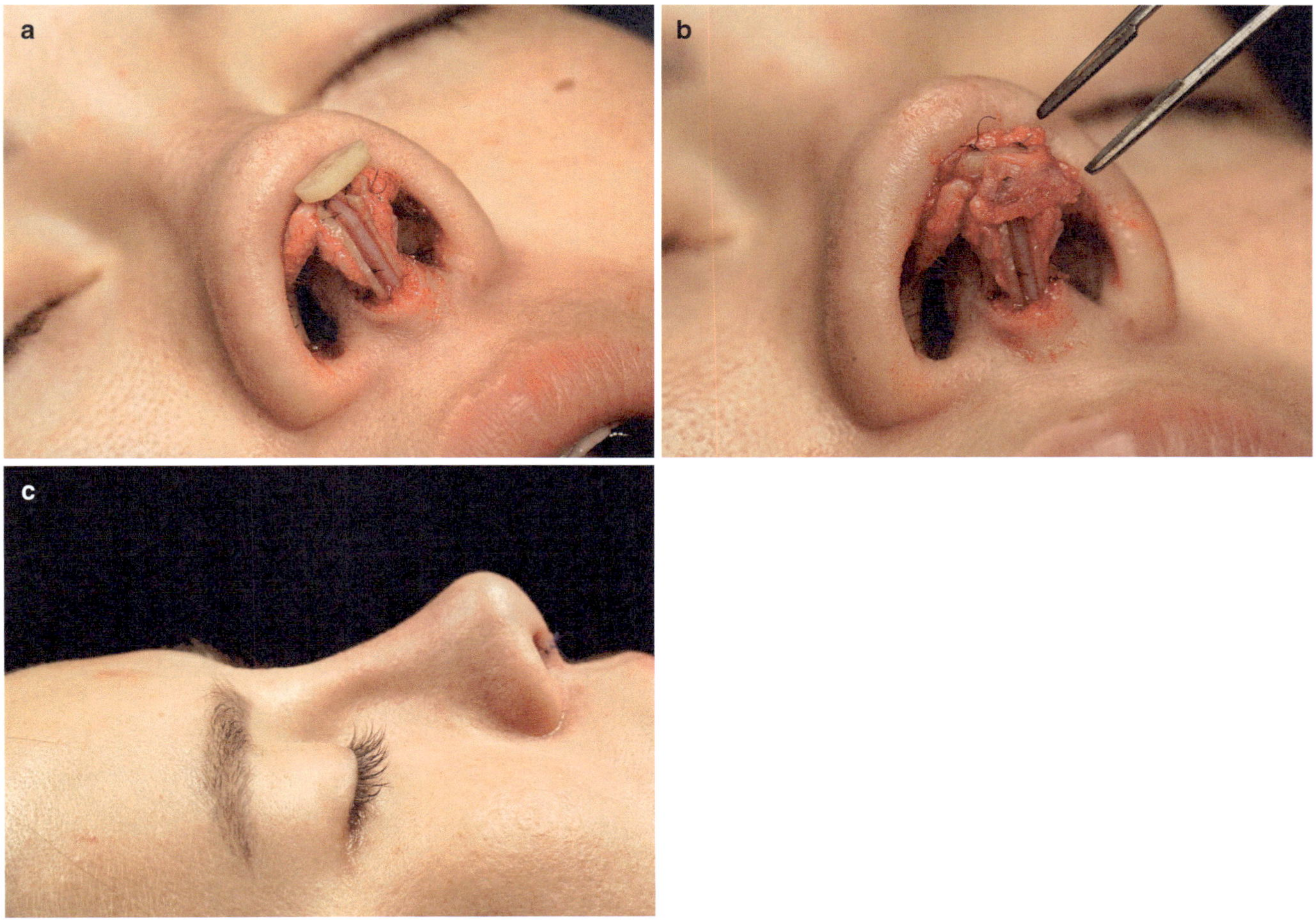

Fig. 15.73 (**a**, **b**) Cap and camouflage grafts placement. (**c**) Immediately after surgery

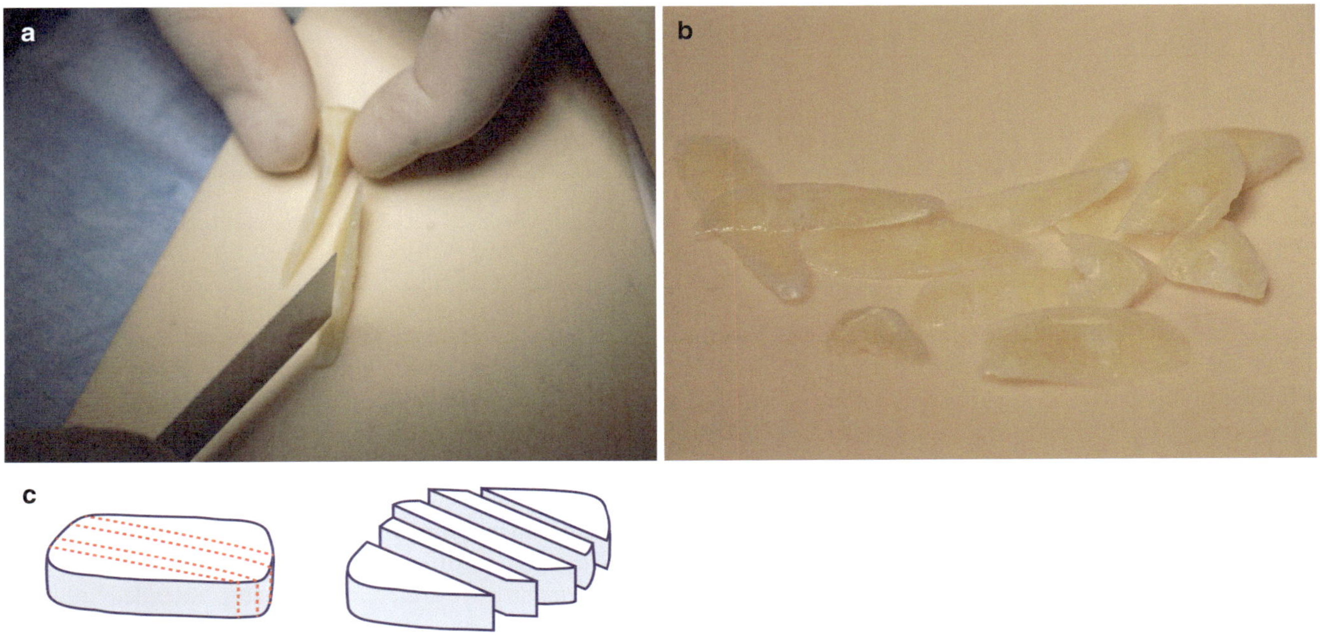

Fig. 15.74 (**a**–**c**) The oblique split method

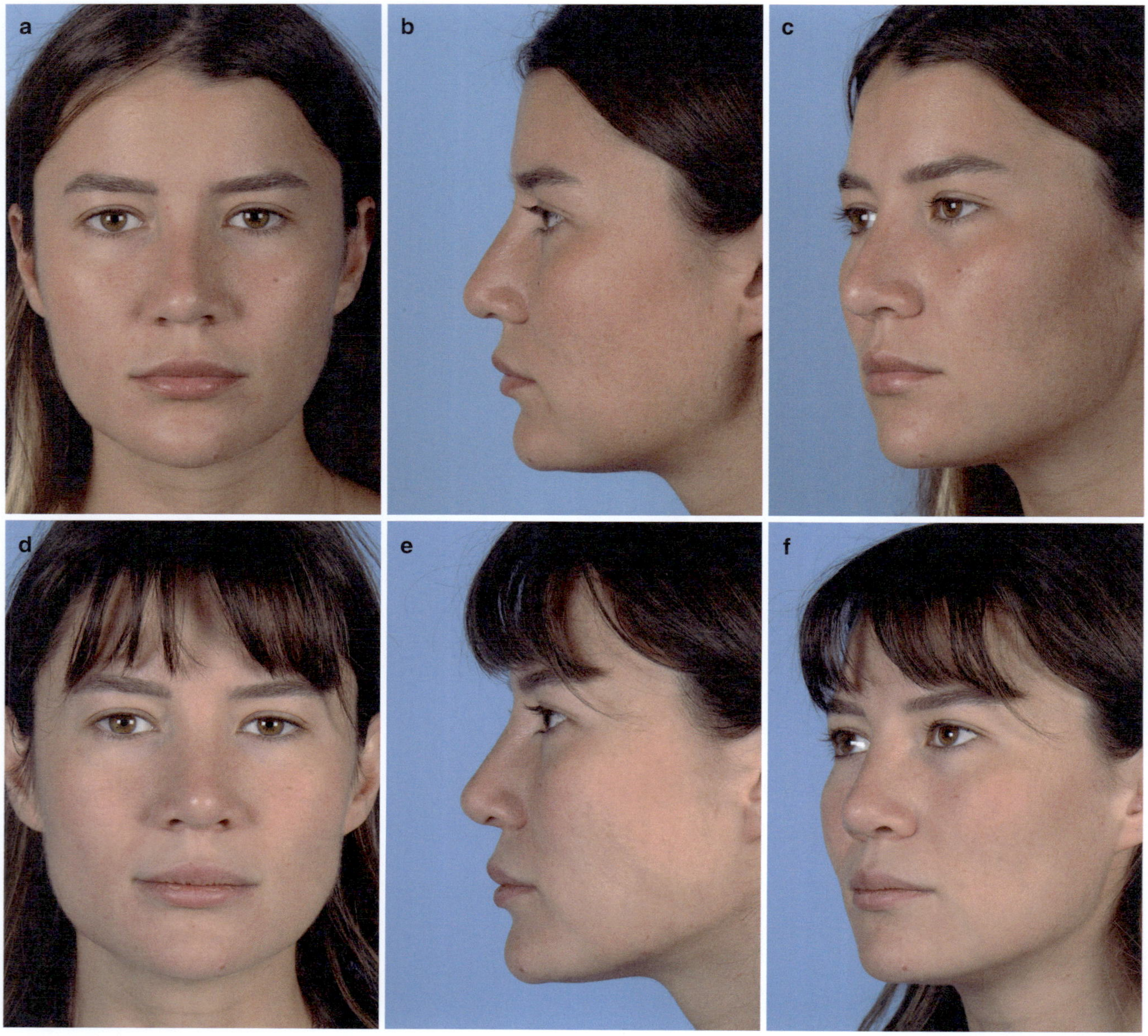

Fig. 15.75 (**a–f**) Pre- and postoperative photographs. Lengthening with augmentation of the caudal septum and reconstruction of alar cartilages corrected the columella-labial angle, retracted columella, and tip projection

autologous septal cartilage may not be sufficient to correct all of the underlying deficiencies; the patient must be informed of this and the surgery should be planned with consideration of the potential use of costal cartilage (Fig. 15.76).

An open rhinoplasty technique should be used in this case. A posterior position of the anterior edge of the septum relative to the nasal spine is noticeable. The shortened caudal septum indicates that the tip has no support; this is the underlying cause of the patient's tip-related problems (Fig. 15.77).

The septoplasty is performed leaving the L-strut as support. The septum is very short and seems to slide posteriorly (Fig. 15.78).

In this case, it may be easier to remove the anterior segment of the septal cartilage and construct a new L-strut, to allow the caudal septum to move more anteriorly (Fig. 15.79).

The technique in Fig. 15.61 was implemented for caudal septal reconstruction.

The cartilage that is removed can then be used as a septal replacement graft to construct a new caudal septum in the required position. The remnant septum and septal replacement graft are connected using extended spreader grafts. The septal replacement graft is then fixed between the two extended spreader grafts and the nasal spine (Fig. 15.80).

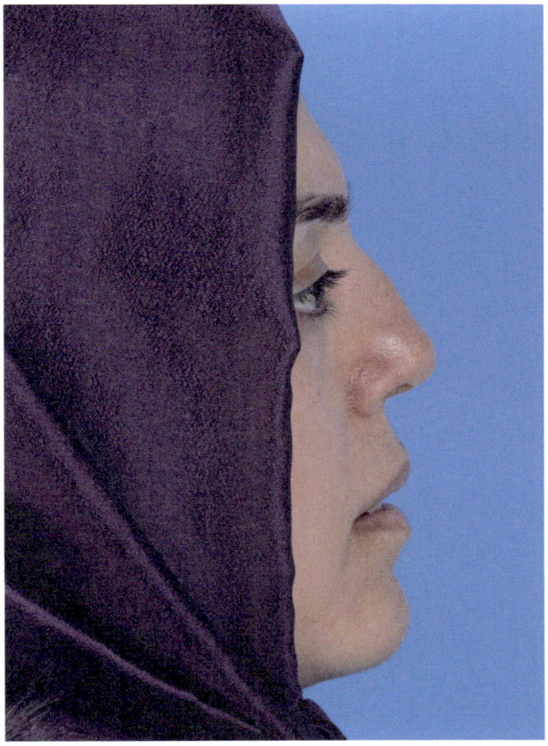

Fig. 15.76 Under-projected nasal tip stems from both caudal septal and alar cartilages weakness

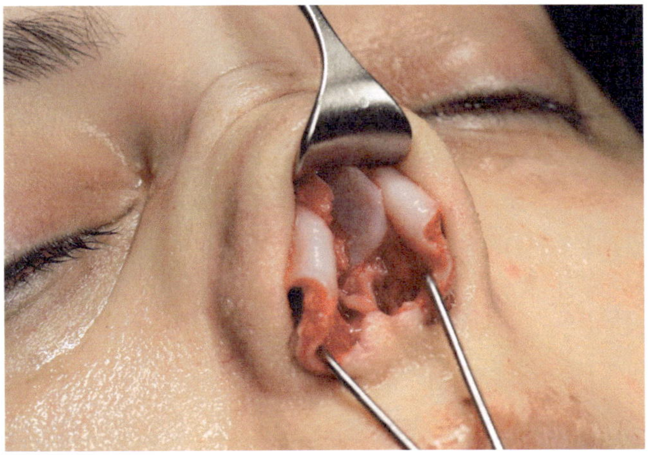

Fig. 15.77 The caudal septum was found previously resected or partially resorbed

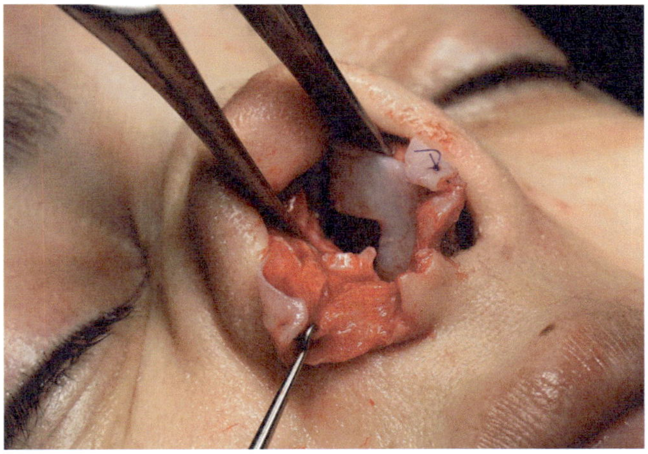

Fig. 15.78 Septoplasty with L strut preservation

The tip plasty is completed using a transdomal suture, cap graft, and lateral crural graft (Fig. 15.81).

The addition of premaxillary cartilage grafts at the end of the procedure can substantially increase tip projection. This increase in tip projection may be structural or simply optical. By opening the angle at the columella-lip junction, the tip appears elevated, which can be advantageous for nose surgery in older patients when tip elevation is imperative. In addition, grafts of septal or auricular cartilage can be used for premaxillary augmentation. These grafts are placed through a separate pocket created with curved Stevens scissors at the base of the columella, directly over the premaxilla (Fig. 15.82).

One-year postoperative views of the patient after caudal reconstruction with an irradiated costal cartilage homograft and premaxillary augmentation (Fig. 15.83).

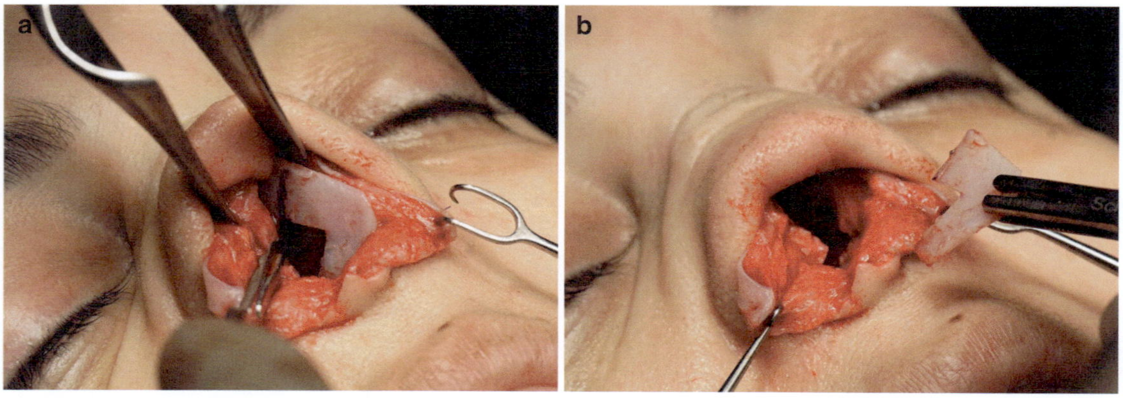

Fig. 15.79 (**a**, **b**) An end-to-end septal incision is made, and remnant cartilage is left at the dorsum while the remaining cartilage is removed

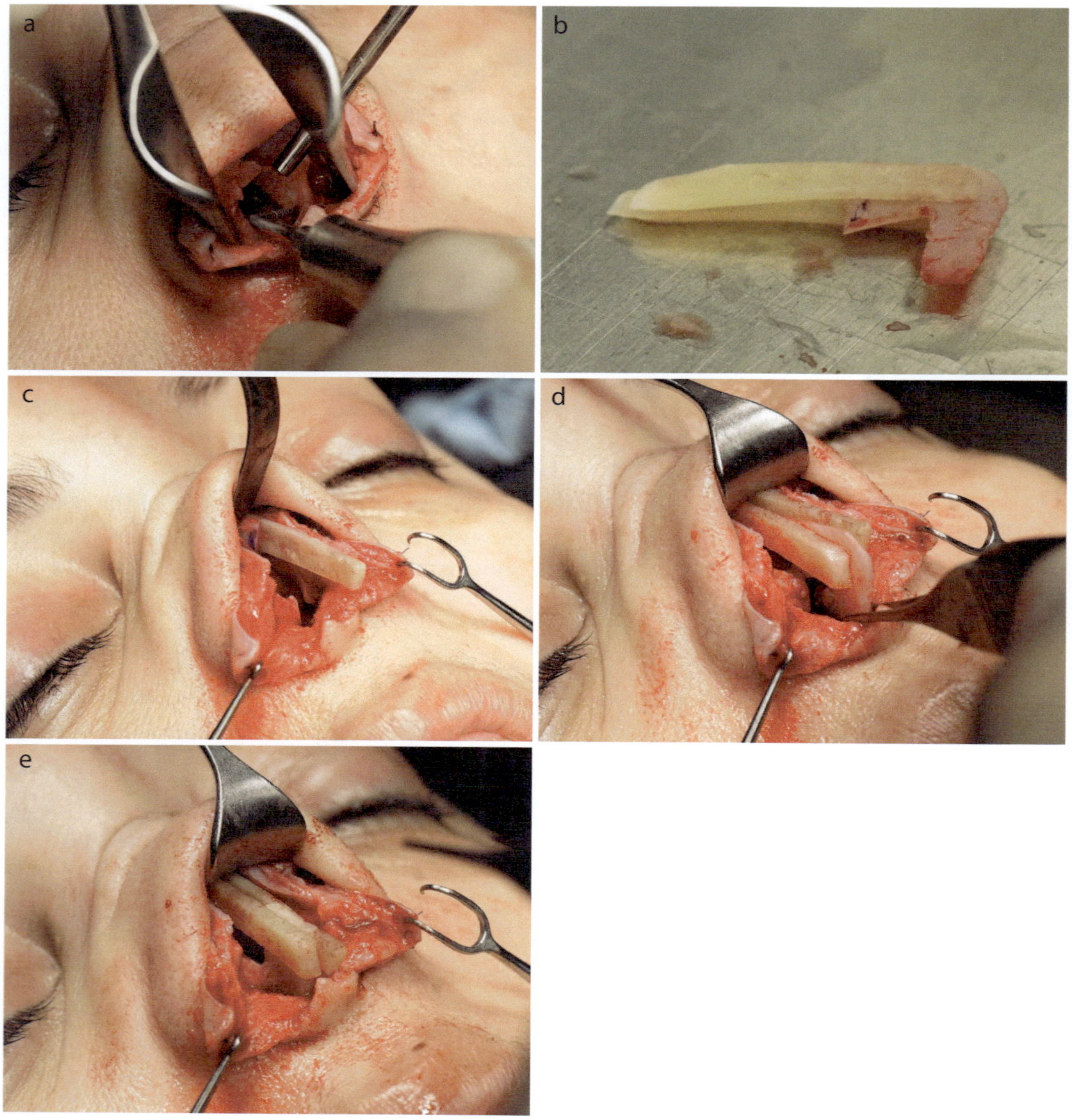

Fig. 15.80 (**a–e**) A piezo device is used to drill a hole in the nasal base before securing the caudal septal replacement graft. Each extended spreader graft is fixed to the remnant septum using 4-0 or 5-0 PDS absorbable suture material. The replacement graft is then fixed to the nasal spine, and then between the two spreader grafts. The newly constructed caudal septum is anteriorly positioned and reinforced for long-term stability

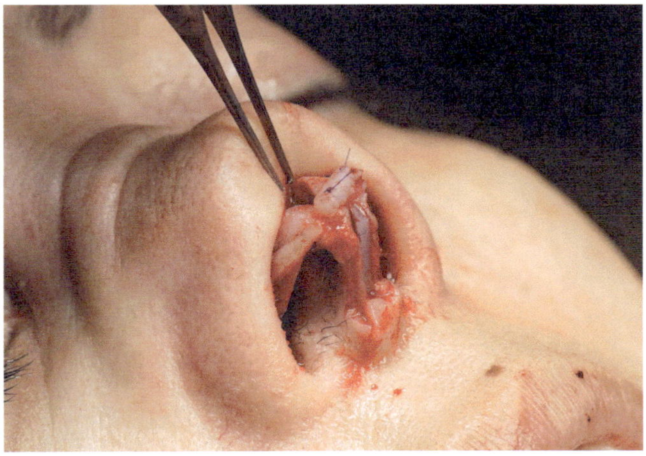

Fig. 15.81 Columellar strut, lateral crural grafts, cap grafts placement

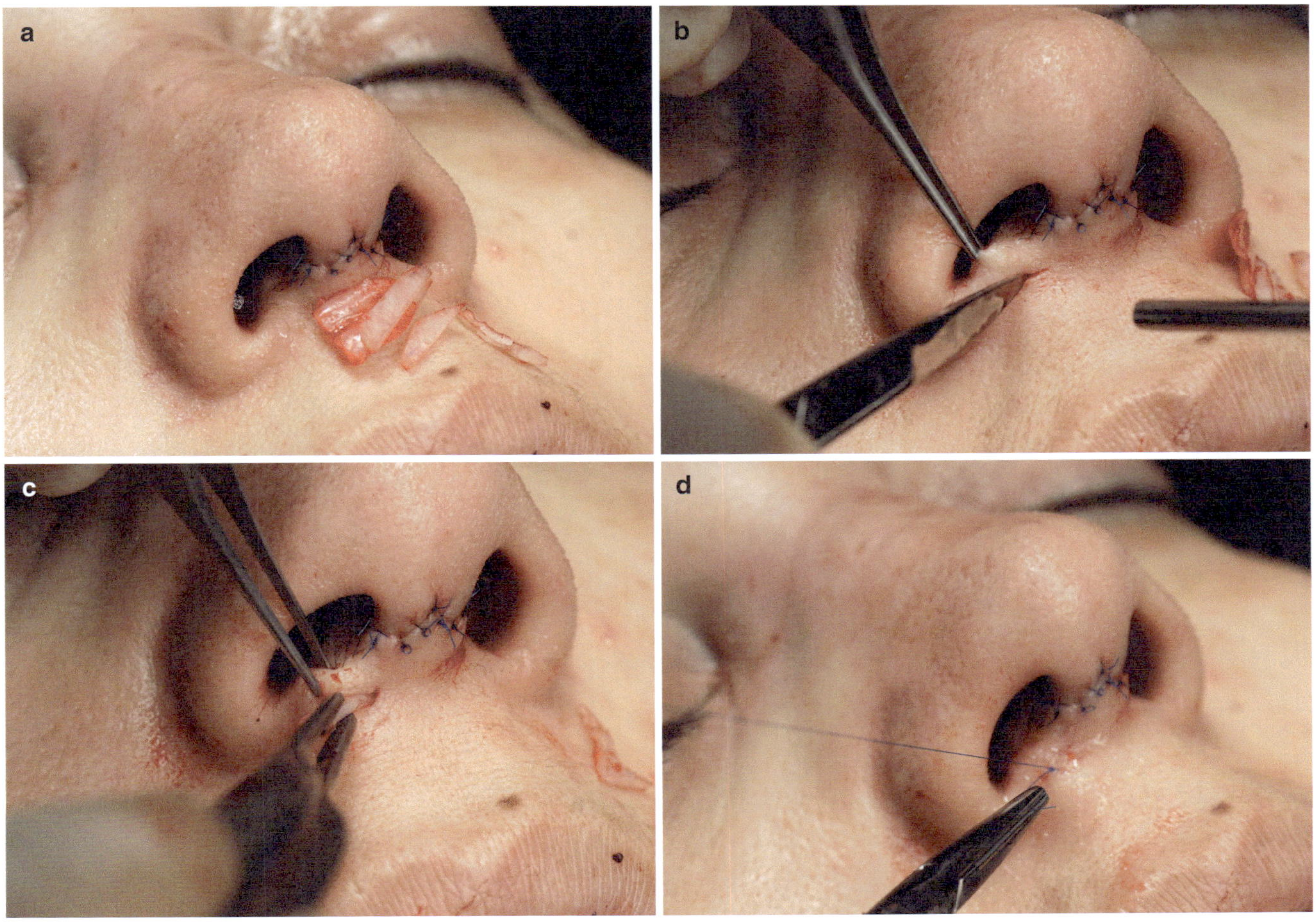

Fig. 15.82 (**a–d**) Premaxillary grafts placement

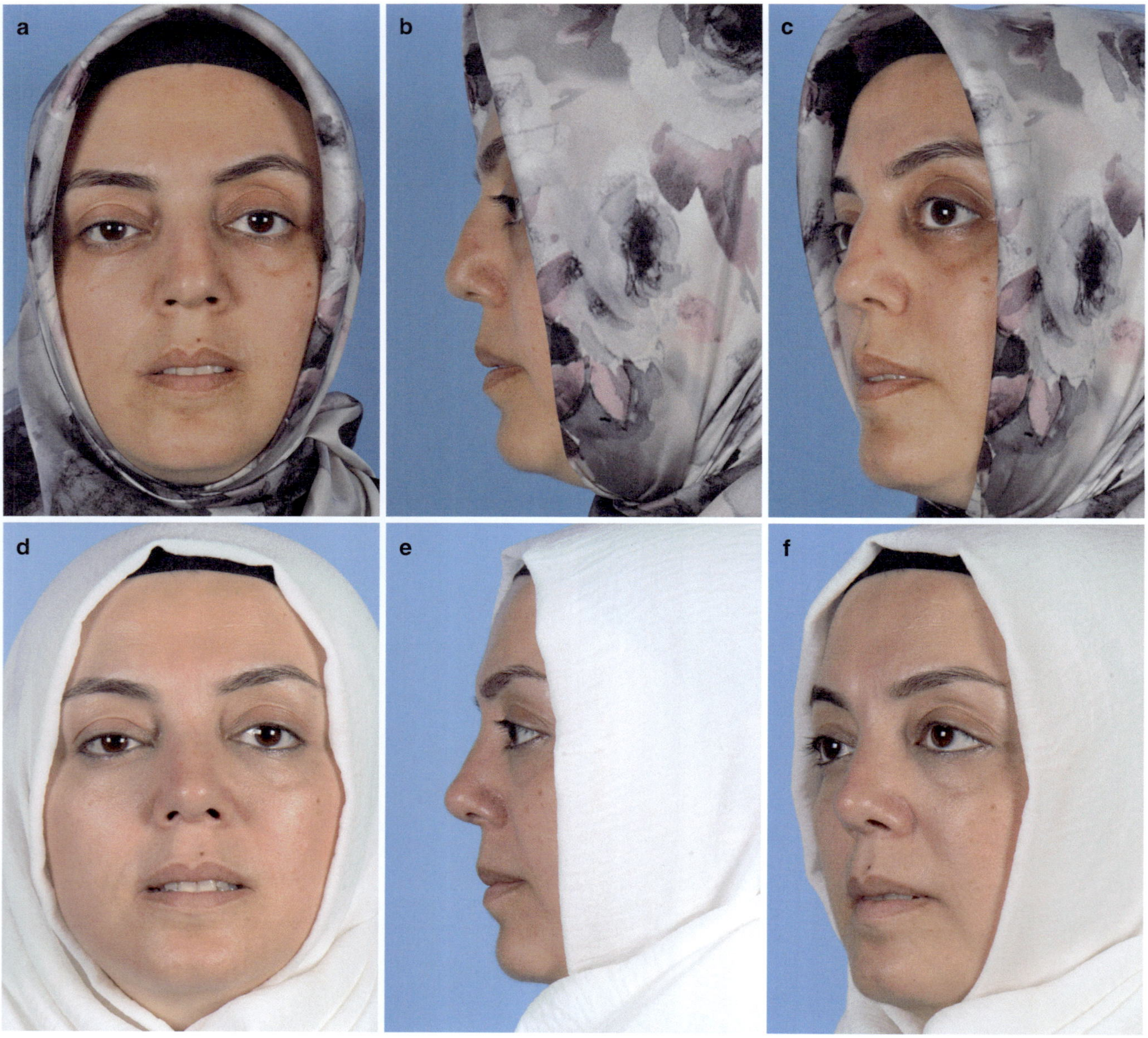

Fig. 15.83 (a–f) The lateral postoperative photograph shows a straight dorsum with increased tip projection and apparent lengthening of the nose

15.6 Conclusion

The essence of rhinoplasty correction is reprojection. First, deficiencies in the septal cartilage and anterior nasal spine, which comprise the nasal pedestal, are corrected, followed by the use of cartilage grafts and suturing techniques to provide strength and support to, and achieve an elegant appearance of, the nasal tip.

The table seen in Fig. 15.84 briefly summarizes all projection-increasing procedures discussed thus far.

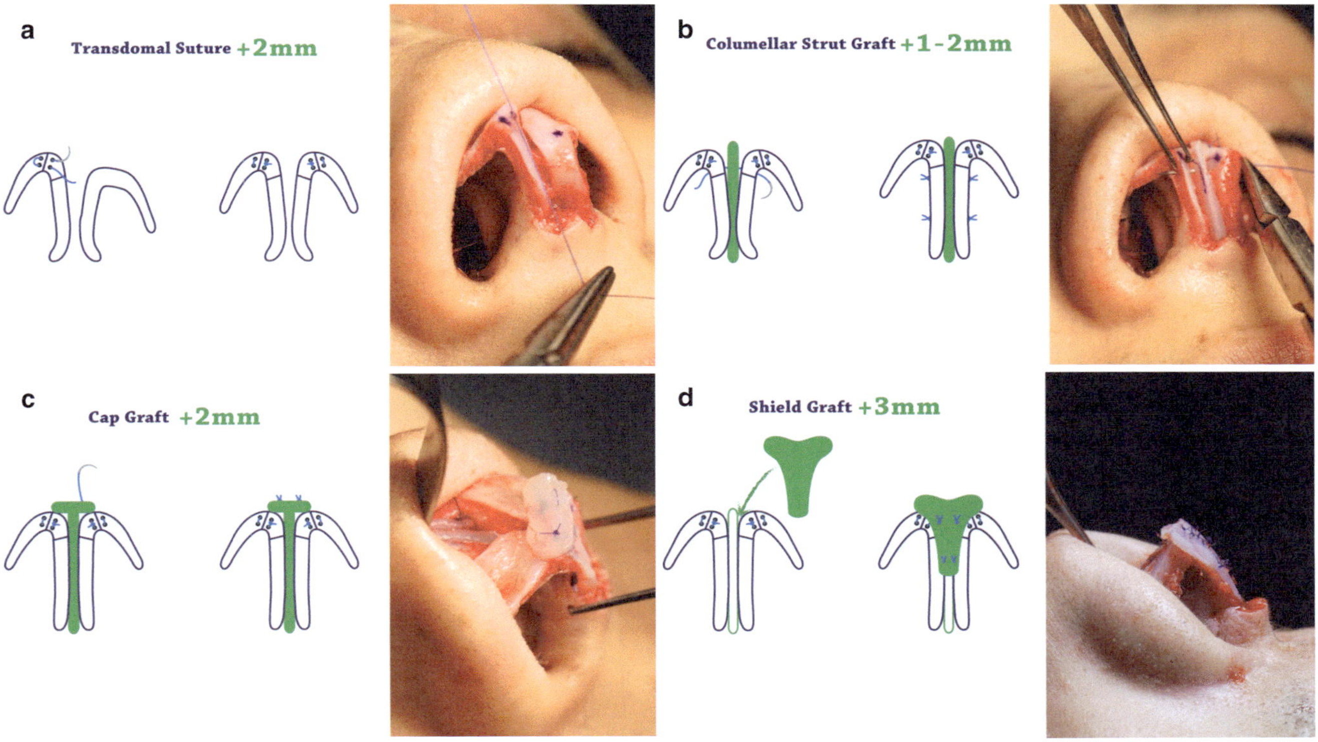

Fig. 15.84 (**a**–**d**) In cases with poor projection, technique selection depends on the needed projection. Each technique increases the millimeter of the tip projection differently

Disclosures The author reports no conflicts of interest or funding requiring disclosure.

Further Reading

Acikel C. Hypoplastic lateral crus causing alar retraction and underprojected nasal tip: correction with multiple grafts. Aesth Plast Surg. 2012;36(4):862–5.

Cerkes N. Nasal tip deficiency. Clin Plast Surg. 2016;43(1):135–50.

Davis RE. Lateral crural tensioning for refinement of the wide and underprojected nasal tip: rethinking the lateral crural steal. Facial Plast Surg Clin North Am. 2015;23(1):23–53.

de la Peña-Salcedo JA, Soto-Miranda MA, Lopez-Salguero JF. Treatment protocol for "Mestizo nose" with open rhinoplasty. Aesth Plast Surg. 2011;35(6):972–88.

Foda HM. Management of the droopy tip: a comparison of three alar cartilage-modifying techniques. Plast Reconstr Surg. 2003;112(5):1408–17; discussion 1418–21.

Ghazipour A, Ghadakzadeh S, Karimian N. The comparison between two different combinations of alar cartilage-modifying techniques: is lateral crural steal the choice? Eur Arch Otorrinolaringol. 2009;266(3):391–5.

Kuran I, Öreroğlu AR, Efendioğlu K. The lateral crural rein flap: a novel technique for management of tip rotation in primary rhinoplasty. Aesthet Surg J. 2014;34(7):1008–17.

Pastorek N, Ham J. The underprojecting nasal tip: an endonasal approach. Facial Plast Surg Clin North Am. 2004;12(1):93–106.

Robinson S, Thornton M. Nasal tip projection: nuances in understanding, assessment, and modification. Facial Plast Surg. 2012;28(2):158–65.

Rohrich RJ, Adams WP Jr, Ahmad J, Gunter JP, editors. Dallas rhinoplasty: nasal surgery by the masters. 3rd ed. Boca Raton FL: CRC Press; 2014.

Sadeghi M, Saedi B, Arvin Sazegar A, Amiri M. The role of columellar struts to gain and maintain tip projection and rotation: a randomized blinded trial. Am J Rhinol Allergy. 2009;23(6):e47–50.

Sen C, Iscen D. Caudal septal advancement for nasal tip projection and support in rhinoplasty. Aesth Plast Surg. 2006;30(2):135–40.

Taştan E, Yücel ÖT, Aydin E, Aydoğan F, Beriat K, Ulusoy MG. The oblique split method: a novel technique for carving costal cartilage grafts. JAMA Facial Plast Surg. 2013;15(3):198–203.

Weinstock MS, Stupak HD. Bony/cartilaginous mismatch: a radiologic investigation into the cause of tension nose deformity. Plast Reconstr Surg. 2018;141(2):312–21.

Yaberi R, Amali A, Emami H, Saedi B. A comparison of the tongue-in-groove and columellar strut in creating and maintaining tip projection and rotation: a randomized single blind trial. Eur J Plast Surg. 2017;41(3):293–8.

Yeşiloğlu N, Sarici M, Temiz G, Yildiz K, Mersa B, Filinte GT. Hezarfen wings: a lower lateral cartilage-based cartilage suspension technique for the adjustment of nasal tip rotation and projection and the correction of supratip deformity. J Craniofac Surg. 2014;25(3):983–7.

Over-Projected Nasal Tip

16

16.1 Introduction

Nasal tip projection refers to the distance from the tip of the nose to the posterior most point of the alar-cheek junction (i.e., the distance that the nose projects from the face) (Fig. 16.1).

Although a number of methods are available for quantitative evaluation of nasal over-projection, the most useful, accurate and practical is Goode's method. Although not perfectly suited to cases of highly unusual facial disharmony, Goode's mathematical formula still provides a useful starting point for pragmatic measurement.

Goode's method involves measurement of the nasal dorsal length from the radix to the tip-defining point and the projection from the alar crease to the tip-defining point. The projection should be between 0.55 and 0.6 of the nasal dorsal length. The nasofacial angle should be between 36° and 40° (Fig. 16.2).

Projection of more than 0.60 is defined as over-projection (Fig. 16.3).

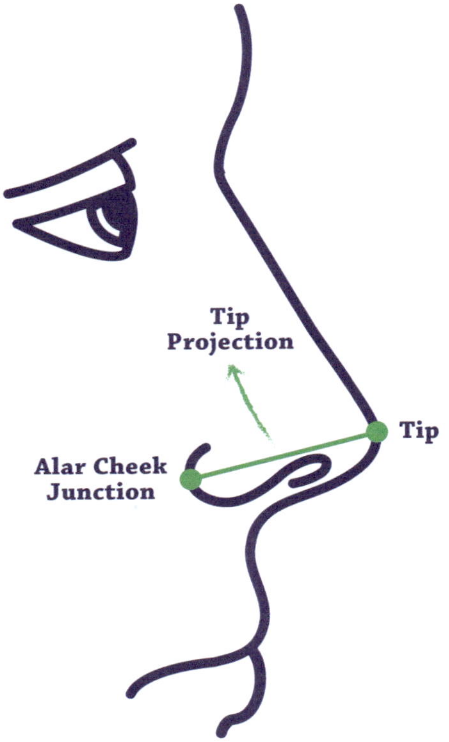

Fig. 16.1 Tip projection

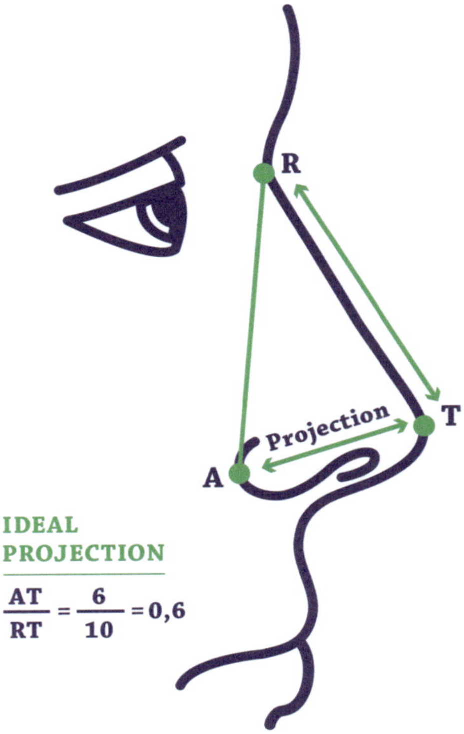

Fig. 16.2 First, a vertical straight line is drawn between the alar sulcus and the nasal tip, with a final line connecting the radix with the nasal tip; Goode's index is then calculated to quantify the degree of projection. Three points are utilized: A (alar–cheek junction), R (radix), and T (nasal tip). Goode's index is the AT/RT projection ratio of 0.55–0.6 corresponding to normal projection

Supplementary Information The online version contains supplementary material available at https://doi.org/10.1007/978-3-031-65619-4_16.

S. Şeneldir, *Photographic Atlas of Rhinoplasty*, https://doi.org/10.1007/978-3-031-65619-4_16

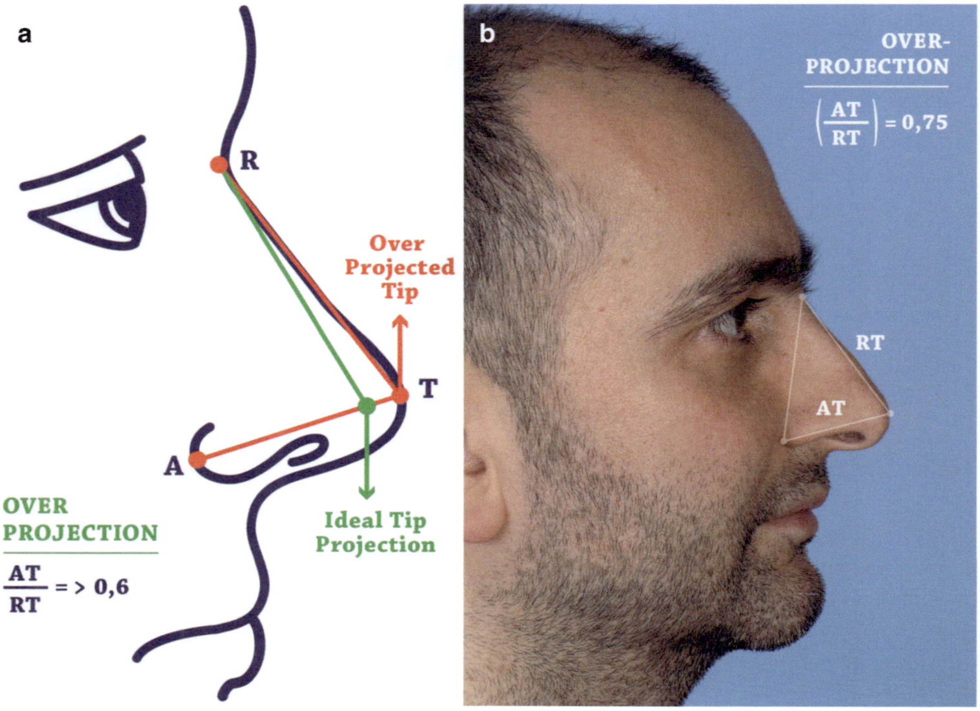

Fig. 16.3 (**a**, **b**) Over-projected nasal tip. The projection is more than 0.6 of the nasal dorsal length

The presence or absence of an over-projected nose resides in the eye of the beholder.

16.2 Potentially Overlooked Over-Projected Tip

Nasal tip over-projection is a common problem but it may often be overlooked during preoperative analysis. There are two reasons for this: (1) The overall size of the nose, and (2) the presence of a droopy nasal tip.

16.2.1 Size of the Nose

The nose may be too big in all dimensions, i.e., the dorsum, nasal base, nasal tip, etc. Over-projection of the dorsum in particular may cause tip over-projection to go unnoticed by the observer.

16.2.1.1 Case 1

In this case, the over-projected dorsum seemed to be responsible for the large nose. However, not only the dorsum, but also the tip, showed over-projection such that the nose was too large in all dimensions. Therefore, both the dorsum and the tip must be lowered to achieve a harmonious facial profile (Fig. 16.4).

Outcome at 5 years postoperatively is shown in Fig. 16.5. During surgery, dorsal reduction and deprojection were performed to achieve the ideal dorsal and tip projection simultaneously.

Lowering only the dorsum and leaving the tip untreated may result in an imbalanced profile, causing the tip to appear "to jump out of the face."

16.2.1.2 Case 2

The patient had previously undergone rhinoplasty, where her primary surgeon lowered the nasal dorsum but did not alter the tip. The nasal tip appeared "to jump out of the face" (Fig. 16.6).

Satisfied dorsal profile after deprojection surgery is shown in Fig. 16.7.

16.2.2 Presence of Droopy Nasal Tip

A droopy nasal tip may also result in an existing over-projection going unnoticed. In such cases, deprojection techniques should be used when increasing rotation. Otherwise, the hidden over-projection can become more prominent. This is even more critical in cases with a droopy nose where the over-projection is due to a long lateral crura. Use of a steel suture to correct the droopy tip makes the projection even more prominent. A previously unnoticed over-projection may emerge if surgery concludes without resolving this problem.

16.2.2.1 Case 3

Patient with a drooping nasal tip and dorsal hump presenting with an over-projection hidden by the drooping tip (Fig. 16.8).

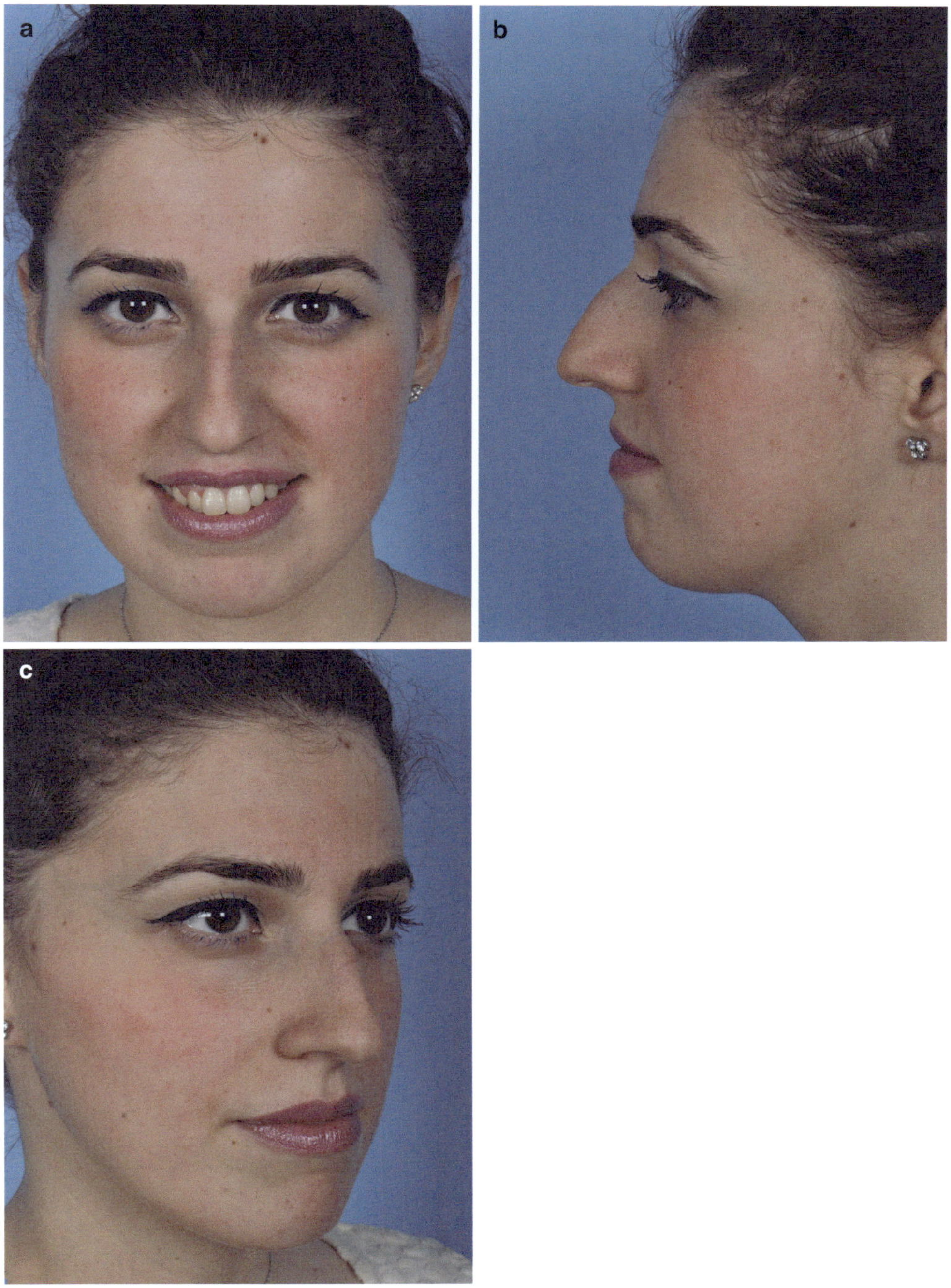

Fig. 16.4 (**a–c**) The patient with over-projection of the dorsum and the tip together

When steel sutures were used only to correct the rotation, thus ignoring the projection, the existing over-projection became even more prominent. With the effect of the suture being compounded by an already existing projection, the tip had an extremely over-projected appearance (Fig. 16.9).

In such cases, the surgeon must change strategy and use techniques that can simultaneously address both rotation and projection. VAR is the technique of choice to achieve this (Fig. 16.10).

Ideal projection and definition were achieved by placing a small cup graft after deprojection (Fig. 16.11).

Outcome 1-year postoperatively is seen in Fig. 16.12. After simultaneous dorsal and tip deprojection, the rotation was ideal.

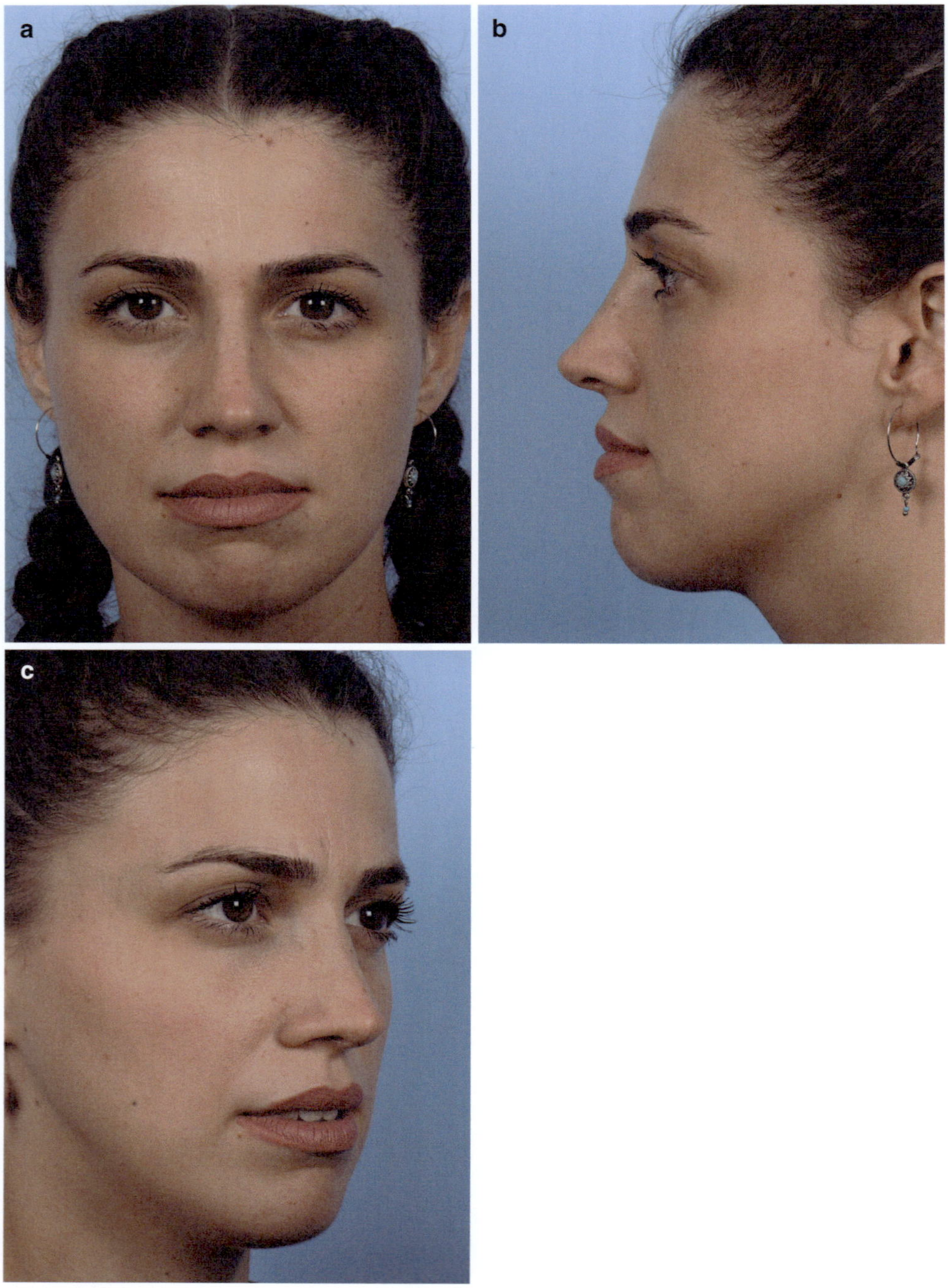

Fig. 16.5 (**a–c**) Correction by reduction of all overdeveloped components, including tip projection by Var technique

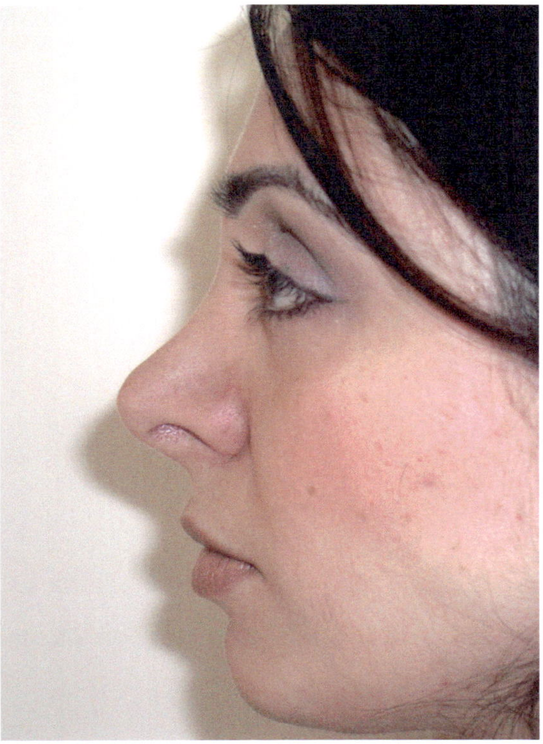

Fig. 16.6 Over-projected tip with "jump out of the face" appearance. While dorsum projection has been reduced, tip projection has not altered

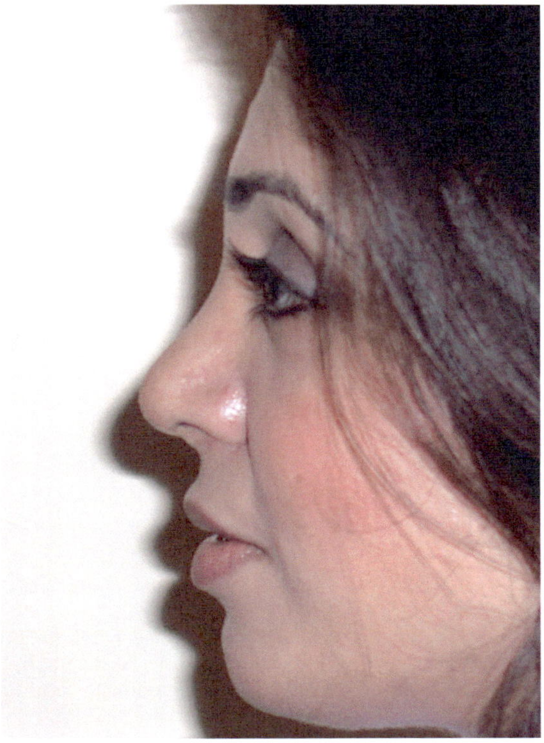

Fig. 16.7 After tip deprojection, the nasal tip was in balance with the rest of the face

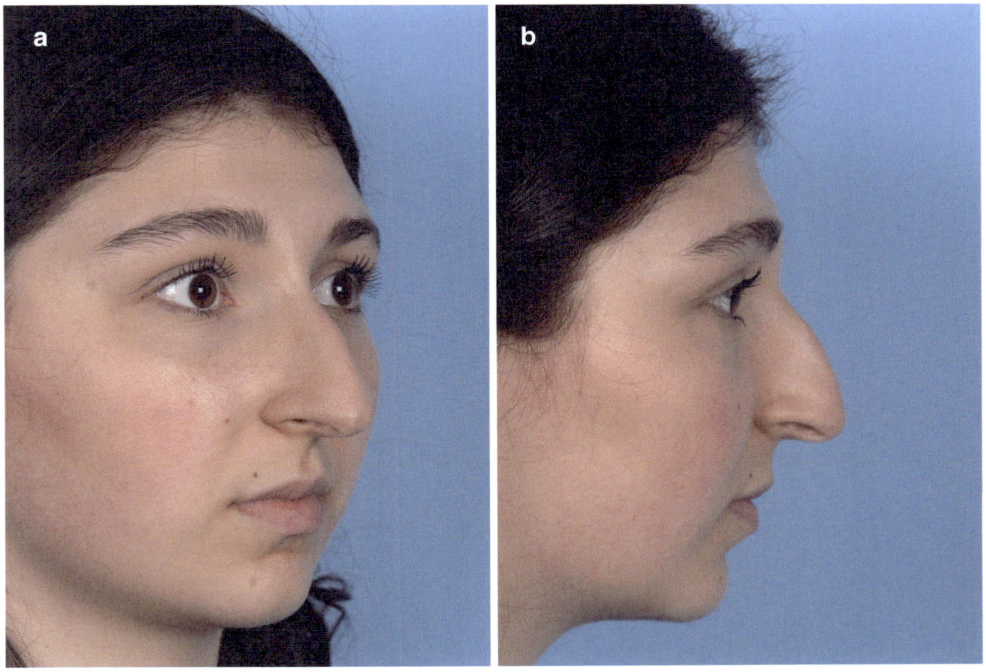

Fig. 16.8 (**a**, **b**) Over-projected and droopy nasal tip, droopiness hides the over-projection of the tip

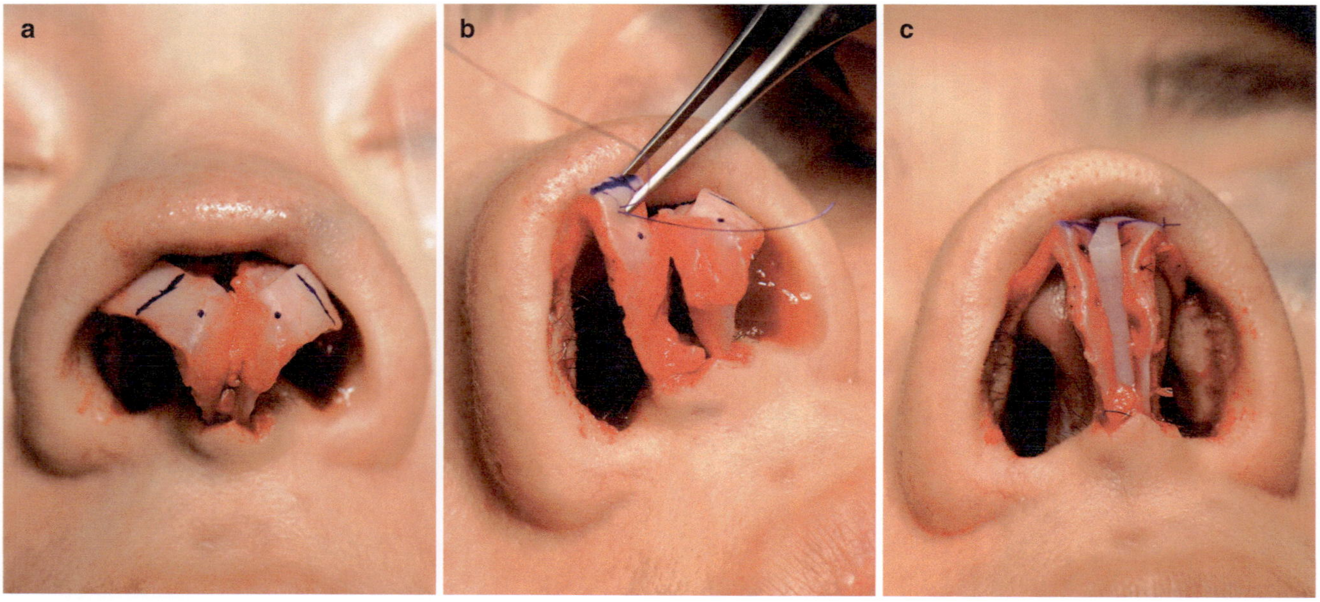

Fig. 16.9 (**a**) The lateral crura are long and strong. For this reason, the tip is droopy. (**b**) Planning of the lateral crural steal technique by suture is commonly known as the best choice to fix a droopy nasal tip with long lateral crura. (**c**) After suturing and fixing the columellar strut, hidden over-projection became more prominent

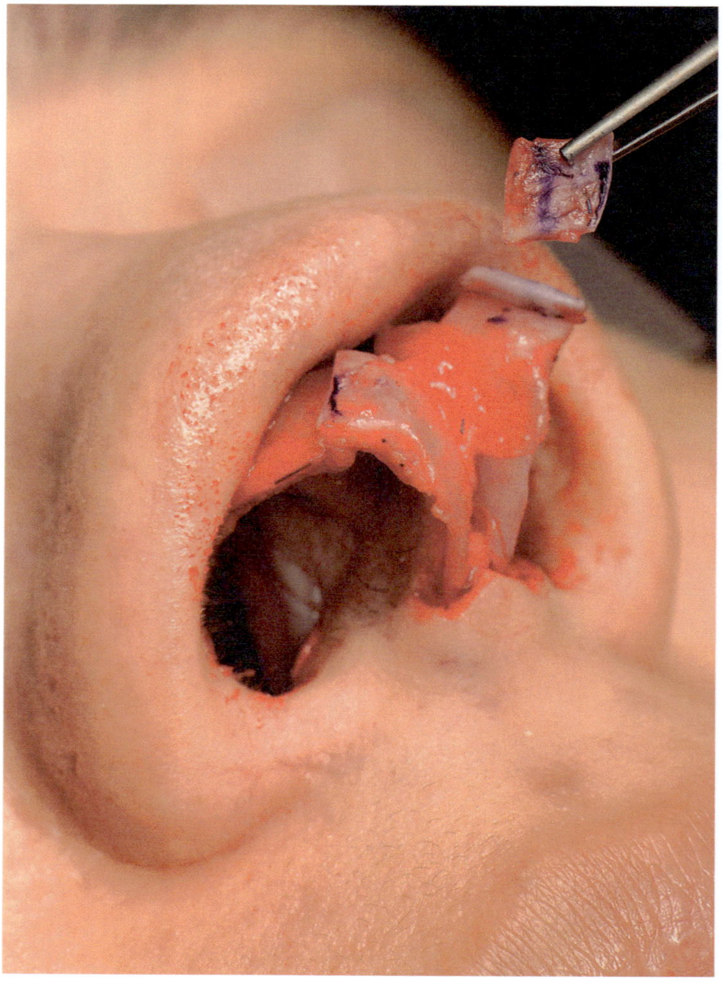

Fig. 16.10 The surgery should not finish like this. It needs an alternative strategy. The technique was changed. The sutures were cut, the alar arch divided, and the vertical excess lateral crura removed. The two ends were then sutured together

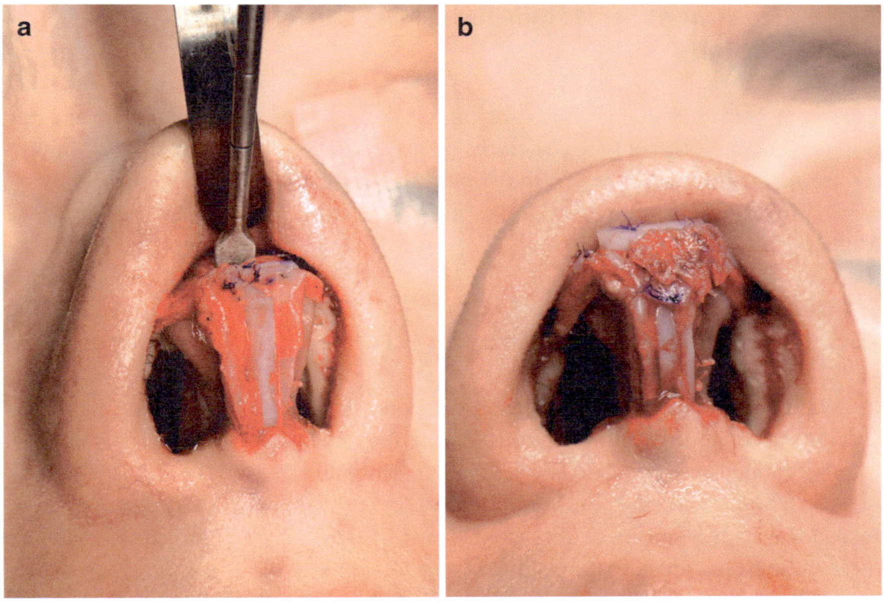

Fig. 16.11 (**a**) Columellar strut, cap graft placement. (**b**) This is the altered alar cartilage anatomy

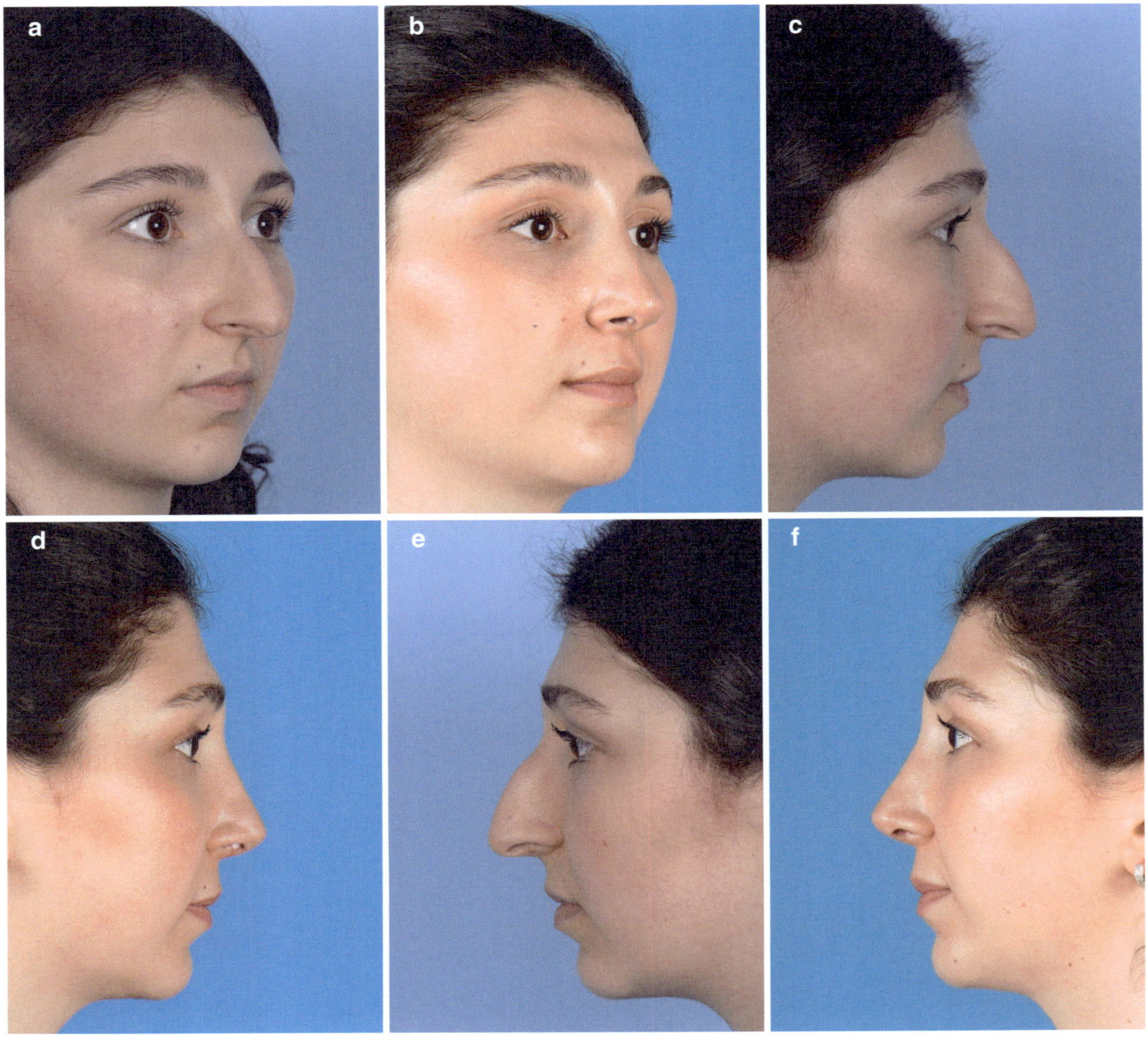

Fig. 16.12 (**a**–**f**) Pre- and postoperative photographs. Deprojection and counter-rotation of the tip simultaneously achieved resection of the excess part of lateral crura

16.3 Treatment Strategy/Clinical Outcome/ Etiology

There are basically two reasons for nasal tip over-projection or long nasal tip: (1) the structures adjacent to the nasal tip are underdeveloped; or (2) the structures that form the nasal tip are overdeveloped (Lee et al. 2014; Papel and Mabrie 1999).

16.3.1 Underdeveloped Nearby Structures

In patients presenting for rhinoplasty, surgeons should specifically examine factors known to influence the appearance of projection. These can be divided into non-nasal and nasal factors, which give the illusion of nasal over-projection (pseudo-over-projection). Decreasing nasal projection in these patients may lead to worsening of facial and nasal harmony, thus emphasizing the importance of appropriate analysis and diagnosis.

16.3.1.1 Non-nasal Causes

Non-nasal factors include a sloping forehead, anterior maxilla, and deficient chin; these factors may be addressed at the time of rhinoplasty if the patient desires. Patients with poor chin projection may be candidates for genioplasty or implantation. Aberrant occlusion with midfacial or mandibular malposition warrants consideration for orthognathic referral.

Case 4

Underdevelopment of the chin caused the nasal tip to appear more projected than it actually was. Surgical planning should include advancement of the chin, rather than deprojection of the tip, to improve the nasal tip pseudo-over-projection (Fig. 16.13).

A transdomal suture and columellar strut were applied to the nasal tip. No deprojection was performed (Fig. 16.14).

A chin prosthesis was applied during the same session (Fig. 16.15).

The deprojected appearance of the nose at 1 year postoperatively was due to jaw advancement contributing to a balanced profile (Fig. 16.16).

16.3.1.2 Nasal Causes

An illusion of nasal over-projection, i.e., pseudo-over-projection, may result from nasal factors such as (1) low radix, (2) over-resected bony dorsum, and (3) saddle nose deformity.

Low Radix

A nose with a low radix has an over-projected appearance despite having a normal tip projection. Therefore, tip projection should be adjusted after taking the radix to its ideal height.

Case 5

Preoperative and postoperative photographs of the patient clearly illustrate a deprojected appearance of the nose,

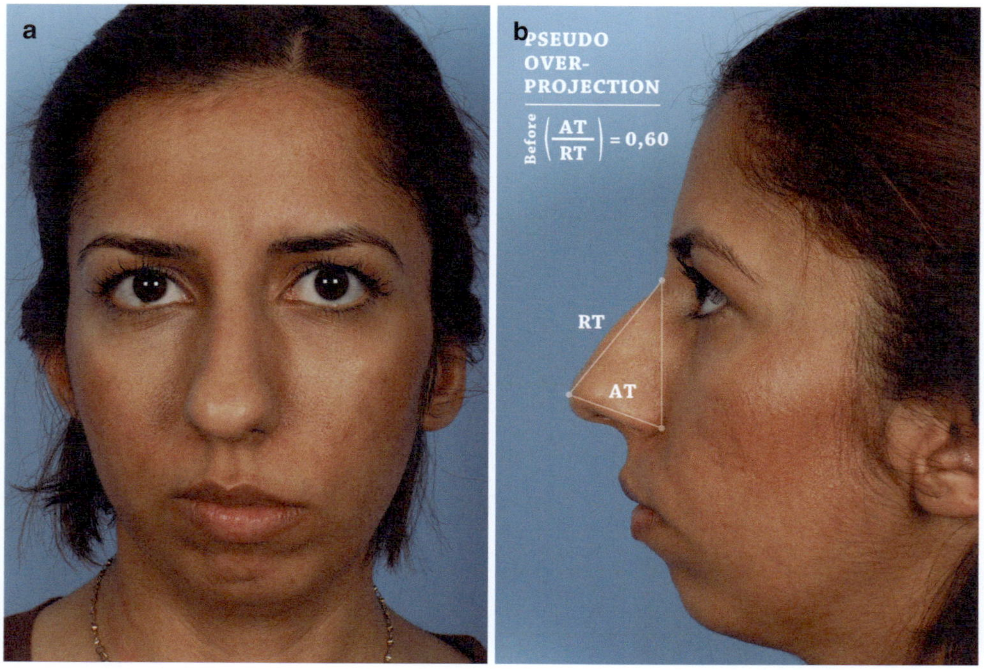

Fig. 16.13 (**a**, **b**) Over-projected tip appearance but not real. Underdevelopment of the chin is shown as the nasal tip is more projected (pseudo-over-projection)

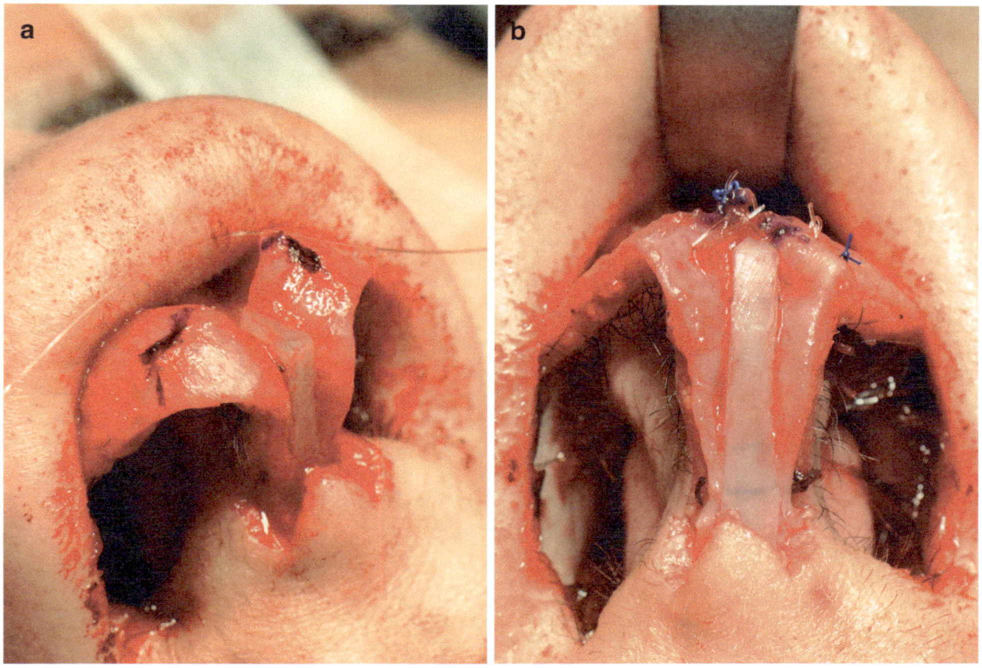

Fig. 16.14 (**a**, **b**) The tip shaped with basic tip techniques (transdomal suture, columellar strut, etc.). No deprojection techniques were performed

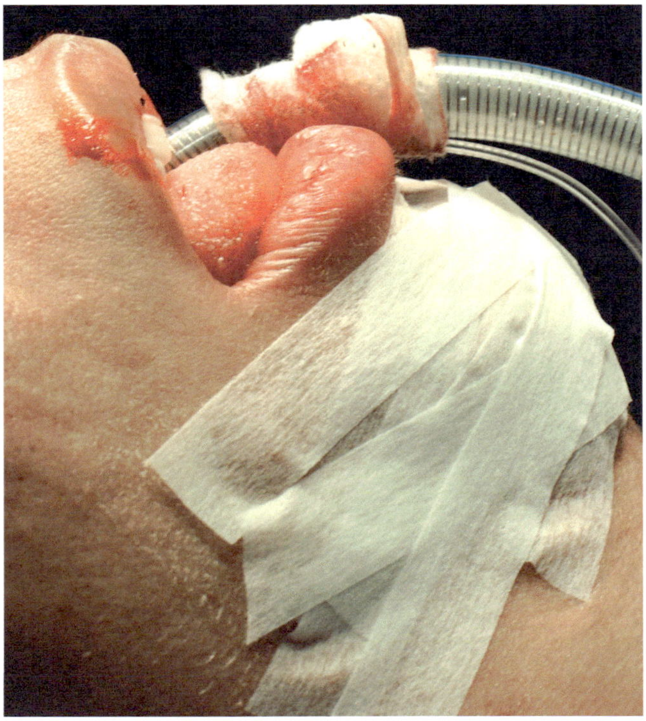

Fig. 16.15 Chin augmentation was performed

although no tip deprojection procedure was applied. Filling of the radix was sufficient to achieve this result, as the root cause of the over-projected nose was the illusion created by the low radix (Fig. 16.17).

Following hump resection, ideal dorsal height was achieved by filling the radix with diced cartilage. Transdomal suture and a columellar strut sufficed for the tip (Fig. 16.18).

Over-Resected Dorsum

Even if the tip is in the ideal position, dorsal deficiency creates an over-projected appearance of the tip. Elevating the dorsum to its ideal position corrects the over-projected appearance of the tip.

Case 6

Outcome at 1 year postoperatively is shown in Fig. 16.19. In her previous rhinoplasty operation, the dorsum was over-resected. Therefore, the tip was over-projected relative to the dorsum. The over-projected appearance was corrected by compensating for the deficient dorsum rather than by deprojection of the tip.

A dorsal onlay graft obtained from costal cartilage was laid through the dorsum, fixed with absorbable sutures (Fig. 16.20).

16.3.2 Overdeveloped Tip Framework (True Over-Projection)

Two anatomical structures underlie the dome of the nasal tip, constituting the caudal third of the nose:

- Septum–nasal spine complex
- Two pairs of alar cartilage

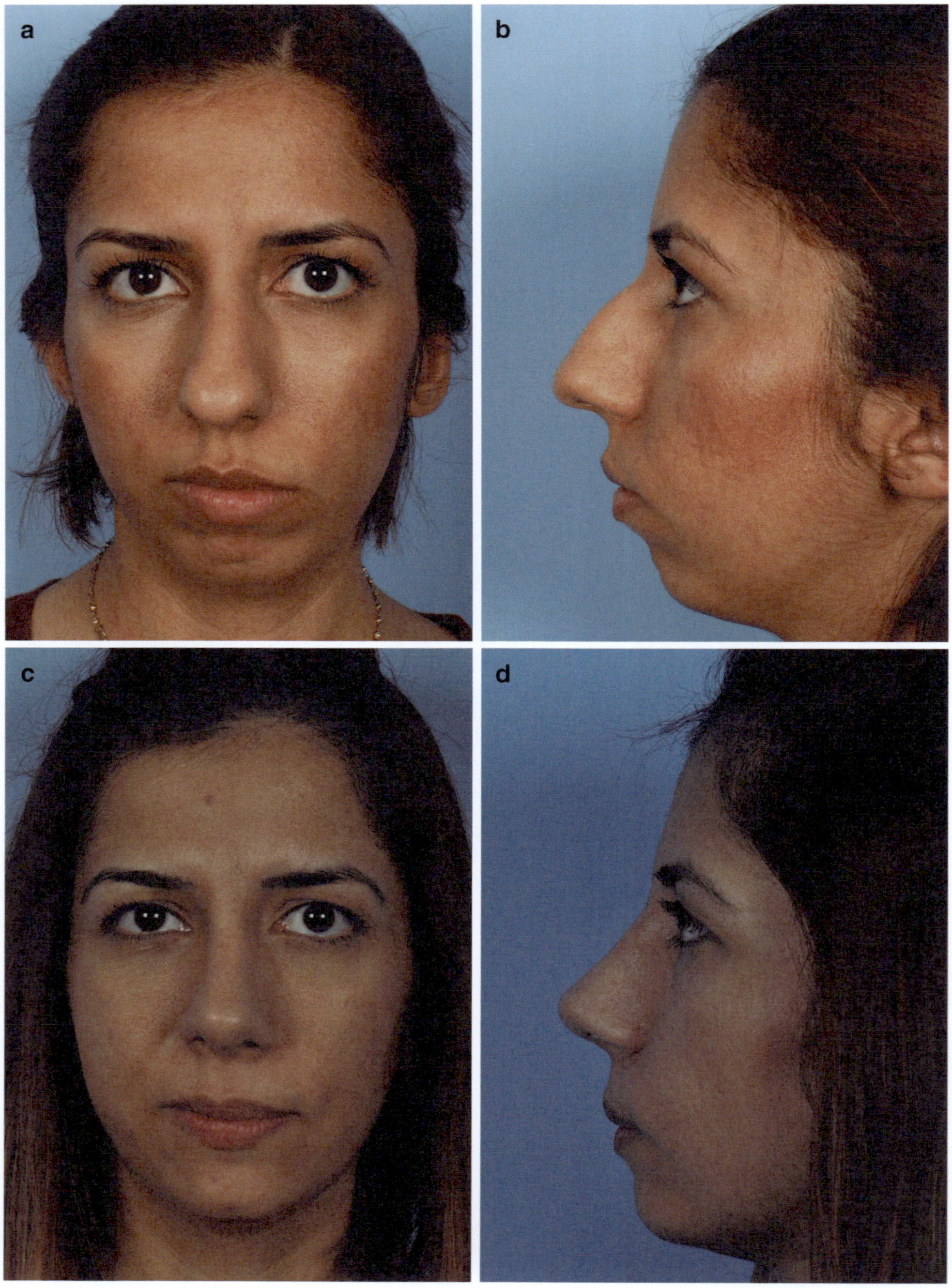

Fig. 16.16 (**a**–**d**) Compare profile pictures: deprojected tip appearance comes from chin augmentation

Any overdevelopment of these structures, either collectively or separately, can cause an over-projected nasal tip.

The septum nasal spine complex can be conceived of as a pedestal, with the alar cartilages acting as a statue resting thereon (Johnson and Godin 1995). Overgrowth of the pedestal and/or the statue will cause over-projection. Volume reduction of the overdeveloped anatomical component will resolve this problem (Fig. 16.21).

16.3.2.1 Over-Projection Due to the Septum–Nasal Spine Complex

An overdeveloped quadrangular cartilage and nasal spine (pedestal) component may elevate the tip to an abnormally forward-projecting position, even when the tip anatomy is otherwise normal. The nose will appear as if it has been pulled forward from the plane of the face (Fig. 16.22).

The following findings are relatively common: overgrowth of the pedestal and anterior displacement of the naso-

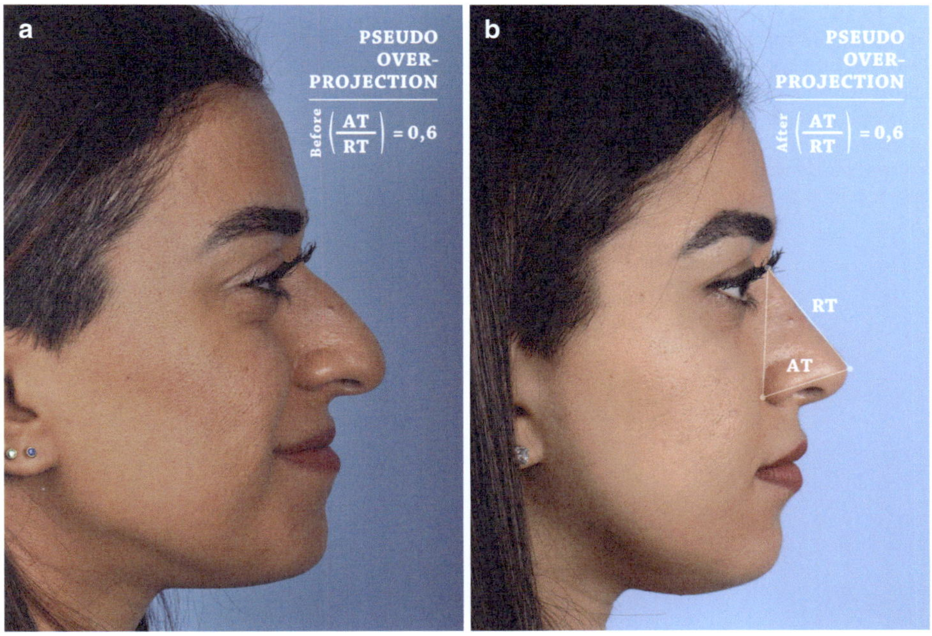

Fig. 16.17 (**a**) Tip appeared over-projected but it was not real. Unbalanced dorsum with low radix is shown as the nasal tip is more projected. (**b**) No deprojection techniques were performed on her tip. The profile is well balanced with decreased dorsal height and increased radix projection. Deprojected tip appearance comes from the balanced dorsum

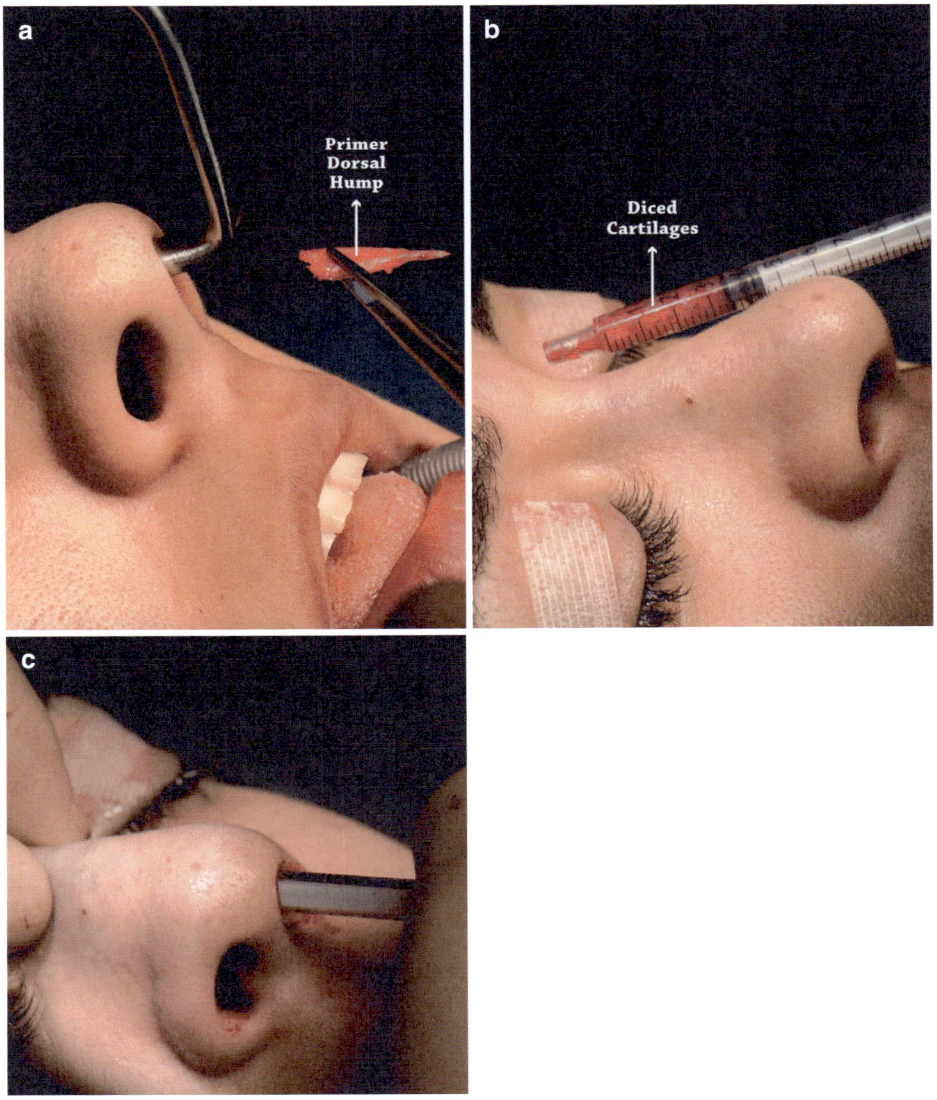

Fig. 16.18 (**a–c**) Intraoperative pictures of this patient. (**a**) Removal of primer dorsal hump. (**b**, **c**) Diced cartilage was filled with syringe used for radix augmentation

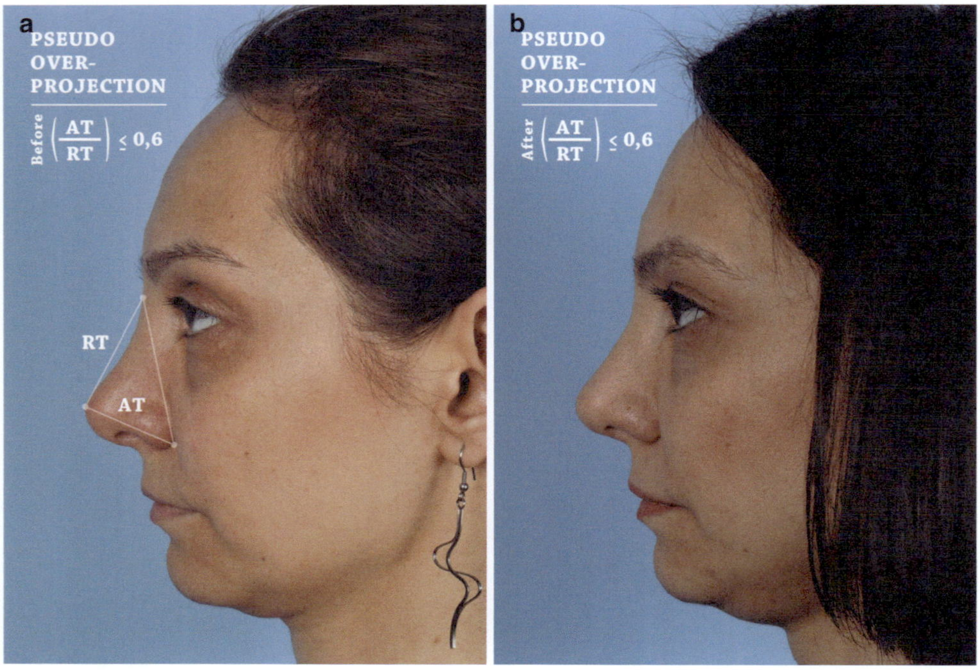

Fig. 16.19 (**a**) Overprotected tip but only in appearance. Over-resected dorsum is shown as the nasal tip is more projected (pseudo-over-projection). (**b**) Deprojected tip appearance was caused by augmentation of the dorsum

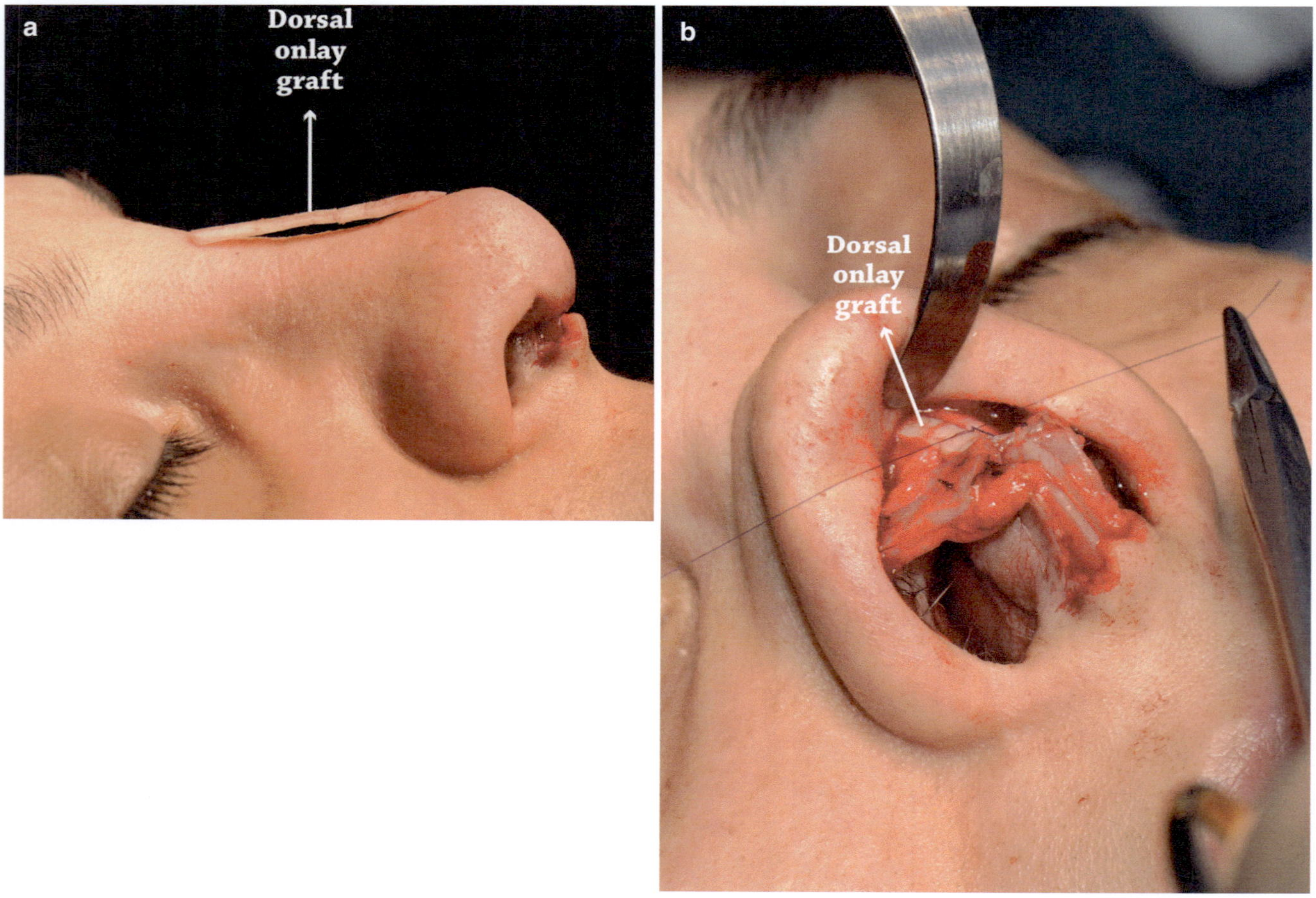

Fig. 16.20 (**a**, **b**) Standard technique was used for tip reshaping, desired dorsal height is achieved with an onlay dorsal grafting

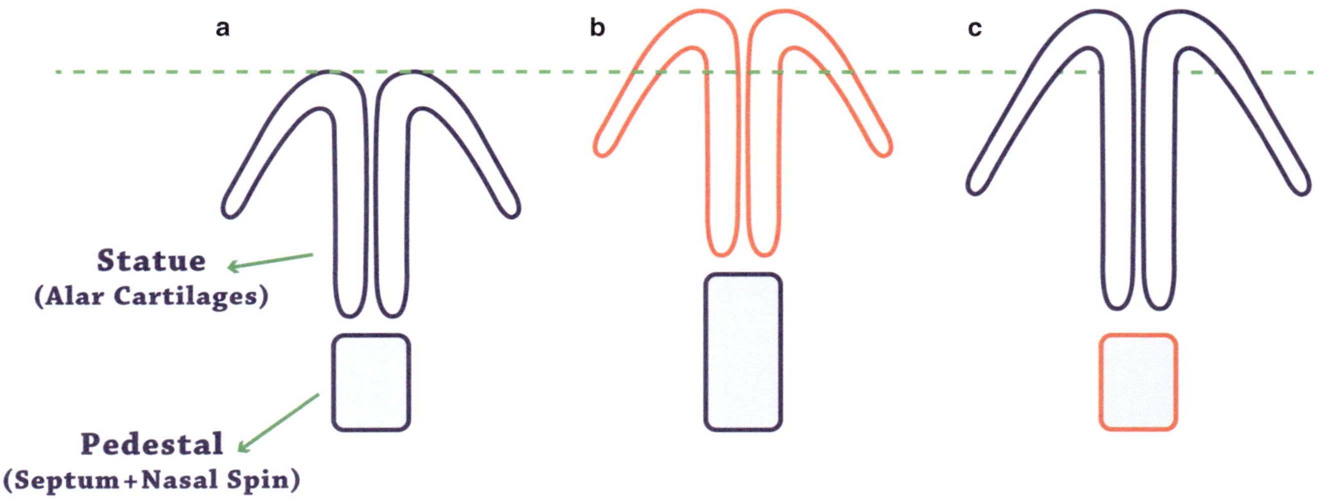

Fig. 16.21 The pedestal effect is defined in 1995 firstly by Calvin M. Johnson. (**a**) Normal relation of the pedestal and "statue." (**b**) Over-projection caused by enlargement of the pedestal, as seen in tension nose. The statue is of normal size. (**c**) Over-projection due to enlargement of the statue. The pedestal is of normal size. The statue is overdeveloped relative to the alar cartilages

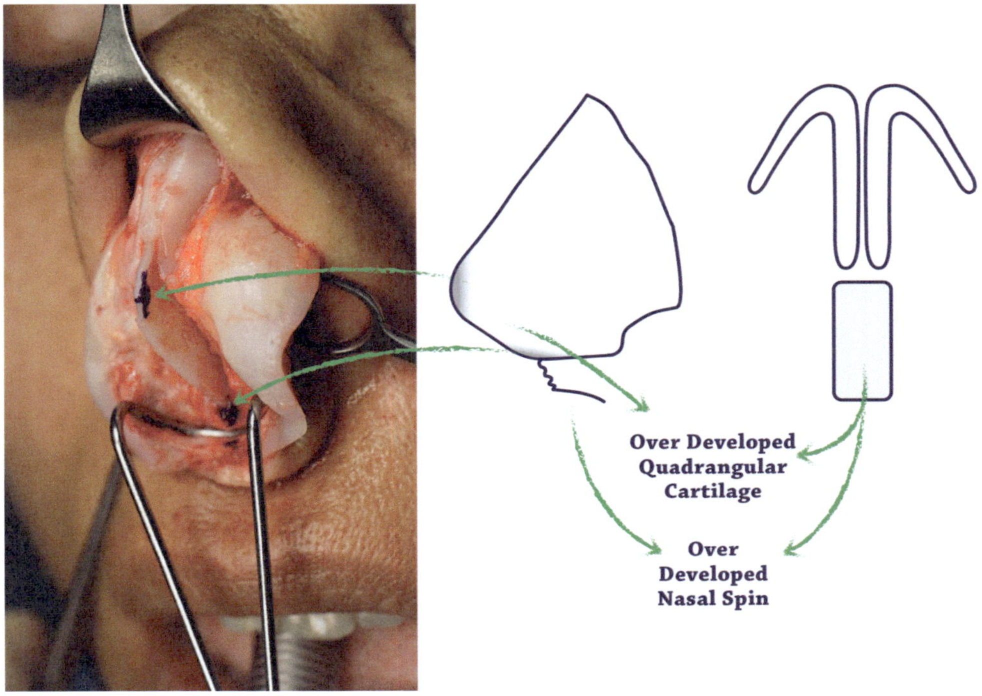

Fig. 16.22 Illustration showing the clinical presentation of the overdeveloped quadrangular cartilage and nasal spine

labial angle, which may appear full, webbed, and excessively obtuse, with no obvious demarcation between the lip and columella (Fig. 16.23). The upper lip may appear short, tethered, and tense (Fig. 16.24).

Excessive anterior growth of the caudal septum pushes the nasal tip cartilages forward, exerting a "tent pole" effect on the nasal alae. This results in narrowing of the nostrils and flattening of the alar curvature. In severe cases, the narrowing is sufficient to cause partial nasal airway obstruction (Fig. 16.25).

An overdeveloped pedestal can displace the medial crura inferiorly, sometimes resulting in enhanced columellar show.

16.3.2.2 Over-Projection Due to Overdeveloped Alar Cartilage

Medial, intermediate, and lateral crura may all be involved in over-projection but each can also be overdeveloped in isolation. The cartilages are often buckled at the dome region, creating marked asymmetries and irregularities (Fig. 16.26).

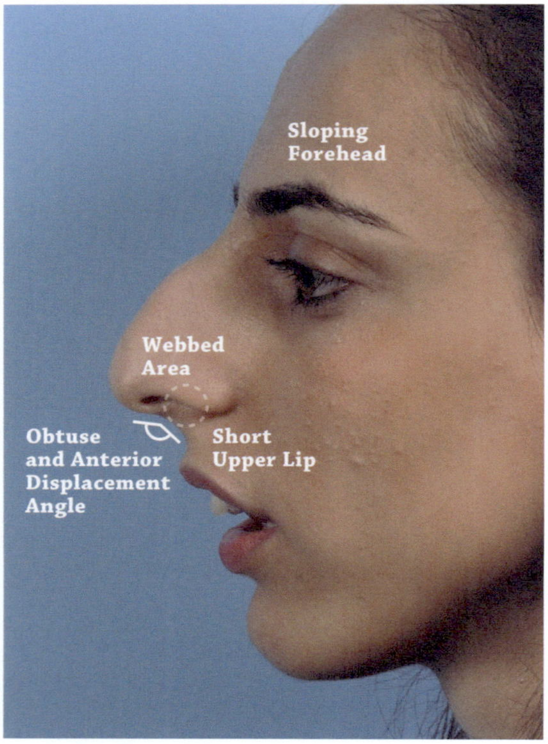

Fig. 16.23 A typical finding in patients with over-developed quadrangular cartilage and nasal spine is shown

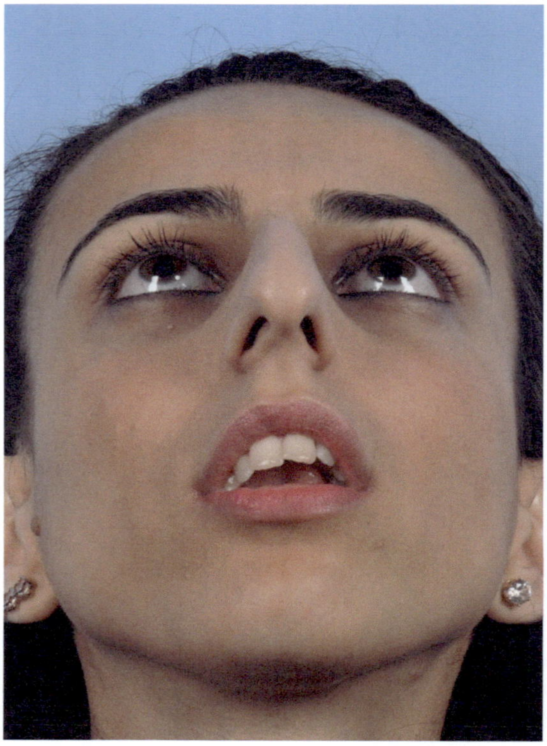

Fig. 16.25 "Tent pole" effect on the nasal alae

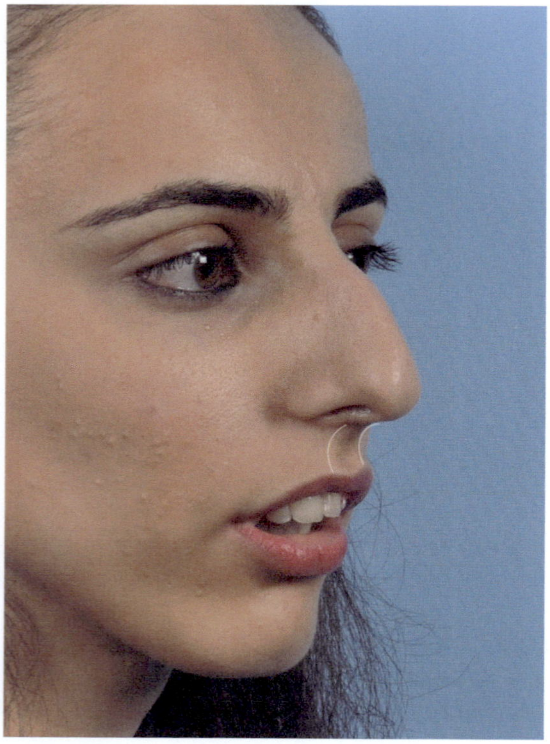

Fig. 16.24 In an oblique view, the philtral columns are pulled forward

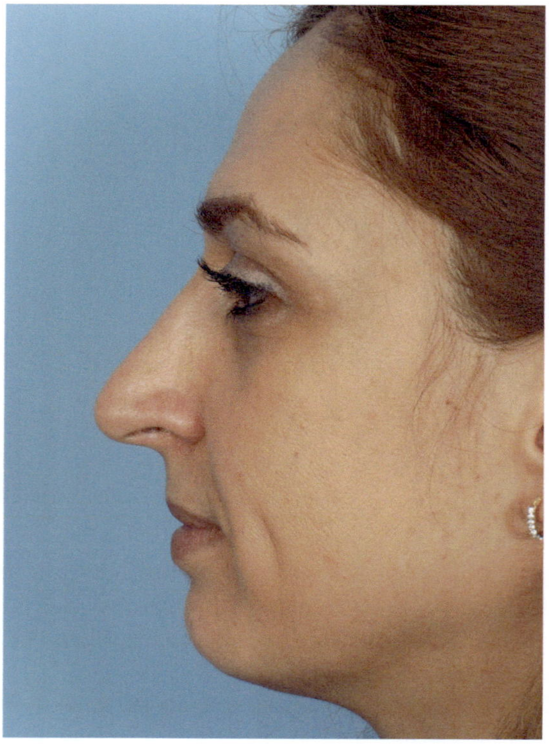

Fig. 16.26 Nose appears over-projected because of overdeveloped alar cartilages. Caudal septal hypertrophy does not contribute to the projection. Notice that there are no signs of hypertrophic septum such as obtuse columella labial angle and short lip

Once true over-projection has been determined, the surgeon can perform an objective analysis. Combinations of the above hypertrophic anatomical problems may contribute to the overall nasal tip over-projection. In preoperative analysis, each component must be comprehensively identified and analyzed; only then can a definitive plan for natural correction be made. Each factor should be addressed in turn, and the desired tip projection should be decided on.

16.4 Surgical Techniques

Over-projected tip surgery should be performed once radix and dorsum projection have been brought to the ideal level. Surgical correction of the over-projected nasal tip is achieved by a deprojection–reprojection operation, which consists of three steps (Johnson and Godin 1995):

1. Deprojection

Over-projected tip surgery is a type of reduction surgery in which hypertrophic structures are resected to achieve deprojection. At this point, if needed, tip rotation can be changed with techniques for decreasing projection.

2. Reprojection

The need for deprojection in cases of nasal tip over-projection is obvious. Reprojection is normally performed because, in the course of deprojection, the important support mechanism of the tip is weakened. It is essential to reestablish support for the nasal tip; failure to do so would result in loss of definition and projection.

3. Alar base reduction

Upon completion of deprojection, it is necessary to attend to the nasal base. In some cases, the nasal base is widened (Fig. 16.27).

It is generally agreed that reduction of the nasal base should be considered when the interalar distance exceeds the intercanthal distance (Figs. 16.28 and 16.29).

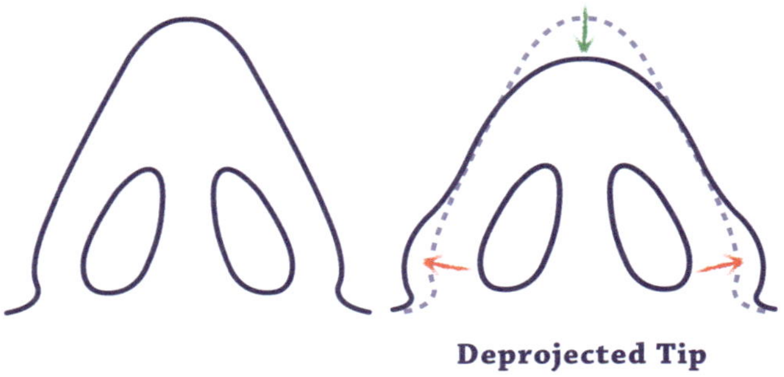

Fig. 16.27 Wide nasal base

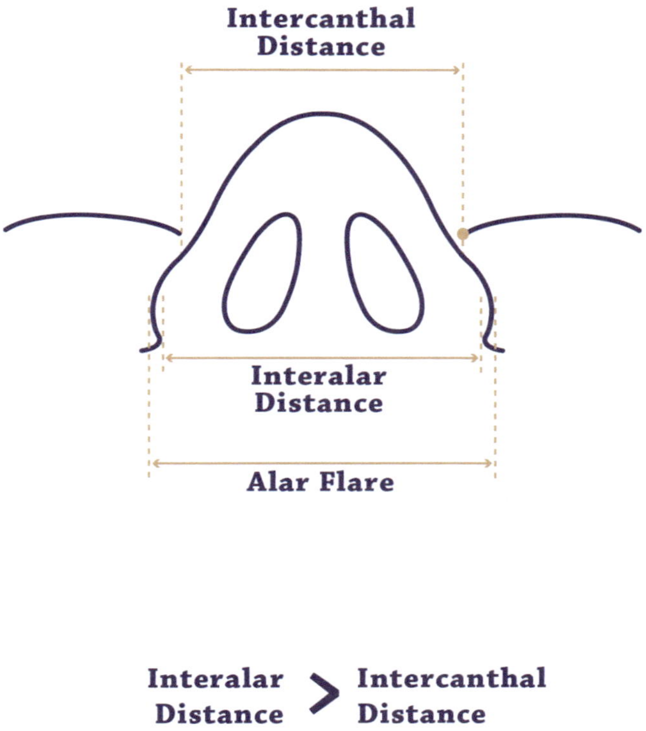

Fig. 16.28 Interalar distance is bigger than intercanthal distance

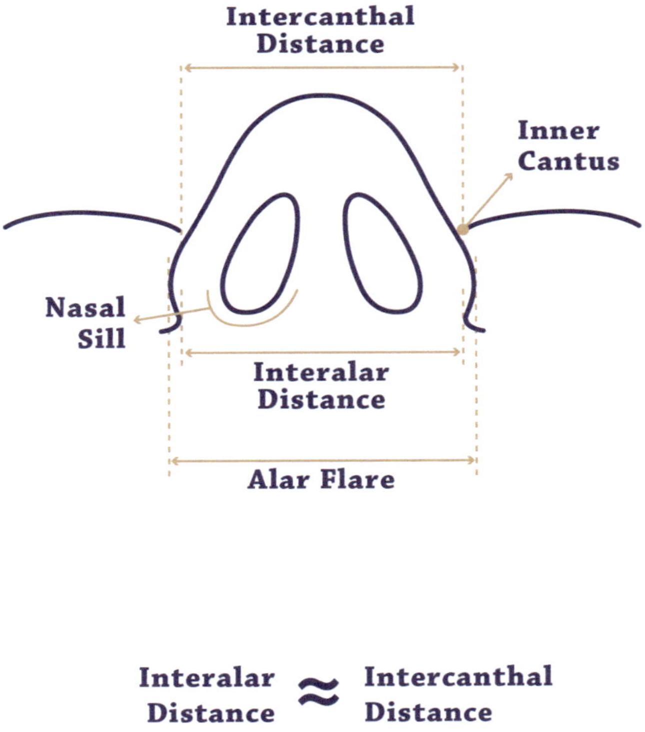

Fig. 16.29 Interalar distance is equal to intercanthal distance

Technical Note: The surgeon should decide to perform nasal base surgery only after having completed tip surgery. If in doubt, we do not perform excision at the time of initial rhinoplasty. In such cases, it is best to wait until the nose has healed and then to perform excision in the office setting with the patient's consent after several weeks or months.

Effective nasal base narrowing can be achieved only by combining internal vestibular floor excision and nostril sill excision with external alar wedge excision, if the surgeon decides to perform nasal base reduction. A crescent-shaped excision is very effective for this purpose. This excision also allows maximum preservation of the natural curvature of the alar rim. The internal vestibular floor piece of the excised crescent should correspond to one third of the total piece, with the remaining two thirds composed of the sill and the alar base (Fig. 16.30).

The starting point of the crescent on the alar base should not go beyond the 9 o'clock position and should finish on the vestibular side of the nasal sill after being detached from the base as a bow with a 45° opening. The lower incision should not sit on the alar crease, but rather should pass a few millimeters from the alar crease (Fig. 16.31).

16.4.1 Over-Projection Surgery Due to Septum/Nasal Spine

Over-projection can be caused merely by the septum and/or the nasal spine. The tip will be deprojected by resection of the excessive portion of the caudal septum and/or the nasal spine that pushes in the upward direction (pedestal) (Fig. 16.32).

This resection not only decreases projection, but also shortens the nose. If some increase in rotation is desired, extra resection can be performed anteroseptally, whereas the posterior septal angle should be used for extra resection when the aim is to achieve a decrease in rotation (Fig. 16.33).

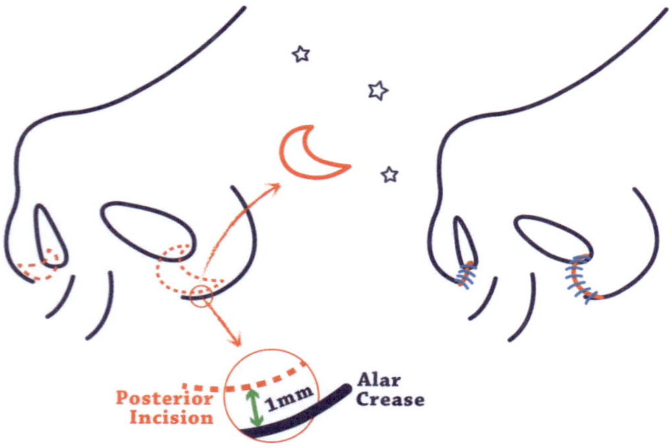

Fig. 16.30 Crescent-shape alar base reduction

An inverted "V" resection in the anterior septal direction, as indicated by **A** in Fig. 16.33, increases rotation, whereas resection from the posterior septal angle and nasal spine, as indicated by **P**, drops the tip downward.

Although the amount of resection depends on the case, care should be taken to avoid over-resection. Once the tip surgery has been completed, the columella should lightly touch the caudal septum when pushed in the cranial direc-

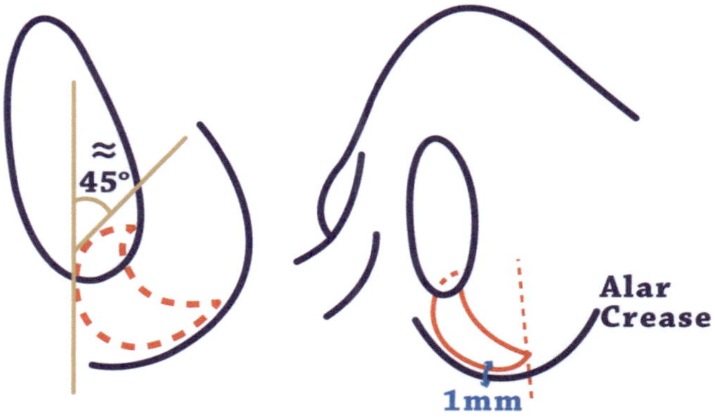

Fig. 16.31 The lower incision of external alar wedge excision should not sit on the alar crease or sill. The external incision then should be turned internally, being detached from the base, like a bow with a 45° opening

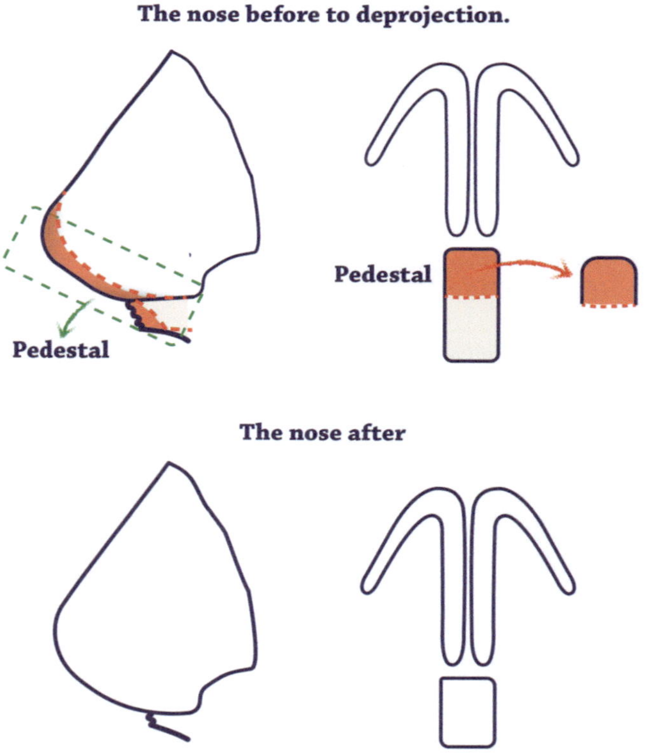

Fig. 16.32 Resection of the excess part of septum nasal spin complex (pedestal) normalized the tip projection. The red areas to be reduced are shown. (Supplementary Video 16.1)

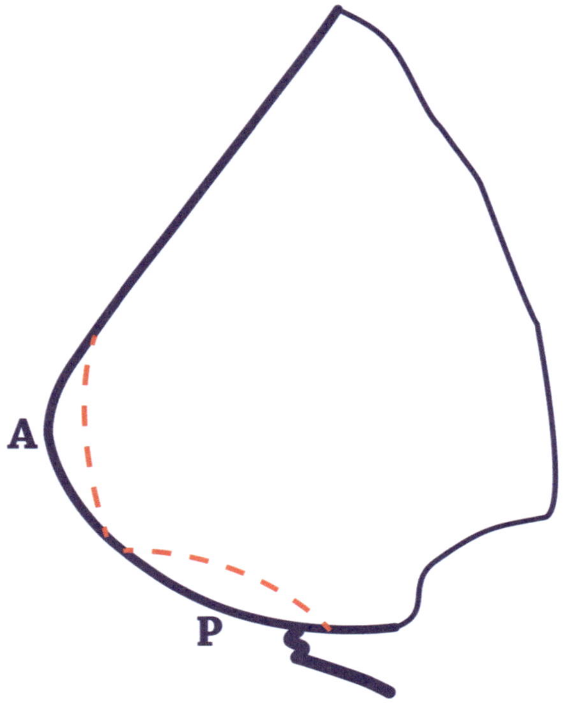

Fig. 16.33 After resection from "A" line, the rotation increases, whereas after "P" line, the tip drops downward

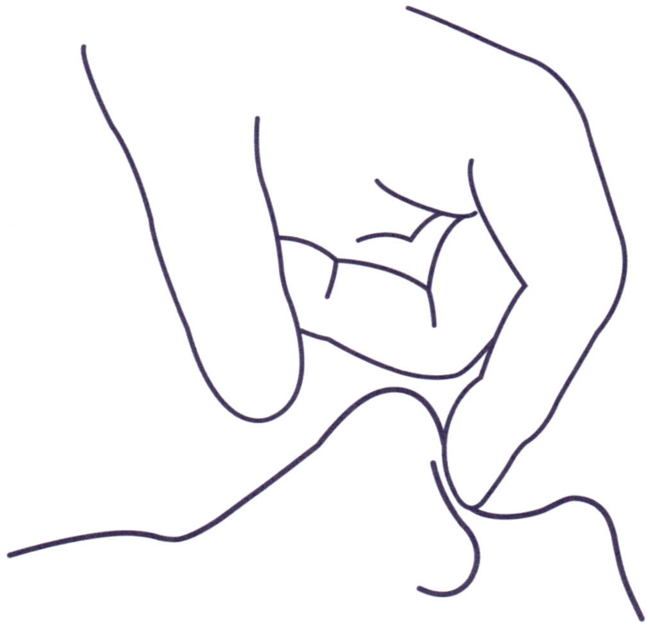

Fig. 16.34 Caudal septal excess should be checked meticulously. (Supplementary Video 16.2)

tion. The surgeon should avoid leaving too much space between the columella and the septum. The tip–septum association is checked intraoperatively by pushing the tip in the cranial direction with the index finger (Fig. 16.34).

Any septal hypertrophy can be resected with the closed or open approach.

The following section takes a closer look at both of these approaches, with examples.

16.4.1.1 Case 7: Resection with the Closed Approach

The closed approach is preferred in cases with an over-projected nose due to a pedestal, i.e., septum/nasal spine hypertrophy (Fig. 16.35).

Once tip deprojection has been achieved by septum and nasal spine resection, as well as nasal hump resection, the surgeon proceeds to the second stage. Reprojection, i.e., achievement of tip stability and definition, is done in the second stage. In the case with endonasal access shown in Fig. 16.35, a columellar strut and cup graft sufficed for this purpose.

Although the patient still had a slightly over-projected appearance due to problems with the forehead and chin (pseudo-over-projection), the projection was obviously in the ideal position (Fig. 16.36).

16.4.1.2 Case 8: Resection with the Open Approach

In the case presented in Fig. 16.37, over-projection was caused by caudal septal hypertrophy. The open approach was preferred in this case.

16.4.1.3 Case 9

The extreme tip projection, stem from caudal septal hypertrophy, has led to a "tension tip" deformity, causing the upper lip to be pulled anterosuperiorly. Tip rotation is appropriate. A significant part of the dorsal hump is cartilaginous. Resecting the excess parts of cartilaginous septum (dorsal and caudal) was the cornerstone to achieving ideal dorsal profile. The long-term result shows that the diagnosis and treatment are right (Fig. 16.38).

16.4.2 Over-Projection Surgery in Cases with Alar Cartilage Hypertrophy

Although hypertrophy of the entire alar cartilage represents a major cause of over-projection, isolated hypertrophy of only the lateral or medial/middle crus may also be responsible for over-projection (Fig. 16.39).

In all three cases, surgery was performed to resect the hypertrophic segments. The vertical alar resection (VAR) technique is an effective method for deprojection.

Evaluation of the preoperative and postoperative photographs based on four parameters (projection, rotation, symmetry, volume) showed that the VAR technique is effective for correction of both over-projected and broad, under-

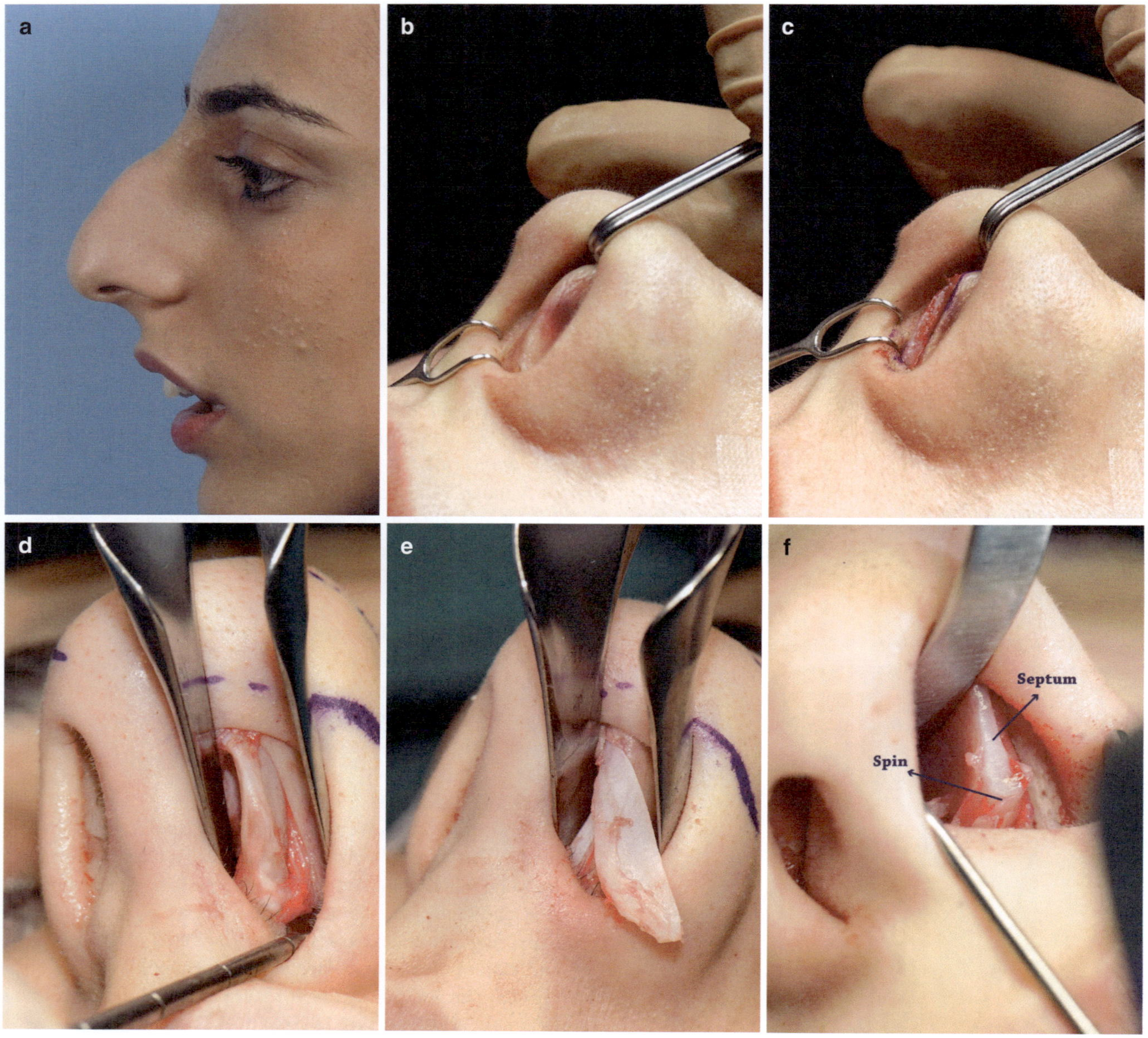

Fig. 16.35 (**a**) The tip is dramatically over-projected due to over development caudal septum. (**b**, **c**) The procedure begins with complete transfixion incision. (**d**) This incision is preferred as it interrupts the ligamentous attachment between the caudal septum and the feet of the medial crura releasing some of the anterior support on the tip. This step is followed by bilateral elevation of the septum from the mucoperichondrium. (**e**) Caudal septal excess is resected. (**f–i**) Then, the nasal spine is resected. A rongeur, osteotome, or drill may be used for spine resection

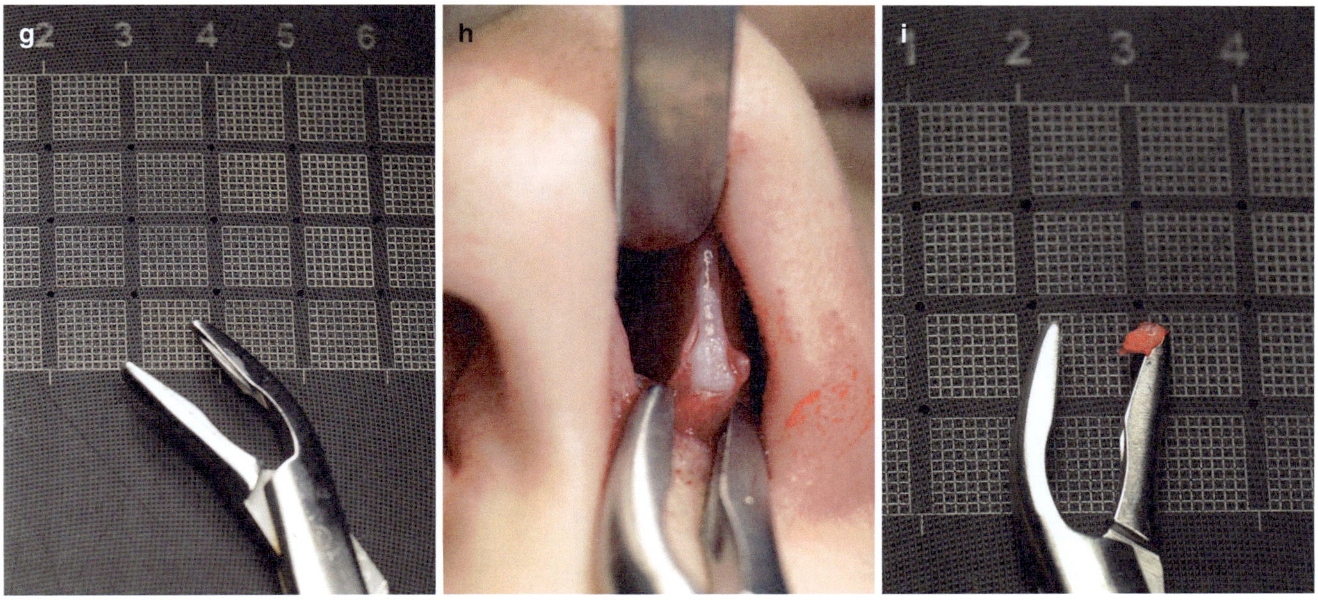

Fig. 16.35 (continued)

rotated nasal tips, and that it produces long-lasting results with respect to the projection, rotation, and shape of the tip.

We have successfully used the VAR technique with both open and closed approaches to correct over-projection of the nasal tip secondary to overdeveloped alar cartilage.

Regardless of the cause of overdevelopment, the VAR technique can be used in all types of alar cartilage hypertrophy as long as certain differences are taken onto account. The following section describes how the technique can be applied to three different types of alar cartilage hypertrophy.

16.4.3 Over-Projection Due to Entirely Hypertrophic Alar Cartilage

In cases where all segments of the alar cartilage that constitute the nasal tip are hypertrophic, the lateral crus and middle/medial crus segments should be shortened individually. Choosing the domal arch as the resection site allows simultaneous shortening of the lateral crus and the middle crus. Any excess of the middle crus under the dome point and the lateral crus to the lateral aspect is resected with the dome (VAR). A greater amount of resection would lead to a greater degree of tip deprojection. Therefore, gradual resection should be preferred over aggressive resection. The tip–dorsum relation should be respected during resection and the tip should never be deprojected to below the caudal dorsal level (Fig. 16.40).

Technical Note: Radix and dorsum projection should be brought to the ideal level before VAR. The shape of the resection must be a trapezoid; that is, the caudal edge of the resected alar cartilage should be designed to be shorter, while the cranial edge should be longer. The caudal edge of the lateral crus will be projected upward as soon as the flaps remaining after resection are sutured, bringing the caudal edge level with the cranial edge (Fig. 16.41).

As discussed in the previous chapters, bringing the caudal edge level with the cranial edge leads to a good anatomical configuration to the tip; a nasal tip with this configuration becomes more stable in the lateral nasal wall and the alar rim, creating a broad surface where the skin will sit. This is particularly important for achieving tip stability in patients with thicker skin (Fig. 16.42).

Resection not only decreases the projection, but also resolves any configuration disturbance in the lateral and middle crus (excessive convex or concave lateral crus, elongated columella, etc.).

One of the most important advantages of VAR is the removal of tension on the alar cartilage. Resection removes tip-malpositioning propulsive forces from hypertrophic areas, and thus makes the tip more stable.

Technical Note: As the amount of material removed from the lateral crus increases, the tip bends backward, i.e., the rotation increases. The surgeon must keep in mind any need for extra rotation (Fig. 16.43).

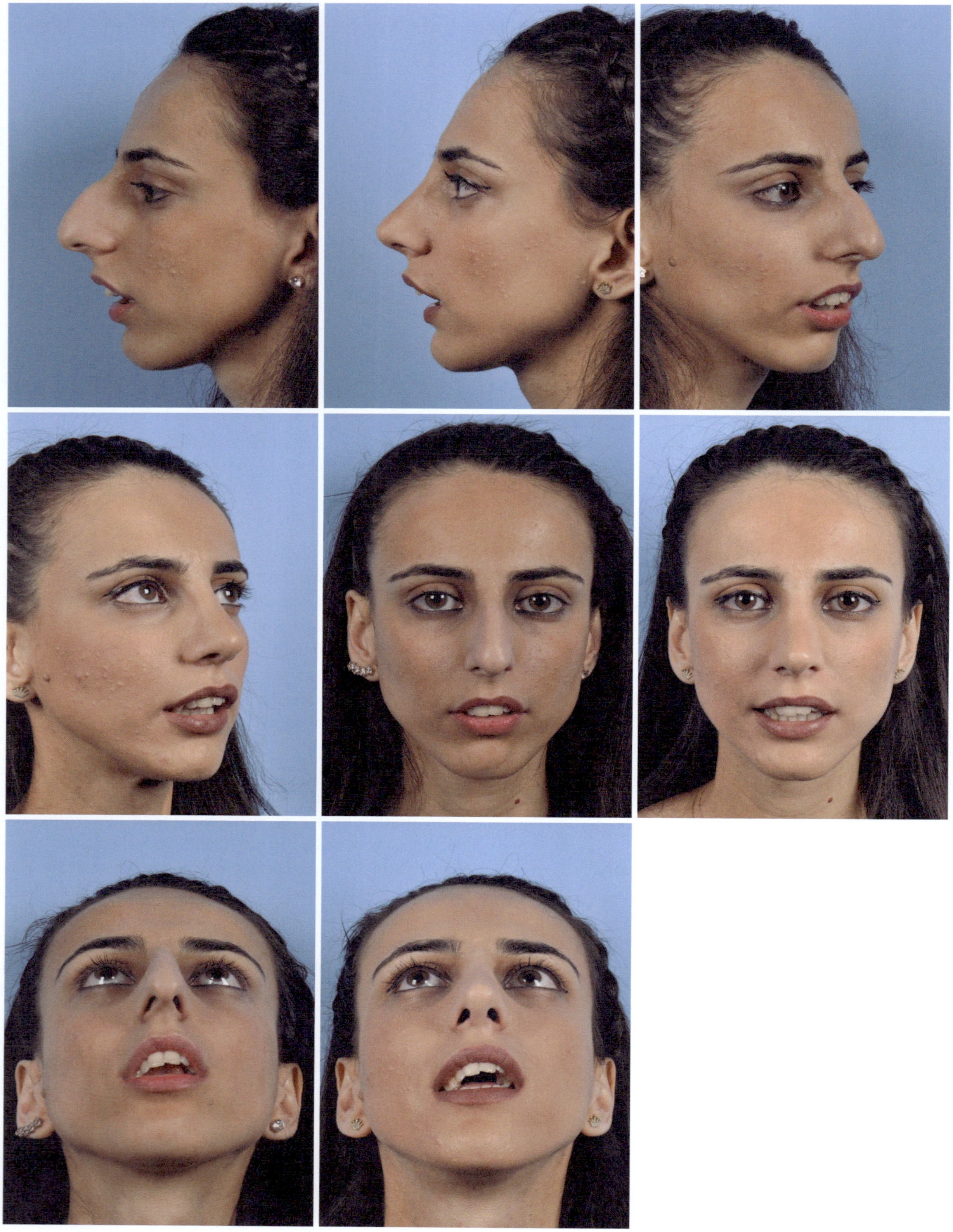

Fig. 16.36 (**a–h**) Preoperative and postoperative photographs: the dorsal hump has been corrected. This is classic tension tip by a large caudal septum and spin that pulls the lip and columella forward. The excess caudal septum was resected. In this way, the tip was deprojected and then reprojected with a strut and transdomal suture. The result is a nose that is well shaped but seems slightly larger because of deficiency of the chin and sloping forehead

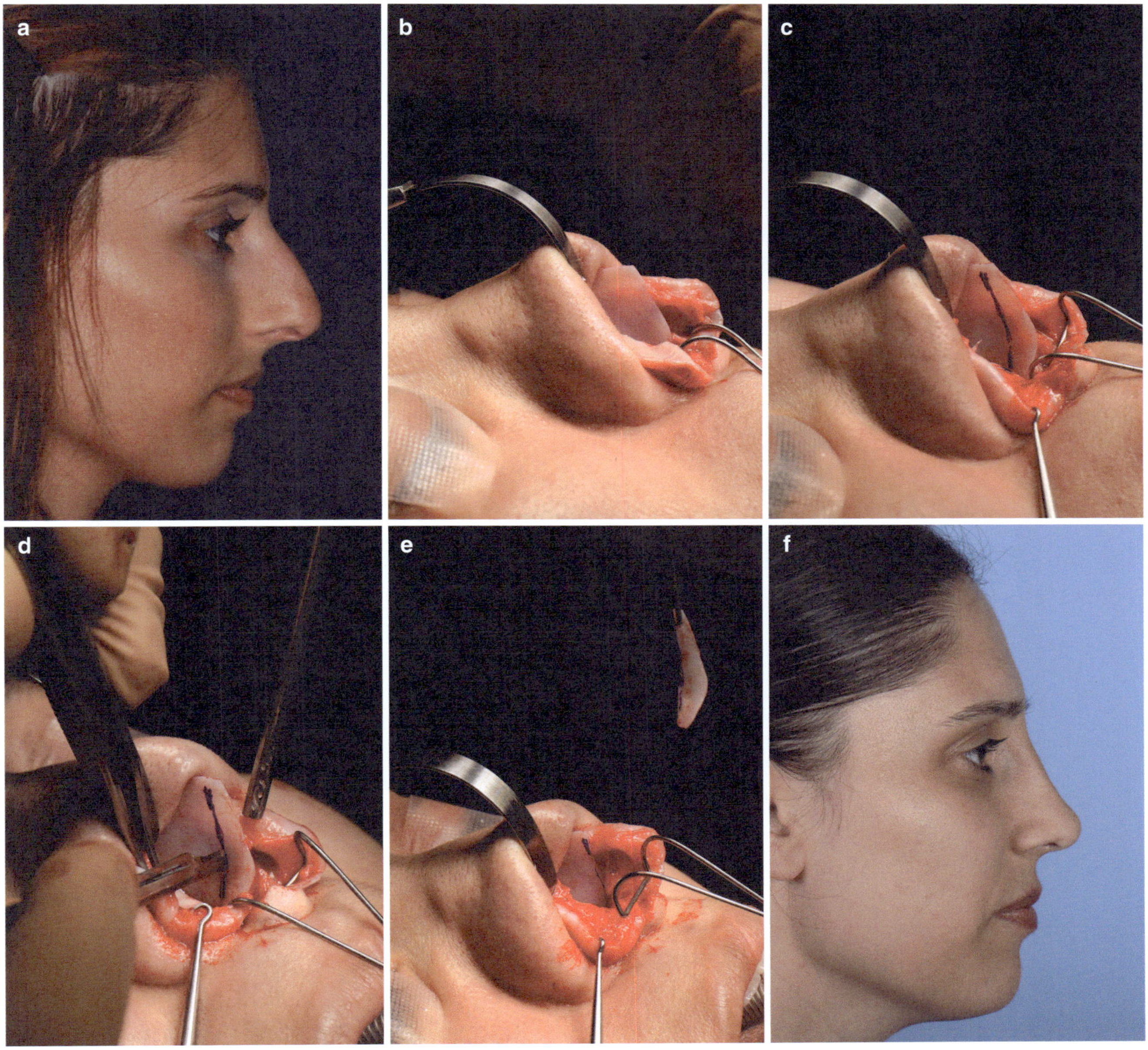

Fig. 16.37 (**a**) A patient with an overdeveloped pedestal who underwent rhinoplasty. (**b**) The septum is accessed from between the crura. The mucoperichondrium is elevated on both sides. (**c**) The excision was designed to be parallel to the anterior aspect of the caudal septum. (**d**) Then, the excessive septal cartilage and nasal spine were resected. (**e**) Excised part of the septum. (**f**) Postoperative lateral view. The tension tip deformity has been corrected, and improved upper lip position and subnasale

If the medial and lateral crura on one side are longer (taller dome), it will be necessary for the surgeon to resect more cartilage from this side, thus reducing the height of the lateral crura more thereon, such that the two lateral crura are equalized after the operation.

Regarding the stability and definition of the new tip formed after deprojection, final projection is achieved by complementary procedures, including columellar strut, cap graft, alar batten graft, etc. (reprojection) (Fig. 16.44).

16.4.3.1 Case 10

This case presented with an over-projected and wide nasal tip and hanging infratip lobule due to hypertrophy of the entire alar cartilage and caudal septal hypertrophy. The tip was markedly over-projected, and the nasolabial angle was full and anteriorly oriented. The skin permits alar cartilage to show through in relief, resulting in a bifid tip and infratip lobule (Fig. 16.45).

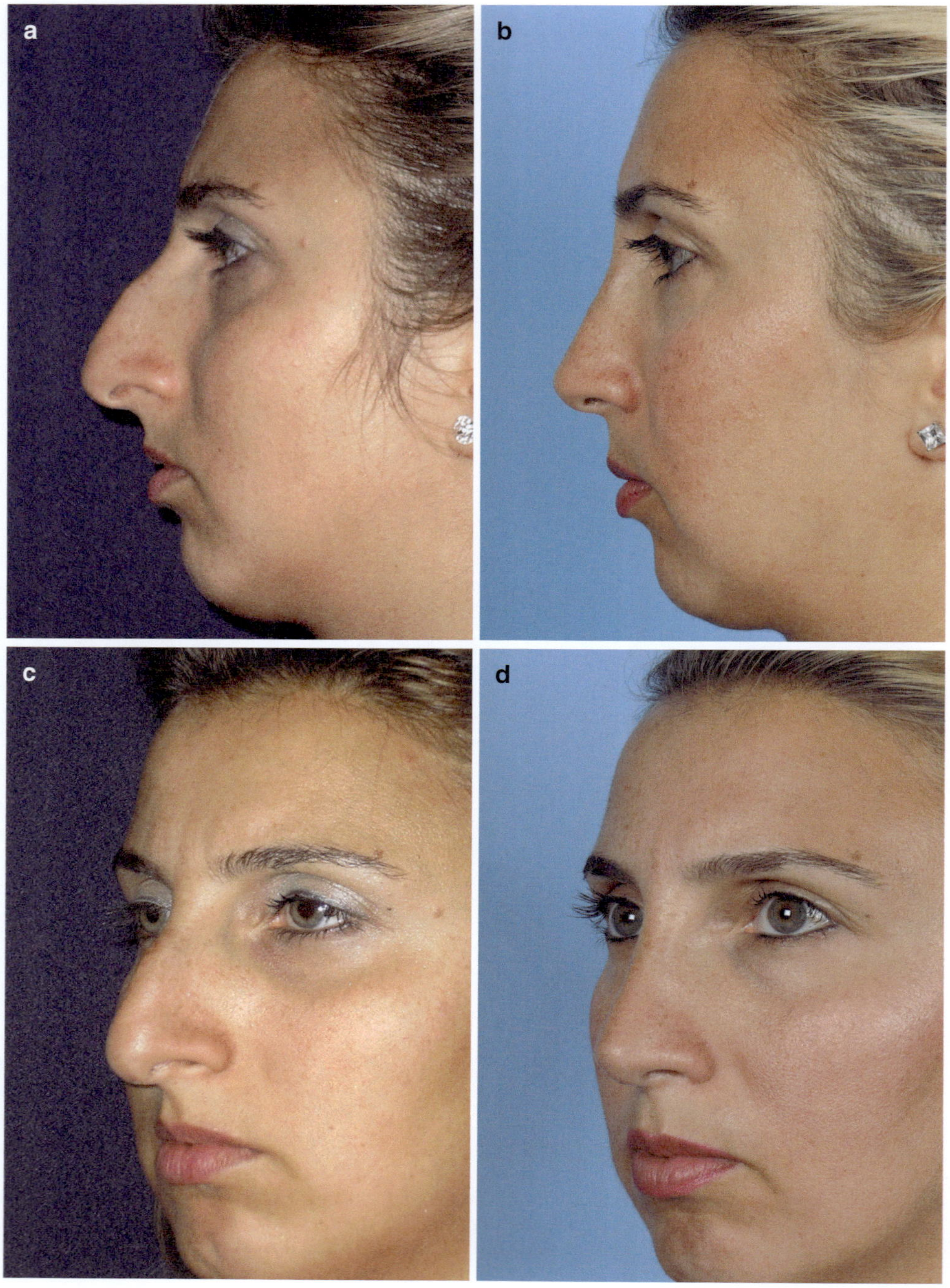

Fig. 16.38 (**a**–**d**) Long-term result. Preoperative and 7-year postoperative photographs

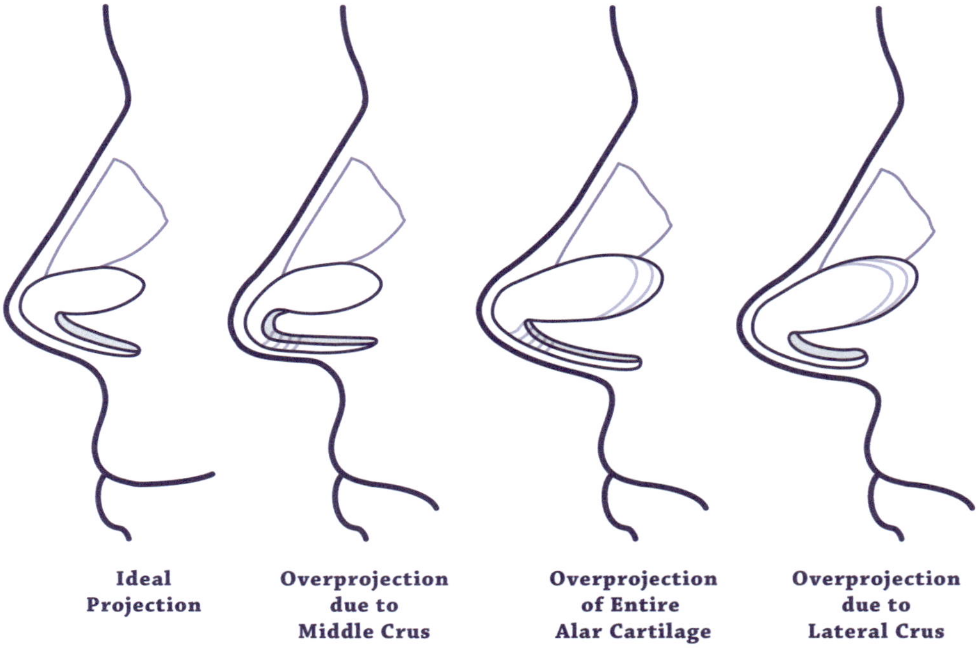

Fig. 16.39 Types of over-projected tip due to alar cartilages

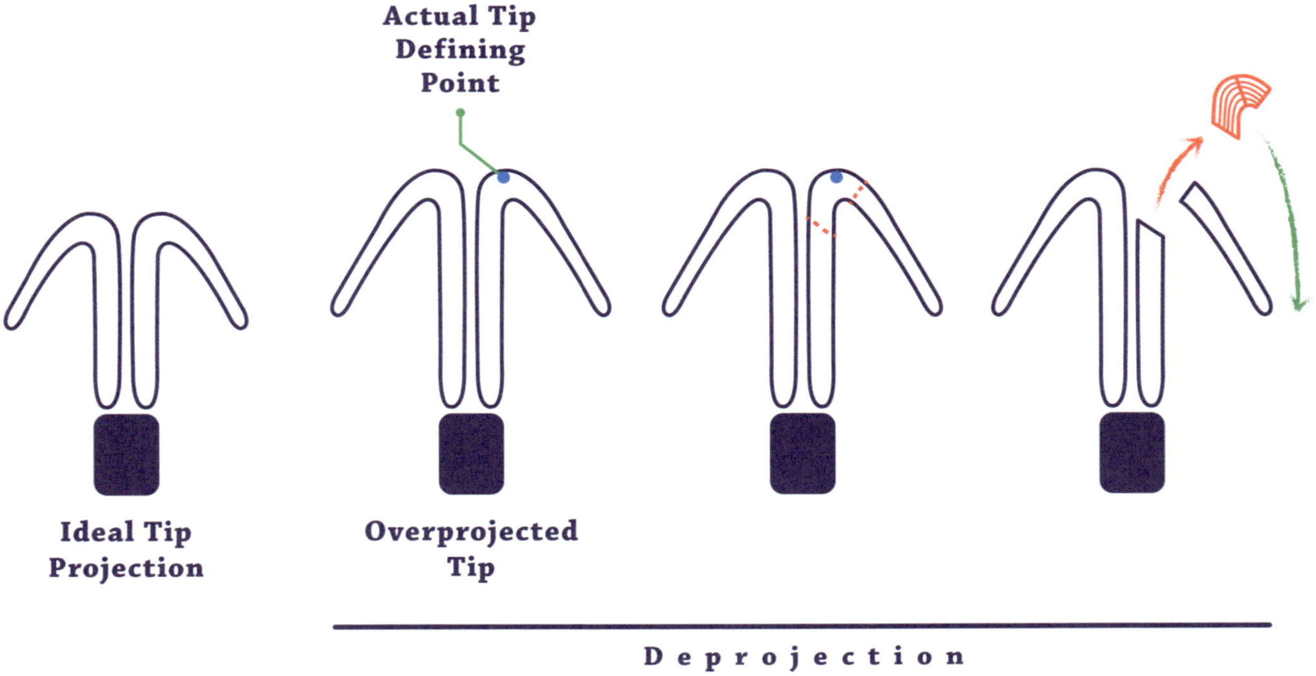

Fig. 16.40 Simultaneous shortening of the lateral crus and the middle crus

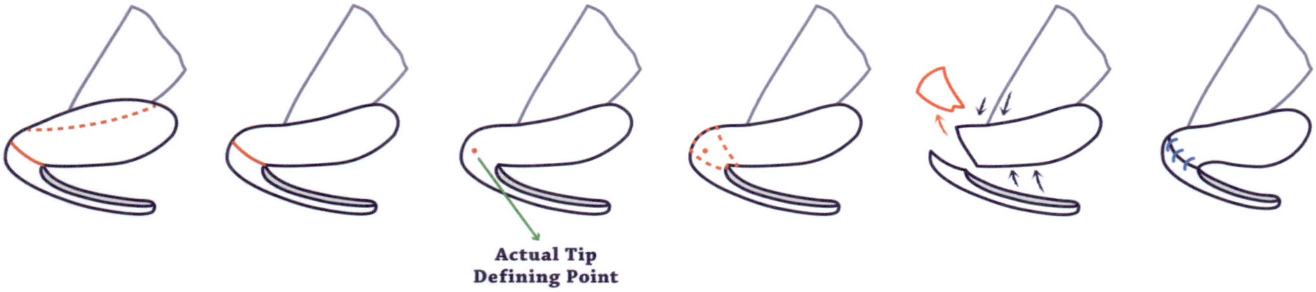

Fig. 16.41 Both projection and rotation can adjust with the same maneuver. (Supplementary Video 16.3)

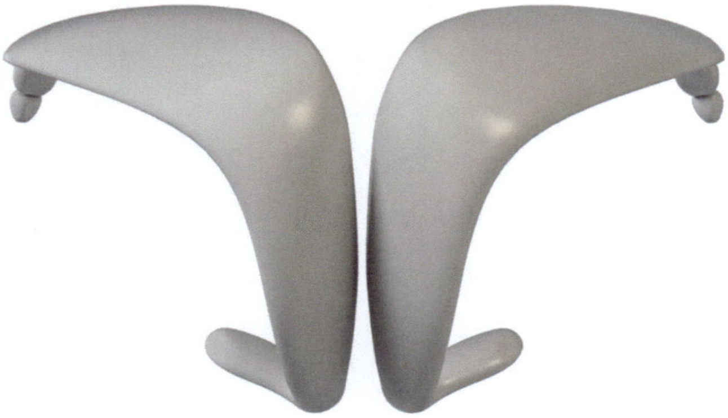

Fig. 16.42 The caudal aspect of the lateral crus should ideally be in the horizontal plane with the cephalic margin at the same level to it

Fig. 16.43 Any need for extra rotation can be achieved with trimming of lateral crura

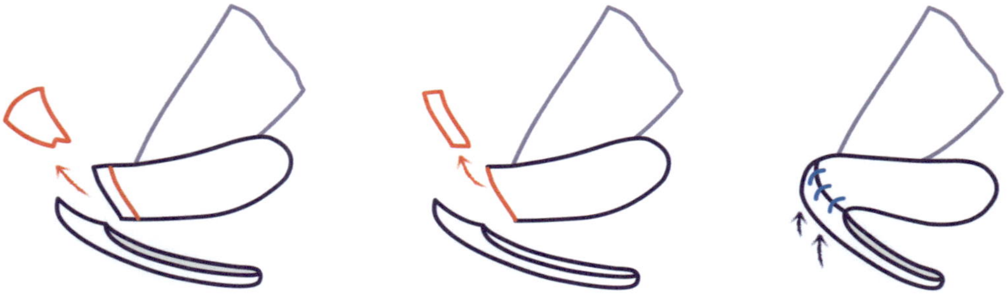

Fig. 16.44 Complementary procedures of resection, including columellar strut, cap graft, alar batten graft, etc. (reprojection)

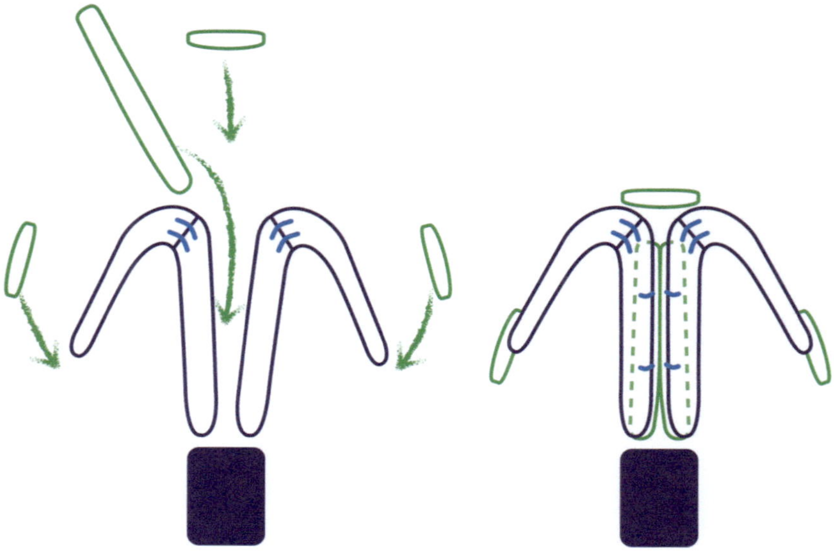

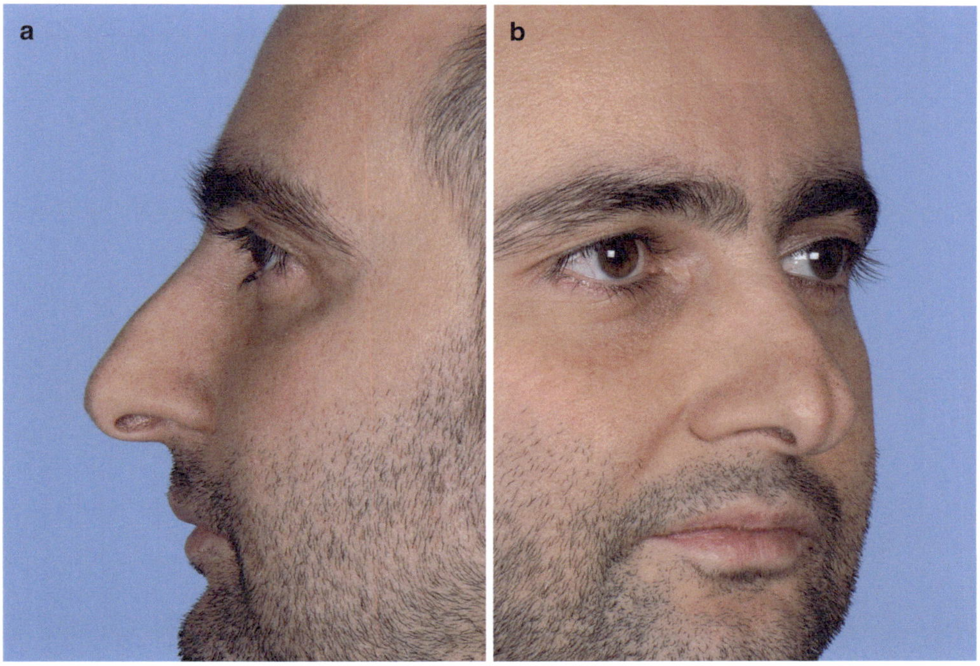

Fig. 16.45 (**a**, **b**) The tip is over-projected, bulbous, and bifid. Large pedestal with caudal excess pushing the tip. This is typical deprojection–reprojection rhinoplasty for an overprotected tip

As discussed above, correction of the over-projected tip proceeds according to two main steps: (1) deprojection and (2) reprojection.

In terms of deprojection, in this case, both the medial and lateral crura and the hypertrophic septum were shortened. Then, the alar cartilages were reconstructed to increase the stability and strength of the tip complex (reprojection). The details of each step are presented here:

1. Deprojection

In this case, the open approach was used to initially resect the overgrowth of the posterior septal angle (Fig. 16.46).

Figure 16.47 shows a view of the nasal tip cartilages after elevating the soft tissue envelope, showing the convexity and the entire overdeveloped alar cartilages.

The dotted point shows the most projected point of the alar cartilages (dome point) (Fig. 16.48).

Both of the alar cartilages were transected from a point 5 mm under the dome point (Fig. 16.49).

Alar cartilages were dissected from the vestibular skin by a minimum of 10 mm up to the dome point. It is necessary to include the more lateral aspect in the dissection (Fig. 16.50).

After dissection, the excessive part of the lateral crus can always be seen. The lateral crus should then be cut obliquely (Fig. 16.51).

Excess trapezoid alar cartilage is shown in Fig. 16.52.

The same excision was performed on the contralateral side (Fig. 16.53).

After VAR of the alar cartilages, the two stumps were sutured together. This suture was similar to the transdomal mattress suture. For this purpose, 5-0 PDS suture represents a good choice (Fig. 16.54).

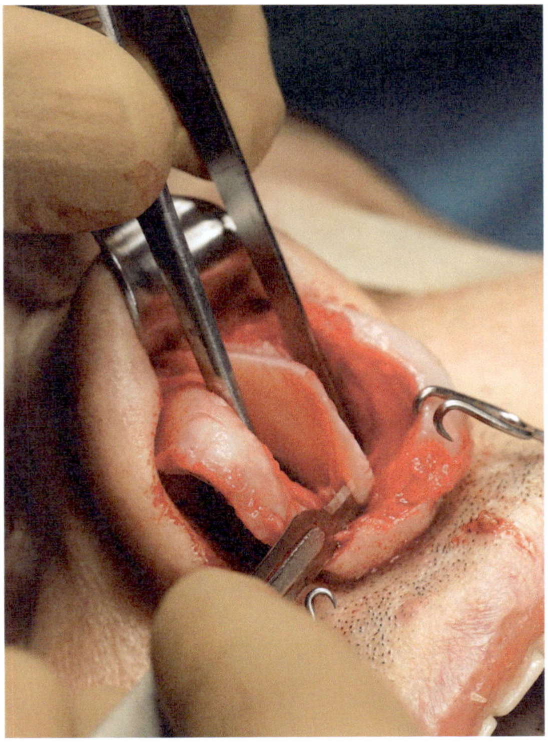

Fig. 16.46 Caudal septal trimming

Figure 16.55 presents side views of both deprojected tip cartilages after suturing. Configuration defects of alar cartilages were also improved.

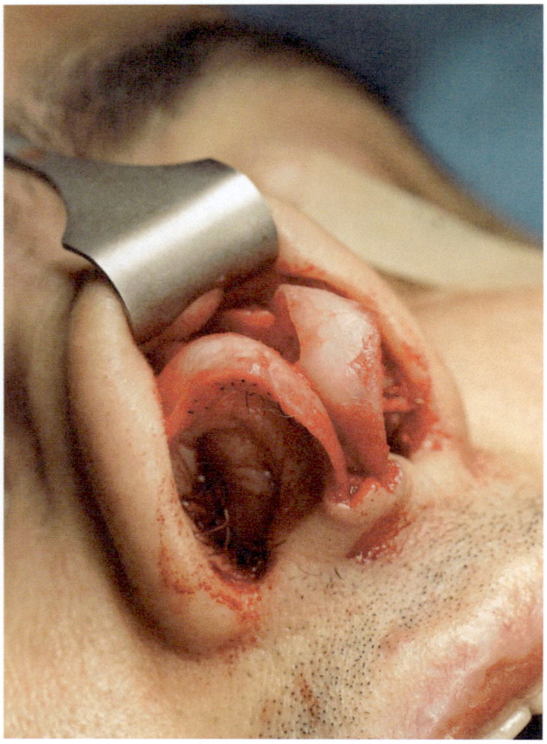

Fig. 16.47 Open approach revealing large alar cartilages

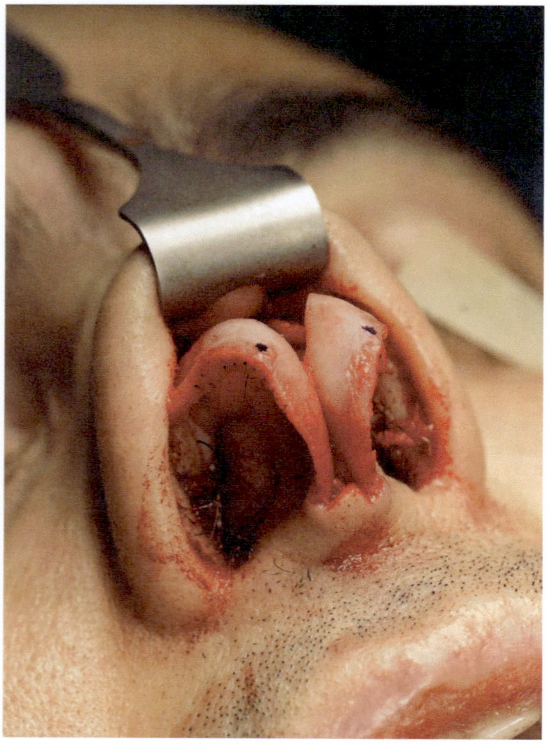

Fig. 16.48 Actual dome points marked

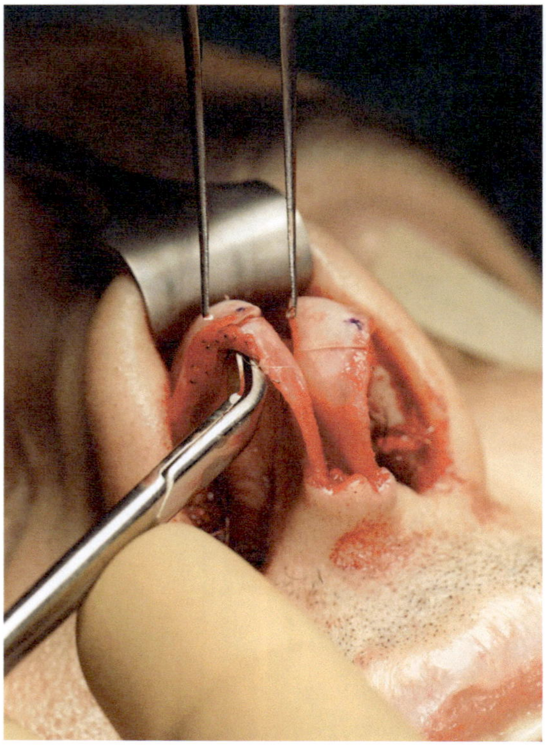

Fig. 16.49 Alar cartilages divided transversely just below the domes

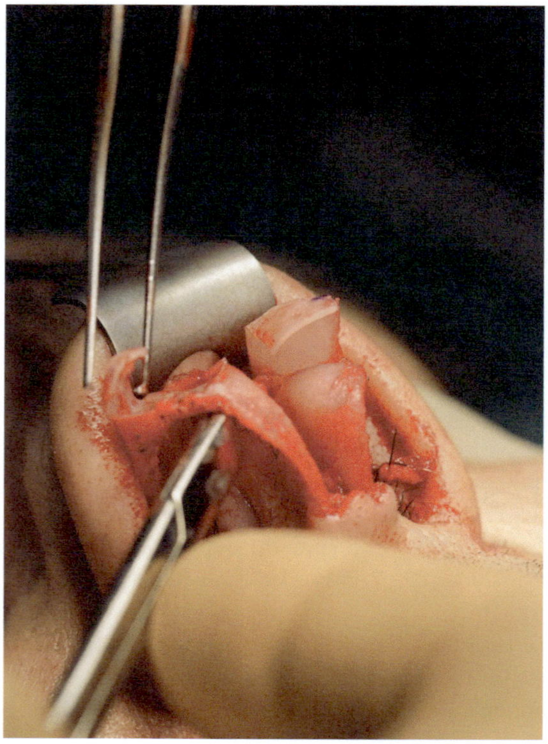

Fig. 16.50 Lateral segments dissected free

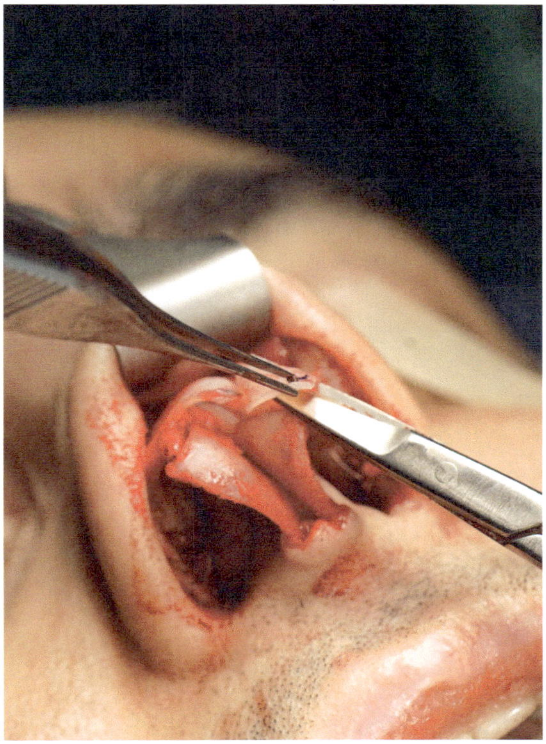

Fig. 16.51 Segment dissected and then cut obliquely

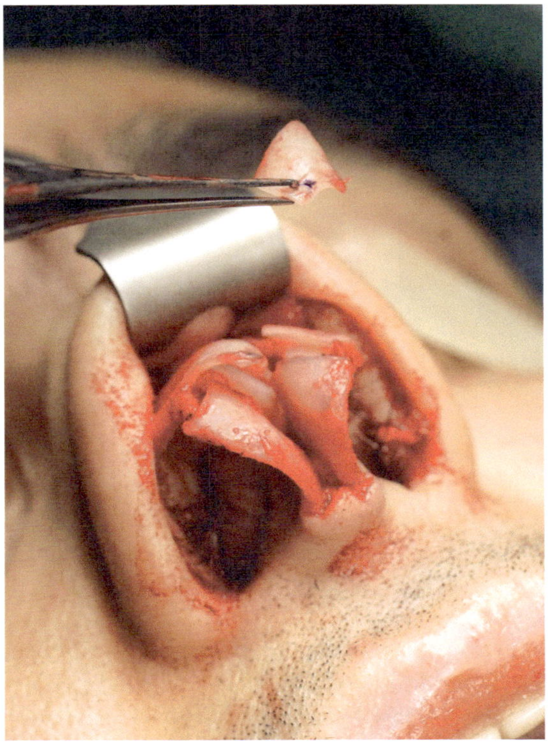

Fig. 16.52 Excess trapezoid alar cartilage contains both middle and lateral crus

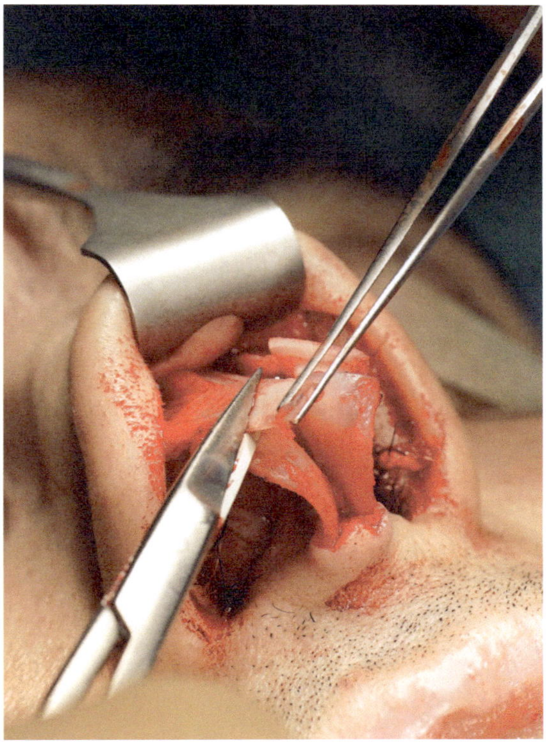

Fig. 16.53 Same procedure contralateral side

2. Reprojection

To achieve stability of the newly formed alar cartilage from the base to the lateral crus, resulting in the final definition and projection result, we apply an alar batten graft, columellar strut, dome-equalizing suture, and onlay tip graft in all VAR cases.

Placement of bilateral alar batten grafts strengthen the alar side walls. Pockets are created for alar batten grafts in the alar sidewalls below the alar groove. Alar batten grafts are placed in pockets along the alar sidewalls. The trapezoidal excess of alar cartilage represents an ideal source of alar batten grafts. Before inserting these grafts, a flat surface should be obtained by crushing (Fig. 16.56).

A columellar strut is essential to strengthen the alar base (Fig. 16.57).

The two domes are now brought together via a single suture (dome-equalizing suture). This suture connects the caudal corners of the domes, which should be bound together tightly. Permanent suture material should be used for this suture.

The dome-equalizing suture serves three main purposes:

- Equalizes the dome.
- Achieves the ideal interdomal angle.
- Consolidates the ideal relation between the caudal cranial edges of the lateral crus.

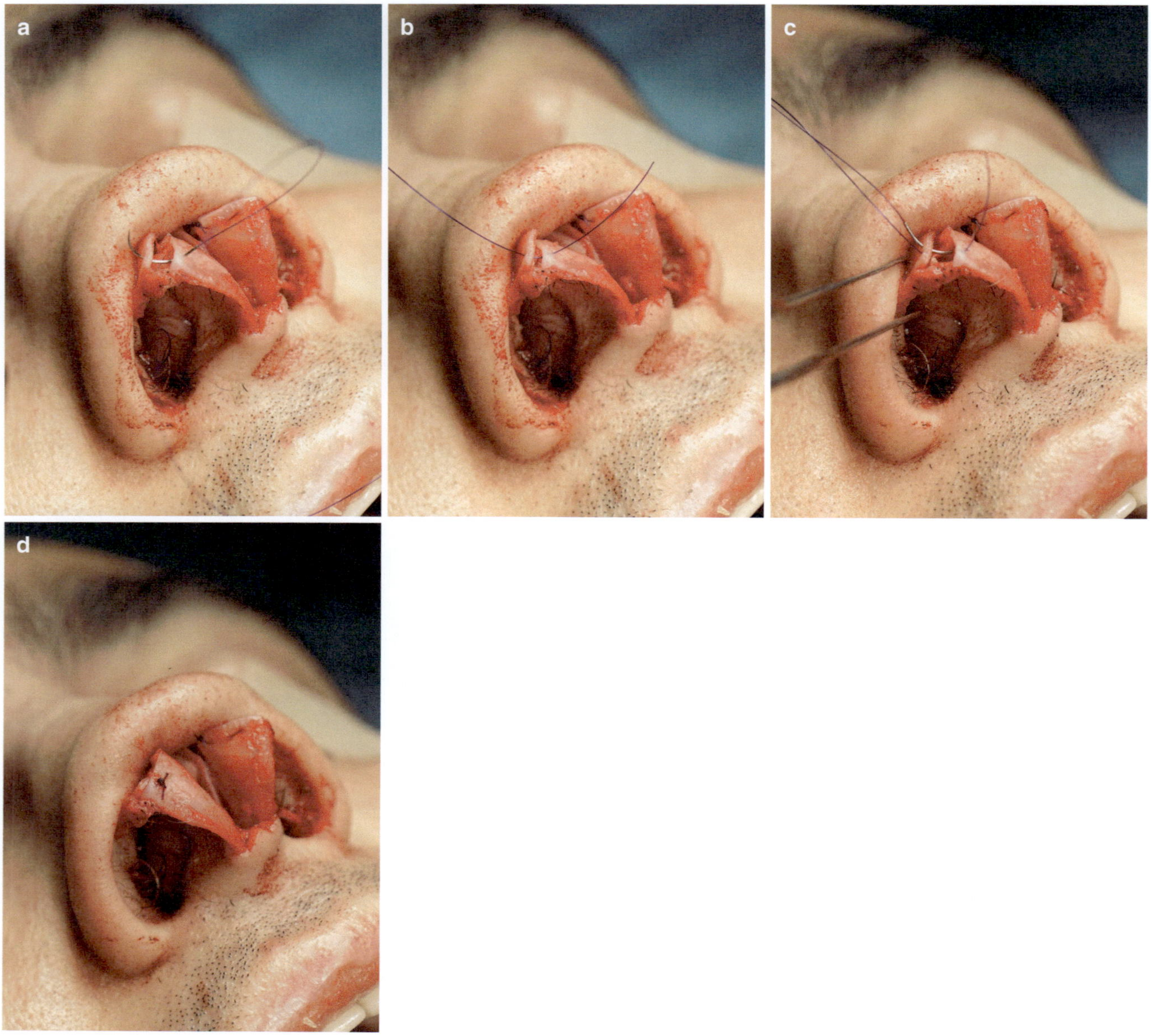

Fig. 16.54 (**a–d**) Free edges reapproximated; domes recreated with 5-0 absorbable suture

The surgeon must then create the final projection. The ideal relationship between the tip-defining point and the dorsum should provide a guide. In an ideal relation, the newly created tip-defining point should be 8 mm higher than the caudal end of the dorsum in men, and 10 mm higher in women. To achieve this, some projection should be applied to the tip at this stage using an onlay tip graft. A cap graft is the graft of choice, as it provides extra projection. A shield graft may be used as an alternative in thick-skinned patients, or when over-projection is needed. Onlay grafts not only allow for projection of the tip, but also provide definition (Fig. 16.58).

Oblique view showing an onlay tip graft. The graft is fixed with 6/0 absorbable sutures and the new dome points form the surface of the cup graft (Fig. 16.59).

Technical Note: In thick-skinned patients, the ideal relation created between the tip and the dorsum may be lost in the mid- to long-term, possibly due to thick skin. To avoid such problems, the movable tip must be associated with the septum (Fig. 16.60).

The posterior part of the newly created nasal tip and the nasal septum were sutured with 5/0 Prolene sutures. The suture starting from the medial edge of the lateral crus was knotted on the midline passing through the top of the septum and extending from the medial aspect of the lateral crus. In thick-skinned patients, increasing the alar support is a prerequisite for achieving a refined tip. For this purpose, the septum may be used to prepare a lateral crural graft 1 mm thick and 18–20 mm long.

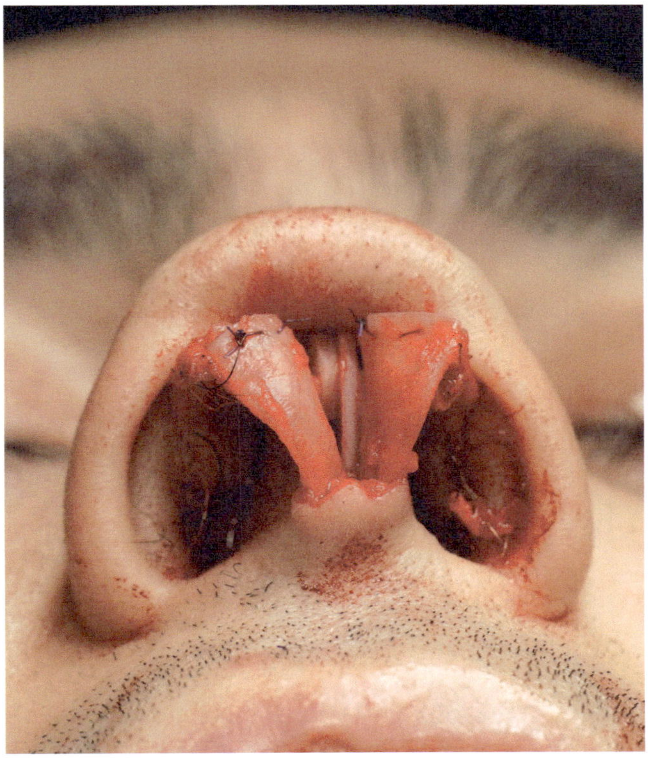

Fig. 16.55 Deprojected alar cartilages

The graft immediately adjacent to the cup graft terminates in a small pouch opened in the lateral nasal wall (Fig. 16.61).

The graft also camouflages the onlay tip graft. The pouch must be directed toward the outer canthus (Fig. 16.62).

The graft is placed on the contralateral side (Fig. 16.63).

The graft is sutured onto the lateral crus. As the suture passes through the vestibular skin, it must be absorbable. The caudal edge of the lateral crus must be properly aligned to avoid extending out of the edges. The operation is finished by correcting the width of the nasal base according to the decreased projection (Fig. 16.64).

A crescent-shaped resection is the best choice for narrowing the nasal base (Fig. 16.65).

After resection, the subcutaneous layer is approximated with 5-0 PDS sutures (Fig. 16.66).

Mattress sutures are preferred to close the skin (Fig. 16.67).

The dorsum is straight. Tip projection has been lessened to a more aesthetic level. The tip is also rotated slightly, and the pedestal has been narrowed. The bifidity is also corrected (Fig. 16.68).

16.4.3.2 Case 11

We can use the VAR technique in thin-skinned patients if there is no risk of resection. It is important to note that if an

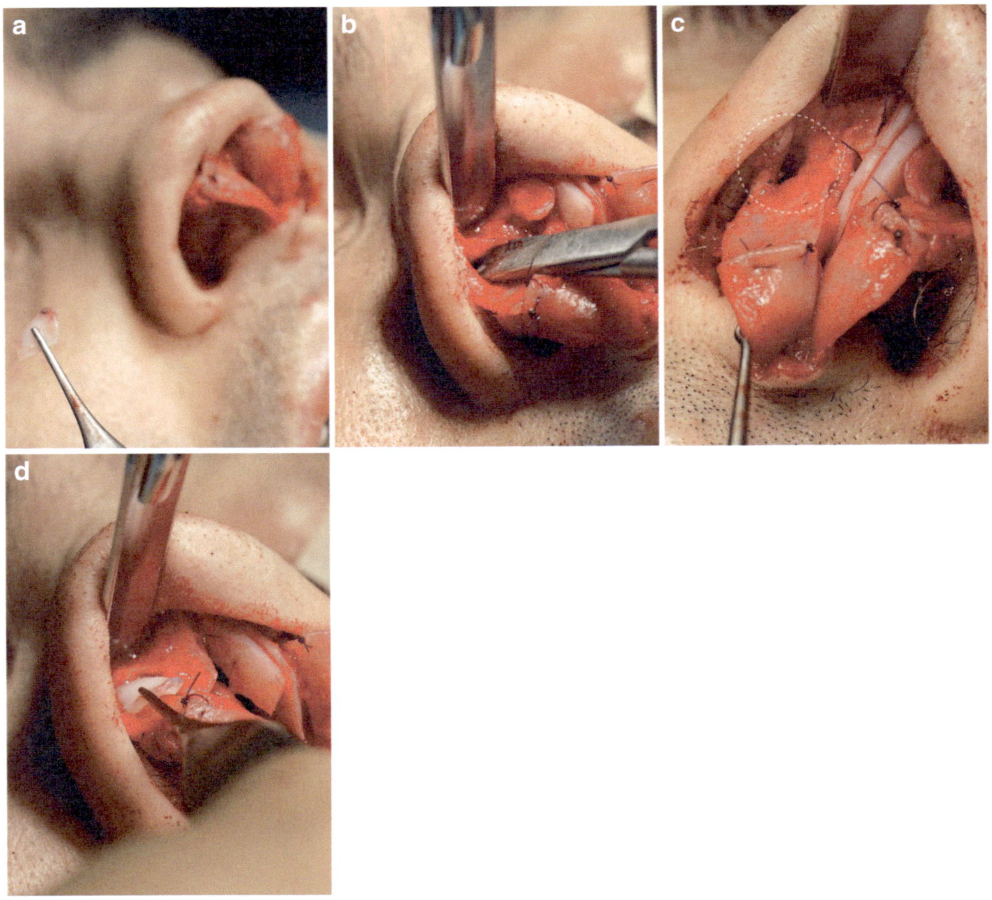

Fig. 16.56 (**a–d**) Placement of alar batten graft

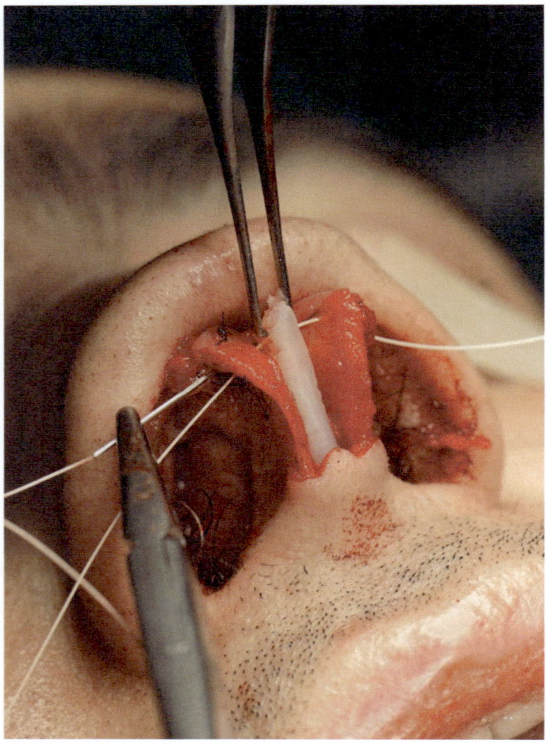

Fig. 16.57 Columellar strut fashioned from septal cartilage

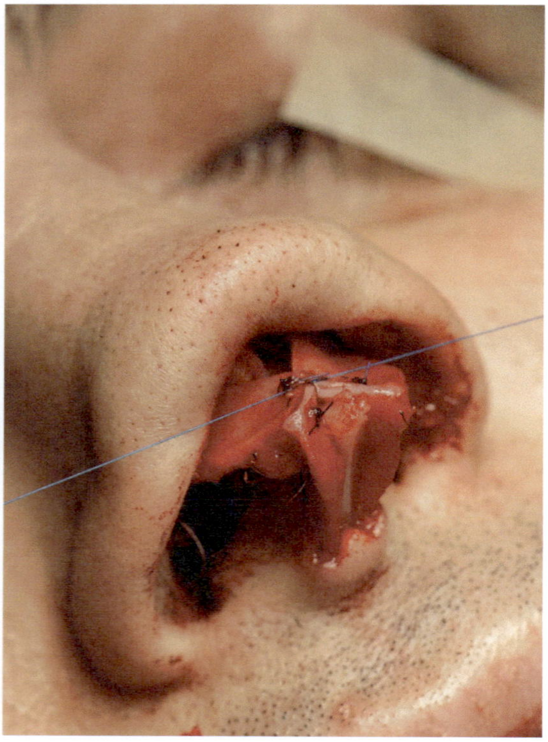

Fig. 16.58 Dome-equalizing suture

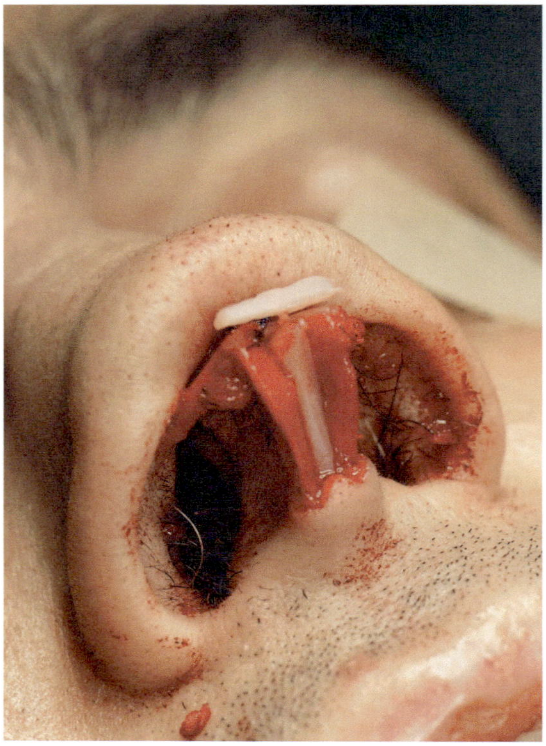

Fig. 16.59 Cap graft sutured over domes with absorbable suture

onlay tip graft is used, it must be camouflaged. This figure shows an example of a patient with over-projection and thin skin. The VAR technique was used, as described below, to cut a predetermined length of the medial and lateral crus that was then tucked to reduce projection of the tip (Fig. 16.69).

The VAR technique involved vertical dome division and modest excision of the lateral and medial crural elements for nasal tip deprojection. The medial/middle crura were then sutured together with a columellar strut. The excess part of the lateral crus was used for tip definition. Crescent-shaped alar base reduction surgery was then performed (Fig. 16.70).

Over-Projection Due to Hypertrophic Lateral Crus: The overdeveloped lateral crus pushed the nasal tip in the anterior and inferior directions, resulting in an over-projected tip with a drooping appearance.

The lateral crura were shortened for rotation and projection of the nasal tip. The VAR technique is an excellent choice for shortening the lateral crus. Removing a segment of the lateral crus lateral to the dome will fix both over-projected and drooping nasal tip pathologies.

Here, alar cartilages were divided vertically just lateral to the dome-defining point. Then, the overdeveloped

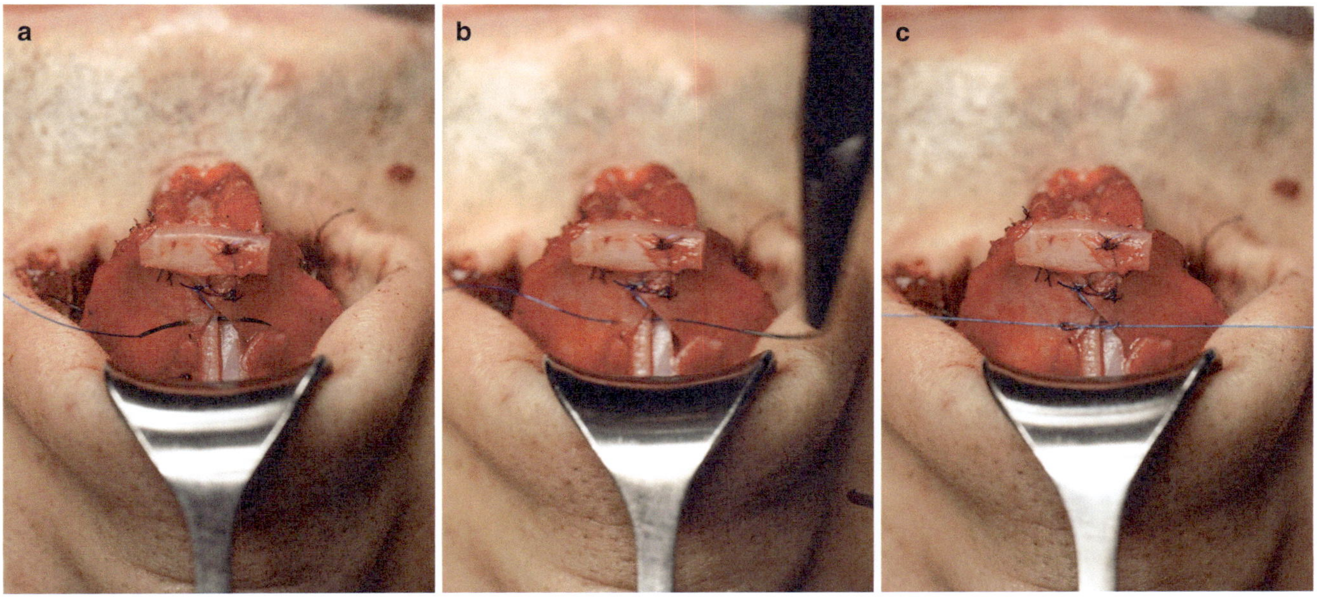

Fig. 16.60 (**a**–**c**) Newly formed alar arches fixed to septum with permanent suture

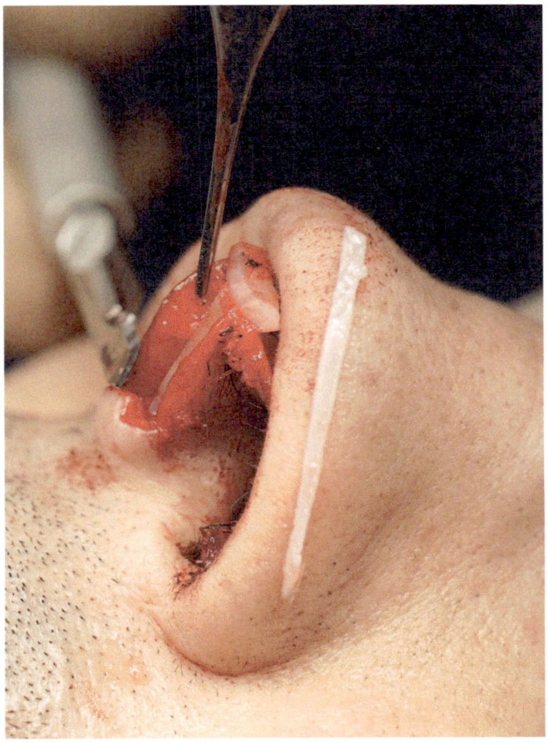

Fig. 16.61 A thin lateral crural graft

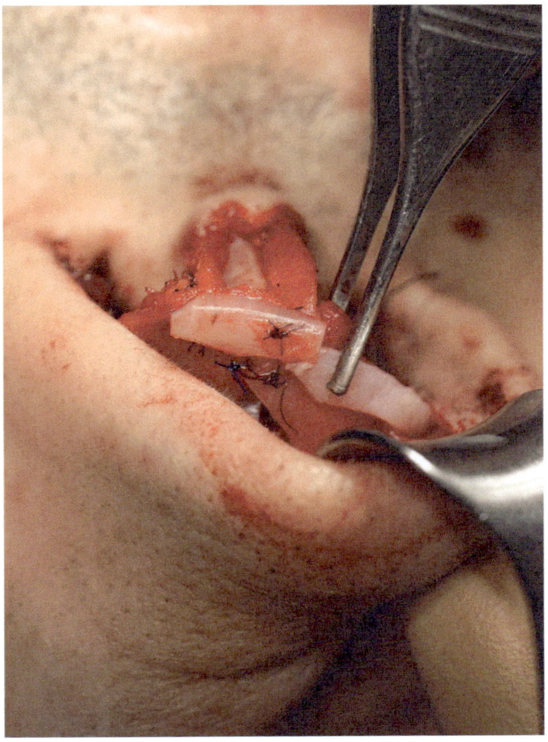

Fig. 16.62 Graft placed over the lateral crura

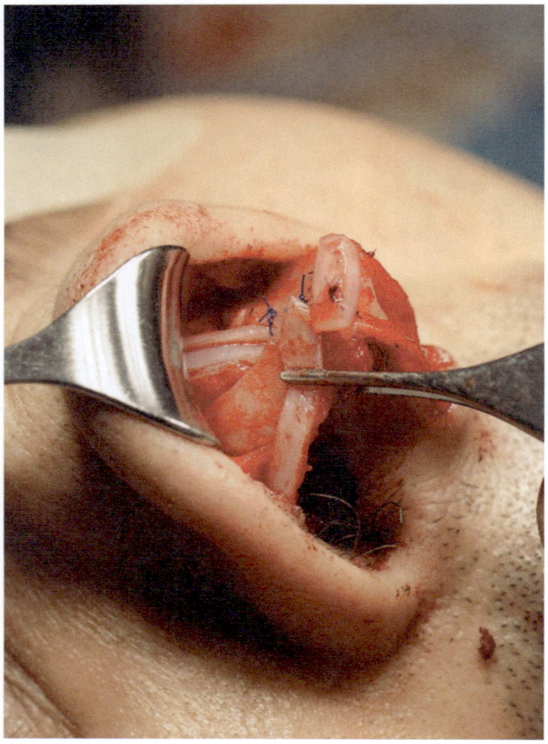

Fig. 16.63 Contralateral side

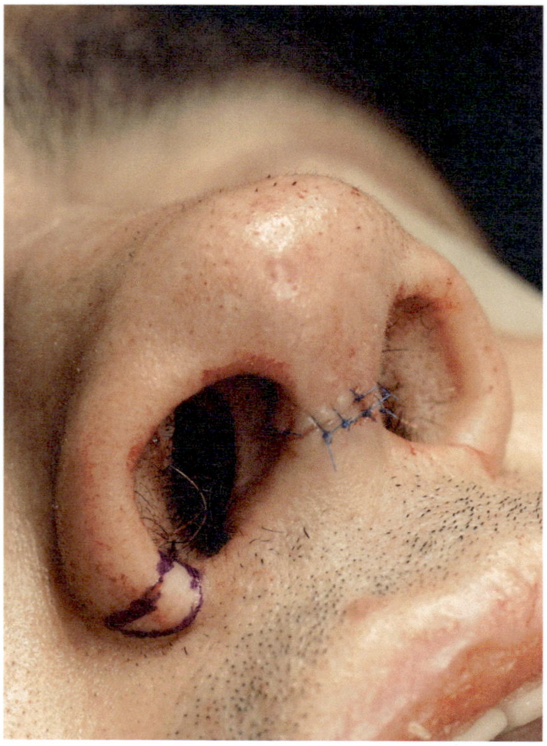

Fig. 16.65 After tip narrowing and deprojection, alar base flared; crescent-shape incisions marked

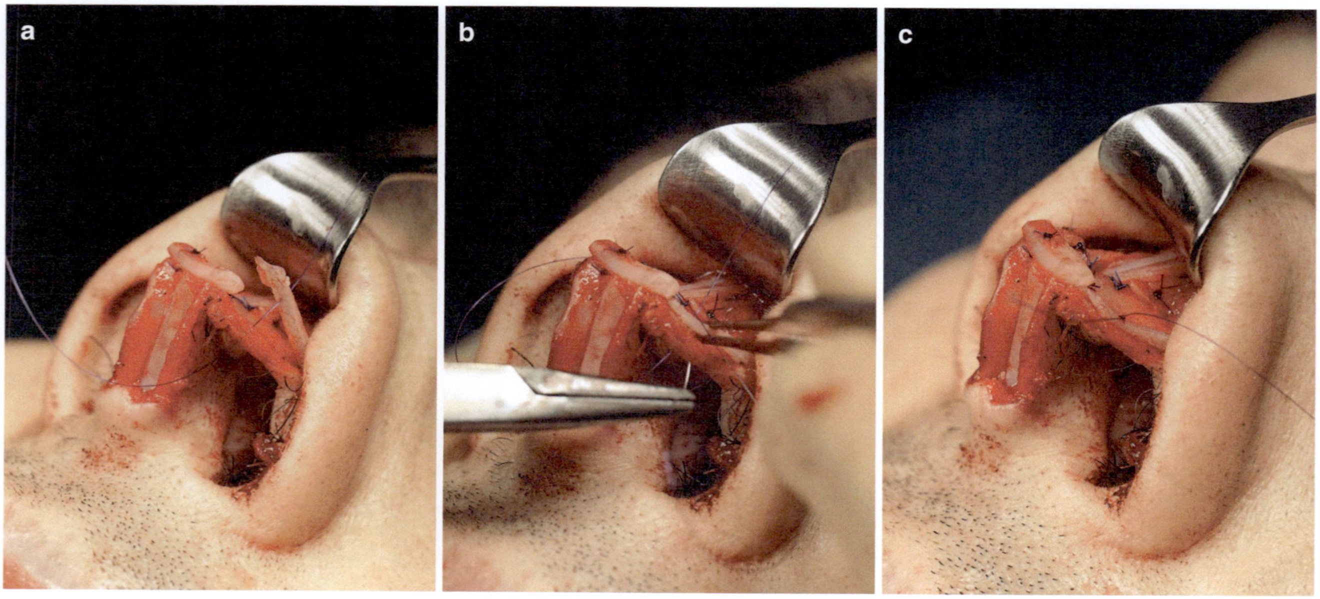

Fig. 16.64 (**a**–**c**) Absorbable suture was used

part was excised in a trapezoidal shape, and the two stumps were sutured together (retro-projection) (Fig. 16.71).

For reprojection and definition, a columellar strut, alar button graft and cup graft were inserted. While the septum is a good source of alar button and cap grafts, the trapezoidal piece was excised as a button graft (Fig. 16.72).

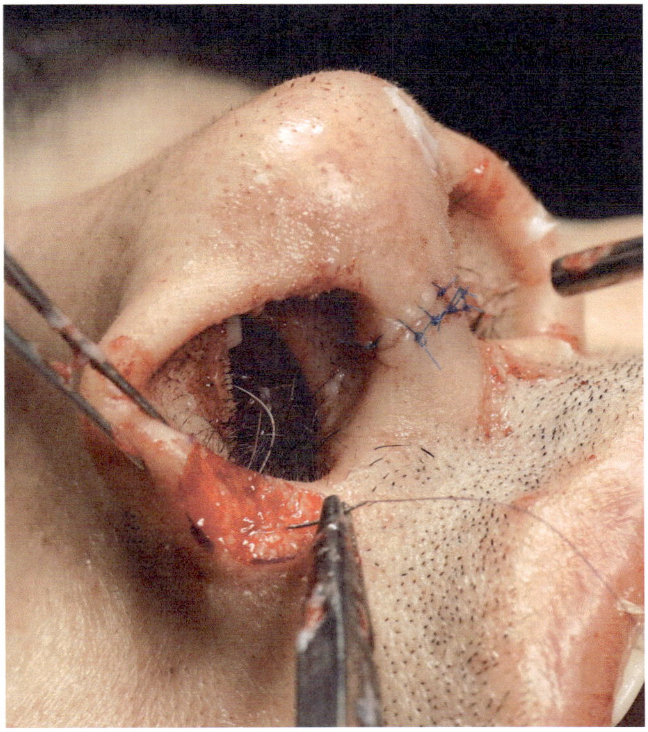

Fig. 16.66 Marked segment excised. After resection, the subcutaneous layer is approximated with 5-0 PDS sutures

This technique can also be used with an endonasal rhinoplasty approach, where marginal and transfixion incision is performed for delivery of the alar cartilages. With this approach, the surgeon can accurately estimate the shape, size, and resistance of the lower lateral cartilages by using the VAR technique for correction of tip abnormalities.

16.4.3.3 Case 12

In this case, the overdeveloped lateral crus pushed the tip anteroinferiorly. The main consideration is the disproportion between the large tip and smaller dorsum, which is evident profile view (Fig. 16.73).

The lateral crura must be shortened. There are two alternatives to reduce the lateral crura: lateral crural steal suture and vertical alar resection. Steal suture was not planned in this case because it would create extra projection. To avoid this, the Var technique was preferred. The operative steps were as follows:

Closed rhinoplasty approach via marginal and transfixion incisions is performed (Figs. 16.74 and 16.75).

As can be clearly seen after exposure of the alar cartilages, the lateral crura are quite long, pushing the tip anteriorly (Fig. 16.76).

Cephalic margins of the lower lateral crura are conservatively trimmed to promote tip refinement, with the surgeon taking care to preserve a complete strip 5–8 mm in width. Overaggressive resection of the alar cartilages could compromise tip support, potentially giving rise to future alar pinching, alar collapse, or bossa formation (Fig. 16.77).

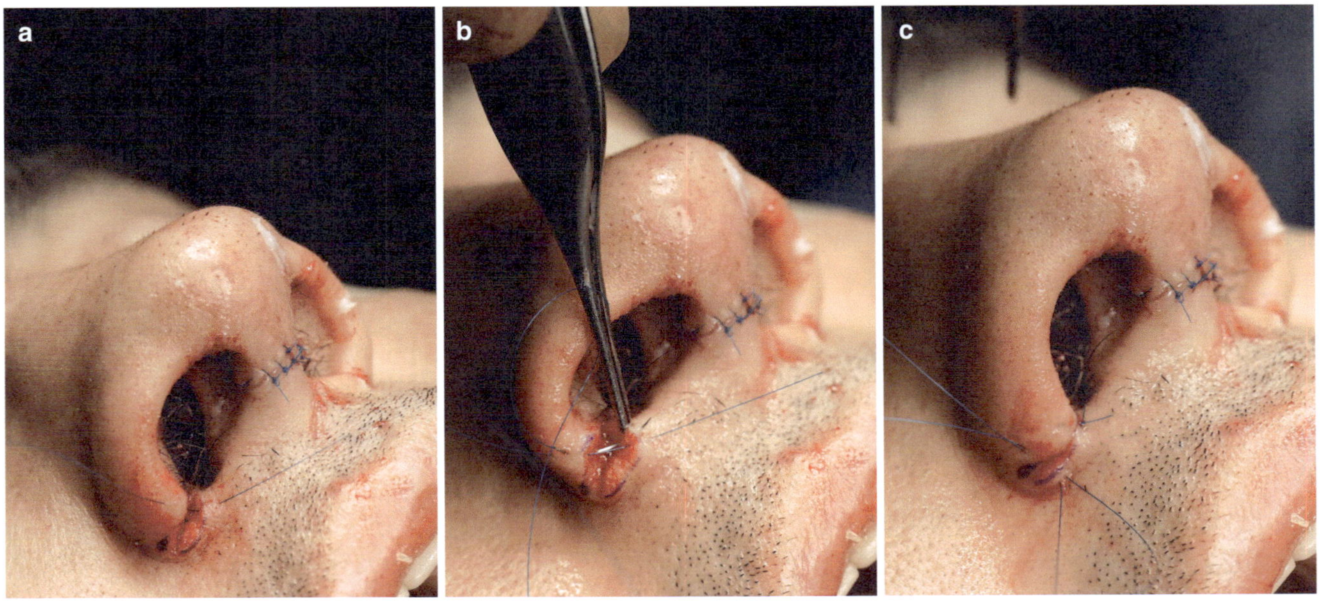

Fig. 16.67 (**a**–**c**) Wound closed with interrupted mattress suture

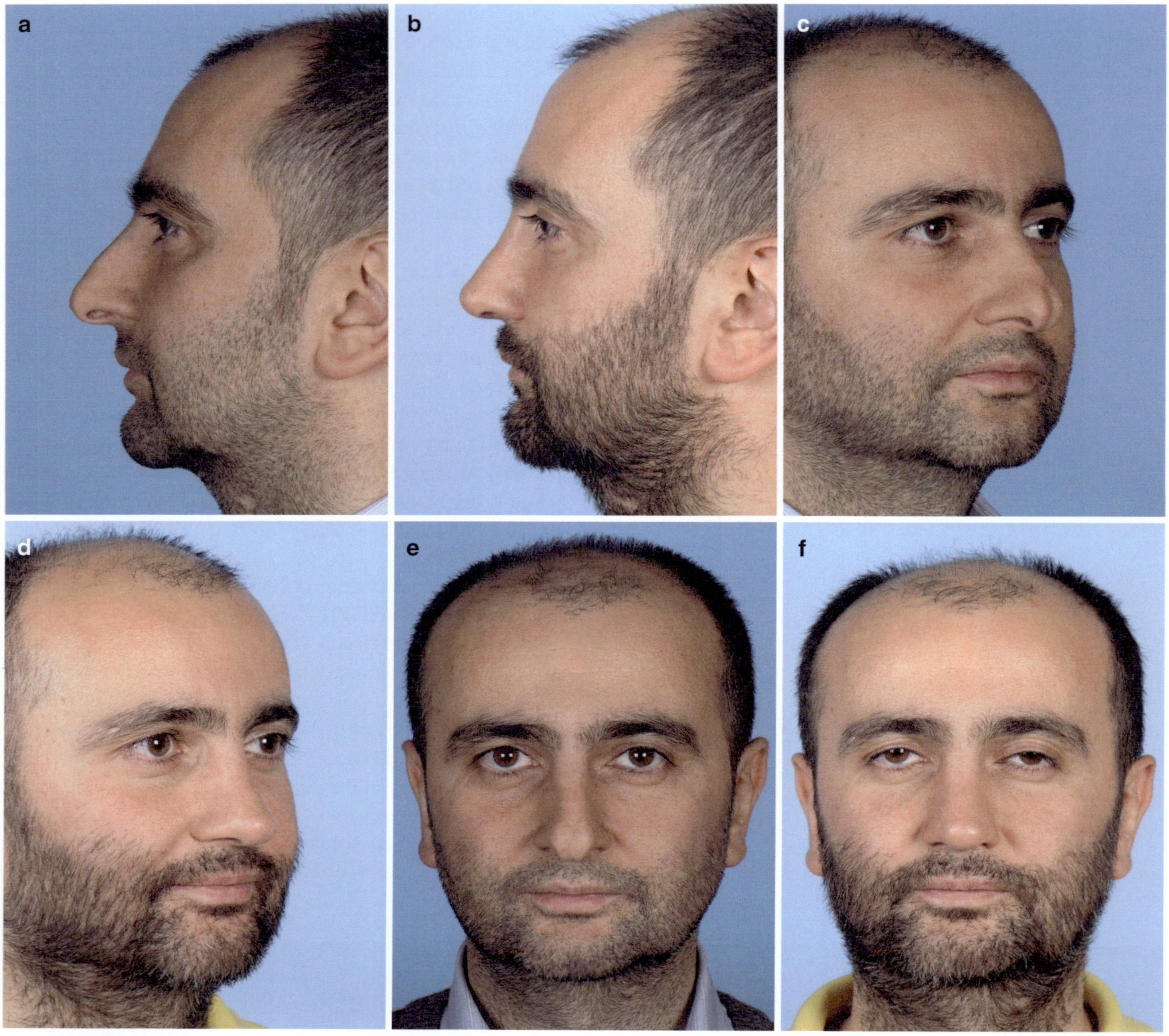

Fig. 16.68 (a–j) Pre- and postoperative photographs. The overall size of the nose has been significantly reduced

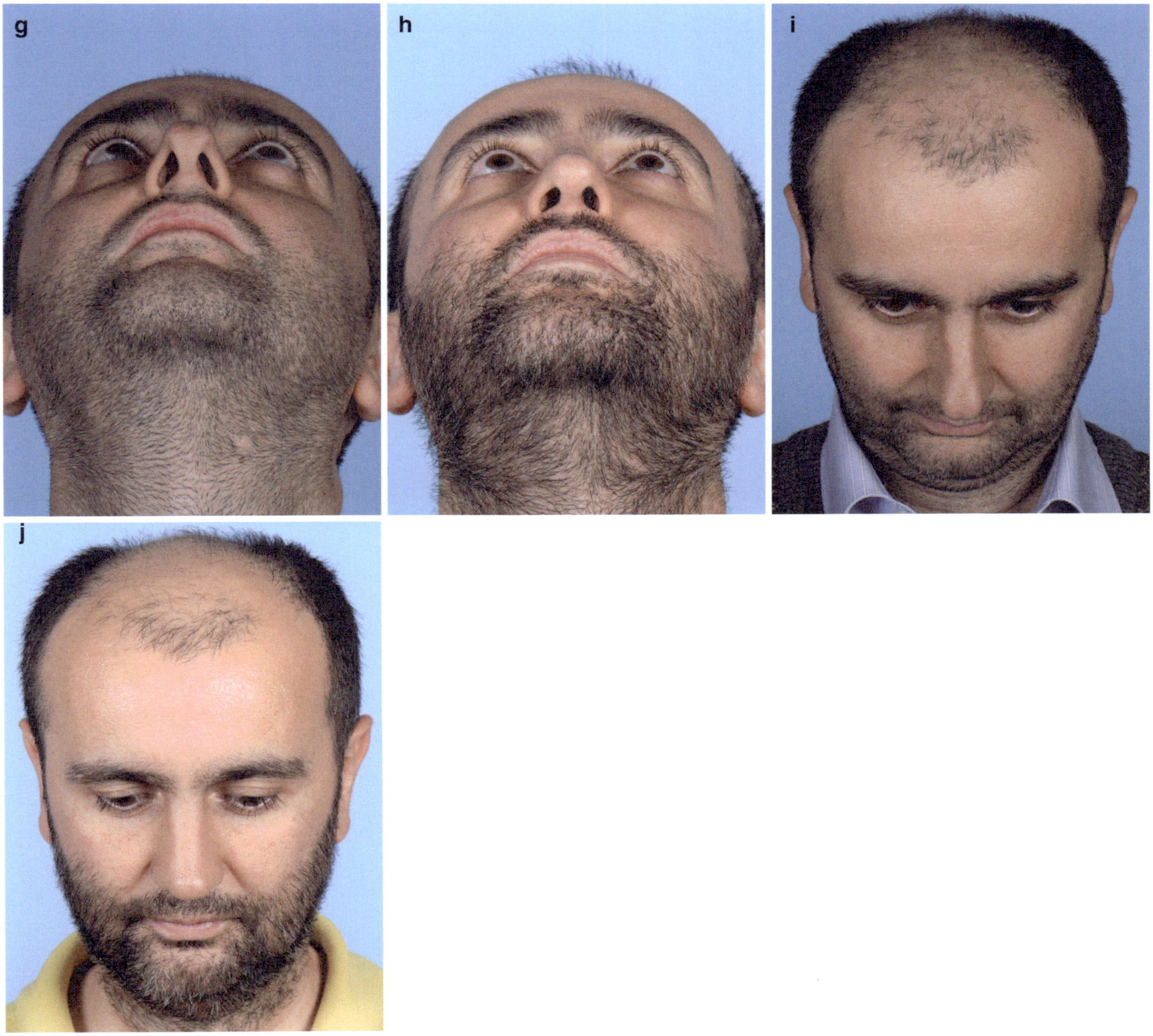

Fig. 16.68 (continued)

The excess part of the lateral crus is resected. Resection from the lateral crus results in more rotation. Next, the surgeon marks the apex of the domes of the lower lateral cartilages and vertically divides the alar cartilages; then, the lateral crus is dissected with the underlying skin. After dissection, the excess lateral crus is always revealed (Fig. 16.78).

The two medial crura are then sutured together with absorbable 5-0 PDS sutures placed 0.2–0.3 cm below the apex of the medial crura, to maintain the normal curvature of the domes and avoid formation of an unnaturally thin or pinched tip (Fig. 16.79).

The same procedure is also applied to the contralateral side. An average of 15 cm was vertically resected on both lateral crura (Fig. 16.80).

In cases with excessive resection, trimming may be necessary, from the upper surface of the vestibular skin (Fig. 16.81).

End-to-end suturing of the cartilages with PDS suture would suffice in this case (Fig. 16.82).

The sutured area constitutes the new dome point. Now, the alar cartilage segments are brought to their ideal length. With this resection, the nasal tip is deprojected and rotated (Fig. 16.83).

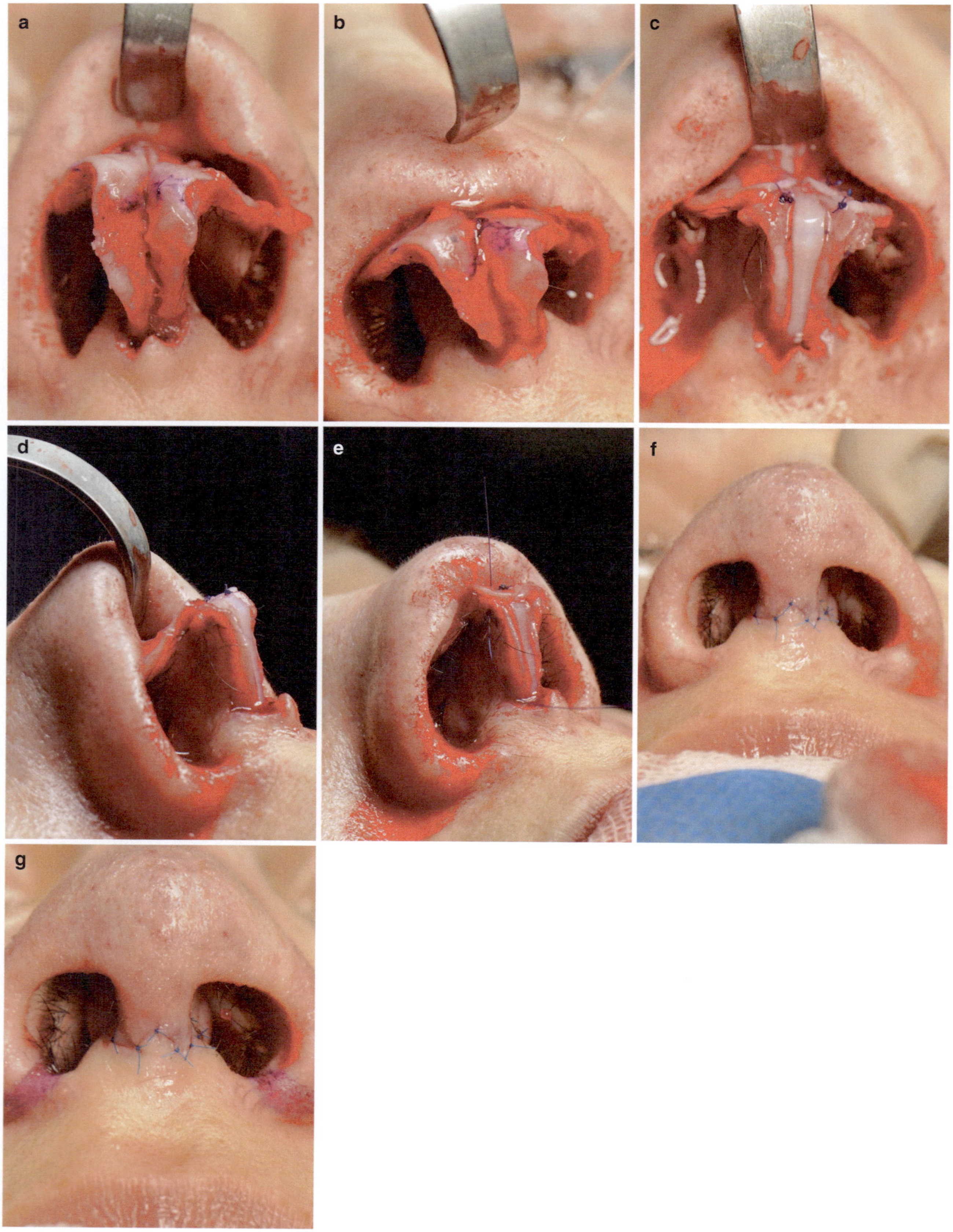

Fig. 16.69 (**a–g**) The alar cartilages were entirely hypertrophic in this case. VAR technique was suitable in this case. This provided decreased tip projection without rotation. After deprojection, alar base reduction was required. (Supplementary Video 16.4)

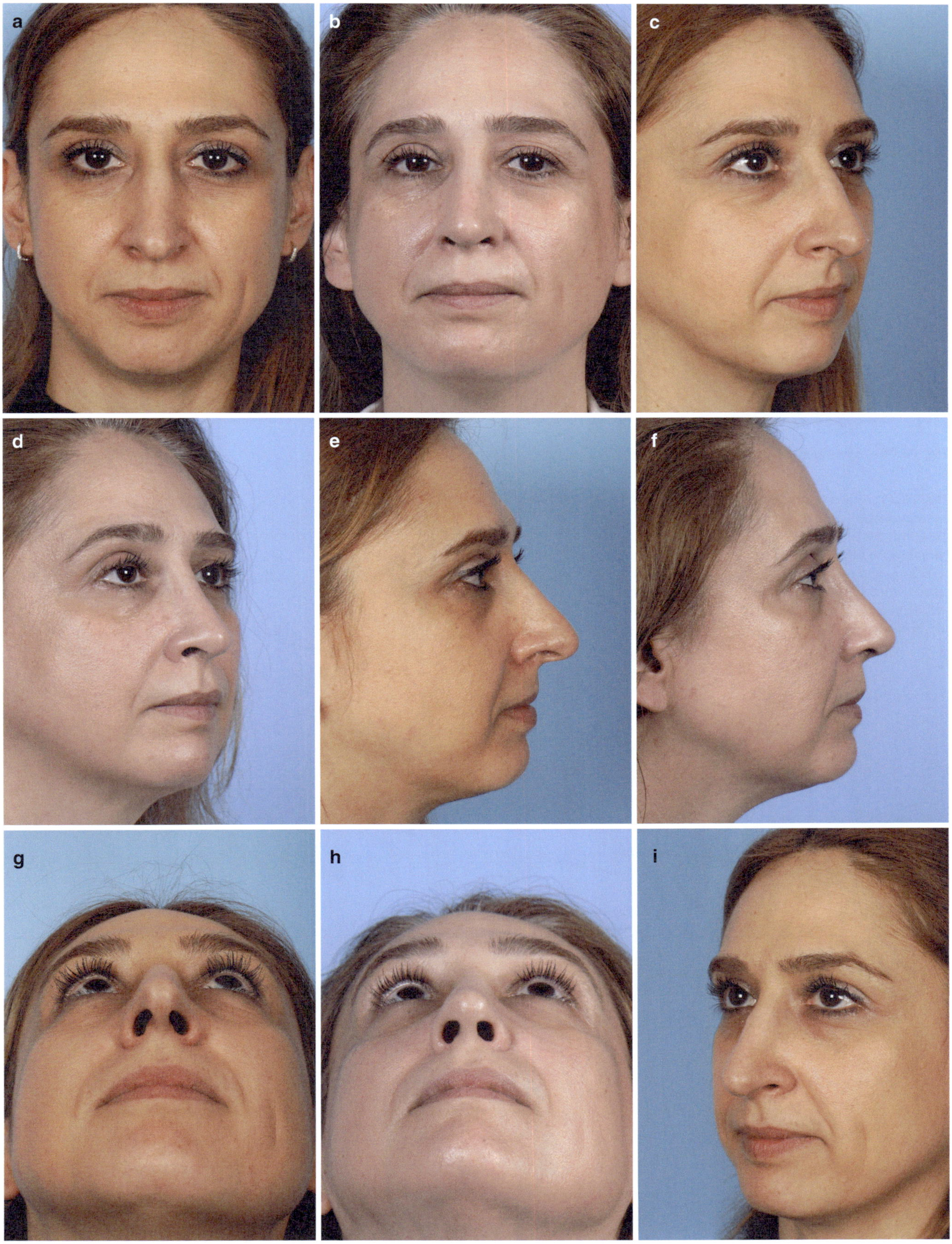

Fig. 16.70 (**a**–**I**) Photographs taken 8 years after the operation showed that the nasal projection was reduced and there was no distortion of the nasal tip. The dorsal hump is reduced

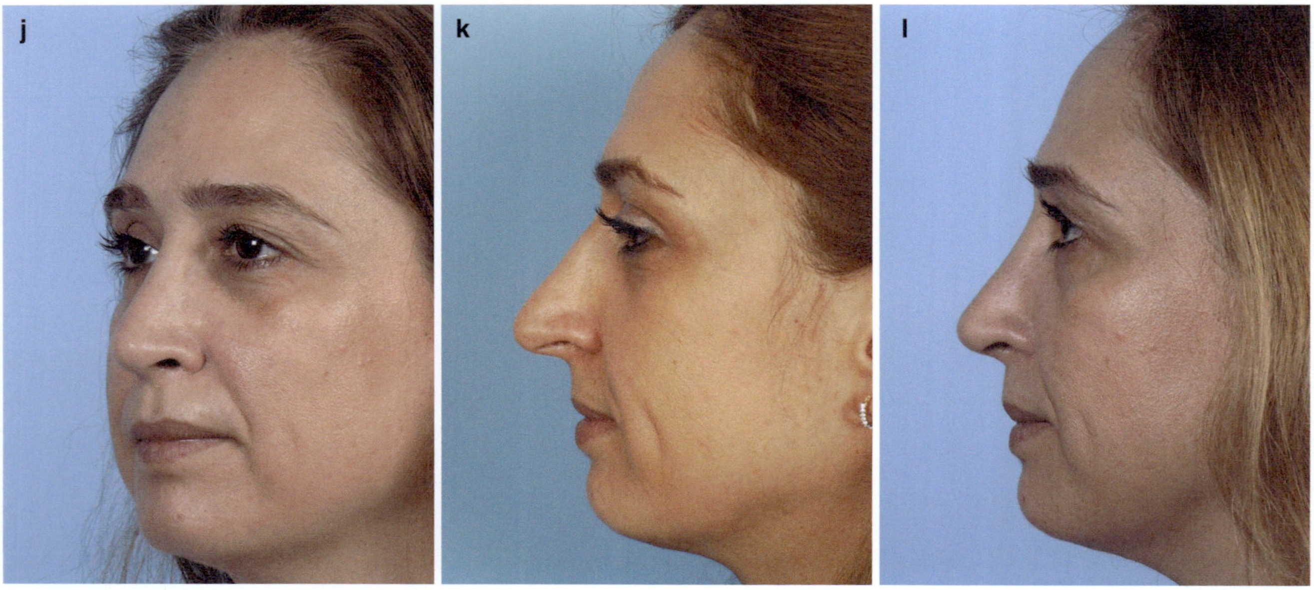

Fig. 16.70 (continued)

Fig. 16.71 When correcting overdeveloped lateral crura, the cartilages are divided just lateral to the domes. Dividing, resecting, and repairing the lateral crura allow us to shape and decrease the projection (de-projection)

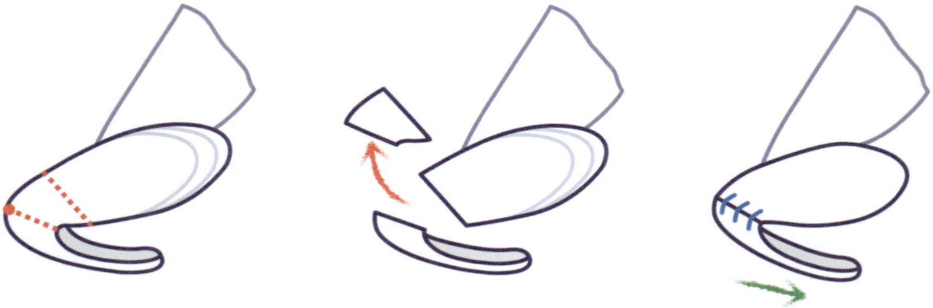

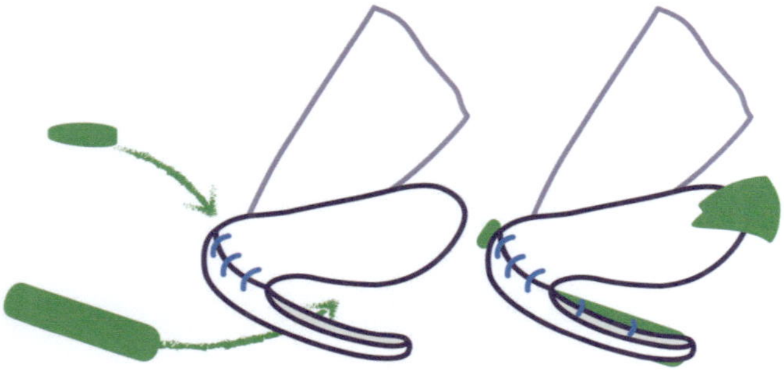

Fig. 16.72 Columellar strut, cap graft, and alar batten grafts provide support and structure to the repair (re-projection and definition)

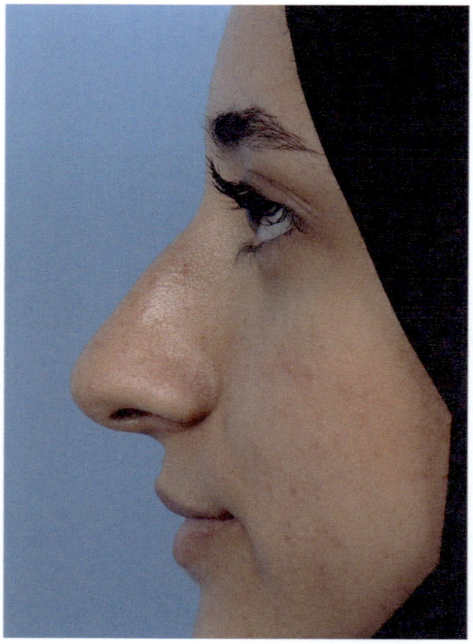

Fig. 16.73 Over-projected, wide, and underrotated nasal tip. (Supplementary Video 16.5)

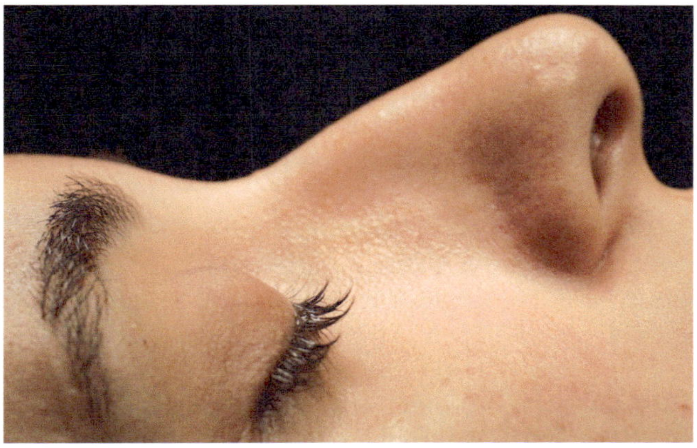

Fig. 16.74 Just immediately before surgery

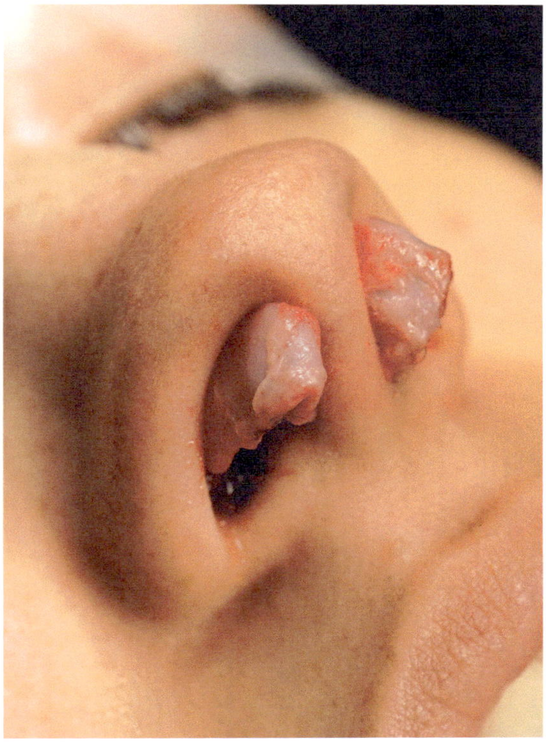

Fig. 16.75 Marginal and transfixion incisions are performed for delivery of the alar cartilages

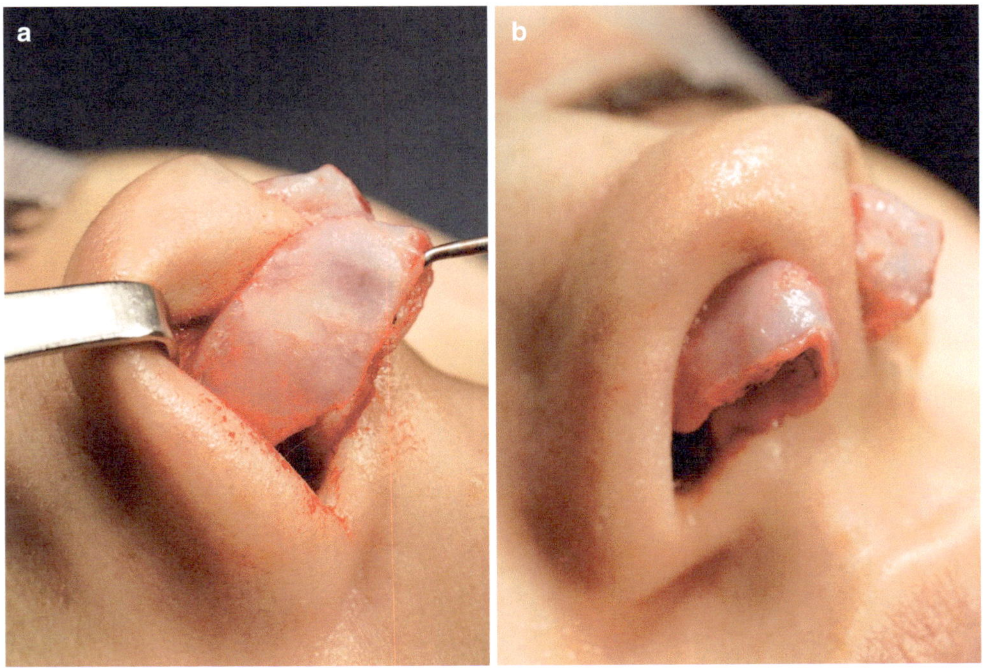

Fig. 16.76 (**a**, **b**) As can be clearly seen after exposure of the alar cartilages, the lateral crura are quite long, pushing the tip anteriorly

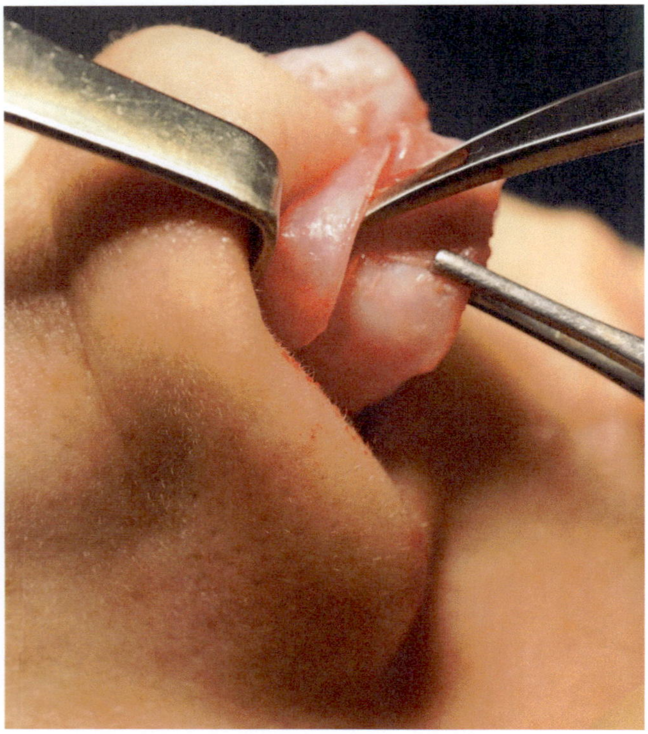

Fig. 16.77 Cephalic margins of the lower lateral crura are conservatively trimmed to promote tip refinement, with the surgeon taking care to preserve a complete strip 5–8 mm in width. Overaggressive resection of the alar cartilages could compromise tip support, potentially giving rise to future alar pinching, alar collapse, or bossa formation

Attention now turns to defining and stabilizing the newly created anatomy (reprojection). For this purpose, a columellar strut (r), dome-equalizing suture (s) and cup graft (t) are used for the nasal base. The excess part of the lateral crus is used as an alar button graft (u) to strengthen the lateral nasal wall (Fig. 16.84).

The final result on table is shown in Fig. 16.85.

Preoperative and 1-year postoperative photographs are presented in Fig. 16.86. The tip is deprojected and rotated upward.

16.4.3.4 Over-Projection Due to Hypertrophy of the Medial and Middle Crura

Hypertrophic medial and middle crura can push the tip anteriorly (over-projection), causing columellar deformation due to configuration deformity. When the cause of nasal tip over-projection is an enlarged medial and intermediate cartilage complex, some form of cartilaginous reduction procedure must usually be performed to bring the protruding tip into balance with the rest of the nose and face.

We have successfully utilized the VAR technique to correct over-projection of the nasal tip secondary to an overdeveloped middle/medial cartilage complex (Fig. 16.87).

Alar cartilages transect the most prominent part of the middle/medial crus complex. Then, the vestibular skin is dissected from the crus up to the dome, and the rectangular-shaped deformed and overdeveloped part will finally be removed

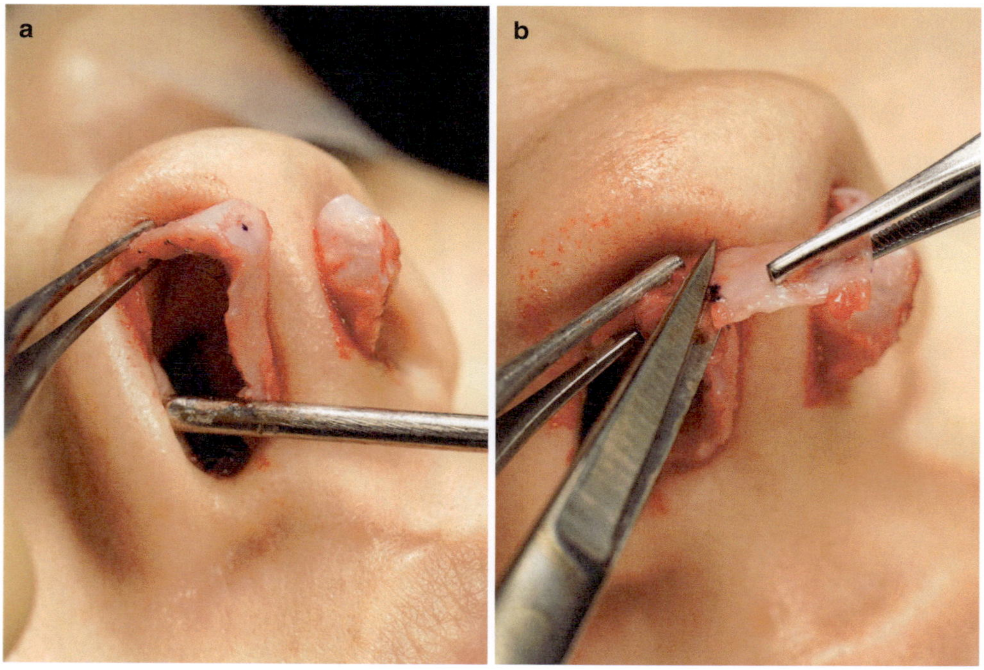

Fig. 16.78 (a, b) The excess part of the lateral crus is resected. Resection from the lateral crus results in more rotation. Next, the surgeon marks the apex of the domes of the lower lateral cartilages and vertically divides the alar cartilages; then, the lateral crus is dissected with the underlying skin. After dissection, the excess lateral crus is always revealed

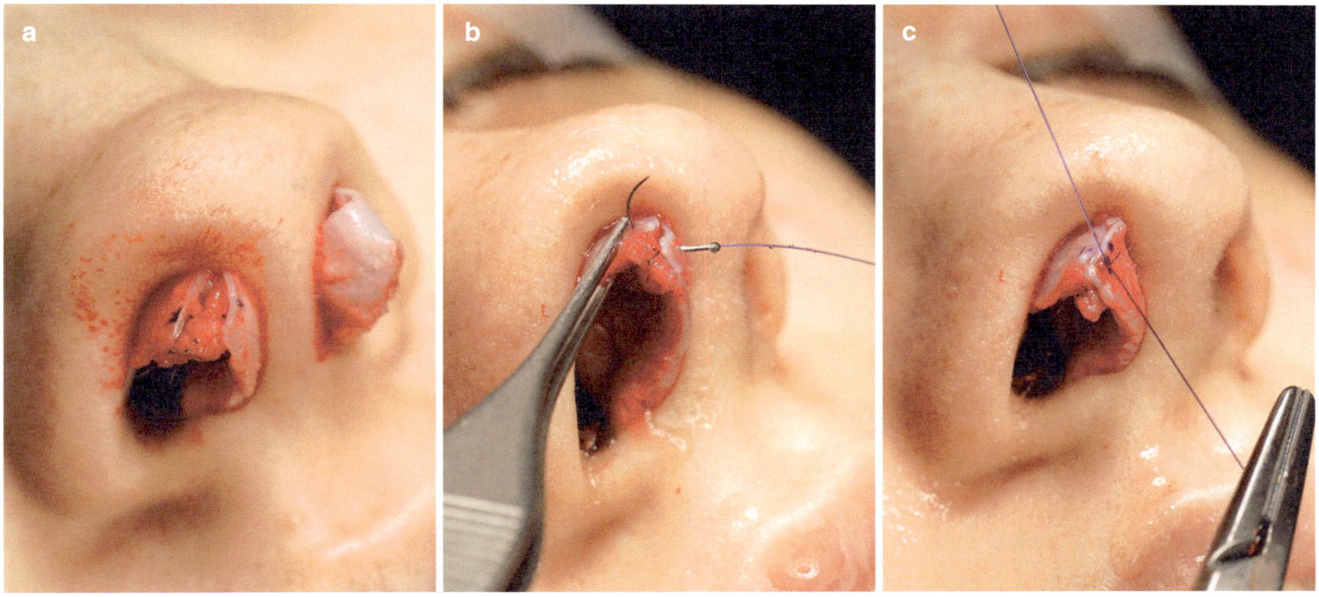

Fig. 16.79 (**a**–**c**) The two medial crura are then sutured together with absorbable 5-0 PDS sutures placed 0.2–0.3 cm below the apex of the medial crura, to maintain the normal curvature of the domes and avoid formation of an unnaturally thin or pinched tip

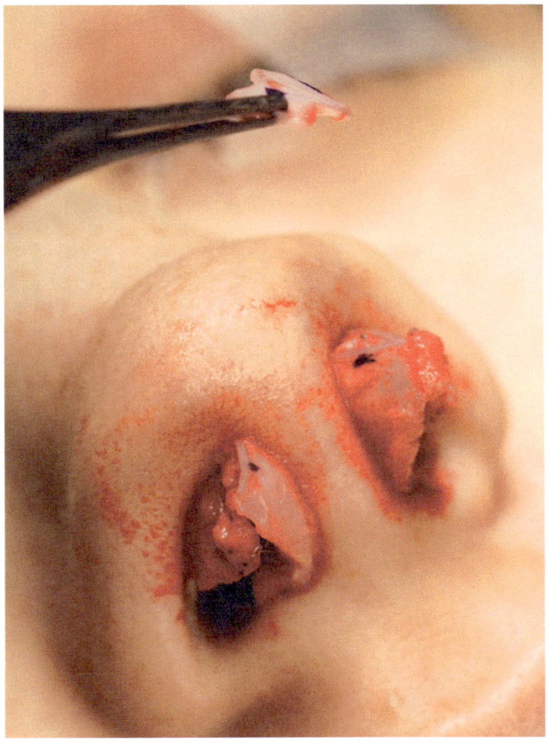

Fig. 16.80 The same procedure is also applied to the contralateral side. An average of 15 cm was vertically resected on both lateral crura

from behind the dome point. Resecting the overdeveloped part not only decreases projection, but also corrects the misconfiguration. Although resection may be expected to reduce the rotation, appropriate resection will not affect it. If we were to resect the medial/middle crus according to a normal length, the tip would of course be derotated. However, restoring a malformed and long crus to normal length will not significantly affect the rotation. To increase or decrease rotation, extra resection will be needed outside the malformed areas.

For stabilization and definition, on the other hand, a columellar strut, cup graft, and alar button graft will suffice (Fig. 16.88).

Case 13 is typical example for over-projection due to hypertrophy of the medial and middle crura.

16.4.3.5 Case 13

This case had severe hanging columella and alar columellar disharmony, as well as nasal tip over-projection. VAR technique can be chosen in the endonasal (closed) approach (Fig. 16.89).

As mentioned above, the VAR technique can be applied via an open or closed approach, with no difference in the results. In this case, the procedure was performed via the endonasal (closed) approach. The surgery was again comprised of three basic steps:

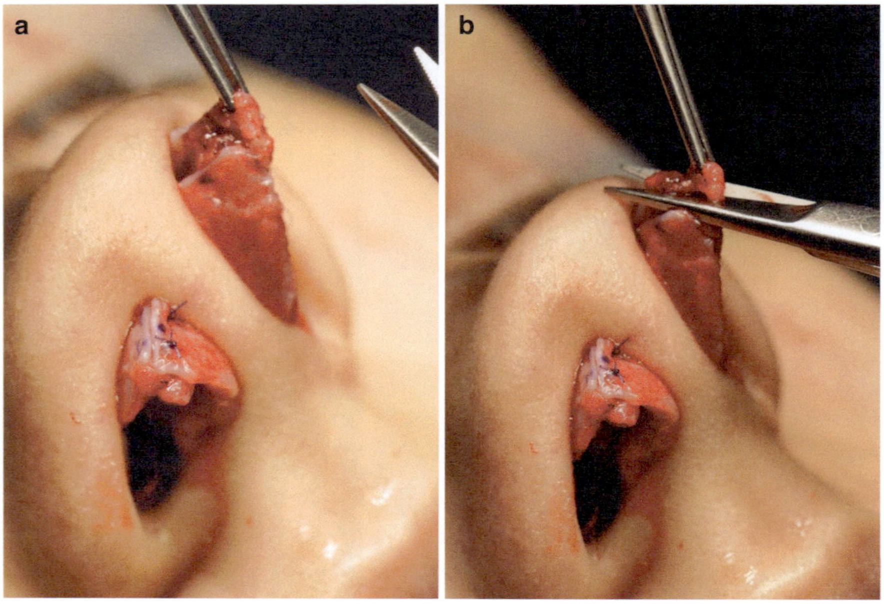

Fig. 16.81 (**a**, **b**) In cases with excessive resection, trimming may be necessary, from the upper surface of the vestibular skin

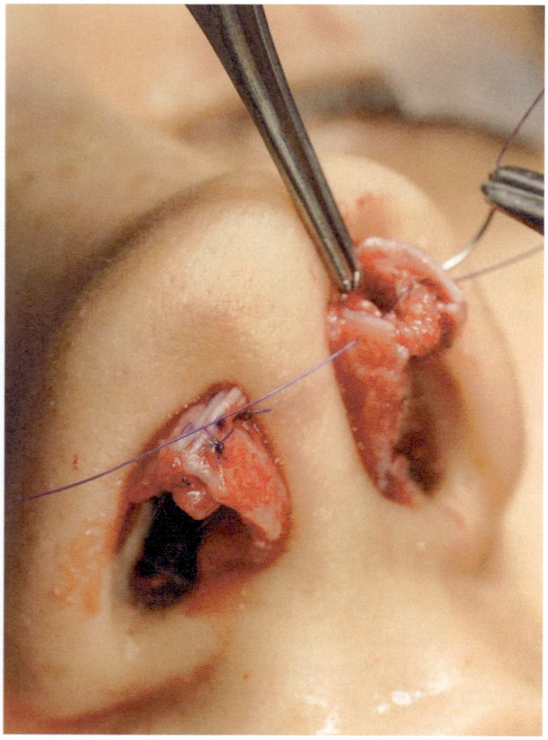

Fig. 16.82 End-to-end suturing of the cartilages with PDS suture would suffice in this case

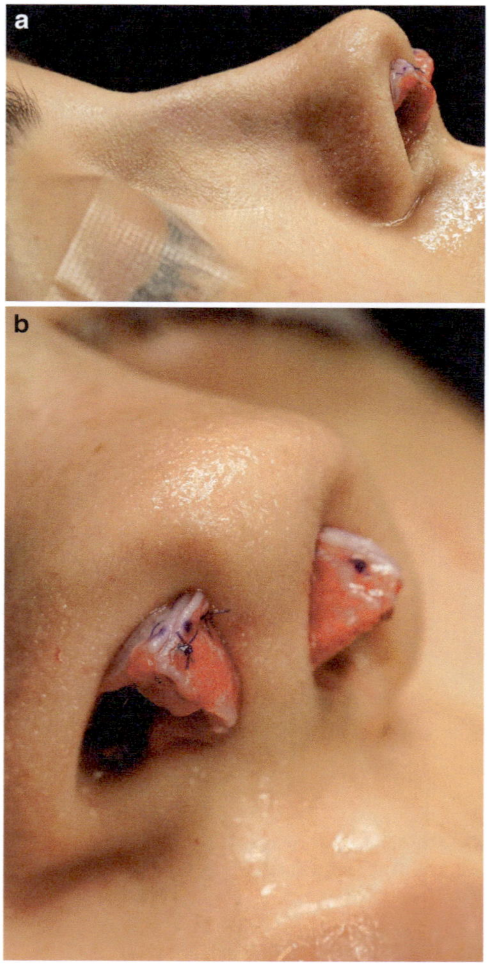

Fig. 16.83 (**a**, **b**) The sutured area constitutes the new dome point. Now, the alar cartilage segments are brought to their ideal length. With this resection, the nasal tip is deprojected and rotated

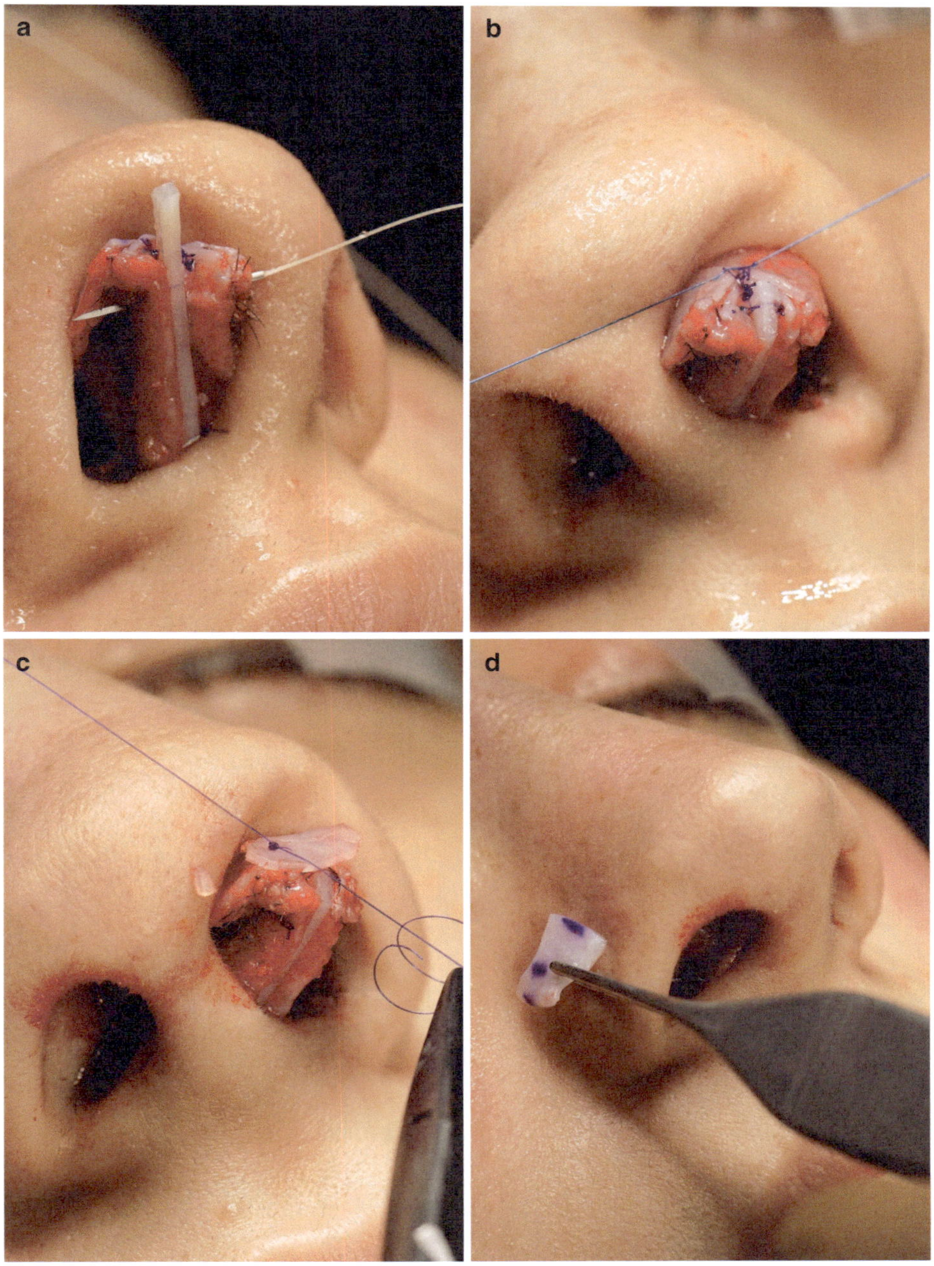

Fig. 16.84 (**a–d**) Attention now turns to defining and stabilizing the newly created anatomy (reprojection). For this purpose, a columellar strut (r), dome-equalizing suture (s), and cup graft (t) are used for the nasal base. The excess part of the lateral crus is used as an alar button graft (u) to strengthen the lateral nasal wall

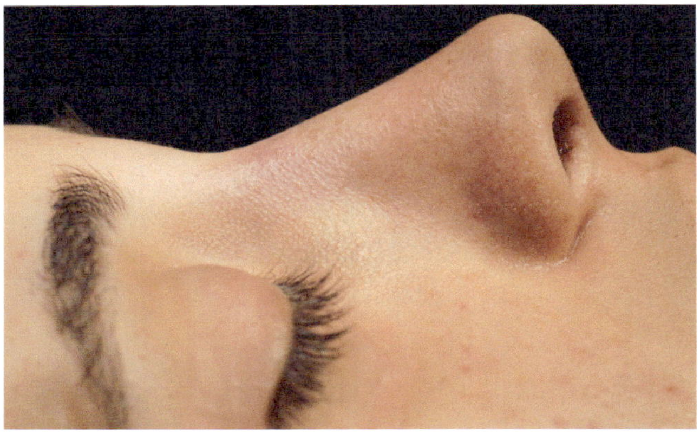

Fig. 16.85 Final result on table

1. **Deprojection:** The procedure begins by correcting septal irregularities through a hemitransfixion incision (Fig. 16.90).
2. Then, alar cartilages are delivered endonasally. Interdomal fibrous connections are severed, allowing additional delivery of the cartilages. At this time, the surgeon assesses the location of the natural dome and the amount of redundant and excessive middle crus cartilage. Volume reduction is carried out by cephalic trimming of the superior margin of the lateral crus (Fig. 16.91).
3. Next, an incision is made at the junction of the middle and medial crura only through the cartilage. This produces a lateral unipedicled cartilage flap. A second

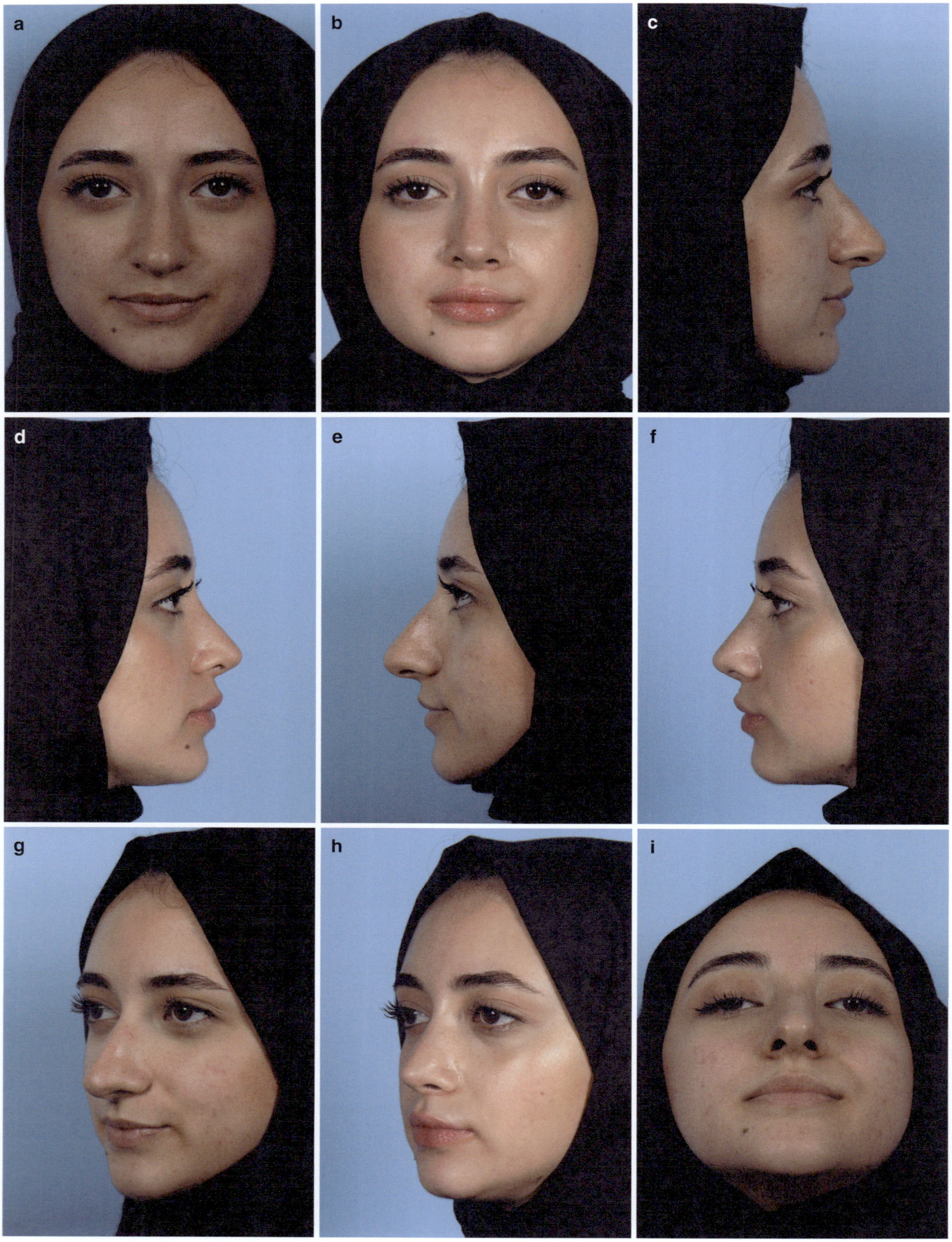

Fig. 16.86 (a–l) Pre- and postoperative photographs. Resecting a segment of the long lateral crura reprojected the tip, allowed tip rotation, and corrected the lateral fullness of the tip

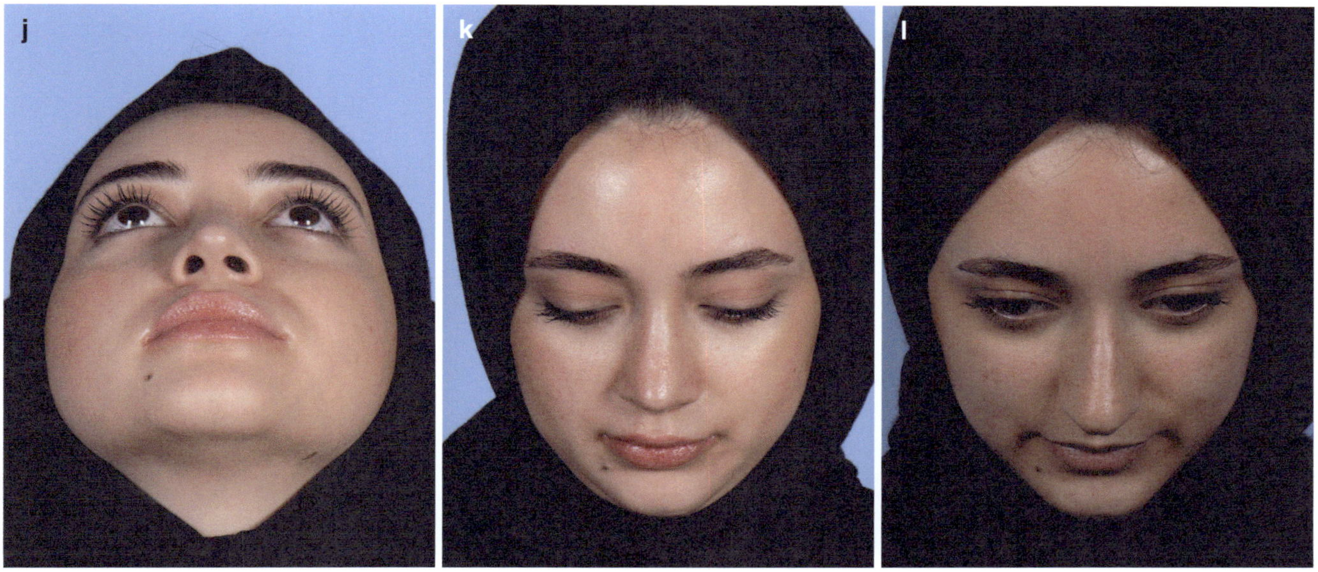

Fig. 16.86 (continued)

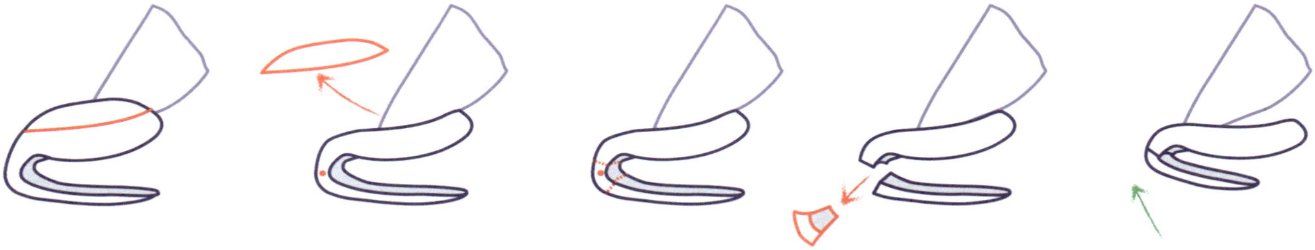

Fig. 16.87 VAR technique should be chosen in over-projection based on hypertrophy of the medial and middle crura cases

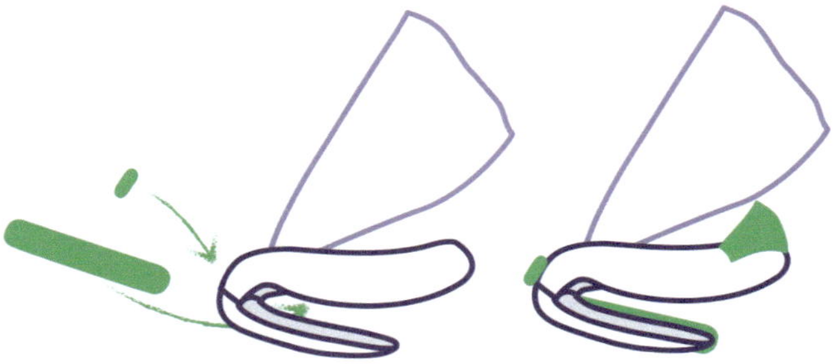

Fig. 16.88 Columellar strut, cap graft, and alar batten grafts provide support and structure to the repair (re-projection and definition)

cartilage incision is made 6–8 mm more proximal to the initial incision according to the amount of tip reduction or narrowing desired. A trapezoid section of cartilage is then excised between the two incisions, leaving the vestibular mucosa intact (Fig. 16.92).

The resection not only decreases projection, but also resolves the hanging columella problem. The next step is to create a new dome by suture placement. This is accomplished by placing a horizontal mattress suture through the proximal end of the lower lateral crural flap (Fig. 16.93).

After deprojection, restabilization and refinement are performed, which we call "reprojection." A columellar strut, cup graft, and alar button graft are placed. A dome-equalizing suture is used (Fig. 16.94).

Postoperatively, the nasal tip projection is shorter and in better balance with the rest of the face. The alar columellar disharmony has been corrected (Fig. 16.95).

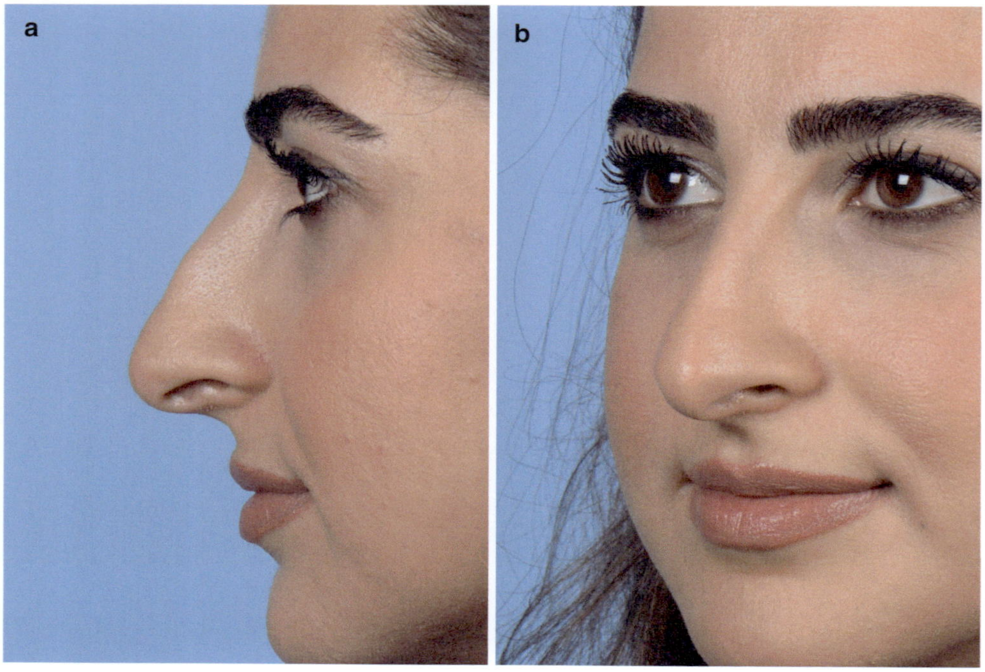

Fig. 16.89 (**a**, **b**) The tip is overprotected by the length of the medial crus and the excess caudal septum. The columella is positioned caudally, this is seen especially well on the oblique view. The thick skin is the limiting factor in this case. Thus, the aim in this case is not to significantly reduce the overall size of the nose but rather to improve the hanging columella and reduce tip projection

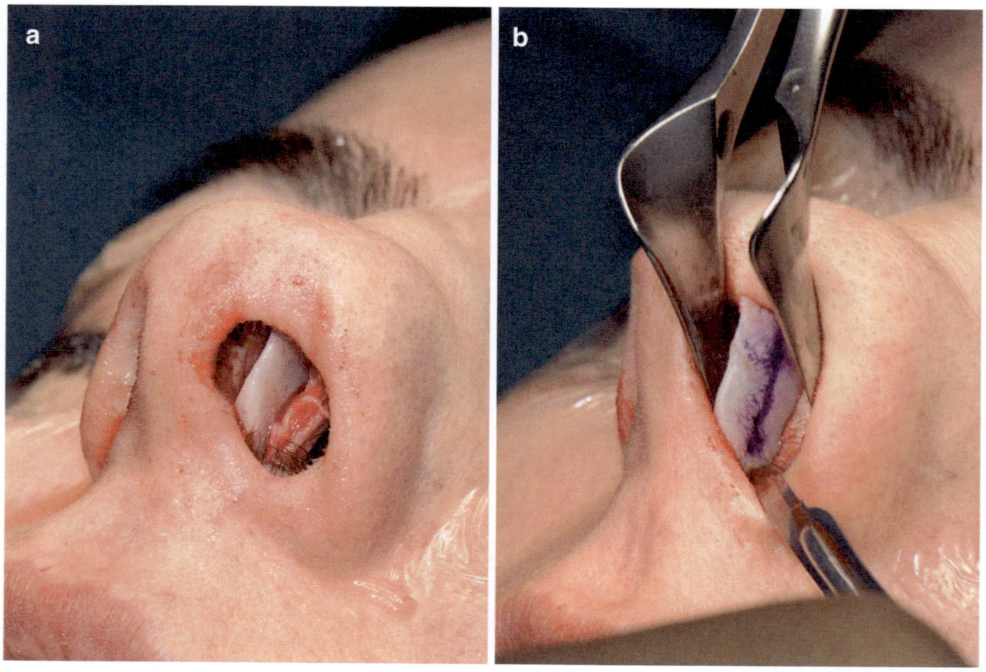

Fig. 16.90 (**a**, **b**) Resection of the excess caudal septum

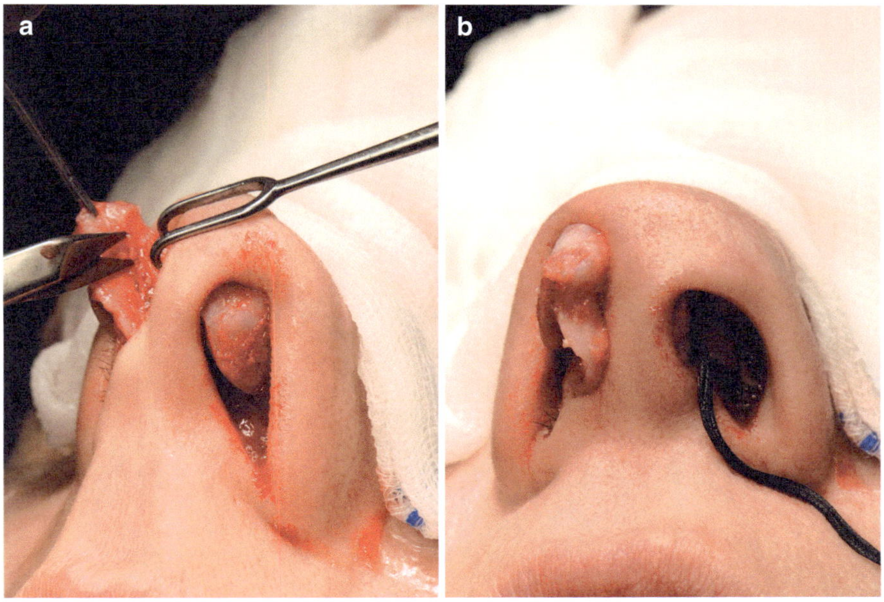

Fig. 16.91 (**a**, **b**) Closed approach revealing the overdeveloped and buckled middle/medial crura

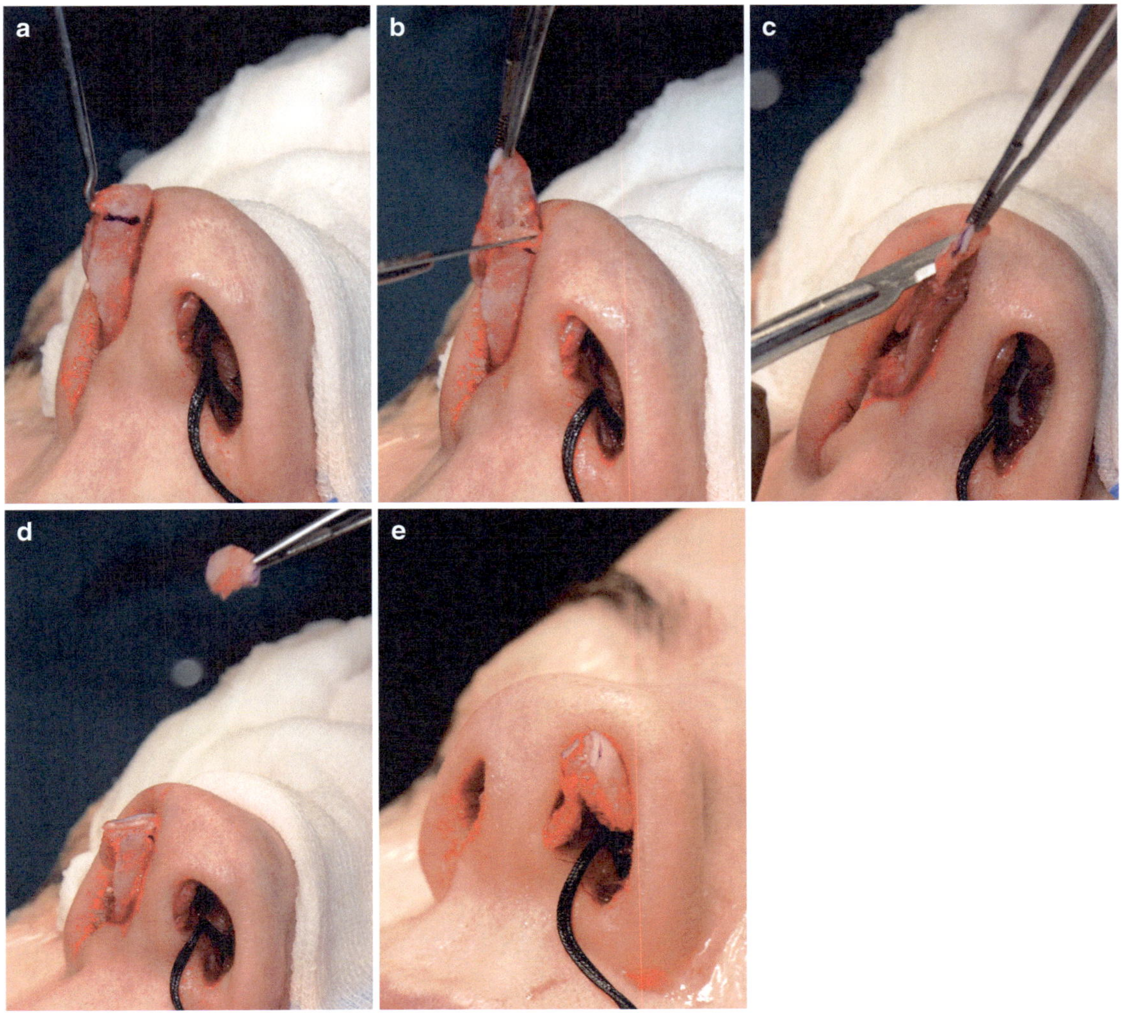

Fig. 16.92 (**a**–**e**) Deprojection: medial crus divided transversely; edges raised from underlying mucoperichondrium and the excess portions resected; free edges reapproximated with 6-0 suture

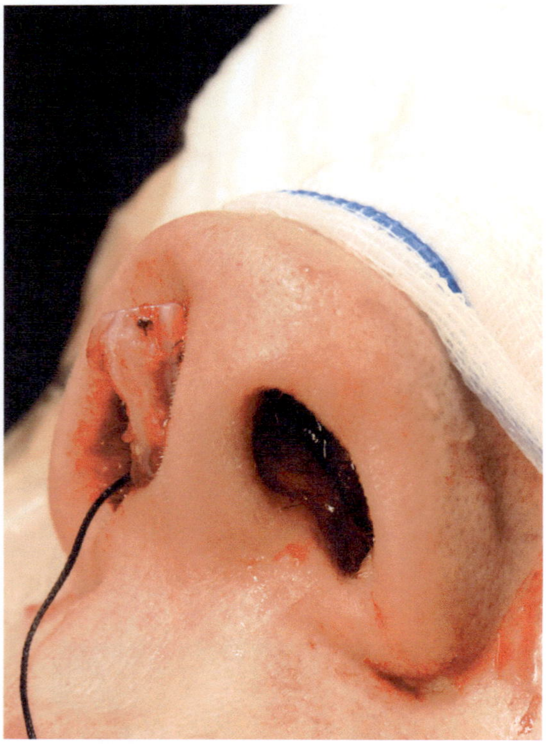

Fig. 16.93 Reprojection: a columellar strut, cup graft, and alar button graft are placed

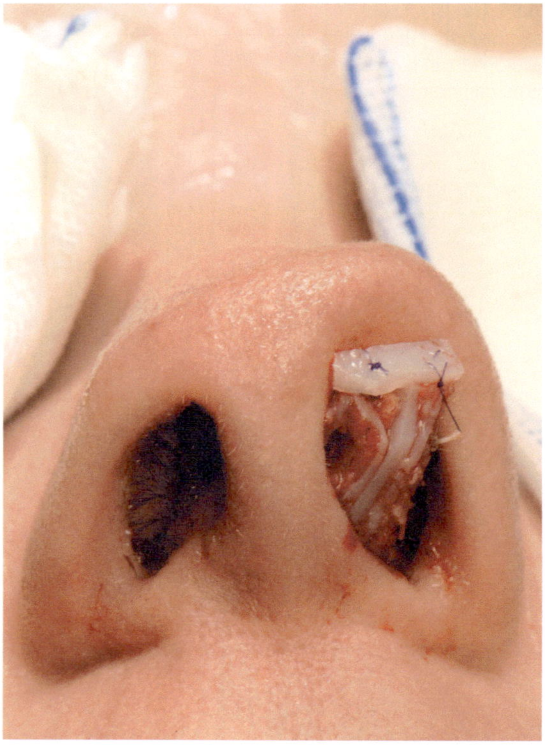

Fig. 16.94 Enhanced nasal tip anatomy

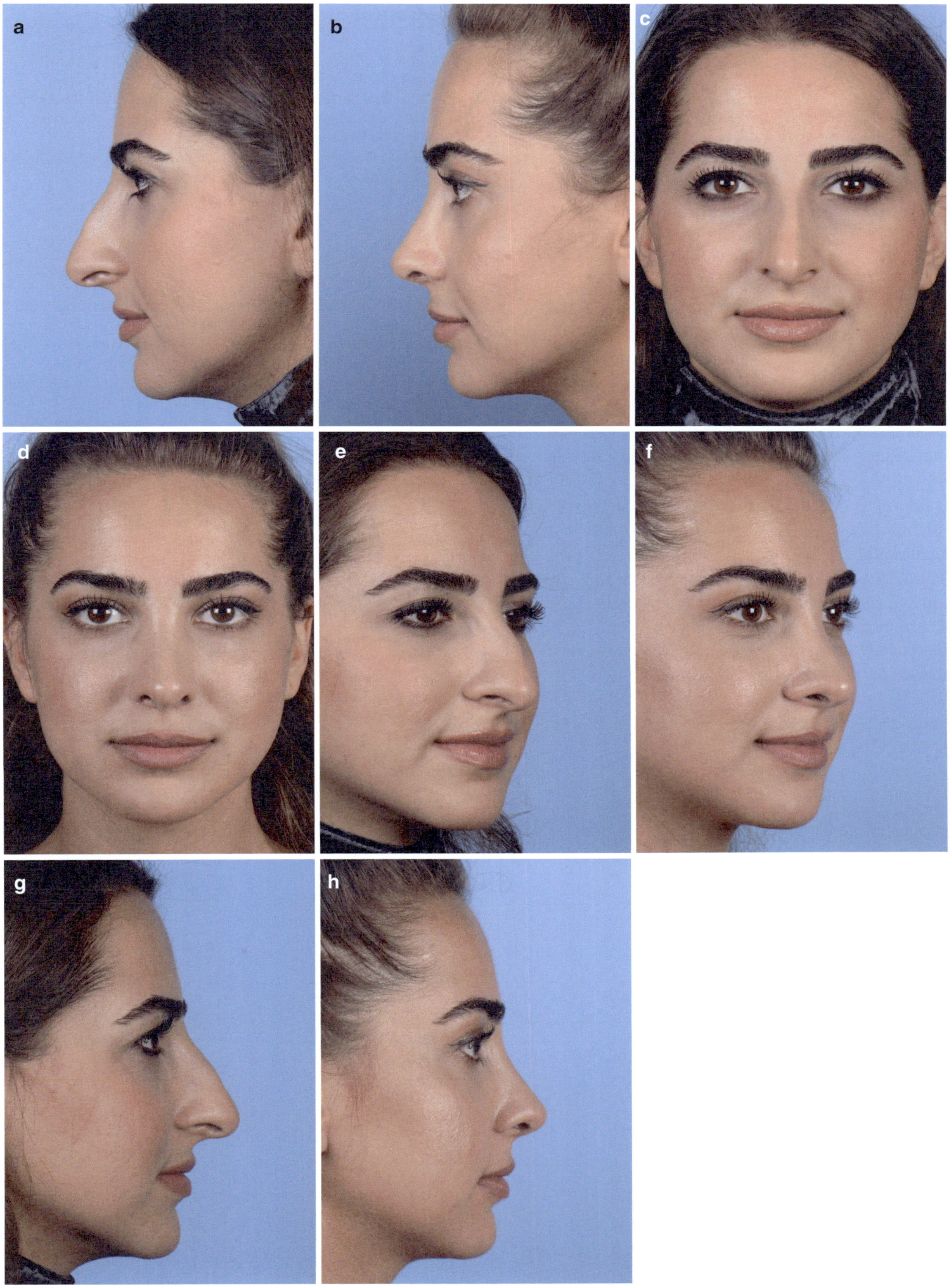

Fig. 16.95 (**a**–**h**) The result is good; however, the columella is a little flared because of excessive skin

16.5 Conclusion

Preoperative evaluation of the nasal tip is extremely important because every over-projected tip pathology requires a different technique.

True over-projection can include (1) overdeveloped alar cartilages, including the lateral crura, medial crura, middle crura, or a combination thereof; (2) a tension nose with overdeveloped quadrangular cartilage; or (3) a combination of these two. Having completed analysis of the nasal projection, the next step is to determine whether rotation is adequate or will need to be addressed, as many projection techniques can alter rotation. The adjacent structure of the tip is further examined for underdevelopment, which can give the appearance of an over-projected nose (pseudo-over-projection).

Over-projected tip surgery starts by resecting overdeveloped, hypertrophic, and elongated structures. Restabilization, recontouring, and refinement may be performed after deprojection.

If the cause of nasal tip over-projection is hypertrophy of the alar cartilage tip, the VAR technique would be effective and achieve better long-term results.

The VAR technique can have a short learning curve for a young surgeon if training with an experienced surgeon who is accustomed to using the technique.

In conclusion, the VAR technique remains a very powerful tool in the surgeon's armamentarium.

Disclosures The author reports no conflicts of interest or funding requiring disclosure.

References

Johnson CM, Godin MS. The tension nose: open structure rhinoplasty approach. Plast Reconstr Surg. 1995;95(1):43–51.

Lee MR, Geissler P, Cochran S, Gunter JP, Rohrich RJ. Decreasing nasal tip projection in rhinoplasty. Plast Reconstr Surg. 2014;134(1):41e–9e.

Papel ID, Mabrie DC. Deprojecting the profile. Otolaryngol Clin N Am. 1999;32(1):65–87.

Further Reading

Crumley RL, Lanser M. Quantitative analysis of nasal tip projection. Laryngoscope. 1988;98(2):202–8.

Friedman WH, Rosenblum BN, Krebs FJ. The Goldman tip in secondary rhinoplasty. Plast Reconstr Surg. 1987;79(3):339–45.

Gubisch W, Eichhorn-Sens J. The sliding technique: a method to treat the overprojected nasal tip. Aesth Plast Surg. 2008;32(5):772–8.

Kridel RW, Konior RJ. Dome truncation for management of the overprojected nasal tip. Ann Plast Surg. 1990;24(5):385–96.

Sands NB, Adamson PA. Nasal tip deprojection with crural cartilage overlap: the M-arch model. Facial Plast Surg Clin North Am. 2015;23(1):93–104.

Silver WE, Zuliani GF. Management of the overprojected nose and ptotic nasal tip. Aesthet Surg J. 2009;29(3):253–8.

Skouras A, Asimakopoulou FA, Skouras G, Divritsioti M, Dimitriadi K. Use of the Goldman technique to correct both the overprojected and the broad nasal tip. Aesth Plast Surg. 2012;36(1):54–61.

Soliemanzadeh P, Kridel RW. Nasal tip overprojection: algorithm of surgical deprojection techniques and introduction of medial crural overlay. Arch Facial Plast Surg. 2005;7(6):374–80.

Tardy ME, Walter MA, Patt BS. The overprojecting nose: anatomic component analysis and repair. Facial Plast Surg. 1993;9(4):306–16.

Tobias GW. Modified universal tiplasty: closed structure rhinoplasty as it pertains to the overprojected and the broad tip. Facial Plast Surg. 1994;10(4):389–98.

17 Alar–Columellar Relationship in Rhinoplasty: Relationship Between the Alar Rim and Columellar Border of the Nose

17.1 Introduction/Brief Clinical History

Nostrils are shaped by the central part of the nose called a columella and the arched "wing-like" areas known as alae (Fig. 17.1).

In an ideal alar–columellar relationship, the two alae are symmetrical to the central columella in the profile view. Observed from the bottom view, each nostril has an elliptical shape. The height of the ellipse (i.e., nostril height) should be about 3–4 mm at the widest point (Fig. 17.2).

From the frontal view, the ideal relationship between the ala and the columella is described as a "gull wing in flight" configuration (Fig. 17.3).

Alar–columellar anomalies are common in patients seeking rhinoplasty. Such anomalies can present in two ways: the so-called excessive nostril show and reduced nostril show from the profile view (Fig. 17.4).

This chapter describes these in detail, with special emphasis on the former type of anomaly.

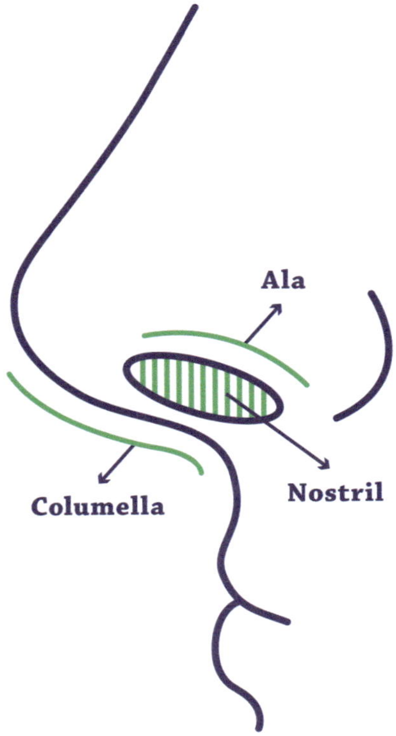

Fig. 17.1 Ideal alar–columellar relationship

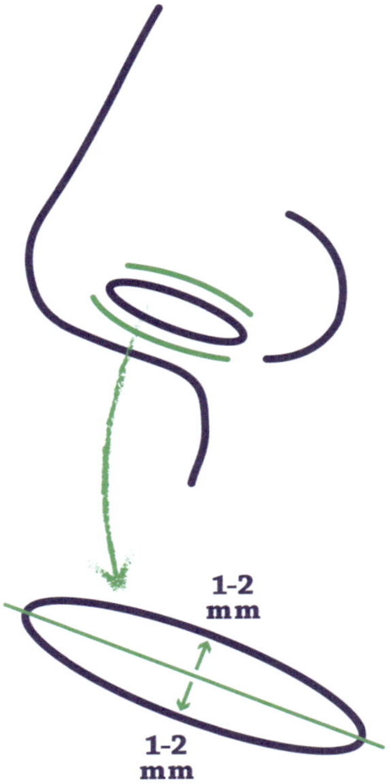

Fig. 17.2 Illustration showing ideal nostril size

Supplementary Information The online version contains supplementary material available at https://doi.org/10.1007/978-3-031-65619-4_17.

S. Şeneldir, *Photographic Atlas of Rhinoplasty*, https://doi.org/10.1007/978-3-031-65619-4_17

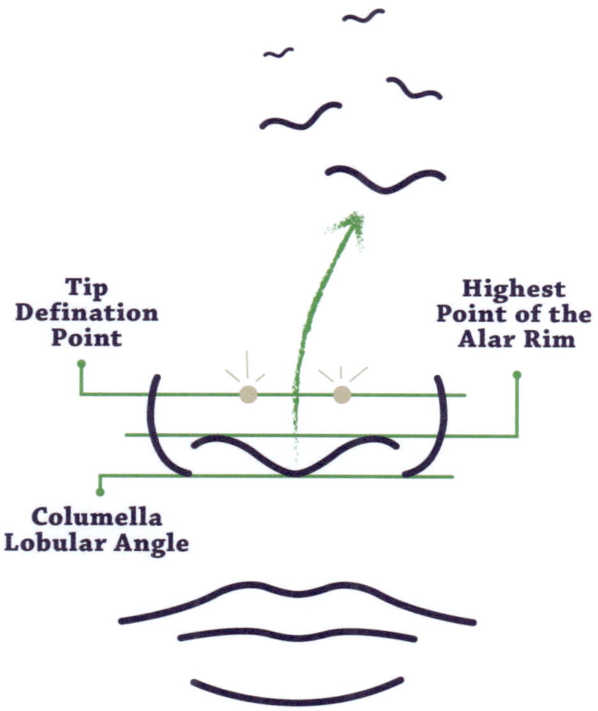

Fig. 17.3 Illustration showing "gull wing in flight"-shape on frontal view

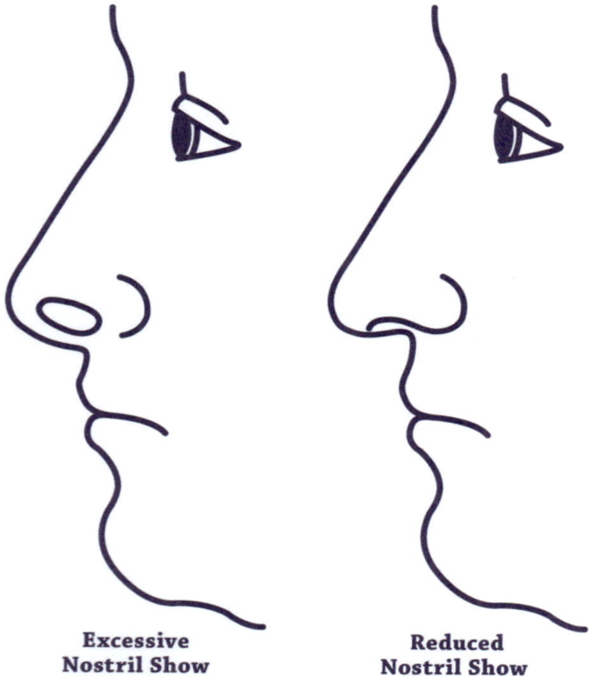

Fig. 17.4 Unfavorable alar–columellar relationship results in excessive or reduced nostril show on the lateral view

17.2 Excessive Nostril Show

There are two reasons for excessive nostril show: the ala may be retracted in the cranial direction (retracted ala), or the columella may "hang" in the caudal direction (hanging columella, also referred to as "columellar show"). In some cases, these two problems can make the nostrils appear abnormally large. Differential diagnosis of the two root causes is critical, as this will guide treatment. Excessive nostril show may be characterized by one or both of the following features (Fig. 17.5):

- Columella curvature that is greater than that of the alar rim, resulting in "wide nostrils" (due to a hanging columella). The gull's body appears to hang in the downward direction from the frontal view.
- Alar rim curvature that is greater than that of the columella in the profile view (due to alar retraction). The "wings" of the "gull" appear to be retracted in the upward direction.

When both curvatures are excessive, deviation from the ideal gull wing sign is visible in both directions from the frontal view.

The causes of each of these features, and solutions for correcting them, are provided below.

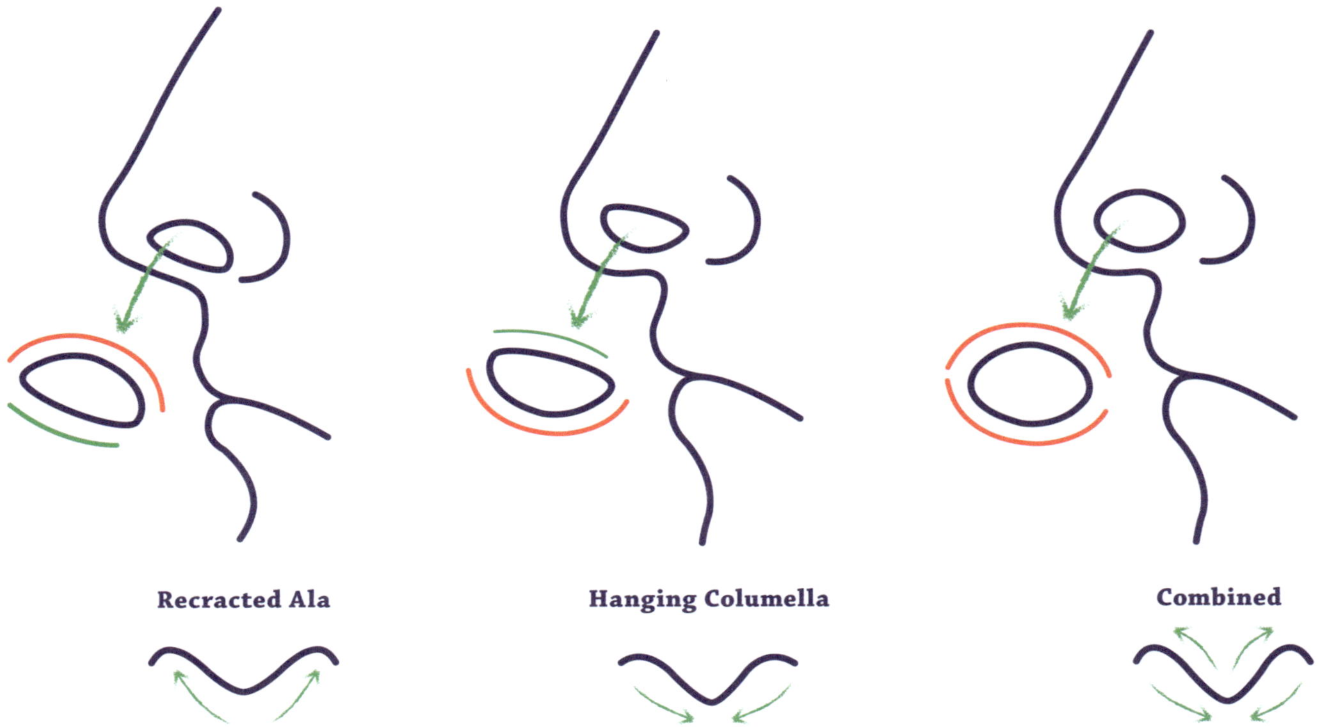

Fig. 17.5 Retracted ala: excessive nostril shows on lateral view without evidence of hanging columella. Hanging columella: excessive nostril shows on lateral view without evidence of alar retraction. Combined type: excessive nostril shows on lateral view combined with retracted ala and hanging columella

17.3 Hanging Columella

In a hanging columella, the columella hangs in the caudal direction, increasing the alar–columellar distance. The curvature of the columella is greater than that of the alar rim. The phenomenon may be due to hypertrophy of the caudal septum and the nasal spine, and/or to a medial crural deformity.

17.3.1 Cause 1: Hypertrophy of the Caudal Septum and Nasal Spine

The caudal septum plays an important role in the cephalocaudal position of the columella, affecting the length of the nose and the nasolabial angle. Anatomically, it lies adjacent to the cephalic portion of the medial crura with a varying amount of membranous septum in between. An overdeveloped caudal septum causes the columella to appear more caudally, resulting in a hanging columella and larger nostrils and usually accompanied by an obtuse columellar-labial angle (Fig. 17.6).

The contribution of the caudal septum to the hanging columella can easily be identified by digital palpation of the columella (Fig. 17.7).

When the problem is due to septal hypertrophy, it can be simply resolved by resecting the hypertrophic segment. If the problem is entirely due to the septum, it will be immediately resolved after resection (Fig. 17.8).

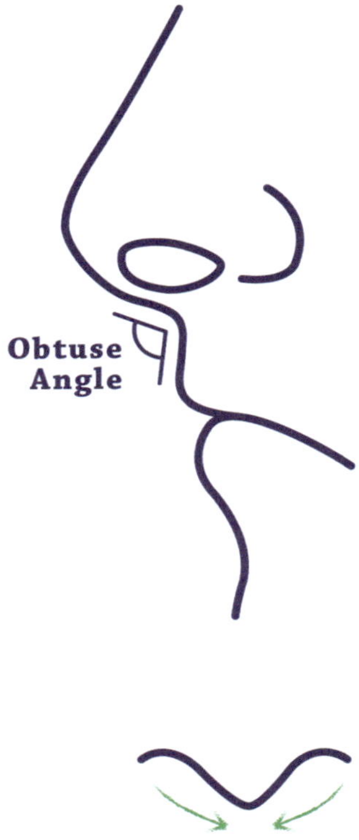

Fig. 17.6 An obtuse subnasal angle characterizes a hanging columella due to caudal septal hypertrophy

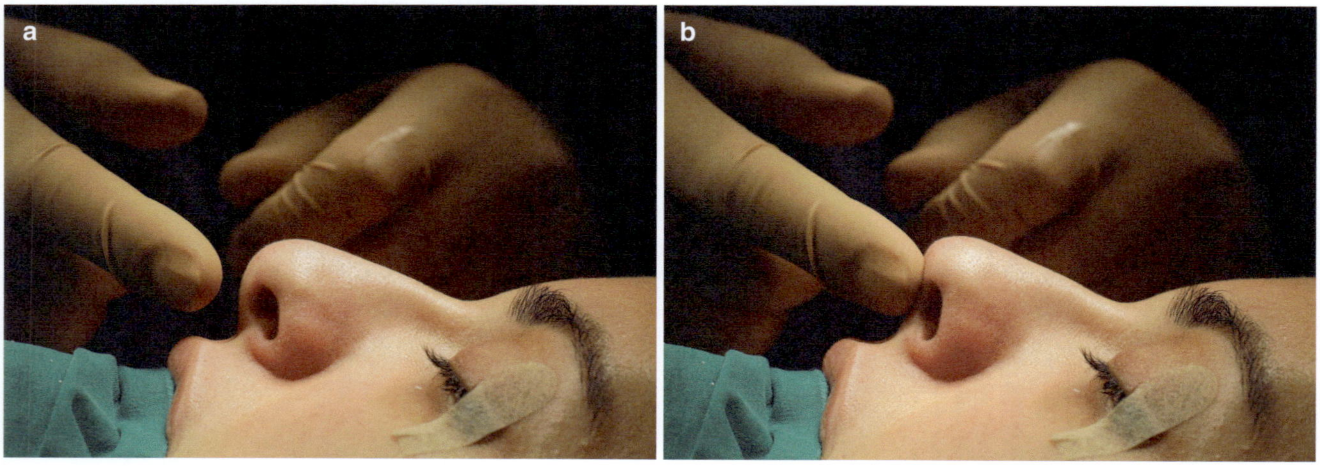

Fig. 17.7 (**a**, **b**) Nasal spine can easily be noted when the philtrum is pushed cephalically. Intraoperatively, palpation of the hanging columella can help to identify overdeveloped caudal septum

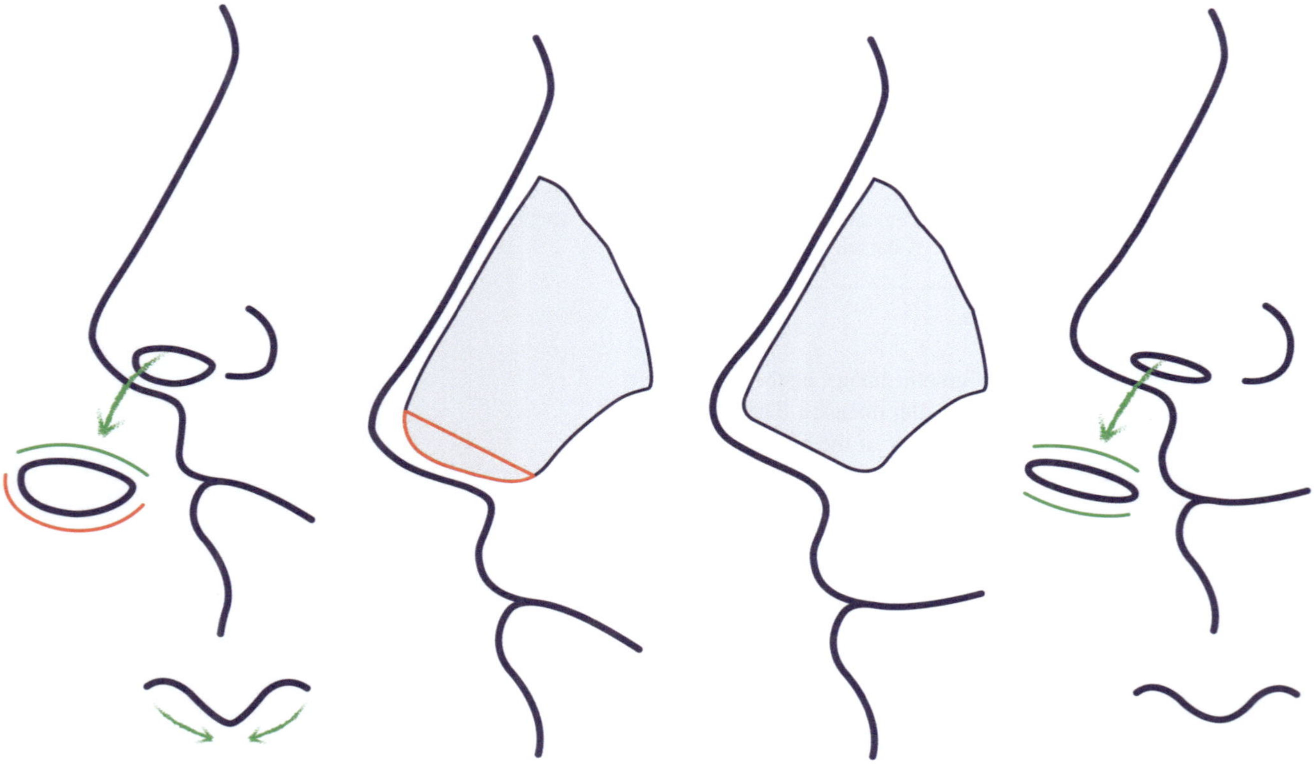

Fig. 17.8 If the only reason for the hanging columella is hypertrophic caudal septum, resecting the excessive part is sufficient

17.3.1.1 Case 1

The photographs in Fig. 17.9 show a patient with large nostrils due to hypertrophy of the caudal septum.

The columellar border has greater curvature than the alar rim. The posteroinferior perimeter of the nostril does not have the desired oval shape. This case was treated via open septoplasty to resect the excess septum (Fig. 17.9c, d).

The surgery reduced the columellar curvature and decreased the gap between the alar rim and the caudal columella, making the septal mucosa less visible from the profile view (Fig. 17.9e, f).

17.3.1.2 Case 2

Figure 17.10a shows a case of large nostrils caused by hypertrophic caudal septum. The septal mucosa is visible

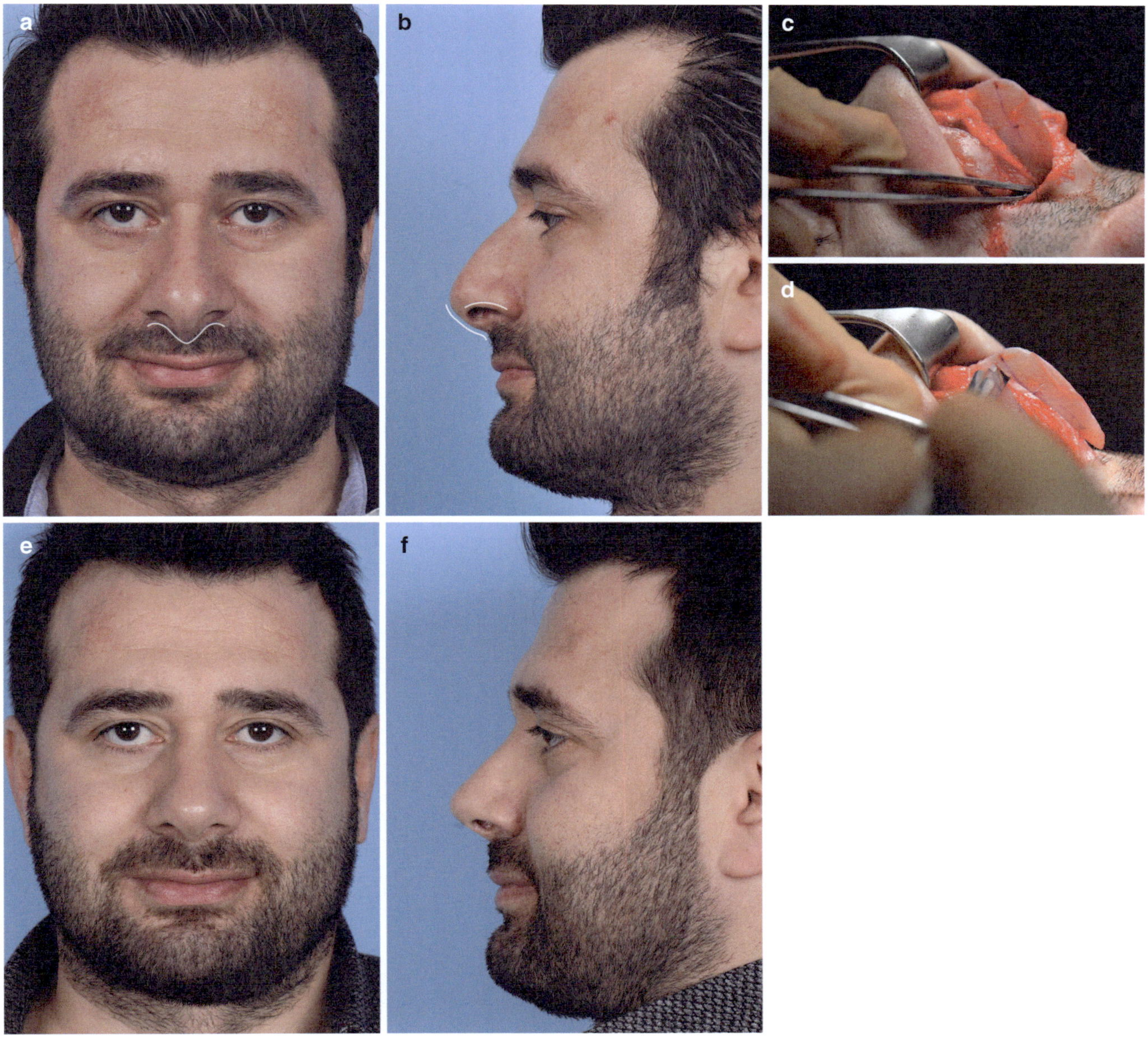

Fig. 17.9 (**a**–**f**) Hypertrophy of the caudal septum resulting in hanging columella can be seen on frontal and lateral view. Notice obtuse angle. Resection of the excess caudal septum was performed. Ideal alar–columellar relationship is achieved postoperatively. (Supplementary Video 17.1)

from the profile view, due to severe curvature of the caudal septum. The patient has an obtuse columellar-labial angle. Resecting the excess caudal septum resolved the problem.

17.3.1.3 Case 3

When such treatment does not resolve the problem, it may be due to under-resection or another underlying condition (e.g., a hypertrophic footplate). Hence, septal resection would not necessarily resolve the problem and would in fact increase the risk of over-shortening the nose. This risk can be mitigated by performing step-by-step septal resection, pushing the nose tip toward the septum at each step to achieve the ideal position.

Figure 17.11 shows a patient with hypertrophy of both the caudal septum and the footplate, resulting in a hanging columella. Both conditions pushed the columella anteriorly.

In this case, closed rhinoplasty was used to resect the excess septal part through a hemitransfixion incision (Fig. 17.12).

The hypertrophic footplate was accessed through an incision made directly into it. The overlying skin was dissected, and the excess portion touching the caudal septum was resected (Fig. 17.13).

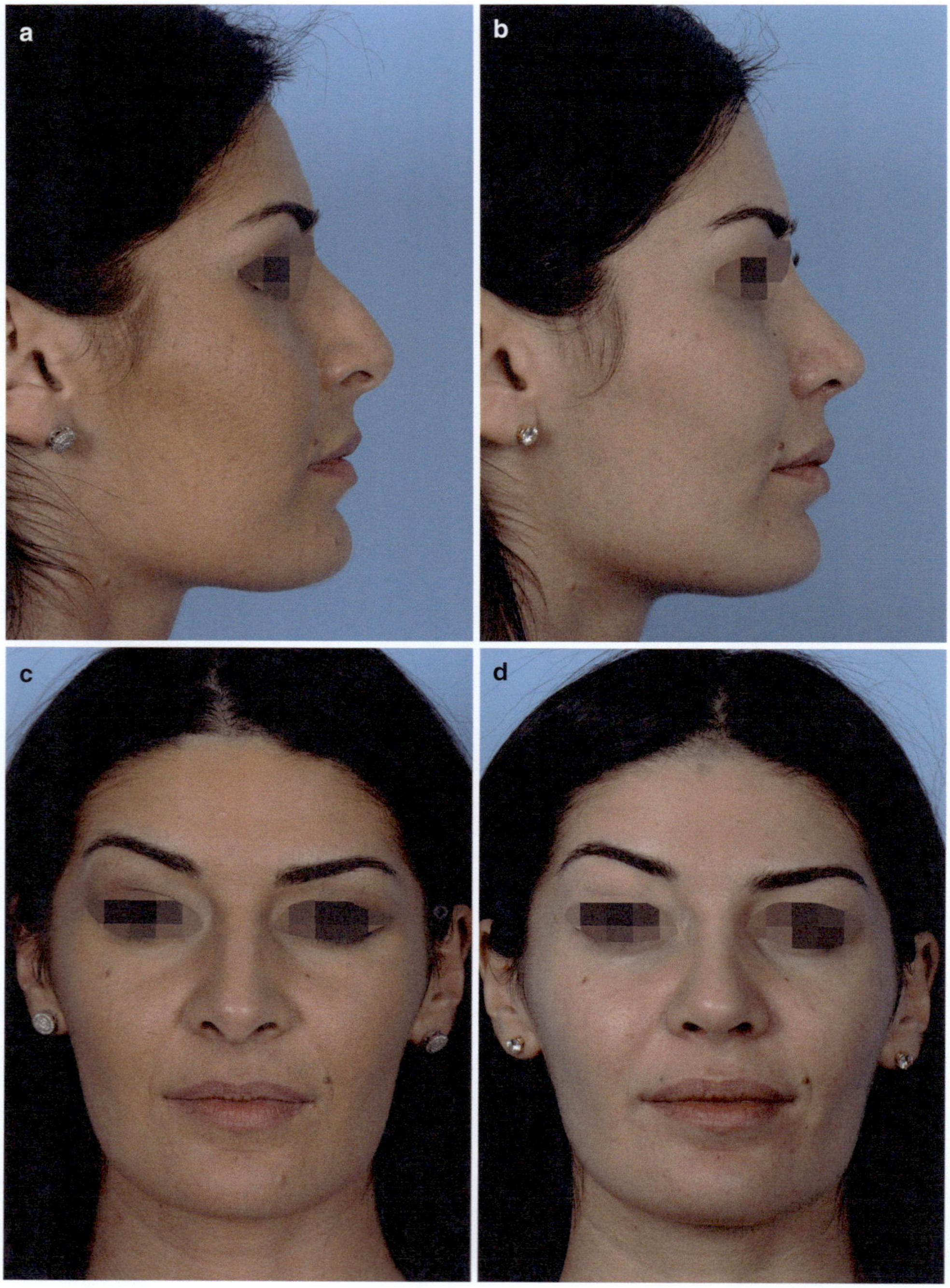

Fig. 17.10 (**a–d**) Pre- and postoperative views: just caudal septal resection solved excessive nostril shows

The surgery corrected the hanging columella, with less of the nostrils being visible from all directions (Fig. 17.14).

It is important to note that redundant membranous septal mucosa can be a problem following caudal septal resection. In such cases, a portion of the membranous septum can easily be resected.

17.3.1.4 Case 4

A 32-year-old woman requested improvement in her prominent dorsum and columella area. Caudal septal excess and a hanging columella are seen in profile (Fig. 17.15).

The caudal septum is dissected, and 5-mm strip of cartilage is excised. Spreader graft is placed (Fig. 17.16).

A small 5-mm strip of excess vestibular mucosa is excised (Fig. 17.17).

Two-year postoperative photographs are shown in Fig. 17.18. The hanging columella is improved. The columella labial angle is more acute and is positioned more caudal.

Also, surgeons may prefer not to shorten the septum if the sizes of the nostrils are due to a hypertrophic caudal septum. Excess septum can be used for the tongue-in-groove technique.

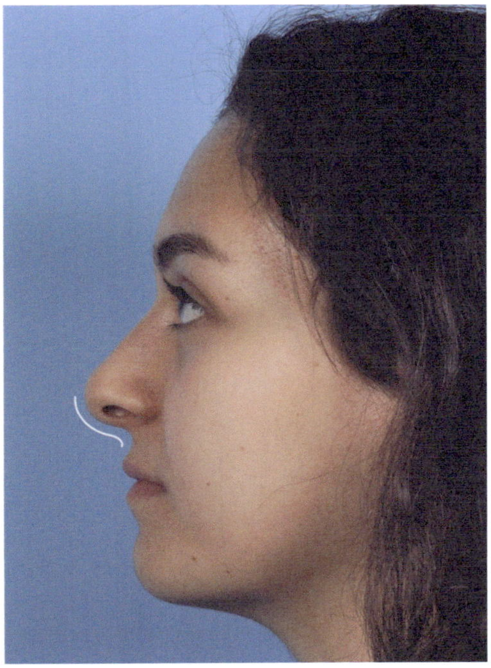

Fig. 17.11 Patient with excessive nostril show

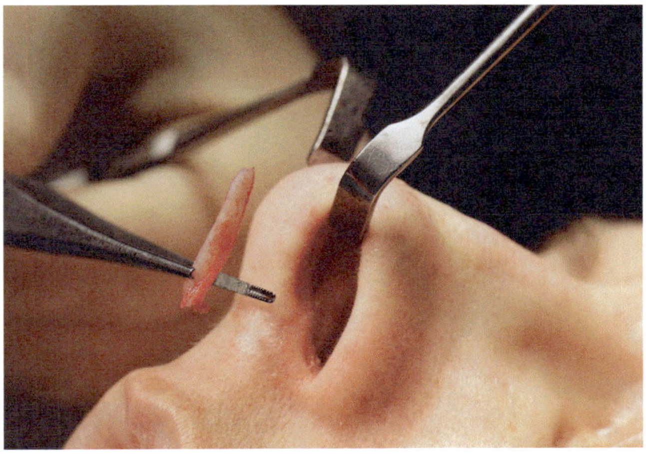

Fig. 17.12 Caudal septal trim and vestibular skin resection

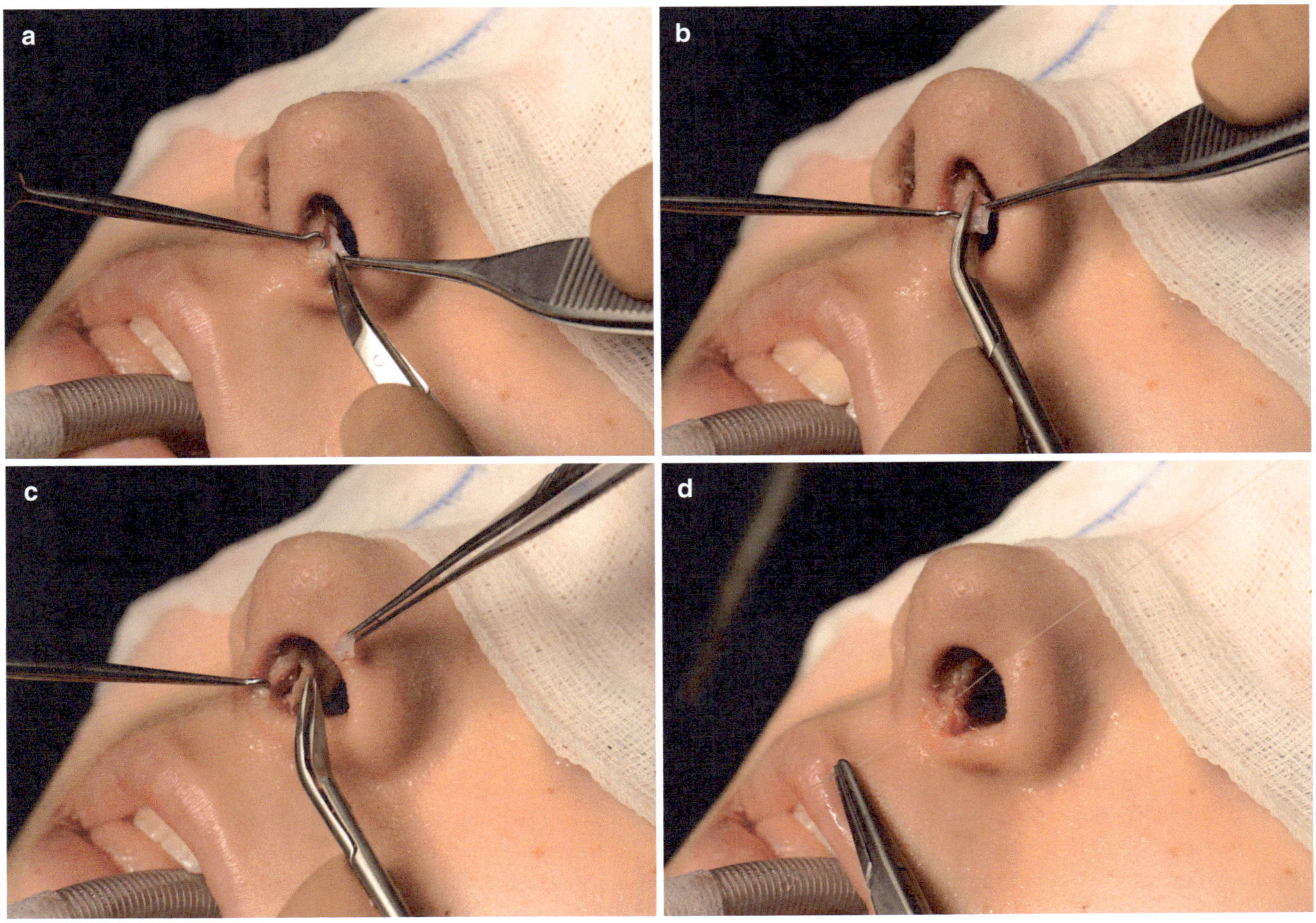

Fig. 17.13 (a–d) Footplate trimming

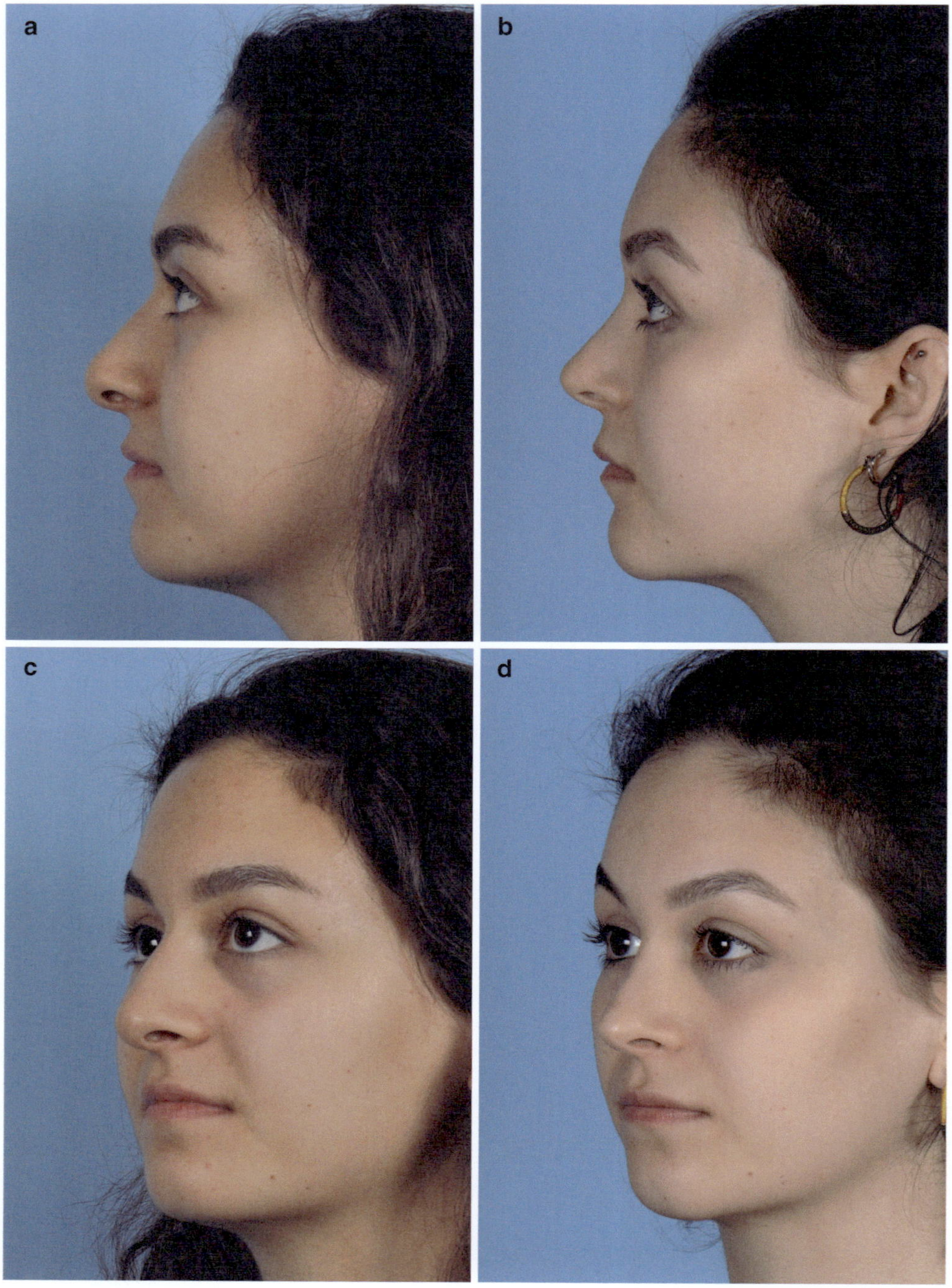

Fig. 17.14 (**a–d**) Pre- and postoperative photographs

In some patients, fullness of the columellar–labial junction may be caused by a so-called pushing philtrum, which in turn can result in an open columellar–labial angle and excessive nostril show. This can result in an unbalanced appearance, with the nose appearing to precede the face. This problem is usually due to a prominent nasal spine, necessitating partial resection. As the caudal septum is normal in length, no changes to the cartilage are necessary. Hence, partial nasal spine resection is performed without resecting the caudal septum to reduce excessive "nasolabial show."

17.3.1.5 Case 5

In this case, hanging columella and open columella labial angle is due to a prominent nasal spine; so again, partial resection of the spine should be performed. The length of the caudal septum is normal, no cartilage resection is necessary (Fig. 17.19).

17.3.2 Cause 2: Anomalies of the Medial Crura

Caudal flaring or downward protrusion of the medial crura results in large nostrils due to a hanging columella. This may result from an abnormal structural configuration of the medial crus or may emerge secondary to surgical manipulation. The hanging columella results from caudal bowing of the medial crural cartilage, characterized by more severe curvature of the caudal alar rim than the columella, and is usually accompanied by an acute columellar–labial angle (Fig. 17.20).

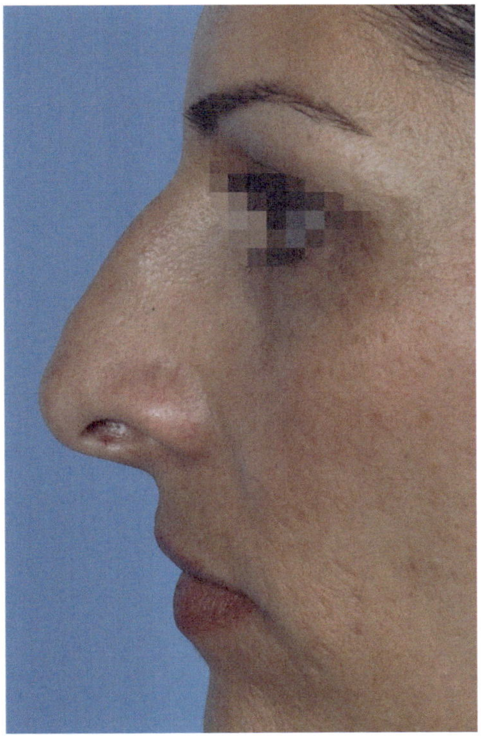

Fig. 17.15 The long caudal septum pushes the columella caudally, creating excessive nostril show

Two treatment approaches for this type of hanging columella have been described. In mild cases, a columellar strut can be placed and a crescent-shaped portion of tissue can be trimmed out from the caudal border of the medial crura of the alar cartilage (Fig. 17.21).

More severe cases are best treated with the medial crural overlapping technique, in which both medial crura are divided at their junctions with the middle crura, overlapped, and then stabilized with sutures to a cartilage strut placed between the two medial crura (Fig. 17.22).

17.3.2.1 Case 6

In the case shown in Fig. 17.23, wide nostrils were accompanied by an acute columellar labial angle and excessive bowing of the medial crura.

Open approach rhinoplasty was used to expose the alar cartilages. It was necessary to pay attention to the bowing of the medial cartilages. The crura were brought together using a columellar strut following transdomal suturing, which partially corrected the misconfiguration in the medial crura, although the bowing persisted. Wide (in a cranial-to-caudal direction) crura were treated by excising a crescent of medial crural cartilage (Fig. 17.24).

The approach (columellar strut placement and caudal trimming of medial crura) resolved the mild hanging columella (Fig. 17.25).

17.3.2.2 Case 7

In the case shown in Fig. 17.26, there was an imbalance between the alar rim and the columella border, contorting the aesthetic features and resulting in excessive nostril show.

Closed approach rhinoplasty was used to access the alar cartilages. A lateral crural steal suture was used to increase the projection of the tip, but this resulted in the problem

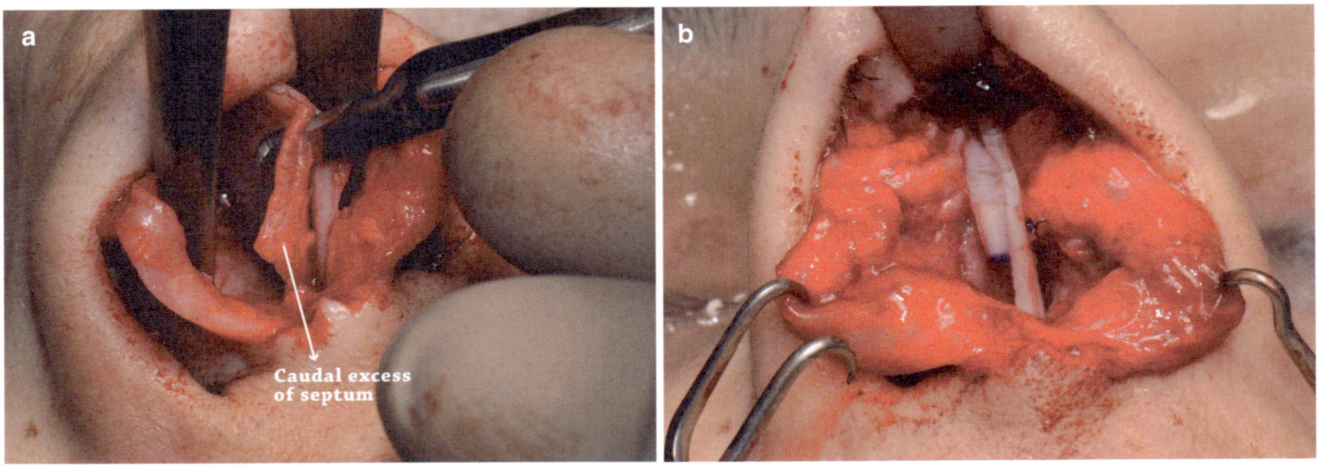

Fig. 17.16 (**a**) Caudal septal excision. (**b**) Spreader graft placement for stability

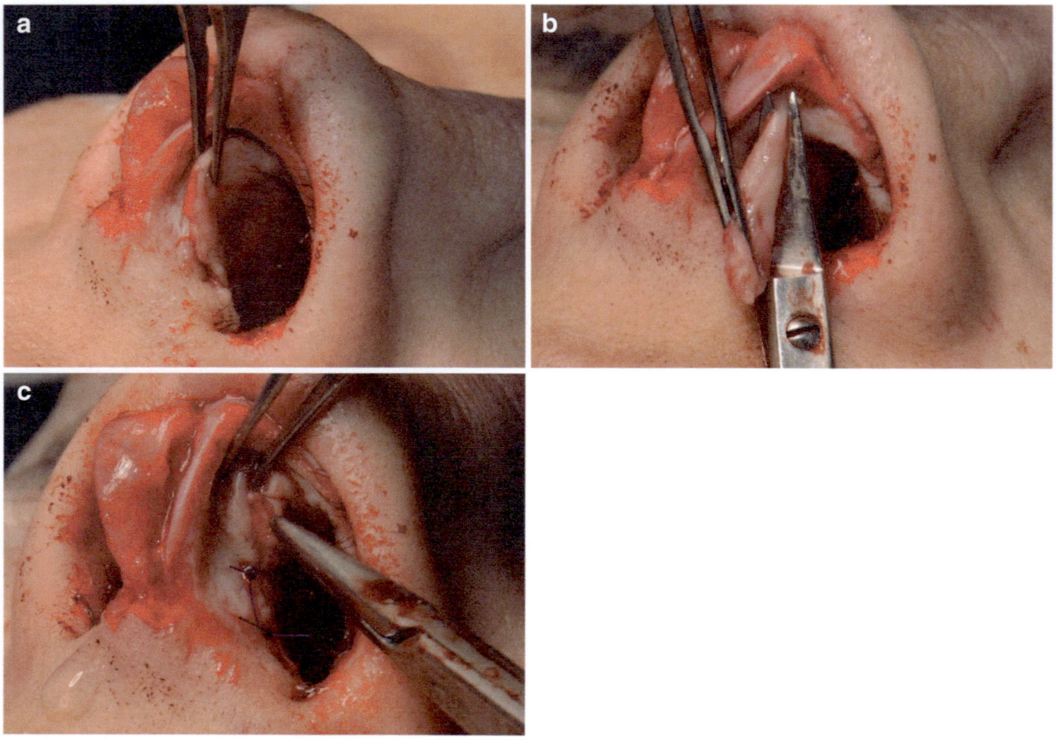

Fig. 17.17 (**a**–**c**) Excess mucoperichondrium at the transfixion incision excised

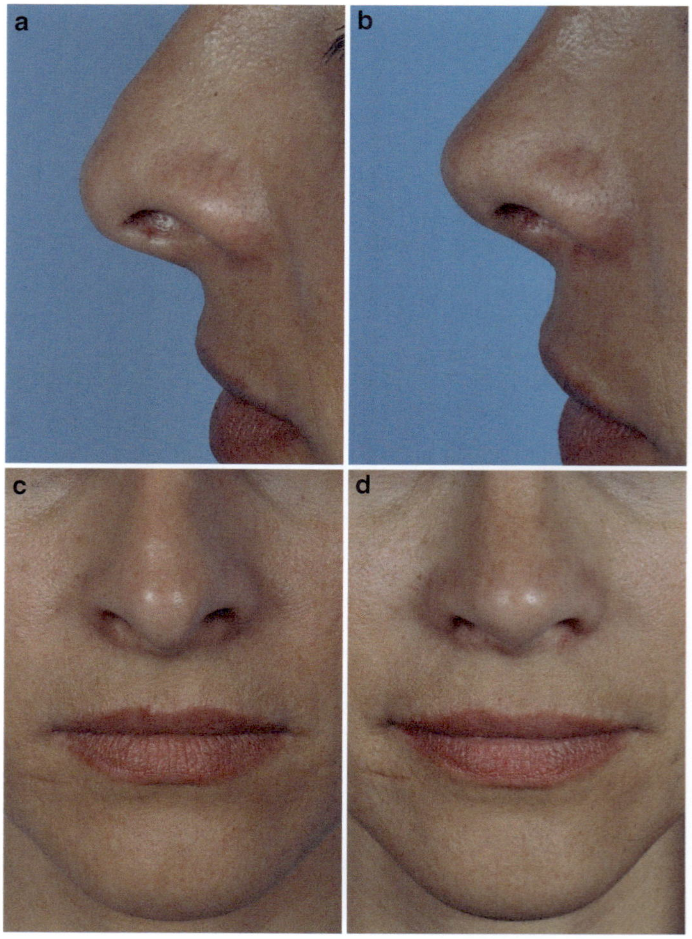

Fig. 17.18 (**a**–**d**) Pre- and postoperative photographs, reduced nostril shows on lateral view. On frontal view, the alar/columellar discrepancy has been corrected

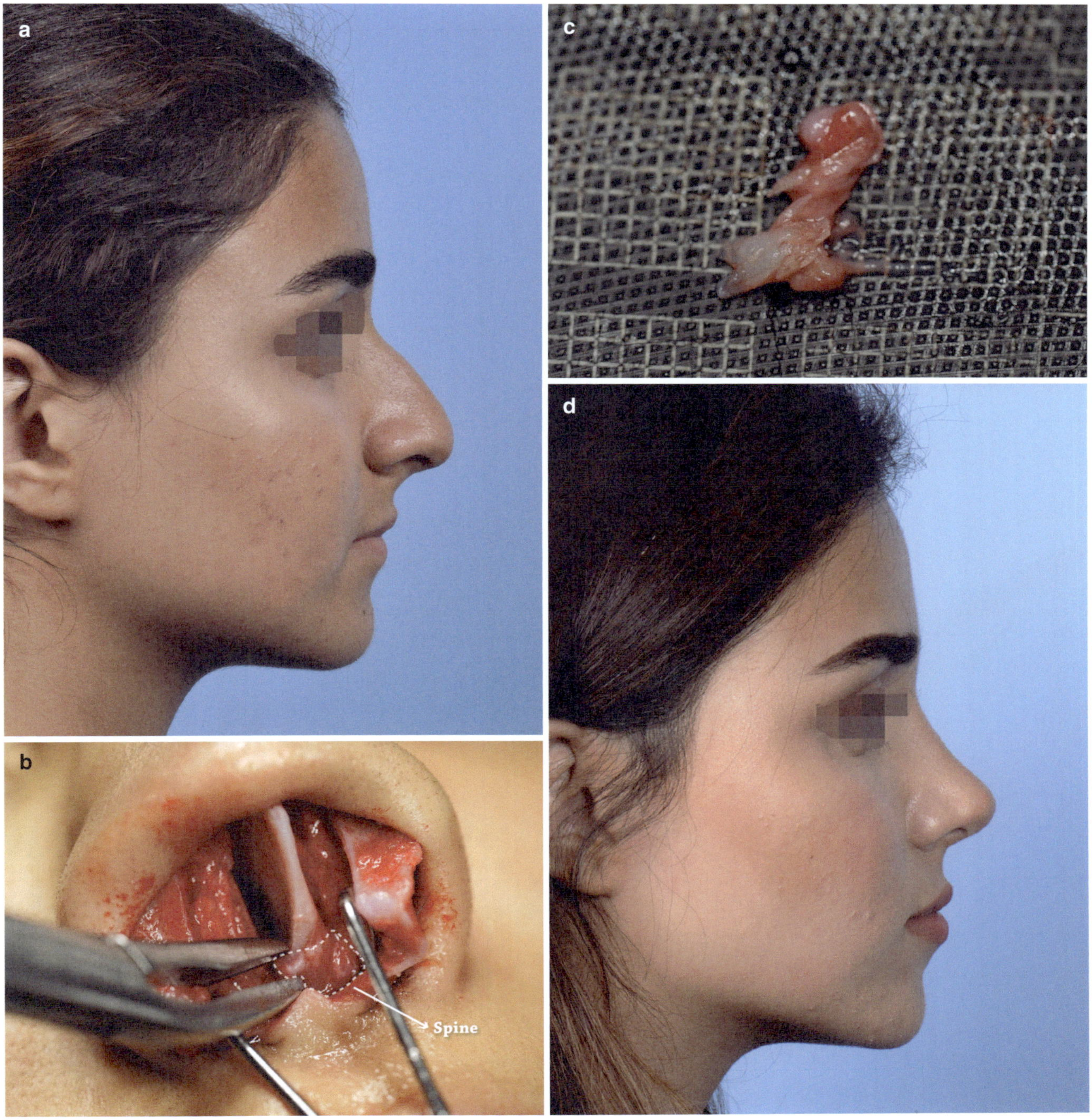

Fig. 17.19 (**a**) Preoperative photograph. (**b**) Partial resection of the nasal spine. (**c**) Excess part of the nasal spine and surrounding soft tissue. (**d**) Nostril show was reduced. The columella labial angle is more acute and is positioned more caudally

becoming even more pronounced. To resolve this problem, the medial crura were cut at their most prominent points without harming the vestibular mucosa. Each upper flap was elevated from the skin to the dome and slid over the distal flap to correct the misconfiguration. A 6-0 absorbable suture was placed to overlap the two segments. As cutting the medial crura inevitably weakens it, stability was achieved by fixing columellar strut. A cap graft was used to create the final projection of the nose tip (Fig. 17.27).

The approach (medial crural overlap) resolved the moderate hanging columella. The treatment of hanging columella adds a subtle beneficial enhancement to the results of rhinoplasty (Fig. 17.28).

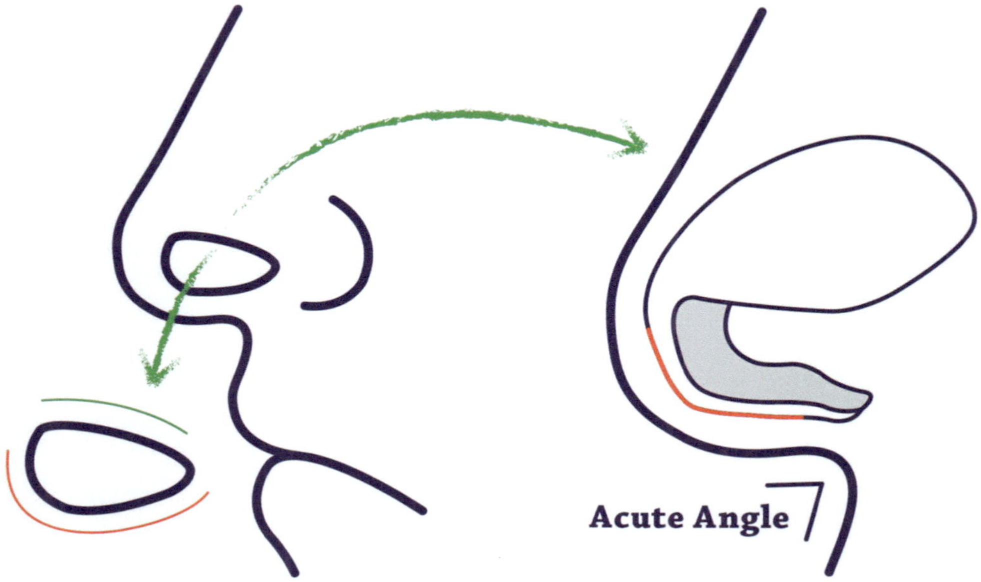

Fig. 17.20 An acute subnasale angle and severe curvature of the caudal alar rim characterizes a hanging columella due to medial alar hypertrophy

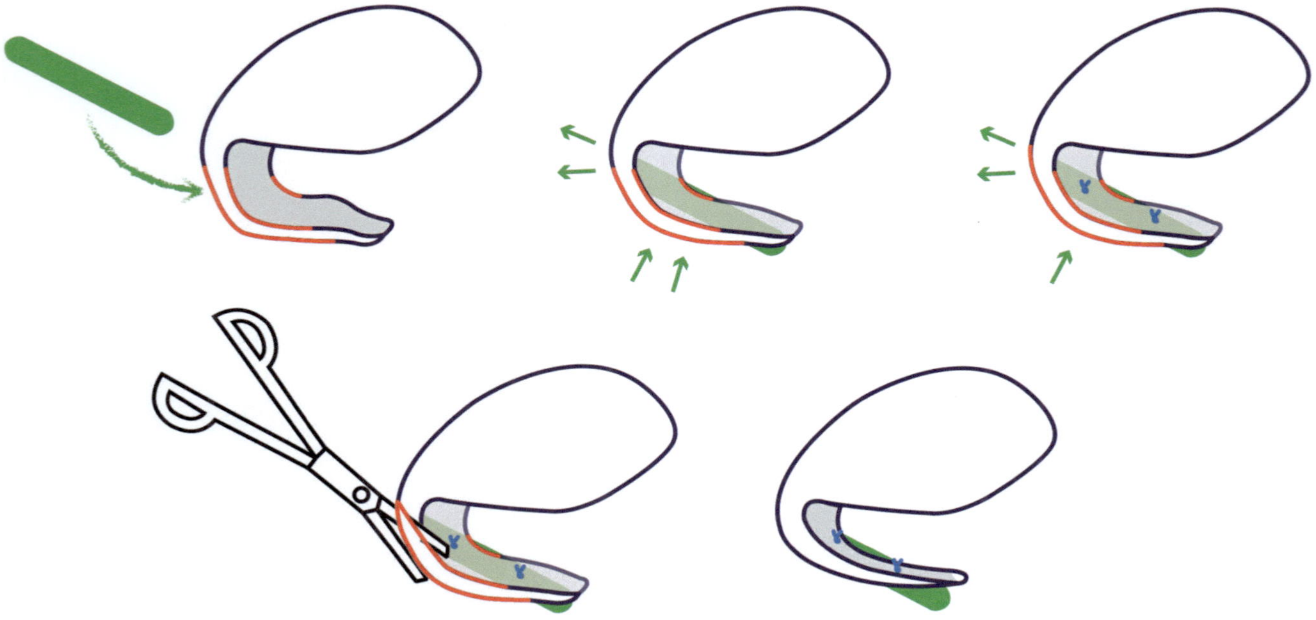

Fig. 17.21 Dependency of the infratip lobule improved by trimming the caudal aspect of the medial crura. (Supplementary Video 17.2)

17.3.2.3 Case 8

Case 8 features a different patient from Case 7, but with the same anatomical problem. Medial crural overlap was used for treatment. A columellar strut was used to increase tip stability. A shield graft and cap graft were used to lengthen the infratip lobule, providing more definition and projection to the nose tip. The footplate was also found to be pushing the columella anteriorly and thus was removed through a separate incision (Fig. 17.29).

Preoperative and postoperative photographs are shown in Fig. 17.30.

17.3.2.4 Case 9

Finally, it may be necessary in some cases to use all of the above techniques, as in the example seen in Fig. 17.31. This case shows an example of disfigurement of the acute nasolabial angle and columellar misconfiguration.

Closed approach was used. First, the columella was pushed cranially to determine the contribution of the septum to the hanging columella. There was limited septal resistance and thus the excess caudal septum tissue was resected. Transdomal suturing resulted in prominent flaring of the medial crura in the caudal direction, which was corrected

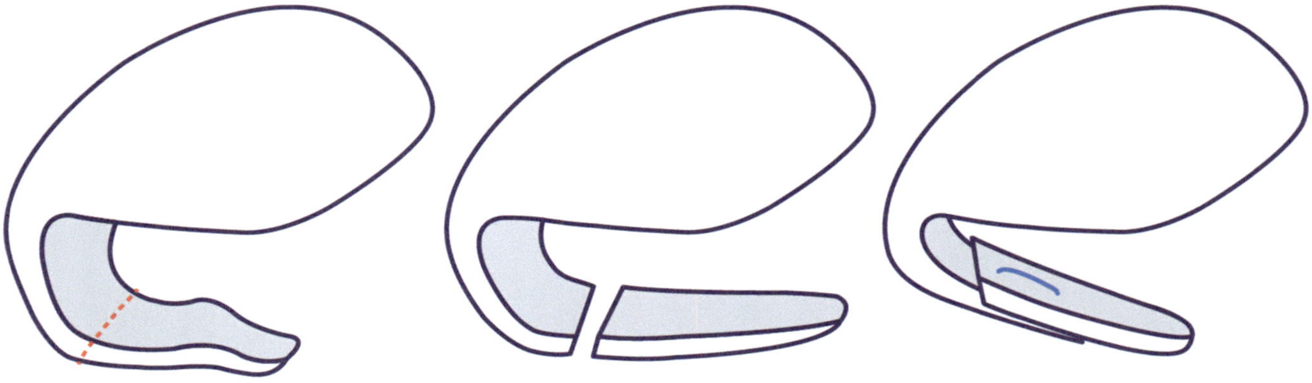

Fig. 17.22 Division and overlap of the medial crus reduces nostril show

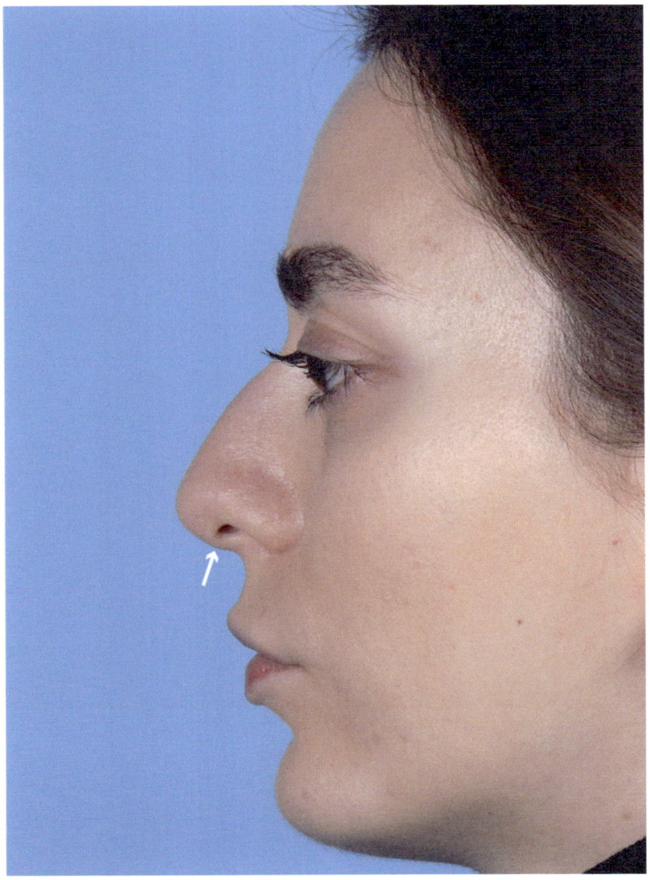

Fig. 17.23 Excessive nostril show stems from medial crura

using the overlapping technique. However, a slight excess of medial crura tissue remained after the overlap was trimmed. Hence, hypertrophic footplates were resected through a separate incision (Fig. 17.32).

Ultimately, the excessive nostril show was corrected and an ideal alar–columellar relationship was restored (Fig. 17.33).

In some situations, hypertrophic and strong lateral crura may have been responsible for the hanging columella pushing away the medial crura. In that case, cutting and shortening the lateral crus next to the dome brought the medial crus to the ideal position, resolving all other pathologies affecting the nose tip.

Case 10 is a typical example of excess nostril size due to a long lateral crus.

17.3.2.5 Case 10

The patient had presented with a wide nasal tip and large nostrils resulting from the hanging columella. Both problems stemmed from long and strong lateral crura (Fig. 17.34).

The hypertrophic segment of the lateral crus was resected via vertical alar resection (VAR technique) (Fig. 17.35).

This resulted in deprojection and mild cephalic rotation while shortening the elongated nostril (Fig. 17.36).

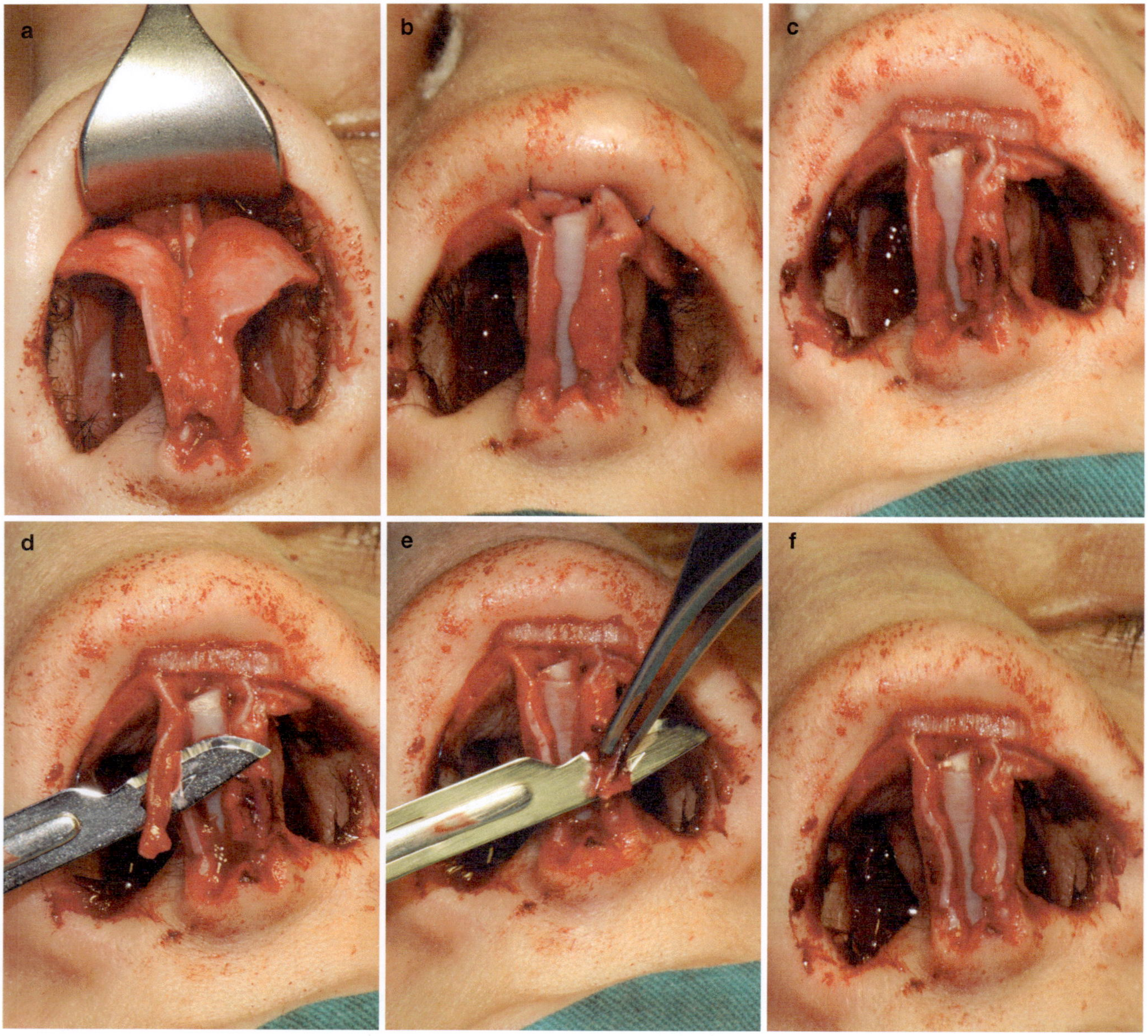

Fig. 17.24 (**a**–**f**) Trimming of the medial crus through the external approach

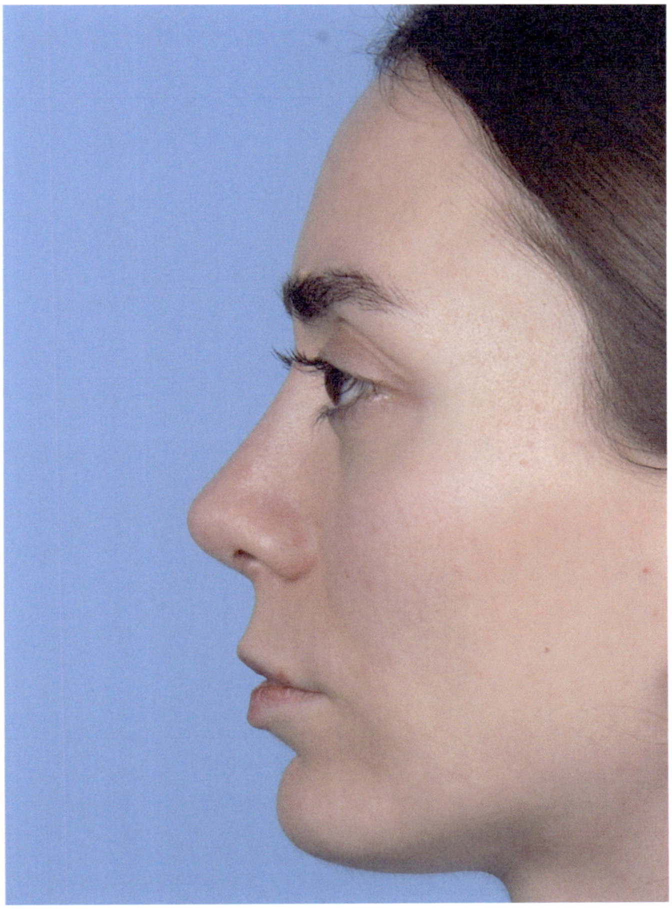

Fig. 17.25 Postoperative lateral view

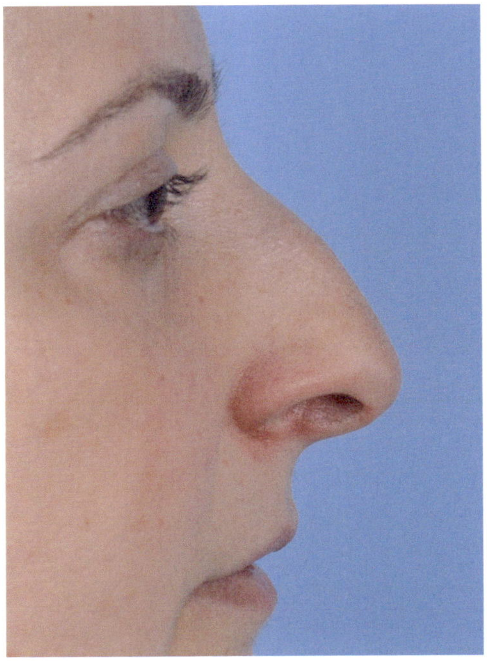

Fig. 17.26 Buckled medial crura and caudal septal hypertrophy resulted in hanging columella

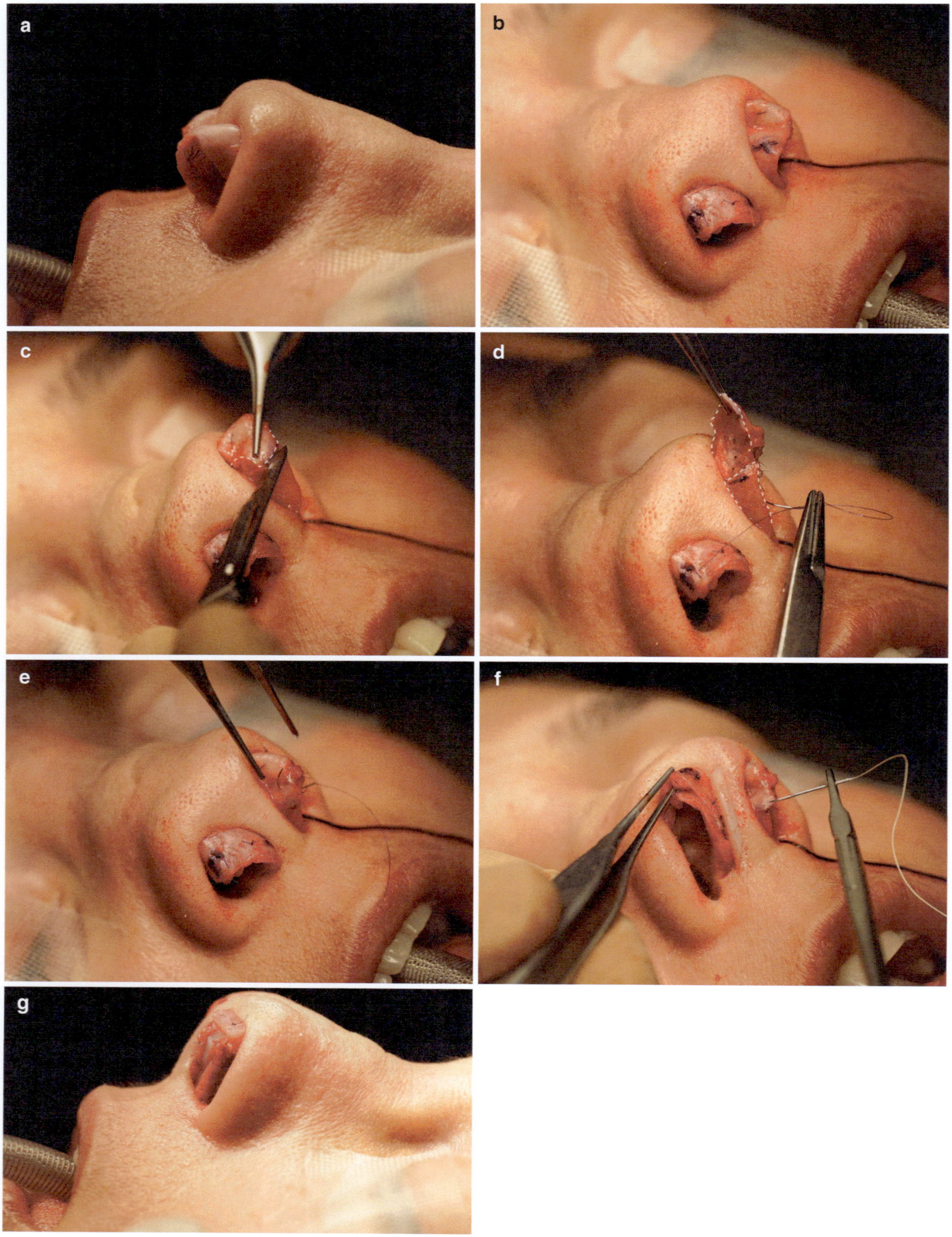

Fig. 17.27 (**a–g**) Caudal septal trimming and medial crural overlap were done

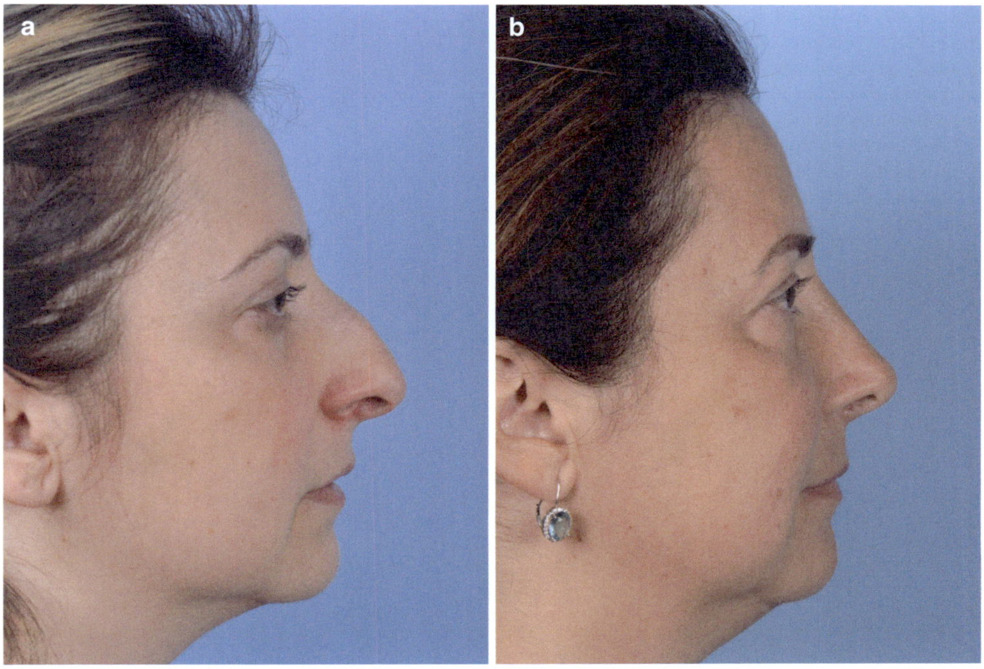

Fig. 17.28 (**a**, **b**) Pre- and postoperative profile views demonstrate improved nostril show

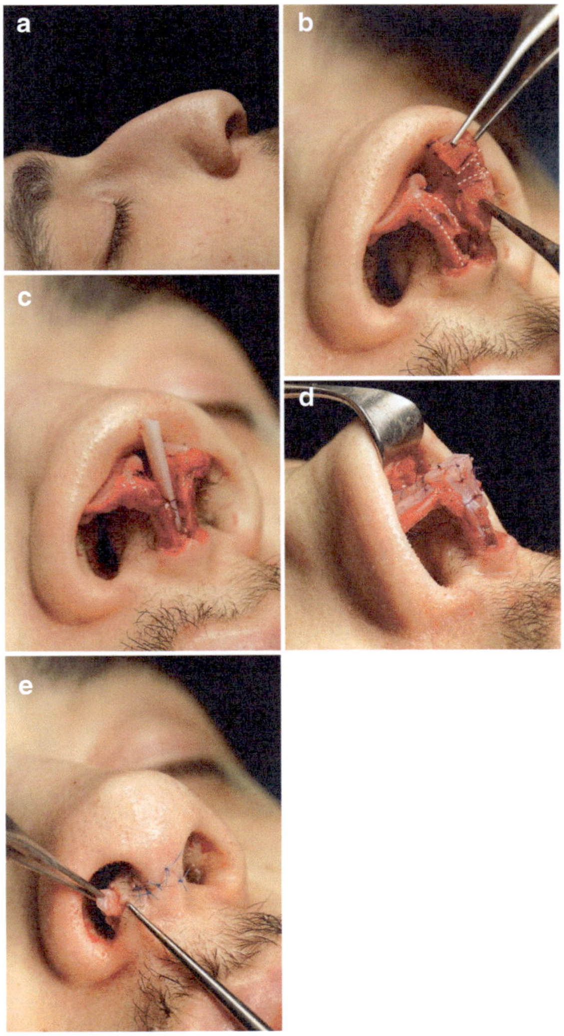

Fig. 17.29 (**a**–**e**) Medial crural overlap and trimming of footplate were used for treating hanging columella. Shield graft, cup graft, columellar strut, and lateral crural graft were placed for rebuilding the tip

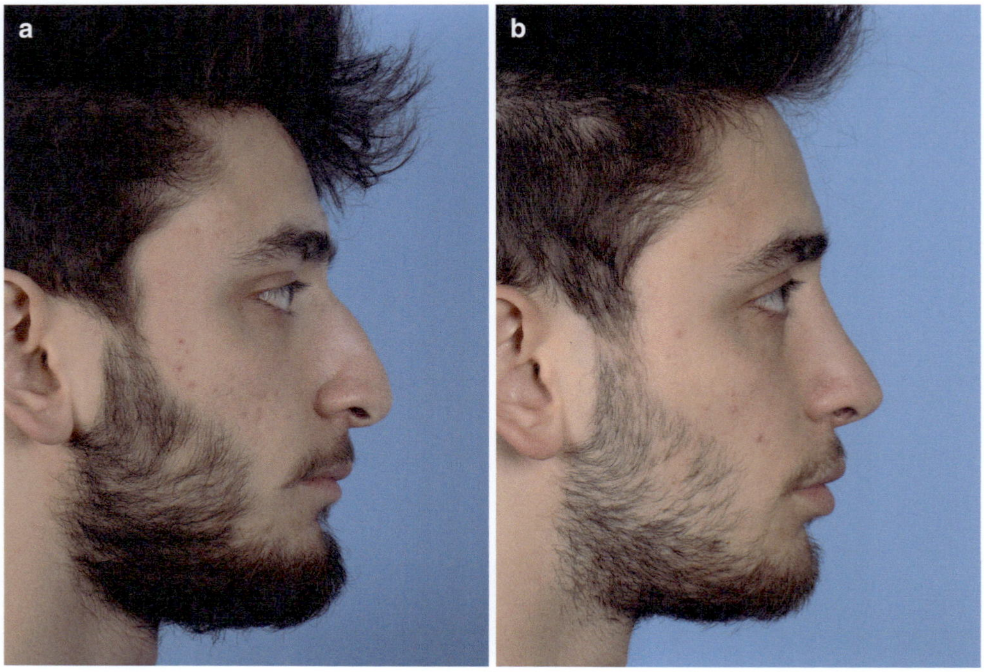

Fig. 17.30 (**a**, **b**) Both medial crura protrude caudally, giving the infratip an unattractive, loop-like appearance on lateral view. (**b**) The hanging columella is improved. Favorable alar–columellar relationship is achieved

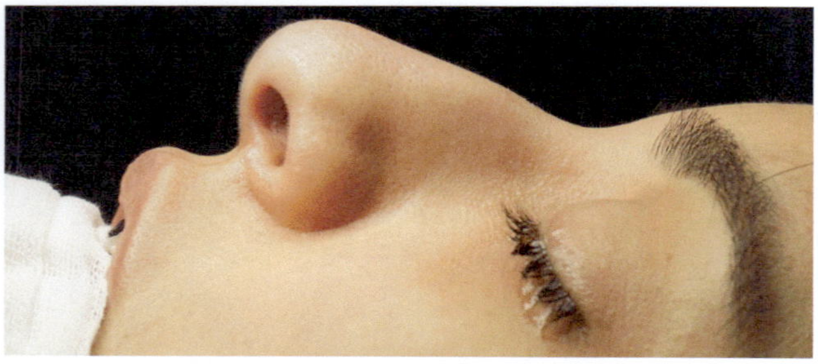

Fig. 17.31 Excessive nostril show; immediately before surgery

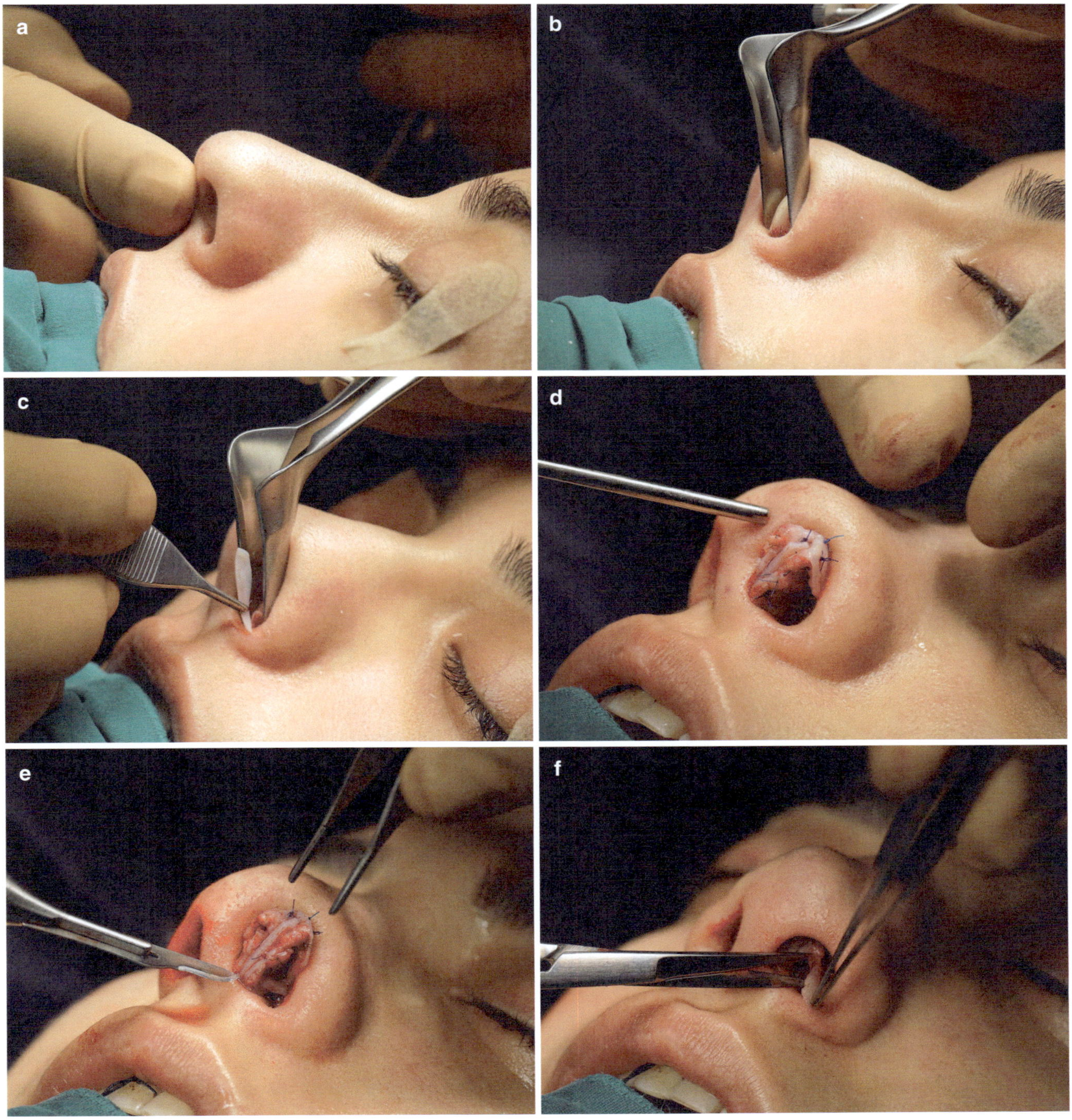

Fig. 17.32 (**a–c**) Caudal septal trimming. (**d**) Medial crural overlap was finished. (**e**) Caudal medial crura trimming. (**f**) Footplate trimming

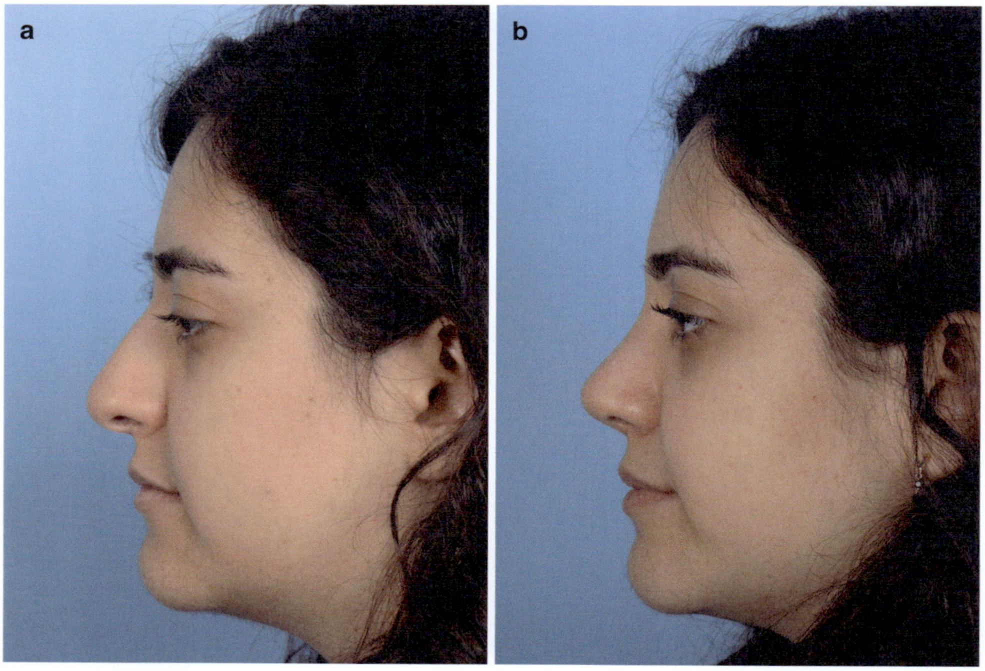

Fig. 17.33 (**a**) On preoperative lateral view, excess nostril show is seen. (**b**) Proportional alar–columellar relationship was achieved

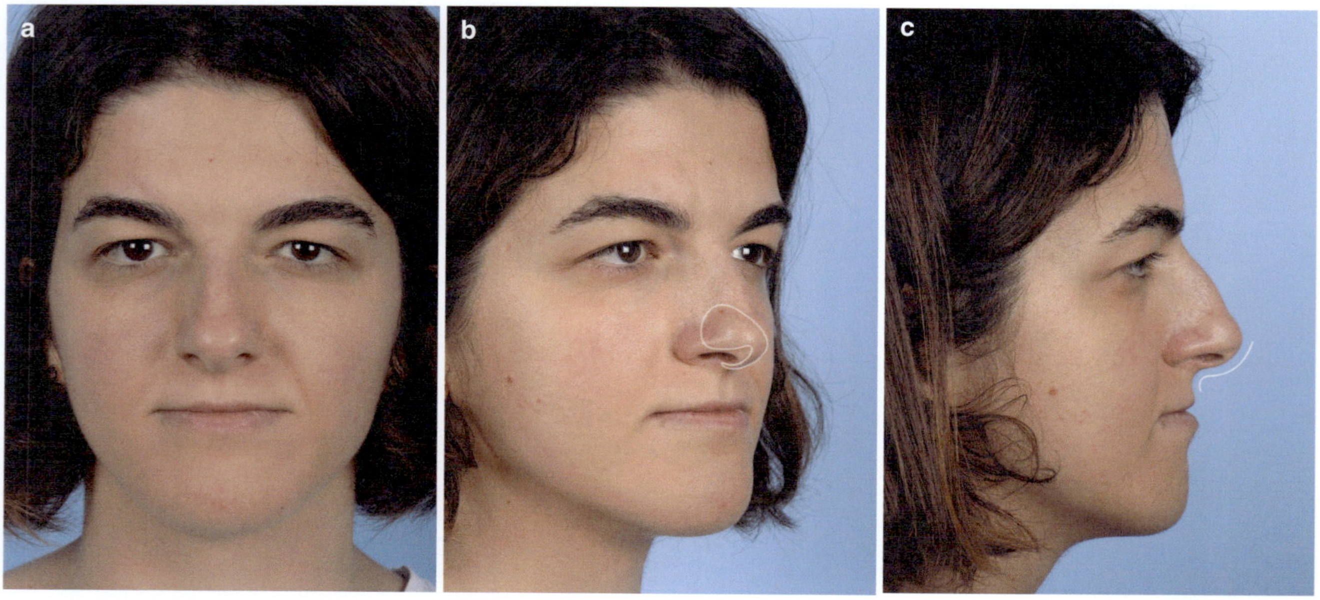

Fig. 17.34 (**a**) Unfavorable alar–columellar relationship on profile view. (**b**) The overdevelopment lateral crus are outlined in the white line. Both lateral crus are pushing the columella caudally. (**c**) Excessive nostril show

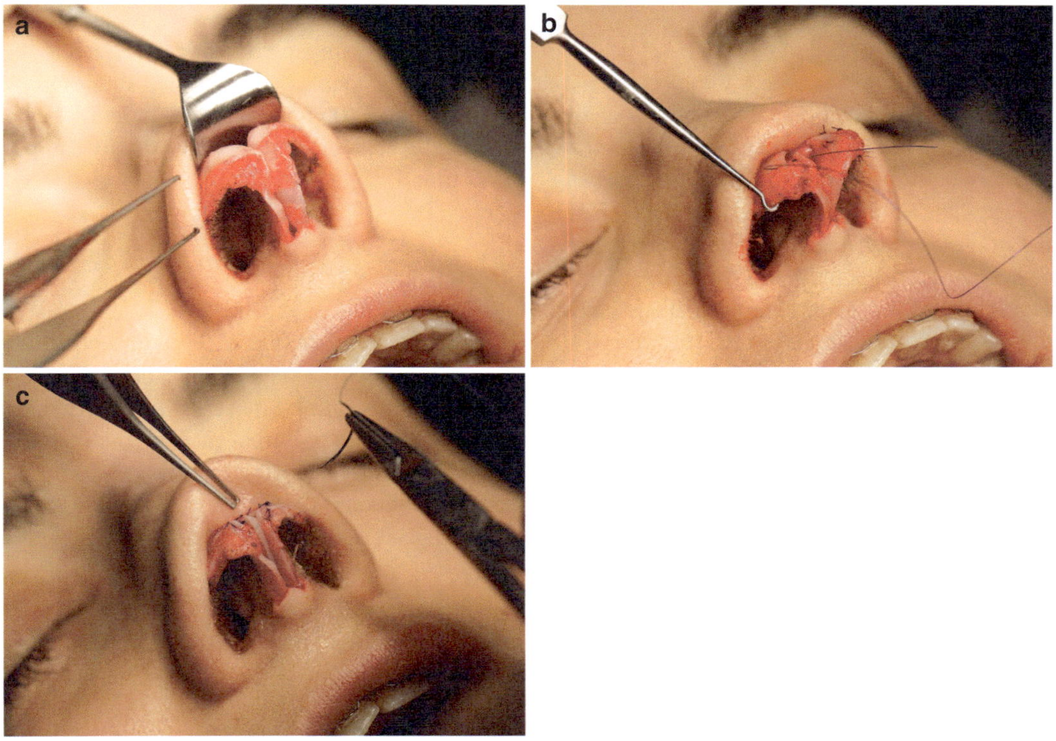

Fig. 17.35 (**a**–**c**) To remove the excess part of lateral crura, alar cartilages were divided, excised, sutured, and reconstructed

Fig. 17.36 (**a**–**c**) Reconstruction of the alar cartilages fixed excessive nostril show and other tip problems

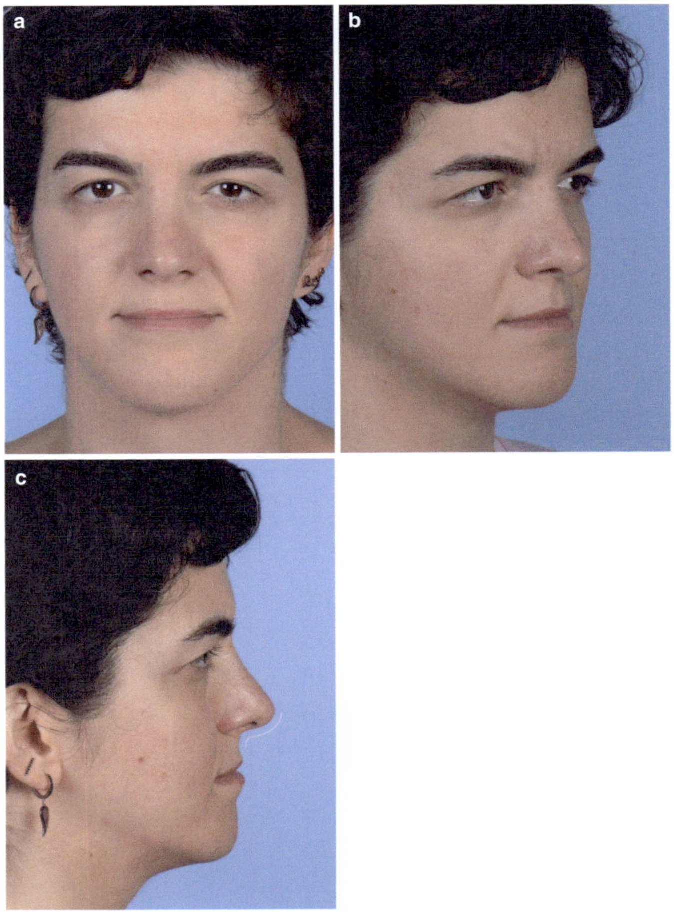

17.4 Retracted Ala

In a retracted alar rim, the nostrils appear too big, and nasal hair can be seen from oblique and lateral views. It is characterized by the presence of alar notching and/or an excessively curved alar rim margin. The oval shape of the nostril is disfigured, and cephalic edges are longer and convex (Fig. 17.37).

The various etiologies can be congenital or iatrogenic. Iatrogenic alar retraction occurs when aggressive resection of the cephalic portion of the lower lateral cartilage leads to weakening of the cartilage, causing it to retract superiorly. A central tenet of rhinoplasty surgery involves the preservation of a critical width of the lateral crura typically >7 mm to maintain the structural integrity of the cartilage framework. However, moderate cephalic resection may sometimes result in alar retraction even with a transdomal suture. The dead space that remains may cause the remaining lateral crus to migrate cephalically. If the patient has a normal alar/columellar relationship preoperatively, there is a good chance that limited cephalic resection and suture will not aggravate the condition. If, however, the patient has borderline alar retraction, cephalic resection may easily cause alar retraction over time.

17.4.1 Case 11

The case depicted in Fig. 17.38 represents a good example of this condition. The patient had borderline alar retraction, which was aggravated by cephalic resection and transdomal suture of the lateral crus, making the alar retraction more prominent.

Conventional prophylactic treatment under these circumstances is added to lateral crural graft or rim graft.

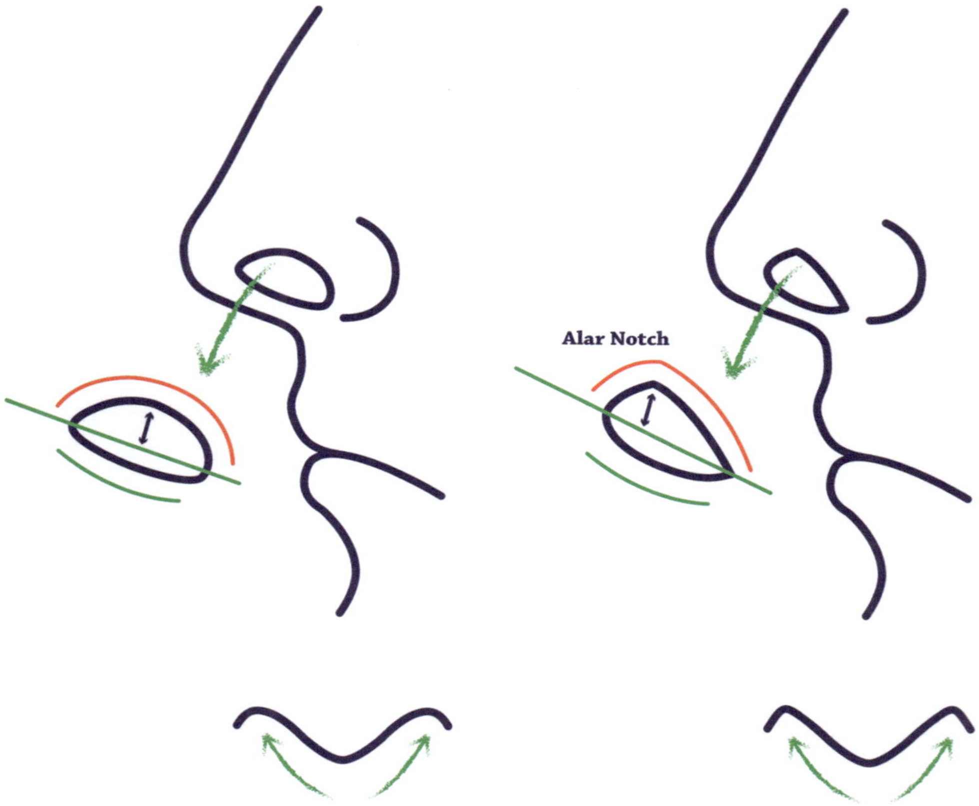

Fig. 17.37 Alar retraction, also connected with septal mucosa show on profile, can be identified by a more severe curvature of the alar rim

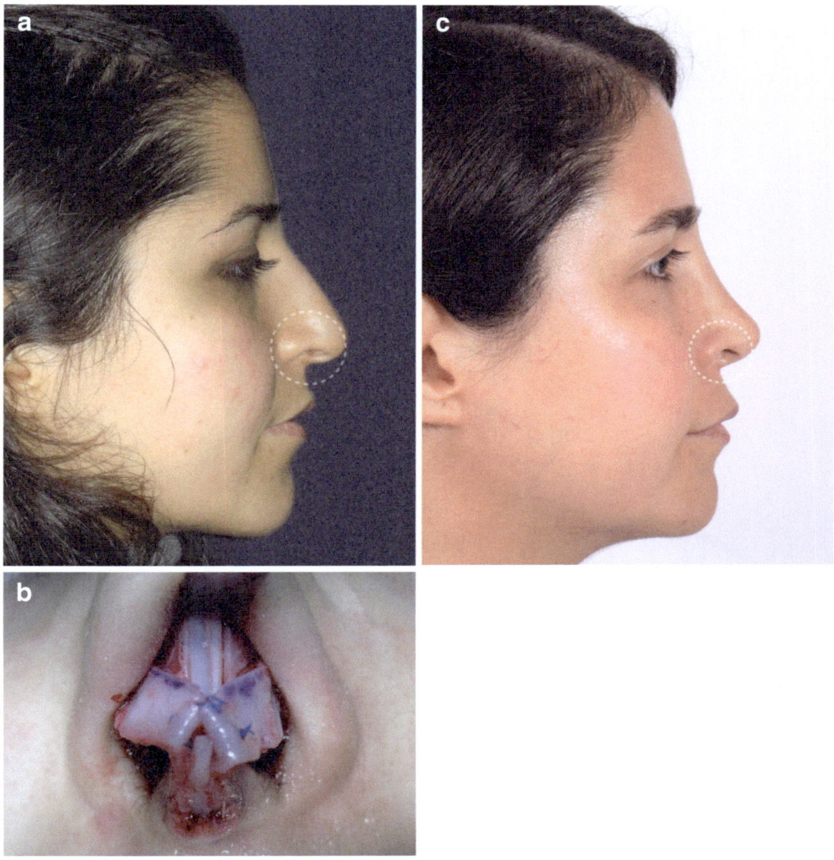

Fig. 17.38 (**a**) Preoperative photograph. The right ala slightly retracted. It can be overlooked. (**b**) Minimal cephalic trim of lateral crura, transdomal suture, dome-equalizing suture. There is no aggressive resection. (**c**) Ten years after surgery; tip projection and rotation are ideal but evident alar retraction is seen

17.5 Treatment Strategy

There are three different grafts that can be used to correct this case: alar rim, lateral crural, and auricular composite grafts. Each of these, with case examples, is discussed below.

17.5.1 Alar Rim Graft

The alar rim graft is a nonanatomical graft that is useful for preventing or correcting alar retraction; it provides structural support to the alar margin. It can be used unilaterally or bilaterally to straighten alar notching and to treat mild alar retraction by pushing the alar margin down 1–2 mm. These grafts are typically cut in a rectangular shape measuring 10–15 mm in length and 2–3 mm in width. They can be placed via open or closed rhinoplasty, a marginal incision, or a small stab incision at the alar margin, and in a floating fashion within the soft tissue envelope or in a secured manner at a right angle to the dome using sutures (Fig. 17.39).

17.5.1.1 Case 12

Figure 17.40 shows an example of excessive nostril show due to a mildly retracted ala and an excessive caudal septum.

Figure 17.41 shows a postoperative view indicating improvement in the alar rim following placement of an alar rim graft and a 2 mm resection of the caudal septum.

17.5.1.2 Case 13

Figure 17.42 shows another primary patient with alar notching. Caudal septal trimming and alar rim grafting were applied during septoplasty, which markedly improved the deformity.

17.5.2 Lateral Crural Graft

Malpositioning of the lateral crus can cause a wide tip lobule and excessive nostril show due to alar retraction. When unsupported by a misdirected lateral crus, the alar rim slips in the cranial direction.

17.5.2.1 Case 14

Figure 17.43 shows a preoperative oblique view of a patient with severe alar retraction due to malpositioning of the lateral crus.

When the lower lateral cartilages are cephalically malpositioned, caudal repositioning of the lateral crura can be performed to bring the cartilage to a more anatomical position;

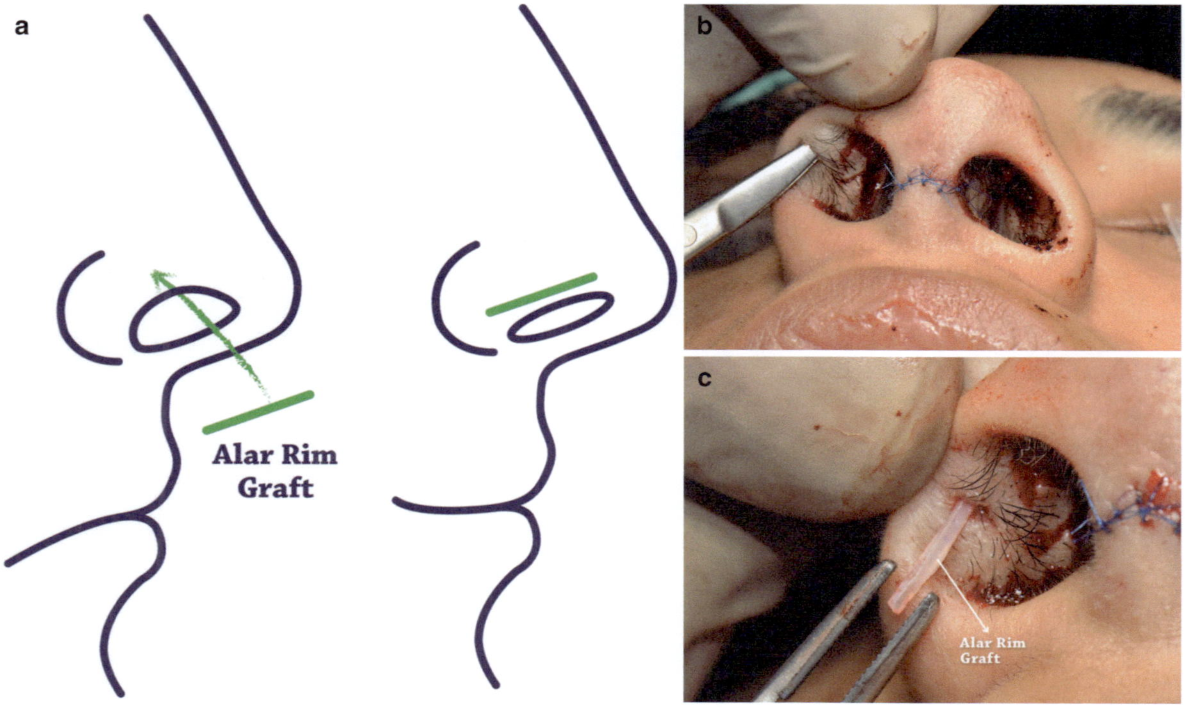

Fig. 17.39 (**a–c**) Alar rim graft is a useful tool to treat a mild degree of alar rim retraction

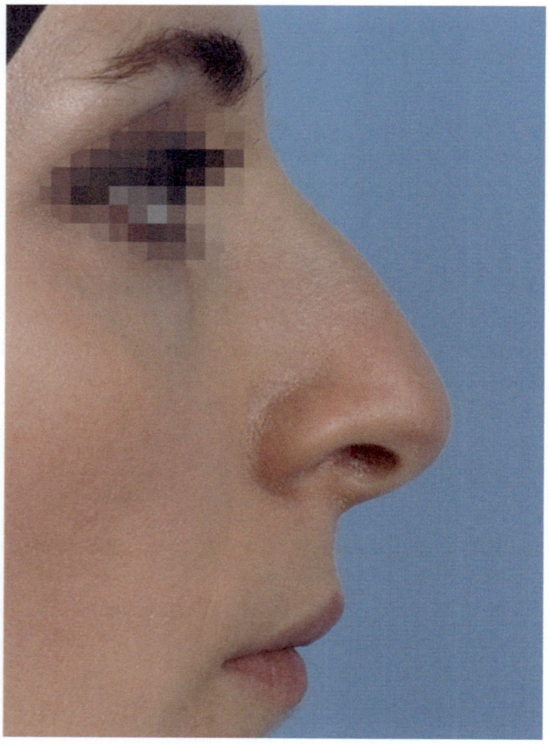

Fig. 17.40 Close-up lateral view of mild alar retraction

a lateral crural graft may be placed concomitantly to lend structural support to the repositioned lateral crus (Fig. 17.44).

In this patient, the angle between the lateral crura and midline was measured to confirm the lateral crural malposition (Fig. 17.45). Then the lateral cartilages were exposed by separating them from their points of attachment to accessory cartilage (Fig. 17.46).

Next, the lateral crus was cut down its long axis and the cephalic segment was folded outward, and then was sutured together with 6-0 absorbable sutures. The folded segment functioned as a lateral crural graft by stabilizing the lateral crura and resolving the configuration disorder (Fig. 17.47).

Next, bilateral pockets were opened at the anterior caudal region of the accessory cartilage, and lateral crura were inserted into them (Fig. 17.48).

New dome-defining points were established via transdomal suture, which also served to obtain cephalocaudal inter-rotation of the lateral crura (Fig. 17.49).

In all patients undergoing repositioning surgery, the tip of the nasal tip must always be fixed to the septum. A septocolumellar strut is an effective graft that can be used for this purpose (Fig. 17.50).

In this case, an 8–20 mm graft was prepared from the septum as a septocolumellar strut. One end of the graft was fixed

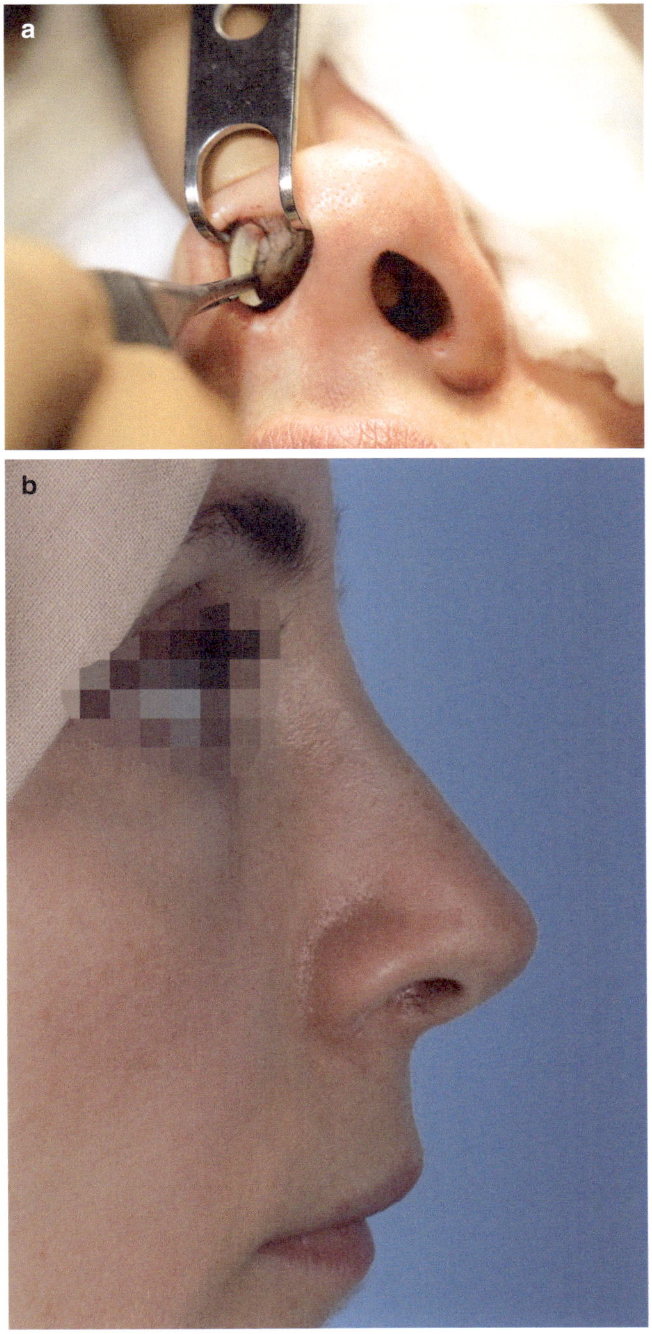

Fig. 17.41 (**a**) Create pocket along alar margin and place alar rim graft. (**b**) Two-years postoperative photograph; the alar retraction is improved

to the septum, and the other was connected to the columellar strut. Then the two medial crura, columellar strut, and septo-columellar strut were sutured together at several points using absorbable sutures (Fig. 17.51).

At the end of surgery bilateral nostril sill excision was performed. Nostril sill excision reduces "nostril show" on anterior or oblique view (Fig. 17.52).

Preoperative and postoperative photographs are shown in Fig. 17.53. The alar columellar relationship was improved by lateral crural repositioning technique.

17.5.2.2 Case 15

The patient presented requesting secondary rhinoplasty to correct excessive nostril show due to alar retraction and a hanging columella. Both of these problems stemmed from malpositioned and weak lateral crura. Both nostrils had severe retraction, but the left one was arched higher than the right and required more correction (Fig. 17.54).

Intraoperative assessments of the cartilage revealed that the lateral crura were malpositioned, and the caudal margin of the lateral crus was well below the cephalic margin of the lateral crus. In addition, the medial crura were flared in the caudal direction. The primary surgeon of a previous surgery made two main mistakes in this patient: the malpositioned lateral crura were not repositioned, and transdomal suturing was incorrect (the dome sutures pinched the domes) (Fig. 17.55).

To correct these issues, the lateral crus of the lower lateral cartilage was dissected free from the vestibular skin, cutting horizontally from the middle point. The cranial segment was turned in and sutured to the caudal segment. This portion acted as a lateral crural strut (auto-lateral crural strut). Then the strong lateral crura with improved inner configuration were repositioned (Fig. 17.56).

After repositioning, the transdomal sutures and the columellar strut were used. This procedure improved both the configuration of the lateral crus and that of the entire alar arch (Fig. 17.57).

A septocolumellar suture was used to fix the alar arch to the septum in this patient. Starting at the medial aspect of the medial crus, a 5-0 nonabsorbable suture was passed through the caudal aspect of the septum and turned in a U shape. After emerging from the medial aspect of the other medial crus, the suture was tied at the midline (Fig. 17.58).

After repositioning and creating a stable alar arch, final tip definition and projection were achieved using a cap graft. Alar retraction was more pronounced on the left side, and thus repositioning alone was not sufficient to correct the deformity. Alar rim graft was used to overcome the deformity (Fig. 17.59).

Preoperative and postoperative photographs are shown in Fig. 17.60. The alar–columellar relationship is corrected.

17.5.3 Auricular Composite Graft

Significant alar notching caused by a loss of tissue requires composite grafting to fill a retraction pocket. This graft is harvested from the lateral concha and contains cartilage and overlying skin on one side only. There is an equal amount of

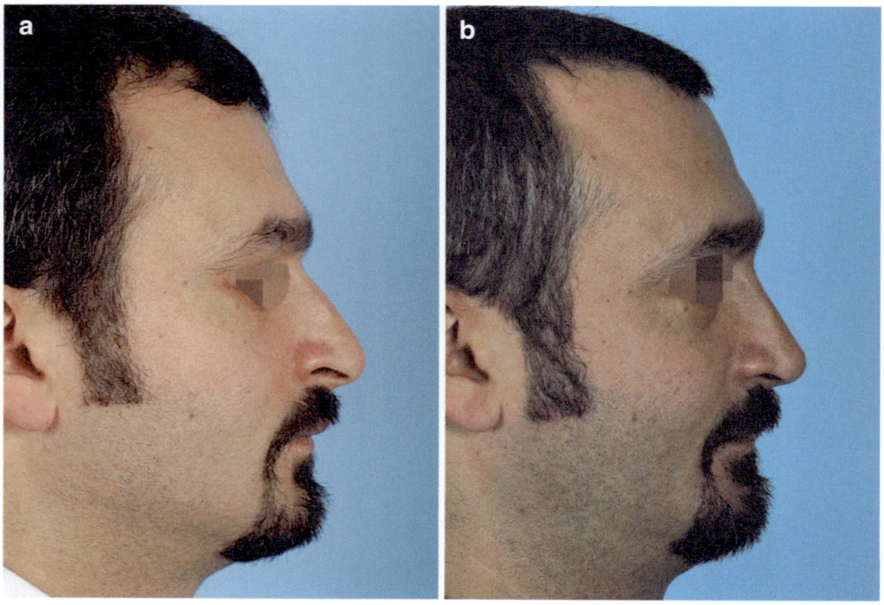

Fig. 17.42 (**a**, **b**) Mild alar retraction was treated with alar rim graft

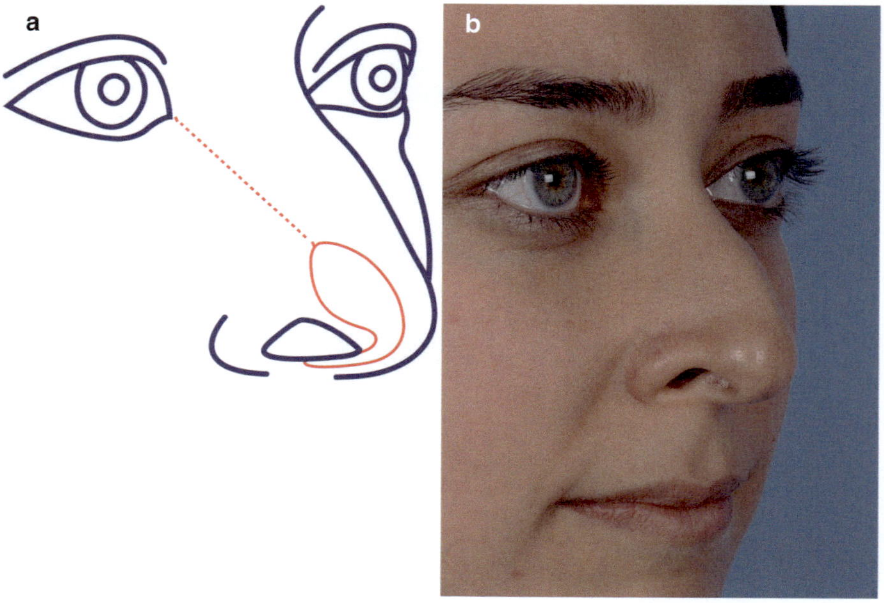

Fig. 17.43 (**a**, **b**) Malpositioned lateral crura are a more common reason for severe retraction than the previous case

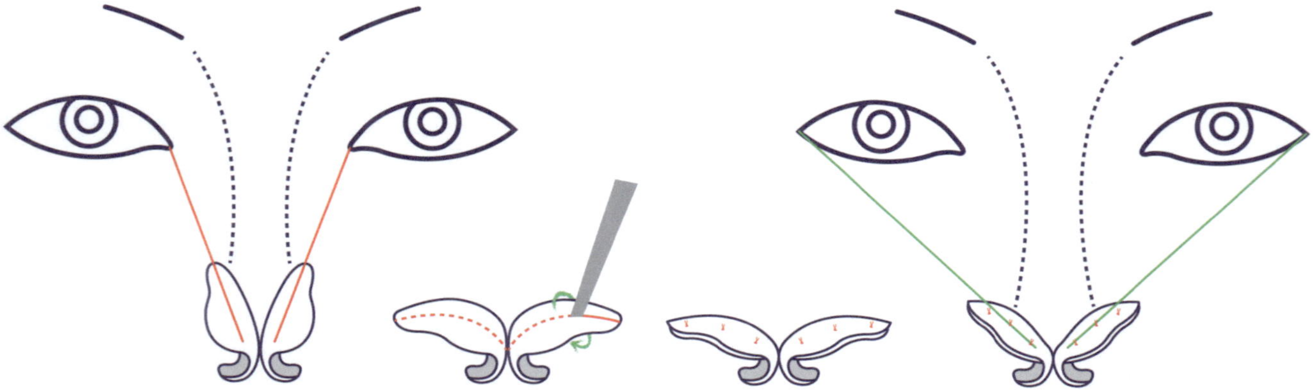

Fig. 17.44 The illustration demonstrates lateral crural repositioning combined with cephalic turn flap

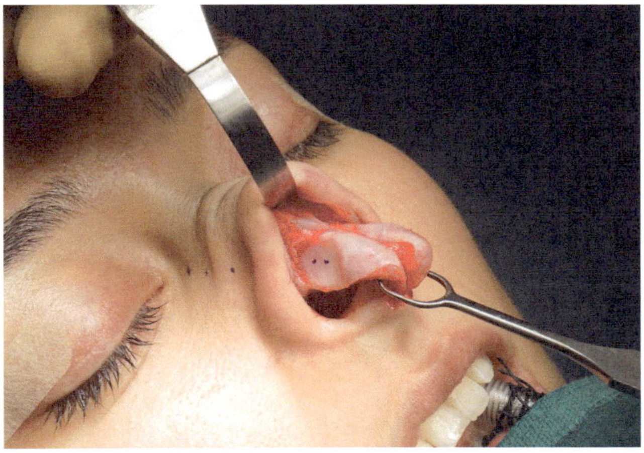

Fig. 17.45 Open approach revealing alar cartilages. The lateral crura are malpositioned, buckled, and concave

cartilage and skin in the graft. The donor site is closed; if the defect is too large, a postauricular full-thickness skin graft or a postauricular island flap is used. The composite graft is then transposed to the recipient site to create a downward thrust of the retracted alar margin (Fig. 17.61).

While a number of donor sites may be used for auricular grafts, the anterolateral surface of the auricle is commonly preferred. This anatomical site is a good source for composite grafts that makes it possible to comfortably accomplish direct primary closure without distorting the auricle. It should be noted that when harvesting the graft, it is important to keep the skin cartilage intact upon removal. Local anesthetic infiltration into the graft site may separate the skin from the cartilage, and thus must be avoided (Fig. 17.62).

Then the composite graft was transferred to the internal alar tissue void, ensuring that the overall graft dimension

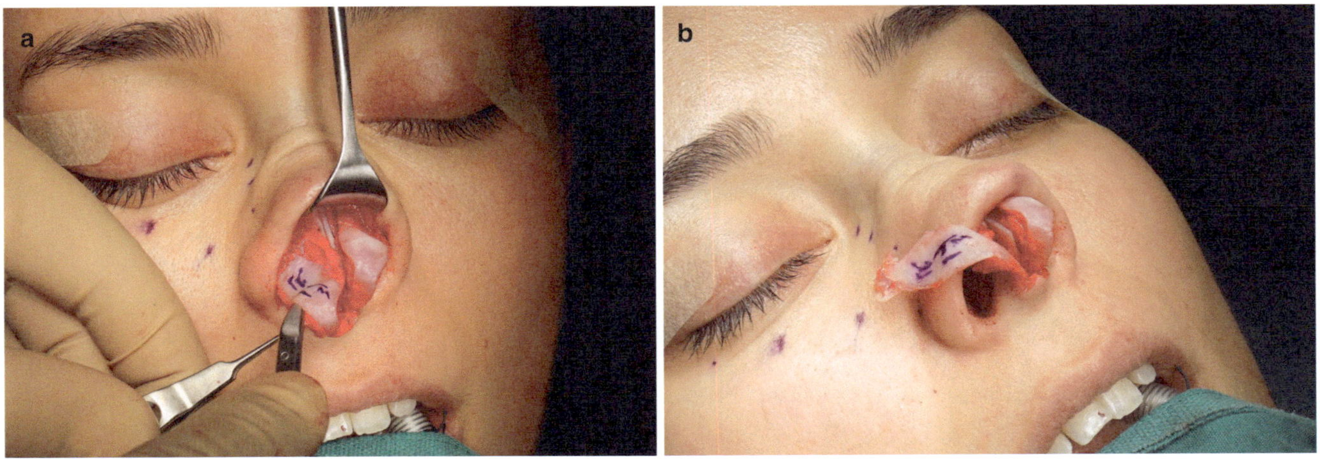

Fig. 17.46 (**a**, **b**) Freeing the vestibular skin from the lower lateral crura

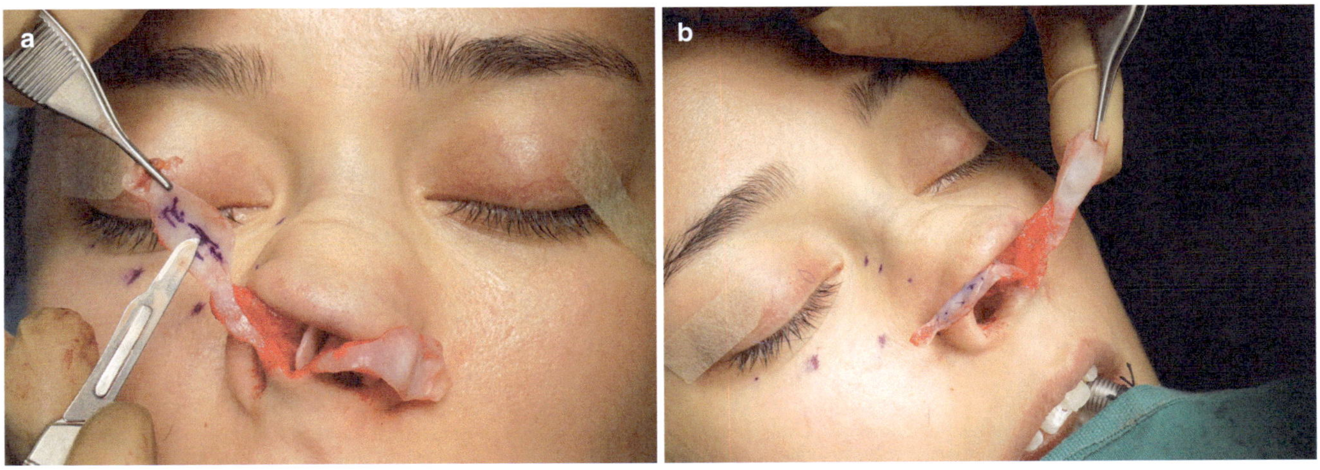

Fig. 17.47 (**a**, **b**) Lateral crus divided horizontally, then the cephalic part turned out finally sutured to caudal part with absorbable sutures

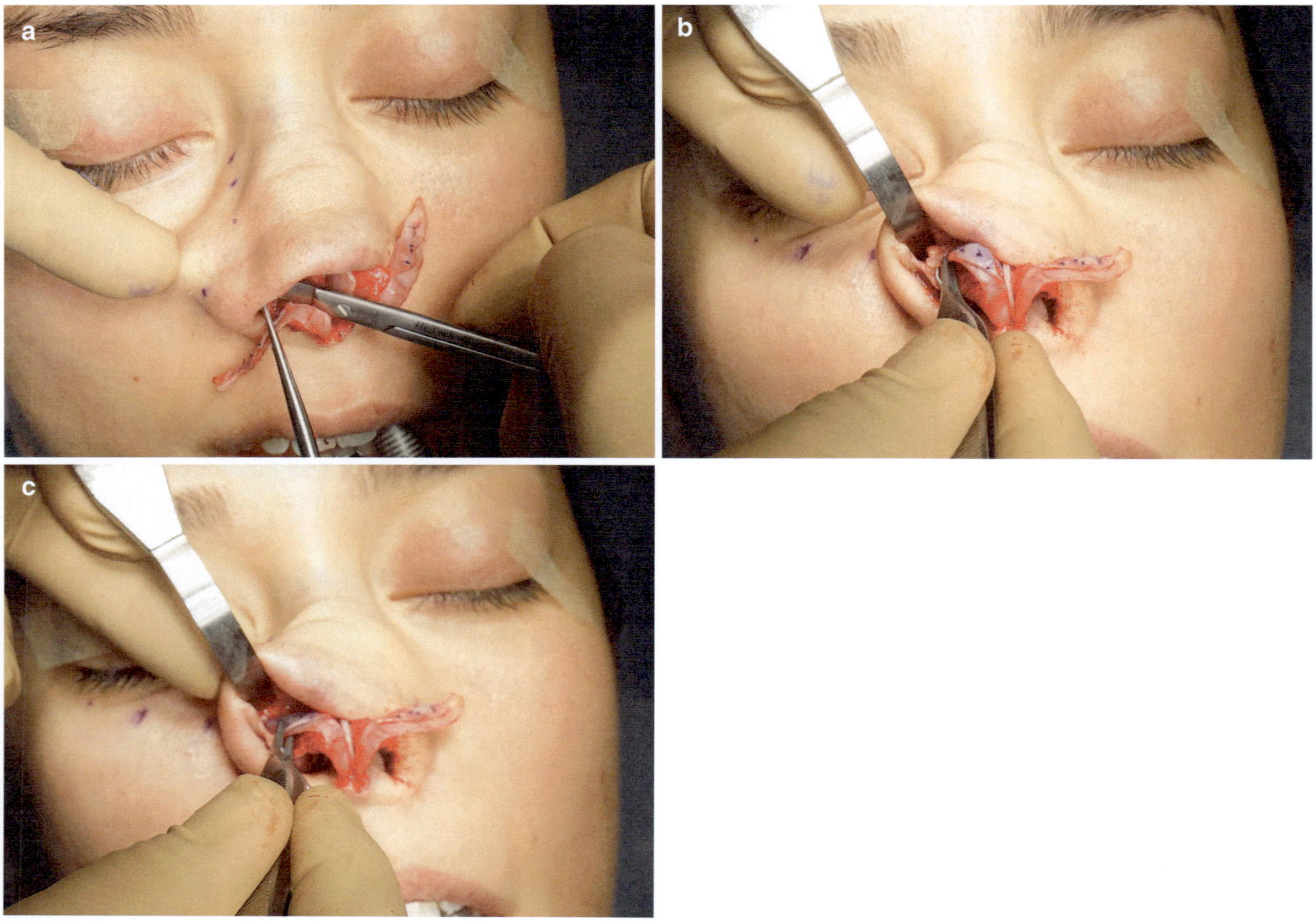

Fig. 17.48 (**a–c**) A more caudal alar pocket was then formed between the vestibular and external skin with a scissor. The lateral crus was then repositioned into the isolated area

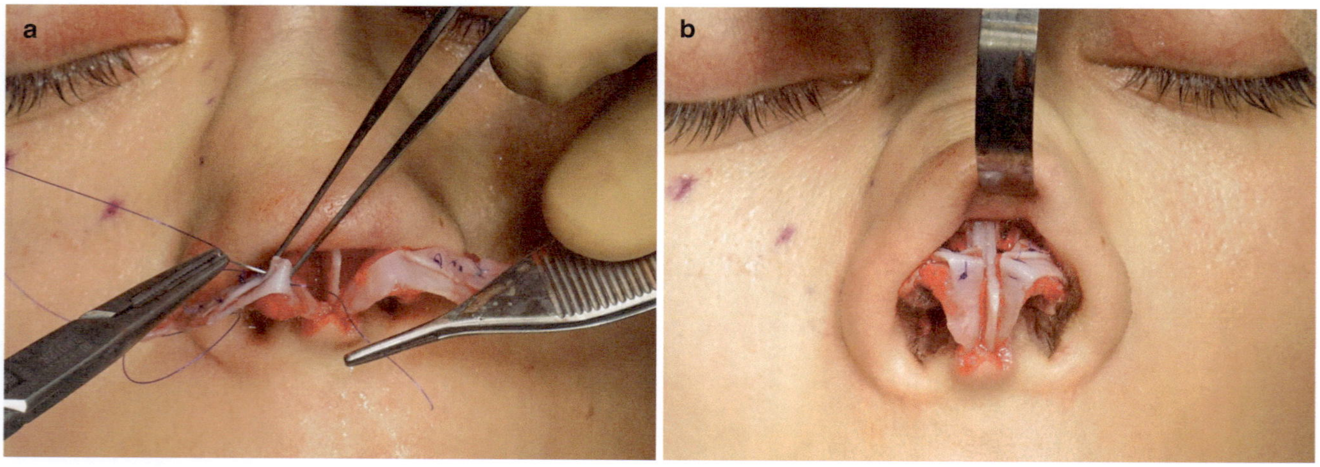

Fig. 17.49 (**a**, **b**) To maintain tip projection and rotation, it is crucial to set the exact place of transdomal suture and to refrain from advancing the lateral crura too far into their newly dissected pockets and shortening the length of the conceptual tripod legs

Fig. 17.50 Once repositioning was completed, the septocolumellar strut secured to stabilize the position of the tip

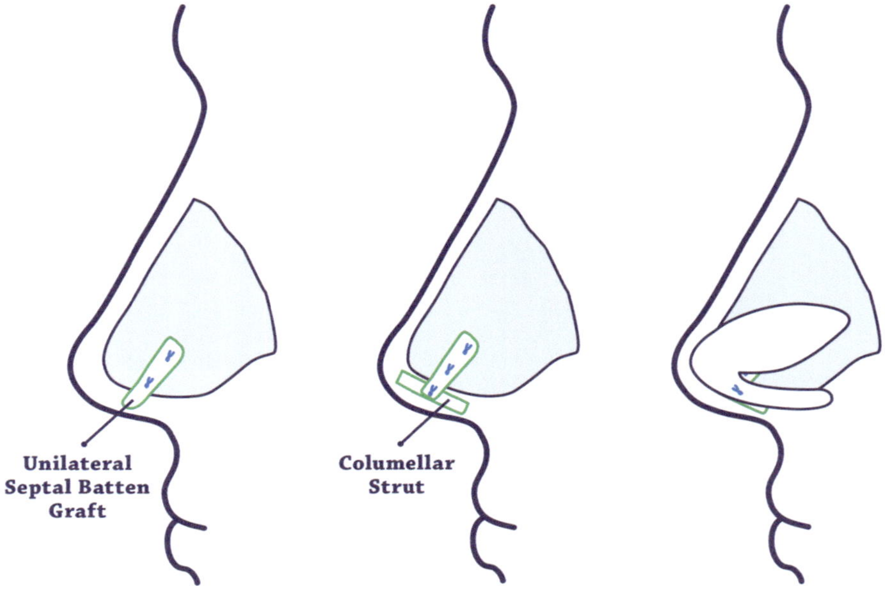

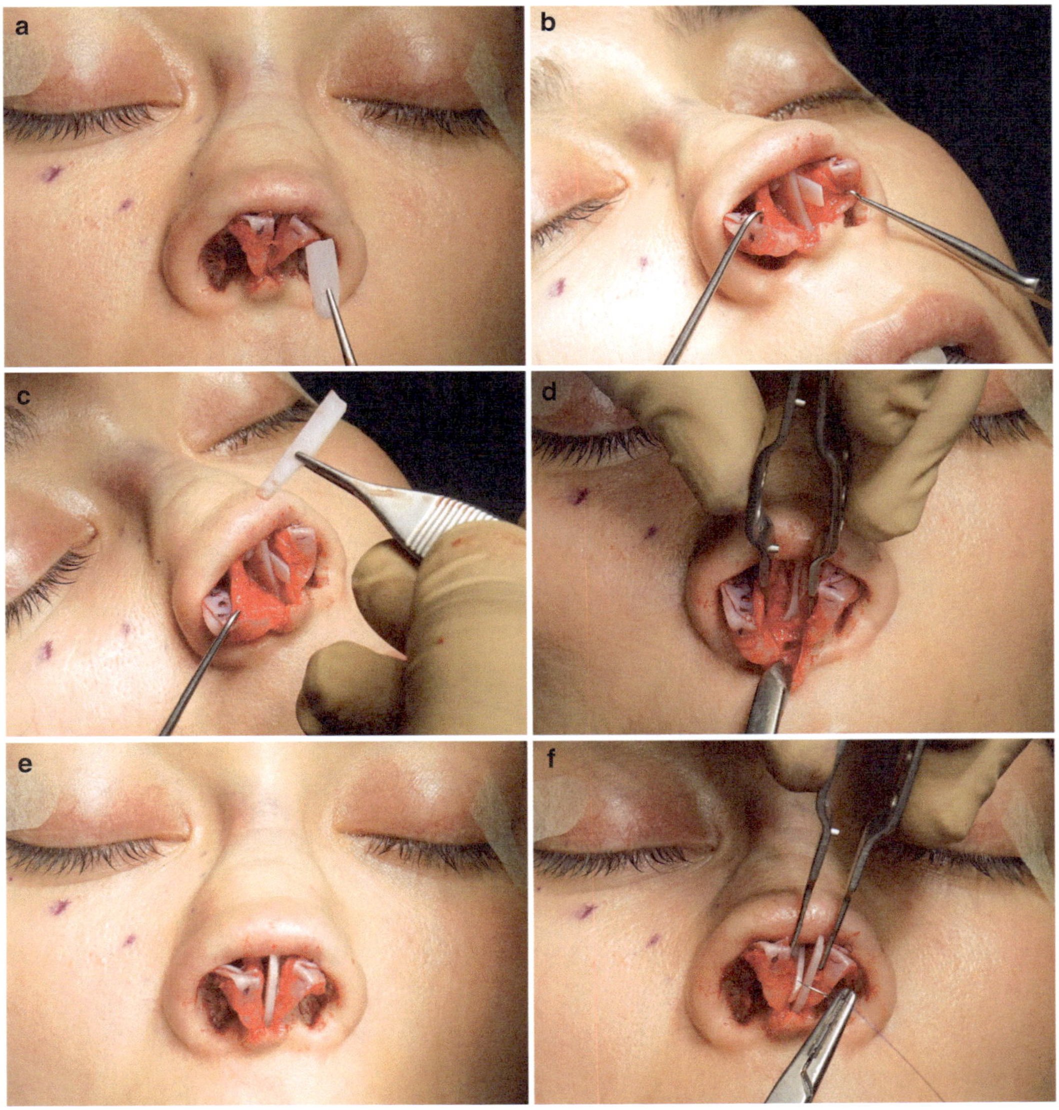

Fig. 17.51 (**a**–**i**) Septocolumellar strut placement

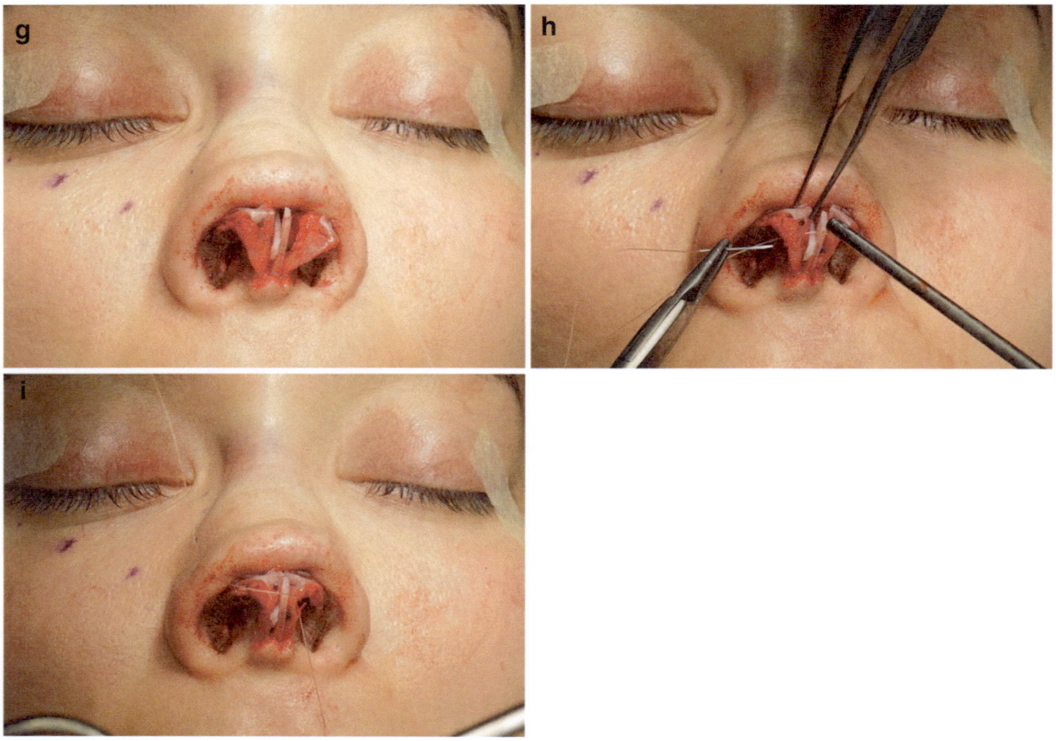

Fig. 17.51 (continued)

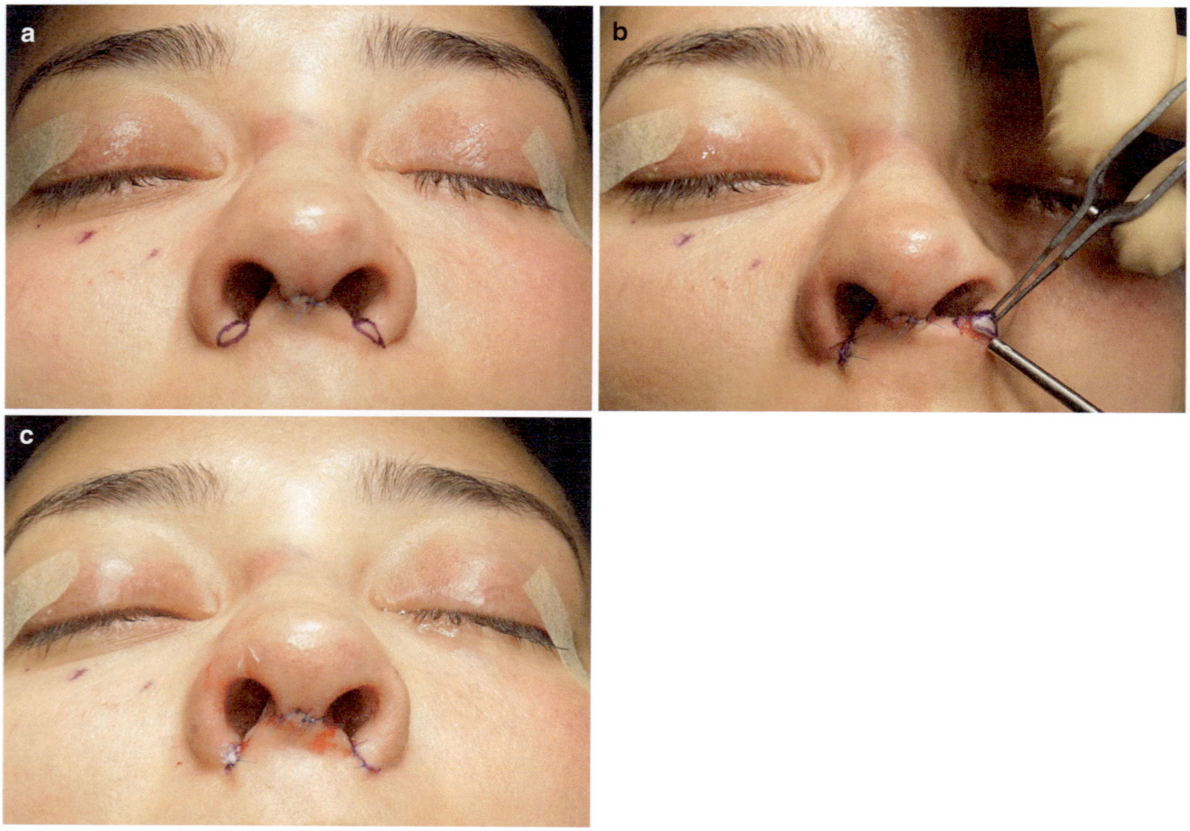

Fig. 17.52 (**a**–**c**) Nostril sill excision

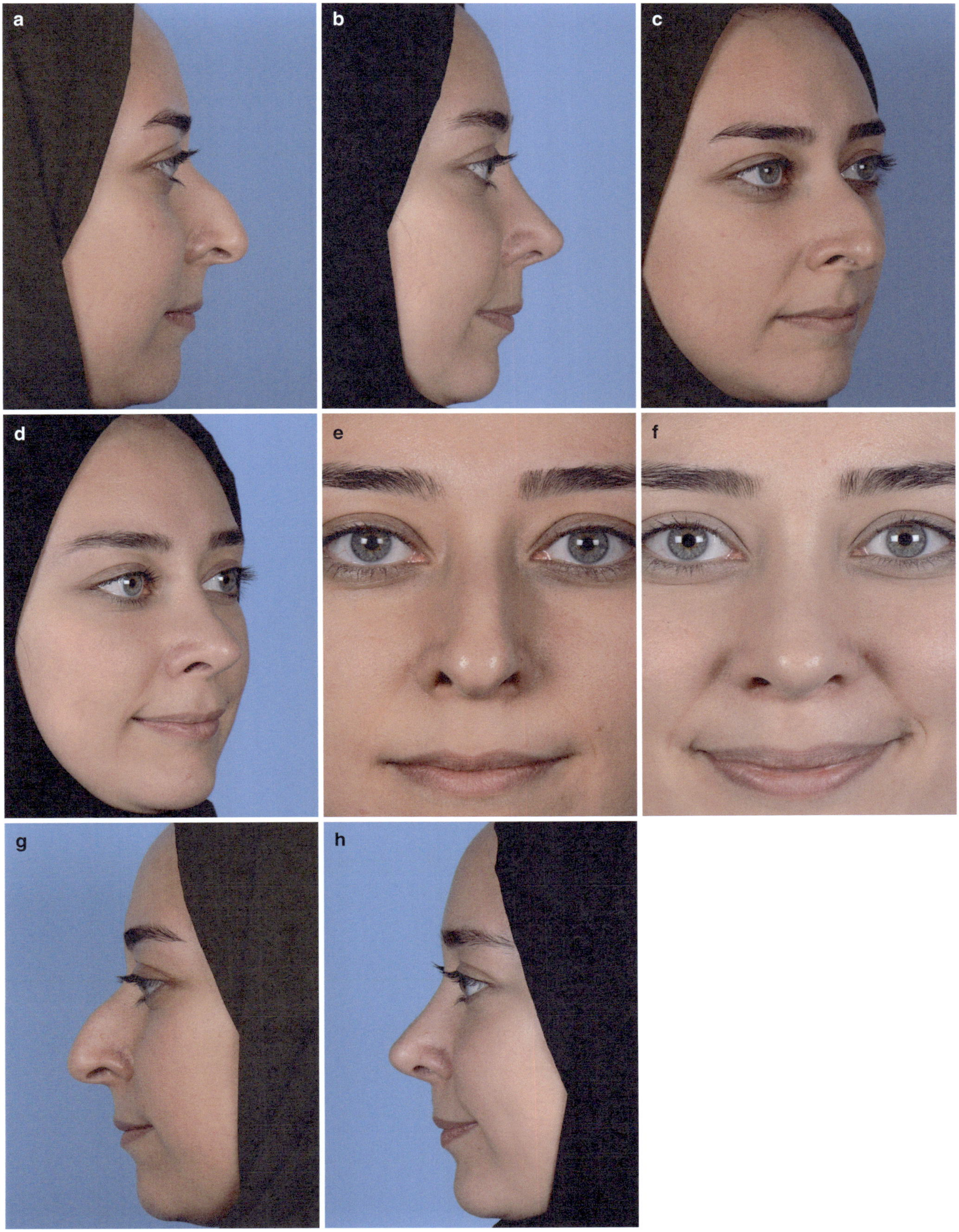

Fig. 17.53 (**a**–**h**) Notice how to improve an alar–columellar relationship, pinched appearance, and wide tip lobule after reposition surgery

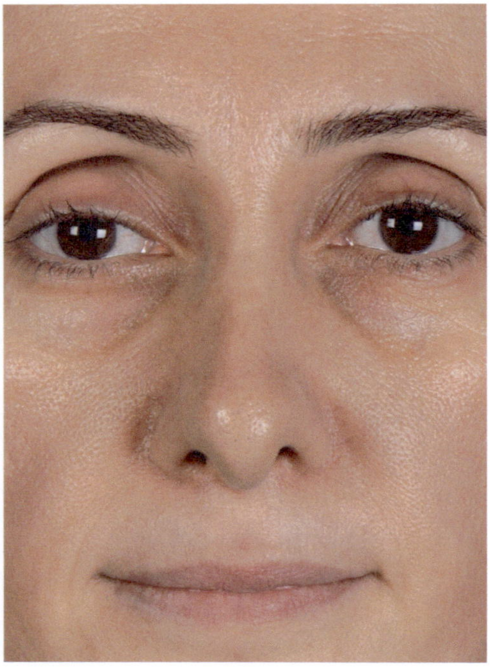

Fig. 17.54 Unfavorable alar–columellar relationship

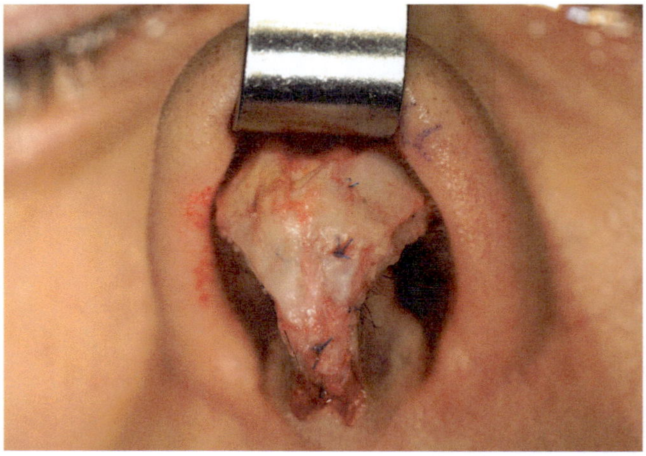

Fig. 17.55 Open approach revealing malpositioned, deformed lower lateral cartilages, and also an unfavorable relationship of edge lateral crus

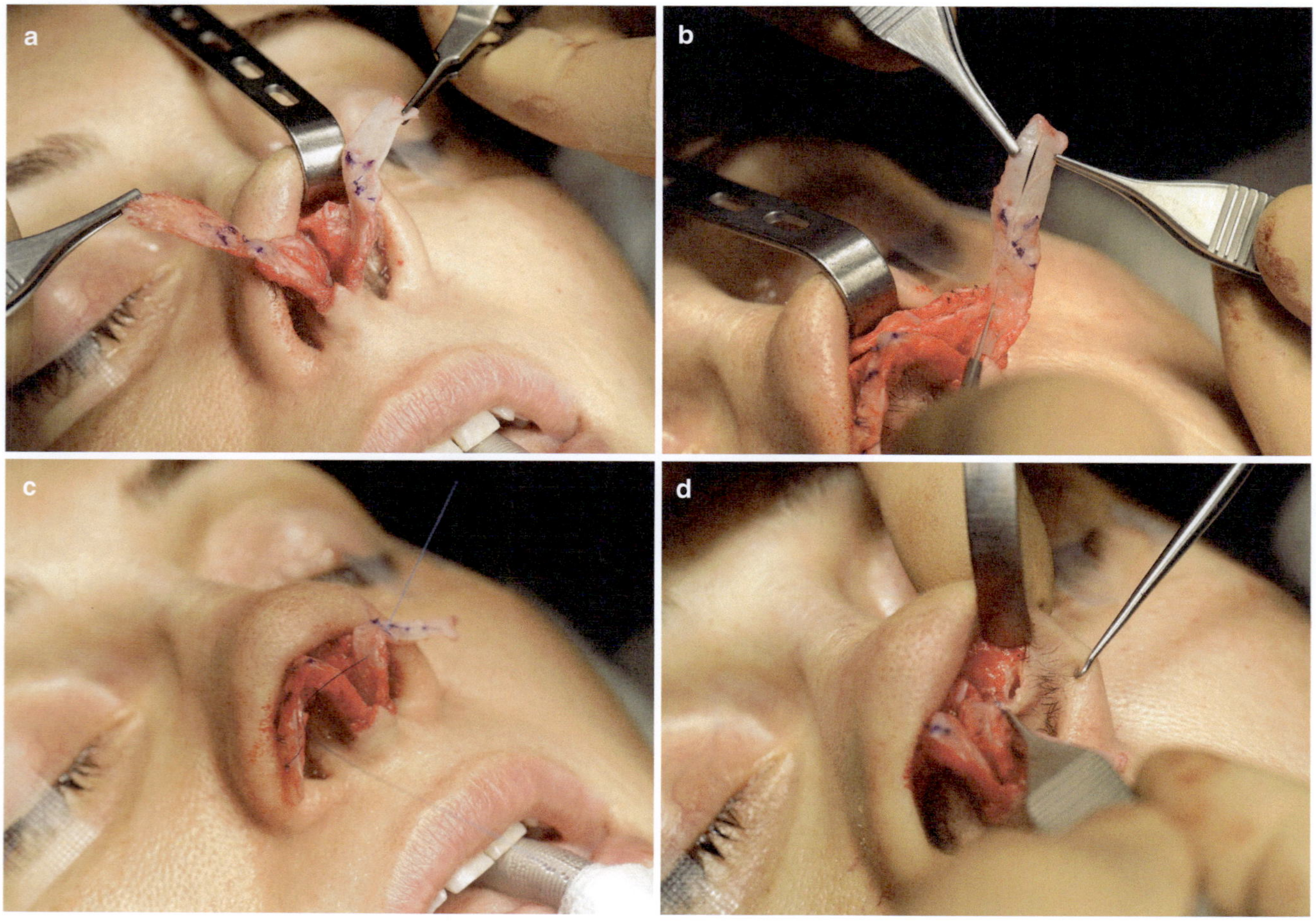

Fig. 17.56 (**a**) Demonstration of cephalically malpositioned lower lateral cartilages. (**b–d**) View after freeing the vestibular skin from the lower lateral cartilages and divided, cephalad turn in the underside to the caudal and repositioning of the lateral crus in a caudally positioned pocket

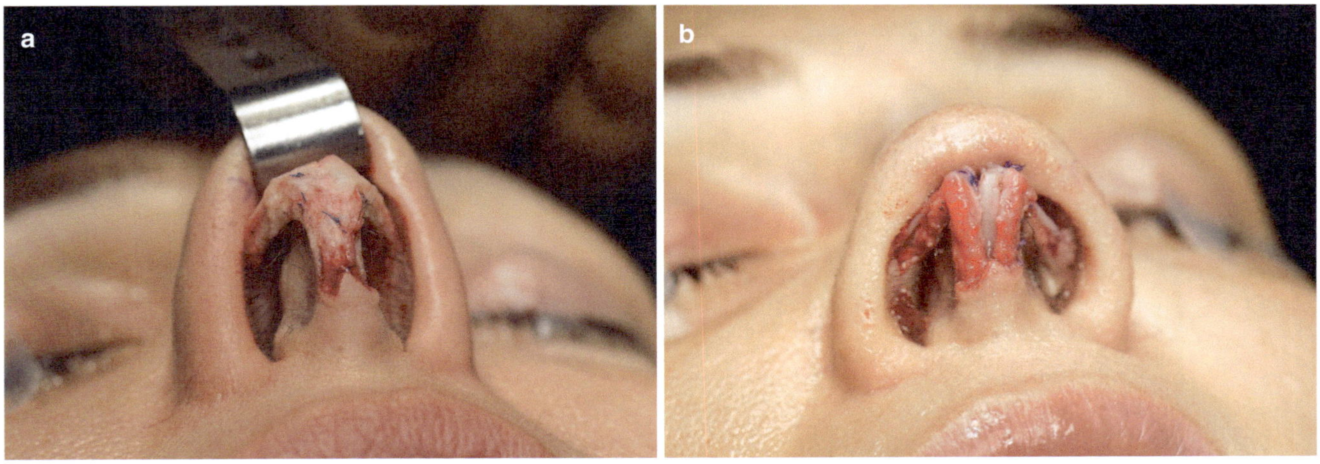

Fig. 17.57 (**a**) Before repositioning. (**b**) Immediately after repositioning

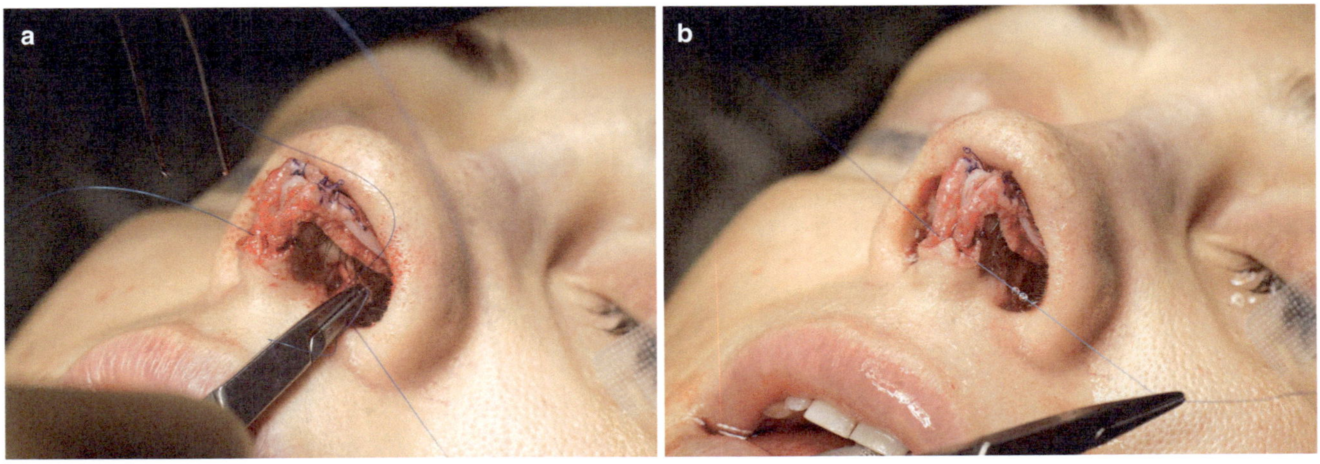

Fig. 17.58 (**a**, **b**) Septocolumellar suture for tip stabilization

imparted a slight inferior thrust on the unfurled alar margin. Once the graft was in place, it was sutured with 6-0 absorbable sutures at several points (Fig. 17.63).

17.5.3.1 Case 16

The patient had severe alar notching and alar retraction after a previous rhinoplasty performed by a different surgeon (Fig. 17.64).

Open rhinoplasty revealed that the lateral crus was completely deformed on the right side. A lateral crural graft prepared from the septum was fixed to the domal segment of middle crus. A graft next to the dome was placed in the pocket opening toward the outer canthus (Fig. 17.65).

The composite graft, which has been sculpted to fill the supra-alar internal defect accurately, is then transposed to the recipient site to create a downward thrust of the retracted alar margin. The procedure resolved the alar retraction (Fig. 17.66).

Preoperative and 1-year postoperative photographs are shown in Fig. 17.67. The nose is longer with correction of over-rotated tip and saddle nose deformity. Improved symmetry of the nasal tip is seen, and right alar retraction is also improved.

17.5.3.2 Case 17

In some cases, the excessive nostril show may be caused from retracted ala together with hanging columella. Here is an example.

A 40-year-old woman underwent rhinoplasty 15 years earlier. Her tip became more deformed over time. She had severe alar–columellar disharmony (Fig. 17.68).

While the malposed lateral crus cause retracted ala, overdeveloped septal cartilage and medial crural bowing cause hanging columella (Fig. 17.69).

Preoperative and 3-year postoperative photographs are shown in Fig. 17.70.

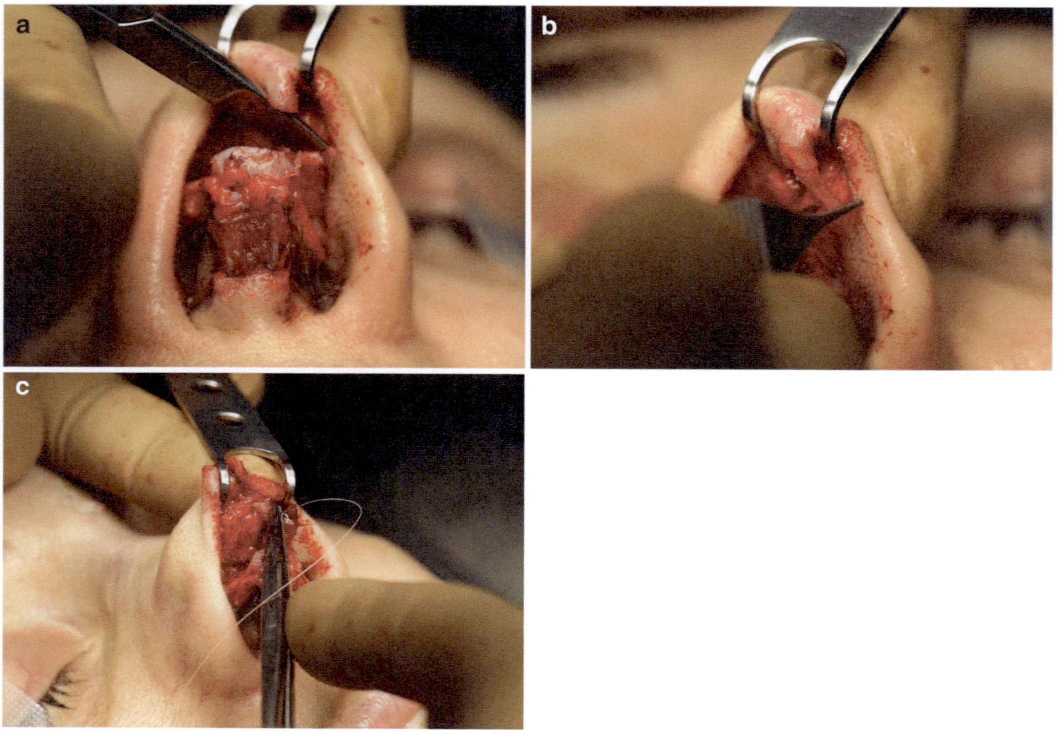

Fig. 17.59 (**a–c**) The rim graft placement on the left side to push the alar rim more inferiorly

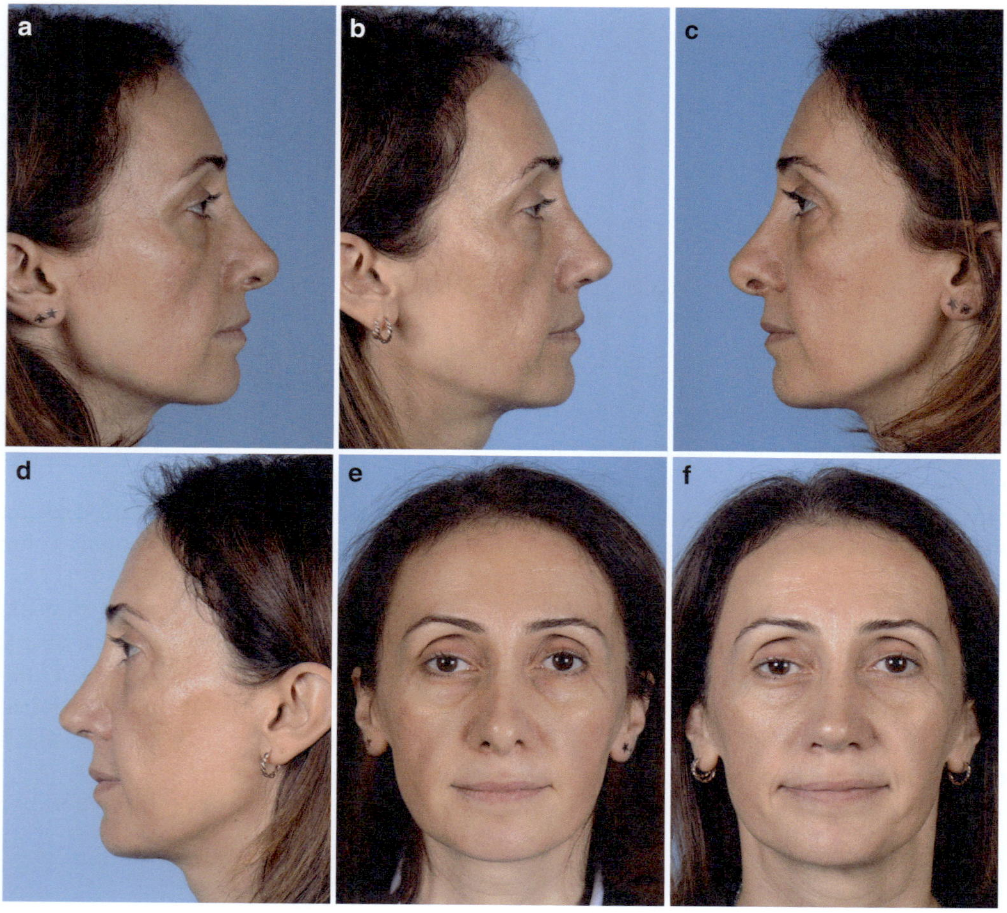

Fig. 17.60 (**a–f**) Pre- and postoperative pictures demonstrate how powerful the repositioning of the lateral crura and placement of left alar rim graft maneuvers together is for the treatment of rim retraction and nostril symmetry

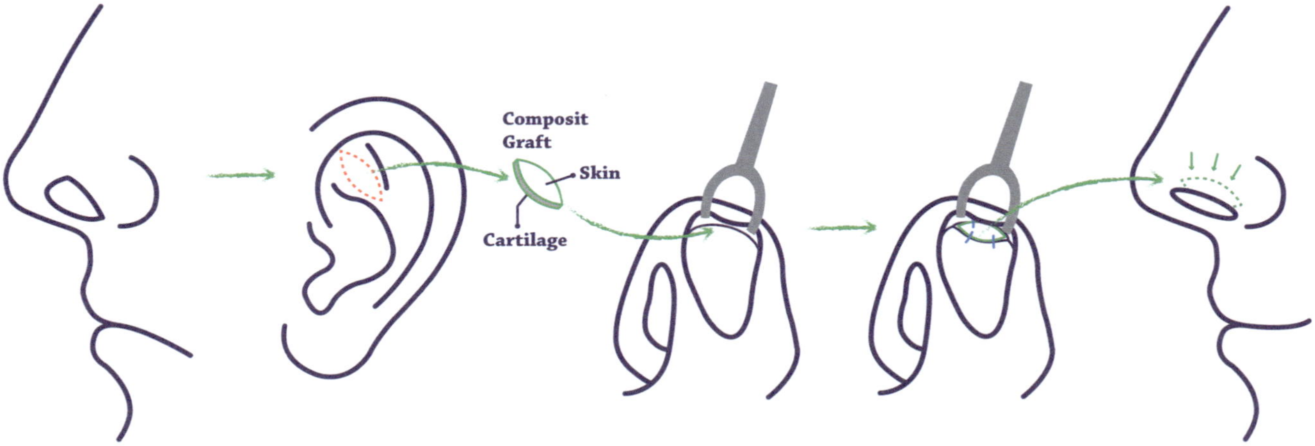

Fig. 17.61 Surgical correction of alar notching with auricular composite grafts. (Supplementary Video 17.3)

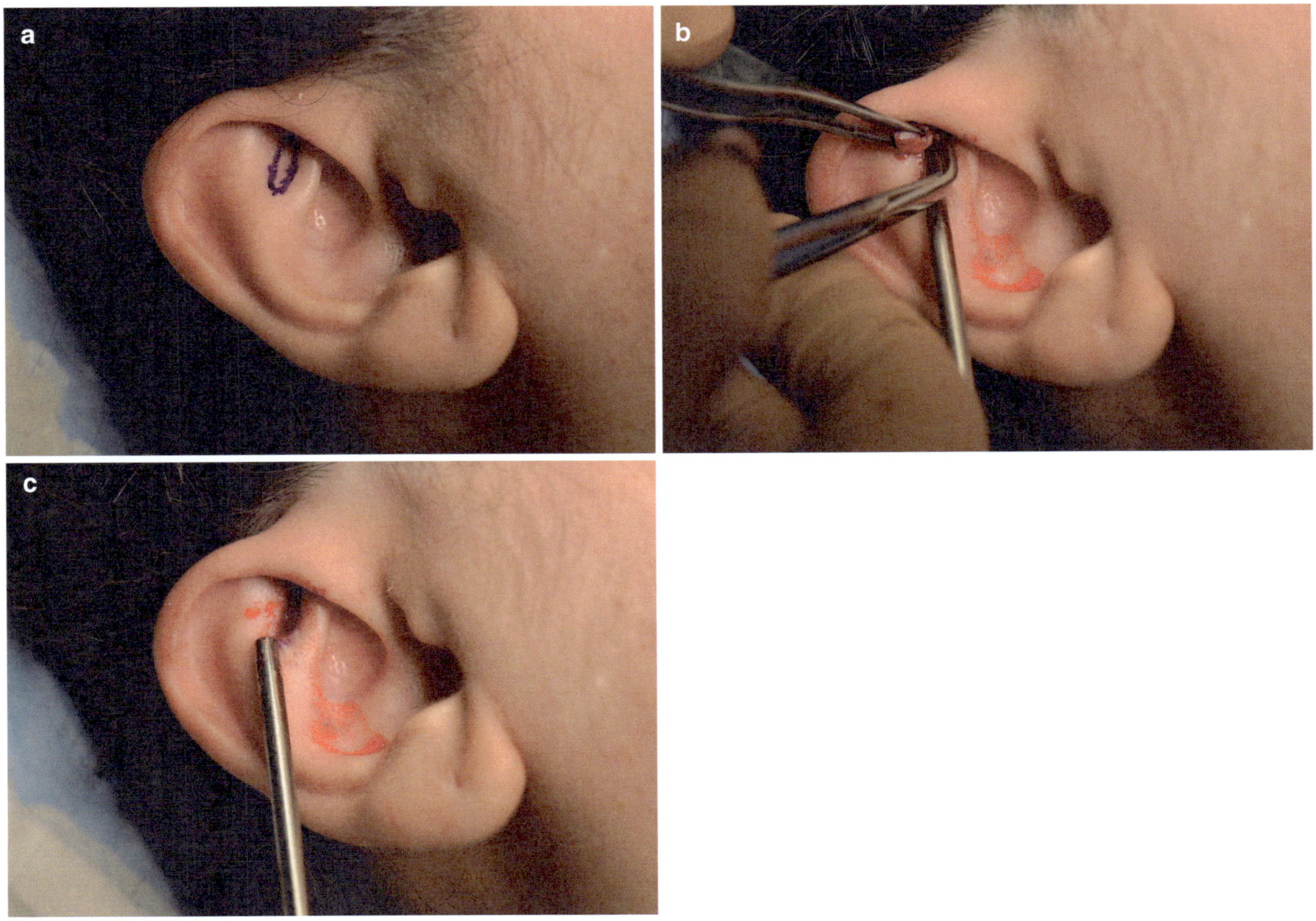

Fig. 17.62 (**a–c**) Surgical procedure. The donor site of the auricular composite graft. The composite graft is harvested to match the intraoperative design of the recipient site. The donor area is closed with nonabsorbable suture

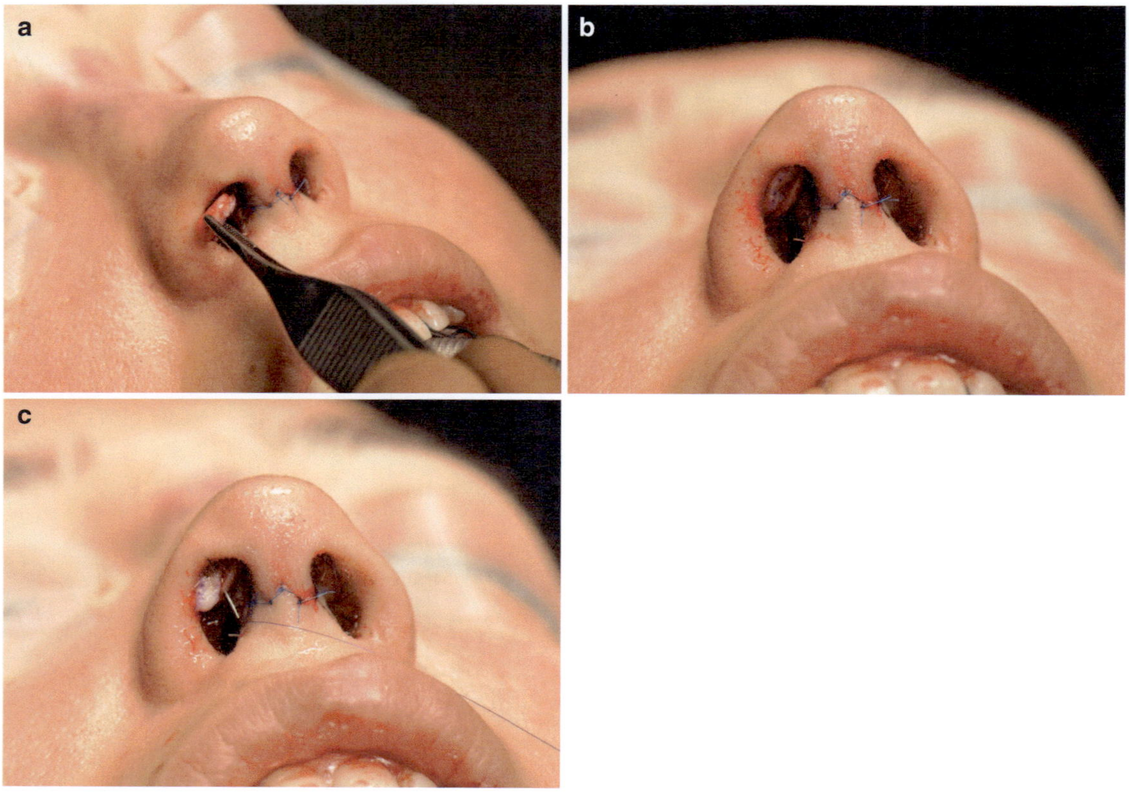

Fig. 17.63 (**a**–**c**) The composite graft was sutured to the recipient site with 6-0 absorbable sutures

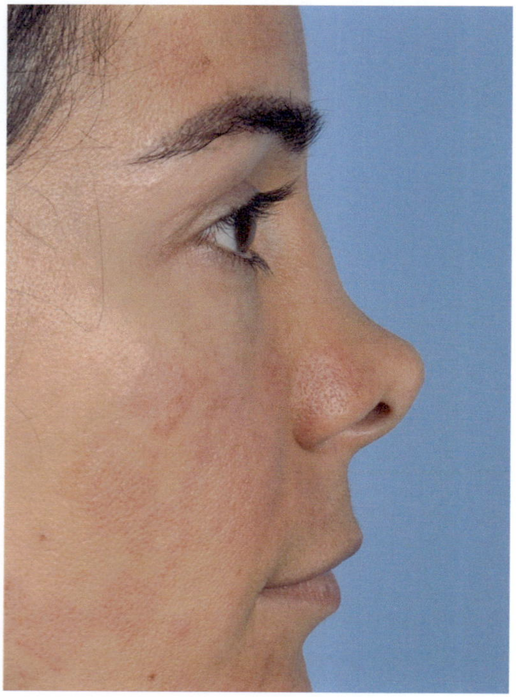

Fig. 17.64 A typical appearance after reductive rhinoplasty. Over-resected tripod cartilages resulting in collapsed tip and alar retraction. The alar cartilages and dorsum require reconstruction

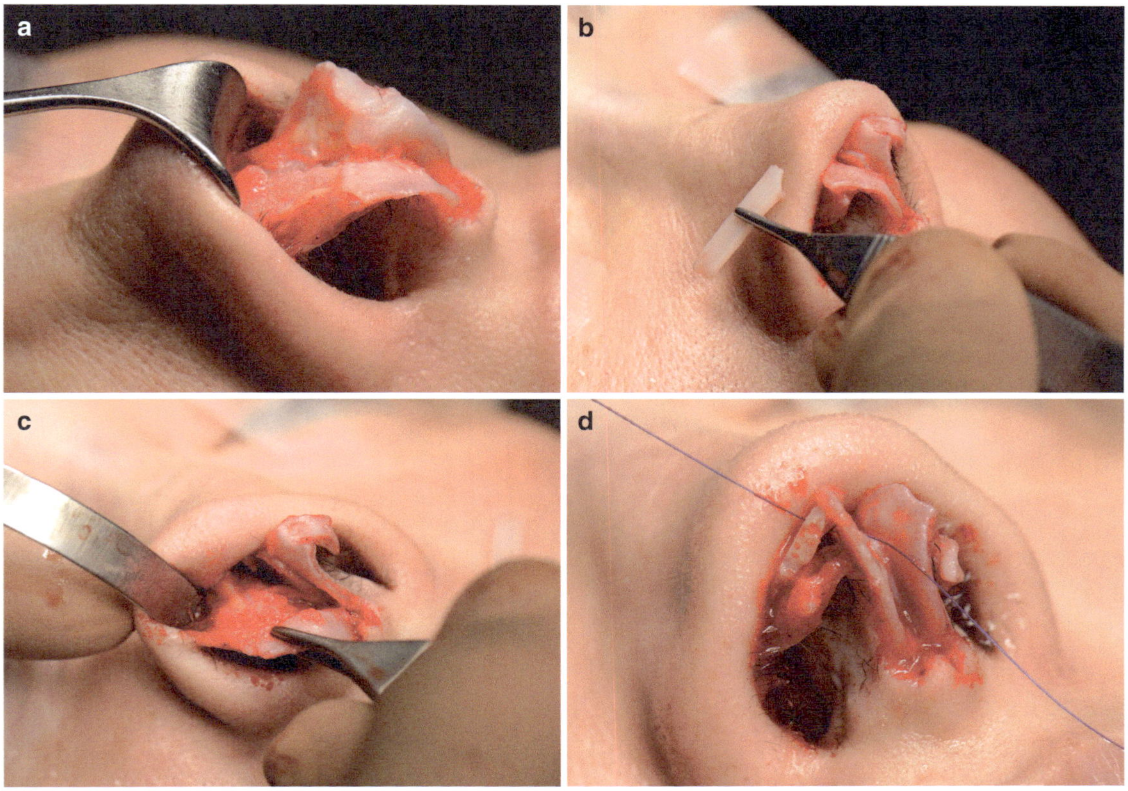

Fig. 17.65 (**a**) The lateral crura appear buckled and collapsed. (**b–d**) The costal cartilage onlay grafts sutured over the lateral crura

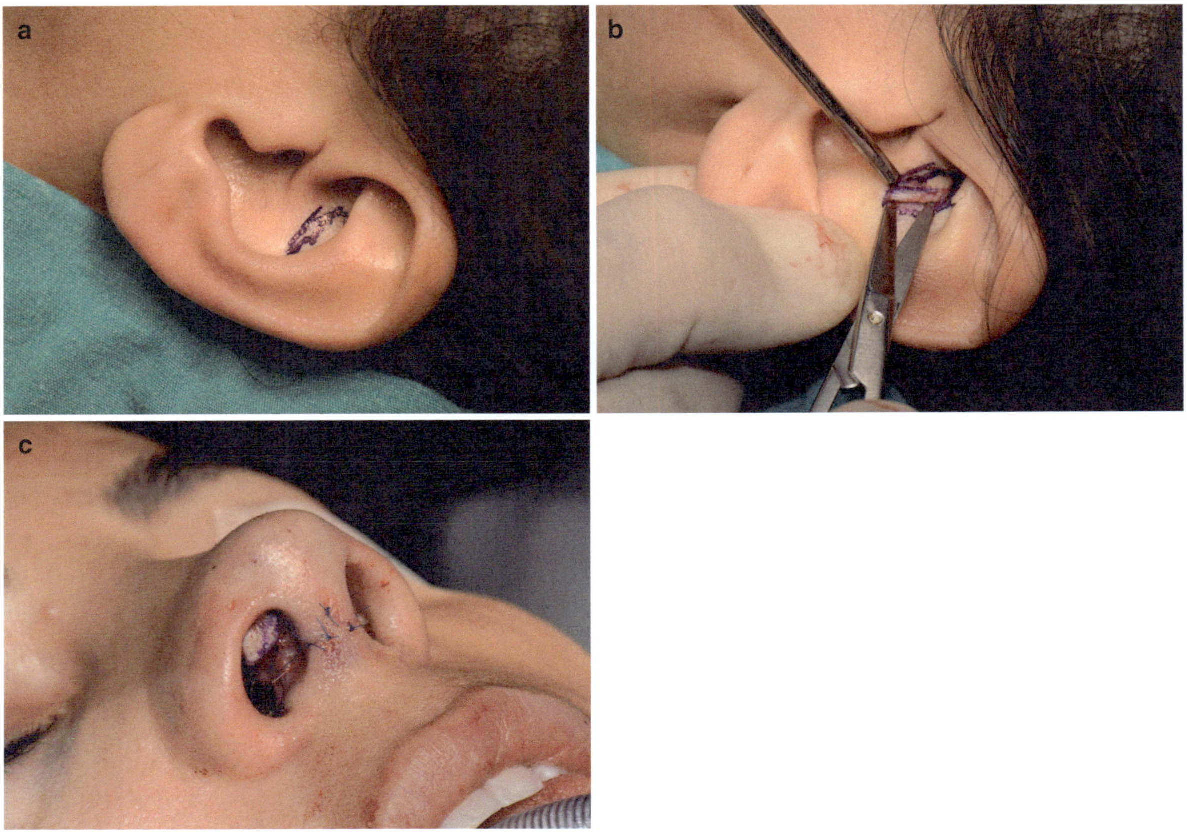

Fig. 17.66 (**a–c**) In this case, retraction has been accompanied by scar contracture and lack of mobile tissue. Extra tissue must be obtained to "push" the alar rim inferiorly. The mainstay for solving is the composite auricular skin–cartilage graft

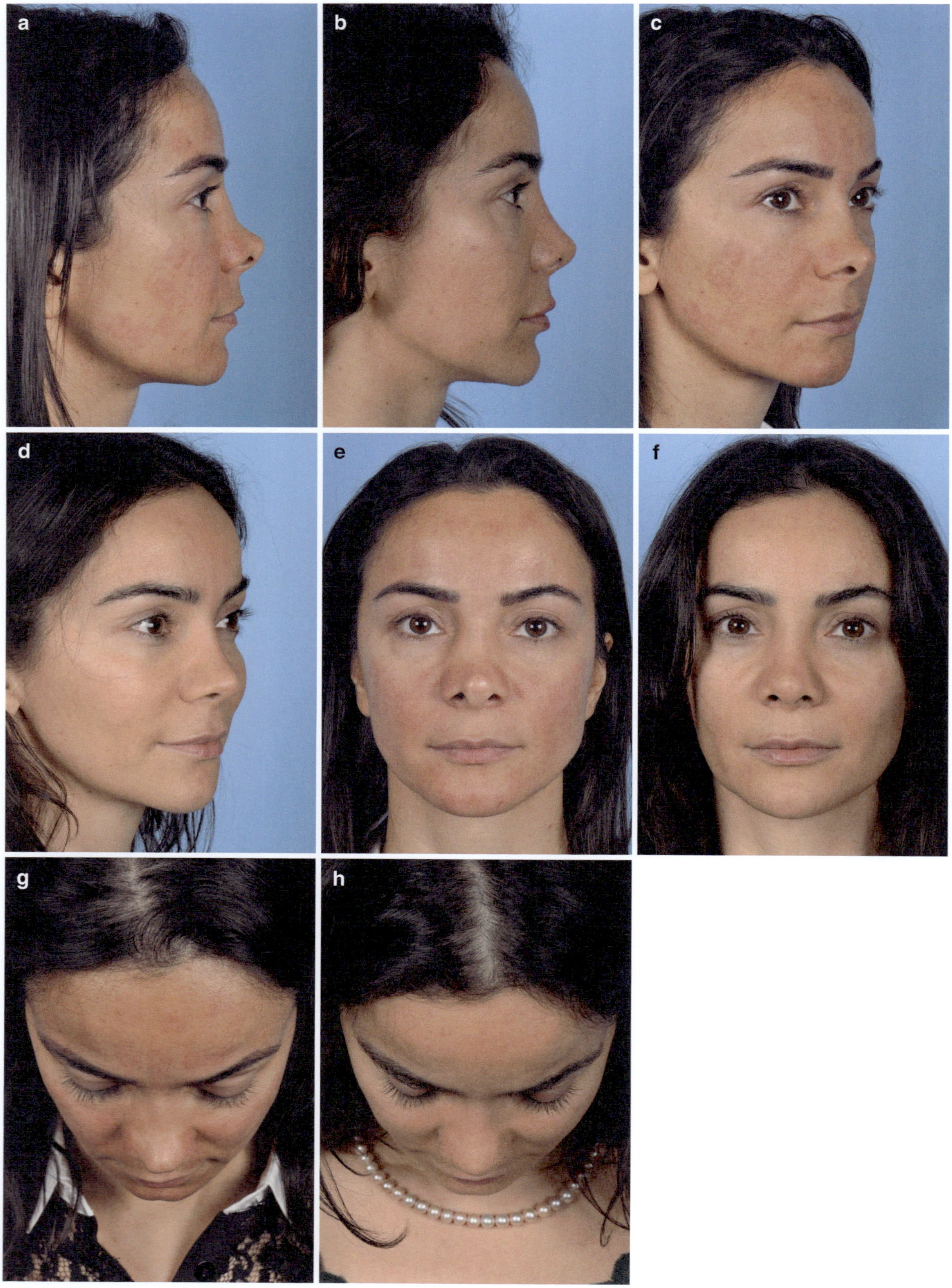

Fig. 17.67 (**a**–**h**) Pre- and postoperative pictures, the tip was reconstructed bilateral costal lateral crural graft, columellar strut, and cap graft. Lateral views showing markedly improved alar rim position following composite auricular cartilage grafting. Collapsed middle vault was reconstructed with bilateral extended spreader and septal replacement graft. Dorsal augmentation was necessary to bring the dorsum up to the level of the newly reconstructed tip

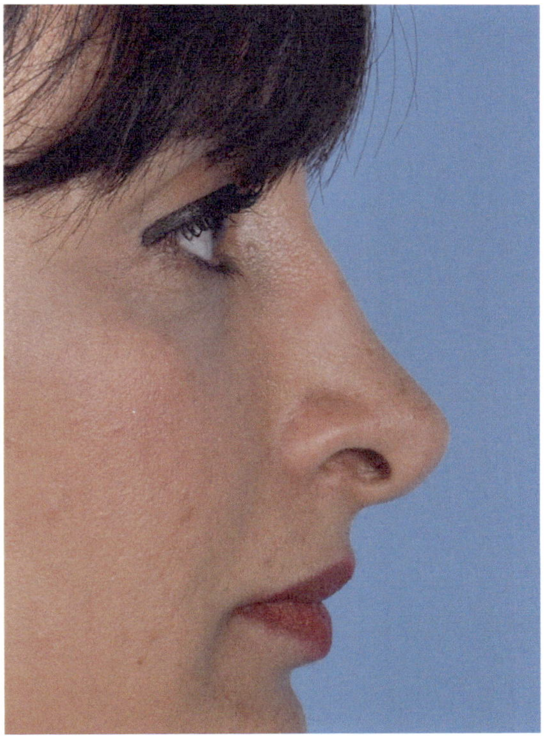

Fig. 17.68 Close-up lateral view, excessive nostril show caused by both alar retraction and hanging columella

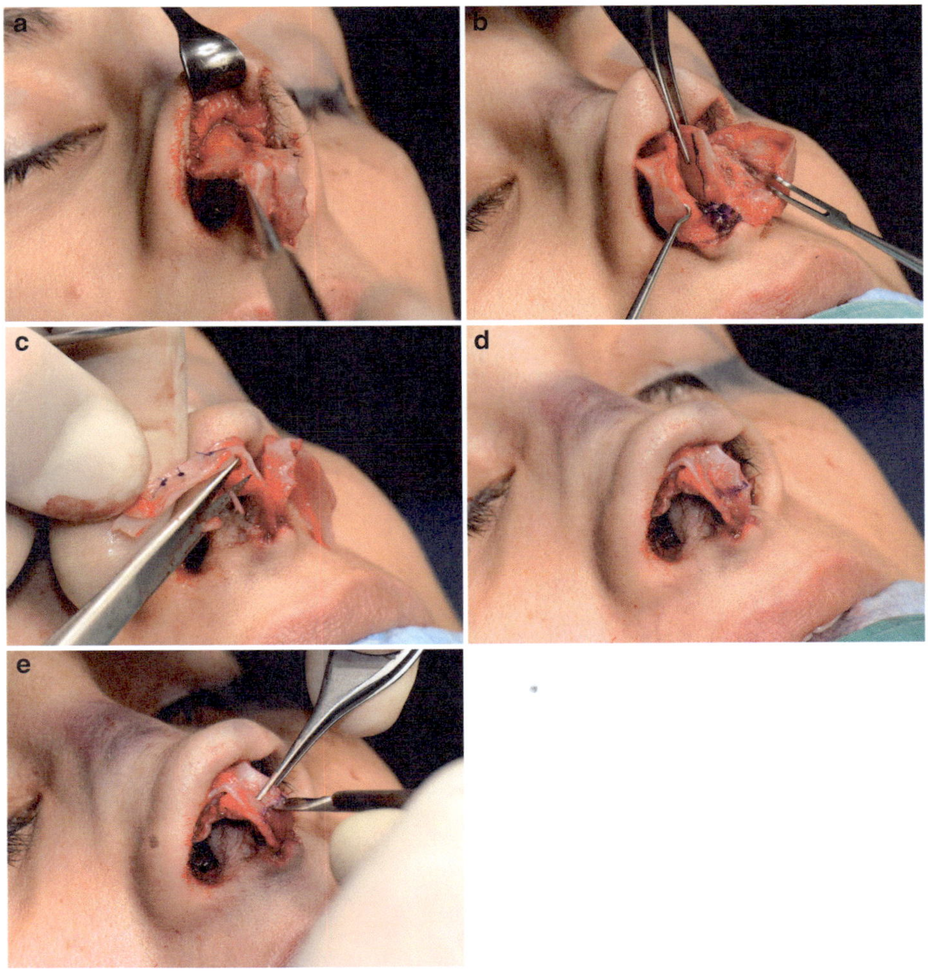

Fig. 17.69 (**a**) Lateral crural cartilages showing cephalic malposition. (**b**) Trimming overly long caudal septum. (**c**) After dissection of lateral crura from underlying vestibular skin, placement of bilateral lateral crural graft sutured to the undersurface of the lateral crura then place into the new pockets. (**d**, **e**) Planned medial crus incision for medial crural overlap

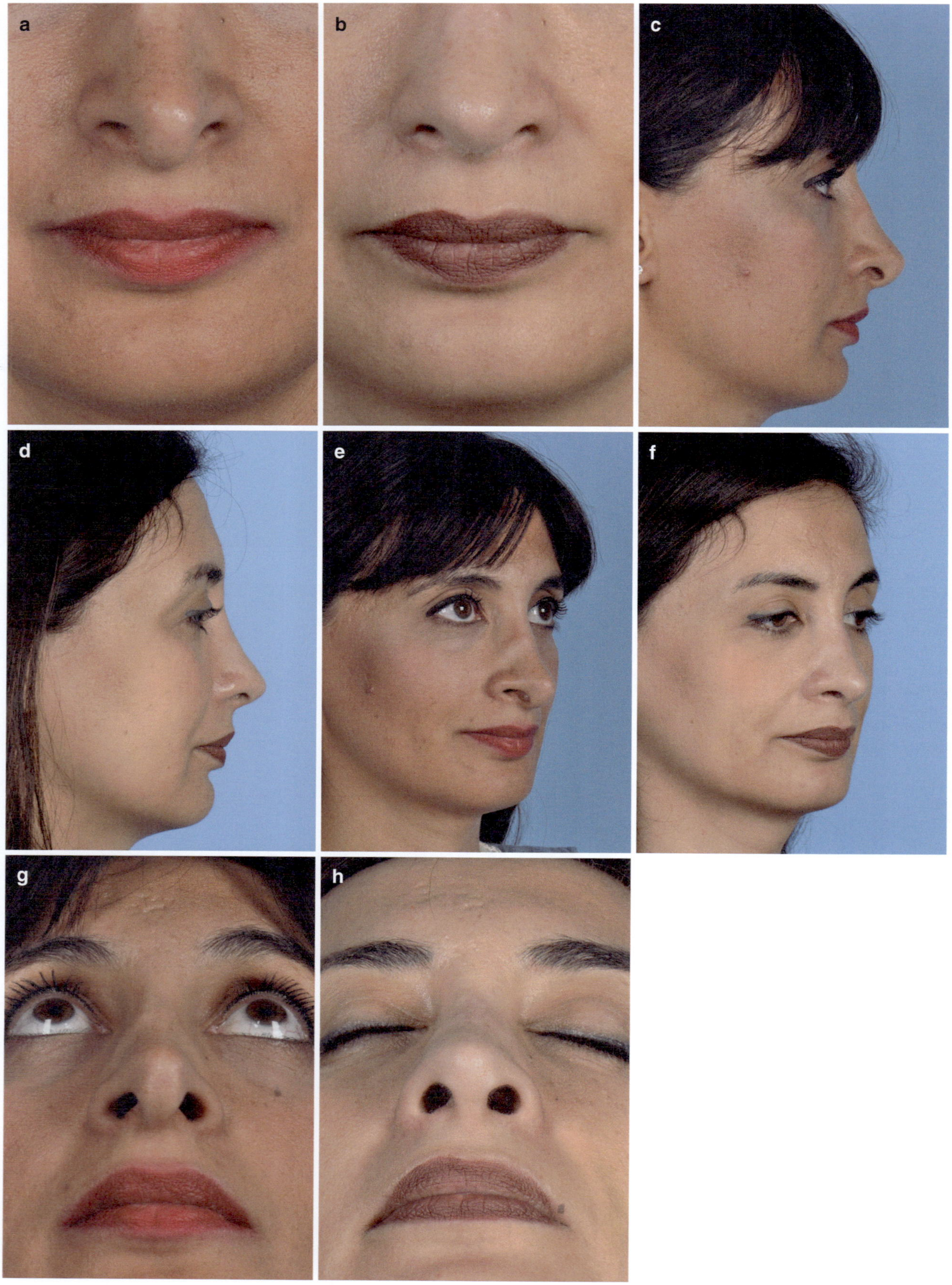

Fig. 17.70 (**a**, **b**) From the frontal view, the ideal relationship between the ala and the columella ("gull wing in flight") is achieved. (**c**, **d**) From the profile view, excessive nostril show is reduced. (**e**, **f**) The nose is shorter and upper lip is longer. Less infratip lobule prominence. (**g**, **h**) Nostril symmetry noted postoperatively

17.6 Reduced Nostril Show

A less common alar–columellar anomaly is reduced nostril show, which is defined as a <2 mm opening in the profile view. Reduced nostril show may result from retraction of the columella in the cranial direction (retracted columella) or from a hanging ala. These are discussed below.

17.6.1 Retracted Columella

There is loss of septal support to the columella due to some deficiency in the caudal septum or severe deviation of the anterior septum, resulting in columellar retraction in the cranial direction. The alar–columellar relationship is impaired and nostril show is reduced. This condition is mostly encountered after previous surgery or following septal trauma. Patients present with a retracted columella accompanied by decreased tip projection and rotation as well as an acute subnasal angle (Fig. 17.71).

The main objective of treatment is to rebuild the deficient or deformed caudal septum and compensate for any deficiency in the spine or premaxilla. A variety of techniques are available to straighten and/or reposition the caudal septal cartilage. Endonasal or open approach can be used, although the open approach is particularly helpful for septal replacement because of the exposition advantage.

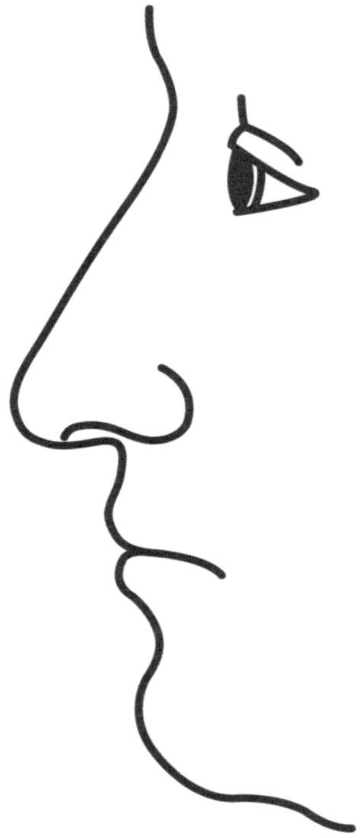

Fig. 17.71 Less or no columellar show because columella retracted

17.6.1.1 Case 18

A typical example is shown in Fig. 17.72. The patient had previously undergone septoplasty. In preoperative assessments, a retracted columella, an under-projected and droopy nose tip, and an acute subnasal angle were observed. Intraoperative assessments revealed deformation at the caudal and dorsal aspects of the septum (Fig. 17.72).

The most effective tool for strengthening a deformed septal dorsum is a spreader graft. A strong spreader graft prepared from costal cartilage is fixed at the concave aspect of the remnant septum. It is extended up to the radix on the cranial side and up to the anterior septal angle on the caudal side. The graft is fixed at three different points (Fig. 17.73).

Once a strong dorsal septal segment has been created, the caudal septum must be reinforced. A batten graft made of costa is sutured to the caudal septum to create a straight, resistant, and strong septal L-strut. Then the caudal septum and batten are fixed to the periosteum of the anterior nasal spine (Fig. 17.74).

As soon as a strong septum is achieved, it is necessary to create a strong columella. Therefore, a fairly thick columellar strut is prepared and placed inside the pocket opened between the two medial crura. The cranial aspect of the columellar strut is sutured to the caudal aspect of the septum using an absorbable suture. Thus, the columella is repositioned to the newly created septum (Fig. 17.75).

Figure 17.76 shows the results for this patient. The retracted columella improved, and the nostril sizes were ideal. The strong septum and columella helped increase nose projection and rotation.

17.6.1.2 Case 19

Overtightening of the septocolumellar suture is also a rare reason of retracted columella.

A 24-year-old woman desired improvement of her droopy nasal tip. Septocolumellar suture was preferred due to her thick skin and tip stabilization. Overtightening of the stitch was missed during surgery (Fig. 17.77).

17.6.2 Hanging Ala

The ala must arc with its peak at the midpoint. A hanging ala is noted when the arc is not present or is not high enough to result in nostril show. It may be necessary to also raise the alar rim (Fig. 17.78).

This problem can be resolved via marginal resection. This consists of removing the excess alar border and restoring a more symmetrical and harmonious curve. This maneuver allows artistic shaping and thinning of the alar rim beyond the reach of the standard approach (Fig. 17.79).

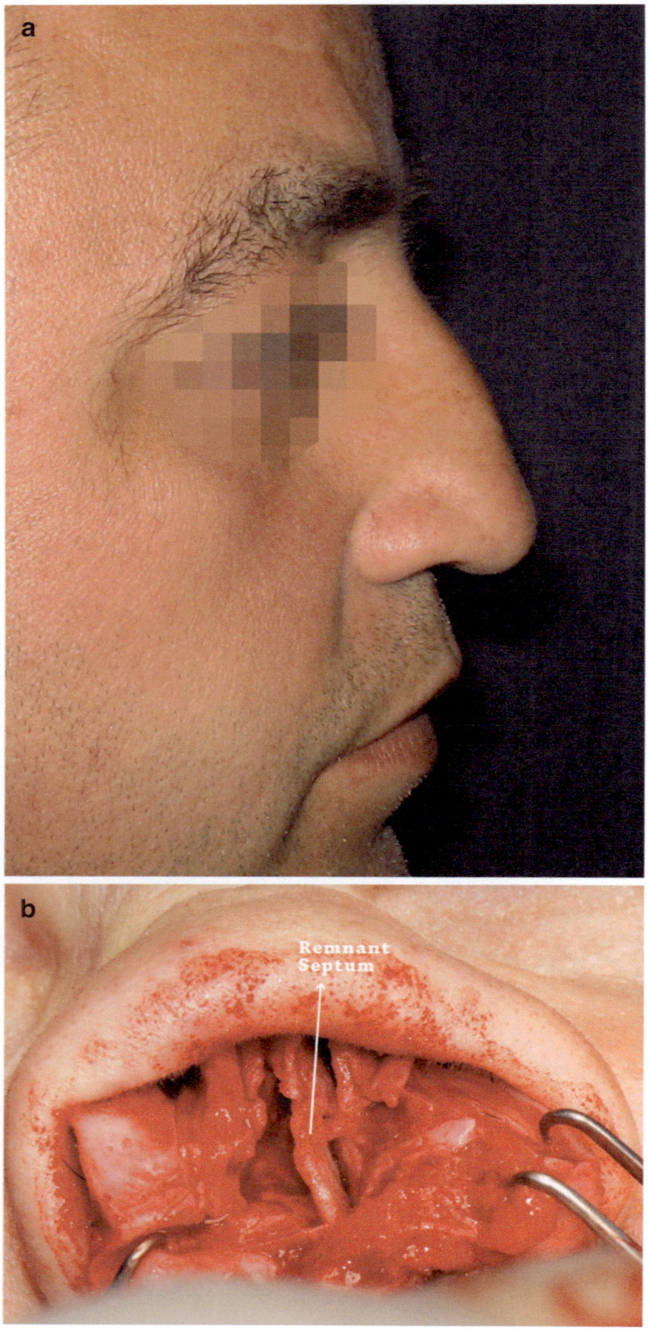

Fig. 17.72 (**a**) The patient with retracted columella had septoplasty anamnesis. (**b**) Open approach revealing deficient and deformed septal cartilage

17.6.2.1 Case 20

A 32-year-old woman had rhinoplasty operation 10 years ago. She was happy with her nose but desired improvement of the reduced nostril show. She had another surgery for the hanging ala problem under local anesthesia. The resection margin was marked with a 15-blade scalpel and carefully carried out. The new open margin was meticulously closed using 6-0 nonabsorbable over-and-over sutures. The alar contour was outlined using a gentian marker pen with the area to be excised colored to aid artistic planning. The marking was checked anteriorly and modified as necessary. A 15-blade scalpel was used to incise the external skin and complete the cut through the mucosa at the same level. Minimal undermining of the external skin rotated the external skin inward. A 6-0 nonabsorbable running closure was used to complete the operation (Fig. 17.80).

As shown in Fig. 17.81, the scar healed nicely and the nostril show was improved.

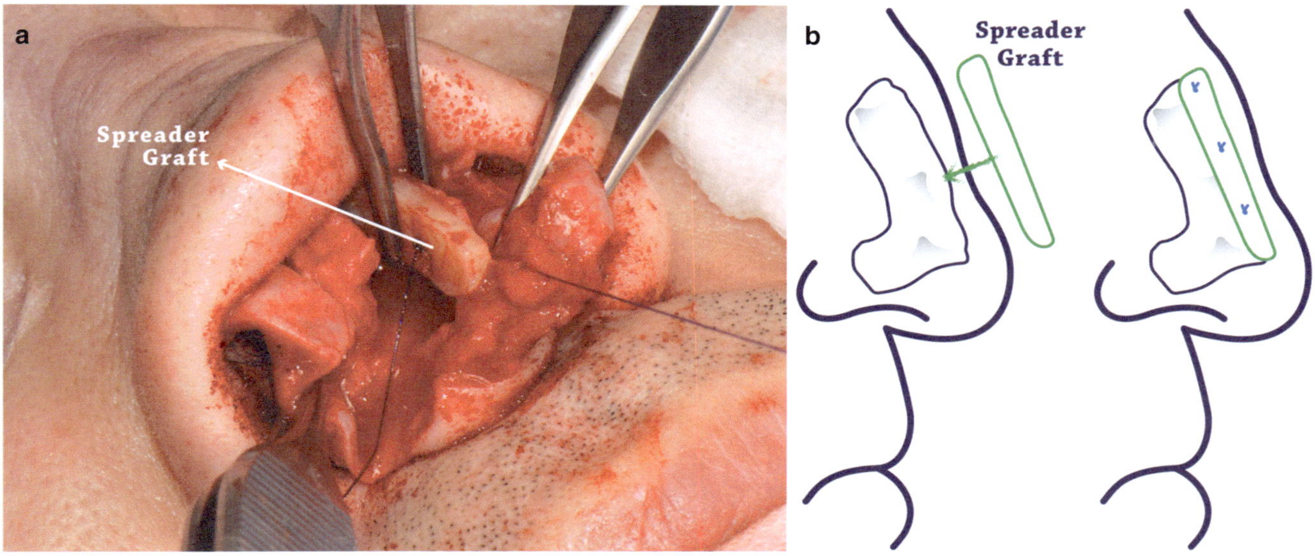

Fig. 17.73 (**a**, **b**) Unilateral costal spreader graft was placed for dorsal reconstruction

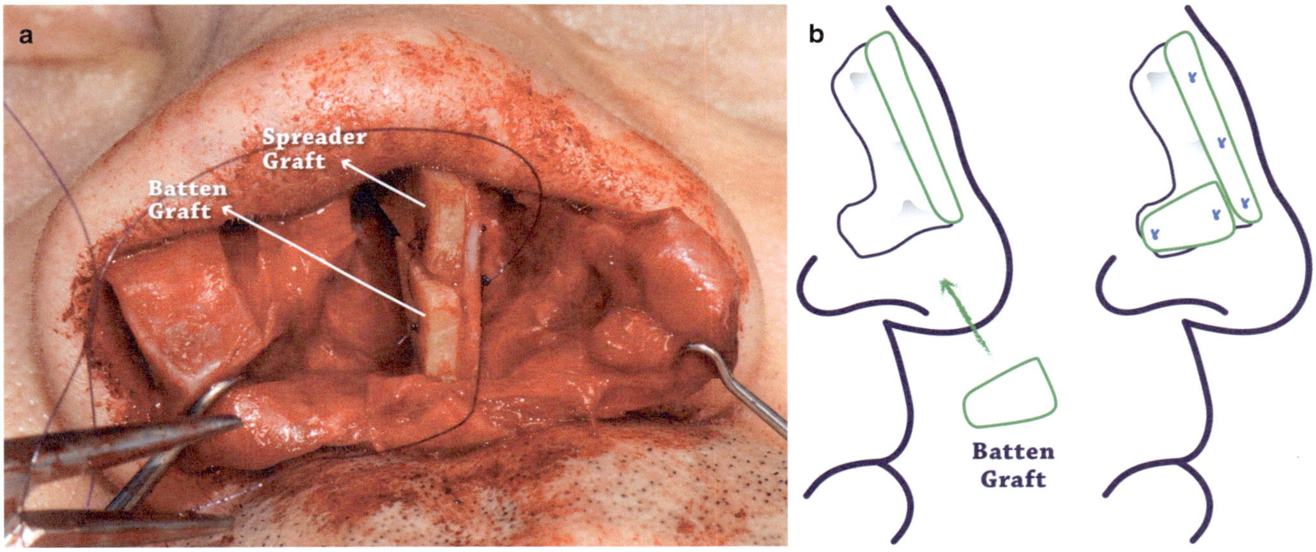

Fig. 17.74 (**a**, **b**) Septal batten graft rebuilt the caudal septum

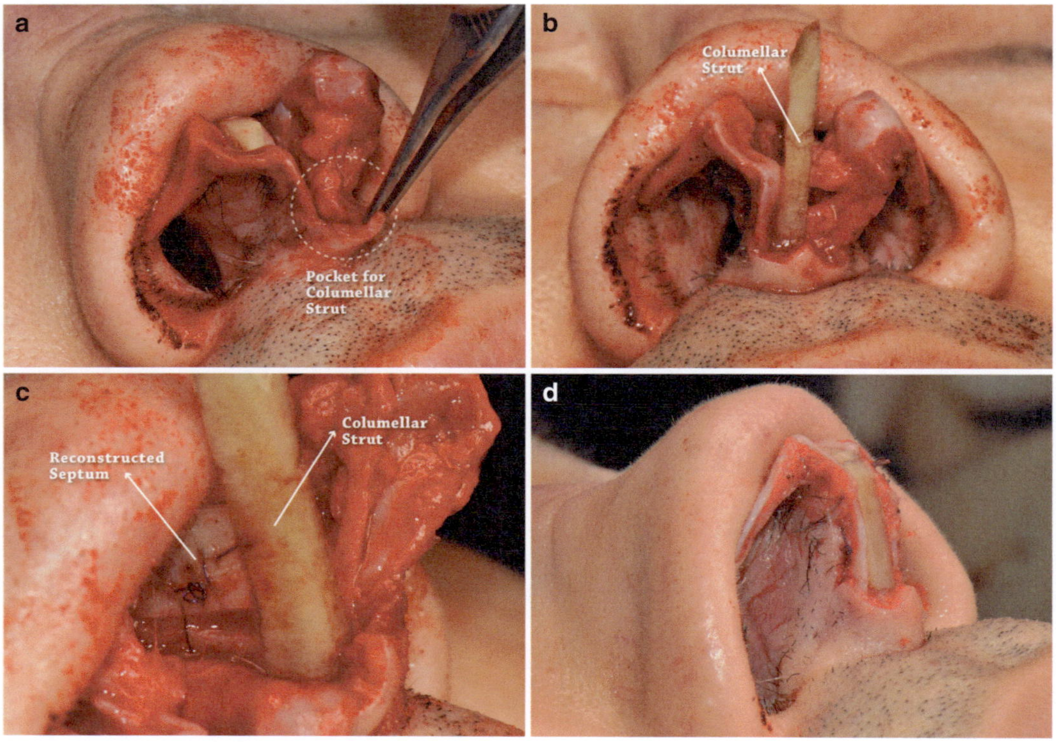

Fig. 17.75 (**a–d**) Strong and sizeable columellar strut is inserted between two media crura and then it sutured the septum and middle-medial crura

Fig. 17.76 (**a–f**) Postoperative views are showing improvement in columellar position after reconstruction of the septum and placement of a strong columellar strut

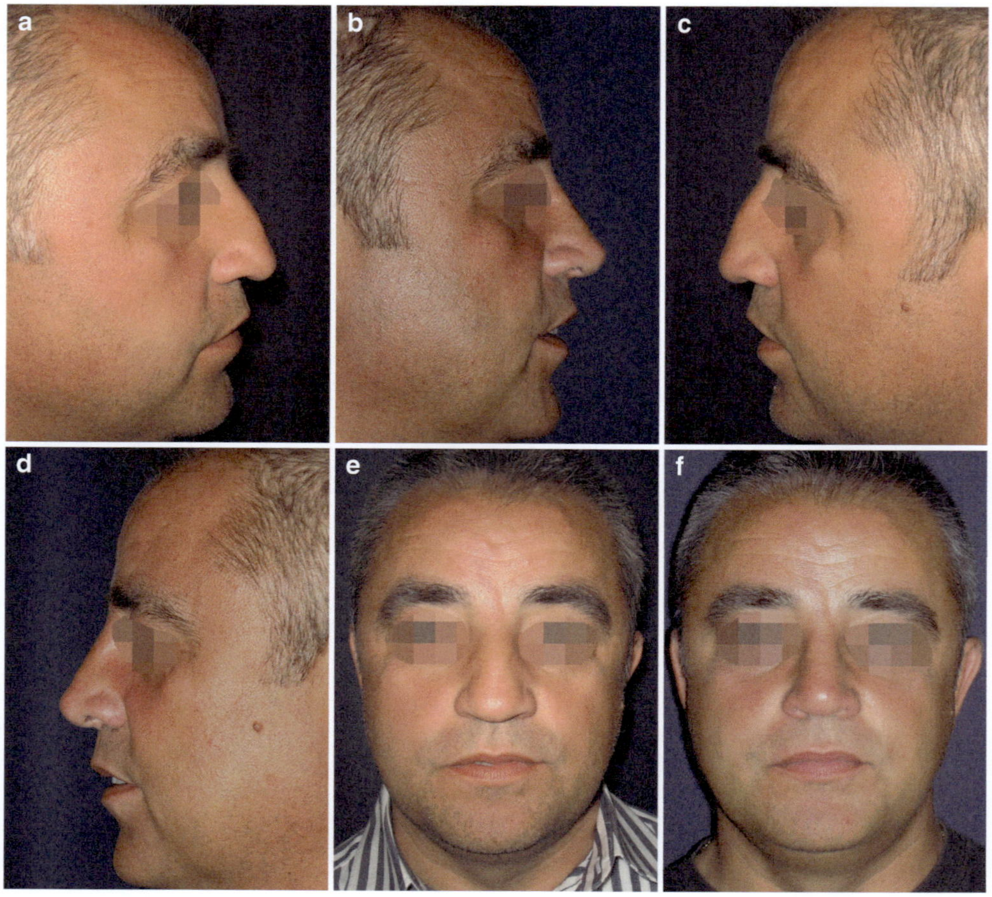

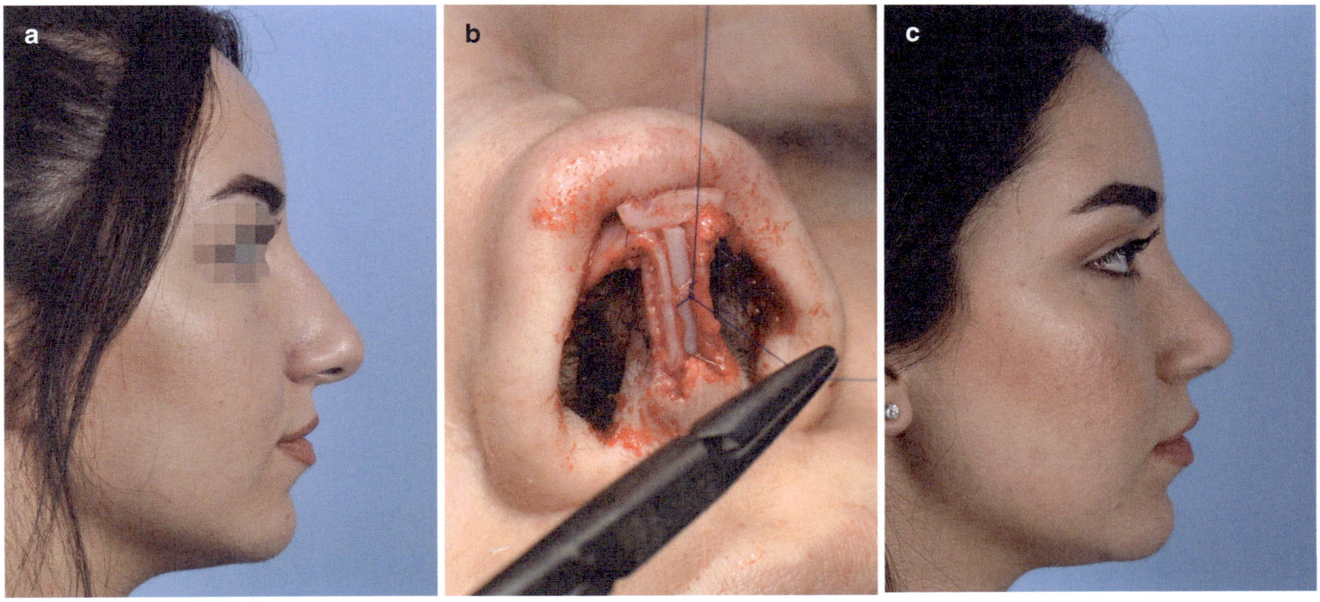

Fig. 17.77 (**a**) Preoperative profile photograph. (**b**) Intraoperative view: transdomal suture, cap, and strut grafts are used. Septocolumellar suturing is seen. (**c**) Slightly retracted columella noted postoperatively

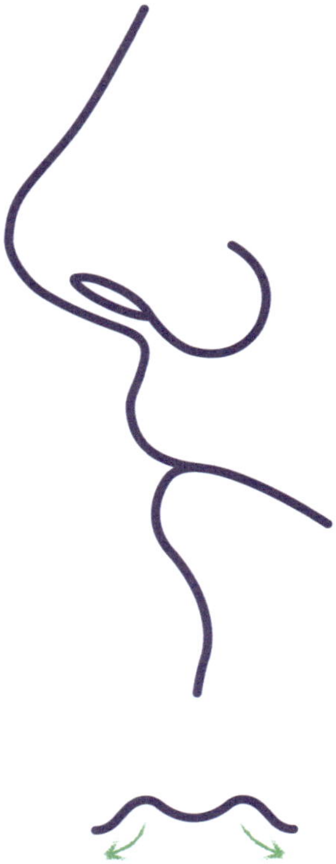

Fig. 17.78 A pure hanging ala deformity. Small round nostril is noted

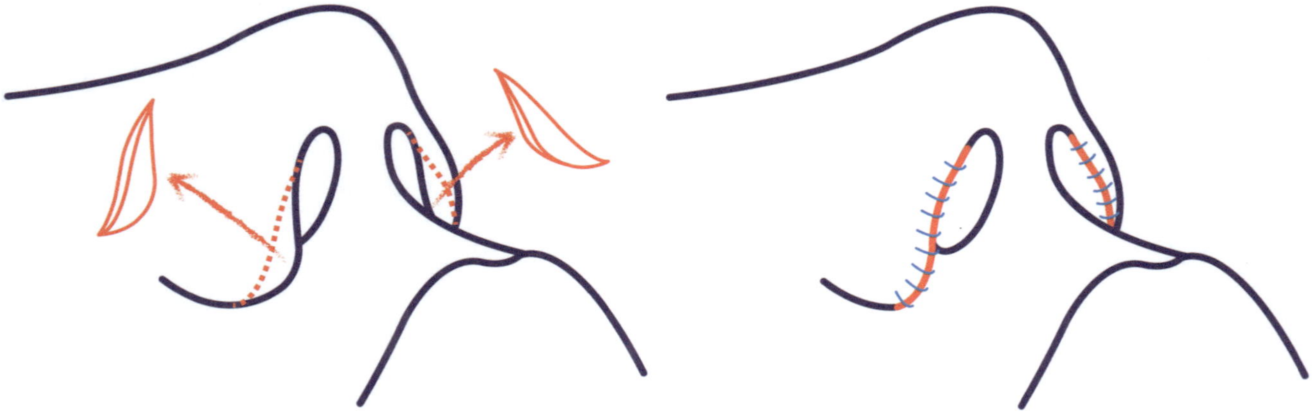

Fig. 17.79 The alar contour is outlined (*red line*) with the area to be excised. (Supplementary Video 17.4)

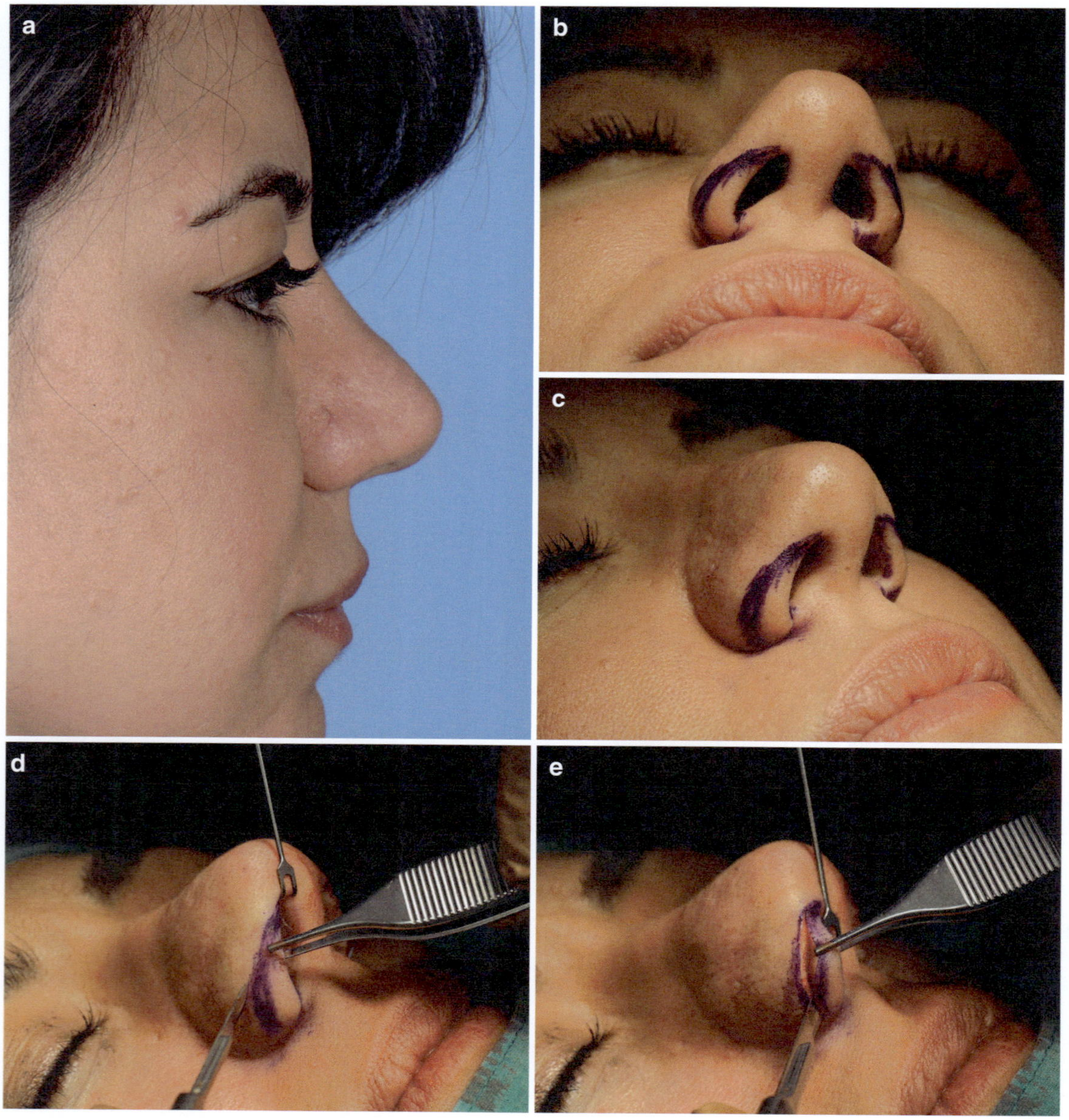

Fig. 17.80 (**a**) The ala is low in relationship to the columella. (**b**, **c**) Excision starts at the top of the nostril and ends at the base with expansion. (**d**–**f**) No. 15 blade incises the external skin and completes the cut through the mucosa at the same level. (**g**–**i**) 6-0 propylene running closure completes the procedure. (**j**) Alar rim raising immediately after resection

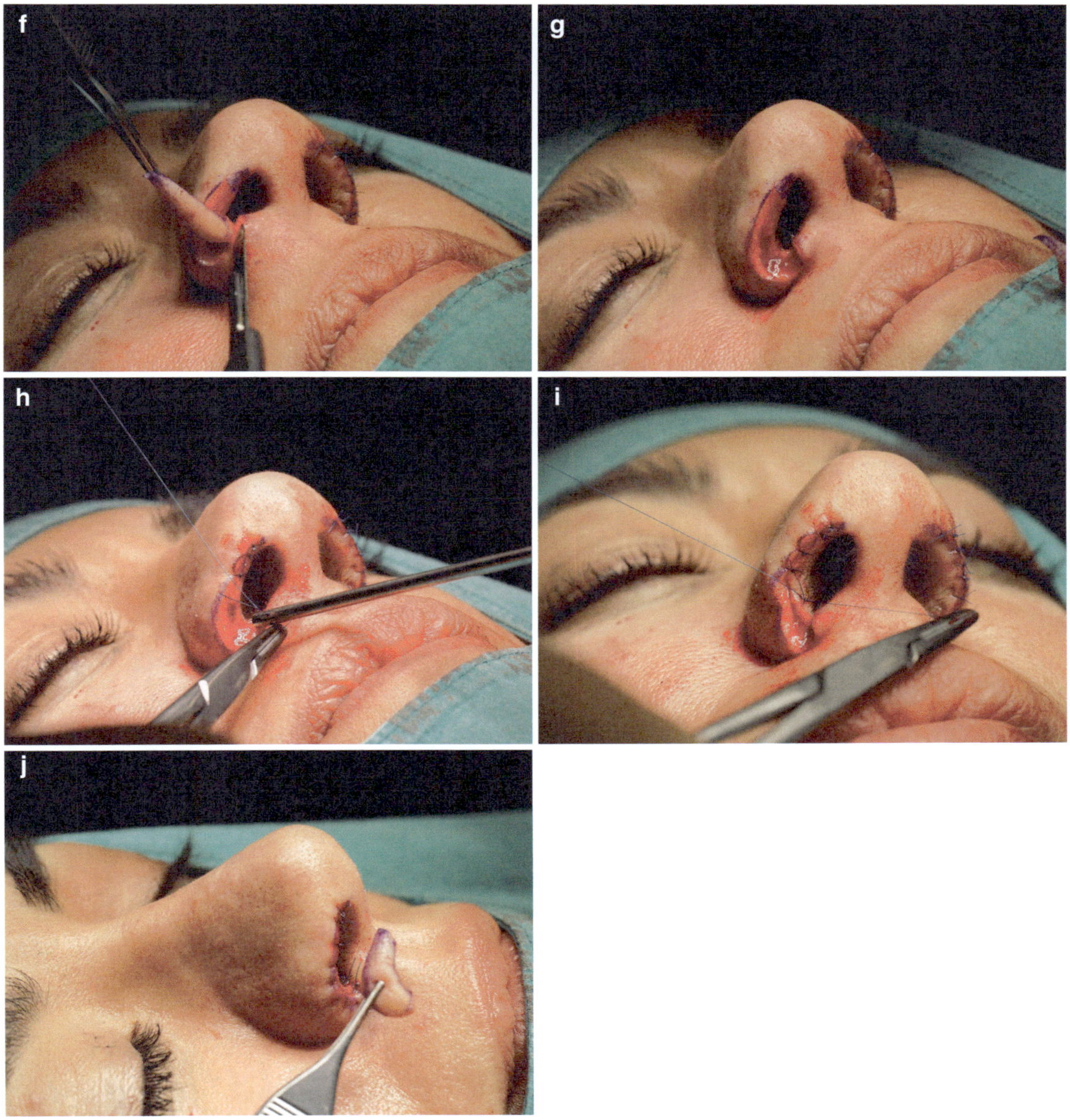

Fig. 17.80 (continued)

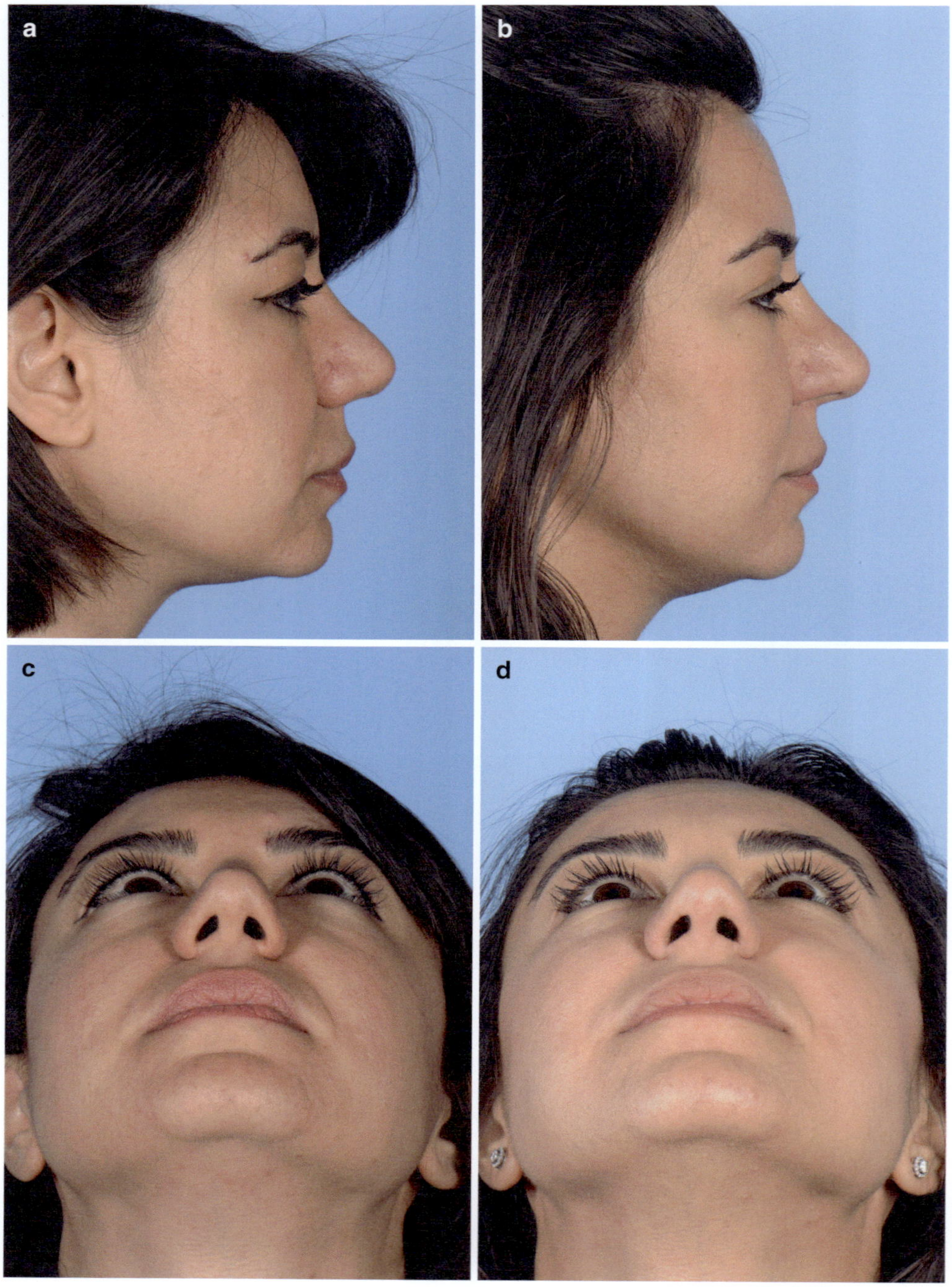

Fig. 17.81 (**a**, **b**) Lateral views: before and after procedure, the alar rim is in a higher position in relation to the columella. Before (**c**) and 6 months after (**d**) base view. Note no noticeable scar in (**d**)

17.7 Conclusion

Asymmetry between the alar rim and the columella border of the nose can constitute an undesirable aesthetic deformity and can manifest in two ways: excessive or reduced nostril show. Alar retraction and a hanging columella are the two causes of excessive nostril show, while columella retraction and a hanging ala result in reduced nostril show. These problems stem from different anatomical variants. For successful rhinoplasty, the surgeon must recognize the underlying causes of an impaired alar–columellar relationship to be able to correct the anatomical variants (Fig. 17.82).

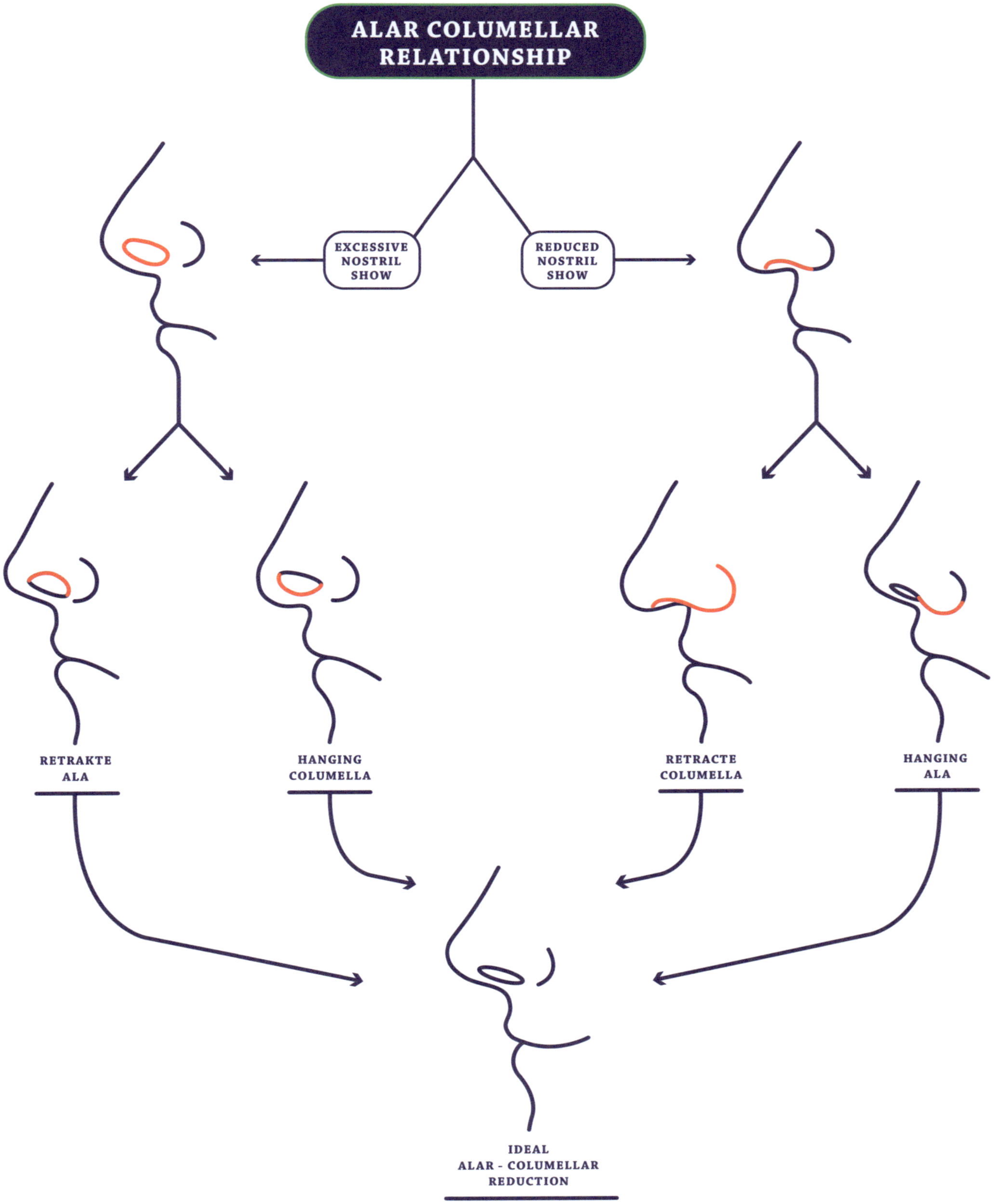

Fig. 17.82 Classification of alar–columella relationship

Disclosures The author reports no conflicts of interest or funding requiring disclosure.

Further Reading

Acikel C. Hypoplastic lateral crus causing alar retraction and underprojected nasal tip: correction with multiple grafts. Aesth Plast Surg. 2012;36(4):862–5.

Adamson PA. Alar base reduction. Arch Facial Plast Surg. 2005;7(2):98.

Adamson PA, Tropper GJ, McGraw BL. The hanging columella. J Otolaryngol. 1990;19(5):319–23.

Alexander AJ, Shah AR, Constantinides MS. Alar retraction: etiology, treatment, and prevention. JAMA Facial Plast Surg. 2013;15(4):268–74.

Armstrong DP. Aggressive management of the hanging columella. Plast Reconstr Surg. 1980;65(4):513–6.

Bafaqeeh SA, Al-Qattan MM. Simultaneous open rhinoplasty and alar base excision: is there a problem with the blood supply of the nasal tip and columellar skin. Plast Reconstr Surg. 2000;105(1):344–7; discussion 348–9.

Bennett GH, Lessow A, Song P, Constantinides M. The long-term effects of alar base reduction. Arch Facial Plast Surg. 2005;7(2):94–7.

Bertossi D, Albanese M, Malchiodi L, Procacci P, Nocini PF. Surgical alar base management with a personal technique: the tightening alar base suture. Arch Facial Plast Surg. 2007;9(4):248–51.

Carniol ET, Adamson PA. Surgical tips for the management of the wide nasal base. Facial Plast Surg. 2018;34(1):29–35.

Choi JY. Alar base reduction and alar-columellar relationship. Facial Plast Surg Clin North Am. 2018;26(3):367–75.

Choi JY, Javidnia H, Sykes JM. New techniques for correction of severe alar retraction using an island pedicled advancement flap of the nasal dorsum. J Plast Reconstr Aesthet Surg. 2013;66(12):1803–4.

Daniel RK, Glasz T, Molnar G, Palhazi P, Saban Y, Journel B. The lower nasal base: an anatomical study. Aesthet Surg J. 2013;33(2):222–32.

Ellenbogen R, Blome DW. Alar rim raising. Plast Reconstr Surg. 1992;90(1):28–37.

Foda HM. Alar base reduction: the boomerang-shaped excision. Facial Plast Surg. 2011;27(2):225–33.

Grinfeld A, Betelli R, Arruda G, Almeida W. How to harmonize the ethnic nose. Facial Plast Surg. 2016;32(6):620–4.

Gryskiewicz JM. The "iatrogenic-hanging columella": preserving columellar contour after tip retroprojection. Plast Reconstr Surg. 2002;110(1):272–7.

Guyuron B, Behmand RA. Alar base abnormalities. Classification and correction. Clin Plast Surg. 1996;23(2):263–70.

Hafezi F, Naghibzadeh B. Prevention of hanging columella in open rhinoplasty. Ann Otol Rhinol Laryngol. 2004;113(10):839–42.

Ilhan AE, Sozen T, Caypinar Eser B, Cengiz B. Association of skin thickness with alar base reduction in patients undergoing lateral crural repositioning and strut grafting. JAMA Facial Plast Surg. 2017;19(6):516–21.

Joseph EM, Glasgold AI. Anatomical considerations in the management of the hanging columella. Arch Facial Plast Surg. 2000;2(3):173–7; discussion 178–9.

Kim JH, Park JP, Jang YJ. Aesthetic outcomes of alar base resection in Asian patients undergoing rhinoplasty. JAMA Facial Plast Surg. 2016;18(6):462–6.

Lima LF, Arroyo HH, Jurado JR. Update in alar base reduction in rhinoplasty. Curr Opin Otolaryngol Head Neck Surg. 2016;24(4):316–21.

McKinney P, Stalnecker ML. The hanging ala. Plast Reconstr Surg. 1984;73(3):427–30.

Ohba N, Ohba M. Preservation of nostril morphology in nasal base reduction. Aesth Plast Surg. 2016;40(5):680–4.

Ponsky D, Guyuron B. Alar base disharmonies. Clin Plast Surg. 2010;37(2):245–51.

Rohrich RJ, Afrooz PN. Components of the hanging columella: strategies for refinement. Plast Reconstr Surg. 2018;141(1):46e–54e.

Silver WE, Sajjadian A. Nasal base surgery. Otolaryngol Clin N Am. 1999;32(4):653–68.

Tellioğlu AT, Vargel I, Cavuşoğlu T, Cimen K. Simultaneous open rhinoplasty and alar base excision for secondary cases. Aesth Plast Surg. 2005;29(3):151–5.

Williams EF. Alar-columellar disharmony using the tongue-in-groove maneuver in primary endonasal rhinoplasty. Arch Facial Plast Surg. 2012;14(4):283–8.

18 Asymmetrical Nasal Tip

18.1 Introduction/Treatment Strategy

There are two main causes of asymmetry at the nose tip: intrinsic deformity of alar cartilage (abnormal alar cartilage anatomy) and deviations of the septum (deviated caudal septum, in particular). In some cases, both exist simultaneously, causing nose tip asymmetry.

18.1.1 Management of Caudal Septal Deviation

Achieving tip symmetry without repositioning the septum in the midline is hardly possible. Deviation of the caudal septum, in particular, may have a direct implication for the tip. Therefore, the first step in asymmetrical tip surgery should be to make sure that the caudal septum rests symmetrically in the midline (Fig. 18.1).

However, it should be noted that, in the presence of an axis deviation affecting the entire nose, it is essential to reposition the entire septum in the midline. Any surgeon who is aware of this requirement will naturally concentrate on the septal pathology.

Once the septal pathology is corrected, the asymmetry at the tip is also corrected along with asymmetry of the other nasal subunits. In Fig. 18.2 asymmetry is remarkable not only on the nose but on the entire face. It would be quite unlikely for a surgeon to overlook nasal asymmetry in such cases. Yet a good proportion of patients present only with caudal septal deviation without axis deviation, which may often be missed by the surgeon.

While taking care of other remarkable problems of the nose, a surgeon may overlook the occult deviation in the caudal septum. This may constitute an intraoperative problem or may result in pronounced postoperative tip asymmetry. If there is any deviation from the midline, although the alar configuration does not appear to have any problem intraoperatively, the caudal septum may be pushing the columella laterally. This must always be kept in mind during tip plasty. Occult caudal septal issues should not be overlooked.

Figure 18.3 shows an intraoperative image of a typical presentation of this problem. Although the alar cartilages are entirely symmetrical, the tip is pushed away unilaterally after the strut is fixed. *This appearance often results from an uncorrected occult caudal septum.*

- Either open or closed approach may be used to correct problems in the caudal septum. In advanced septal problems requiring subtotal or total septal reconstruction, an open approach may be preferred because it offers wide exposure.
- The hump must be removed before correcting the septal deviation.
- Then, septoplasty is performed, leaving a minimum 1 cm of septum at the dorsum and the caudal side. The dorsal and caudal portions are each considered independent units. The caudal segment would not rest in the midline without correcting the deviation in the dorsal segment. Similarly, the dorsal segment could not be corrected without correcting the deviation in the caudal aspect. Each segment can be reconstructed either individually or collectively (subtotal or total septal reconstruction).

Deviations in the dorsal septum are discussed in the chapter related to mid-vault reconstruction. This chapter discusses deviations in the caudal septum.

18.1.2 An Algorithm for Management of Deviations in the Caudal Septum

- In some cases, excess cartilage at the junction between the caudal septum and the nasal spine may be the cause of deflection. The septal base is set back over the spine as soon as the excessive portion is resected, repositioning

Supplementary Information The online version contains supplementary material available at https://doi.org/10.1007/978-3-031-65619-4_18.

S. Şeneldir, *Photographic Atlas of Rhinoplasty*, https://doi.org/10.1007/978-3-031-65619-4_18

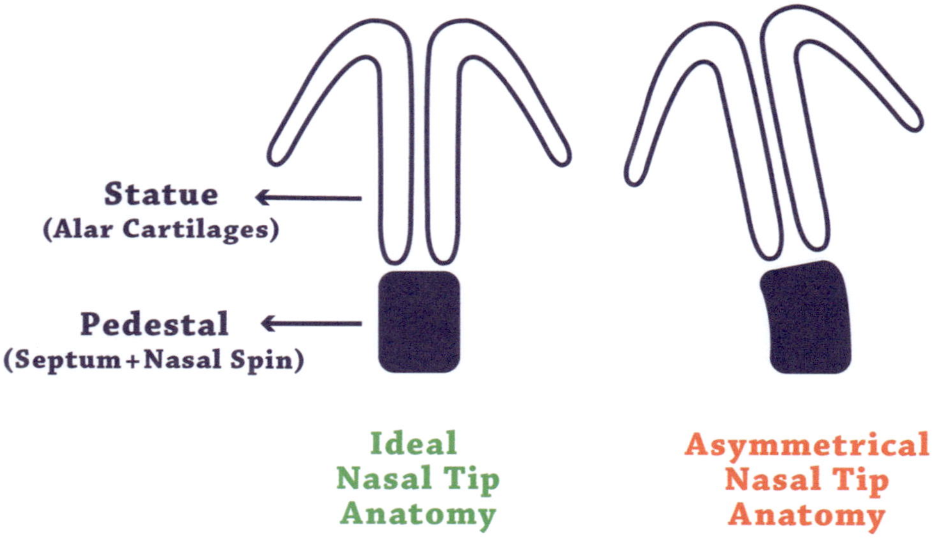

Fig. 18.1 The alar cartilages rest like a statue on a pedestal, which is essentially the caudal septum and nasal spine. The pedestal may deviate in any direction. The alar cartilages are affected accordingly. A deflection of the midline may push the tip sides and give the tip an asymmetrical appearance

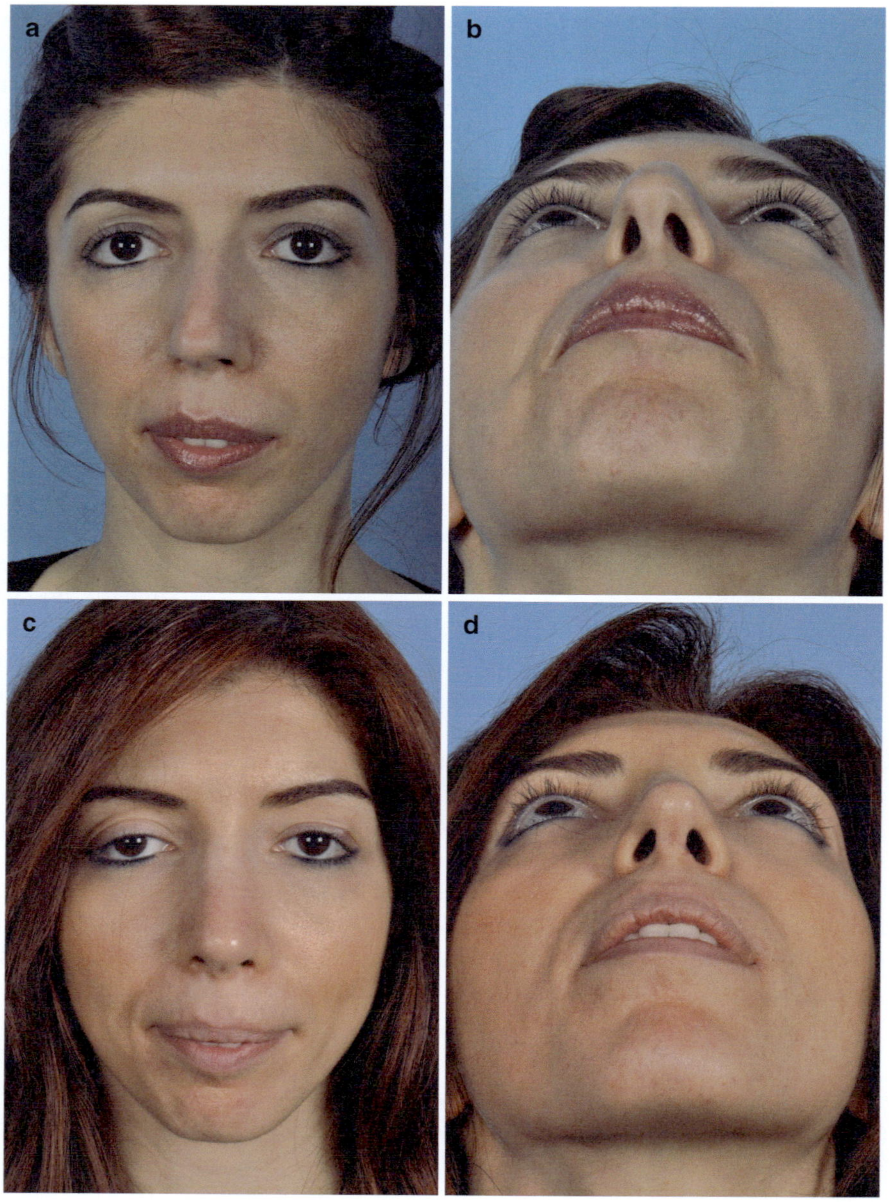

Fig. 18.2 (**a**, **b**) The nose is deviated due to severe septal deviation. Also, the asymmetrical tip stems from the same reason. (**c**, **d**) After septorhinoplasty the nose is straight and the tip is symmetrical

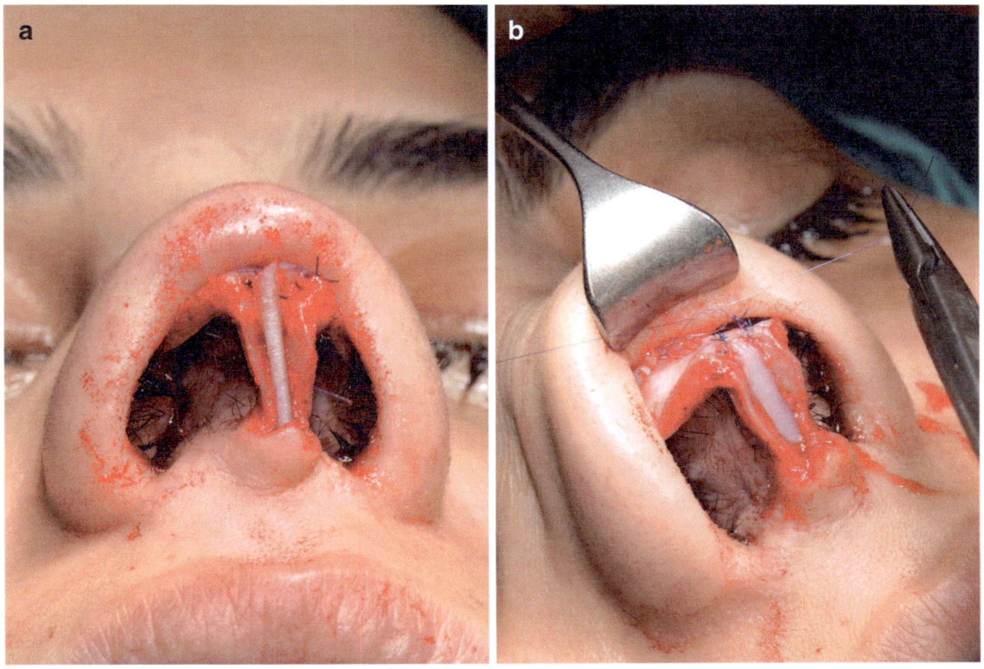

Fig. 18.3 (**a**) Deviated caudal septum pushes the tip side. (**b**) Any maneuvers on the alar cartilages should not be performed. After correction of caudal septum problem, the tip comes midline

the septum in the midline. For a complete setback, a socket can be opened on the spine with a scalpel. If the spine rests in the midline, the socket is opened in the midpoint. Otherwise, it is opened slightly to the right or to the left, depending on the situation. The septum is set back in the socket opened on the spine with the help of a drill or scalpel. Then it is fixed with a figure-of-eight suture (Fig. 18.4).

- If the deviation persists after bringing the caudal septal base to the midline, this is considered an intrinsic deviation of the caudal septum. The septum has an hourglass shape. This configuration can be corrected with a septal batten graft. A septal batten graft serves the same purpose for caudal septal deviation as spreader and autospreader grafts serve for reconstruction of the nasal dorsal segment.
- Inverted triangles are cut off from the convex aspect of the septum before suturing the septal batten graft, which makes the oversized plane of the convex edge smaller. On the concave side, cross-hatching is performed to break resistance. Then a septal batten graft made of septal or costal cartilage is sutured on the caudal septum facing its concave aspect (Fig. 18.5).
- Although rare, septal batten grafts may also be fixed to the convex aspect of the caudal septum to correct configuration deformities. There is no absolute rule. The first attempt must involve the concave aspect. If the desired outcome is not achieved, then the convex aspect is tried (Fig. 18.6).
- The size of the batten graft is versatile. It may extend all of the way along the caudal segment, but may also be smaller in size. The batten graft can also be prepared from the vomer bone. Using an extracorporeal needle, holes are opened on various points of the vomer bone and obliquely sutured on the caudal septum (Fig. 18.7).
- In advanced deviations of the caudal septum that cannot be corrected with the above maneuvers, subtotal septal reconstruction would be a good alternative. These patients often present with crookedness in the dorsal septum. The septum is cut off and removed from the fracture area. The removed portion is analyzed to determine the amount of smooth cartilage to be achieved. If a straight septum can be obtained to fill the gap between the nasal spine and remnant septum, the graft is placed inside this segment. It is sutured to the nasal spine at the nasal base and to the residual septal segment at the cranial side. Thus, a straight septum is achieved. Occasionally, the septal structure created with a unilateral or bilateral spreader graft may need support (Fig. 18.8).

The following sections describe all the steps in a case.

Intraoperative septal views demonstrate that the caudal and dorsal septum are totally deviated. It is quite challenging to correct such a substantially deviated septum intracorporeally. Subtotal septal reconstruction is the best choice for such cases. The surgery starts by leaving behind a straight segment and completely removing the deviated piece (Fig. 18.9).

The distance between the septal stump and the anterior nasal spine is measured. The measurement reveals a 3 cm length and 2 cm height, which is perfectly sufficient. A straight cartilage measuring 3 cm × 2 cm is designed from the removed septum. The graft, termed the Caudal Septal Replacement Graft, is inserted inside the nose (Fig. 18.10).

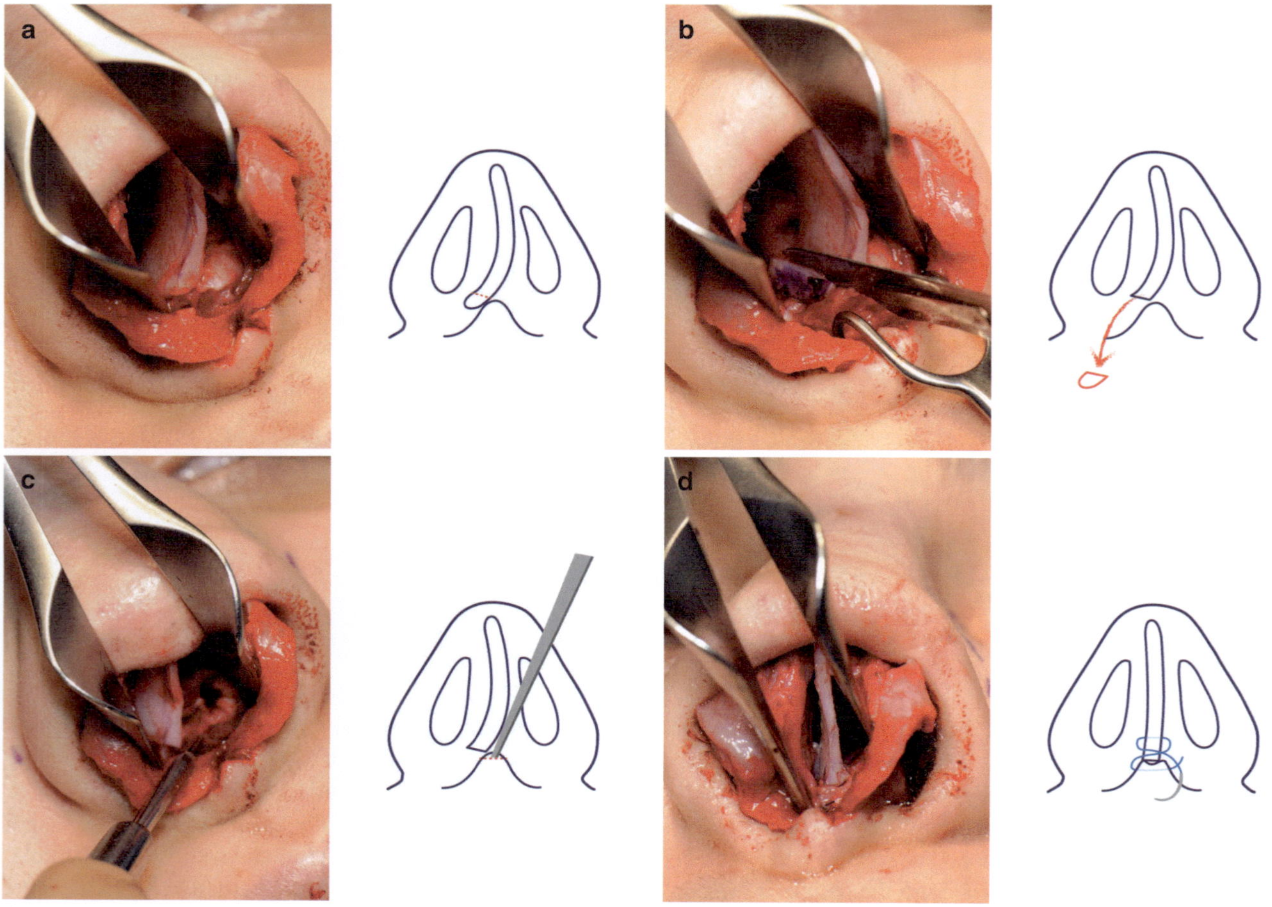

Fig. 18.4 (**a**–**d**) After excising the horizontal wedge of septal cartilage, the septum is repositioned to the midline over the anterior septal spine. Finally, the inferior septum is secured to the spine with a nonabsorbable suture. (Supplementary Video 18.1)

The graft base is first fixed to the nasal spine. To do that:

- A hole is opened in the spine using an injector.
- A 4-0 permanent suture is passed through the spine.
- The suture makes a turn at the point where it exits the skin, passing through the septum in the same direction.
- Once the suture has exited from the septum, the knot is tied by completing a figure-of-eight at the starting point (Fig. 18.11).

Then the graft is fixed at the septal stump at the cranial side (Fig. 18.12).

Thus, a straight septum is achieved. The surgery is standard up to this point. This is followed by a mid-vault reconstruction. In some cases, there is no need for any other technique, whereas in others there may be a need for an extra spreader graft. The spreader graft is sutured to the contralateral side of the septal stump in such instances. A thin graft is placed in between to fill in the forming gap (Fig. 18.13).

It should be noted that there is another way to perform subtotal septal reconstruction, which can be used when it is not possible to fashion a straight graft to fit the exact size of the gap. A caudal replacement graft and two pairs of extended spreader grafts are prepared in a sufficient size to create the caudal septum. Spreader grafts are fixed on the septal remnant at the cranial aspect. The base of the septal replacement graft is fixed at the spine inside the nose. In the dorsal aspect, it is fixed at two pairs of spreader grafts fixated at the septal remnant (Fig. 18.14).

Once symmetry is restored in the caudal septum, the surgeon proceeds with the asymmetries of the alar cartilages.

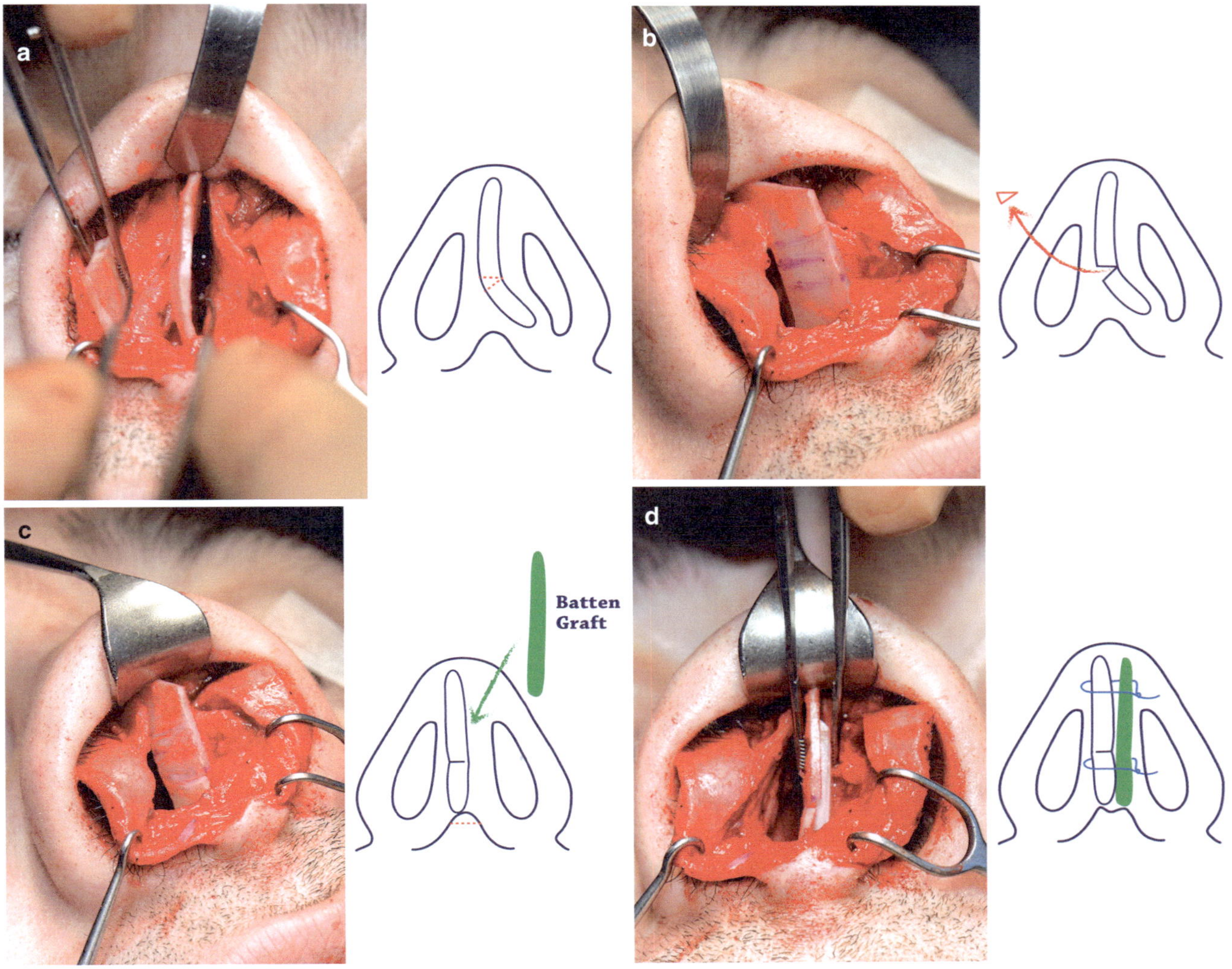

Fig. 18.5 (**a**) Caudal septal deviation. (**b**) A triangular cartilage trim on the convex side. (**c**) Placement of septal batten to the concave side of the septum. (**d**) Sides sutured with absorbable suture. (Supplementary Video 18.2)

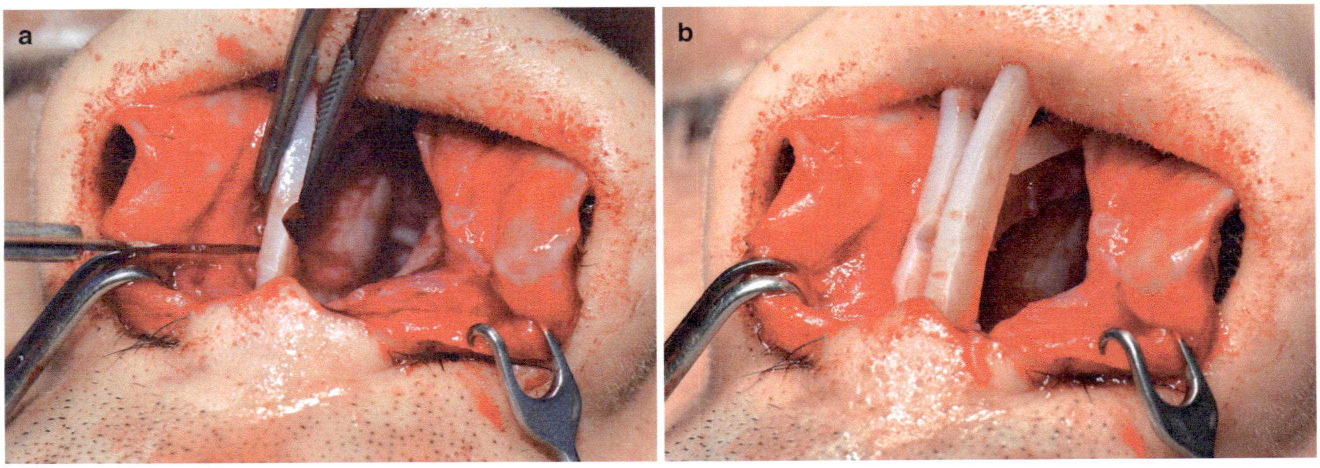

Fig. 18.6 (**a**) Triangular trim on convex side. (**b**) Placement of septal batten on concave side of septum

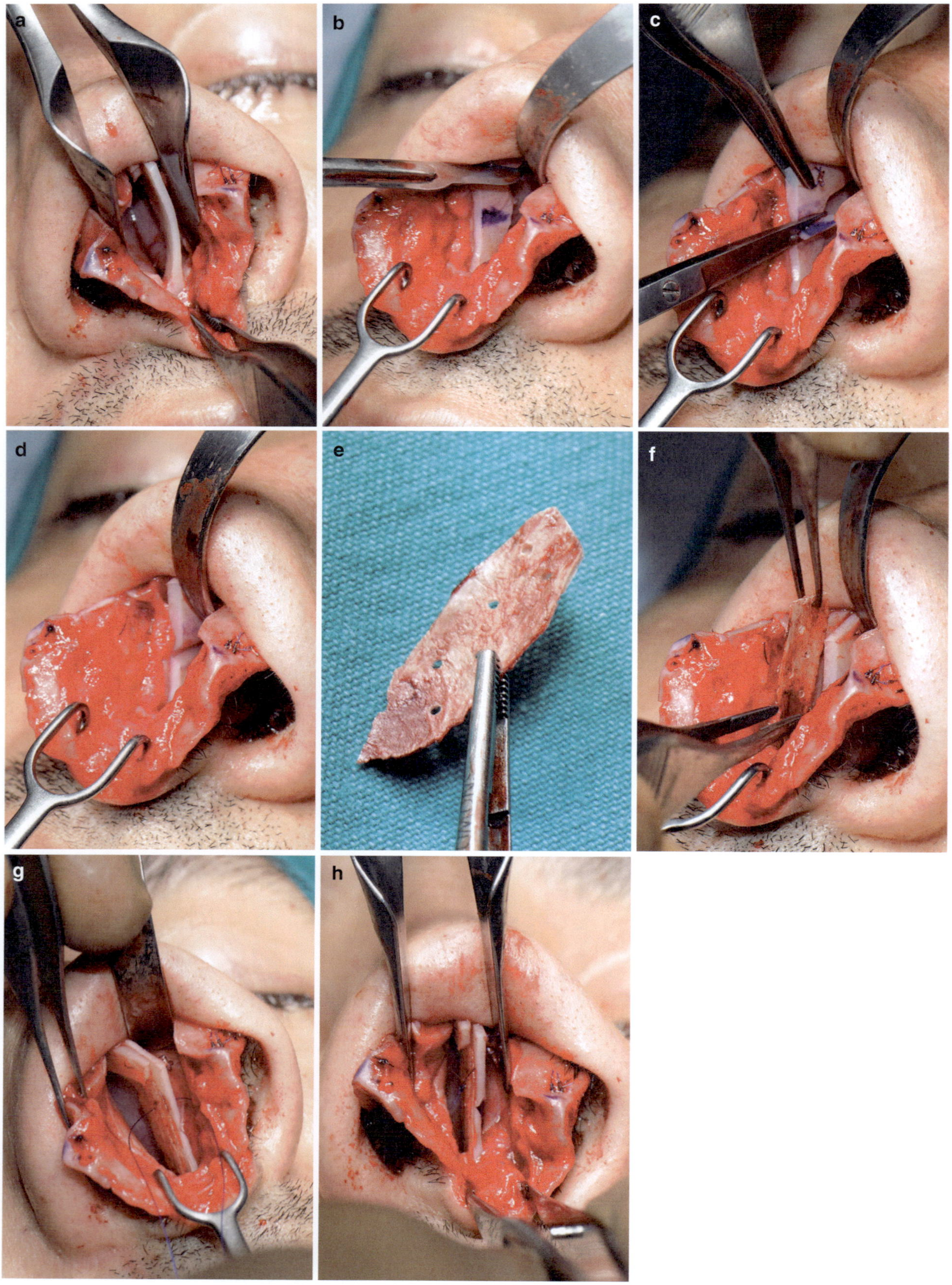

Fig. 18.7 (**a**) Caudal septal deviation. (**b**, **c**) Triangular trim on convex side. (**d**) Bony septal batten graft. (**e–g**) Placement of bony batten graft on concave side. (**h**) The caudal septum is in the midline; notice dorsal septum: right spreader graft has been placed for dorsal septal correction. (Supplementary Video 18.3)

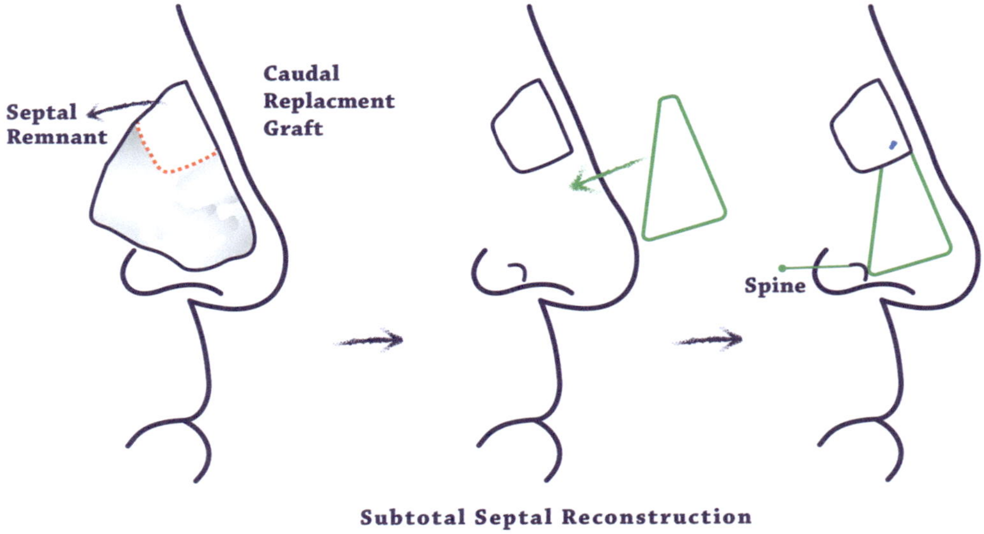

Fig. 18.8 Subtotal septal reconstruction

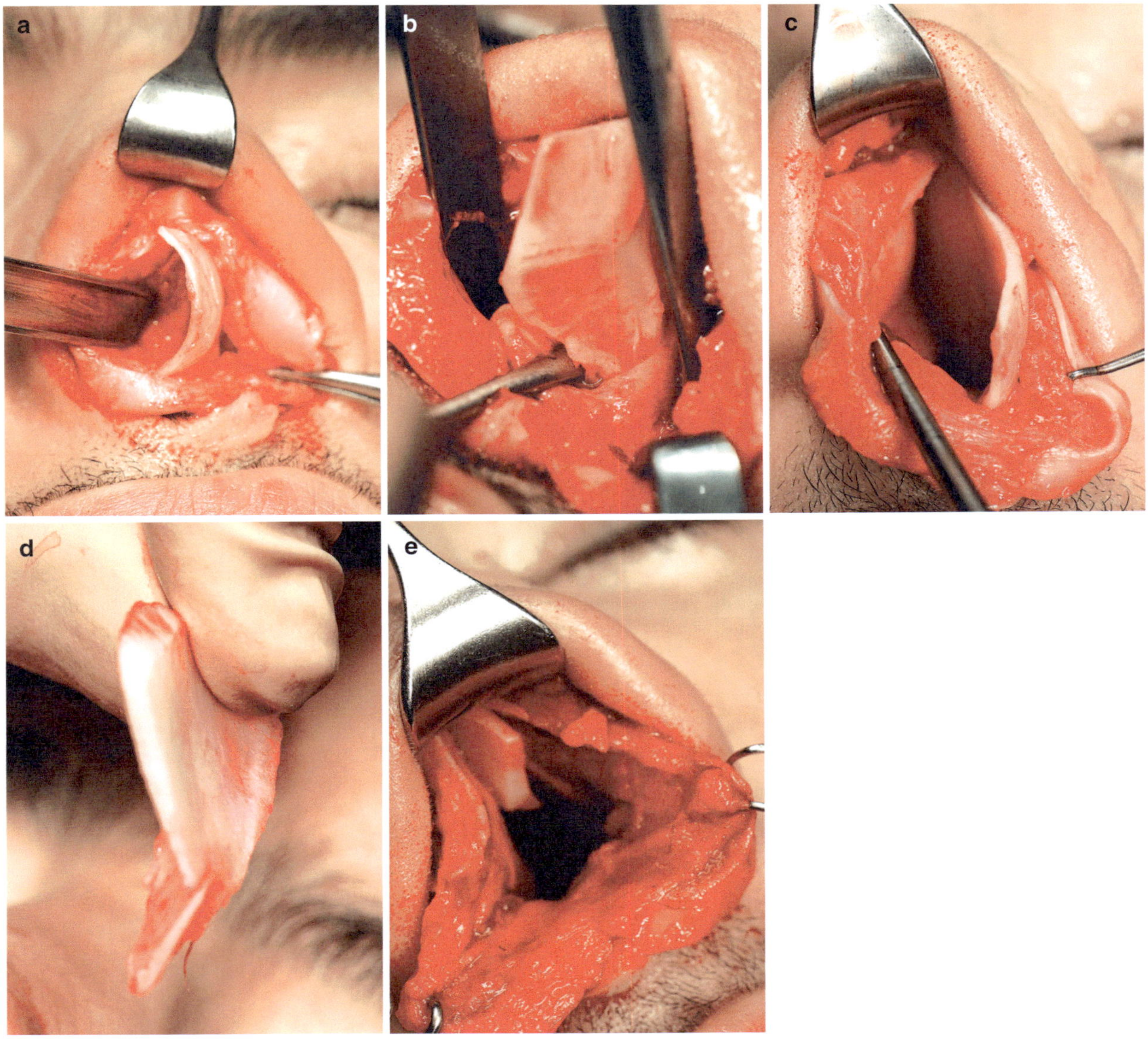

Fig. 18.9 (**a**–**c**) Severely deviated nasal septum. Note the oblique orientation of the septal torsion. (**d**) Distorted part of the septum is excised. (**e**) A remnant of the dorsal strut. (Supplementary Video 18.4)

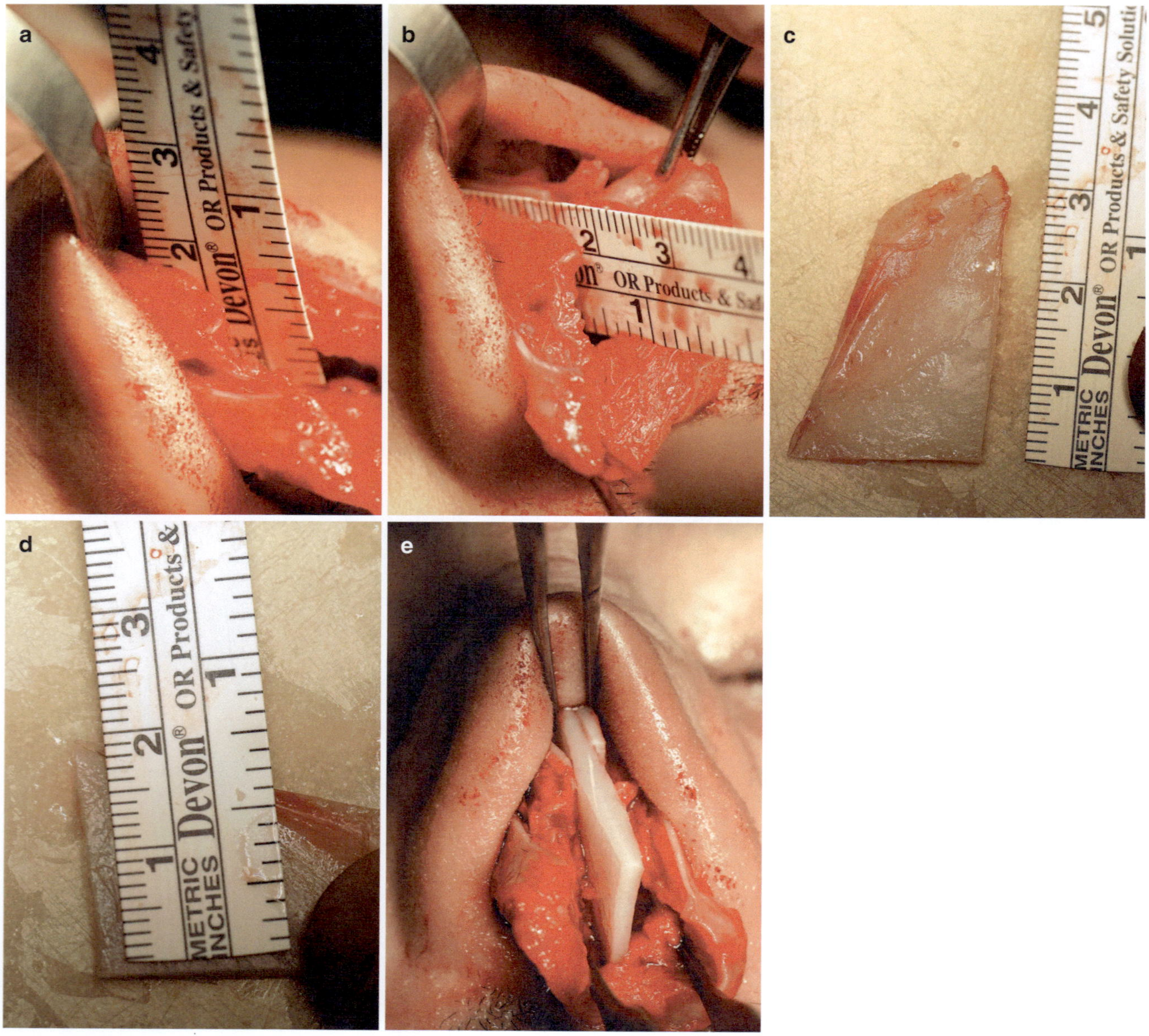

Fig. 18.10 (**a**, **b**) A cartilage graft sized 2 cm vertically and 3 cm horizontally is necessary to fill the gap. (**c**, **d**) Sculpturing the graft from the septum. (**e**) Placement of the septal replacement graft

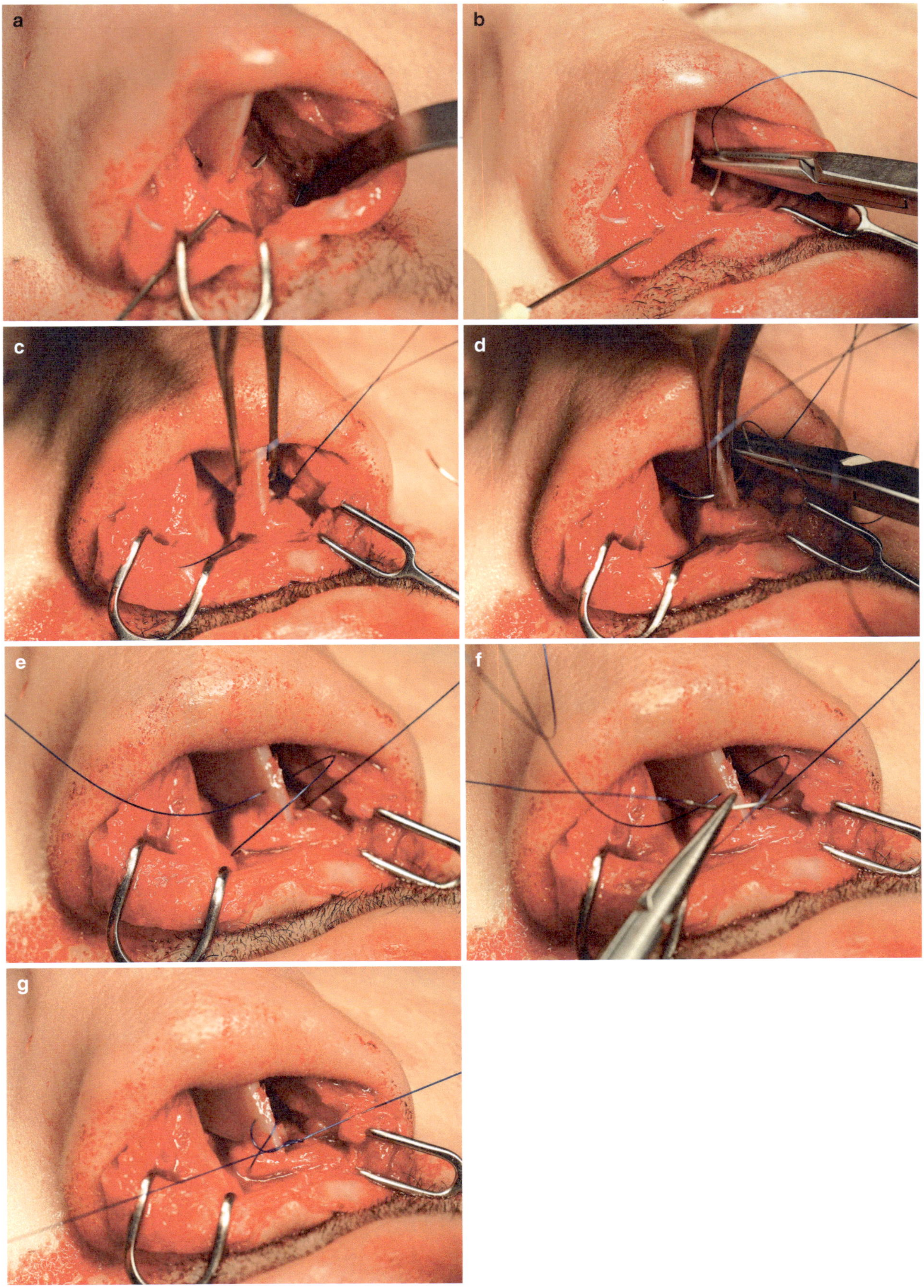

Fig. 18.11 (**a**, **b**) A straight needle to make a hole in the nasal spine. This maneuver must be done carefully to avoid avulsing the nasal spine. (**c**–**g**) A figure-of-eight suture is a method of choice when the graft is fixed to the spine

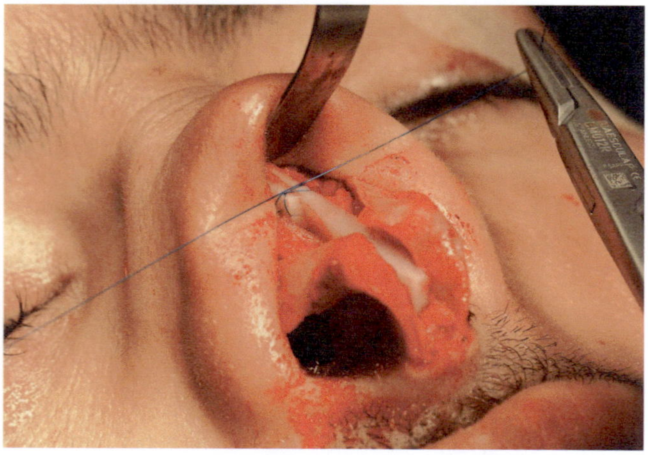

Fig. 18.12 Septal remnant fixed to caudal septal replacement graft

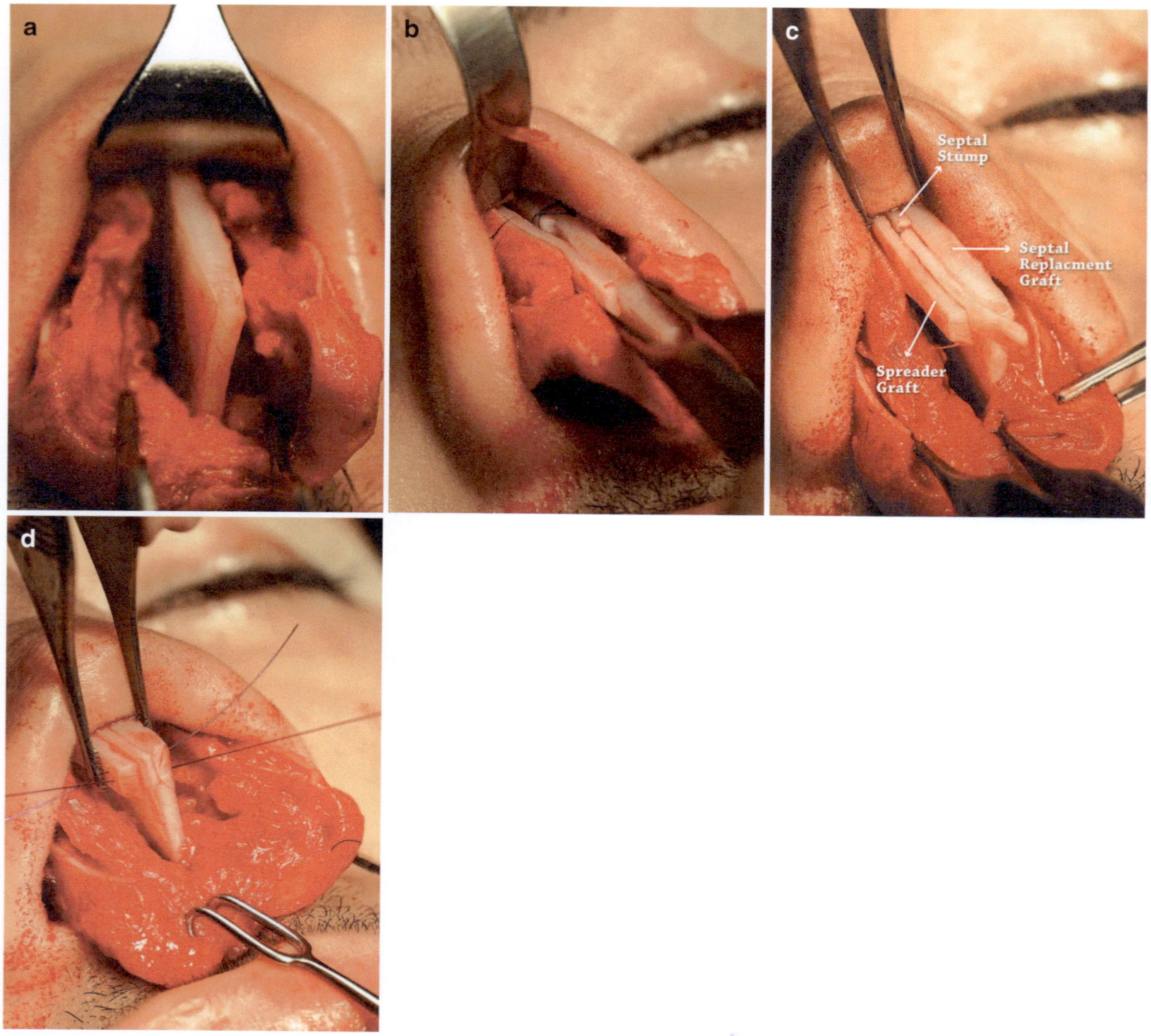

Fig. 18.13 (**a**) Diagram showing straight septum. (**b**) A spreader graft was placed for rebuilding the middle vault. (**c**) At this point, there has been a gap between the caudal septal replacement graft and the spreader graft. This gap was being bridged with a septal strip. (**d**) Oblique view of reconstruction

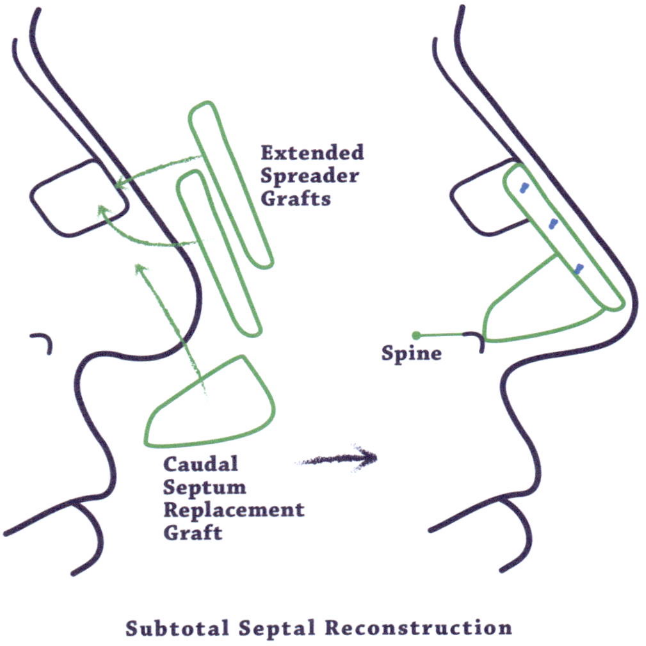

Fig. 18.14 Bilateral extended spreader grafts and caudal septal replacement grafts can be used for septal reconstruction

18.2 Tip Asymmetries Due to Alar Cartilages

Asymmetrical tip surgery can be performed using either an open or closed approach. Whichever method is used, the skin dissection must be performed as widely as possible. The alar cartilage must be skeletonized from all ligaments and connective tissues. Any ligament or connective tissue that remains undissected may cause retraction in the tip during and after surgery.

1. Before starting asymmetrical tip surgery, each of the alar cartilages is assessed separately. The lateral crus and the middle/medial crus are respectively compared according to the length and inner configurations of each segment. This analysis gives the surgeon an idea about the strategy to be followed.
   (a) Dome symmetry is restored by transdomal suture, whereas middle/medial crus symmetry is reinstated by columellar strut. A lateral crural graft is used to correct asymmetries and configuration deformities of the lateral crus (Fig. 18.15).
   (b) Unilateral or bilateral malposition of the lateral crus may also cause an asymmetrical tip. In this instance, unilateral or bilateral repositioning surgery may be necessary to achieve symmetry.
2. It should be noted that the columellar strut to be used for restoring symmetry in the middle/medial crus must be straight. It is necessary to find a straight piece in the septum for a straight columellar strut. However, it may be challenging to do so. Occasionally, the entire septum is curved in an hourglass shape, in which case the septal crest may be quite helpful. Even if the septal crest emerges as curved, its thickness may allow the surgeon to design a straight strut (Fig. 18.16).
3. Another way to achieve a straight septum is to straighten the two septal cartilages carved from the septum in a back-to-back or face-to-face fashion (Fig. 18.17).

   In severe asymmetries, it may be necessary to resect or create overlap in the alar cartilages.
4. If the asymmetry is in the lateral crus, the asymmetrical portion is resected right next to the dome (Fig. 18.18).
5. If the asymmetry lies in the middle/medial crus, it may persist even after transdomal suturing and fixation of the columellar strut. Medial crural overlapping is performed to correct the asymmetry. The medial crus creating the asymmetry is cut, sliding and suturing the proximal stump in the distal direction (Fig. 18.19).

Technical Pearl: It should be noted that resection is preferred in asymmetries of the lateral crus, whereas overlapping is the technique of choice in medial crus pathologies. Why are two different techniques used for the same pathology in two different segments? The medial crus and the middle crus are the load-bearing pillars of the nasal tip. Any resection in this area harms the load-bearing capacity of the pillars. The aim is to regain the lost resistance through overlapping. For this reason, medial crural overlapping is preferred over medial crural resection. The reason why resection is preferred in pathologies of the lateral crus is that overlapping may result in undesired irregularities and stepping in the tip in the mid and long term.

- Once a symmetrical bony frame is achieved in an asymmetrical nasal tip, the surgeon must proceed with the soft tissues. To correct asymmetries of the alar base, alar base reduction may be required. The resection can be made during primary surgery or can be postponed. In the latter case, resection can be performed under local anesthesia in the office setting; this is considered a more rational option by some surgeons because it is performed after healing is complete.

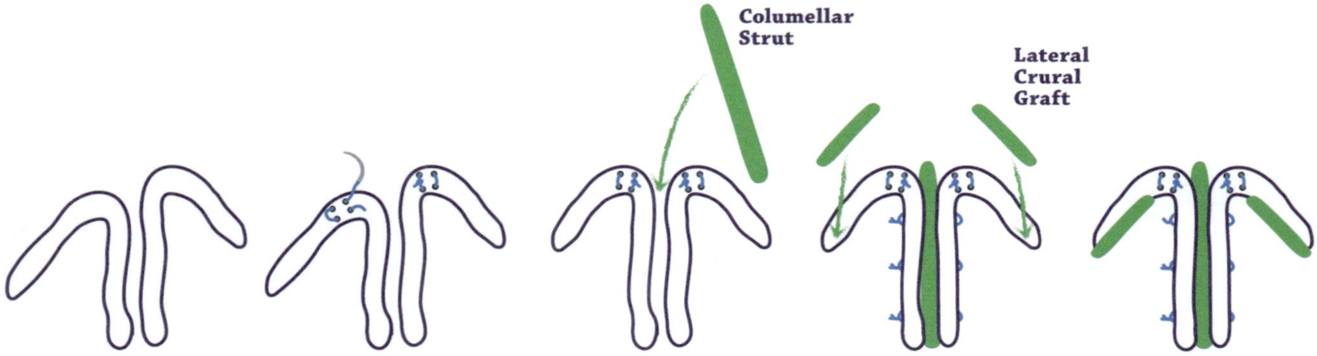

Fig. 18.15 Nasal tip symmetry can be improved utilizing transdomal suture, columellar strut, and lateral crural graft

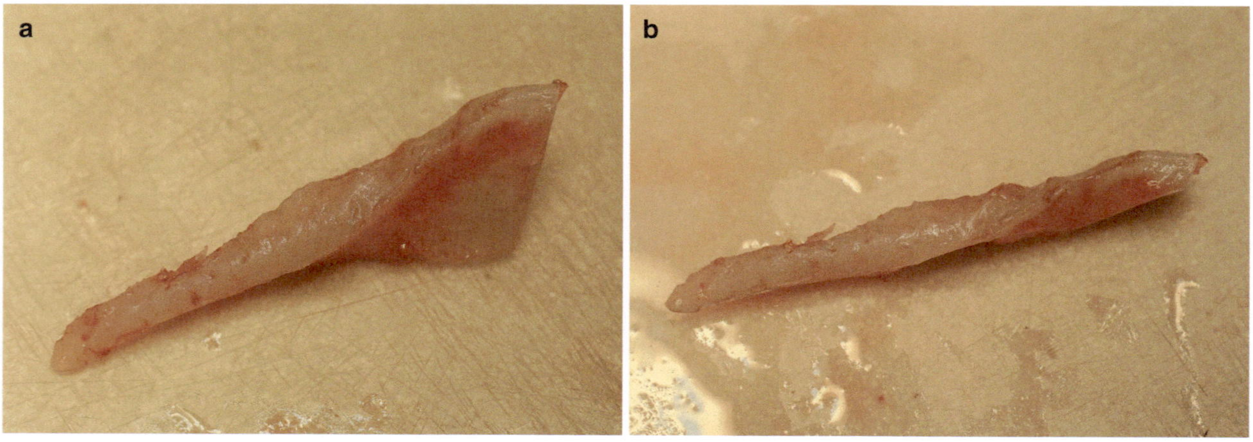

Fig. 18.16 (**a**, **b**) It should be kept in mind that septal crest may be quite helpful for sculpting the columellar strut

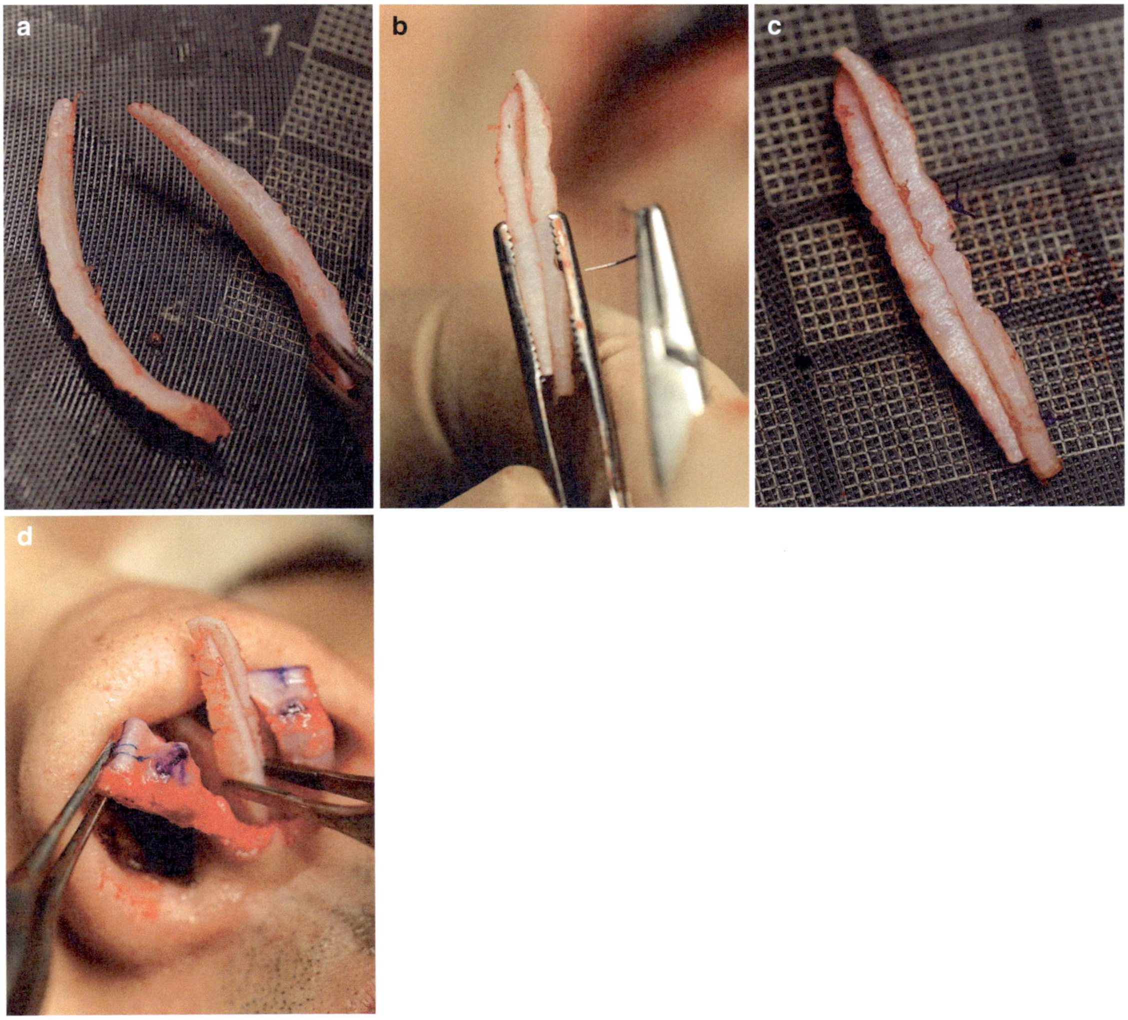

Fig. 18.17 (**a**) Deviated septal cartilage strips. (**b**) Concave sides of the strips are sutured. If necessary the grafts can be lightly crosshatched on the convex side before suturing. (**c**) Laminated columellar strut that is straight. (**d**) Columellar strut placed

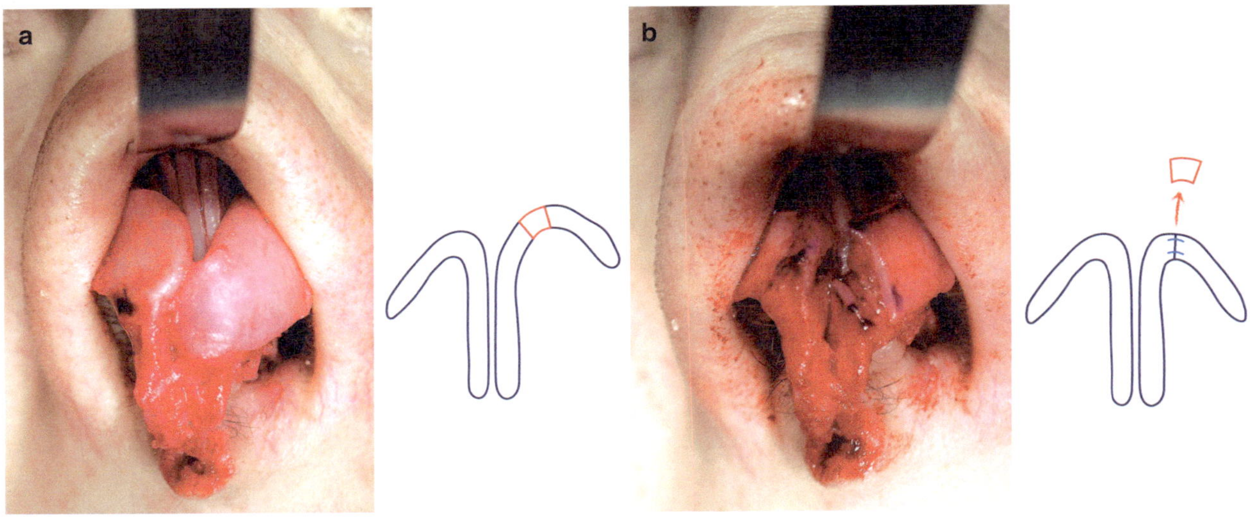

Fig. 18.18 (**a**) Asymmetrical nasal tip. The lateral crura are not symmetrical. (**b**) Excision of the marked segment allows tip symmetry

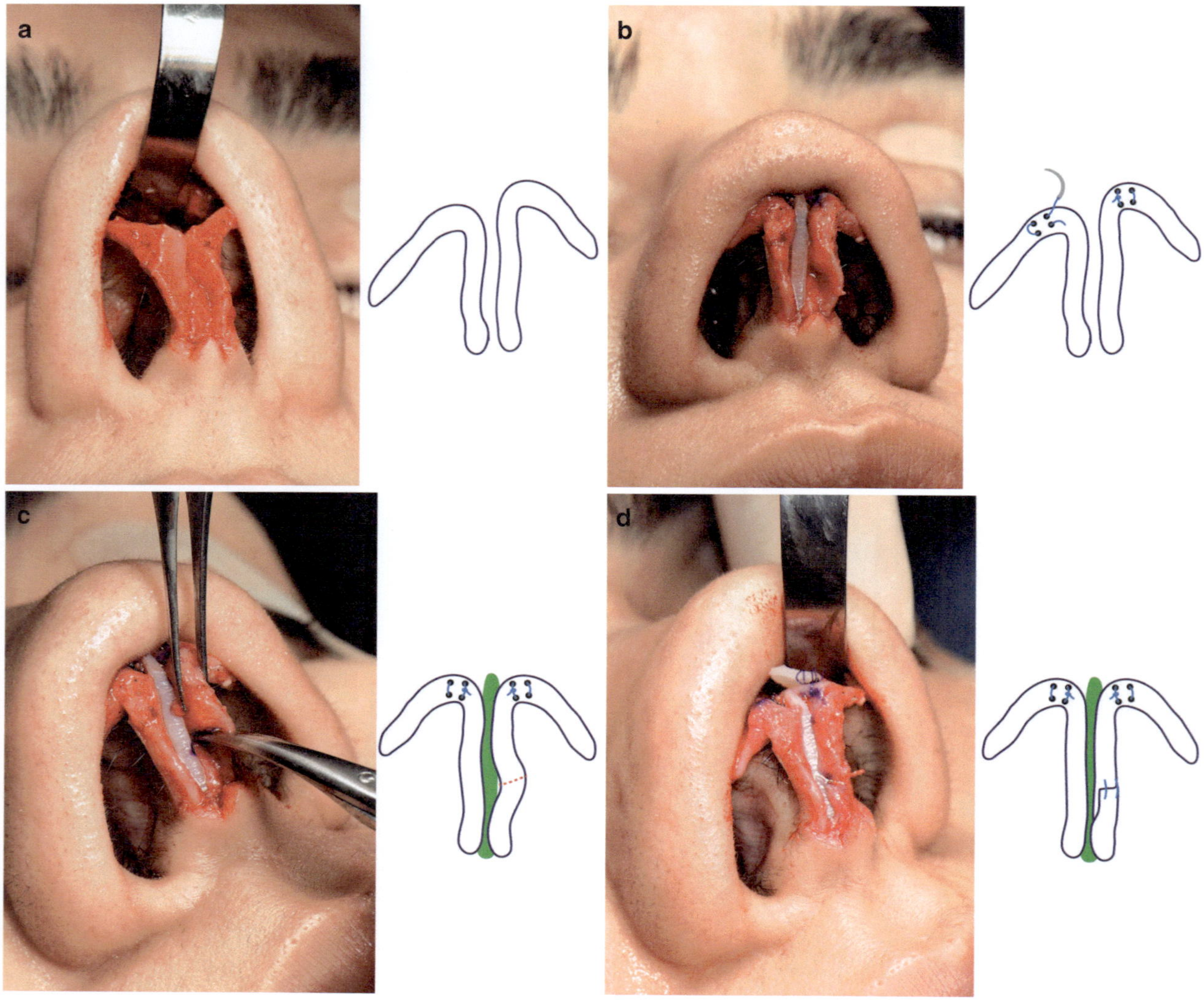

Fig. 18.19 (**a**) Asymmetrical nasal tip. (**b**) Transdomal suture to equalize dome points. (**c**, **d**) Columellar strut was not sufficient for base symmetry. Notice the left medial crus. Overlap of the marked segment allows tip symmetry

18.3 Clinical Outcomes

Patients presenting with an asymmetrical tip must be assessed meticulously. As discussed before, dorsal septal deviations cause crookedness in the tip. The following case is an example of this phenomenon.

18.3.1 Case 1

Comparing the preoperative frontal view versus the intraoperative dorsal view, one may appreciate the cause of tip asymmetry as the dorsal septum. The dorsal septum is repositioned in the midline using spreader grafts. No surgery is performed on alar cartilages. The dorsal septum is moved to the midline through the endonasal route using spreader grafts. Only cephalic resection is performed at the tip through the lateral crura. Through a small marginal incision, crushed cartilage is applied to the tip for definition (Fig. 18.20).

In some cases, as in this one, bringing the deviated dorsal septal segment to the midline corrects the tip asymmetry without the need for an extra maneuver (Fig. 18.21).

18.3.2 Case 2

In this patient, the prominent tip asymmetry at the alar base resulted from the deviation in the caudal septum (Fig. 18.22).

First, the septal excess in the base is removed, and then an inverted triangle is cut off from the convex surface. The caudal septum is taken to the midline by suturing a septal batten graft (Fig. 18.23).

Taking the caudal septum to the midline not only corrects the asymmetry in the tip, but also relieves the nasal passage.

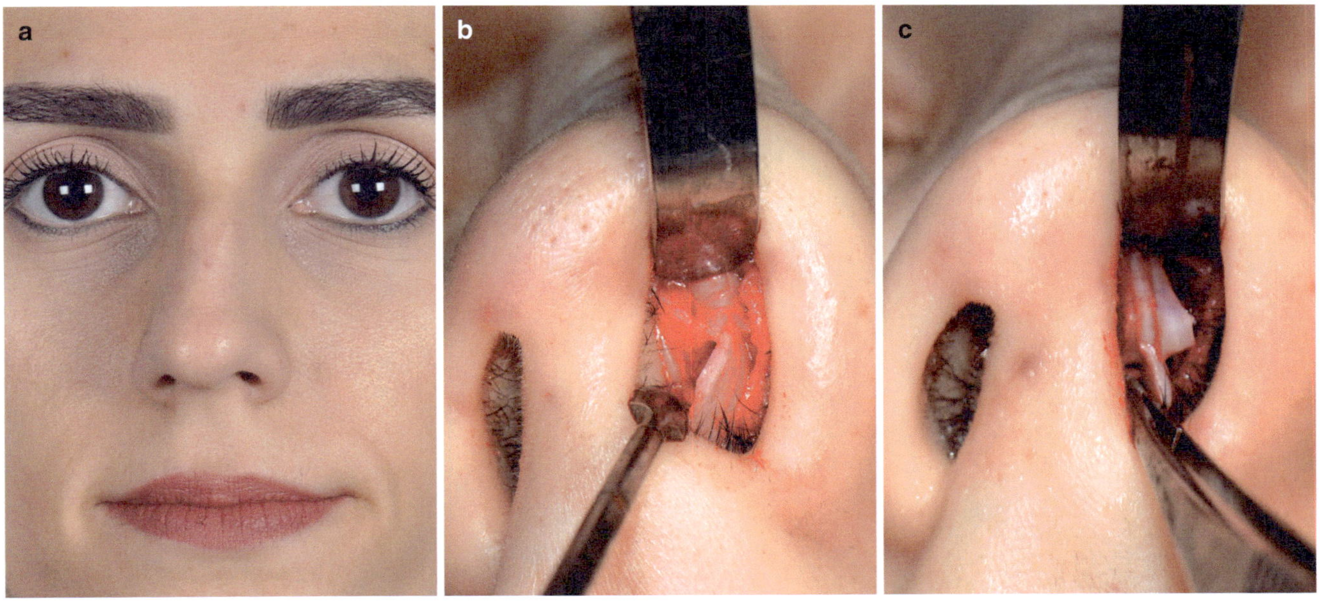

Fig. 18.20 (**a**) Asymmetrical nasal tip due to septum. (**b**, **c**) Spreader graft placement for correcting septal deviation

Fig. 18.21 (**a**–**d**) The nose is straighter and tip complex is on the midline

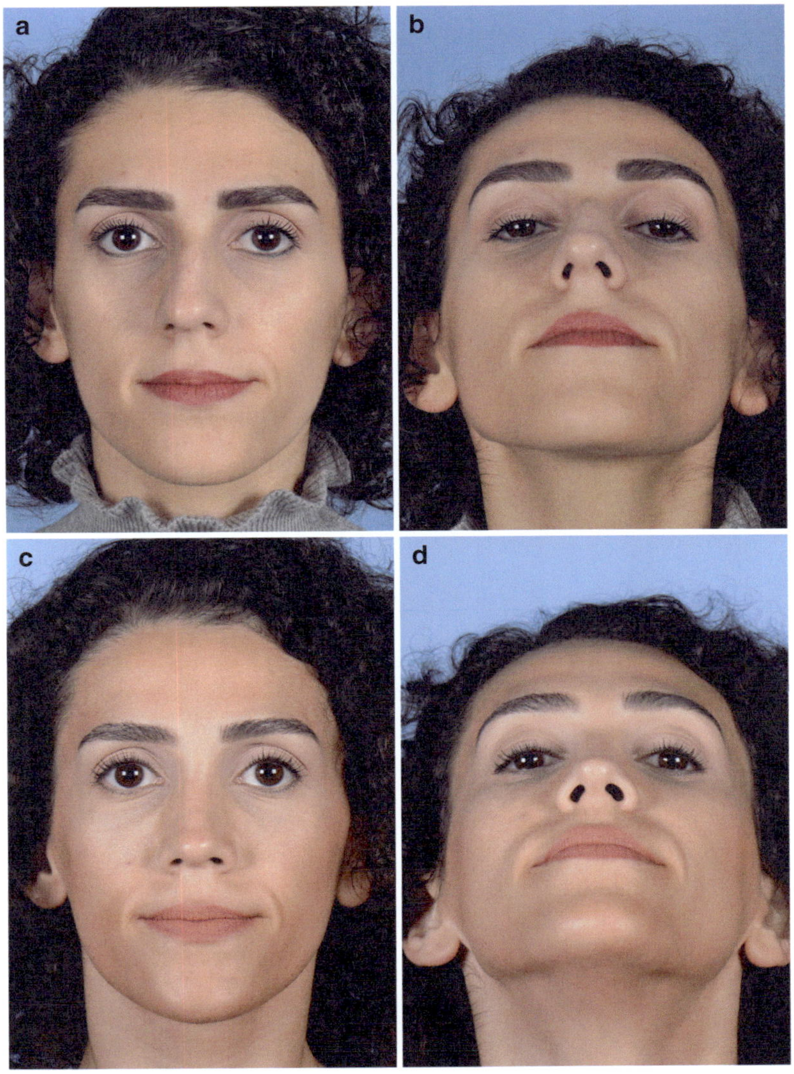

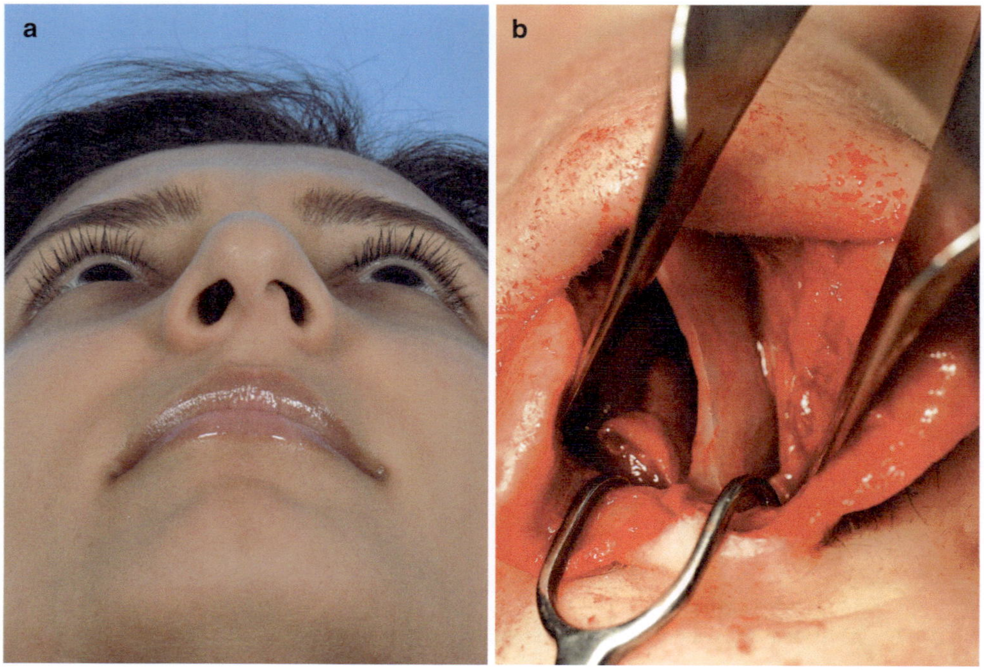

Fig. 18.22 (**a**, **b**) Asymmetrical nostrils stem from caudal septum

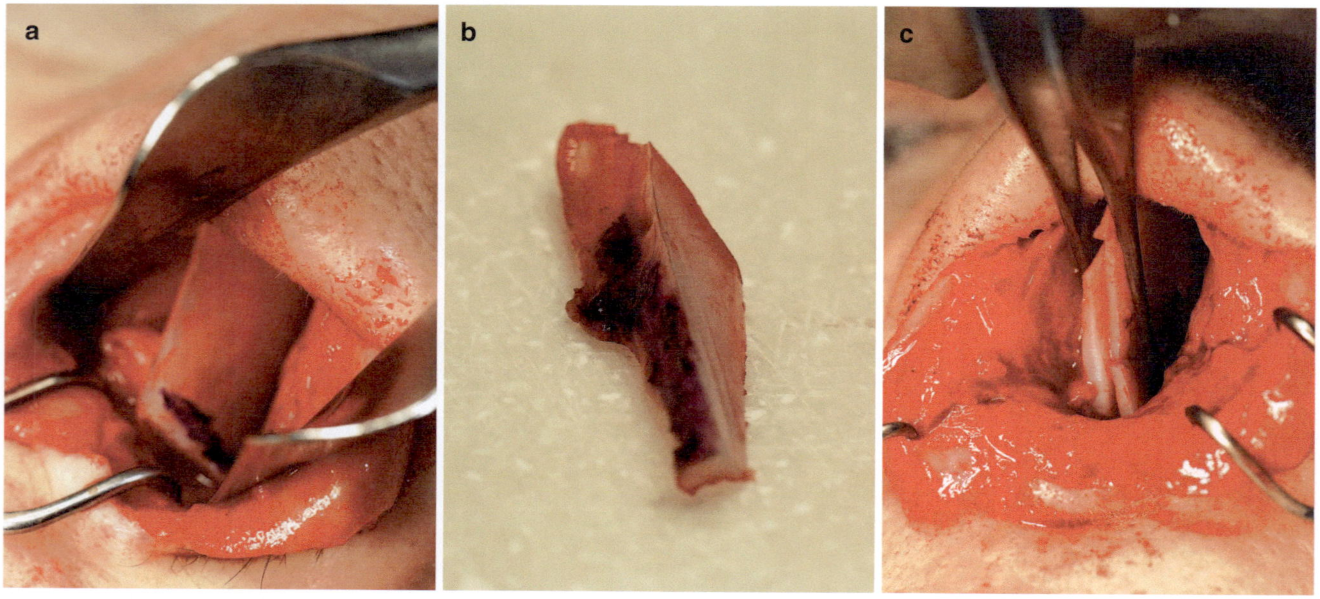

Fig. 18.23 (**a**) Part of the deviated cartilaginous segment is resected. (**b**) Deviated segment. (**c**) The septal batten graft is fixed to the caudal septum remnant to flatten the residual deviation

As one can appreciate from the 8-year postoperative photograph of the patient, the caudal septum would not re-deviate in time, provided that proper techniques are applied to correct the caudal septum (Fig. 18.24).

18.3.3 Case 3

Here is another asymmetrical tip resulting from caudal septal deflection. The basal view is typical in deviated tips caused by twisted caudal septum. In such tip deviations, the basal appearance is typical. The convex portion of the caudal septum averts from one side of the nostrils (Fig. 18.25).

As can be observed in 1-year postoperative images, correcting the caudal septal pathologies provides complete symmetry to the tip (Fig. 18.26).

18.3.4 Case 4

Let us consider another case with a pronounced caudal septal deflection.

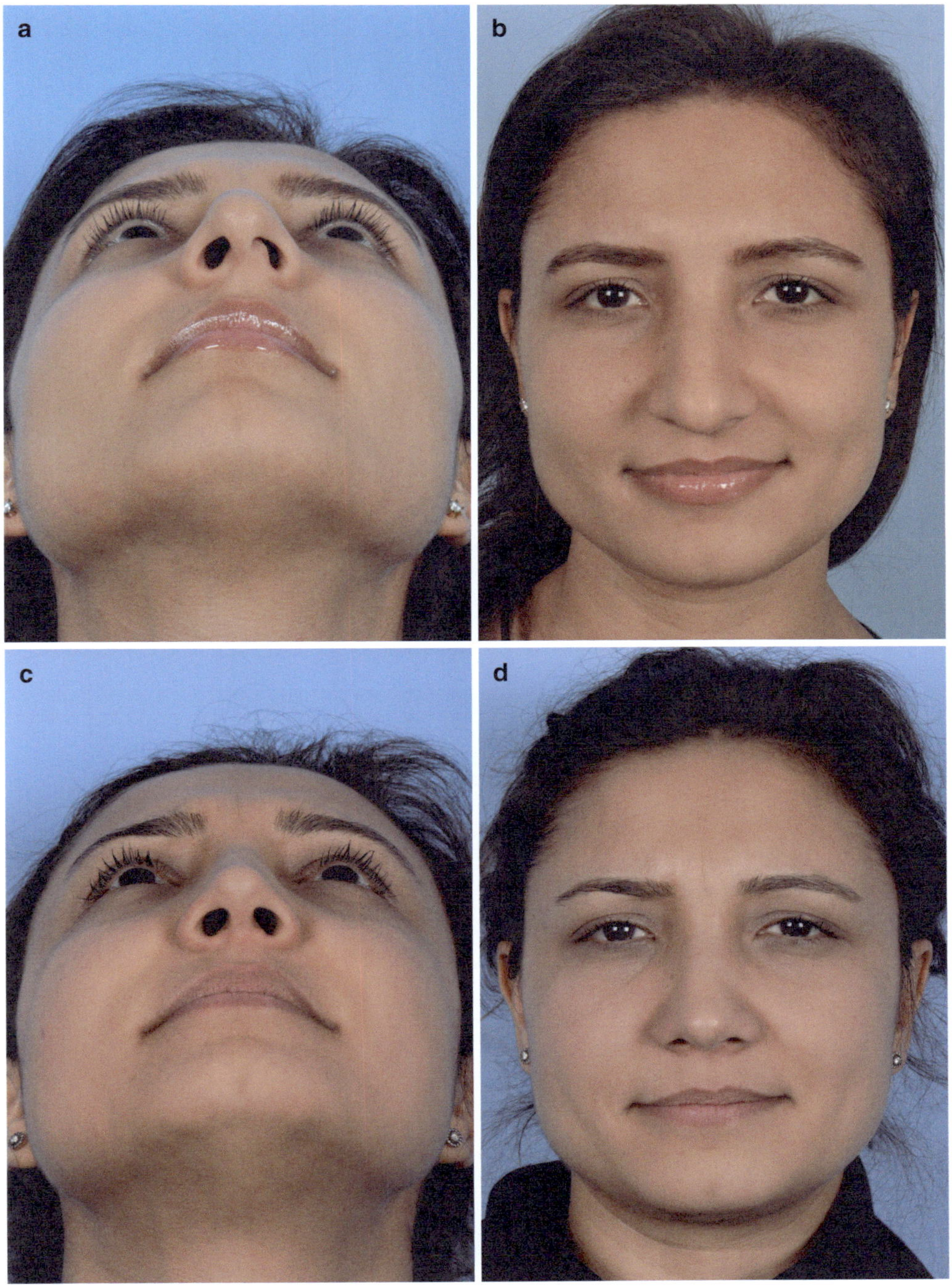

Fig. 18.24 (**a**–**d**) Pre- and postoperative photographs

Prominent tip asymmetry is observed concomitantly with the deviation in the nasal axis. In such cases, achieving a straight septum not only provides tip symmetry but plays a critical role in bringing the entire nose to the midline (Fig. 18.27).

Intraoperative views show a completely deviated dorsum. The deviated caudal septum, in particular, is responsible for the tip asymmetry (Fig. 18.28).

The septum is separated from upper lateral cartilage following dorsal hump resection. Excessive portions are trimmed off leaving an L-strut (Fig. 18.29).

The base of the L-strut is taken to the midline and fixated to the nasal spine by a figure-of-eight suture. Inverted triangles are cut off from the convex segment at the junction of the caudal and the dorsal septum (Fig. 18.30).

A spreader graft is placed at the concave side to correct the convexity at the dorsal septum, whereas a batten graft is used for the caudal septal convexity, taking the septum to the midline (Fig. 18.31).

Preoperative and 2-year postoperative views confirm that symmetry is achieved not only at the nasal base but also in the entire nose (Fig. 18.32).

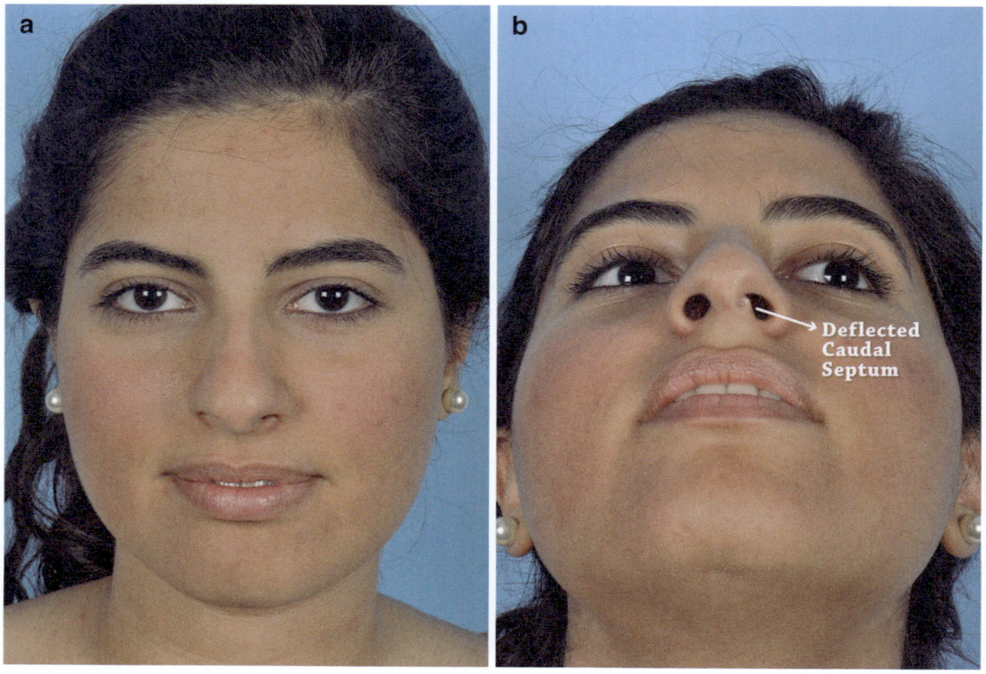

Fig. 18.25 (**a**, **b**) Preoperative views: deviated caudal septum push the tip side. (Supplementary Video 18.5)

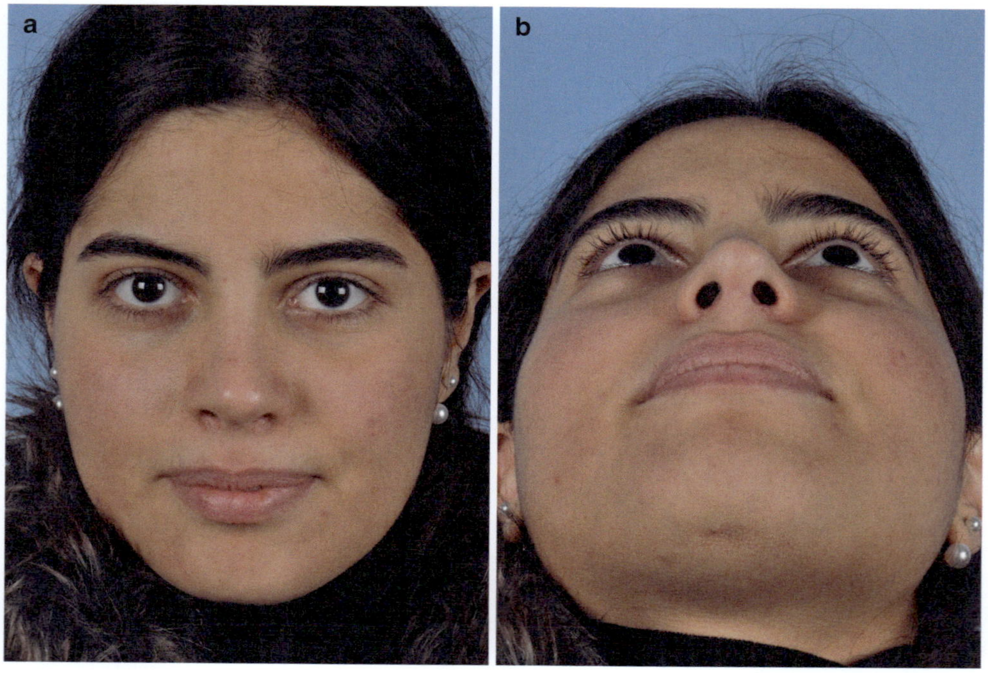

Fig. 18.26 (**a**, **b**) Postoperative views: identifying and addressing the deviated caudal septum was the key to this case. Correcting the caudal septum with a septal batten graft allowed for tip symmetry without violating the integrity of the alar cartilages

Caudal septal deviation may be so advanced that none of the above maneuvers would suffice to correct the problem. In this case, subtotal septal reconstruction may be necessary, as discussed earlier in this chapter.

18.3.5 Case 5

Pay attention to the preoperative profile view and the intra-operative caudal view of the patient shown in this figure. The caudal septum is so twisted that it bends completely to one side. One would expect a more prominent tip asymmetry in such a deeply deviated caudal septum. As explained at the beginning of the chapter, other problems of the tip may become more pronounced than the asymmetry because of the problems of the caudal septum. In this case, the wide tip masks the tip asymmetry (Fig. 18.33).

First, the cartilaginous septum is resected at the mid-segment, followed by complete resection and removal of the L-strut, leaving a straight remnant behind (Fig. 18.34).

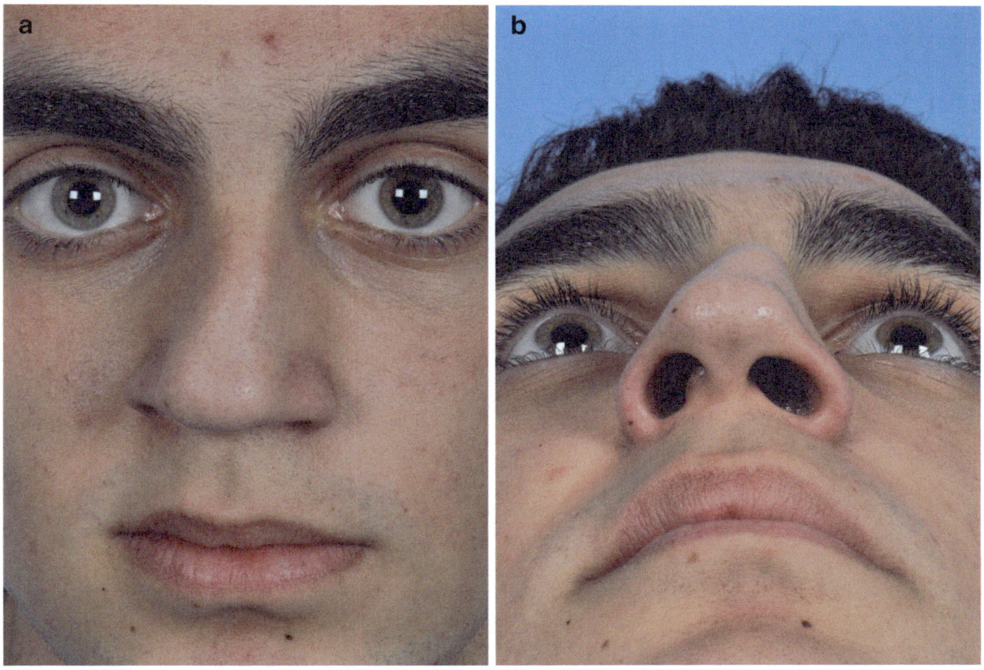

Fig. 18.27 (**a**, **b**) Caudal and dorsal septal deviation resulting in asymmetry of the nasal tip

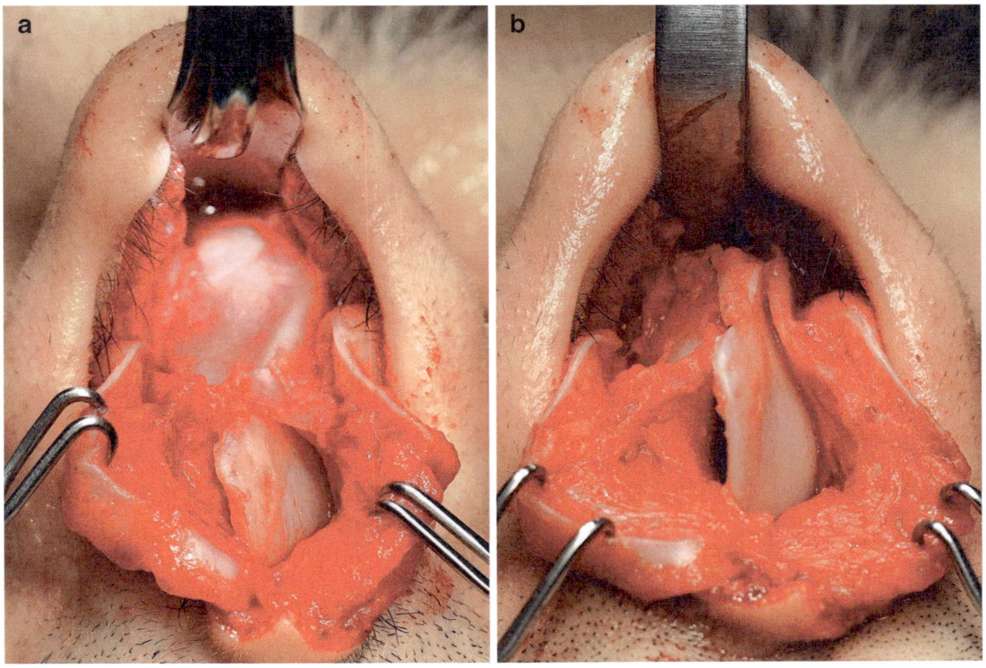

Fig. 18.28 (**a**) Deviated middle vault. (**b**) The septum is divided from upper lateral crus. (Supplementary Video 18.6)

A graft is prepared extracorporeally to fill in the septal gap. The prepared septal replacement graft is sutured to the nasal spine and the remnant septum inside the nose (Fig. 18.35).

Preoperative and 2-year postoperative photographs show that the subtotal septal reconstruction has brought the caudal septum to the midline, solving the problem of tip asymmetry. Only a standard tip suture is applied for alar cartilage (Fig. 18.36).

If the tip asymmetry persists after solving the caudal septal problems, it may be due to asymmetry in alar cartilage. In the presence of alar arch asymmetries, the first option to try should be transdomal mattress suture, columellar strut, and lateral crural graft.

18.3.6 Case 6

In this example, the basal view in particular shows the columella slightly collapsed to the right side. The left dome is slightly higher than the right. The frontal view shows the

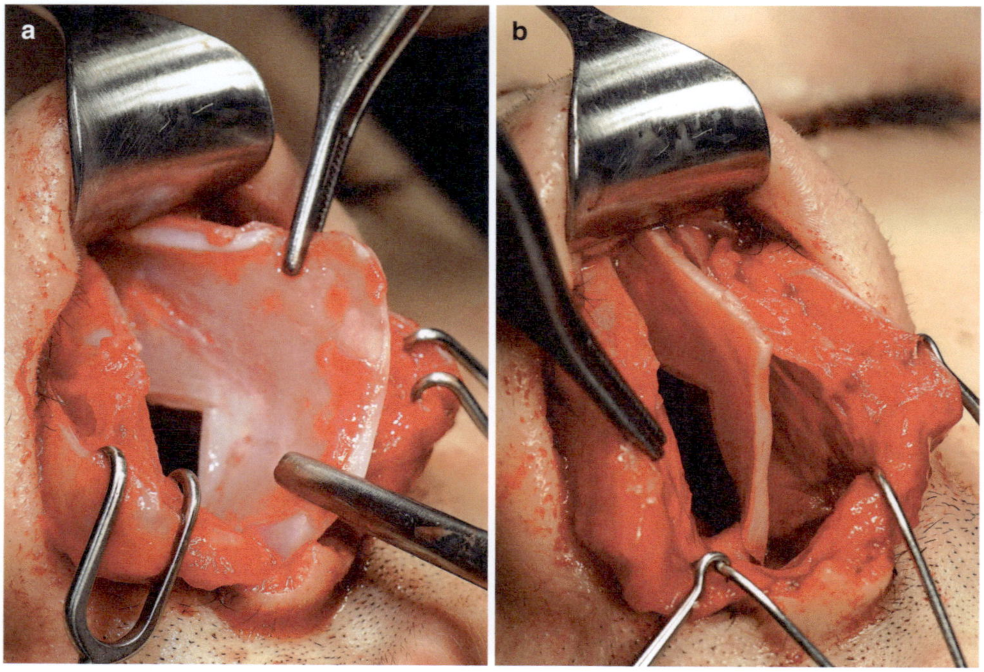
Fig. 18.29 (**a**, **b**) Septoplasty with L-strut

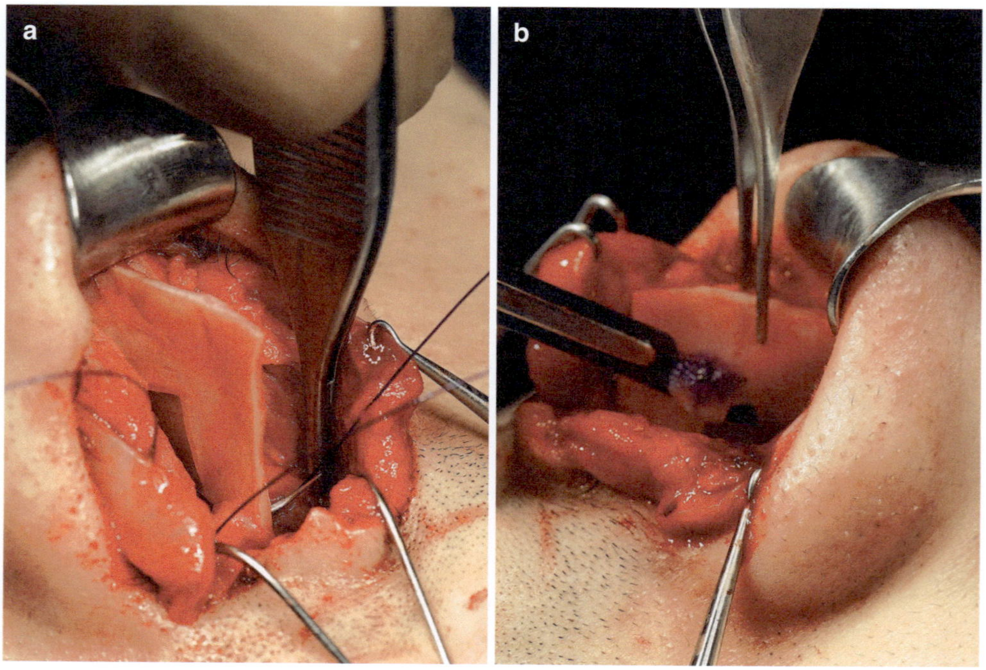
Fig. 18.30 (**a**, **b**) The shaded section shows the convexity from which the inverted triangles are removed

mild asymmetry of the columella and the light reflex at the left dome presenting vaguely higher (Fig. 18.37).

The intraoperative views, on the other hand, reveal a notable asymmetry in the crura, columella, and dome points (Fig. 18.38).

A transdomal suture serves to achieve symmetrical dome points, while the columellar strut helps correct the middle/medial configuration deformity. The lateral crural graft, on the other hand, improves the configuration of the lateral crura, contributing to a symmetrical alar arch. The surgery is finished with a dome-equalizing suture, which has many advantages including improvement of symmetry. The lateral crural graft is placed as an underlay. A cap graft is used for definition (Fig. 18.39).

Preoperative and 1-year postoperative views show well-established tip symmetry (Fig. 18.40).

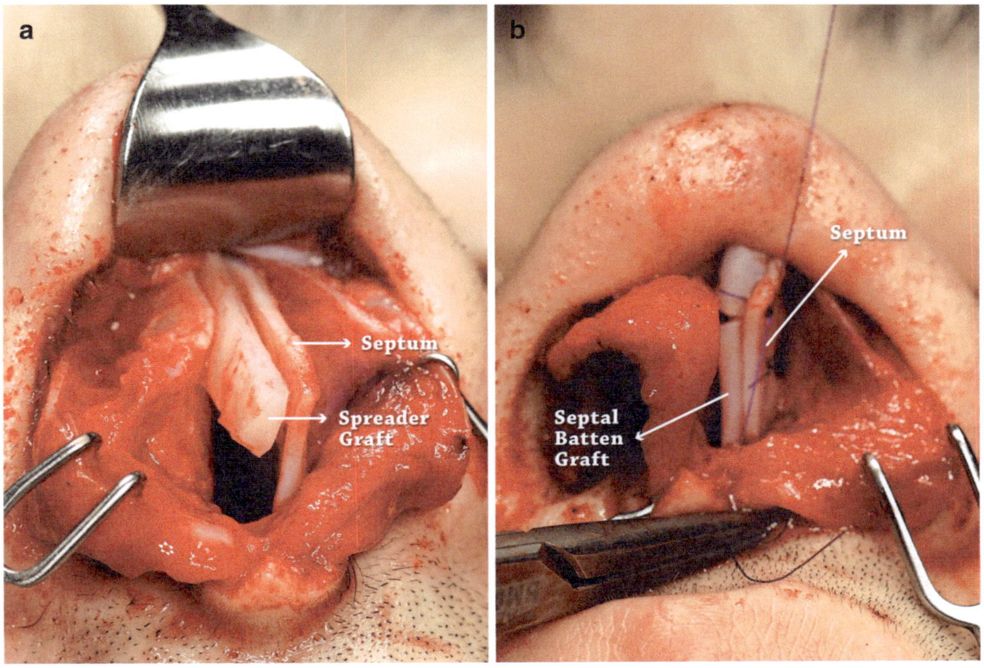

Fig. 18.31 (**a**) Spreader graft placement for dorsal segment of L-strut. (**b**) Septal batten graft placement for flattening the caudal part of L-strut

18.3.7 Case 7

Here is another example for the alar asymmetry.

This patient, who underwent rhinoplasty 10 years ago, mainly complains of tip asymmetry. As noted on the profile and base views, the domes emerge at totally different levels. Both asymmetry and concavity are remarkable on the lateral nasal wall (Fig. 18.41).

Intraoperative views display deflection in the caudal segment, as well as asymmetry in the alar arch. The right lateral crus, in particular, is deformed (Fig. 18.42).

To correct the deviation in the caudal septum, the dorsal septum is first brought to the midline by a spreader graft, followed by a septal batten graft to correct the deflection in the caudal septum. The transdomal mattress suture is used to align the domes. A septal onlay lateral crural graft is used to correct the deformity in the right lateral crus. A cap graft is used to improve projection and to equalize the dome points. Because this is a thin-skinned patient, the cap graft is camouflaged (Fig. 18.43).

Although overall symmetry is achieved postoperatively, minor asymmetry persists in the nostrils in the basal view (Fig. 18.44).

When the alar arch is too asymmetrical to be corrected with sutures and/or grafts, other techniques such as resection or overlapping must be considered. Case 8 is a good example.

18.3.8 Case 8

In this case, the first step is to determine the asymmetrical segment. The columellar strut provides symmetry in the middle/medial crus. The problem emerges from the lateral crura. Asymmetrical lateral crural resection provides symmetry to the tip (Fig. 18.45).

Because this is a thick-skinned patient, lateral crural underlay grafts are used bilaterally to reinforce the nasal wall. The excess portion of the medial crus is trimmed off. Definition and final projection are achieved by cap graft (Fig. 18.46).

Figure 18.47 shows tip symmetry at 1-year follow-up. Lateral crural resection both contributes to the tip asymmetry and narrows the tip.

Vertical alar resection is inevitable in secondary cases with severe asymmetry in the alar arch.

18.3.9 Case 9

A pronounced tip asymmetry is noted in this patient, who underwent rhinoplasty 10 years ago. The goal must be to achieve a straight septum first, followed by symmetry in the alar cartilages. Spreader and septal batten grafts are used to reposition the caudal septum in the midline. Alar arch symmetry is restored by alar cartilage resection (Fig. 18.48).

Alar arch asymmetry is restored using vertical alar resection, a columellar strut, bilateral lateral crural graft, and a cap graft (Fig. 18.49).

As the postoperative view at 1-year follow-up shows, vertical alar resection has been a simultaneous solution to both tip asymmetry and over-projection (Fig. 18.50).

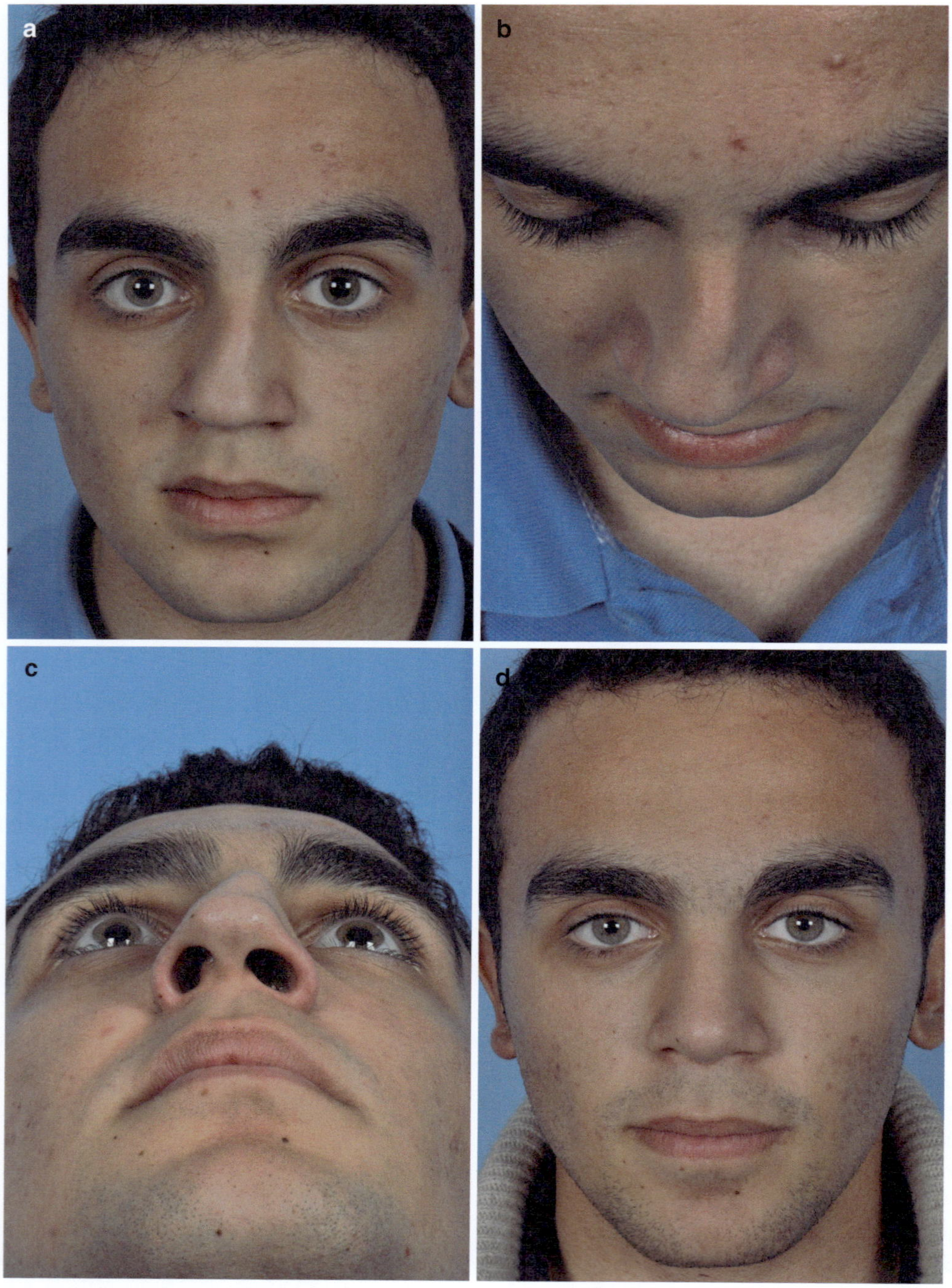

Fig. 18.32 (**a–c**) Deviated dorsal and caudal septum also cause tip asymmetry. (**d–f**) Correcting the septum allowed tip symmetry without violating the integrity of the alar cartilages

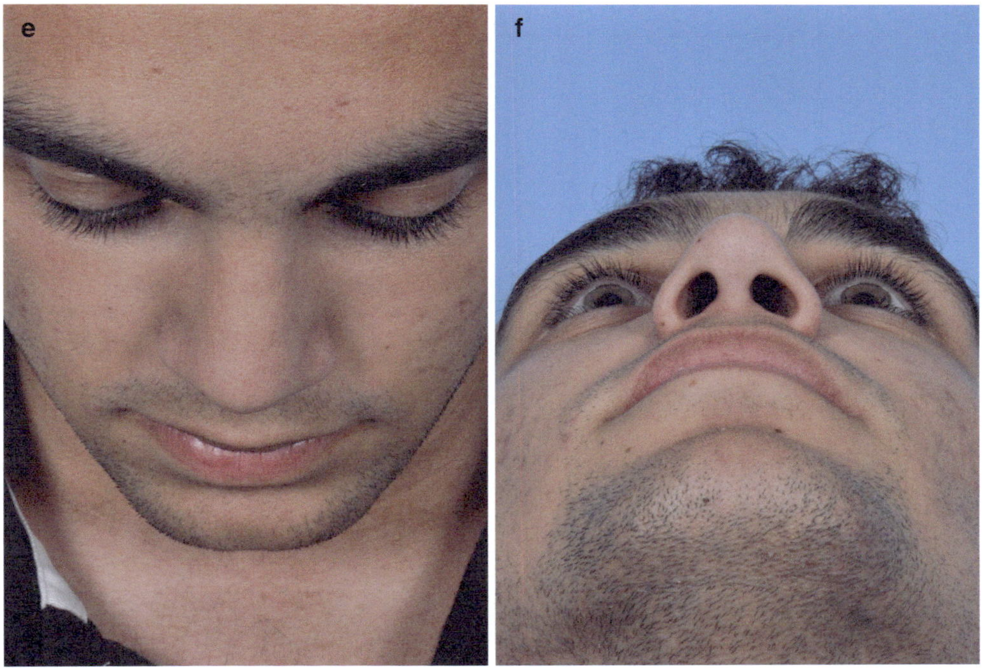

Fig. 18.32 (continued)

Fig. 18.33 (**a**, **b**) Severe buckling of the septum to the right results in a corresponding deviation in the nasal tip

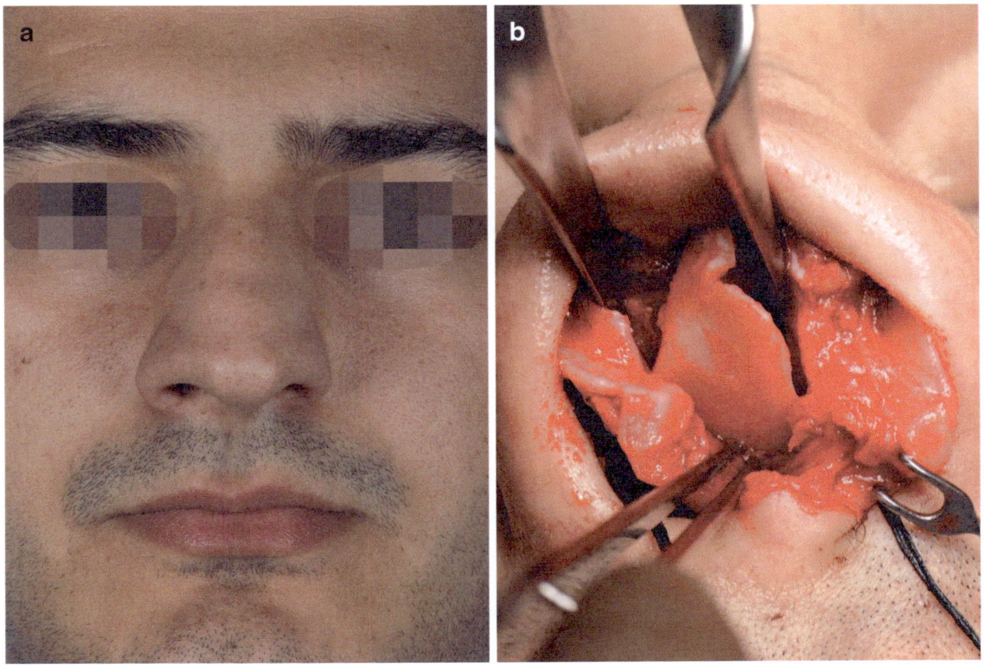

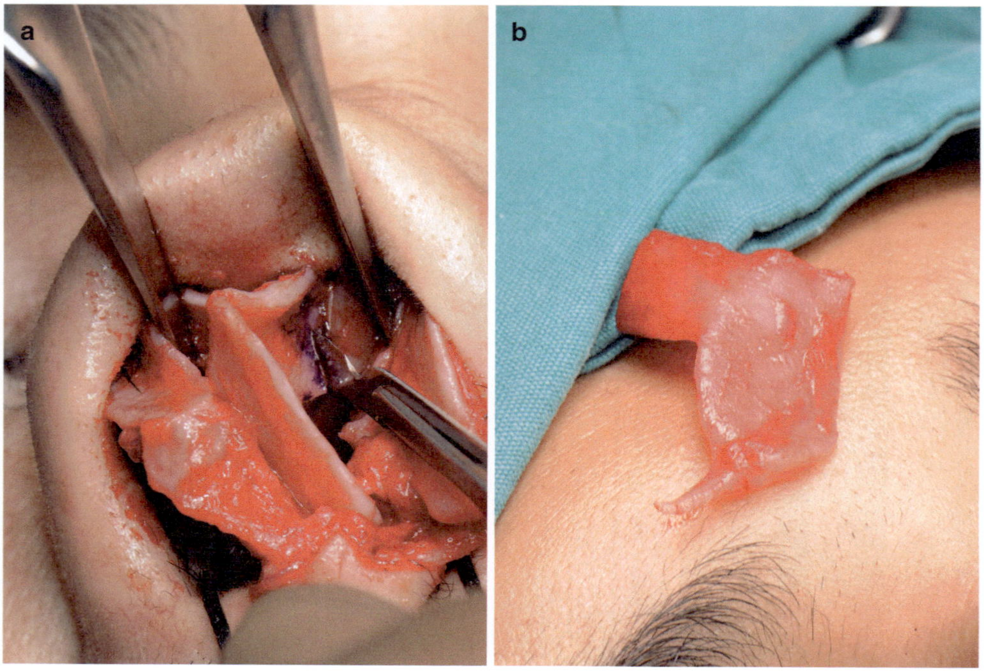

Fig. 18.34 (**a**, **b**) Deviated septum removed

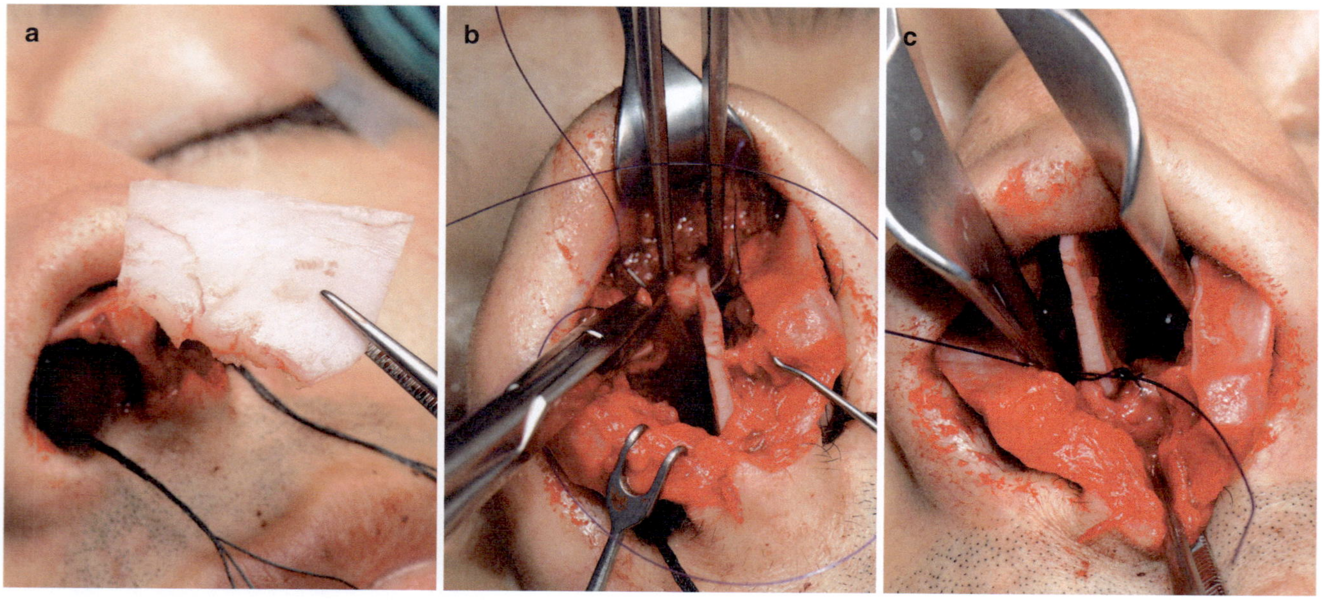

Fig. 18.35 (**a**) Caudal replacement graft harvested from septum. (**b**) Caudal replacement graft in place and sutured to the septal remnant. (**c**) The caudal septal replacement graft is stabilized to the spine with 4-0 PDS sutures

18.3.10 Case 10

Let's have a closer look at another asymmetrical tip case.

The preoperative profile view and intraoperative views demonstrate that the asymmetry emerges from the lateral crura (Fig. 18.51).

Equalized with the help of forceps, the columella points to the origin of the problem as the lateral crura (Fig. 18.52).

Resecting the asymmetrical segments of the lateral crus restores tip symmetry and refines the wide tip resulting from hypertrophy of the crus (Fig. 18.53).

Tip grafts must be used in thick-skinned patients. A shield graft was used for this purpose in this patient. A shield graft helps the surgeon regain projection lost in resection and contributes to tip definition. A lateral crural graft, on the other hand, is used to reestablish alar rim symmetry (Fig. 18.54).

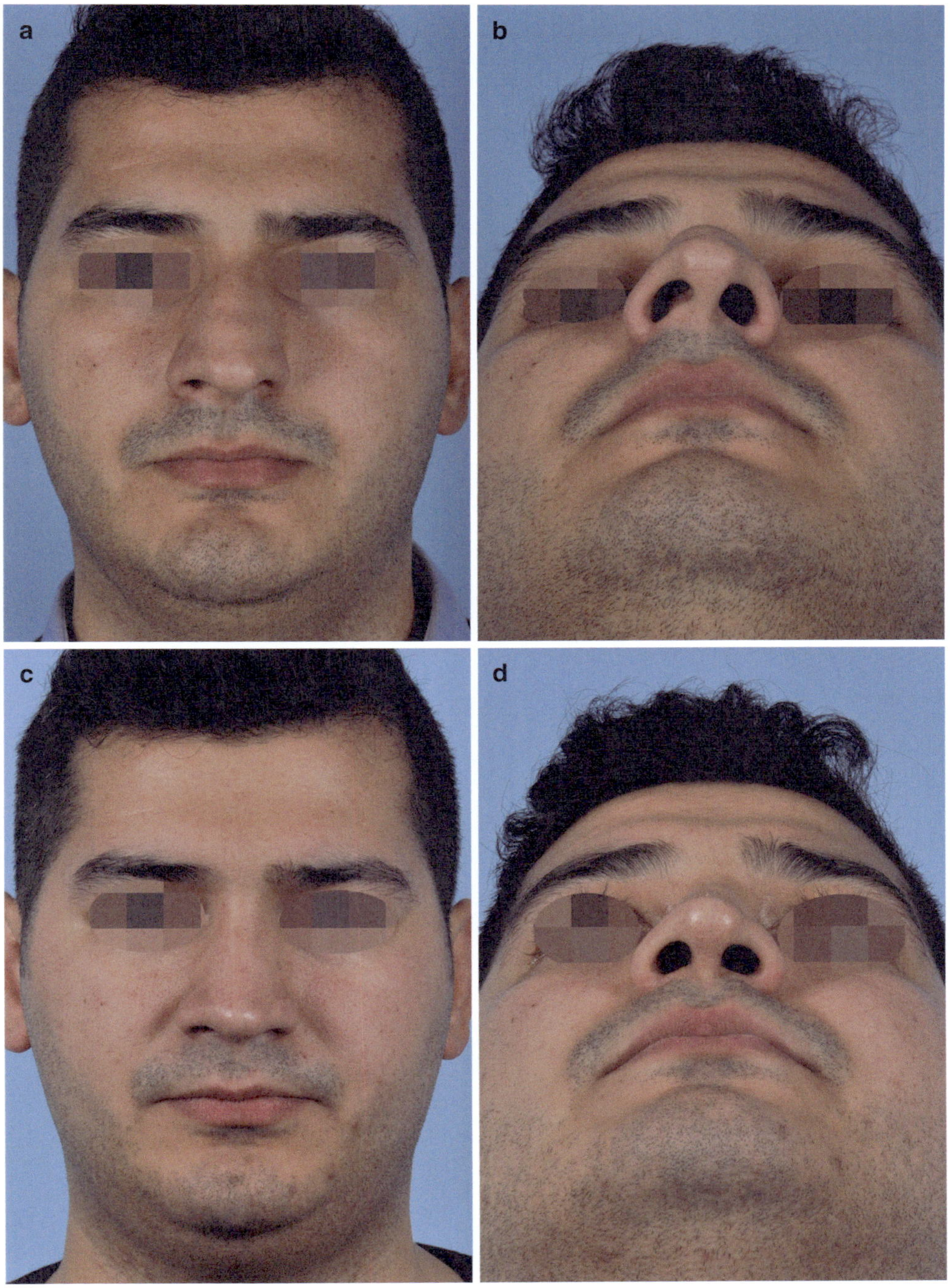

Fig. 18.36 (**a–d**) Correcting the middle vault and caudal septum allowed tip symmetry without violating the integrity of the alar cartilages

In an asymmetrical tip, there may frequently be a need for a unilateral or bilateral alar base reduction. Left nostril resection was performed in this patient to restore symmetry (Fig. 18.55).

A unilateral spreader graft is placed to the left side for dorsal symmetry. Preoperative and postoperative views confirm successful achievement of tip symmetry (Fig. 18.56).

18.3.11 Case 11

When used for the correct indication, lateral crural resection in tip asymmetries resulting from the lateral crus produces satisfactory long-term results.

The photos in Fig. 18.57 are postoperative views of the patient at 2-year follow-up after resection of the lateral crura.

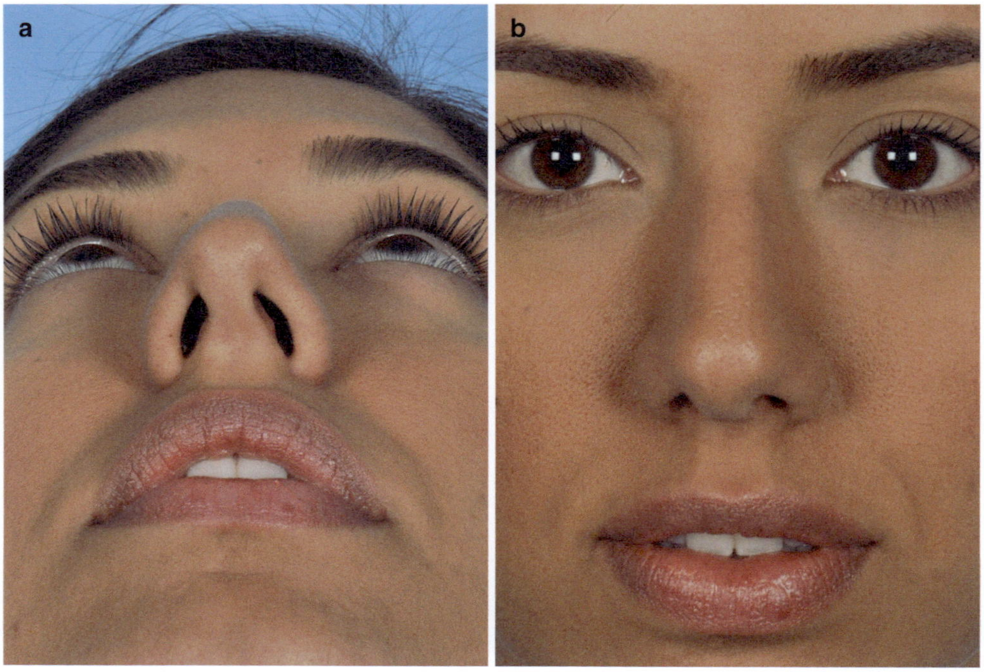

Fig. 18.37 (**a**) Preoperative base view. (**b**) Preoperative frontal view

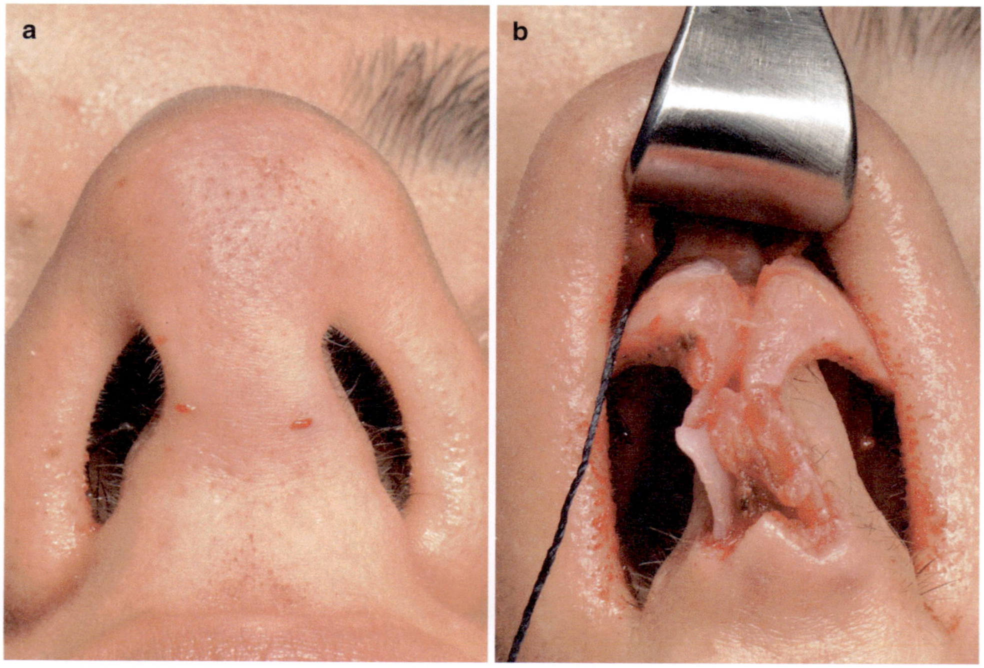

Fig. 18.38 (**a**, **b**) Intraoperative view of asymmetry

When the middle/medial crura are too asymmetrical to be corrected by columellar strut, it would be appropriate to use the medial crural overlap technique. Case 12 is a typical example.

18.3.12 Case 12

As noted on the base view, the tip appears deviated on one side. The photographs from three different perspectives show symmetry in the lateral crura of alar cartilage, whereas severe asymmetry is noted in middle/medial crura (Fig. 18.58).

Symmetrical dome points are first created with a transdomal suture. Achieving symmetry at the dome points restored symmetry in the lateral crura, piling up all of the symmetry to the limb of the alar cartilages (Fig. 18.59).

Cartilaginous division is performed to relieve the tension on the limb of the alar arch and to reinstate symmetry. Of the two emerging stumps, the upper one is elevated from the skin sliding over the distal stump until symmetry is restored (Fig. 18.60).

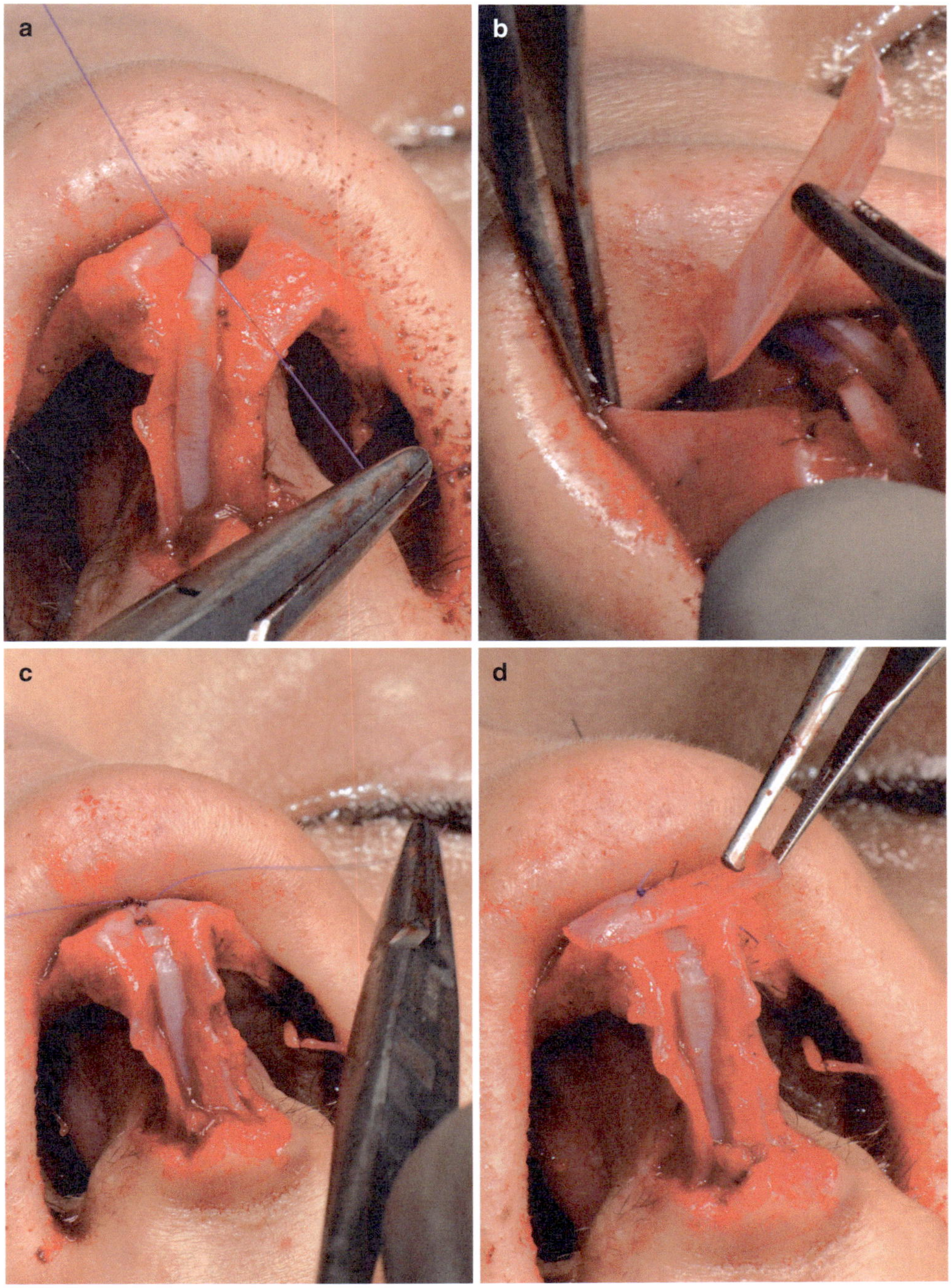

Fig. 18.39 (**a**) Transdomal mattress suture. (**b**) Underlay lateral crural graft placement. (**c**) Dome-equalizing suture. (**d**) Cap graft placement

Symmetry is restored in alar cartilages after the overlap. After overlap, a columellar strut cup graft and lateral crural graft were used to provide stability, projection, and shape of the tip (Fig. 18.61).

Preoperative and 6-month postoperative results are shown in Fig. 18.62.

18.3.13 Case 13

This case is also a good example of asymmetry originating from the medial crus.

Preoperative photos pinpointed asymmetry in the paired medial crura, deflecting the tip in one direction. The tip is repositioned in the midline as soon as the asymmetry in the medial crura is corrected by the overlap technique (Fig. 18.63).

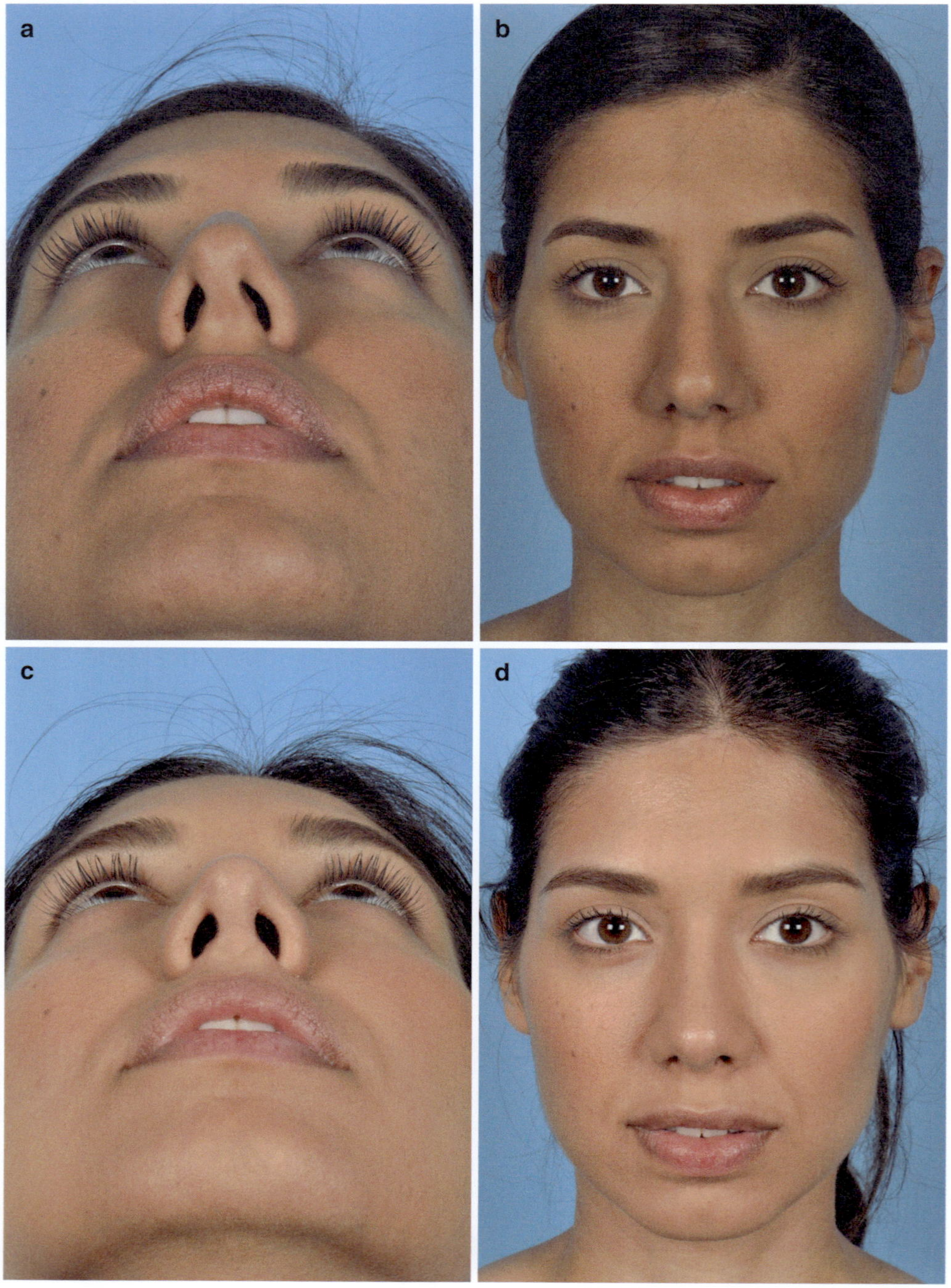

Fig. 18.40 (**a–d**) Mild degree of tip asymmetry fixed with transdomal suture, columellar strut, lateral crucial graft, and cap graft

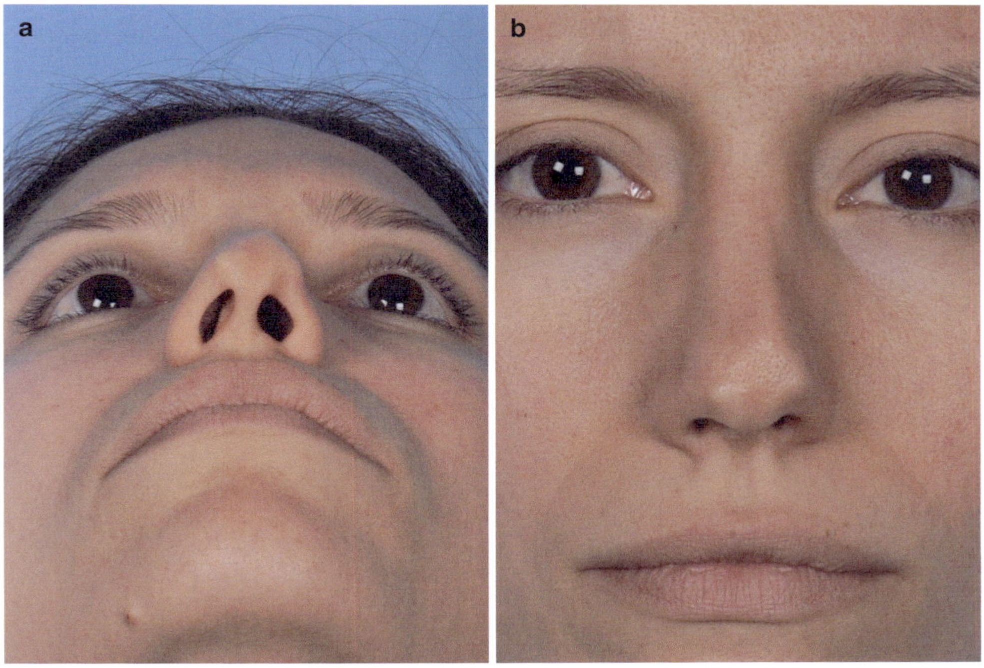

Fig. 18.41 (**a**, **b**) Overexcised alar cartilages resulting in a collapsed, retracted, and asymmetrical tip

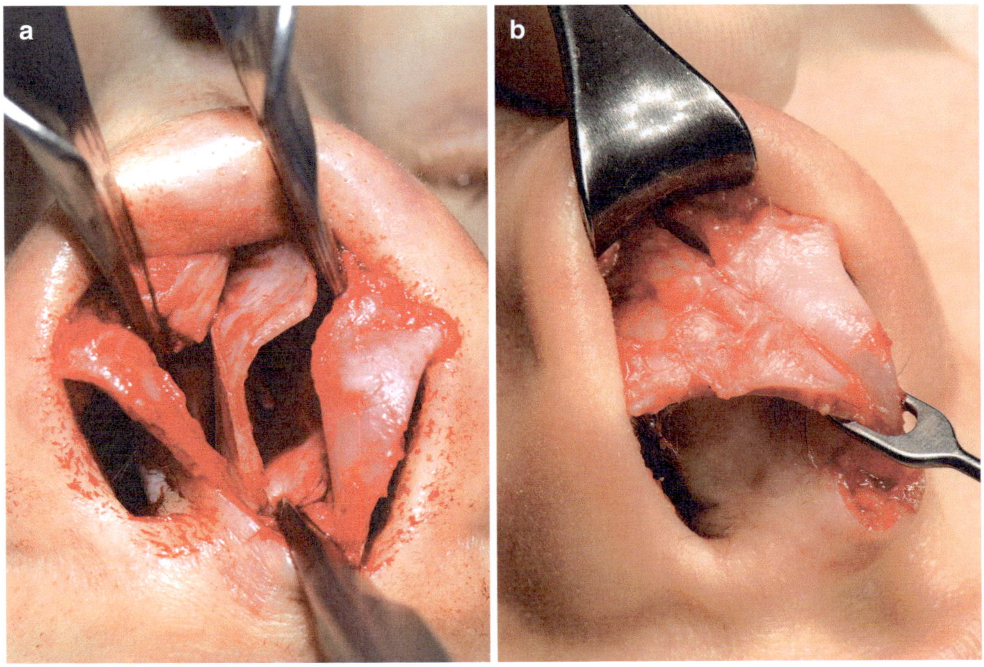

Fig. 18.42 (**a**) The caudal septum is deflected but intact despite previous surgery. (**b**) Deformed lateral crura

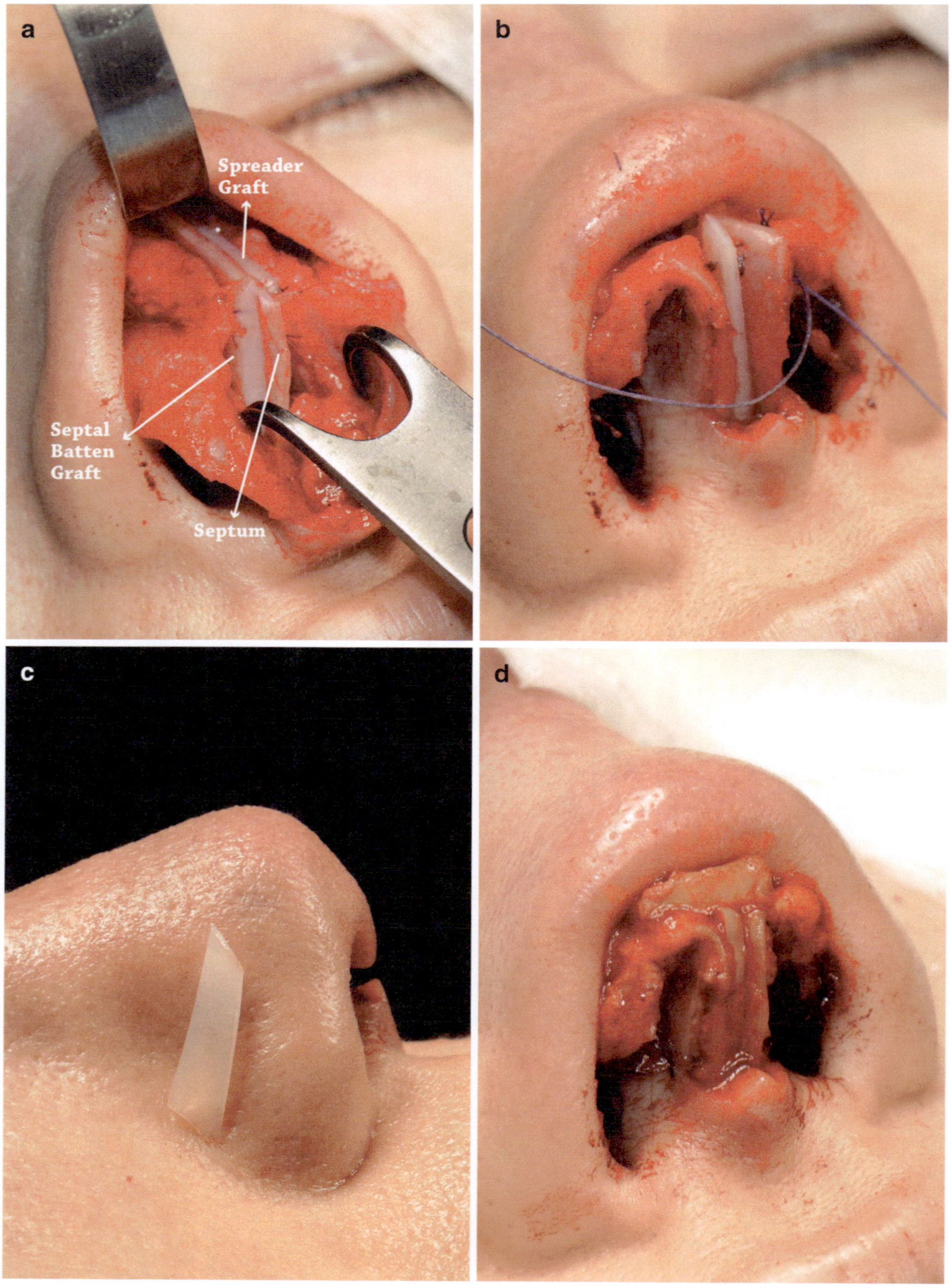

Fig. 18.43 (**a**) Unilateral spreader and septal batten were placed. (**b**) Columellar strut. (**c**) Lateral crural graft was used to restore the lateral crus (**d**) cap graft

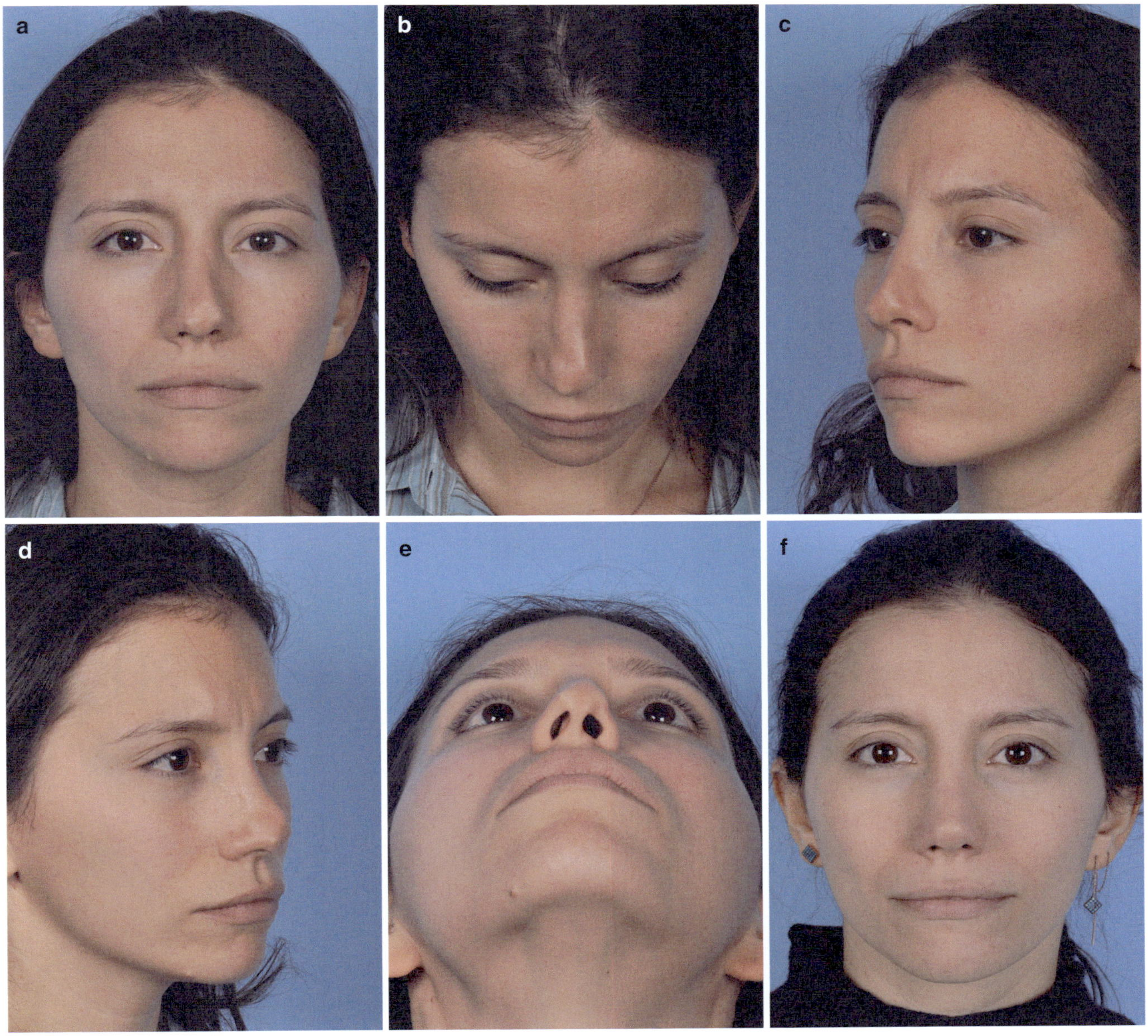

Fig. 18.44 (a–j) Before and after pictures

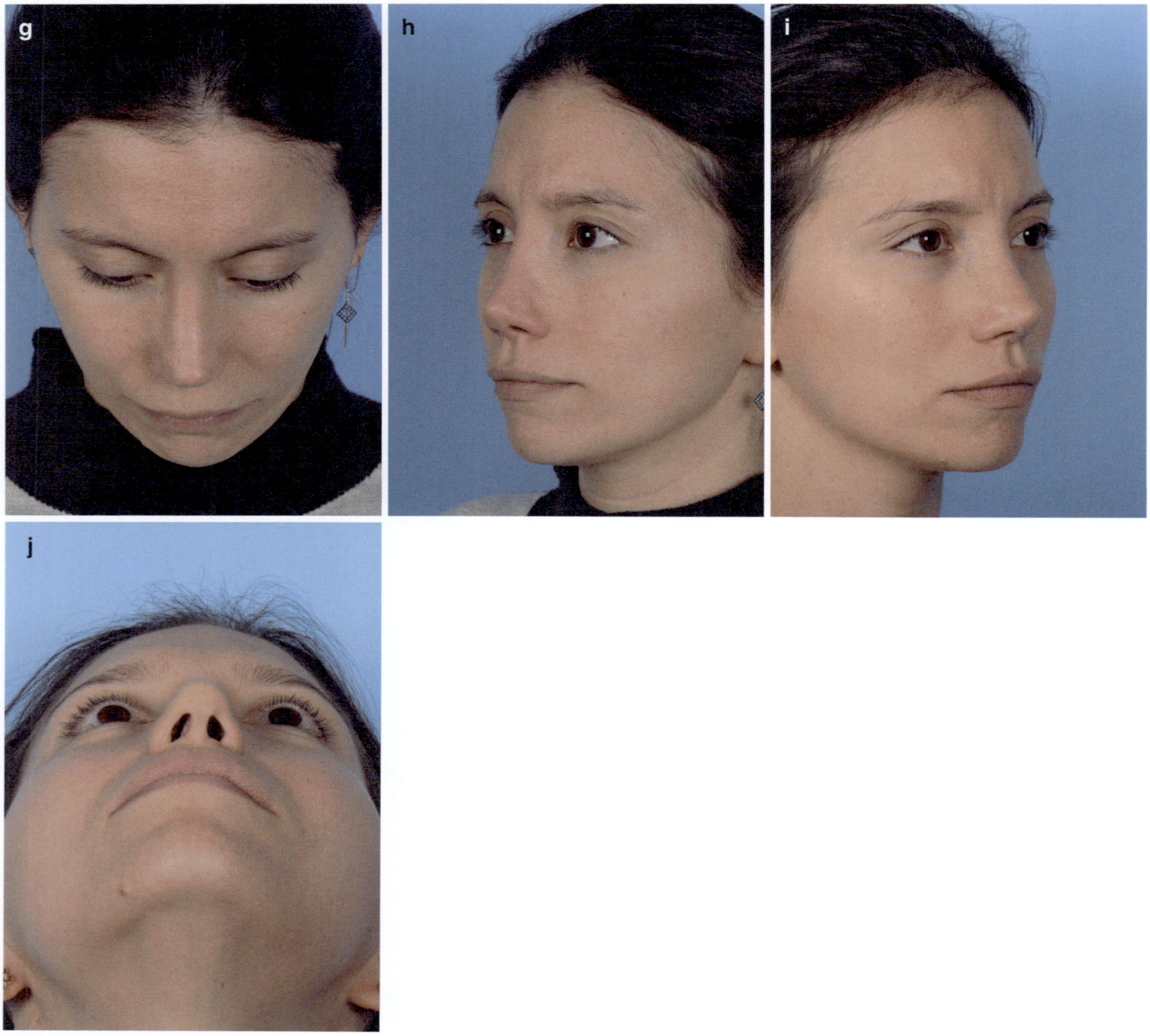

Fig. 18.44 (continued)

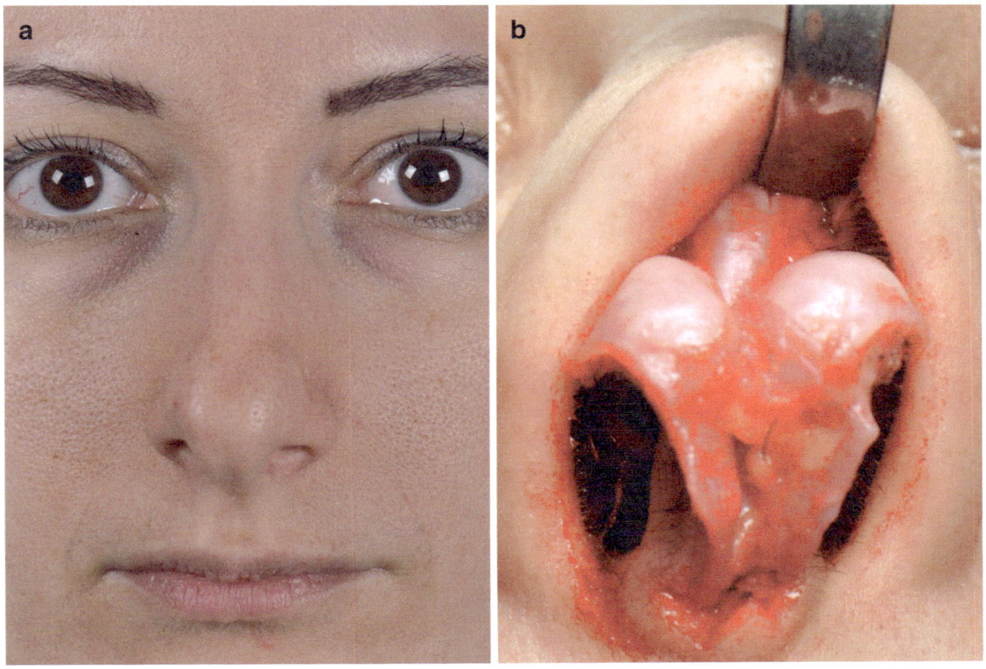

Fig. 18.45 (**a**, **b**) Asymmetrical nasal tip due to asymmetrical lateral crura

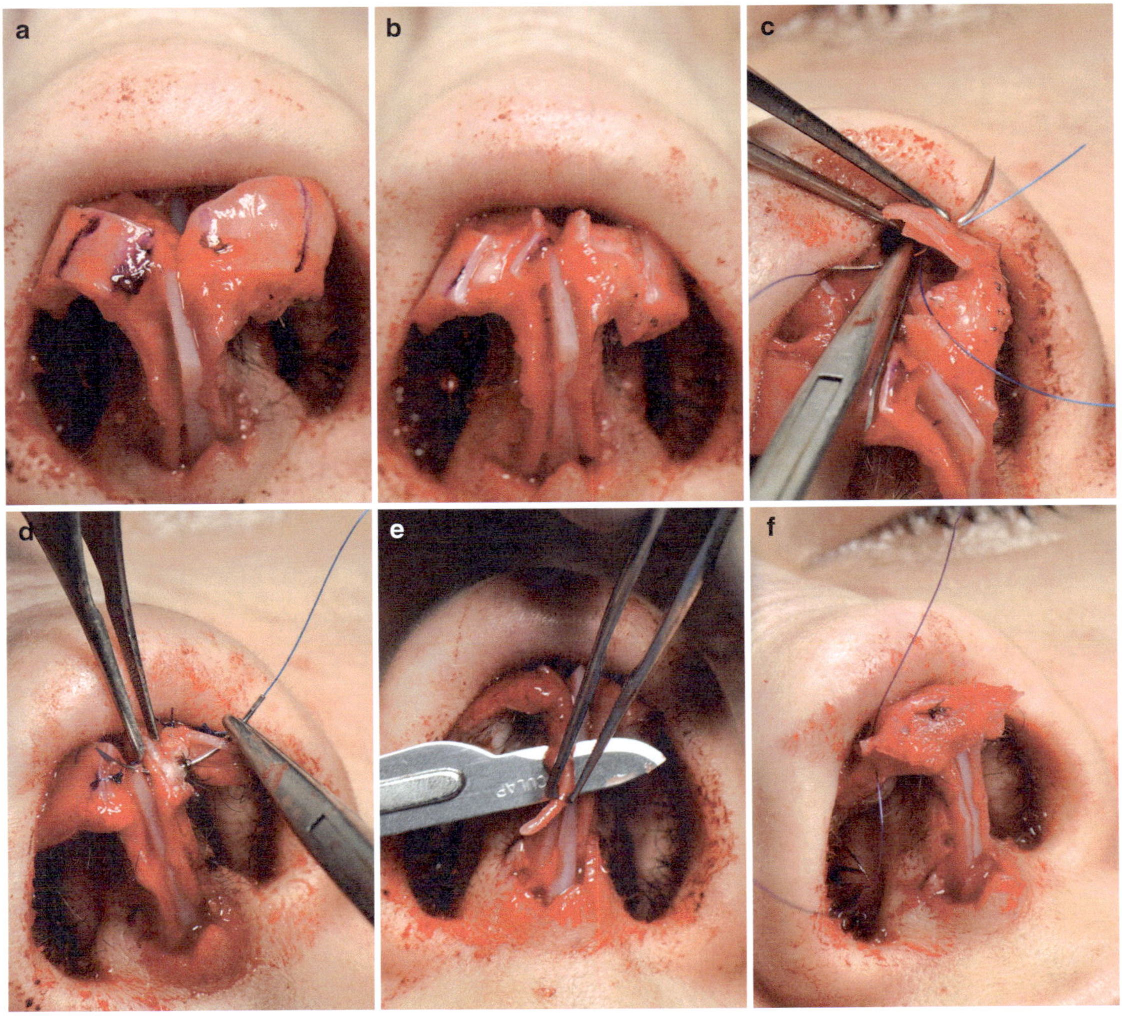

Fig. 18.46 (**a–f**) Domes divided and repaired for symmetry and then sutured up to the tip graft for support and definition

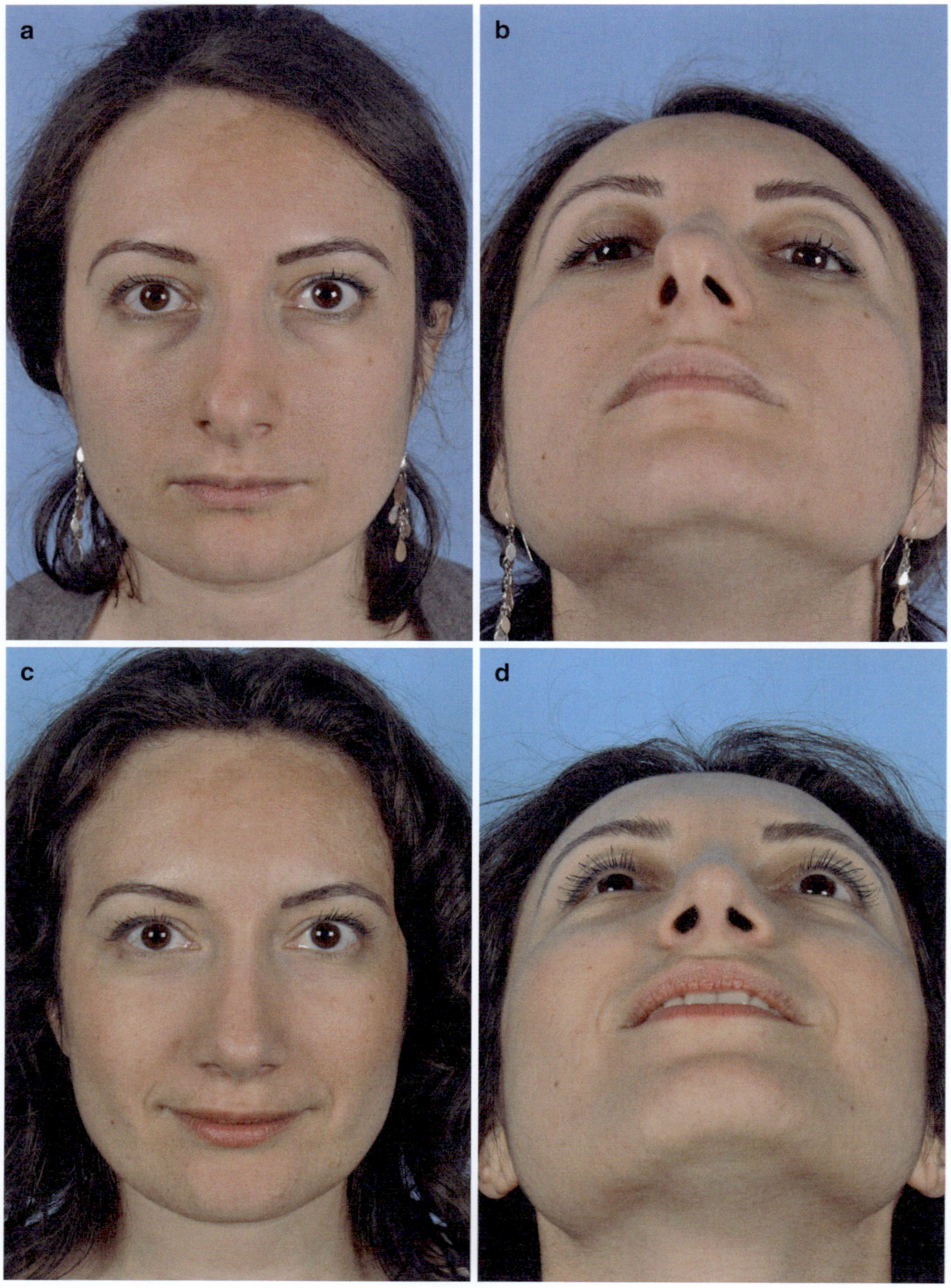

Fig. 18.47 (**a**, **b**) This 28-year-old woman had severe tip asymmetry. She underwent different extents of lateral crural resection to correct the length discrepancy of the lower lateral cartilages. (**c**, **d**) At 2 years postoperatively, the nasal tip is symmetrical and positioned in the midline

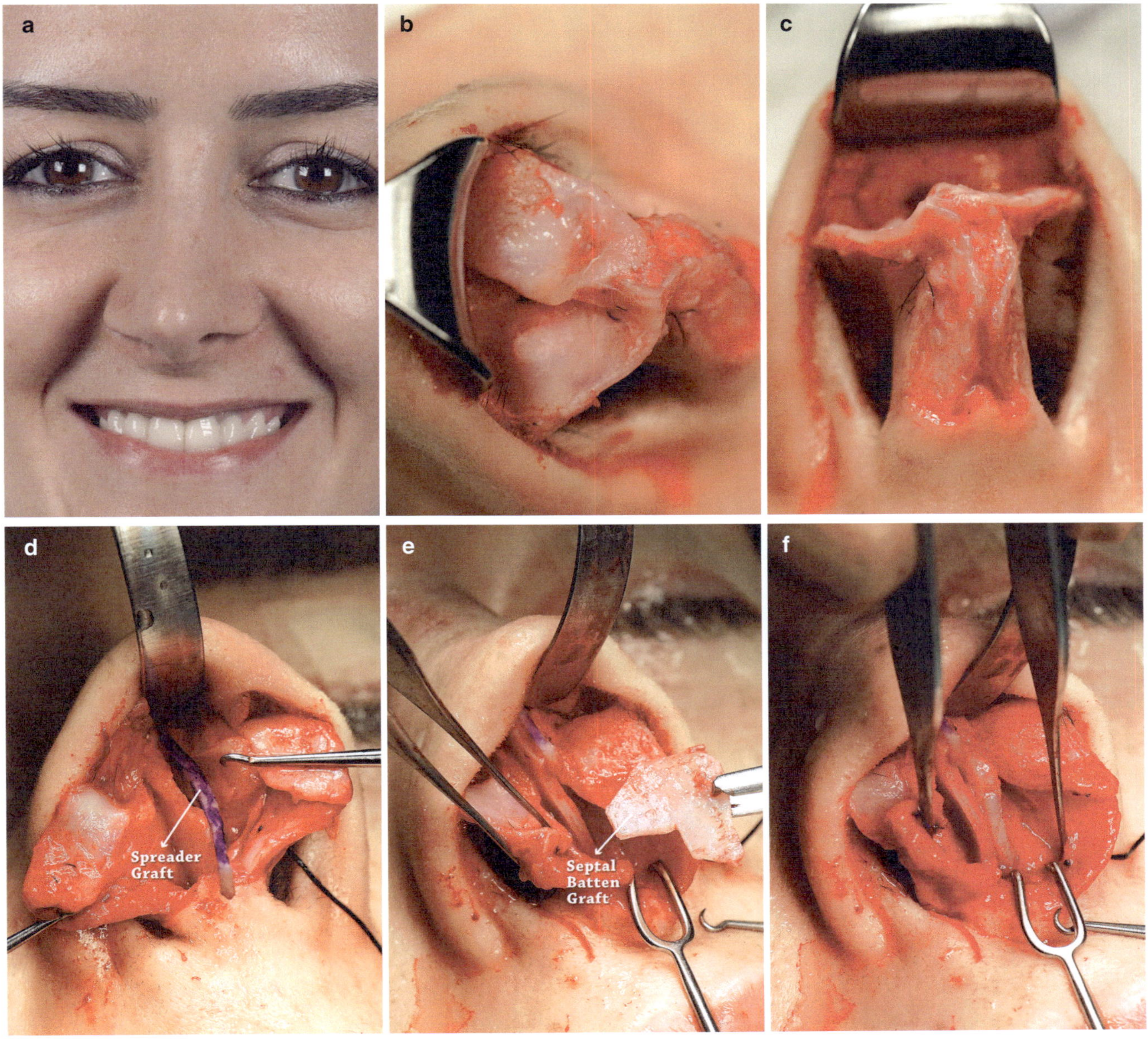

Fig. 18.48 (**a**) Multiple asymmetries and contour irregularities are evident. (**b–f**) Distorted, deformed, and asymmetrical alar cartilages. (Supplementary Video 18.7)

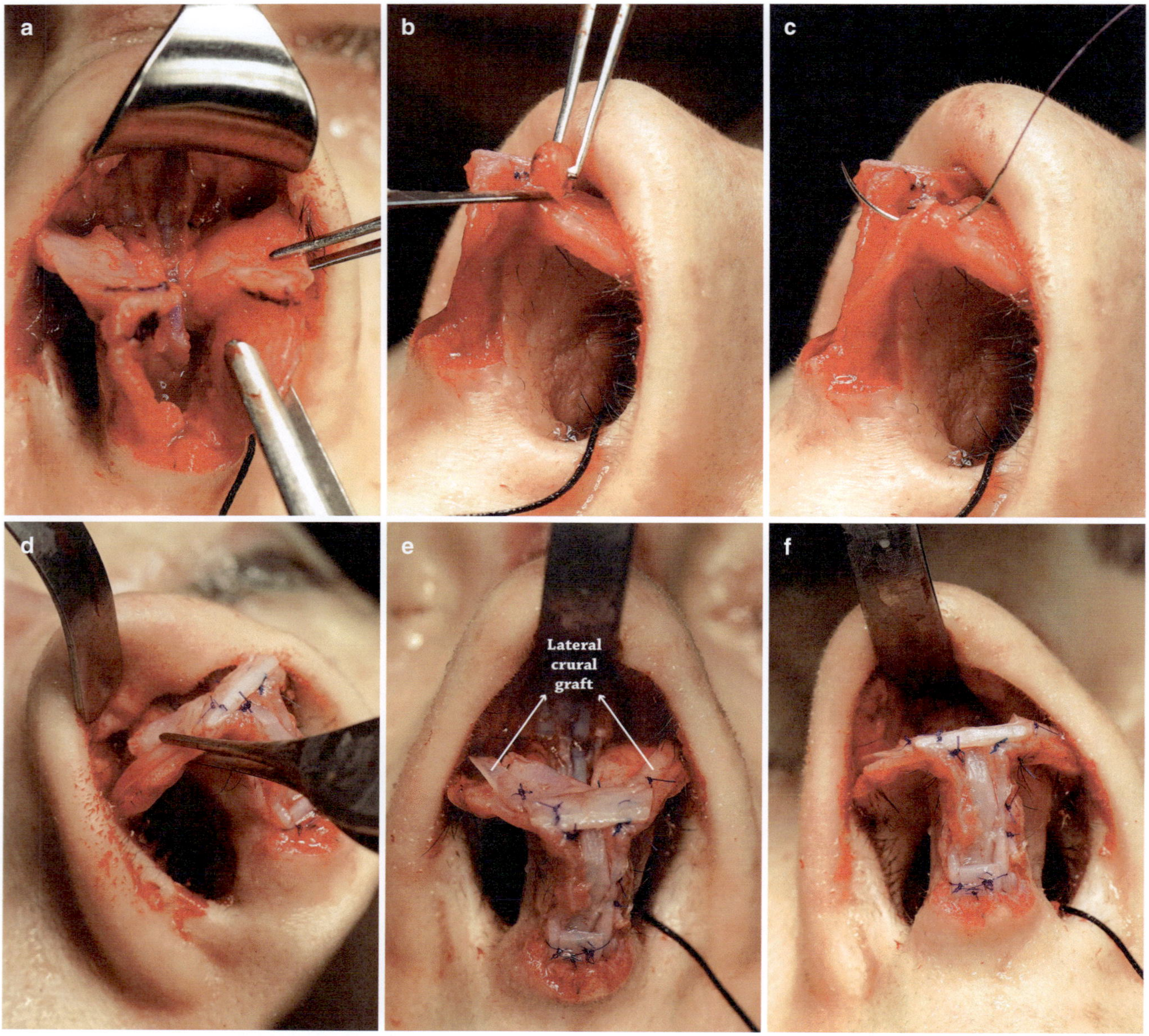

Fig. 18.49 (**a**, **b**) Distorted domes amputated. (**c**) Suture repair of the domes. (**d**) Cap graft placed for tip shape and definition. (**e**) Lateral crural graft to straighten and support lateral crus. (**f**) Appearance of the alar cartilages at the conclusion of the case

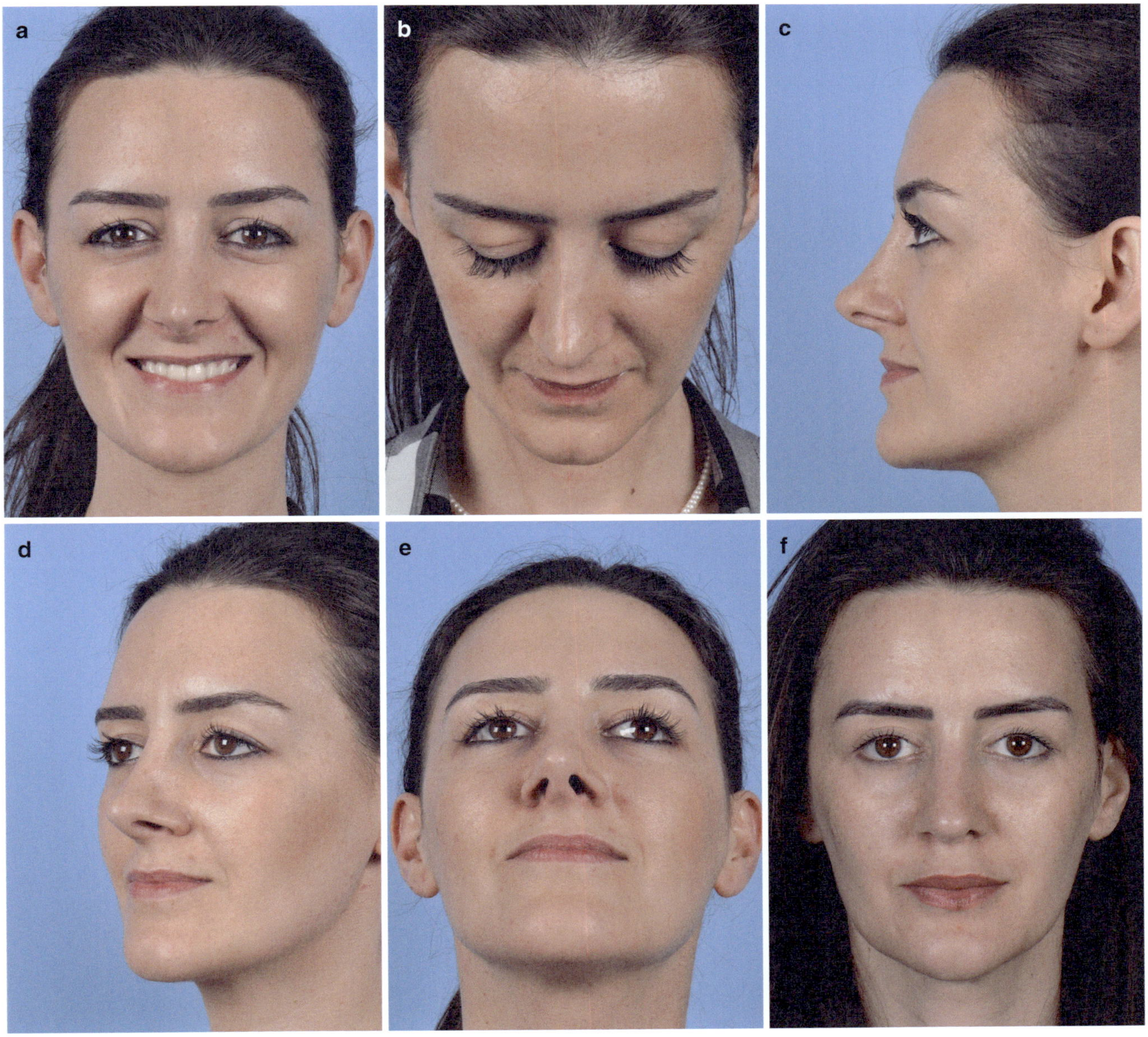

Fig. 18.50 (**a**–**e**) Preoperative photographs. The tip is also asymmetrical, overprotected, and slightly over-rotated. (**f**–**j**) Postoperative photographs: the tip is symmetrical and more softer. The tip projection is more proportional. Improved upper lip position and nasolabial angle

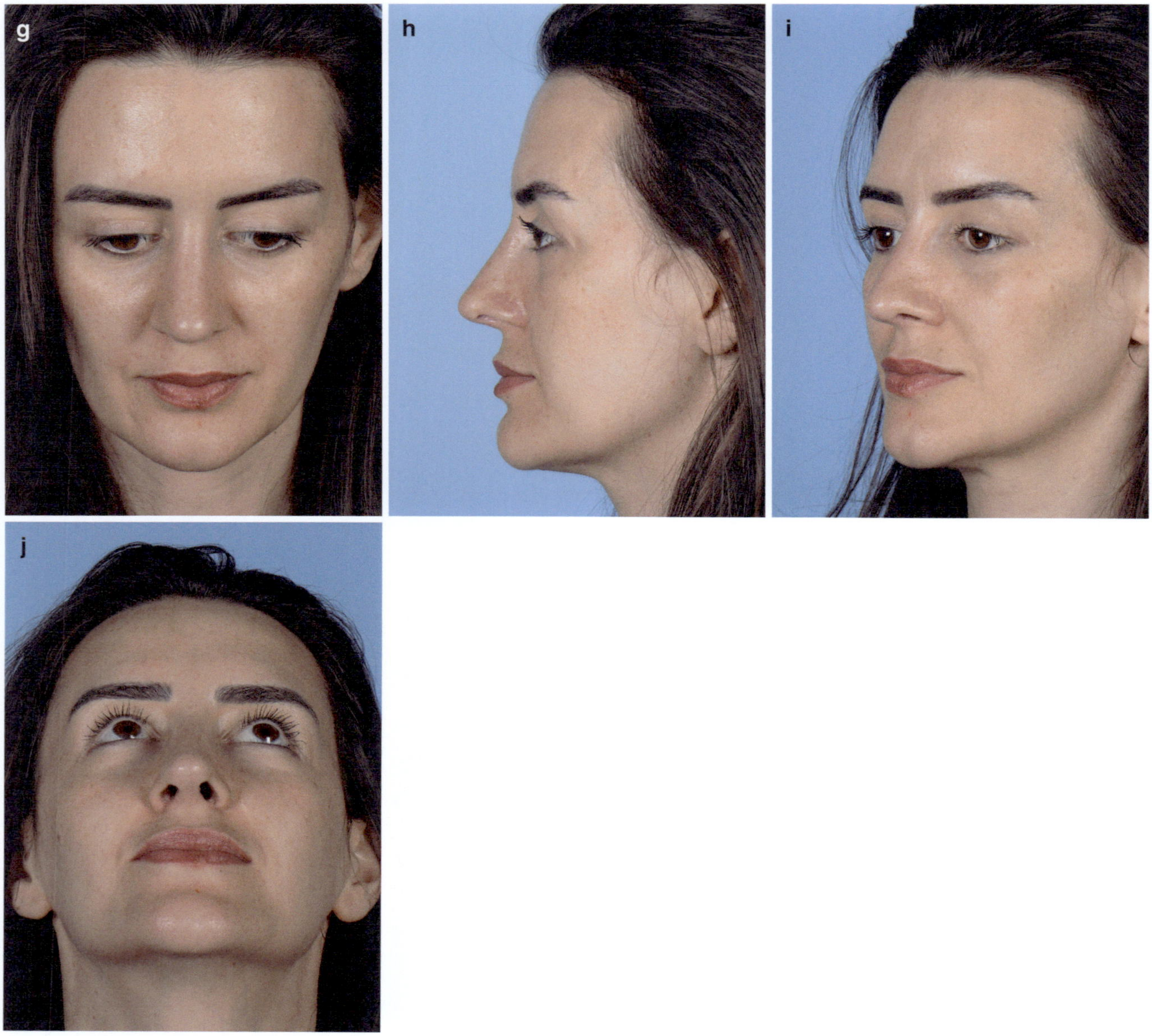

Fig. 18.50 (continued)

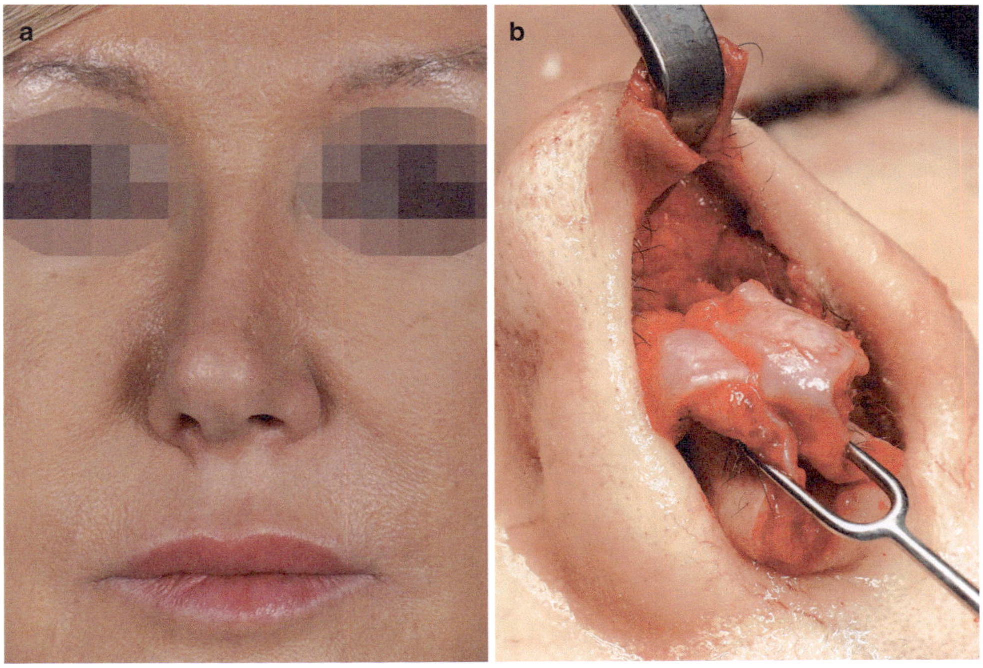

Fig. 18.51 (**a**, **b**) After rhinoplasty by another surgeon, the tip is asymmetrical and deviated to the right

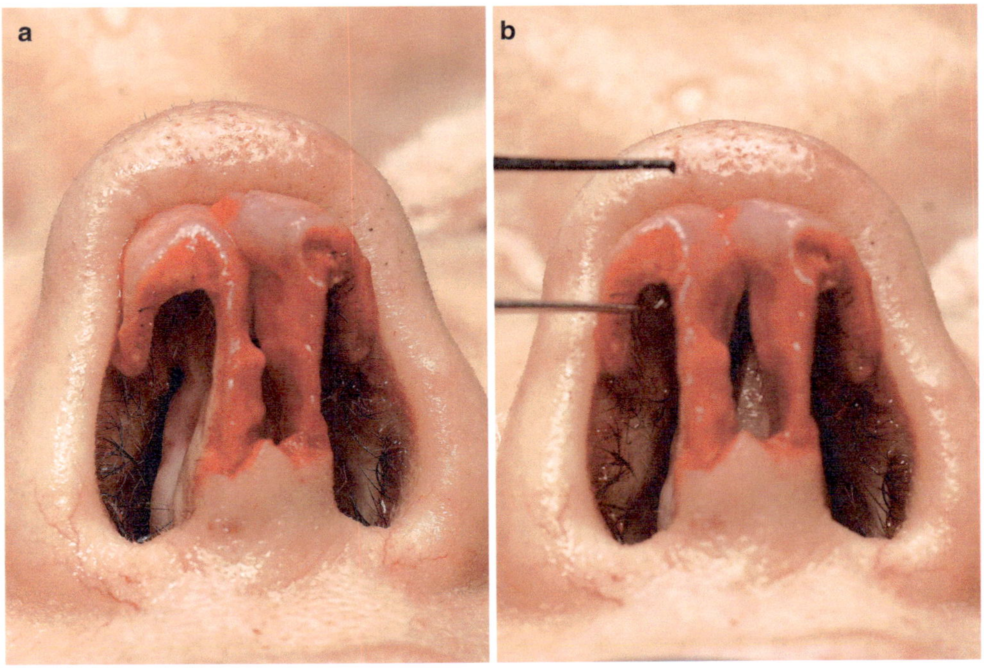

Fig. 18.52 (**a**, **b**) Notice the asymmetry between the lateral crus

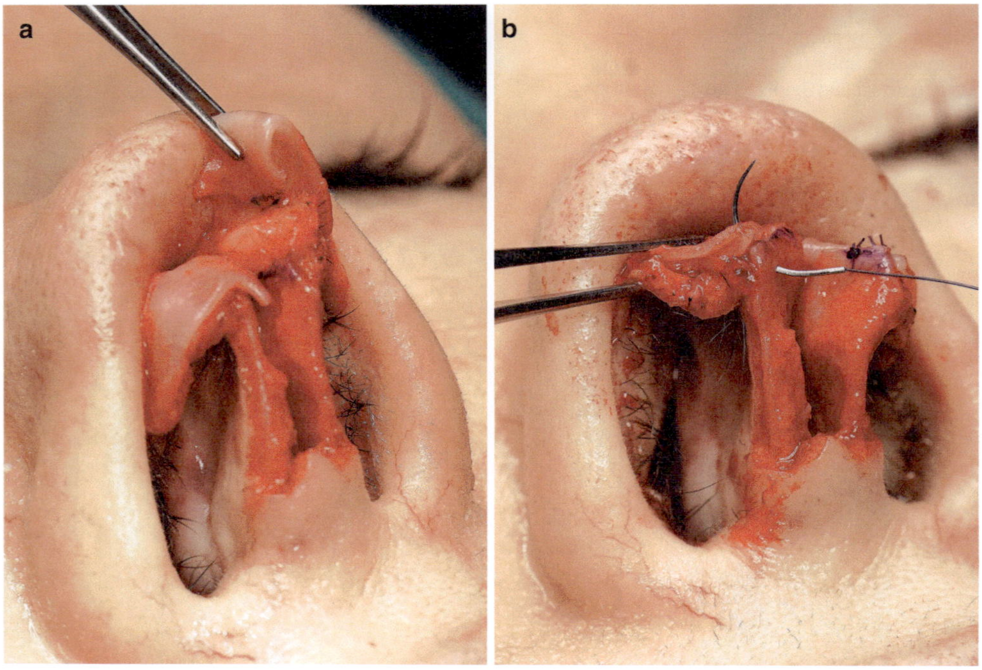

Fig. 18.53 (**a**) Removal of an asymmetrical segment of lateral crus lateral to the dome. (**b**) Continuity of the alar cartilages are reestablished using absorbable sutures

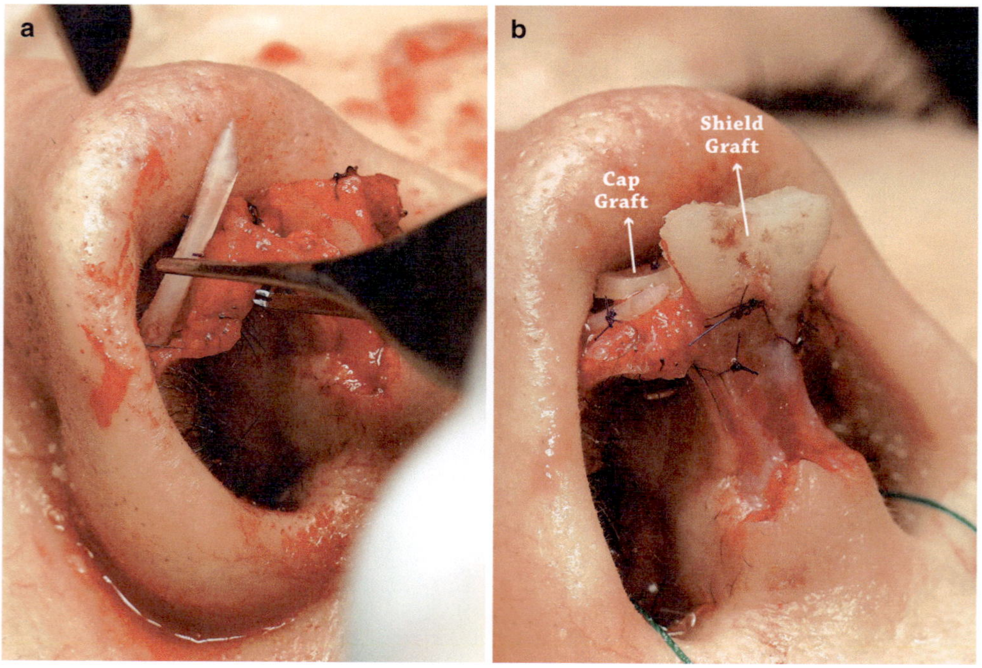

Fig. 18.54 (**a**) Lateral crural graft insertion. (**b**) Shield graft fashioned from costal cartilage and then placed with a cap to prevent cephalad rotation of tip graft

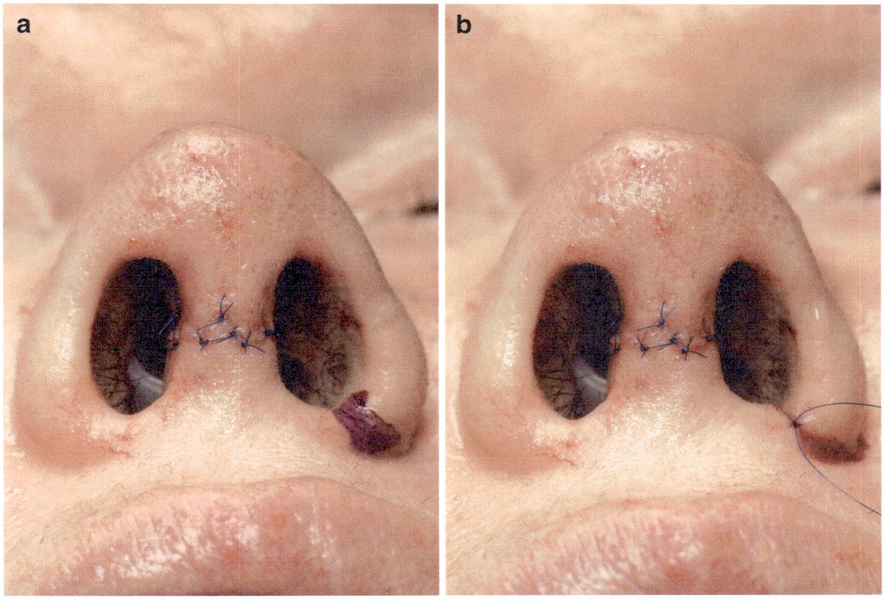

Fig. 18.55 (**a**, **b**) Left sill excision

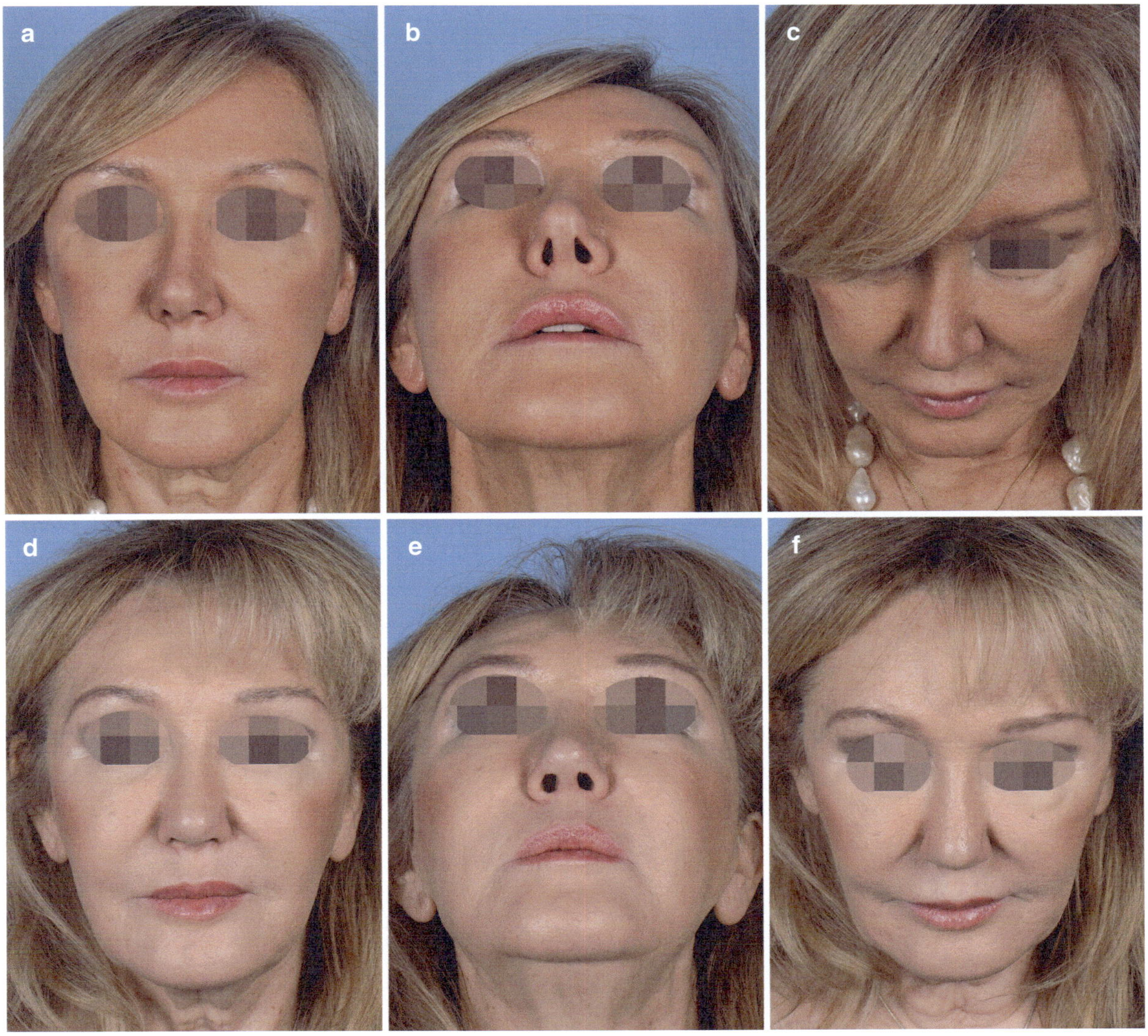

Fig. 18.56 (**a**–**f**) Pre- and postoperative views: the nose is straighter and the tip is more symmetrical. More aesthetically pleasing, tip-defining points. The base of the columella is improved

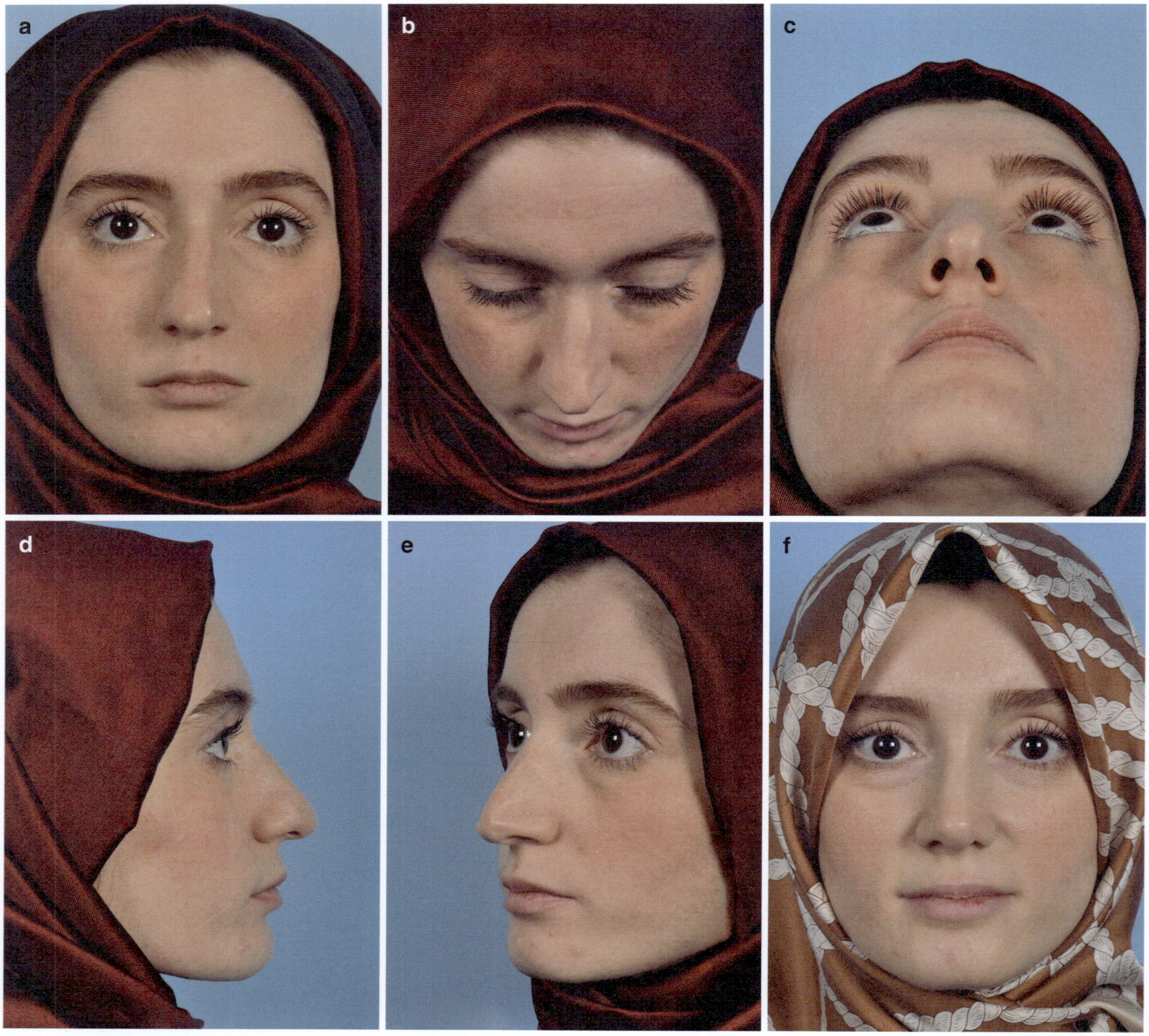

Fig. 18.57 (**a–j**) Tip symmetry and rotation were gained by resection of asymmetrical lateral crura. For left alar sidewall concavity, onlay septal lateral crural graft was used

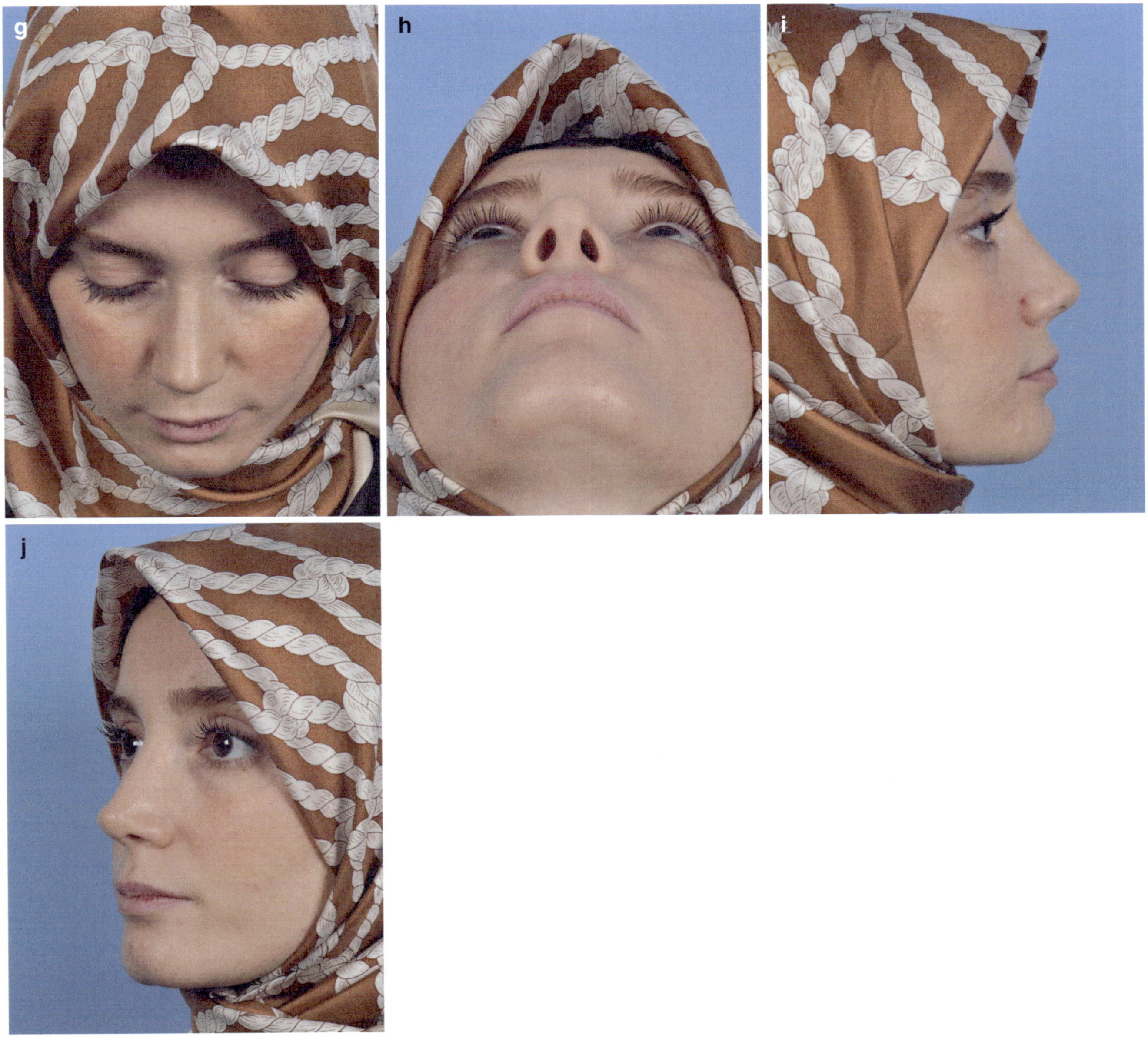

Fig. 18.57 (continued)

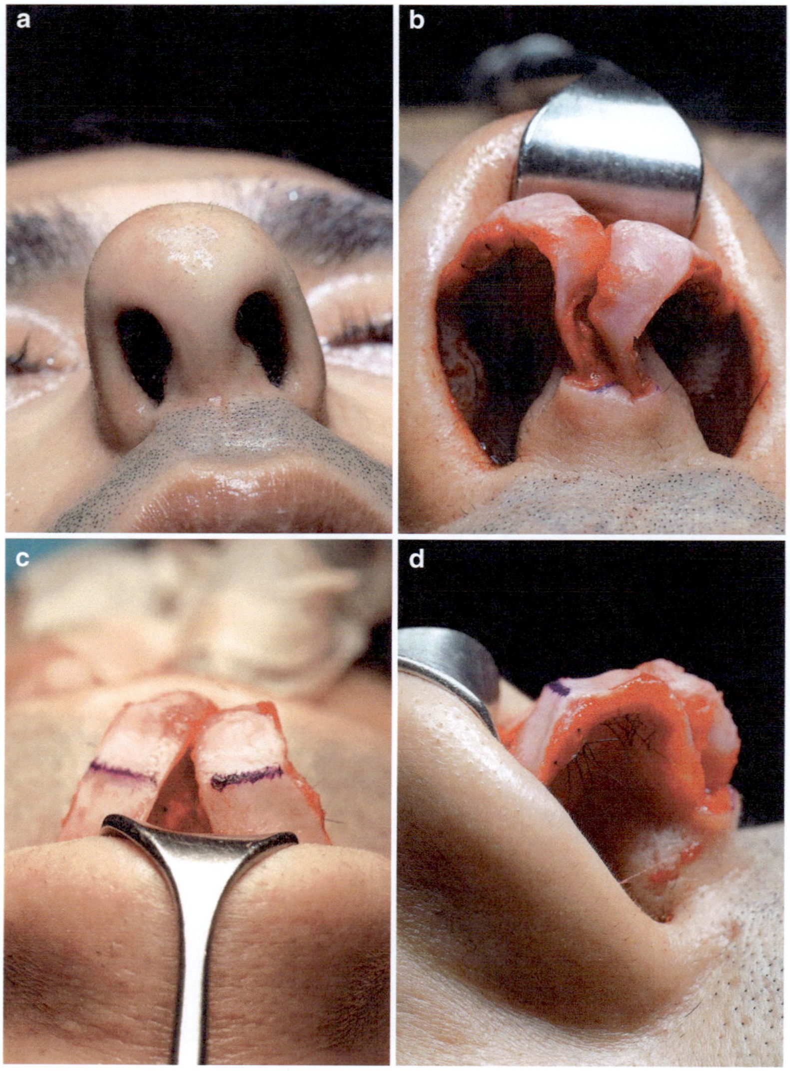

Fig. 18.58 (**a**) Preoperative close-up. (**b–d**) Open approach: note the asymmetrical, buckled medial crura. (Supplementary Video 18.8)

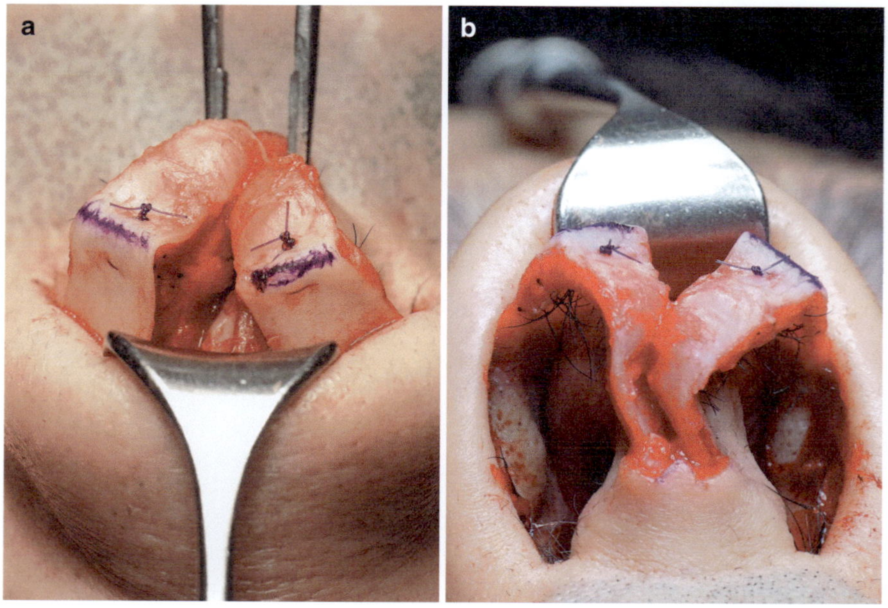

Fig. 18.59 (**a**, **b**) Transdomal mattress suture

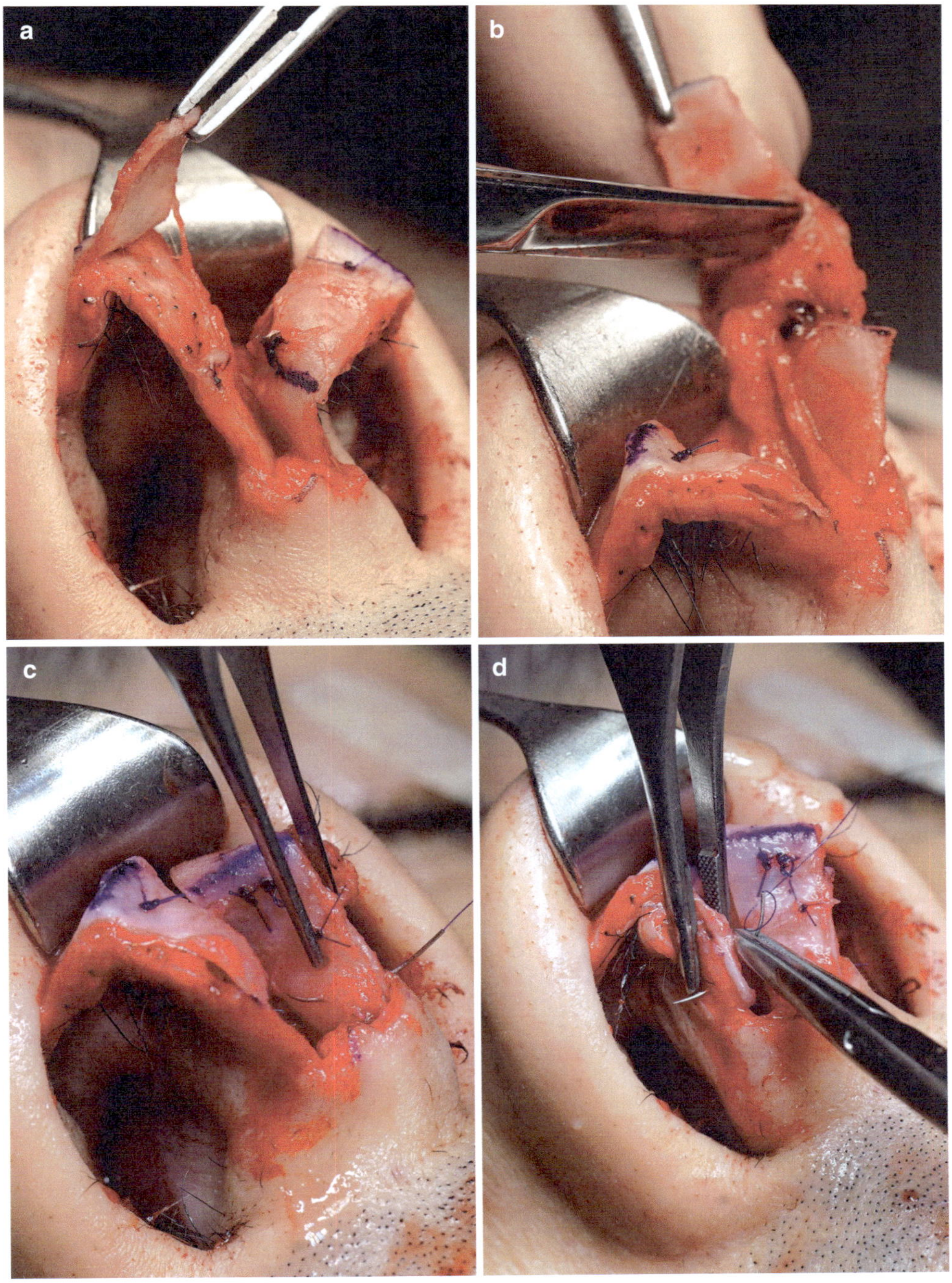

Fig. 18.60 (**a**, **b**) Note the improved alar cartilages symmetry. (**c**) Final appearance of the tip cartilages. (**d**) Medial crura divided, overlapped, and sutured

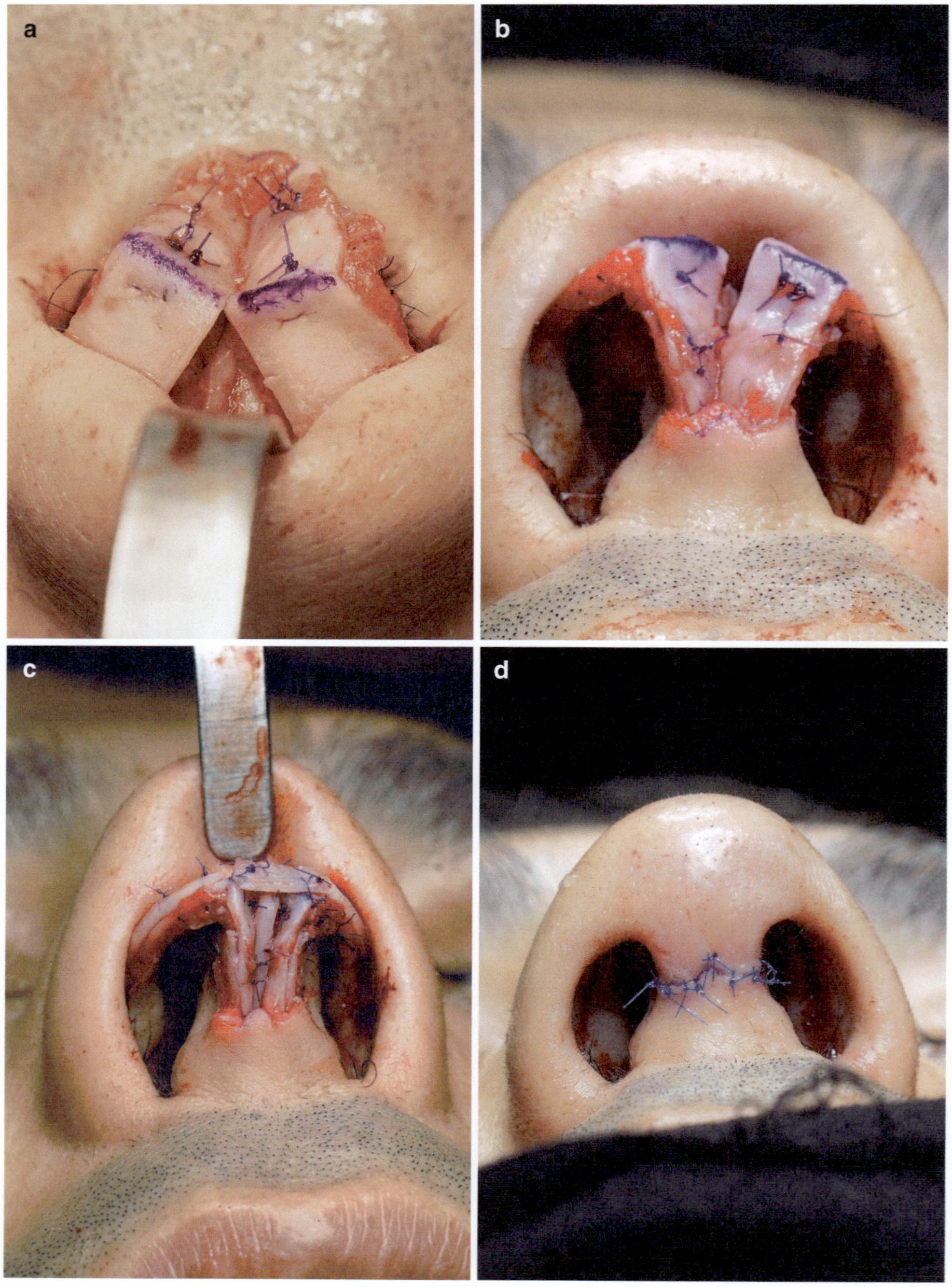

Fig. 18.61 (**a–d**) Note the intraoperative view of the symmetrical alar base

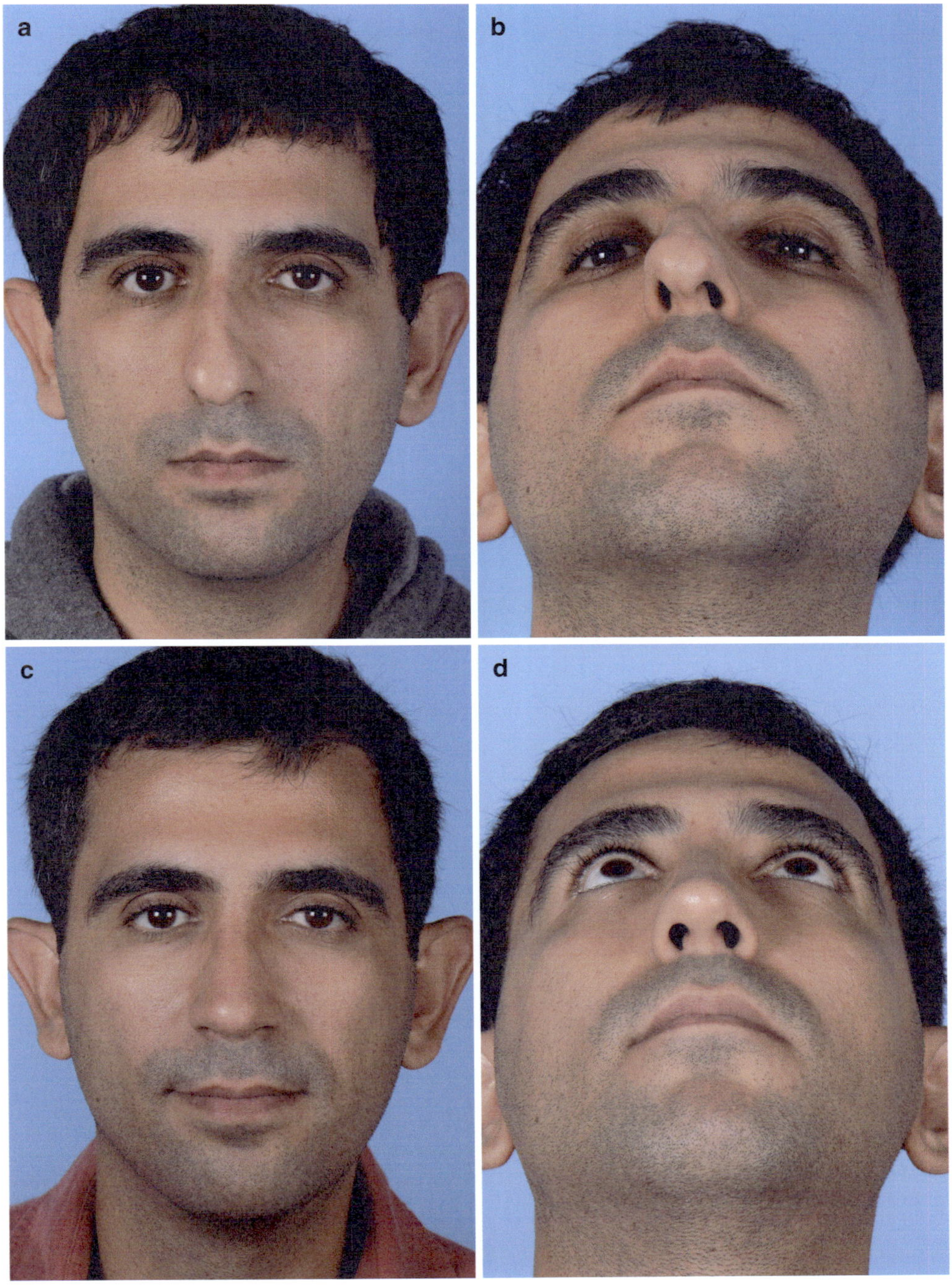

Fig. 18.62 (**a**, **b**) Intraoperative view showing symmetry of alar cartilages after overlap. (**c**) Final anatomy of the tip. (**d**) Pre- and postoperative photographs. The tip is more defined, less bulbous, and more symmetrical

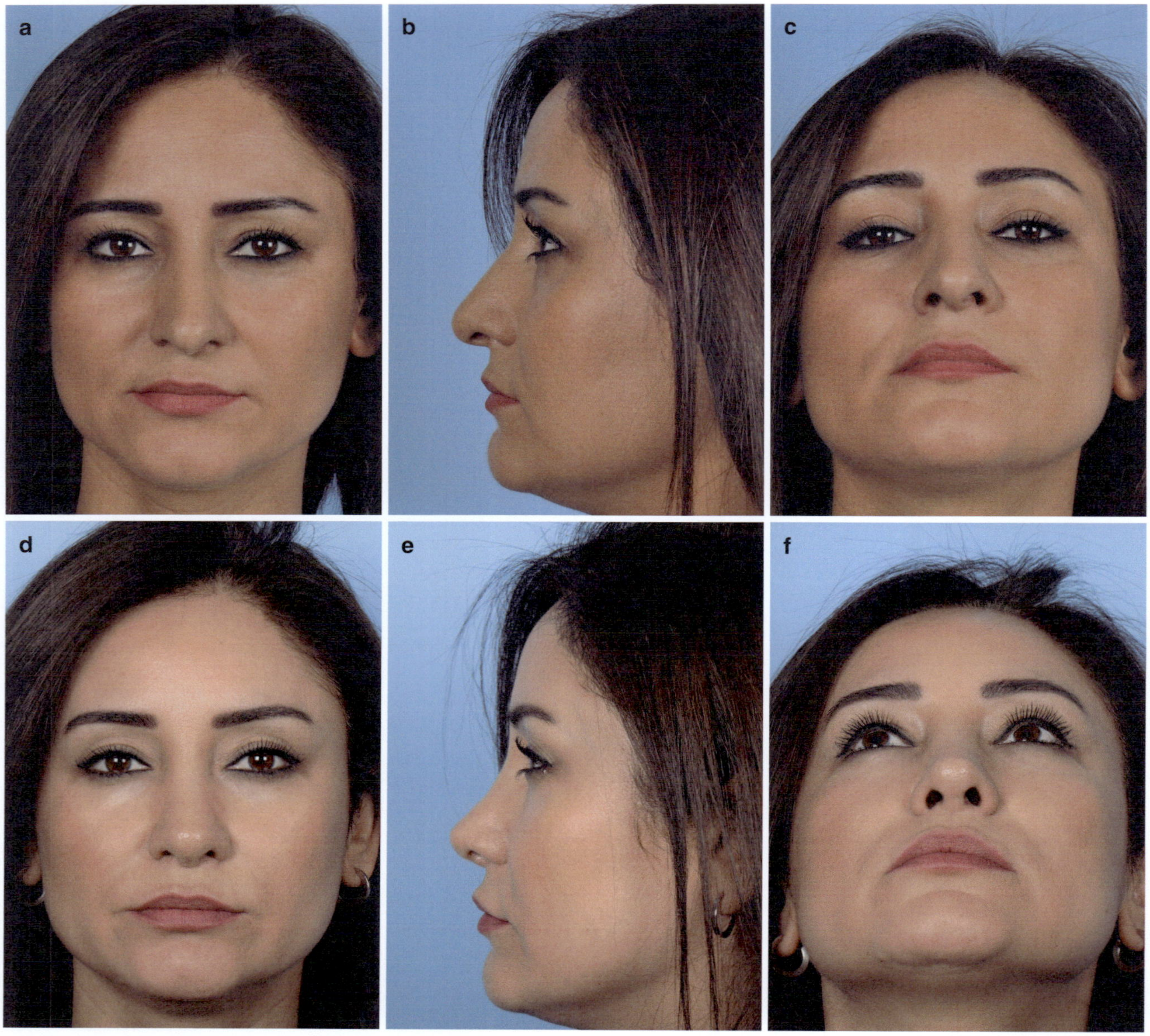

Fig. 18.63 (**a–c**) This 31-year-old woman had severe tip asymmetry. She underwent different extents of medial crural overlap to correct the length discrepancy of the lower lateral cartilages. (**d–f**) At 2 years postoperatively, the nasal tip is symmetrical and positioned in the midline

18.4 Conclusion

Reinstating symmetry, balance, and definition are the three main criteria of success in rhinoplasty. While satisfaction of both the patient and the surgeon lies in a symmetrical nose, the most apparent causes of postoperative dissatisfaction are de novo asymmetries or failures to restore symmetry with rhinoplasty. Although absolute symmetry may be impossible to achieve, at least obvious asymmetries must be avoided. In that regard, it is one of the duties of the surgeon to restore symmetry in the tip, as one of the nasal subunits. The key to tip symmetry is the septum rather than its intrinsic configuration. The way to achieve a straight septum resting in the midline is to reposition the entire septum, particularly the caudal septum in the midline. Clinicians should carefully examine the caudal septum to ensure there is no deflection, deviation, or dislocation, as such caudal septal deformities can lead to nasal base distortion, loss of tip projection, or unequal nostrils with asymmetrical alar flare.

Mild-to-moderate caudal septal deflections can be corrected using batten grafts, while severe ones require subtotal septal reconstruction.

Sutures, columellar struts, and lateral crural grafts can be used to correct mild-to-moderate inner configuration deformities of the alar cartilages. In the presence of severe alar cartilage deformities, vertical alar resection or medial crural overlap technique must be preferred.

Disclosures The author reports no conflicts of interest or funding requiring disclosure.

Further Reading

Constantian MB. An algorithm for correcting the asymmetrical nose. Plast Reconstr Surg. 1989;83(5):801–11.

Daniel RK, Pálházi P. Rhinoplasty: an anatomical and clinical atlas. Cham: Springer; 2018. p. 49–112.

Guyuron B, Behmand RA. Caudal nasal deviation. Plast Reconstr Surg. 2003;111(7):2449–57; discussion 2458–9.

Hafezi F, Naghibzadeh B, Nouhi AH. Applied anatomy of the nasal lower lateral cartilage: a new finding. Aesth Plast Surg. 2010;34(2):244–8.

Rohrich RJ, Griffin JR. Correction of intrinsic nasal tip asymmetries in primary rhinoplasty. Plast Reconstr Surg. 2003;112(6):1699–712; discussion 1713–5.

Şeneldir S, Altundağ A, Dizdar D. Cutting the holy dome: the evolution of vertical alar resection. Aesth Plast Surg. 2018;42(1):275–87.

Şeneldir S, Kırgezen T. Vertical alar folding (VAF): a useful technique for correction of long and concave lateral crura in rhinoplasty. Aesth Plast Surg. 2019;435:1269–78.

Stephan S, Wang TD. Asymmetric nasal tip. Facial Plast Surg. 2012;28(2):177–86.

Step-by-Step Open Approach Rhinoplasty

19

19.1 Introduction

Rhinoplasty surgery requires attention and patience, and the operative time can sometimes be longer than expected. Therefore, general anesthesia is preferred to ensure the comfort of both the surgeon and the patient.

The intubation tube is fixed with the suture passing through the lower incisors and remains on the left side without causing any tension. Corneal abrasion and other potential ocular pathologies are avoided by applying ointment on the eyes and taping from the upper eyelid to the temporal region. The patient is placed in the flexion position, with an angle of 20–30° between the head and the floor. This position helps to decrease venous return and minimize intraoperative bleeding.

Tranexamic acid can be used to minimize bleeding and bruises. At the beginning of the surgery, 250 mg tranexamic acid is administered via slow intravenous push, followed by an additional 250 mg as an intravenous infusion.

The pulse and blood pressure of the patient must be checked prior to local anesthesia and if the levels are elevated, the surgeon must wait until they are normalized. Infiltration must be performed very slowly, and the readings must be attended to closely. A solution containing 20 mg lidocaine hydrochloride and 0.0125 mg epinephrine is used as a local anesthetic.

Supplementary Information The online version contains supplementary material available at https://doi.org/10.1007/978-3-031-65619-4_19.

19.2 Steps for Open Approach Rhinoplasty

The steps for open approach rhinoplasty are as follows.

19.2.1 Step 1

The injection is made into the incision line at the columella and the marginal incision line at the caudal edge of the alar cartilages (Fig. 19.1).

19.2.2 Step 2

Infiltration from the skin on the alar cartilages facilitates dissection of the area (Fig. 19.2).

19.2.3 Step 3

Infiltration occurs bilaterally all the way through the caudal septum.

Technical Pearl: Infiltration of the region superior to the septum is vital for vasoconstriction of the area supplied by the anterior ethmoidal artery. If there is a crest at the septum, infiltration facilitates dissection of the area and prevents mucosal damage (Fig. 19.3).

19.2.4 Step 4

Dorsal infiltration from inside the nose occurs via the anterior septal angle.

Technical Pearl: The surgeon must avoid extrusion from the skin in cases presenting with a high hump (Fig. 19.4).

S. Şeneldir, *Photographic Atlas of Rhinoplasty*, https://doi.org/10.1007/978-3-031-65619-4_19

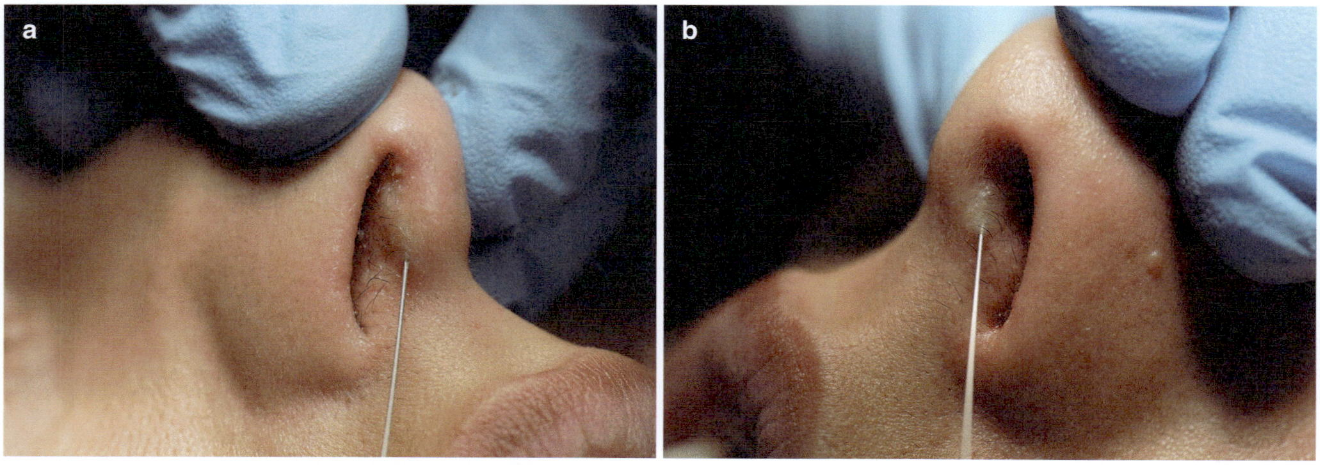

Fig. 19.1 (**a**, **b**) Injection into the columella. (Supplementary Video 19.1)

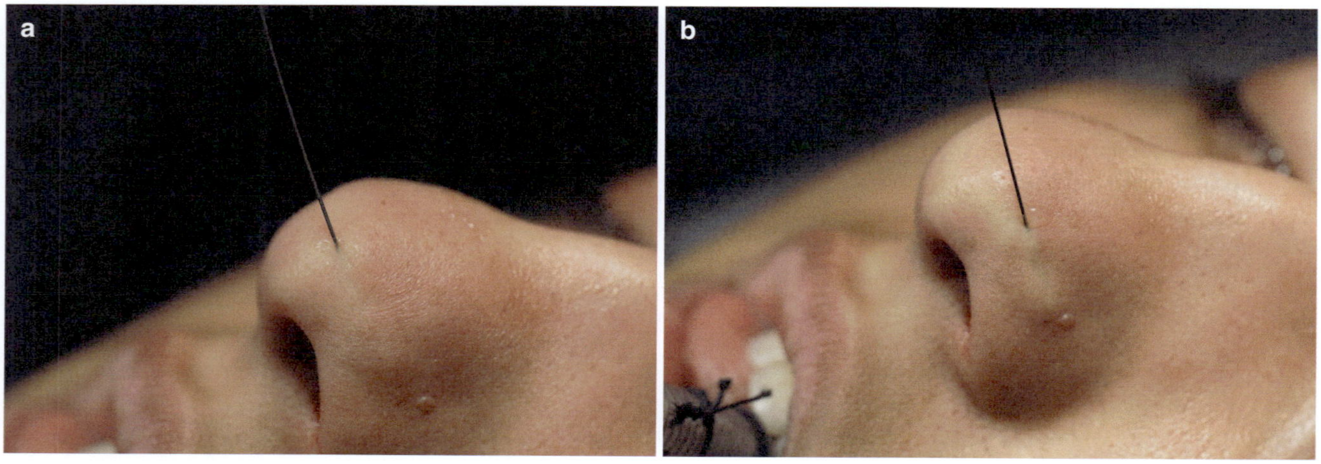

Fig. 19.2 (**a**, **b**) Injection into the interdomal region and tip

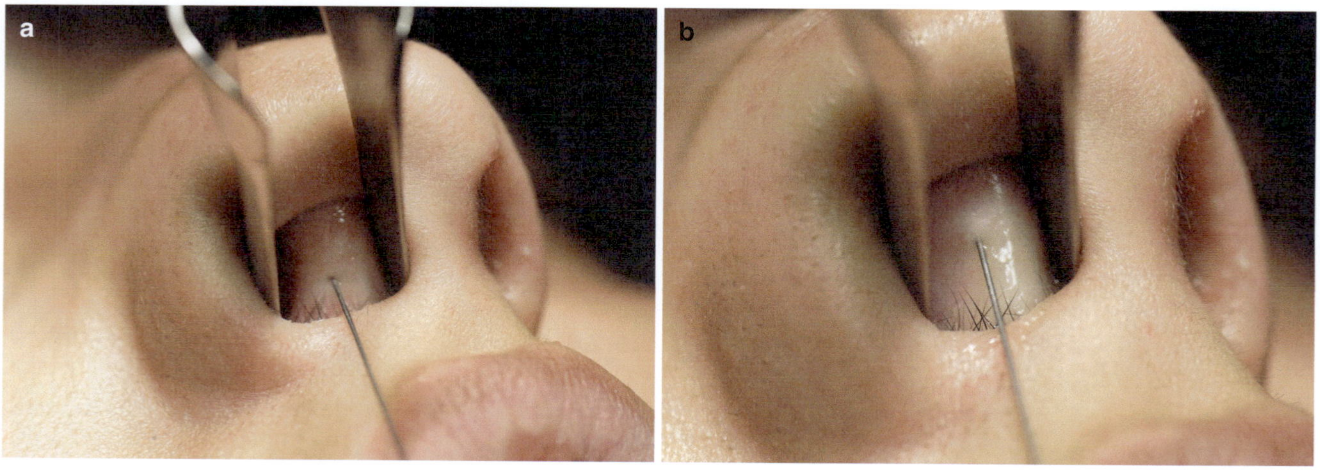

Fig. 19.3 (**a**, **b**) Injection into the septum in a subperichondrial plane

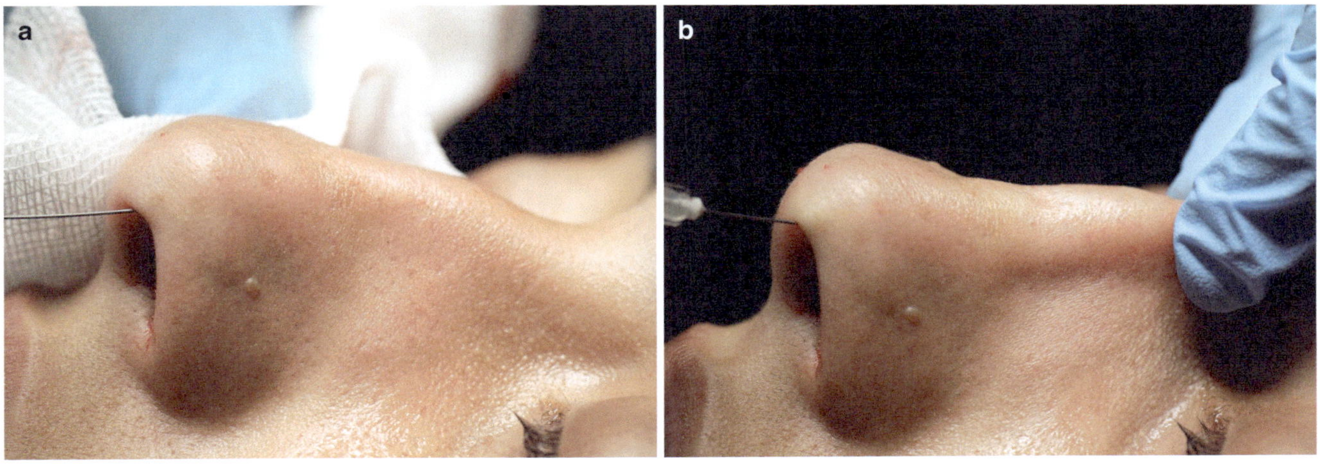

Fig. 19.4 (a, b) Injection into the dorsum

19.2.5 Step 5

Infiltration at the lateral osteotomy line proceeds from the lateral to the anterior end of the inferior nasal concha and then advances through the medial canthus.

Technical Pearl: The surgeon must press down on the medial canthus with one finger to protect the orbit from infiltration (Fig. 19.5).

After infiltration, it takes a minimum of 10 min for the local anesthetics to take effect.

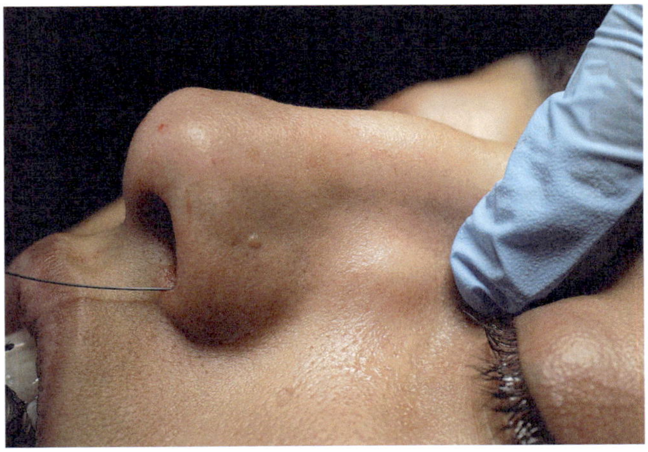

Fig. 19.5 Injection into the lateral nasal wall

19.2.6 Step 6

After the local anesthetics take effect, three points to define the margins of an inverted "V" are marked from the narrowest point of the columella (Fig. 19.6).

19.2.7 Step 7

The inverted "V" is created by connecting the three points described above. The incision must be terminated at the lateral sides, where the caudal edge of the middle crus ends. A mid-columellar incision is made because the mid-columella is the narrowest part of the columella. If an incision is made on wider parts of the columella, there would be a higher risk of scarring due to less cartilaginous support for the flap (Fig. 19.7).

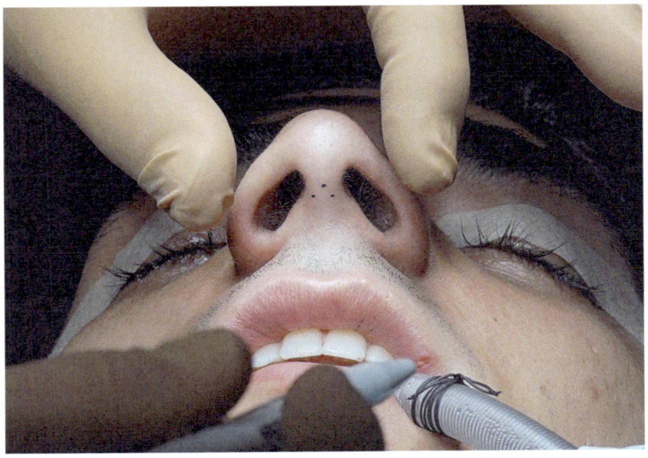

Fig. 19.6 The narrowest part of columella is marked. (Supplementary Video 19.2)

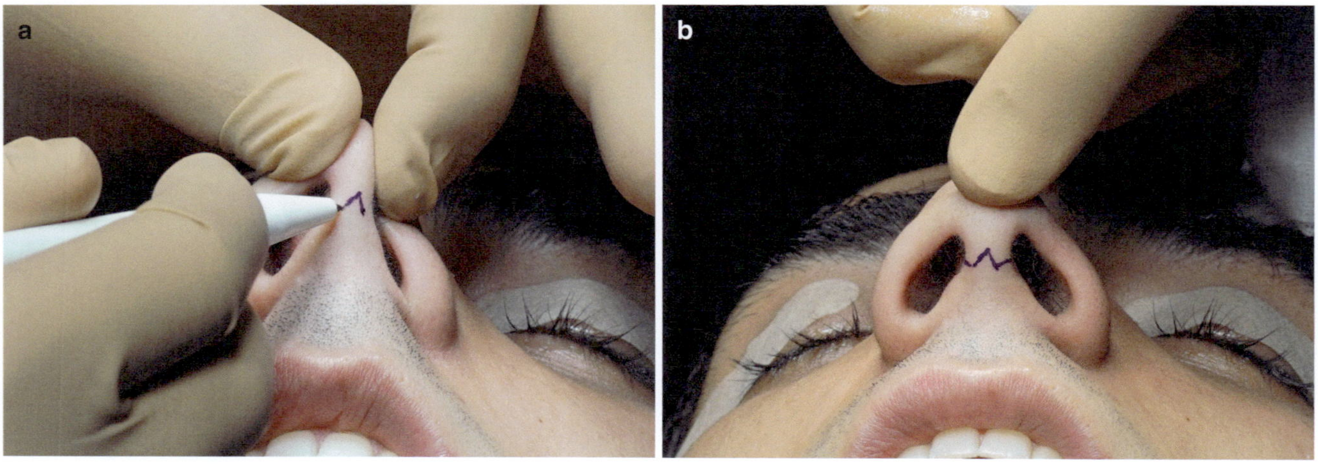

Fig. 19.7 (**a**, **b**) Inverted V incision is marked

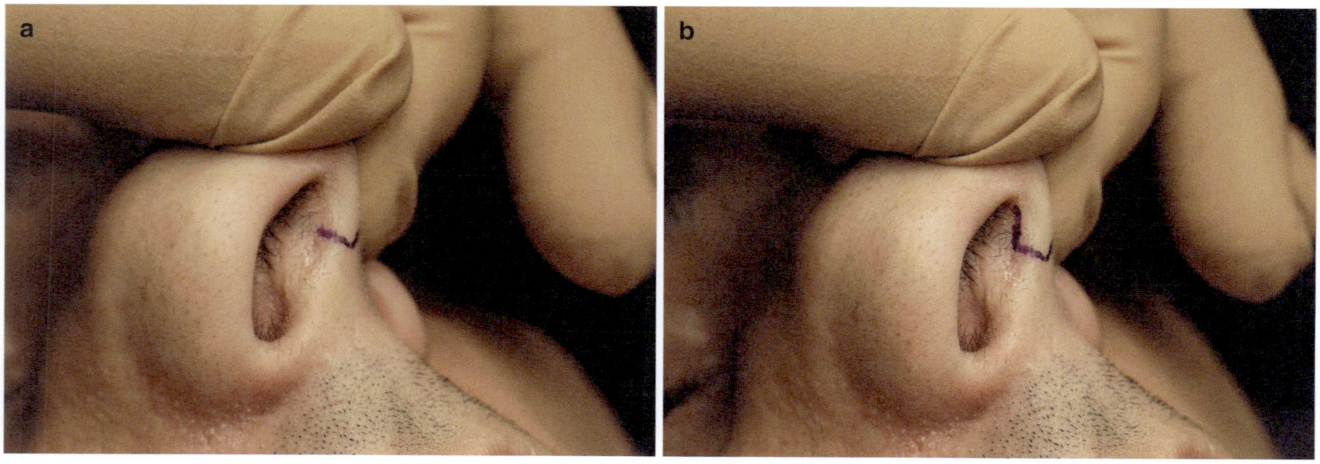

Fig. 19.8 (**a**, **b**) Marginal columellar incision is marked

19.2.8 Step 8

The borders of the marginal incision are marked at the lateral aspect, and are connected to the points marked for the columellar incision (Fig. 19.8).

19.2.9 Step 9

An inverted "V" incision is made with a number 11 blade over the marked points (Fig. 19.9).

Technical Pearl: Because the medial crus lies superficial to the lateral sides of the incision, a superficial skin incision is made rather than a deep incision. Meanwhile, incision of the medial crus must be avoided. In cases of accidental incision of the medial crus, the surgeon must not lose motivation and should proceed with full concentration (Fig. 19.10).

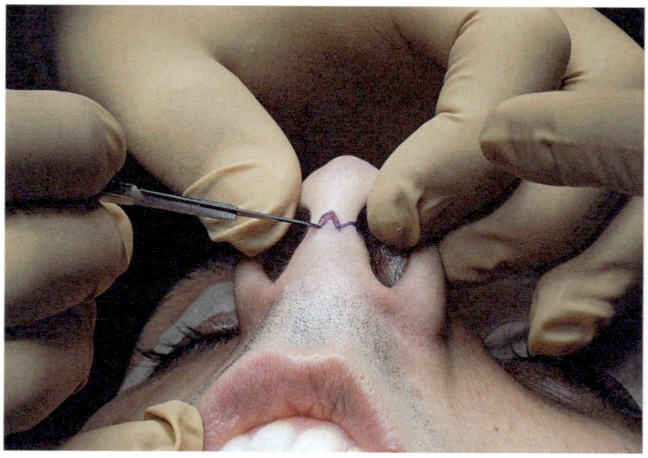

Fig. 19.9 Mid-columellar incision

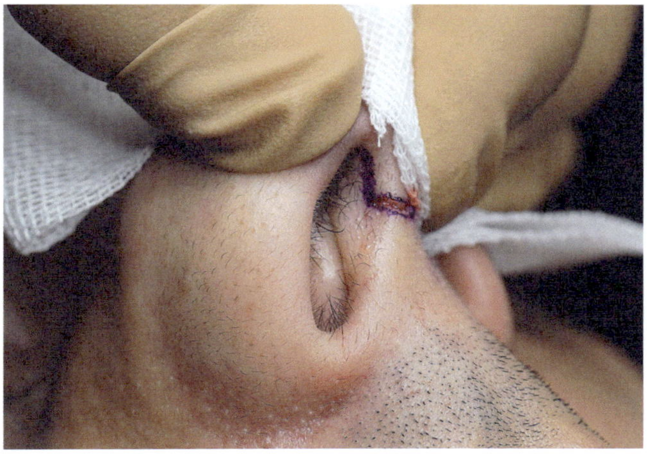

Fig. 19.10 Care is taken to avoid cutting the cartilages

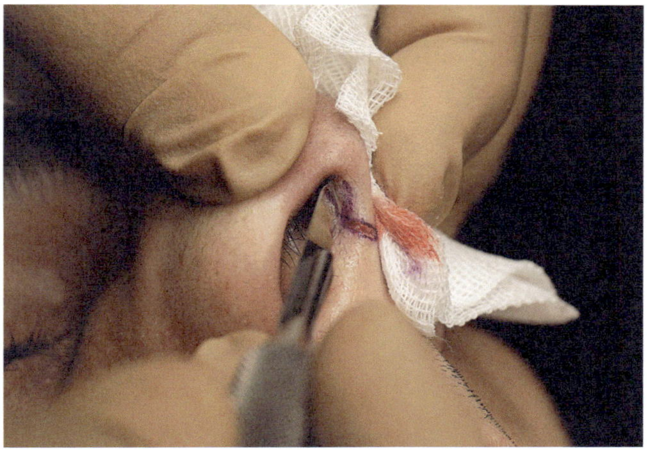

Fig. 19.11 Marginal columellar incisor

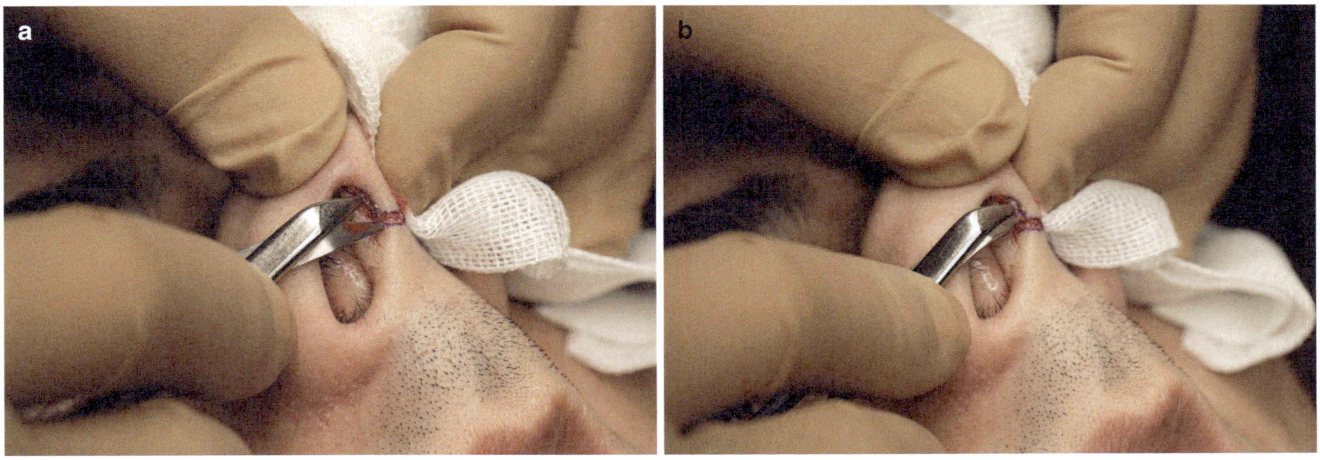

Fig. 19.12 (**a**, **b**) The flap is elevated with Converse scissors (Graefe)

19.2.10 Step 10

A marginal incision is made lateral to the columella with a number 15 blade. The incision is advanced superiorly and is terminated on reaching the infracartilaginous incision made by scissors. The inverted "V" at the columellar connects to the incision (Fig. 19.11).

19.2.11 Step 11

Converse scissors (Graefe) are used to access the incision site at the lateral side. Columellar dissection is performed over the perichondrium of the medial crus, in the plane between the skin and the cartilage (Fig. 19.12).

19.2.12 Step 12

The surgeon advances up to the incision line lateral to the contralateral crus. The columellar vessels are cauterized, and a transcolumellar incision is made (Fig. 19.13).

19.2.13 Step 13

Suspending the columellar flap with a double hook, the surgeon elevates the skin to increase cartilaginous exposure by pressing down the tip with the middle finger (Fig. 19.14).

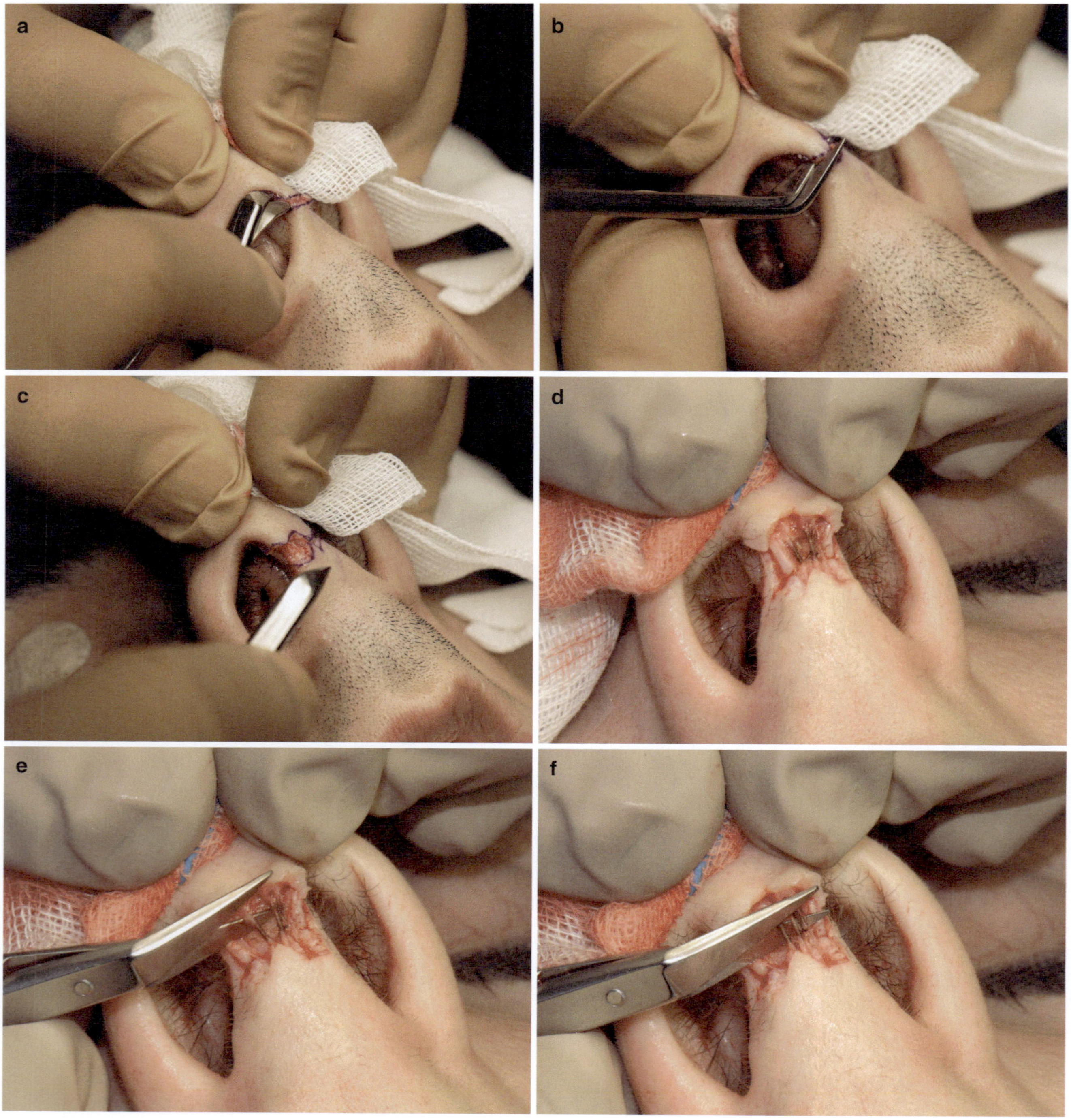

Fig. 19.13 (**a**–**f**) The flap is detached from the middle crus

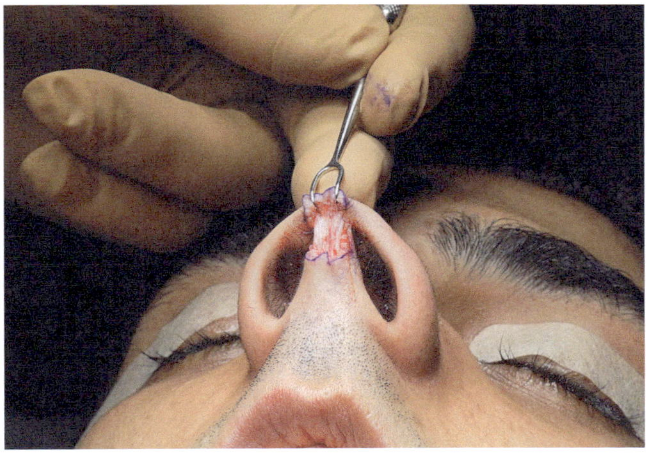

Fig. 19.14 Avascular plane

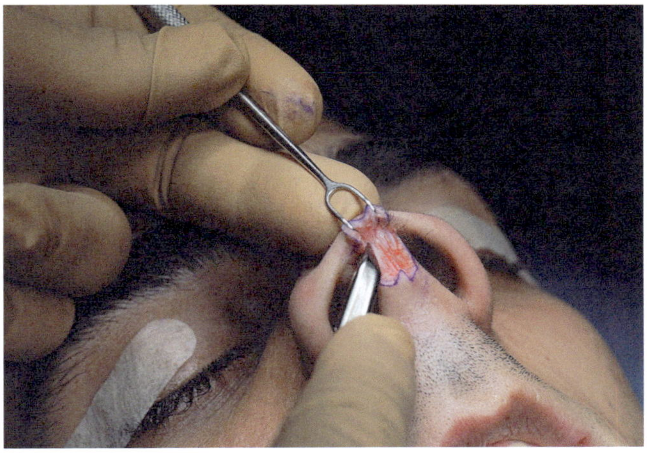

Fig. 19.15 Two-point fixation is used to elevate the skin flap

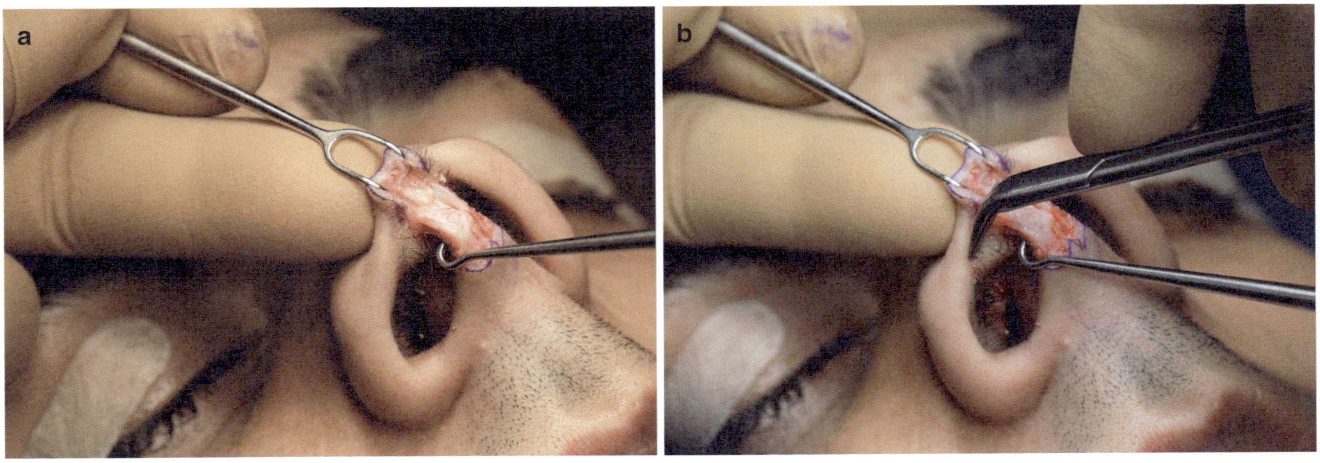

Fig. 19.16 (**a**, **b**) The flap is detached in a plane just supraperichondrial

19.2.14 Step 14

The medial crus is dissected in the supraperichondrial plane (Fig. 19.15).

19.2.15 Step 15

Once the dome is reached, the assistant pulls down the tip with a hook and the columella is suspended with a double hook. The surgeon presses down the supratip with the middle finger to obtain a better view for dissection. The caudal edge of the cartilage must be followed during this dissection (Fig. 19.16).

19.2.16 Step 16

The supraperichondrial plane is reached by moving the scissors back and forth over the cartilage at the caudal edge of the lateral crus. Cartilaginous dissection is performed in this plane via a continuous infracartilaginous incision (Fig. 19.17).

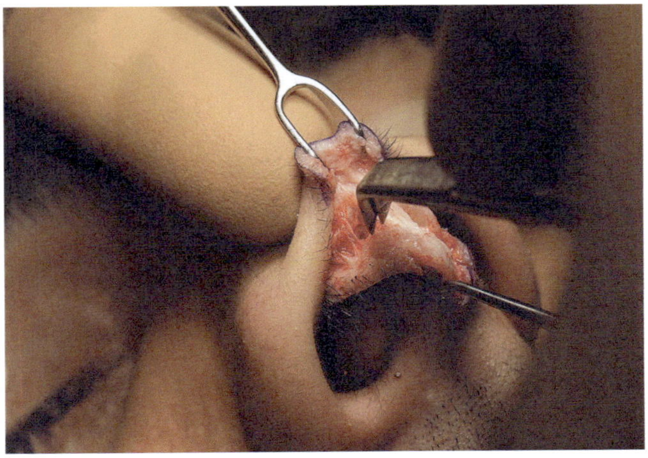

Fig. 19.17 Suprapericondrial dissection of the lateral crura

19.2.17 Step 17

The dissection is advanced up to the accessory cartilages toward the end of the lateral crus. The same procedure is applied to the contralateral crus (Fig. 19.18).

19.2.18 Step 18

Pitanguy's ligament is transected (Fig. 19.19).

Technical Pearl: Why cut Pitanguy's ligament? Pitanguy reported in one of his studies that "once the dermocartilaginous ligament is sectioned, it permits freeing and raising of the nasal tip. Division of this structure improves the overall aesthetic result but also maintains the independence and mobility of the tip." This view is shared by the author.

19.2.19 Step 19

After the lower lateral cartilages are pulled by the assistant, local anesthesia is administered to the anterior septal angle for hydrodissection. Hydrodissection aids advancement at the dorsum (Fig. 19.20).

19.2.20 Step 20

Soft tissues are suspended superiorly using forceps and dissected up to the cartilaginous dorsum (Fig. 19.21).

19.2.21 Step 21

The cartilaginous dorsum is reached via dissection (Fig. 19.22).

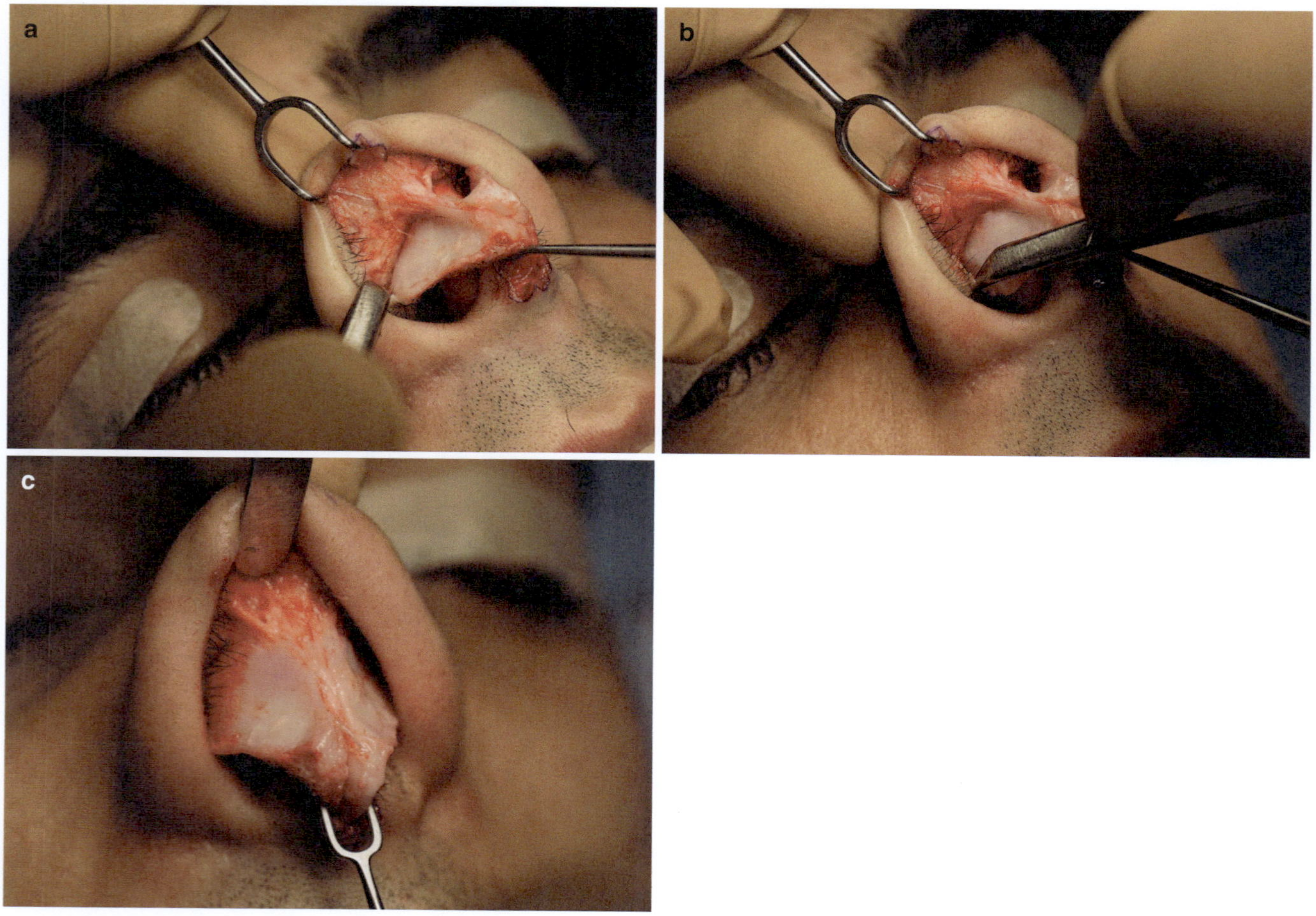

Fig. 19.18 (a–c) The lateral extent of dissection over the lateral crus is to the area of the endpoint of the crus

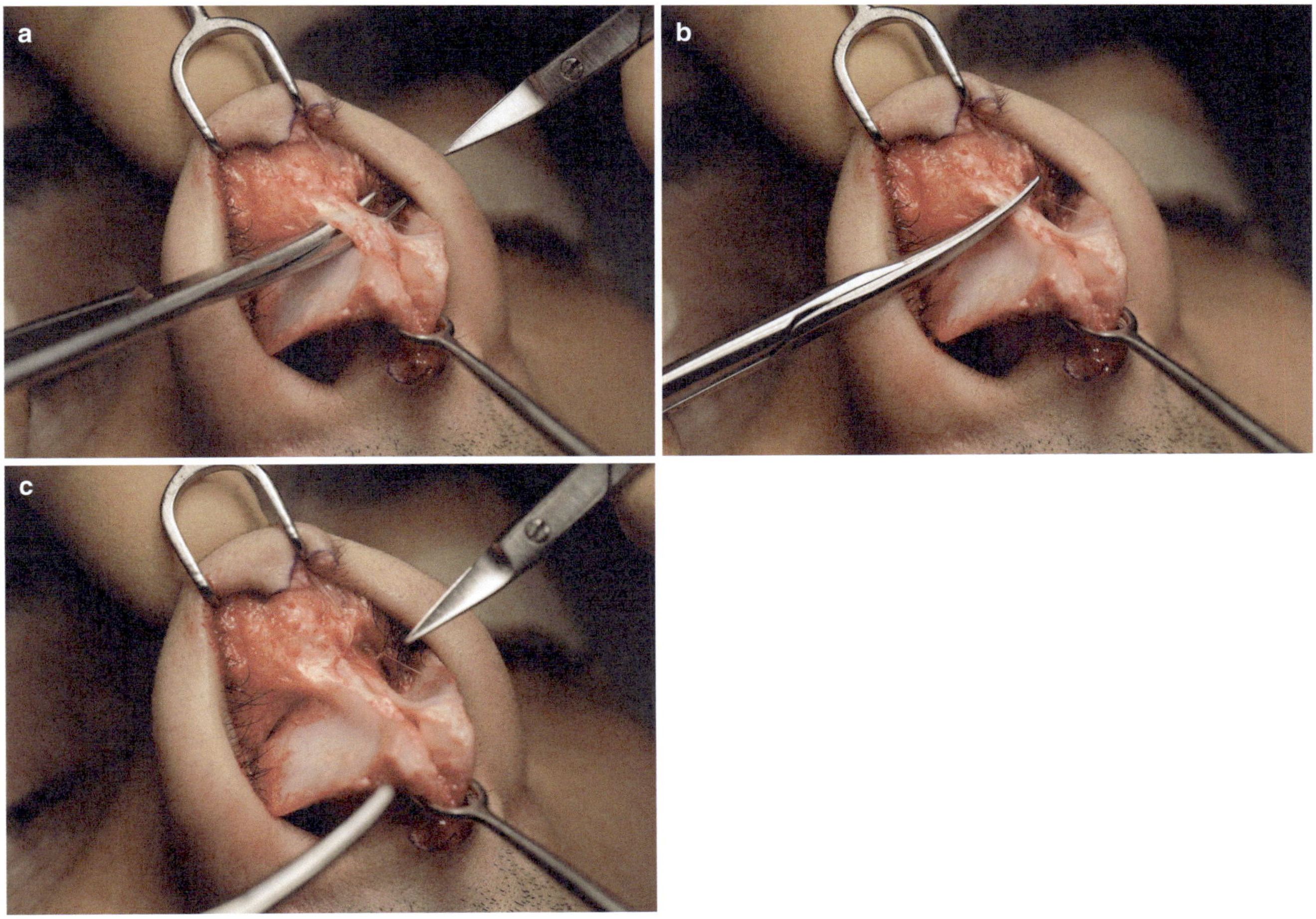

Fig. 19.19 (a–c) Pitanguy's ligament is transected

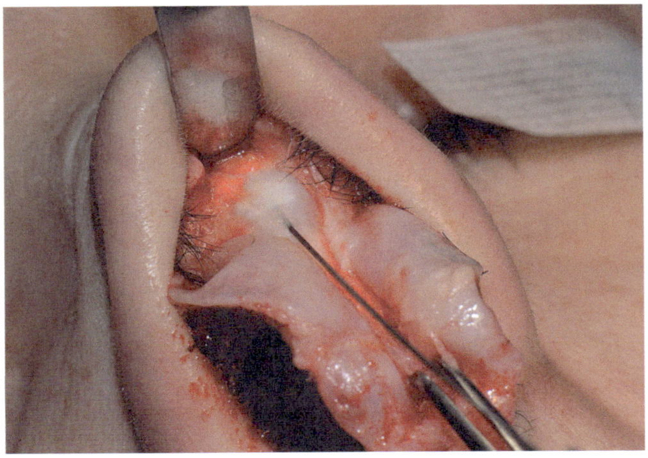

Fig. 19.20 Injection into the subpericondrial plane

19.2.22 Step 22

After the cartilaginous dorsum is reached, the periosteum of the nasal bone is incised at the Keystone area (K area) with a scalpel (Fig. 19.23).

19.2.23 Step 23

A periosteal elevator is used to access the incision and elevate the tissues in the subperiosteal plane (Fig. 19.24).

19.2.24 Step 24

The periosteum, elevated together with the dorsal flap, is divided from the nasal skeleton as a single flap (Fig. 19.25).

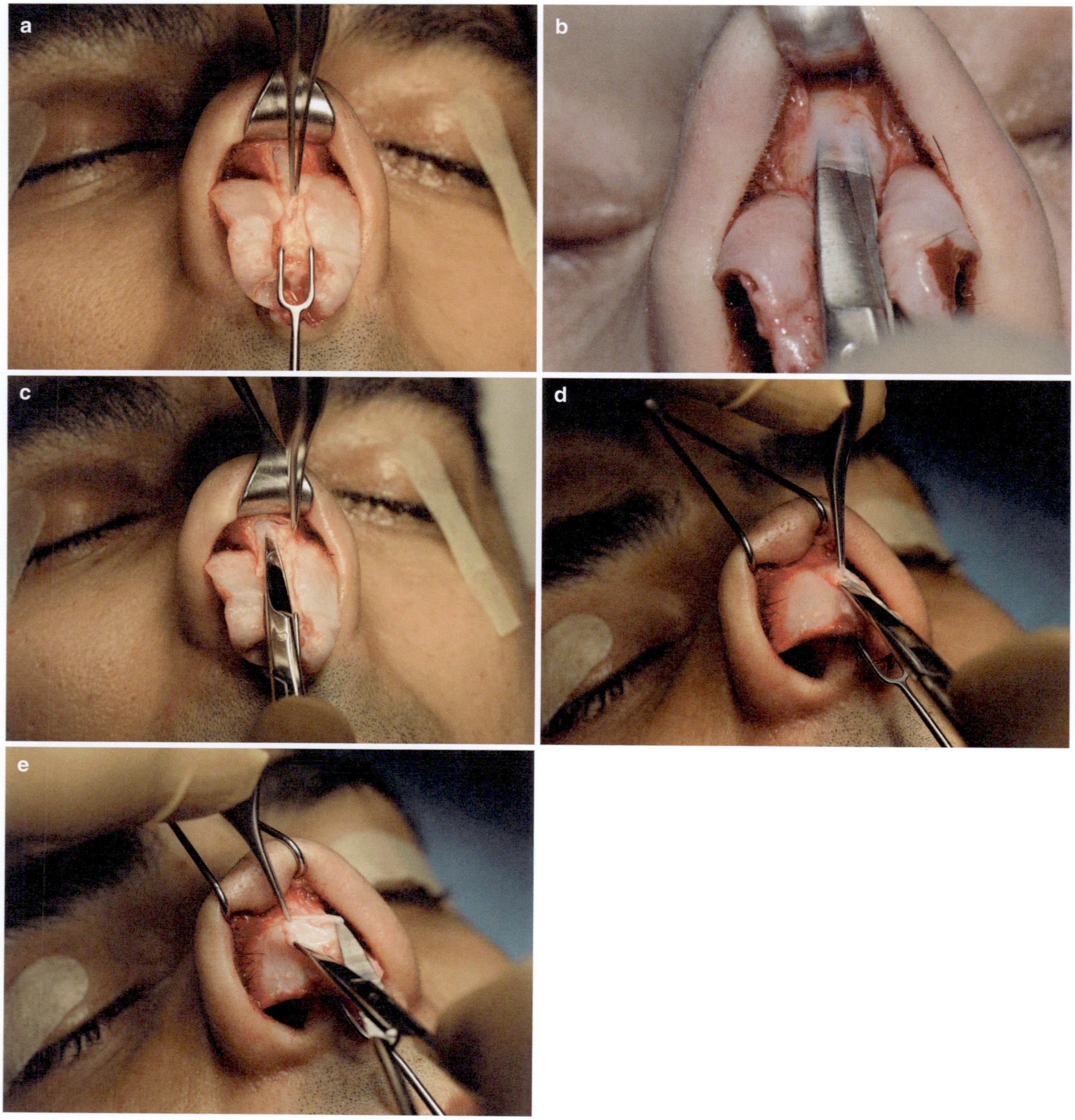

Fig. 19.21 (**a**–**e**) Subpericondrial dissection

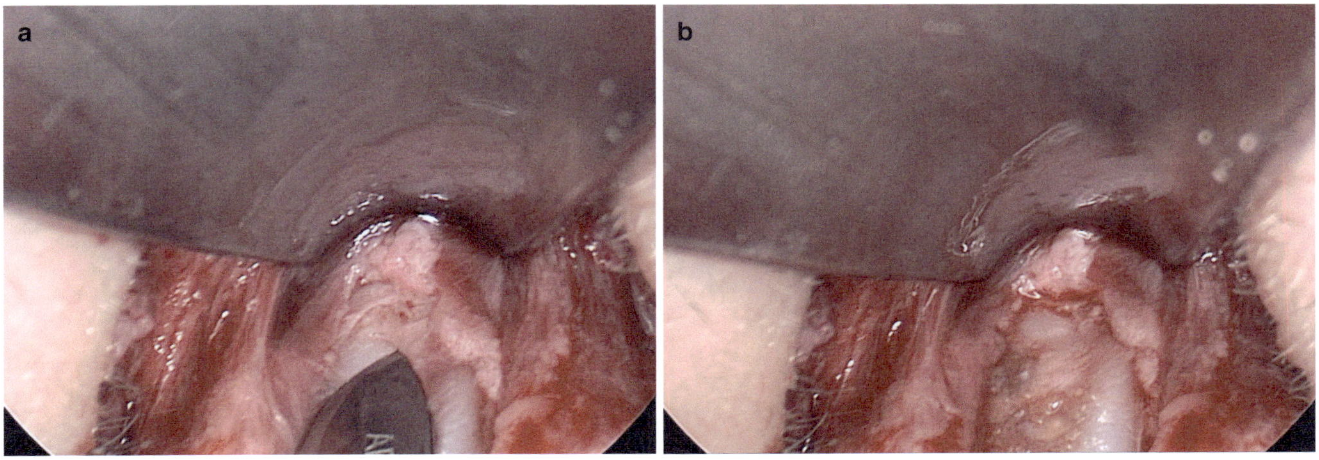

Fig. 19.23 (**a**, **b**) The nasal bone is incised to find the subperiosteal plane

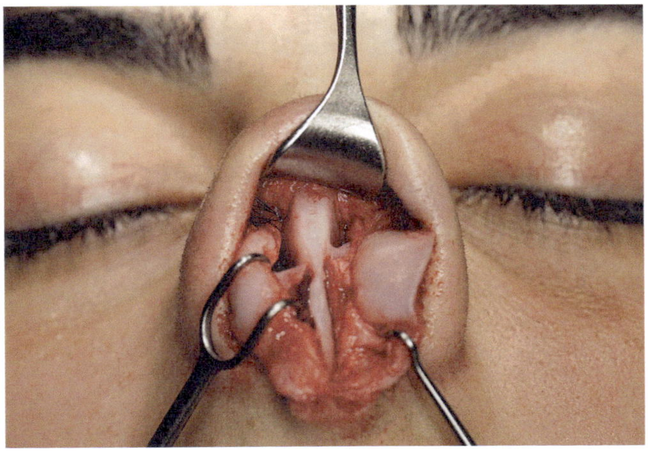

Fig. 19.22 Cartilaginous dorsum

19.2.25 Step 25

While the assistant pulls the left dome in the lateral direction with a hook, the surgeon uses a forceps to pull the right dome toward him or her. Intercrural ligaments between the two crura are dissected, and the caudal septum is thus reached (Fig. 19.26).

19.2.26 Step 26

After the caudal septum is identified, sharp-pointed scissors are moved up and down in parallel to the septum to reach the subperichondrial plane. A purple-blue-colored reflection of the cartilage is seen.

Technical Pearl: Dissection at the subperichondrial plane is easier and bloodless (Fig. 19.27).

19.2.27 Step 27

Mucoperichondrial dissection continues to the base at the anterior. Wide dissection is particularly essential in patients with anterior caudal deflection (Fig. 19.28).

19.2.28 Step 28

The mucoperichondrium is fully elevated from the septum at the subperichondrial plane with an elevator (Fig. 19.29).

19.2.29 Step 29

The same applies for the contralateral mucoperichondrium. The mucoperichondrial flap is elevated from underside of the upper lateral cartilages to prevent any mucosal injury during hump resection.

Technical Pearl: Mucosa must be preserved to the fullest extent possible. Excess mucosa functions as a spreader at the dorsum.

19.2.30 Step 30

After all dissections are completed, hump resection is performed as needed (details are discussed in the relevant chapter).

Technical Pearl: Hump resection must always be performed prior to septoplasty.

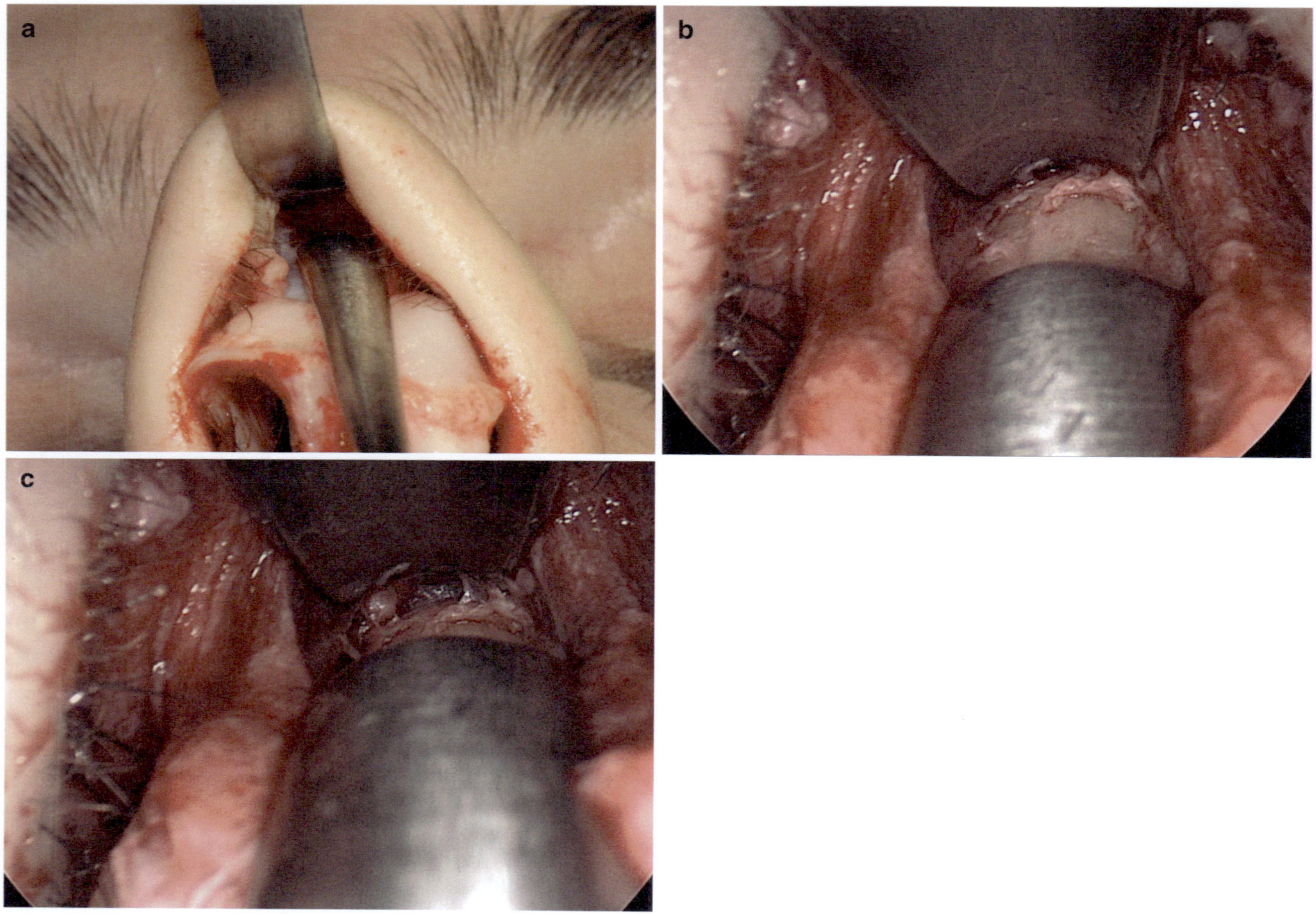

Fig. 19.24 (**a**–**c**) The flap is elevated in a subperiosteal plane with a periosteal elevator

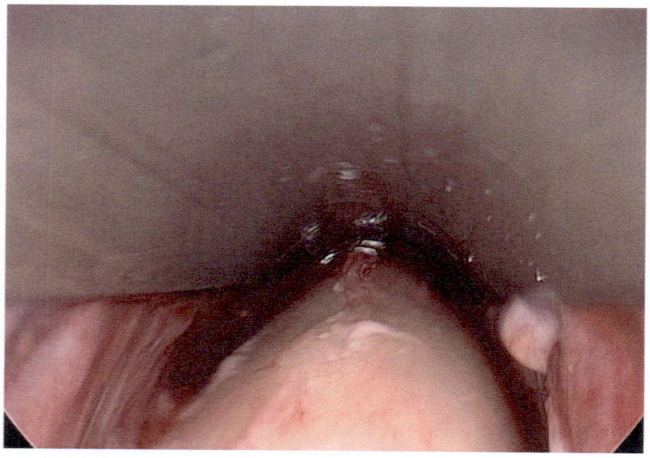

Fig. 19.25 Bony dorsum

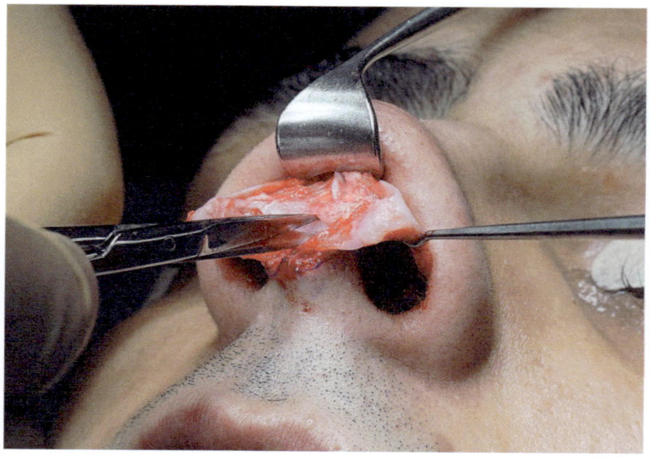

Fig. 19.26 Intercrural dissection is made the caudal aspect of the septum

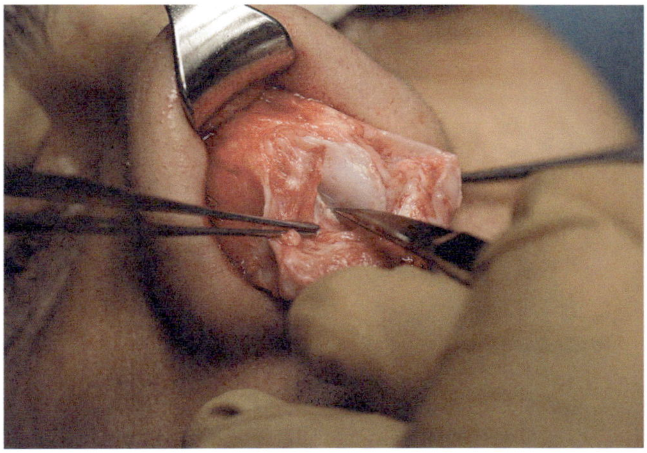

Fig. 19.27 A scissor is used to find the subperichondrial plane

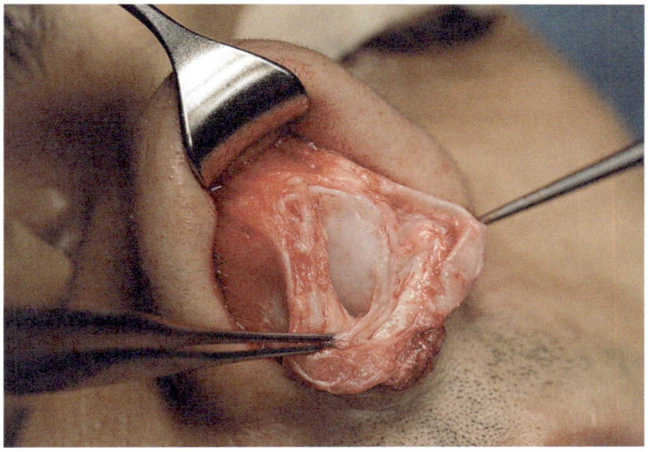

Fig. 19.28 Dissection of the mucoperichondrium

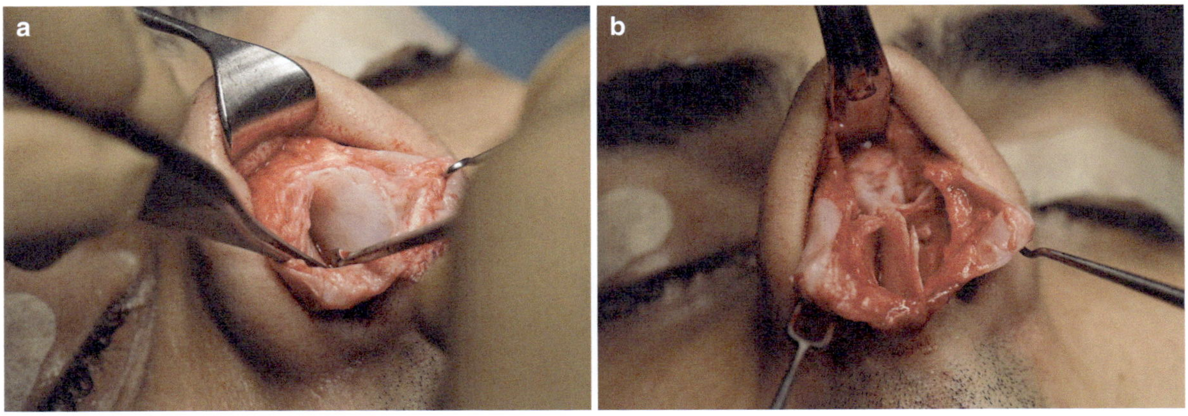

Fig. 19.29 (**a**, **b**) Open approach is completed

19.2.31 Step 31

Septoplasty is performed with preservation of the septal L strut. A large piece of cartilage must be excised en bloc, if possible, for future use as graft material. Then the excised cartilage is put in serum physiologic solution (Fig. 19.30).

19.2.32 Step 32

The maxillary crest at the base is excised with a hammer and gouge osteotome. Once the gouge osteotome is inserted under the crest, it must be advanced parallel to the vestibular base (Fig. 19.31).

19.2.33 Step 33

The dorsum is rechecked after septoplasty; dorsal height may change after septoplasty.

19.2.34 Step 34

The midvault and open roof are reconstructed, if opened (by using a spreader, autospreader, or spreader flap and performing osteotomies as discussed in relevant chapters).

19.2.35 Step 35

Primary tip plasty is performed (as discussed in the relevant chapters). The relationship between the dorsum and the tip is reassessed after tip-plasty to make the necessary corrections, if any.

19.2.36 Step 36

Doyle nasal splints are placed and sutured after surgical corrections have been made.

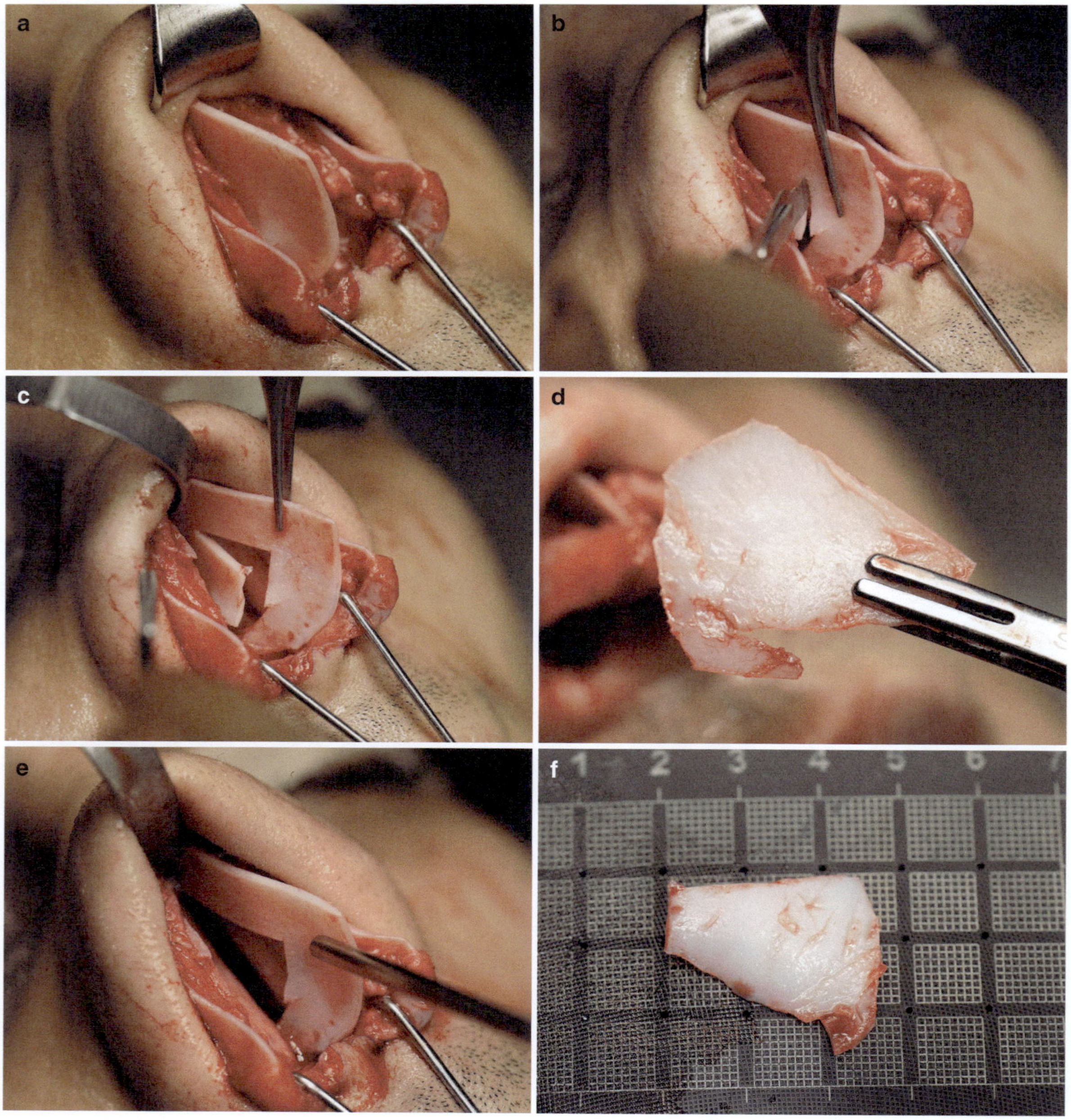

Fig. 19.30 (**a**–**f**) The L-shaped cuts in the septal cartilage are made with a blade, leaving a minimum of 1 cm at the caudal and dorsal support

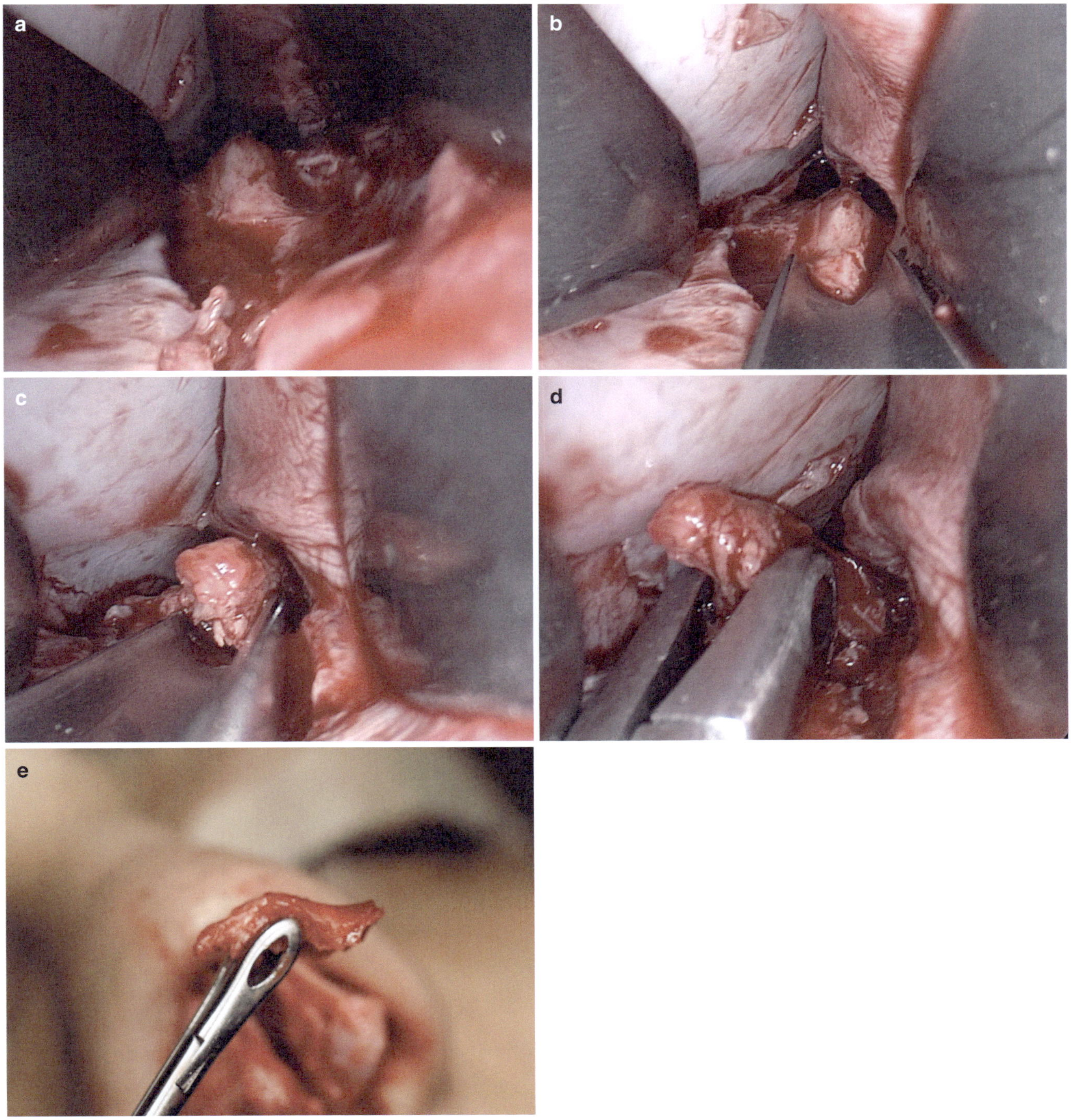

Fig. 19.31 (**a**–**e**) The maxillary crest is removed

19.2.37 Step 37

Skin incisions are sutured end-to-end without applying any tension using 6–0 sharp polypropylene suture material. Sutures must be removed on day 10.

Technical Pearl: As suturing of marginal incisions at the alar region may result in retraction, it is preferable to allow secondary healing to occur.

Technical Pearl: A double-loop mattress suture can be placed in the midline of the columella in cases where the open technique is used to increase projection (Fig. 19.32).

19.2.38 Step 38

The use of benzoin tincture prior to taping the nose improves adherence of the tape, similar to the effect of using an adhesive, and protects the skin from irritation. Porous paper tape must be used for taping. Taping is performed from the tip to the radix. Then, the two ends of the tape are fashioned into a "U" shape at the tip area, starting from the nasal vault, to cover the tip gently and completely (Fig. 19.33).

Technical Pearl: The use of nylon-reinforced strips may later result in edema and cuts in the skin.

19.2.39 Step 39

An aqua thermal nasal splint of sufficient size to cover the nasal bones must be placed on the tape; overtightening of the laterals must be avoided (Fig. 19.34).

Technical Pearl: Although one of the major disadvantages of the open technique is a visible scar at the incision line, the risk of potential scarring and step deformity can be minimized by proper placement of the end-to-end suture, and by supporting the skin flap with a cartilage frame.

Early stage and 5-year postoperative photographs of the columella, properly sutured end-to-end, show barely visible scarring after columellar incision even on close examination (Figs. 19.35 and 19.36).

In open rhinoplasty patients, irregularity of the columella is typically considered to be due to an incision scar. However, the actual cause is uncorrected irregularities of the columellar structure. Lateral view photographs of a case where the open technique was used are presented in Fig. 19.37.

A postoperative photograph (base view) shows seamless restoration of the incision line. Intraoperative photographs show that the irregularity, which seems to be associated with the incision, is actually due to configurational deformities of the columella not being fully corrected (Fig. 19.38).

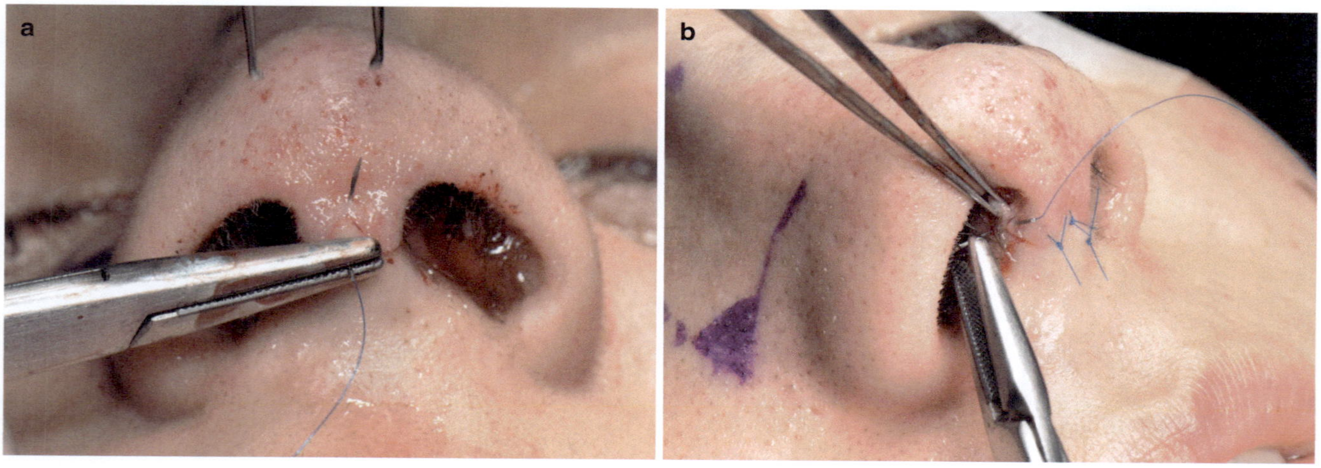

Fig. 19.32 (**a**) Transcolumellar incision is closed. (**b**) The corner is closed meticulously

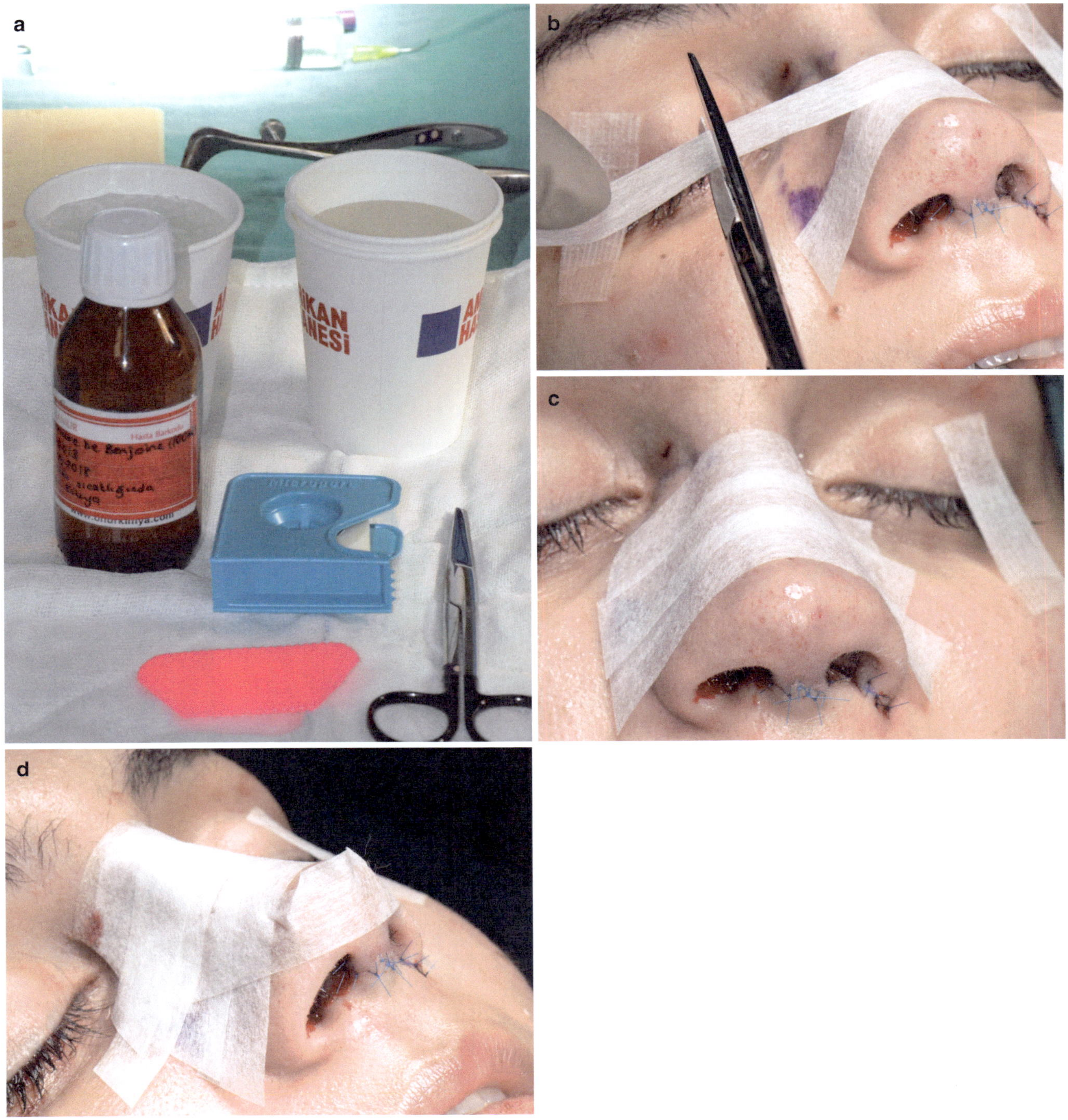

Fig. 19.33 (**a**–**d**) Micropore tape paper helps reduce postoperative edema

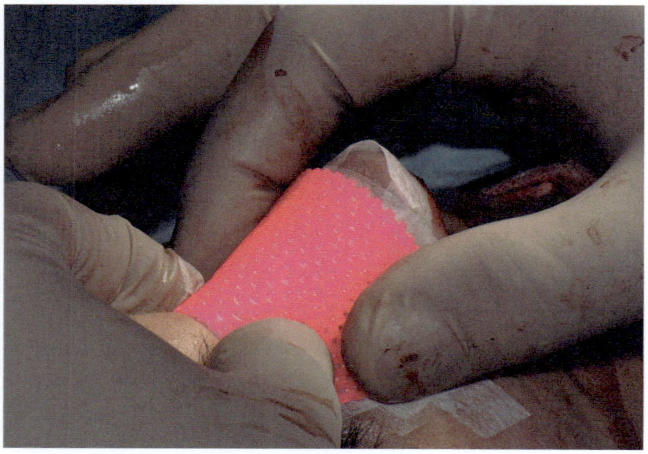

Fig. 19.34 An aquaplast splint is applied

Fig. 19.35 (**a–c**) Preoperative pictures

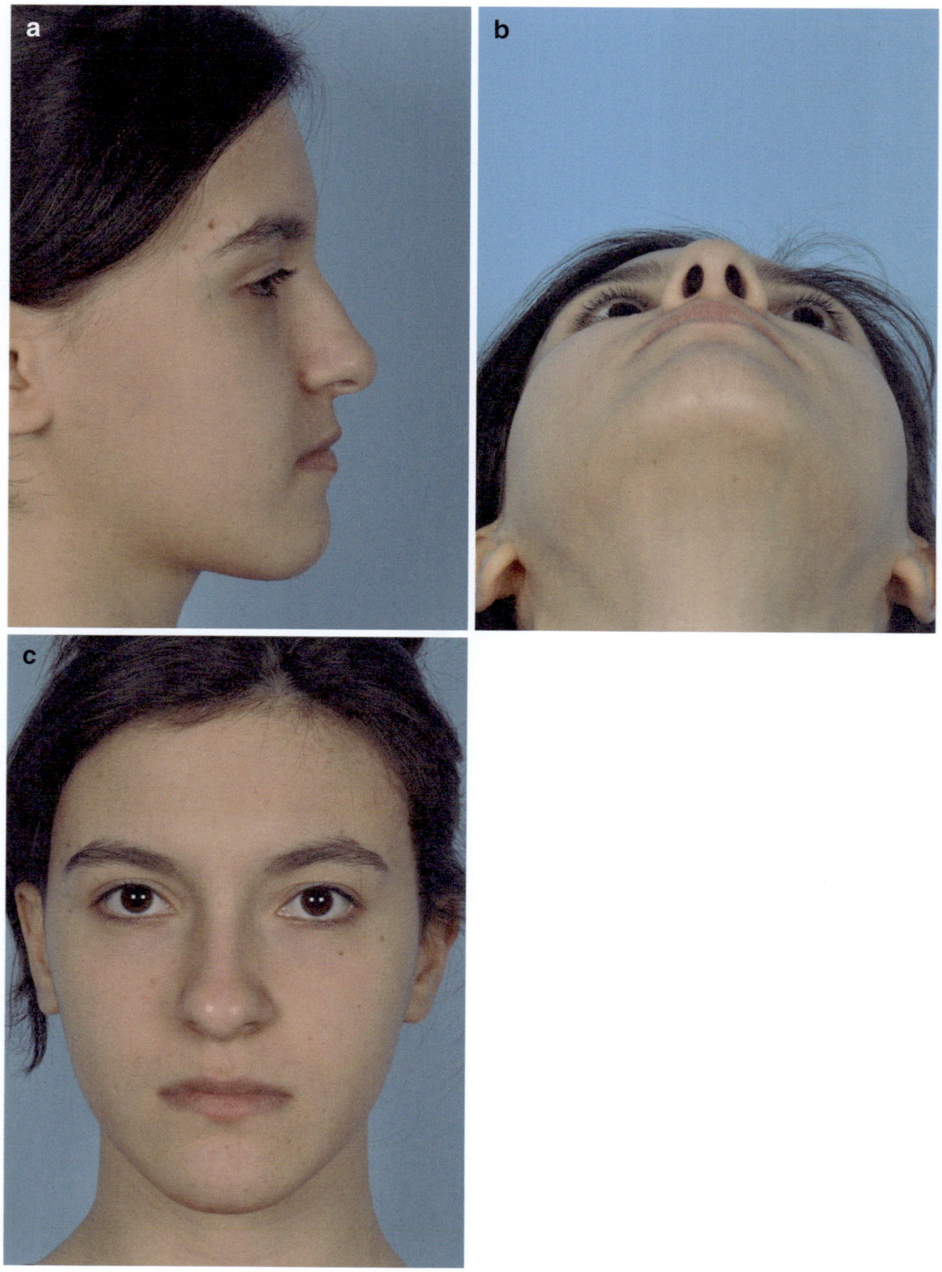

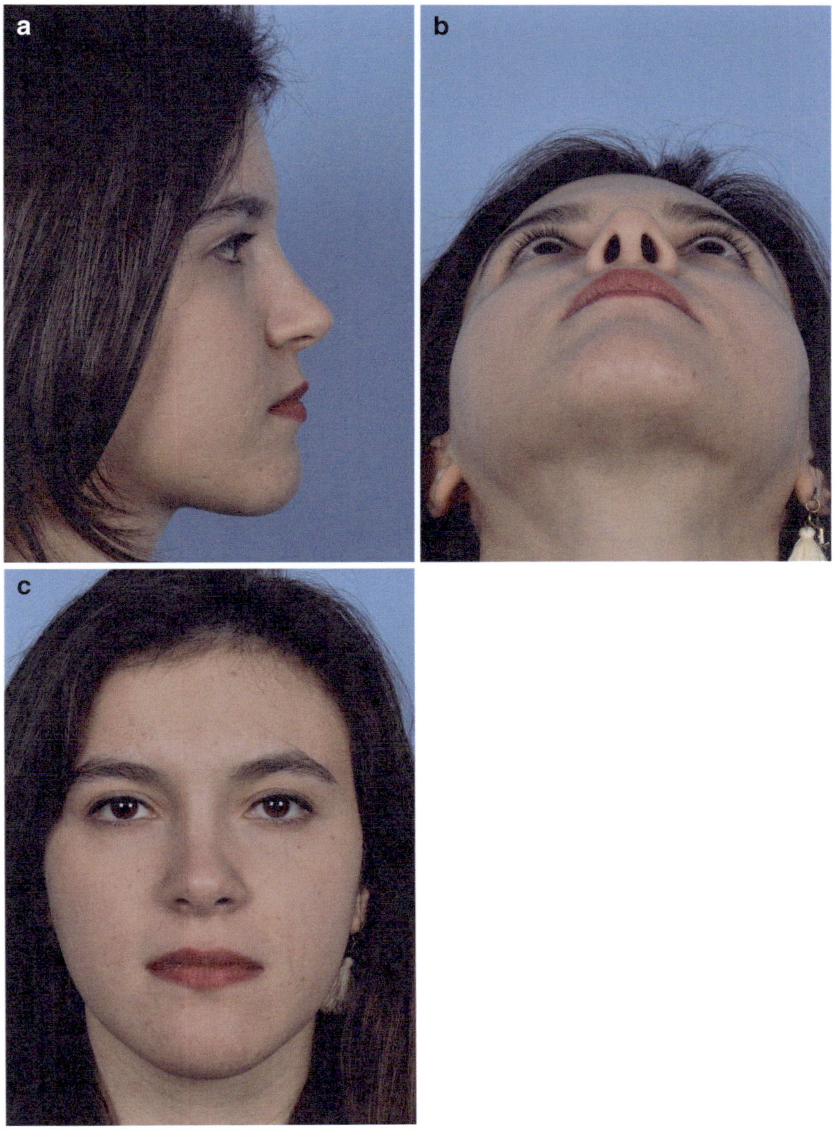

Fig. 19.36 (**a**–**c**) Postoperative pictures: there is no visible scar on the incision line

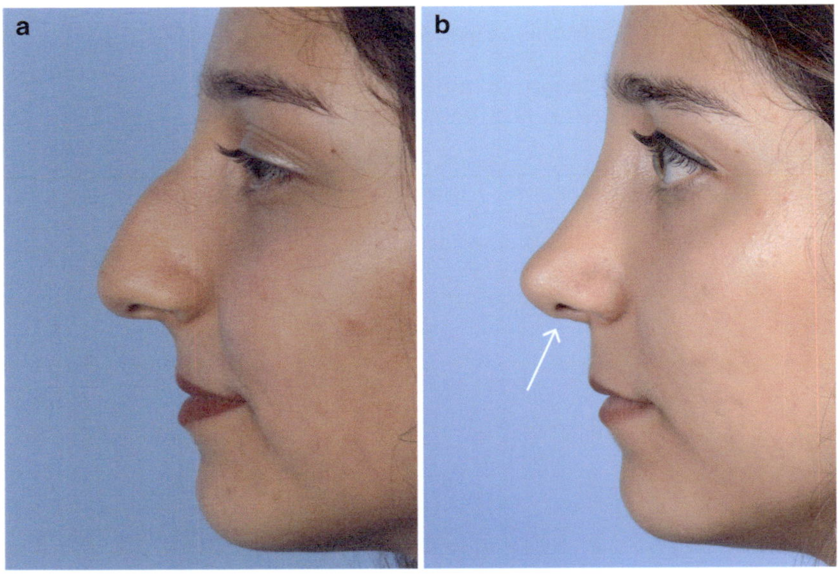

Fig. 19.37 (**a**) Preoperative view. (**b**) Two-year postoperative view

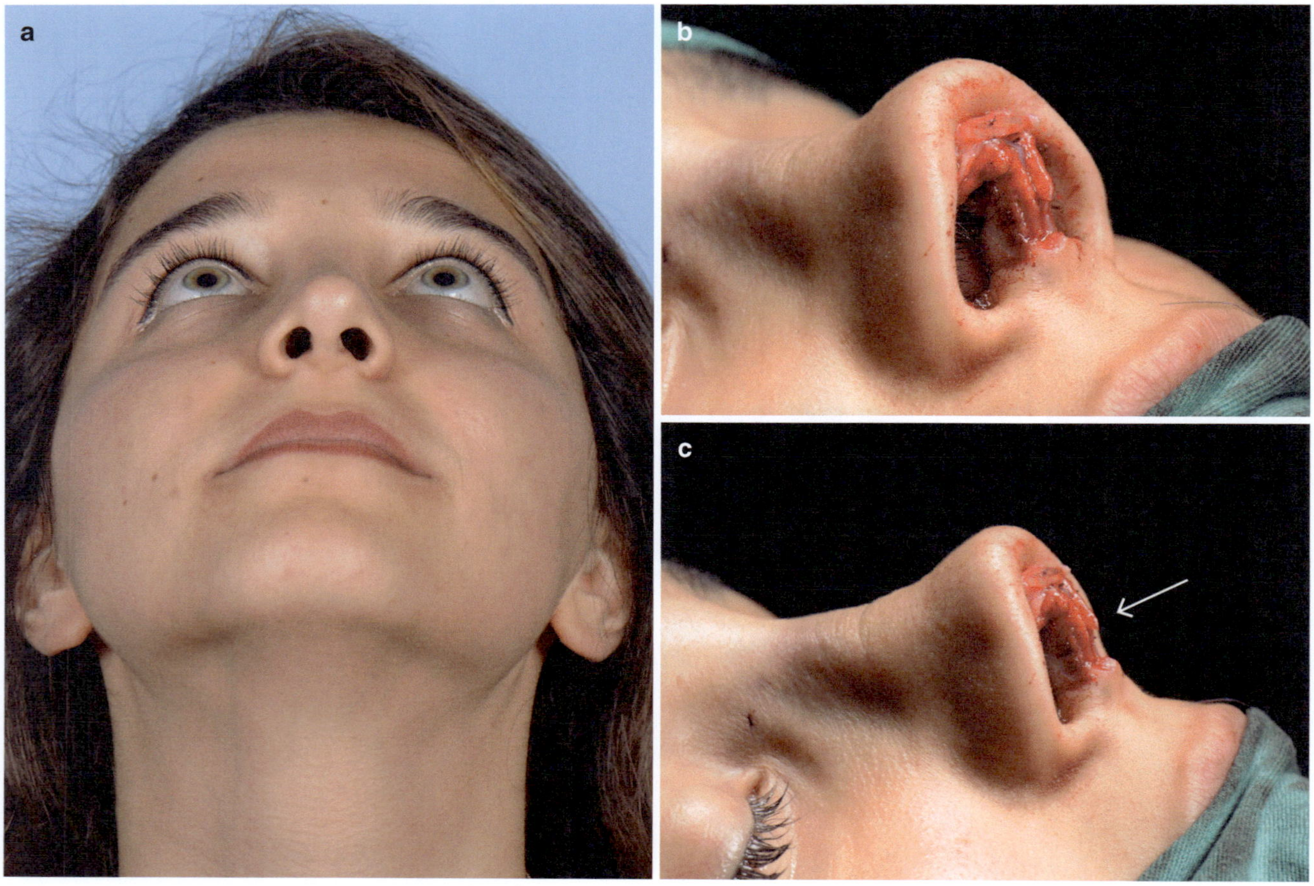

Fig. 19.38 (**a–c**) Postoperative scar-like appearance is not a real scar. Note the intraoperative pictures. It stems from ignored irregularities of the middle crura

Disclosures The author reports no conflicts of interest or funding requiring disclosure.

Further Reading

Adamson PA, Galli SK. Rhinoplasty approaches: current state of the art. Arch Facial Plast Surg. 2005;7(1):32–7.

Adamson PA, Smith O, Tropper GJ. Incision and scar analysis in open (external) rhinoplasty. Arch Otolaryngol Head Neck Surg. 1990;116(6):671–5.

Aksu I, Alim H, Tellioğlu AT. Comparative columellar scar analysis between transverse and inverted-V incision in open rhinoplasty. Aesth Plast Surg. 2008;32(4):638–40.

Cafferty A, Becker DG. Open and closed rhinoplasty. Clin Plast Surg. 2016;43(1):17–27.

Harrison DH. Reflections on the open and closed rhinoplasty. J Plast Reconstr Aesthet Surg. 2013;66(10):1356–9.

Ihvan O, Seneldir L, Naiboglu B, Verim A, Cetiner S. Comparative columellar scar analysis between W incisions and inverted-V incision in open technique nasal surgery. Indian J Otolaryngol Head Neck Surg. 2018;70(2):231–4.

Momeni A, Gruber RP. Primary open rhinoplasty. Aesthet Surg J. 2016;36(9):983–92.

Pitanguy I, Salgado F, Radwanski HN, Bushkin SC. The surgical importance of the dermocartilaginous ligament of the nose. Plast Reconstr Surg. 1995;95(5):790–4.

Rohrich RJ, Afrooz PN. Rhinoplasty refinements: the role of the open approach. Plast Reconstr Surg. 2017;140(4):716–9.

Rohrich RJ, Afrooz PN. Primary open rhinoplasty. Plast Reconstr Surg. 2019;144(1):102e–17e.

Smith O, Goodman W. Open rhinoplasty: its past and future. J Otolaryngol. 1993;22(1):21–5.

Zijlker TD, Adamson PA. Open structure rhinoplasty. Clin Otolaryngol Allied Sci. 1993;18(2):125–34.

20 Step-by-Step Close Approach Rhinoplasty

20.1 Introduction

Preoperative procedures and administration of local anesthetics in the closed technique do not differ from those used with the open technique. Infiltration is performed based on the same principles, and the surgery starts after a minimum of 10 min to allow time for the local anesthetics to take effect.

Meanwhile, hairs on the nasal vestibule skin are removed with a number 15 blade by holding the blade at an angle of around 30–40° to the skin (Fig. 20.1).

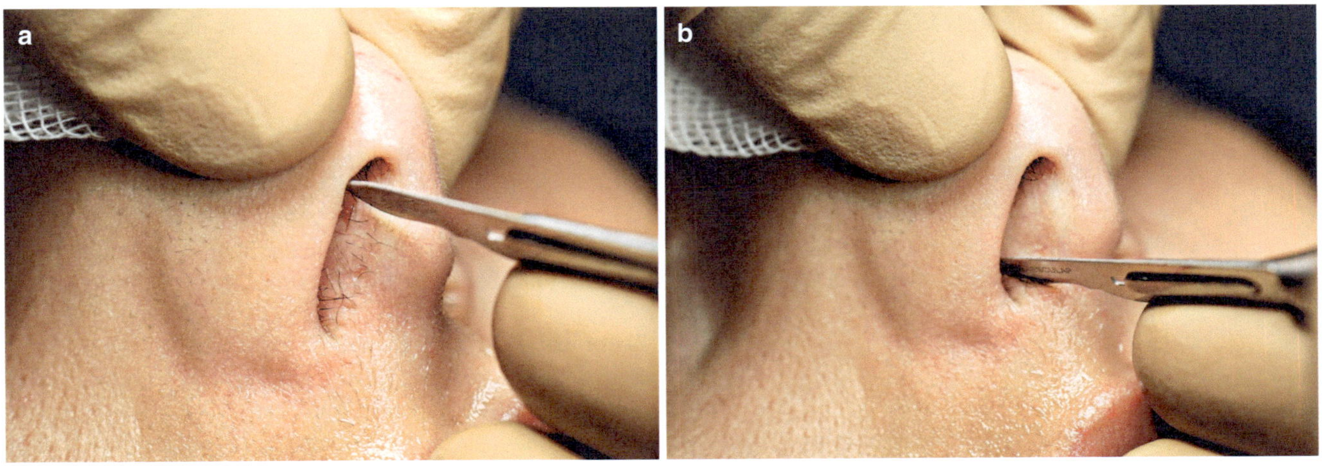

Fig. 20.1 (**a**, **b**) Hairs on the nasal vestibule skin are removed. (Supplementary Video 20.1)

Supplementary Information The online version contains supplementary material available at https://doi.org/10.1007/978-3-031-65619-4_20.

S. Şeneldir, *Photographic Atlas of Rhinoplasty*, https://doi.org/10.1007/978-3-031-65619-4_20

20.2 Steps

After the introductory procedures, the following steps are performed.

20.2.1 Step 1

An incision is made at the left nostril, and the mucosa at the anterior septal angle is slightly stretched to the superior aspect with a retractor. The mucosa is passed through with the help of sharp-pointed scissors (Fig. 20.2).

20.2.2 Step 2

The perichondrium of the dorsal cartilage is reached. Dissection continues at the subperichondrial plane.

20.2.3 Step 3

After subperichondrial dissection of the dorsum, the periosteum of the bone is elevated with a periosteal elevator and a skin flap is created.

20.2.4 Step 4

The hemitransfixion incision is made, and the mucoperichondrium of the septum is elevated with a scissors (Fig. 20.3).

20.2.5 Step 5

The hemitransfixion incision is connected with the dorsal incision at the superior aspect (Fig. 20.4).

Technical Pearl: When necessary, dorsal surgery (reduction or augmentation) is performed. Septoplasty must always be performed after dorsal surgery. (Details are discussed in the relevant chapter.)

20.2.6 Step 6

"L Strut" septoplasty is performed (discussed in the open approach chapter).

20.2.7 Step 7

The lower lateral cartilages are palpated. The caudal margin of the cartilage is identified by sliding the scissors from the cranial aspect to the caudal aspect by applying a slight pressure. Dissection is started by making an incision with a scalpel or directly using converse scissors and is continued at the supraperichondrial plane (Fig. 20.5).

Technical Pearl: The right plane is reached by making a gentle scoring move on the cartilage with sharp-pointed scissors.

20.2.8 Step 8

The assistant retracts the vestibular skin of the cartilage to the inferior aspect using a hook (Fig. 20.6).

Technical Pearl: This maneuver facilitates dissection of the stretched cartilage. Dissection must be performed with due attention and patience. The primary goal here is not to cause any damage to the cartilage. In case of damage, a graft can be used for reconstruction.

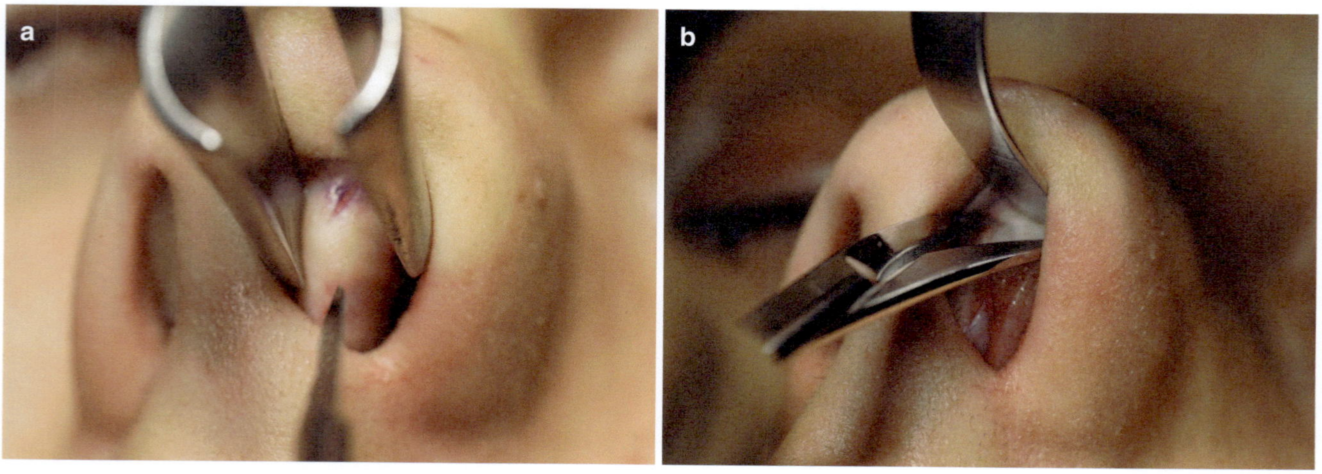

Fig. 20.2 (**a**, **b**) Incision of anterior septal angle and cartilaginous dorsum exposed

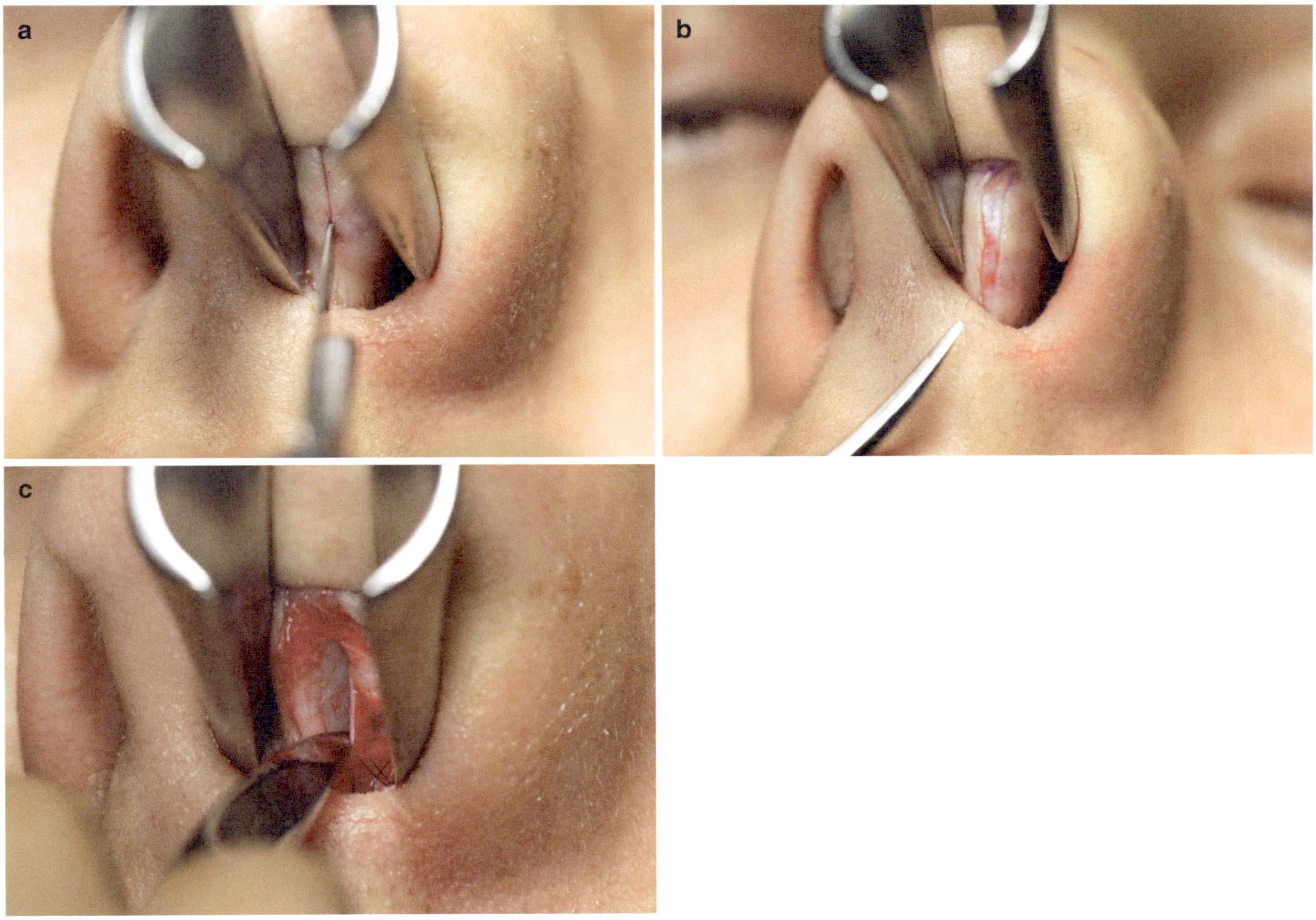

Fig. 20.3 (**a–c**) Hemitransfixion incision is made along the caudal aspect of the septum

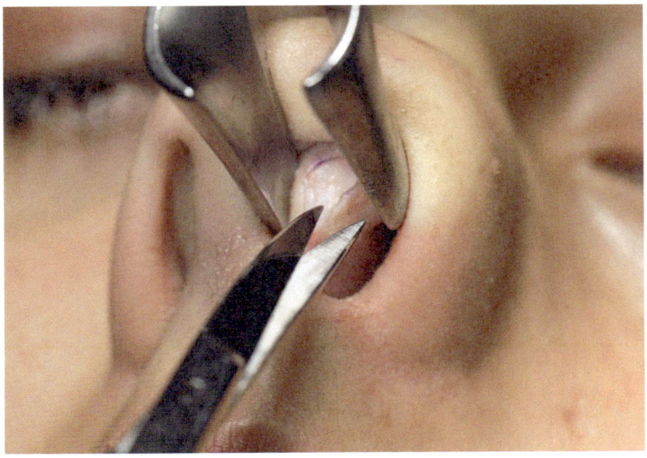

Fig. 20.4 Hemitransfixion incision is connected with the dorsal incision at the superior aspect

20.2.9 Step 9

The skin incision is advanced laterally by saving a cartilaginous portion at the caudal edge of the lower lateral cartilage (Fig. 20.7).

20.2.10 Step 10

While the assistant retracts the dome in the lateral and inferior directions with a hook, the middle crus and medial crus are dissected supraperichondrially (Fig. 20.8).

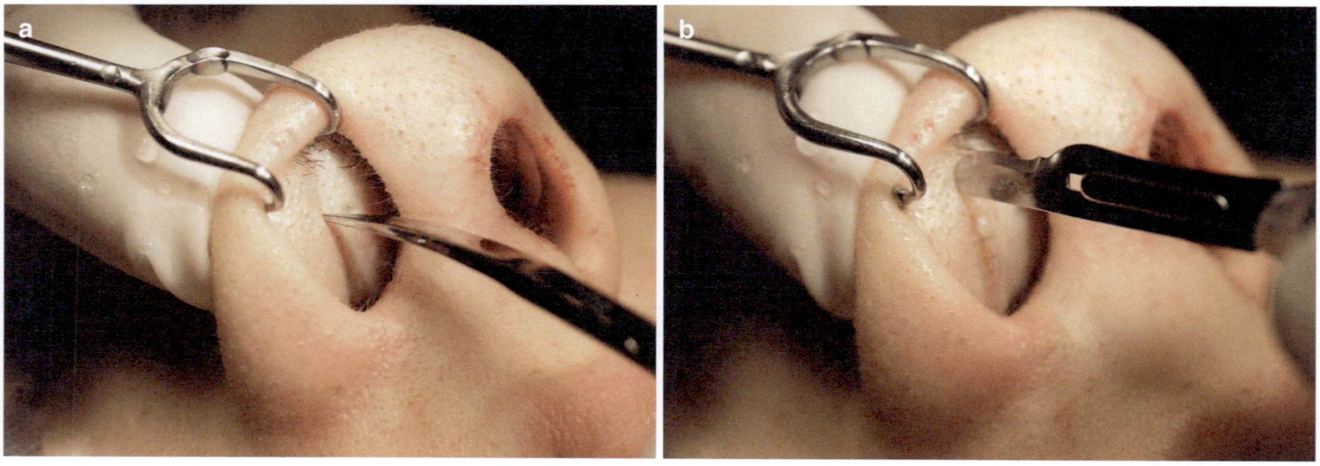

Fig. 20.5 (**a**) Infracartilaginous incision with scissor. (**b**) Infracartilaginous incision with scalpel

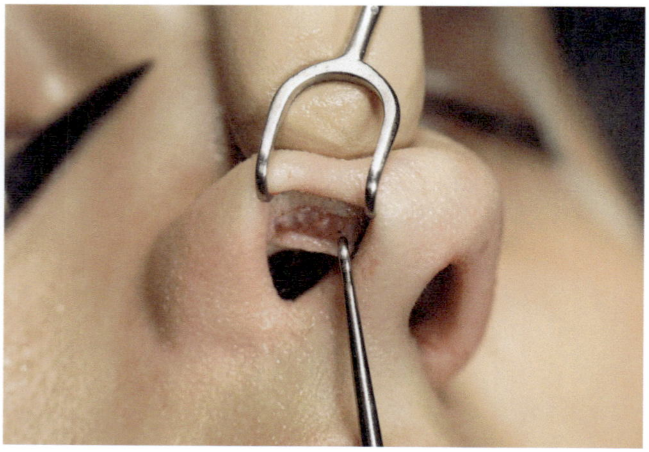

Fig. 20.6 Eversion of the nostril using the double hook provides exposure

20.2.11 Step 11

Following the medial crus dissection, the skin incision is extended to the footplate (Fig. 20.9).

Technical Pearl: The lateral and medial dissections must be performed in a very wide fashion, and the movement of the cartilage must be kept at a maximum. Scroll ligaments or intercrural ligaments are not preserved. On the contrary, they are cut to avoid any traction on the cartilage and skin. Pitanguy's ligament is also cut.

20.2.12 Step 12

Dissection is completed by applying the same procedures on the other alar cartilage (Fig. 20.10).

Technical Pearl: After alar cartilage dissection, both cartilages must be mobilized so they protrude from the contralateral vestibule when manipulated. If any problem occurs, both cartilages must be reassessed, and the surrounding tissues must be fully removed (Fig. 20.11).

20.2.13 Step 13

Primary tip plasty is performed. (Details are discussed in the relevant chapter.)

20.2.14 Step 14

The middle vault is reconstructed, and osteotomies are performed. (Details are discussed in the relevant chapter.)

20.2.15 Step 15

Incisions are individually sutured with absorbable suture material (Fig. 20.12).

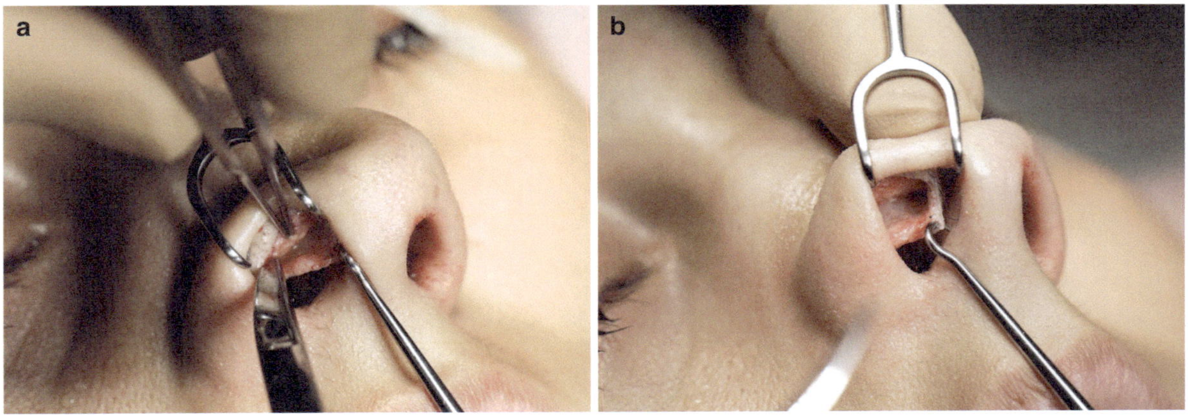

Fig. 20.7 (**a**, **b**) Lateral crural dissection

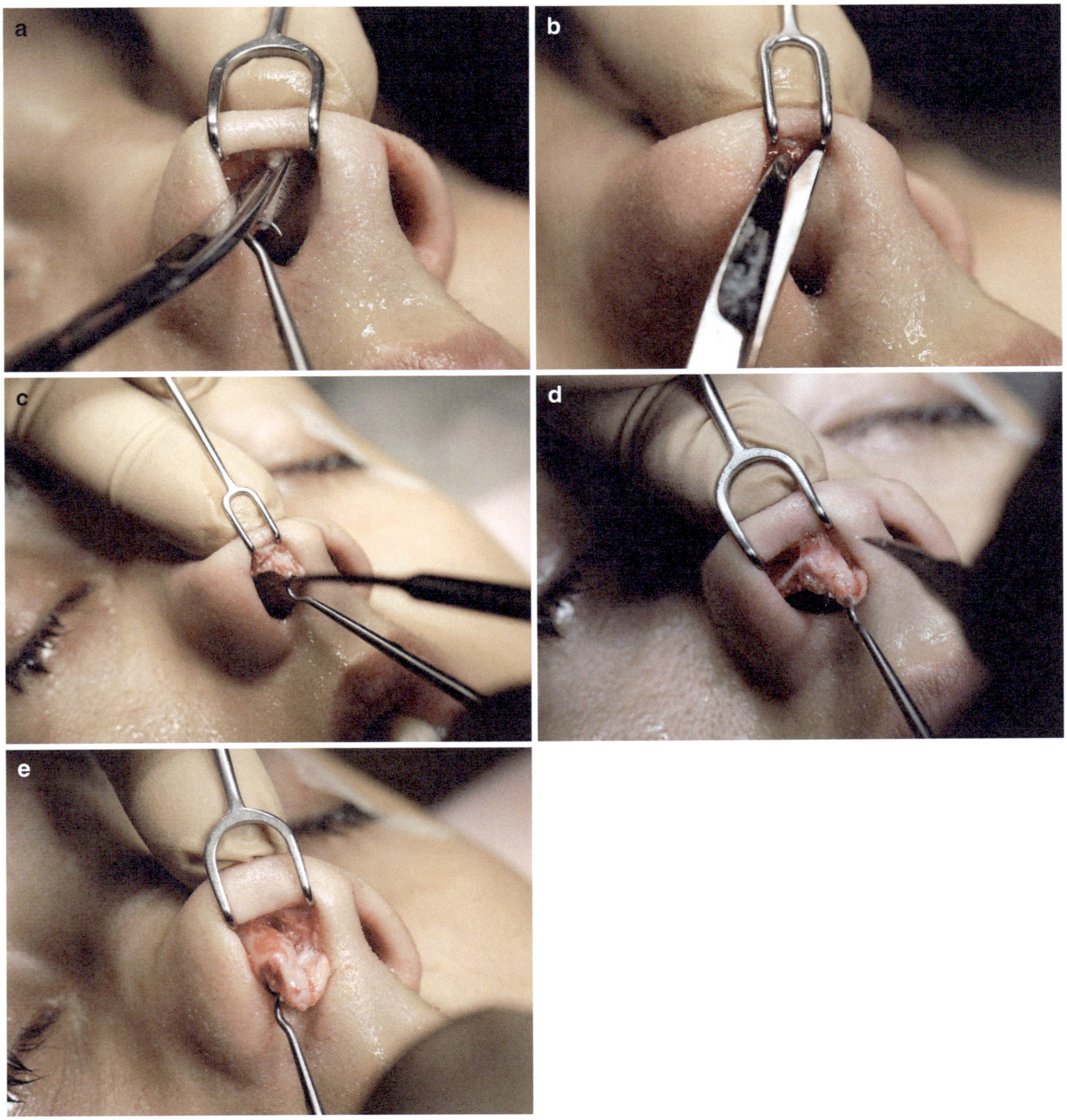

Fig. 20.8 (**a–e**) Medial crural dissection

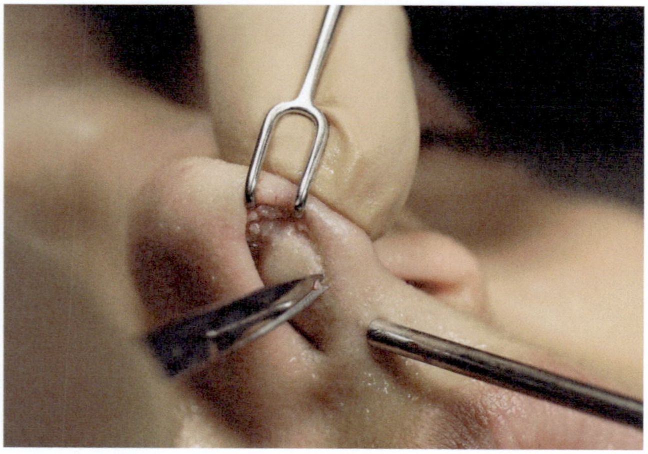

Fig. 20.9 The medial extent of dissection

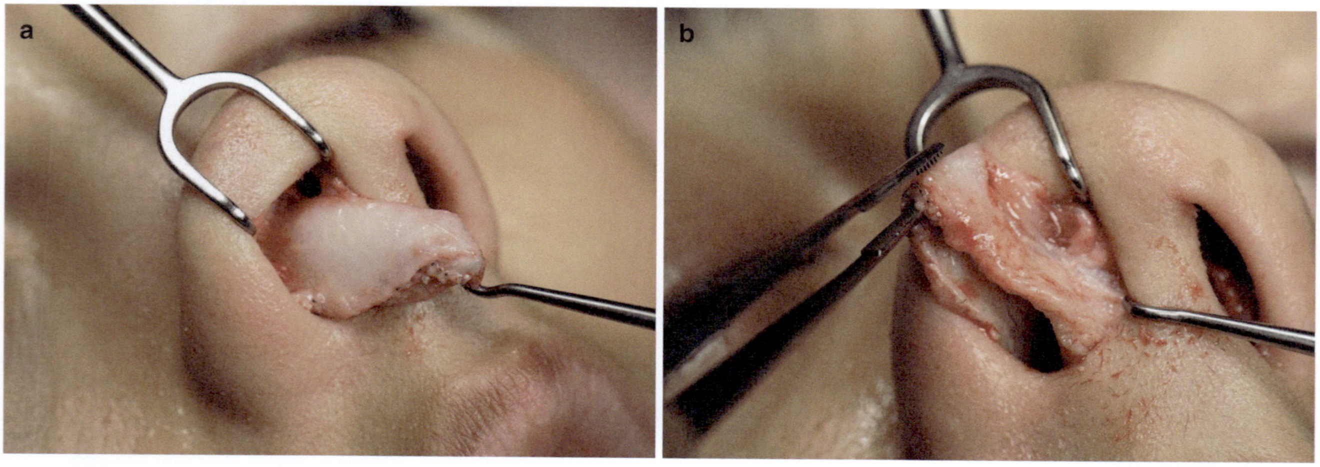

Fig. 20.10 (**a**, **b**) Dissection is completed

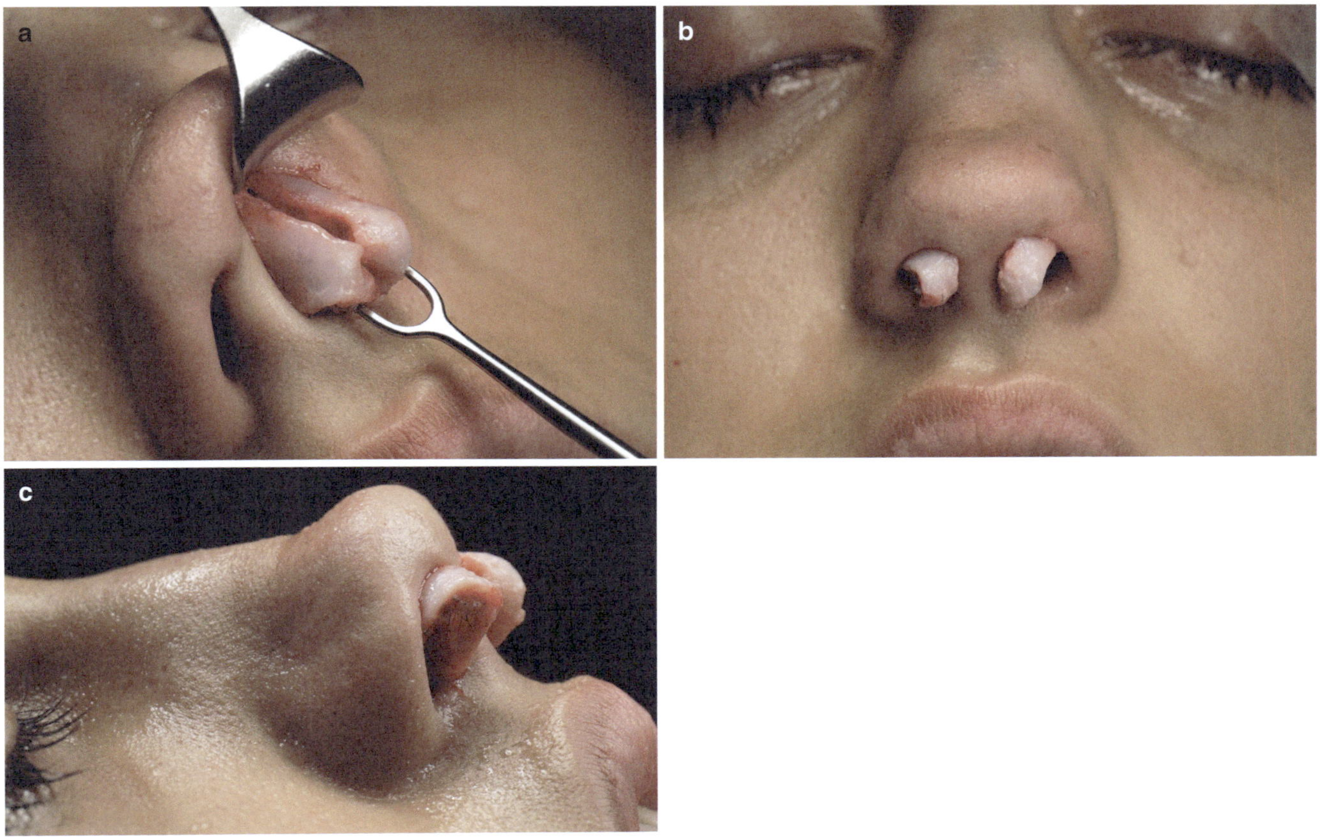

Fig. 20.11 (**a–c**) The alar cartilages in situ

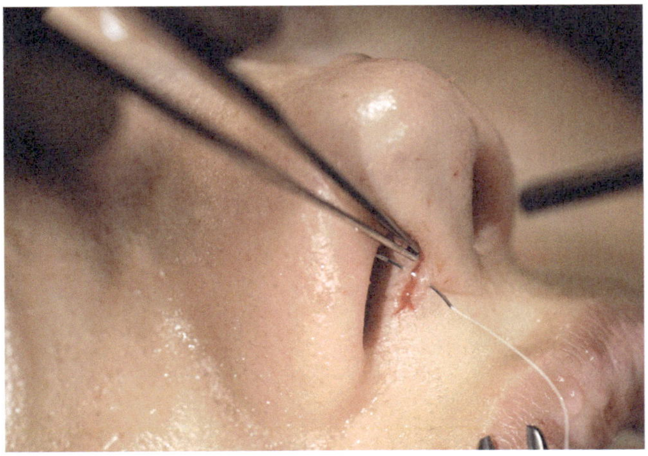

Fig. 20.12 Incisions are individually sutured with absorbable suture material

Disclosures The author reports no conflicts of interest or funding requiring disclosure.

Further Reading

Aksu I, Alim H, Tellioğlu AT. Comparative columellar scar analysis between transverse and inverted-V incision in open rhinoplasty. Aesth Plast Surg. 2008;32(4):638–40.

Bruschi S, Bocchiotti MA, Verga M, Kefalas N, Fraccalvieri M. Closed rhinoplasty with marginal incision: our experience and results. Aesth Plast Surg. 2006;30(2):155–8.

Cafferty A, Becker DG. Open and closed rhinoplasty. Clin Plast Surg. 2016;43(1):17–27.

Harrison DH. Reflections on the open and closed rhinoplasty. J Plast Reconstr Aesthet Surg. 2013;66(10):1356–9.

Ihvan O, Seneldir L, Naiboglu B, Verim A, Cetiner S. Comparative columellar scar analysis between W incisions and inverted-V incision in open technique nasal surgery. Indian J Otolaryngol Head Neck Surg. 2018;70(2):231–4.

Pitanguy I, Salgado F, Radwanski HN, Bushkin SC. The surgical importance of the dermocartilaginous ligament of the nose. Plast Reconstr Surg. 1995;95(5):790–4.

21 Ask the Author: Questions and Answers in Rhinoplasty Surgery

1. **What is your opinion of the dorsum preservation technique?**

   The dorsum preservation technique can be used for the unproblematic dorsum. I used to choose it for cases like the one shown in Fig. 21.1. No problems are observed in the profile or frontal view, except a slight curve.

   In the short term, the results were satisfying. However, in such cases, I experienced two main problems after 6 months:

   (a) Widening of the middle vault over time
   (b) Supra tip depression

   Patients complained of both of these problems and were upset.

   Focus on the depression and splaying expands gradually over time on the midvault, as shown Fig. 21.2.

   As I have observed in my practice, a hump can recur in some cases, especially when a bony hump is apparent. I present an example in Fig. 21.3.

   As you can clearly see, the dorsum appears straight intraoperatively. However, 1 year later, a dorsal hump recurred.

   I also believe that the risk of cerebrospinal fluid (CSF) rhinorrhea is higher than with the dorsal reduction technique.

   Ultimately, I stopped using the dorsal preservation technique.

2. **If the patient has filler in the nose, when is the right time for nasal surgery?**

   If hyaluronic acid is used, the operation can be performed no matter when the filler was made. It is not necessary to soften it with hyaluronidase. At the start of surgery, on performing the incision and dissection, the filling flows out. In noses with filler, it can be difficult to analyze the previous problems preoperatively. This condition may affect our surgical plan (Fig. 21.4).

3. **Do you recommend a cortisone injection for persistent edema in the radix or supratip area?**

   A corticosteroid injection in this area can definitely be beneficial. I base my decision to perform an injection on whether the swelling is edema or bone or cartilage that has not been lowered. Steroids do not work when the fullness is caused by excess cartilage in the supratip area or bone in the radix that has not been lowered sufficiently. In this area, it works well for edema of the subcutaneous tissue. In my practice, I dilute one ampule of triamcinolone acetonide with a patent medicine in 5 mL of serum. For this area, I extract 1 mL of insulin into an injector and inject 2–3 U into the area. I sometimes repeat the process every 3 weeks until I get results.

4. **Do you protect the nose ligaments?**

   The role of the ligaments in a non-operated nose is clear. However, I have found that after the anatomy of the alar cartilage has been changed at surgery, the remaining ligaments can cause two problems:

   (a) They obstruct the settlement of the skin in the newly formed alar-arch anatomy; this can be seen intraoperatively. I observed that if the pots formed by ligaments were not cut when the alar arch was reformed, the cartilage did not settle on the skin.
   (b) I like ligaments in non-operated noses, but I do not rely on them as a carrier in the postoperative period. I do not think that they have enough strength to carry the newly formed structure in operated noses and fulfill the role that they serve in non-operated noses. In my practice, I have observed that the projection and rotation of the nose has been lost in the operations I performed that relied on the strength of the ligaments.

   I will show you a case in Fig. 21.5. In this case, I preserved the ligaments using the closed approach. You can see the short- and long-term postoperative results.

   As seen in the intraoperative photograph, the results are satisfactory. However, note the projection and rotation loss that occurred over time. I believed that the strength of

Supplementary Information The online version contains supplementary material available at https://doi.org/10.1007/978-3-031-65619-4_21.

S. Şeneldir, *Photographic Atlas of Rhinoplasty*, https://doi.org/10.1007/978-3-031-65619-4_21

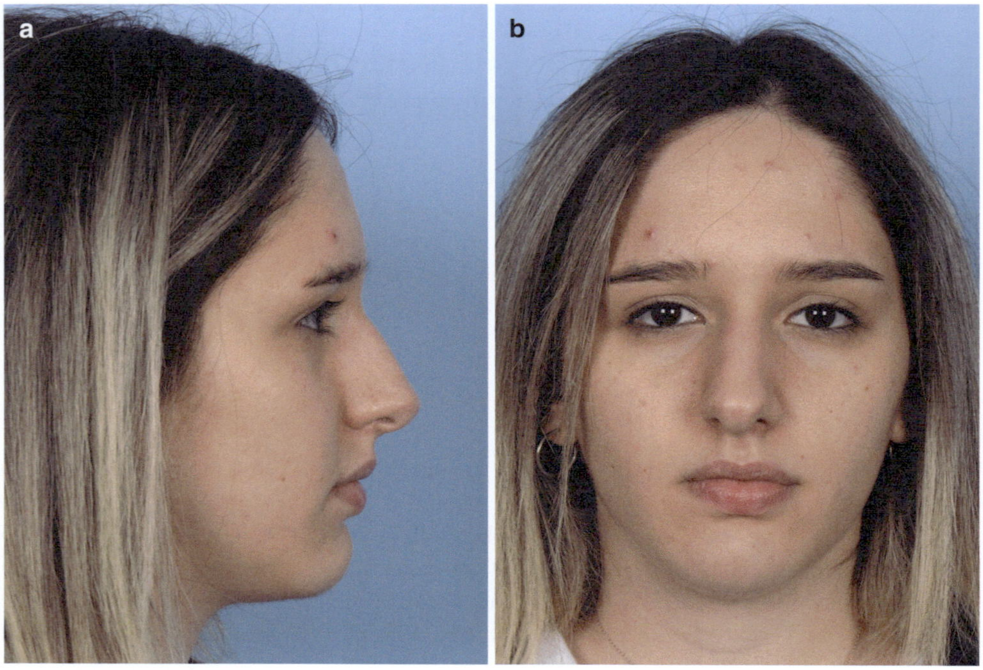

Fig. 21.1 (**a**, **b**) A 21-year-old woman wanted to reduce the size of her nose. The nasal bone, K-point area, and cartilaginous dorsum were all slightly high

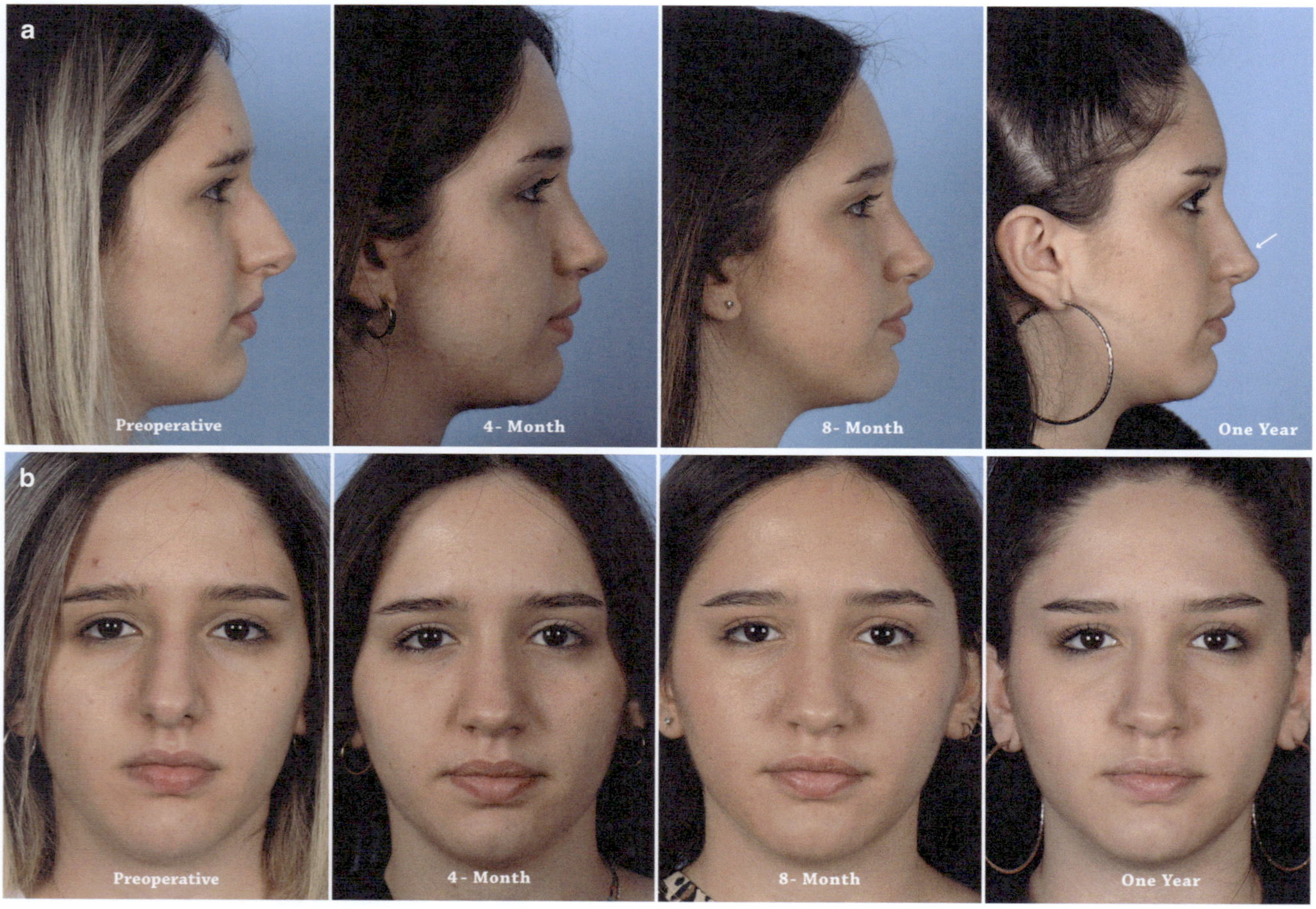

Fig. 21.2 (**a**, **b**) Preoperative and then 4-month, 8-month, and 1-year postoperative images are shown. During this period, supra tip depression in profile views and widening middle vault in frontal view have occurred

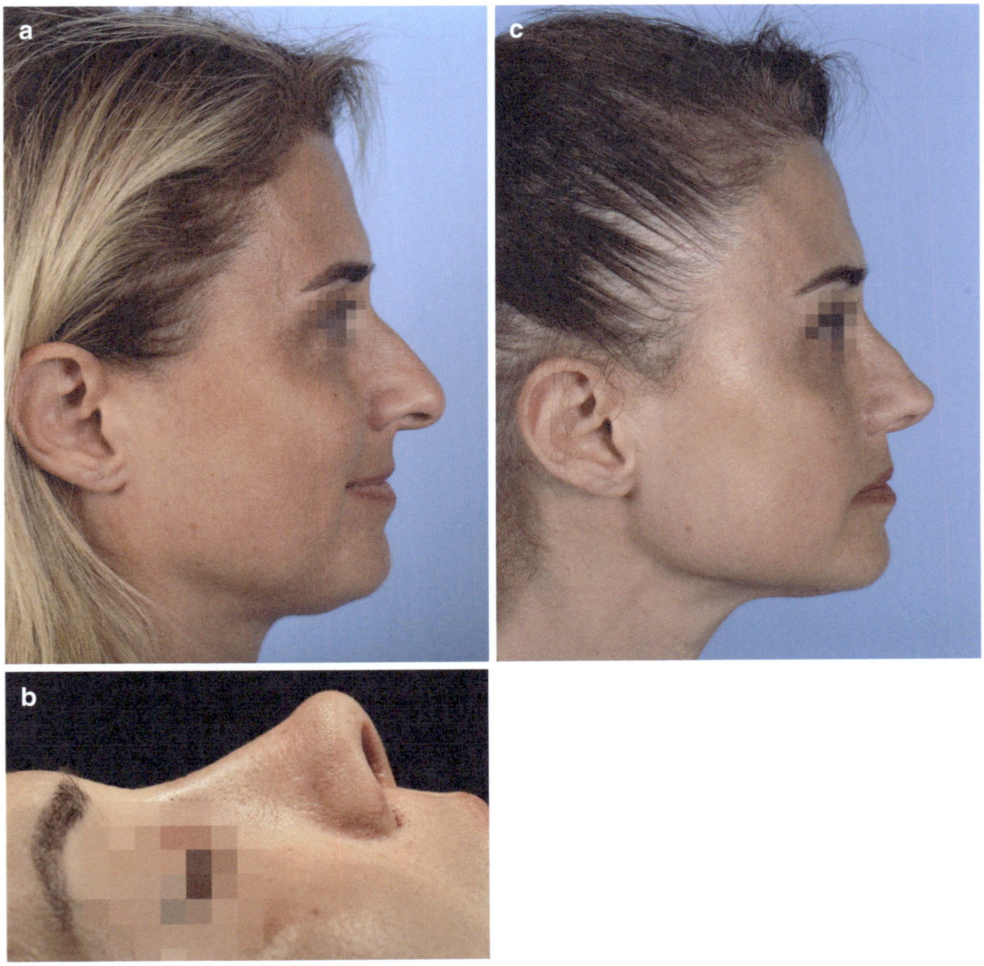

Fig. 21.3 (**a**) Patient complained about nasal bridge. (**b**, **c**) The dorsum preservation technique was used. Immediate postoperative appearance: the hump has been eliminated. (**c**) One year after the dorsal hump has reappeared

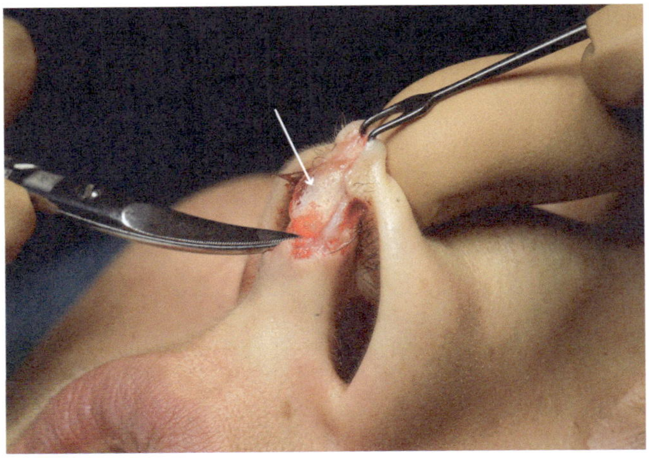

Fig. 21.4 After dissection the filler flows out. (Supplementary Video 21.1)

the ligaments in this case did not meet my expectations. I should have used my own structural techniques.

5. **Which do you prefer: An open approach or endonasal approach?**

   The long-term results are important in rhinoplasty. The results in the first year are early results. One might think that the closed approach is advantageous because the recovery in the first year is faster. However, as I mentioned above, the permanent results are more important, as I have observed in my practice. If the permanent result after 1 year is unsatisfactory, it does not matter which approach you choose. The advantage of the closed technique is the speed of the surgery. The advantage of the open technique is that the operation can be done under direct vision. Beginning surgeons can perform the operation easily under direct vision.

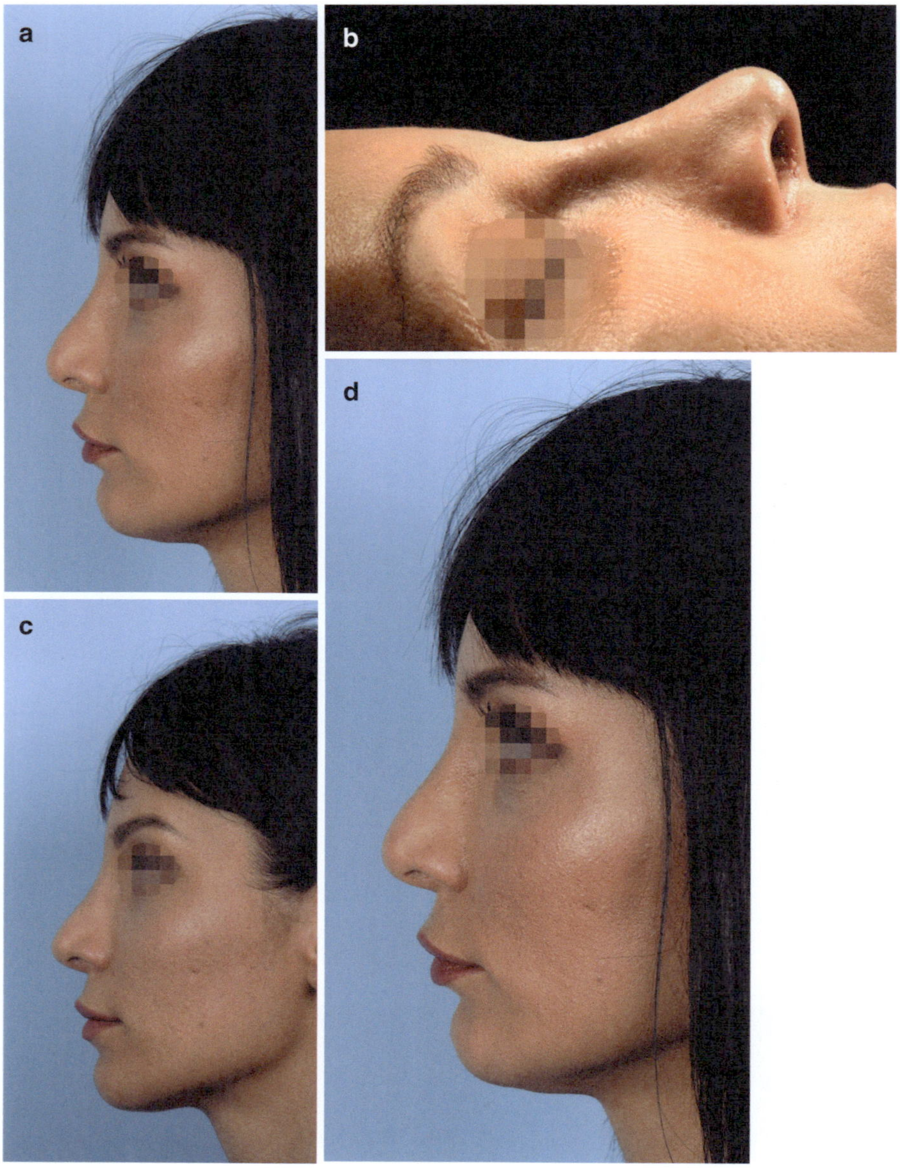

Fig. 21.5 (**a**) Preoperative lateral view. (**b**) The ligament preservation technique was used for shaping the tip. Immediate postoperative appearance. (**c**, **d**) Note the projection and rotation loss that occurred over time

After this brief consideration of the pros and cons, I would like to mention my practice. According to my understanding of rhinoplasty, success does not result from the approach chosen. If we expect a satisfying result, we must analyze the anatomic problems of the nose and learn which techniques can be used as a solution. If we cannot realize a solution, the technique used is not important. If the underlying anatomy is analyzed properly, maximum results can be reached with minor interventions. The main problem is observed with the dorsal hump. The patient in Fig. 21.6 complained of the size of his nose. When the tip of the nose is examined, it is almost perfect. In this nose, neither an open approach nor touching the cartilage at the tip using a delivery approach is needed.

It is sufficient to remove the nasal hump from the anterior septal angle with a small incision and place a one-sided graft at the incision and then perform osteotomies (Fig. 21.7).

Let's look at the postoperative photos (Fig. 21.8). All the problems were solved by closing the dorsum with a limited cut. If the goal is a natural, straight nose, it has been attained completely.

Let us examine another example (Fig. 21.9). In this case, there is a slight dorsal hump and a wide nasal tip that is slightly under-projected. Neither an open approach nor a closed approach is needed in this case. Ideal results are possible with small touches. A two-sided spreader graft is fixed by removing the hump with a small incision in the anterior septal angle. Then, an onlay tip graft is placed in an incision right in front of the dome.

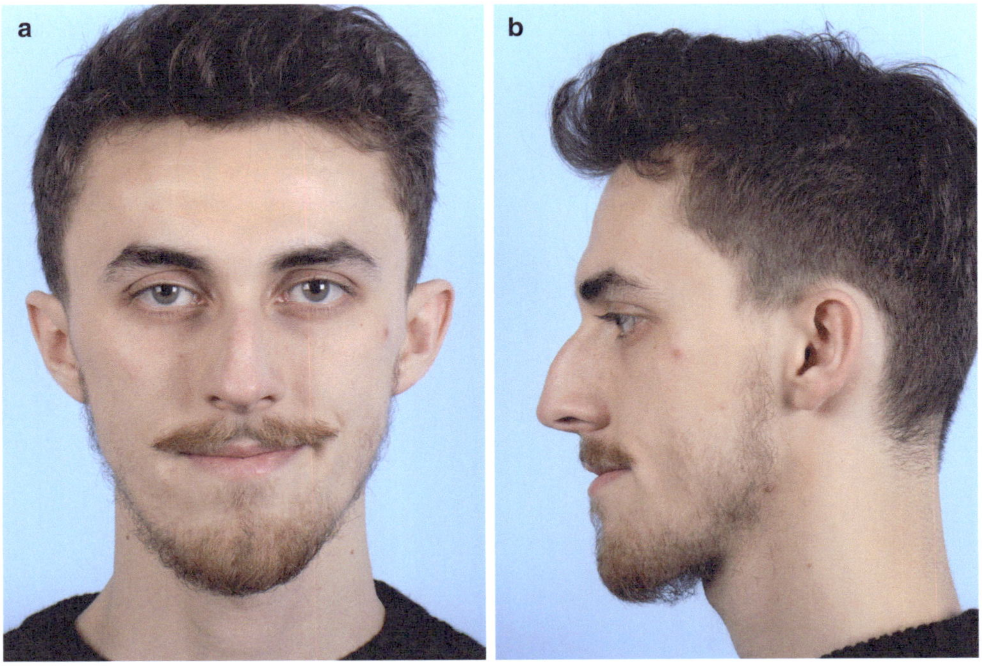

Fig. 21.6 (**a**, **b**) A 25-year-old patient: he has a prominent dorsal hump. The tip projection, rotation, and tip width are aesthetically pleasing

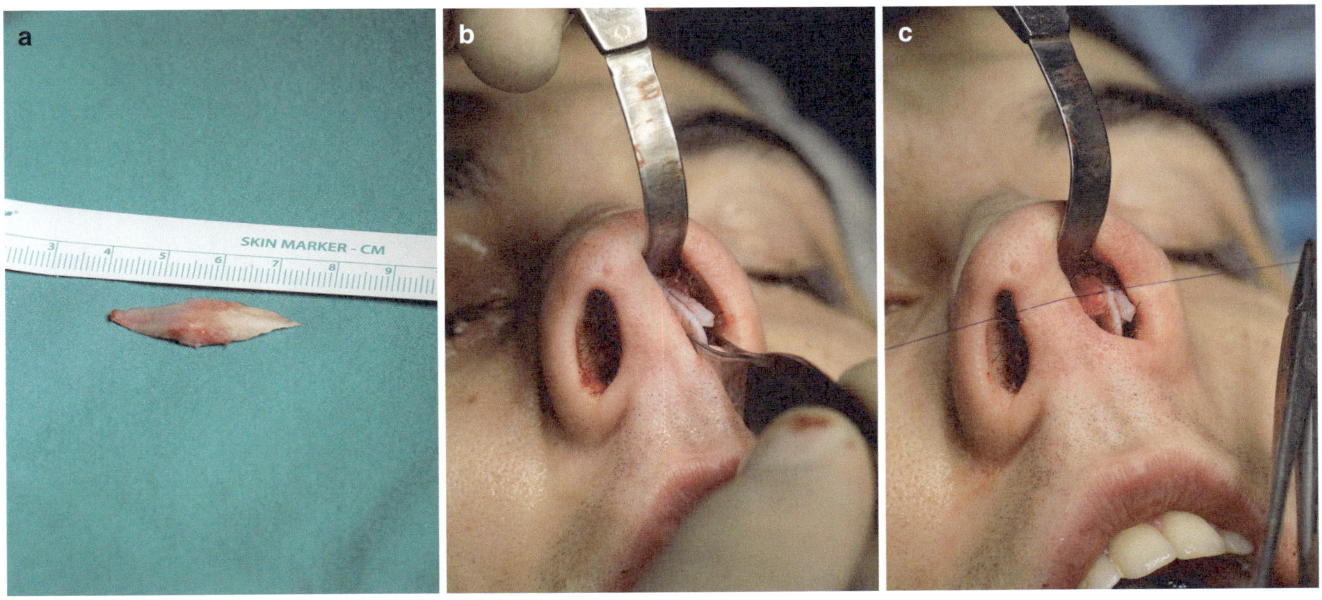

Fig. 21.7 (**a**) Dorsal hump. (**b**, **c**) Spreader graft placement via endonasal approach

6. **Do you irrigate the surgical field intraoperatively?**

   I used to irrigate the surgical field in order to have a cleaner area. However, after realizing that it causes swelling and disrupts my perception, I do it only when closing the skin incisions.

7. **What do you prefer as suture materials?**

   I prefer 5/0 or 6/0 nonabsorbable sutures for shaping the tip. I avoid using absorbable sutures for transdomal and lateral crural steal sutures, which alter the cartilage configuration. I prefer absorbable sutures while fixing any grafts, such as a cup, spreader, or columellar strut graft because they impose no burden or resistance. The most important benefit is that the possibility of absorption by the mucosa or skin does not carry any risks.

8. **Are there any risks when using the VAR technique in thin-skinned cases?**

   Vertical alar resection (VAR) can be performed regardless of the skin type given the proper indications. An onlay tip graft should generally be used after the VAR technique. In thin-skinned cases, the onlay tip

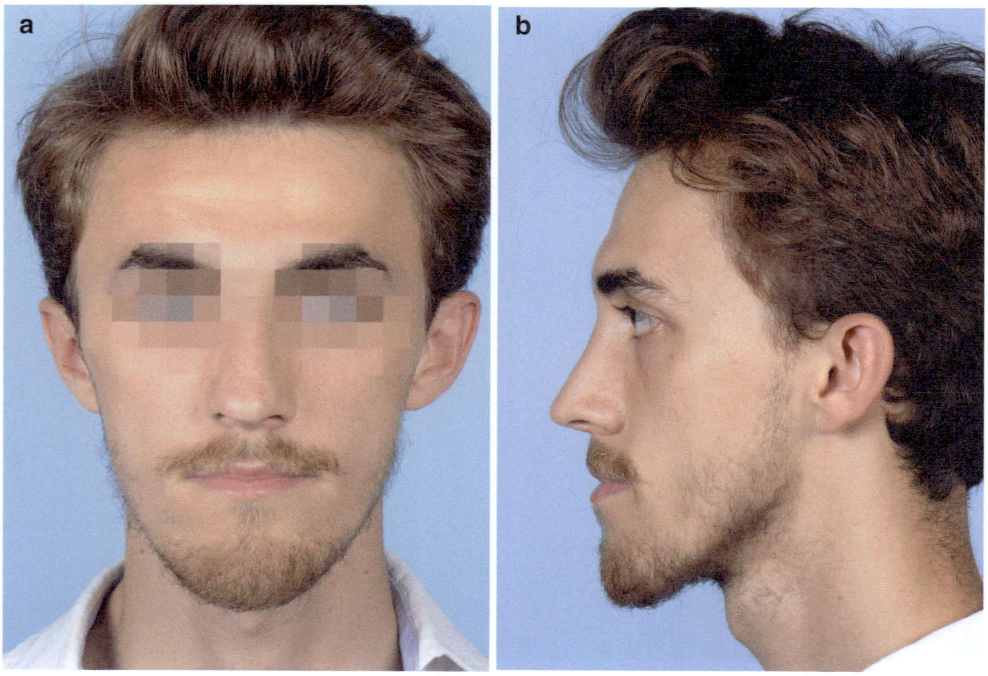

Fig. 21.8 (**a**, **b**) Correcting the dorsum allowed for a natural-looking nose without violating the integrity of the alar cartilages

Fig. 21.9 (**a**, **b**) Preoperative profile and frontal views. (**c**) After hump removal, bilateral spreader grafts were placed. (**d**) Onlay tip graft. (**e**) Small incision. (**f**) Creating small pocket over the dome. (**g**) Onlay tip graft inserted. (**h**, **i**) Postoperative images

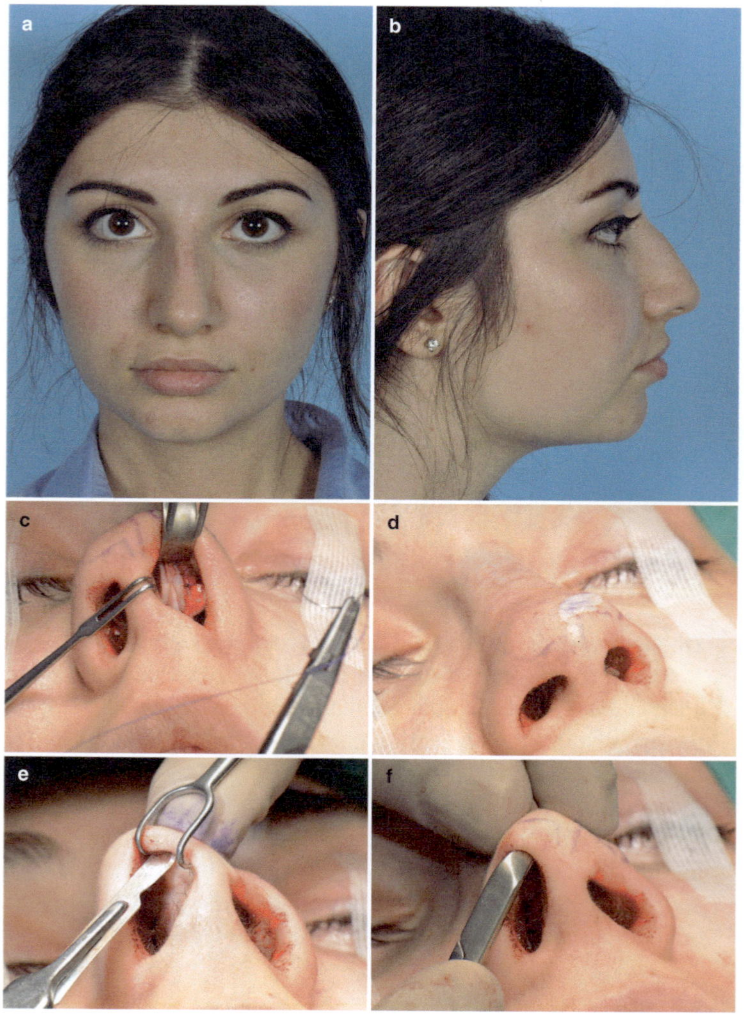

Fig. 21.9 (continued)

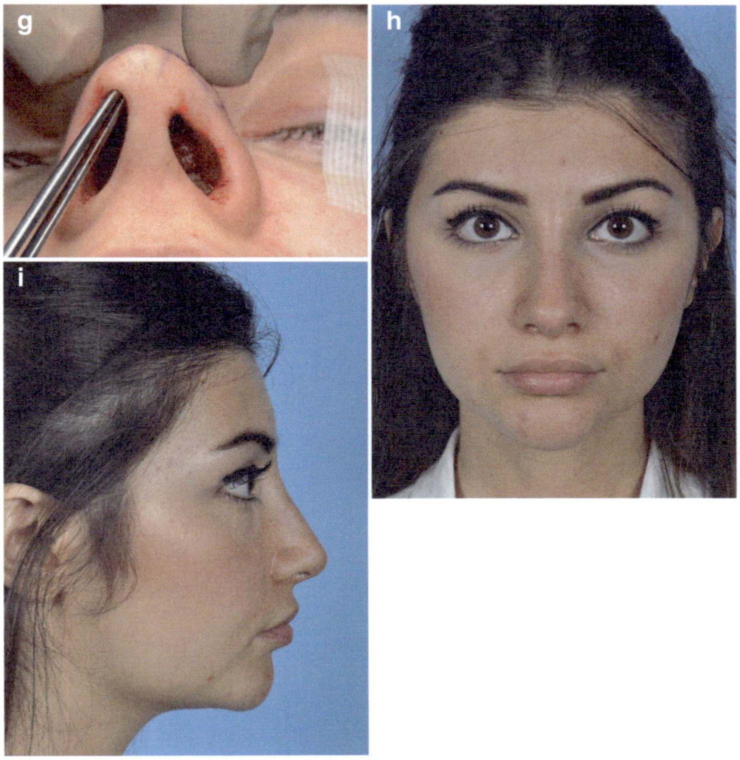

graft should be camouflaged. In thick-skinned cases, camouflage is not necessary. This thin-skinned patient complained that the tip of the nose appeared to droop (Fig. 21.10).

Poor tip rotation secondary to lateral crura excess. The VAR technique was used to shorten the lateral crura (Fig. 21.11).

Photographs 6 years postoperatively show no visible irregularity through the skin/soft tissue envelope (Fig. 21.12).

9. **Should I trim alar rim irregularities after rhinoplasty?**

   In corrective rhinoplasty, the skeletal structures and mucosal lining are reduced leaving only the covering skin without tailoring. In most cases, the skin will adjust; with severe skeletal reduction, wide skin undermining will allow the redistribution of excess skin out onto the cheeks with no unattractive sequelae. Occasionally, however, the excess residual skin after cartilage reduction may be reflected in a strange peripheral pileup. Marginal sculpturing can be used to refine the discrepancies as the postoperative irregularities of the alar rims are symmetrized (Fig. 21.13).

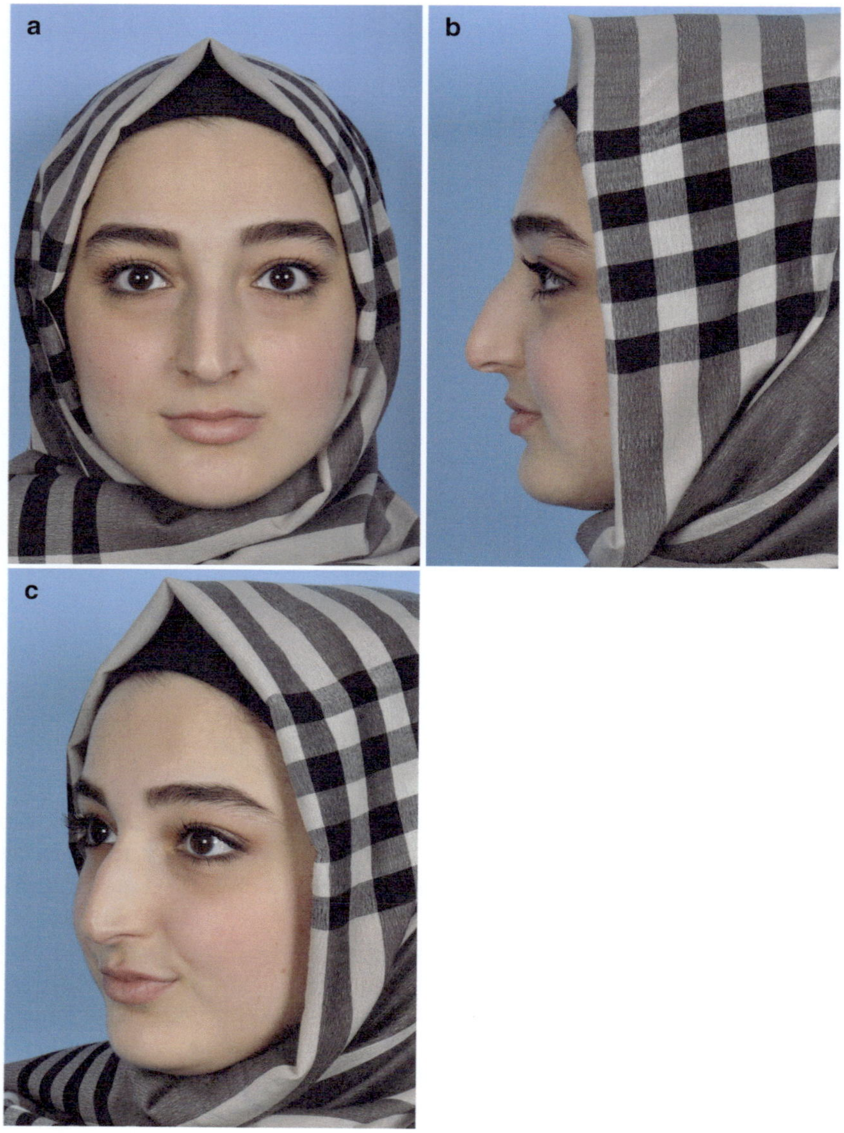

Fig. 21.10 (**a**–**c**) Droopy nasal tip with thin skin

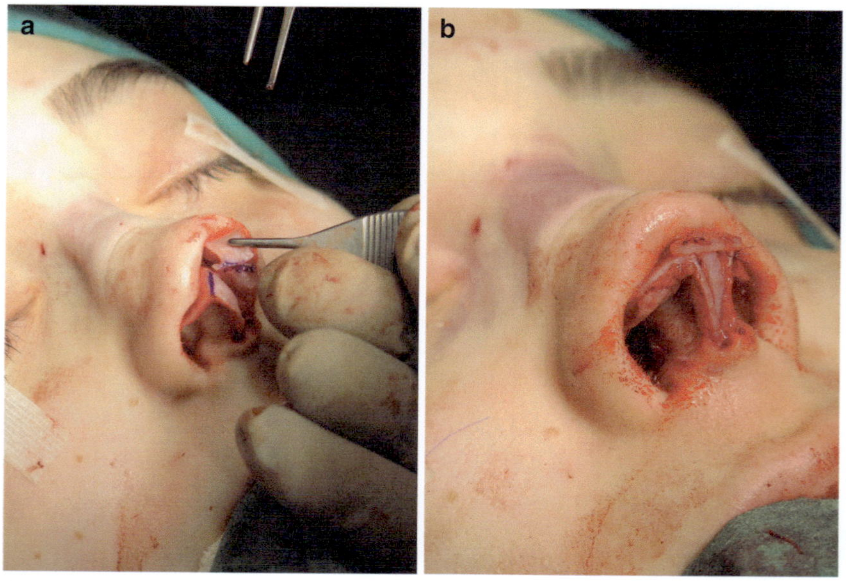

Fig. 21.11 (**a**, **b**) In a patient with such thin skin, it is essential that the tip cartilages be extremely well crafted

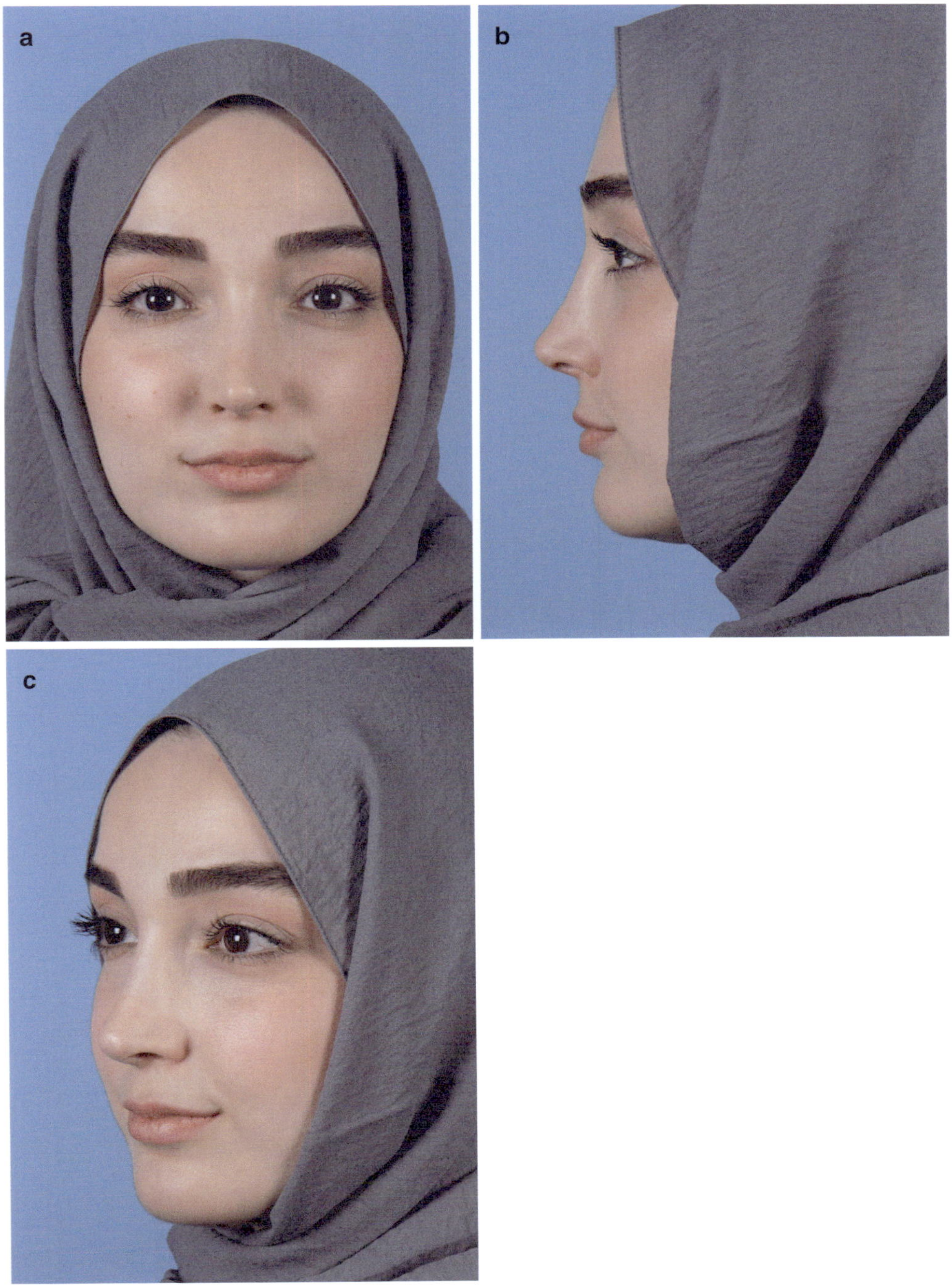

Fig. 21.12 (**a**–**c**) Long-term results are satisfied

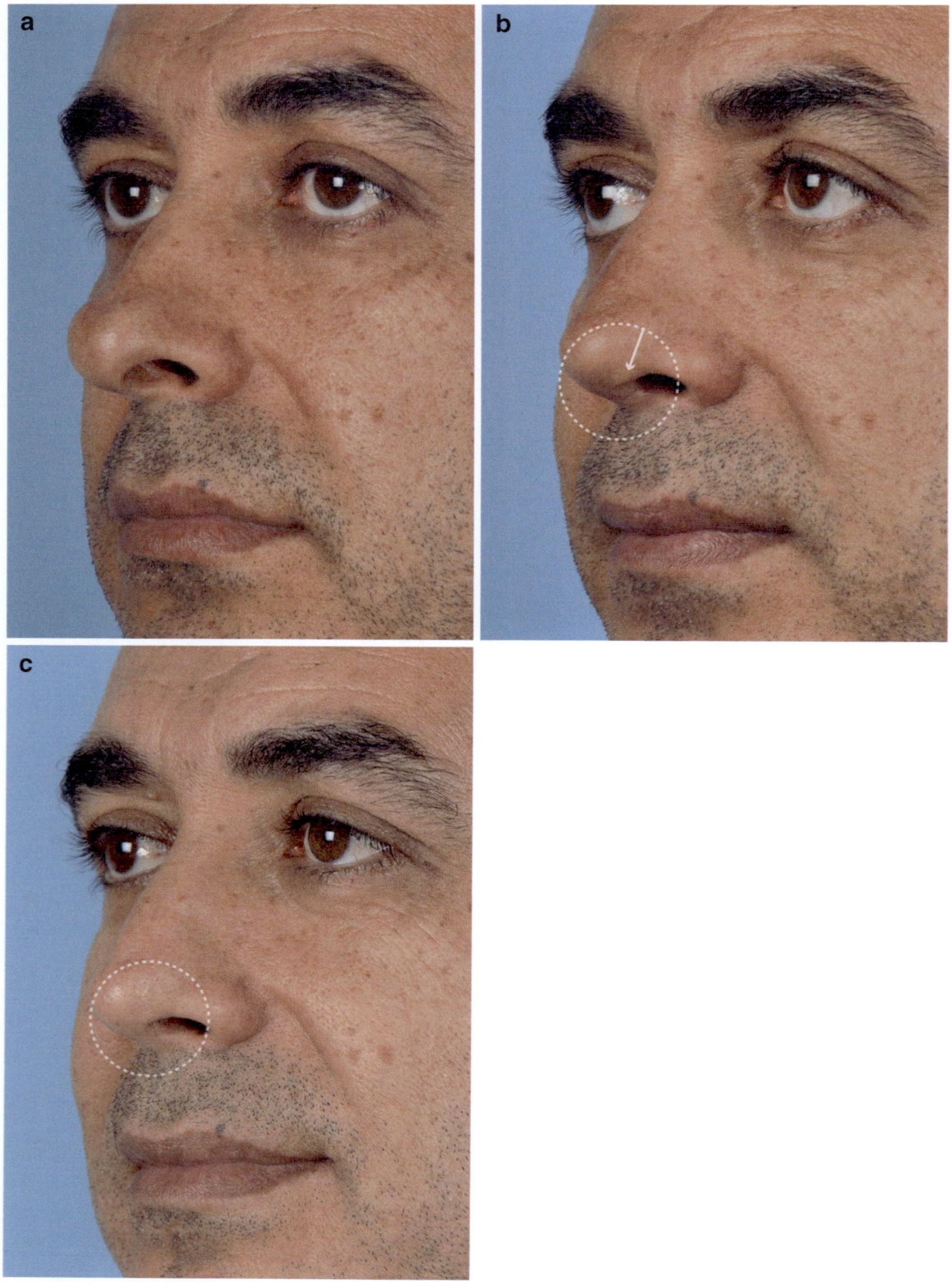

Fig. 21.13 (**a**) Preoperative oblique view. (**b**) Six months after surgery. Notice the residual skin. (**c**) Residual skin was trimmed under local anesthesia. (Supplementary Video 21.2)

Disclosures The author reports no conflicts of interest or funding requiring disclosure.

Further Reading

Millard DR. A rhinoplasty tetralogy: corrective, secondary, congenital, reconstructive. Boston, MA: Little, Brown; 1996. p. 79.

Şeneldir S, Altundağ A, Dizdar D. Cutting the holy dome: the evolution of vertical alar resection. Aesth Plast Surg. 2018;42(1):275–87.

MIX
Papier aus verantwortungsvollen Quellen
Paper from responsible sources
FSC® C105338

If you have any concerns about our products,
you can contact us on
ProductSafety@springernature.com

In case Publisher is established outside the EU,
the EU authorized representative is:
Springer Nature Customer Service Center GmbH
Europaplatz 3, 69115 Heidelberg, Germany

Printed by Libri Plureos GmbH
in Hamburg, Germany